Medical Language

IMMERSE YOURSELF

FIFTH EDITION

SUSAN M. TURLEY

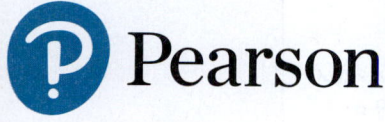

Director of Portfolio Management:
Marlene McHugh Pratt
Courseware Portfolio Manager, Health
Sciences: John Goucher
Development Editor: Laura S. Horowitz /
York Content Development
Medical Illustrator: Anita Impagliazzo
Portfolio Management Assistant:
Cara Schaurer
Vice President, Content Production and
Digital Studio: Paul DeLuca
Managing Producer, Health Science:
Melissa Bashe
Operations Specialist: Maura Zaldivar-Garcia
Creative Digital Lead: Mary Siener
Director, Digital Studio, Health Science:
Amy Peltier
Digital Studio Producer, e-text: Ellen Viganola
Digital Content Team Lead: Brian Prybella

Digital Content Project Lead: William
Johnson
Vice President, Product Marketing:
Brad Parkins
Product Marketing Manager: Rachele Strober
Field Marketing Manager: Brittany
Hammond
Full-Service Project Management and
Composition: Pearson CSC
Project Management Team Lead/Nursing
Sciences: Patty Donovan
Production Project Manager: Joanna Stein
Editorial Project Manager: Emily Tamburri
Inventory Manager: Vatche Demirdjian
Interior Design: Studio Montage
Cover Design: Studio Montage
Printer/Binder: LSC Communications, Inc.
Cover Printer: LSC Communications, Inc.

Two Journeys

In August 2000, I began two journeys—the adoption of children into our family and the writing of this textbook. Although very different, these two journeys shared a common thread of language and communication.

The first journey was the adoption of two beautiful children, Minh and Lien (then ages 8 and 9), who joined our family from an orphanage in Vietnam in 2001. This journey of adoption involved completing much paperwork, doing research, learning a new language and culture, and traveling to an exotic land.

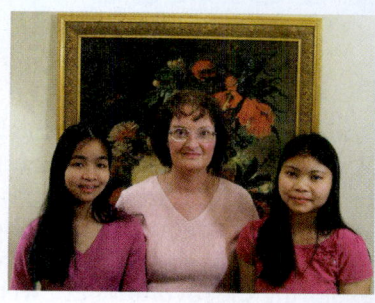

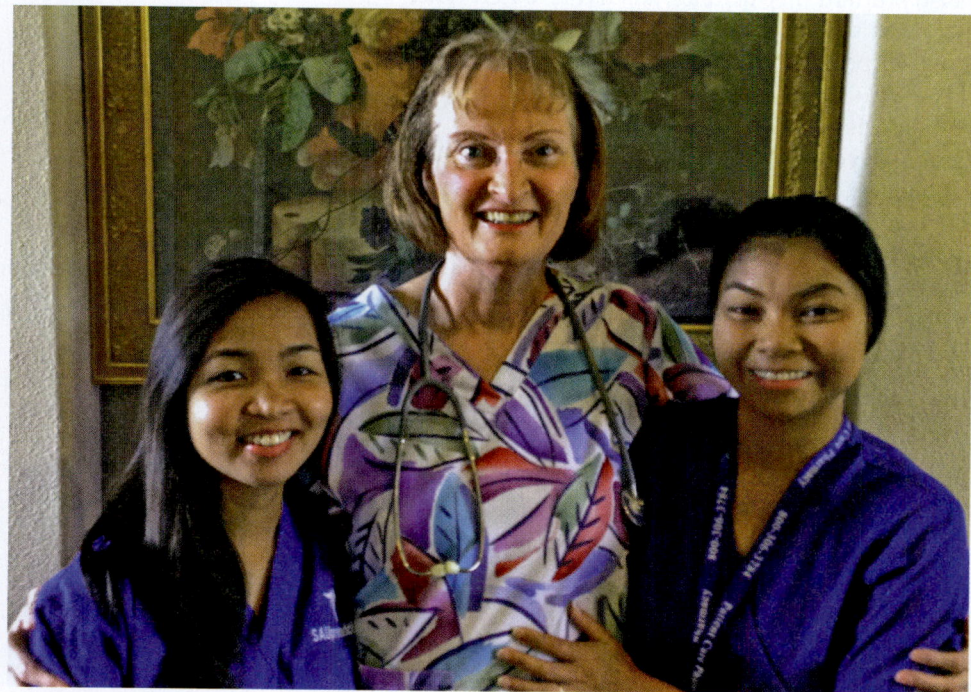

The second journey was the process of writing this textbook. This journey also involved paperwork and research, but I did not need to learn a new language or culture. Because of my many years of experience in the healthcare field, I already understood medical language and culture.

I did, however, need to determine the best way to convey that knowledge to each student who would study this textbook. And so, as I wrote, I drew on my own efforts and struggles to learn a new language and culture during the adoption process. Those insights helped me identify with students who are learning medical language and culture for the first time and encouraged me to include new real-world-of-medicine features that would support and strengthen students' efforts as they learned.

I am thrilled to say that each of my daughters has begun a new journey of her own in that they have chosen to follow in my footsteps and embrace the medical field as their career choice: Minh is a nursing assistant and Lien is a physician's assistant.

Did You Know?

As I write this in late 2018, I am ever mindful of the many children in this country and around the world who are in need of help, food, and homes.

All of the royalties from this textbook are given to provide ongoing financial support to orphanages and feed-and-read school programs for destitute children in several countries, as well as to help poor and hungry children in the United States.

Preface

Something Different

You may have already noticed that there is something different about this book! Perhaps by thumbing through the pages, you have taken note of the abundance of real-world healthcare images. Maybe you have discovered some of the practice exercises that abound within these pages, many of which place you in your soon-to-be-realized role of a healthcare professional. Or perhaps you have already begun exploring the revolutionary web-based student media materials that are rich with highly engaging and interactive activities that add a unique dimension to your learning. As you begin this exciting and important journey into the world of medical language and health care, we offer you this promise—that you will soon be immersed in a new, exciting learning experience.

As a soon-to-be healthcare professional, your knowledge, hard work, and interpersonal skills will have a direct impact on health care throughout your career. Therefore, we do everything we can to help you learn and to empower you, so you can use what you learn to positively impact the lives of others. And so, we encourage you to immerse yourself in this book and the rich variety of resources it offers to help you learn medical language, the language of your chosen career!

Let's start at the beginning and take a close look at the title of this book: *Medical Language: Immerse Yourself.*

Medical Language

Medicine is the drama of life and death, and few subjects are as compelling, profound, or worthy of study. *Language* is a method of communicating and an expression of the people, events, and culture it represents. This book is about *medical language*. As opposed to simply memorizing vocabulary words, this book offers a complete experience—the opportunity to embrace the world of health care, just as if you were learning a foreign language. Like traveling to Tokyo for a year to learn Japanese, the goal here is for you to become immersed in the sights and sounds of your new culture of health care. This book surrounds you with context that brings the medical words to life.

This book is about real medicine that affects real patients—their lives, their families, and their futures. As a healthcare professional, no matter which aspect of health care you choose, you will have important responsibilities. Therefore, we feel it is our responsibility to provide you with as realistic a view as possible of health care today. Here are some examples of how we have done this:

- The chapters in this textbook are titled as medical specialties, not just as body systems (as are other medical terminology books). This reflects the real world. For example, people with skin conditions visit a dermatologist, not an "integumentary system specialist." That's why the related chapter in this book is titled "Dermatology." A patient with heart problems is treated in a hospital's cardiology department and not in a "cardiovascular system department." The decision to present the chapters in this way is an example of our commitment to make this book a realistic reflection of health care as it is in the real world. This distinction was tested extensively, and instructors and students alike overwhelmingly support and validate this way to learn.

- The majority of the images in this book incorporate medical illustrations and photographs that include a diverse array of real people, instead of cartoon-like illustrations. The photographs are of real patients and real healthcare professionals in real healthcare settings.

- The chapter review exercises present real medical reports with related critical-thinking questions. There are also exercises where you play the role of the healthcare professional in interpreting a patient's condition and rephrasing it as medical language.
- The web-based student media will immerse you in the virtual world of MyLab Medical Terminology, where you will explore a variety of fun study opportunities. In one of them, you will listen to real doctors dictating real medical sentences for you to interpret.

Immerse Yourself

You are about to begin an interactive learning experience between you, this book, and your instructor—one that will equip you and inspire you to become an expert in medical language. The goal of this book is to connect with you, to engage your visual, auditory, and kinesthetic senses, to stimulate you, and to fuel your complete understanding of medical language.

You will not be a passive reader of this book. Instead, you will be challenged to listen, speak, write, respond, examine, think, and make connections to medical language. You should consume this book by writing notes in it and filling in your answers. By being an active participant in your own learning process, the concepts presented here will come alive in vibrant color and full texture. This book is a *living* document about a *living* language. Through the features of this book and the accompanying multimedia resources, you will get a true taste of the world of health care in *living* color.

As you engage in the multisensory experience within these pages, remember to *discover*, *learn*, *know*, and *understand* the information. But—even more—experience it and *live it*! So dive in and immerse yourself!

New to This Edition

This fifth edition maintains the best aspects of previous editions while continuing to facilitate the learner's mastery of medical language in new and exciting ways. We have revised this edition so that it provides an even more valuable teaching and learning experience. Here are the enhancements that we have made:

New Book and Chapter Structure

- The book now includes 15 chapters designed to be taught within a 16-week semester course as one chapter per week, leaving the last week for review and the final examination. Much of the content from the three other chapters from the fourth edition (psychiatry, oncology, and radiology) has been incorporated into the 15 chapters and is included in the Index. The full content of the psychiatry chapter is available at www.pearsonhighered.com/healthprofessionsresources.
- The chapter structure now includes numbered sections that correlate with numbered learning outcomes. These new sections are used in Chapters 2–15, giving instructors and students a consistent template that is easy to follow. These new sections include:
  1. Anatomy
  2. Physiology
  3. Diseases
  4. Laboratory, Diagnostic, and Radiologic Procedures
  5. Medical Procedures, Drugs, and Surgical Procedures

- An innovative student-centered learning format evaluates competency after each chapter section with the use of the Practice Laps exercises.
- A new design reinforces the new chapter structure for ease of use.
- A new eText format is compatible with any device that a student might use.

Updates to Existing Content

As in every edition of *Medical Language*, we strive to improve existing content. For the fifth edition, we have:

- Improved the Anatomy and Physiology sections by revising all of the illustrations and text to improve the clarity of details concerning complex structures and functions.
- Emphasized the relationship between different body systems and how they work in conjunction to maintain homeostasis.
- Reorganized Appendix A so that it now combines all word parts and their meanings in alphabetical order to facilitate searching. The types of word parts (combining form, prefix, suffix) are indicated by color shading of the rows and by a column that indicates *CF*, *P*, or *S*. The meaning of each word part has been revised, as needed, and verified that it is consistent across all chapters.
- Provided an Answer Key, as in the fourth edition, that includes every other answer. This encourages students to think for themselves about the answers, rather than just copying them from the Answer Key. A full Answer Key is provided in the Instructor's Manual, which allows the instructor to use any chapter exercise as a homework assignment.

Comprehensive Teaching Package

Perhaps the most gratifying part of an instructor's work is the "aha" learning moment when the light bulb goes on and a student truly understands a concept—when that connection is made. Along these lines, Pearson is pleased to help instructors foster more of these educational connections by providing a complete suite of resources to support teaching and learning. Qualified adopters are eligible to receive a wealth of tools designed to help instructors prepare, present, and assess. For more information, please contact your Pearson sales representative or visit *www.pearsonhighered.com/educator*.

Online Instructor's Resources

- A complete chapter-by-chapter Test Bank with a full variety of test questions. It also allows instructors to generate customized exams and quizzes.
- A comprehensive, turn-key lecture package with fully narrated chapter-by-chapter lectures ("Guided Lectures") in an audio format, as well as an accompanying PowerPoint presentation containing discussion points and images.
- A sample course syllabus.
- A complete image library that includes every photograph and illustration from the book.
- Articles with useful ideas, such as classroom management tips, how to construct test questions, and how to put students at ease on the first day of class.
- Ready-made worksheets that can be used for quizzes or homework assignments.
- An array of teaching pearls and tips.
- Interesting facts and anecdotes.
- Extra content, such as word origins and the stories behind anatomical structures and diseases named for someone (eponyms)—things not covered in the book.
- A complete Answer Key that includes the answers to each of the student questions in each chapter.

What Makes This Book Different?

We Listened

In developing this book over five editions, we have immersed ourselves in the perspective of you, our readers. We have strived to make *Medical Language* a customer-driven text by aggressively and comprehensively researching the needs and desires of current medical terminology students and instructors. We aimed to guarantee that we were "speaking the same language" as those who would ultimately be using this book. To do this, we gathered a highly qualified development team of over 170 reviewers, with over 2,250 years of teaching experience, 4 physician specialists, as well as 11 students from across the United States to help steer us toward success.

Over the past 14 years we sat in classrooms, hosted focus groups, and conducted thorough manuscript reviews. We asked for blunt and uncompromising opinions and insights. We also commissioned dozens of detailed reviews from instructors, asking them to analyze and evaluate each chapter of the textbook. They not only told us what they did and didn't like, but they identified, page by page, numerous ways in which we could refine and enhance our key features. Their invaluable feedback was compiled, analyzed, and incorporated throughout *Medical Language*, Fifth Edition.

We asked our team to imagine their ideal medical terminology book—what it should include, how it should look. We had the author meet personally with several instructors to discuss the specifics of the book's organization, layout, format, and features. We asked question after question. This book is truly the product of a successful partnership between the author, the publisher, and our development team of students and instructors. We listened.

We Learned

Here are some of the recommendations that we heard from our team, responded to, and included in all four editions, now updating and enhancing them even further in the new fifth edition:

- **Design.** Students and instructors alike told us they wanted an appealing, uncluttered design with an abundance of rich medical images and enough white space to allow for notetaking.

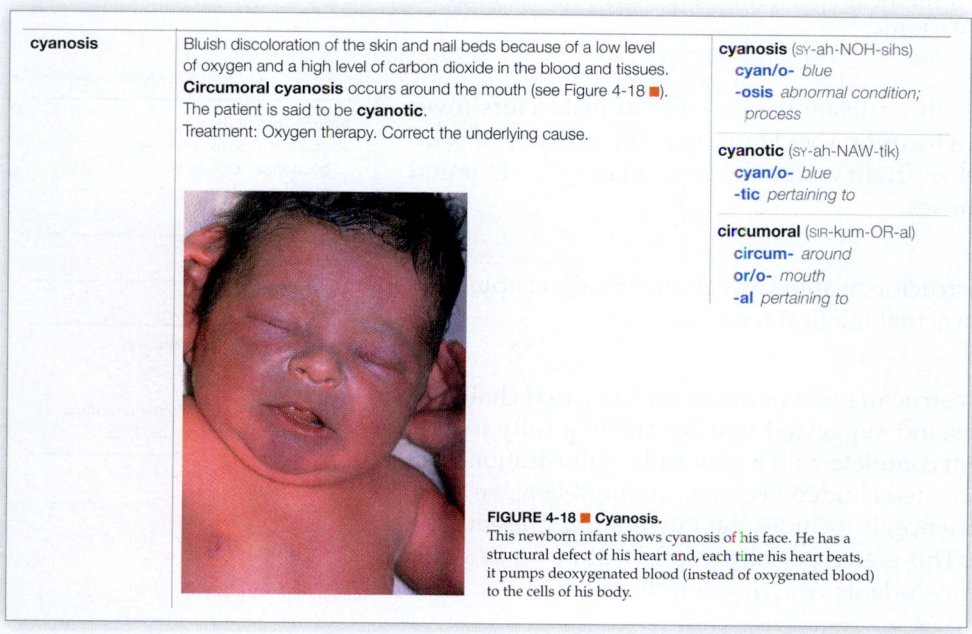

| cyanosis | Bluish discoloration of the skin and nail beds because of a low level of oxygen and a high level of carbon dioxide in the blood and tissues. **Circumoral cyanosis** occurs around the mouth (see Figure 4-18 ■). The patient is said to be **cyanotic**. Treatment: Oxygen therapy. Correct the underlying cause. | **cyanosis** (SY-ah-NOH-sihs)
  cyan/o- *blue*
  -osis *abnormal condition; process*

cyanotic (SY-ah-NAW-tik)
  cyan/o- *blue*
  -tic *pertaining to*

circumoral (SIR-kum-OR-al)
  circum- *around*
  or/o- *mouth*
  -al *pertaining to* |

FIGURE 4-18 ■ Cyanosis.
This newborn infant shows cyanosis of his face. He has a structural defect of his heart and, each time his heart beats, it pumps deoxygenated blood (instead of oxygenated blood) to the cells of his body.

- **Exercises.** Both students and instructors suggested that we provide a greater quantity and variety of exercises than any other book, thus providing maximum opportunities to reinforce learning. Instructors asked that we only provide the answers to some of the exercises so that the exercises could also be used as graded homework assignments. In the fifth edition, we have added a set of Practice Laps exercises after each numbered section to allow students to immediately assess their knowledge of that section.

- **Illustrations.** Students and instructors alike suggested that we display colorful and interesting illustrations as large as possible on the page, with opportunities to label those images as practice opportunities.

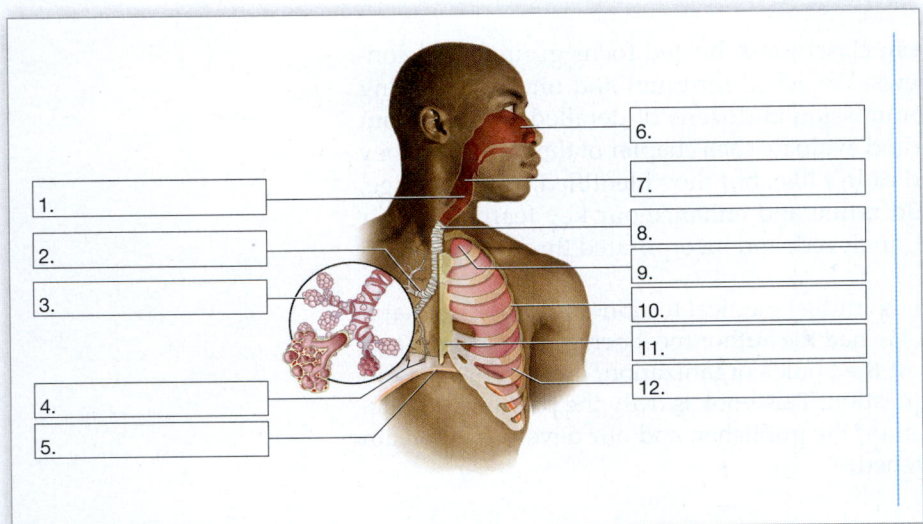

- **Special Feature Boxes.** Students asked for highlighted boxes that would help break up the reading and also provide them with opportunities to learn something new or interesting, thereby providing additional context.

- **Medical Specialties Approach.** A substantial majority (75%) of instructors told us that they wanted a medical specialties approach, rather than an approach based only on body systems.

- **Focus on Word Building.** Another substantial majority of instructors (over 70%) told us that they wanted a focus on word building with analysis of combining forms, suffixes, and prefixes right within the text and not just at the end of each chapter or in isolated boxes.

- **Medical Report Activities.** Instructors wanted an activity in each chapter that challenged students to analyze actual medical reports.

- **Lecture Support Materials.** Instructors told us about the increased challenge of creating interesting lectures and suggested that we create a fully loaded PowerPoint presentation system complete with a multitude of illustrations and photographs. In addition, we created Guided Lectures, a comprehensive auditory and visual learning experience. It includes the PowerPoint presentation coordinated with a full lecture. This is an especially helpful feature for students enrolled in online courses or for students who miss a lecture.

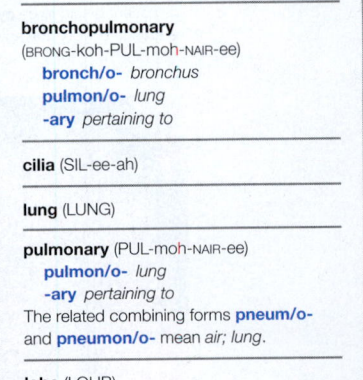

bronchopulmonary
(BRONG-koh-PUL-moh-NAIR-ee)
  bronch/o- *bronchus*
  pulmon/o- *lung*
  -ary *pertaining to*

cilia (SIL-ee-ah)

lung (LUNG)

pulmonary (PUL-moh-NAIR-ee)
  pulmon/o- *lung*
  -ary *pertaining to*
The related combining forms **pneum/o-**
and **pneumon/o-** mean *air; lung.*

lobe (LOHB)

- **Tools for Testing.** Instructors asked for a complete testing package that was customizable to fit their needs. Additionally, they asked for these test items to be available in online course formats.

We Made a Commitment to Accuracy

As part of our respect for real medicine, and the importance of getting it right the first time, we made a commitment to accuracy. It was important to us to attain the highest level of accuracy possible throughout this educational package in order to match the precision required in today's healthcare environment. The author drew on her 30 years of experience in nursing, health information management, medical transcription, and medical publications and as a college instructor to provide accurate and complete information. Our development team read every page, every test question, and every vocabulary word. No less than 11 content experts read each chapter for accuracy and analyzed every bit of content in the ancillary resources. We also engaged the technical editing services of four physician specialists who carefully reviewed the chapters that correspond to their respective practices.

We welcome any and all feedback you may have to help us enhance the accuracy of this book. If you identify any errors that need to be corrected in a subsequent printing, please send them to:

Pearson Health Science Editorial
Medical Terminology Corrections
221 River Street, 4th Floor
Hoboken, NJ 07030

Our Development Team

About the Author

Susan M. Turley, **MA (Educ), BSN, RN, RHIT, CMT,** is a full-time author and editor who has extensive experience in both the medical and educational fields.

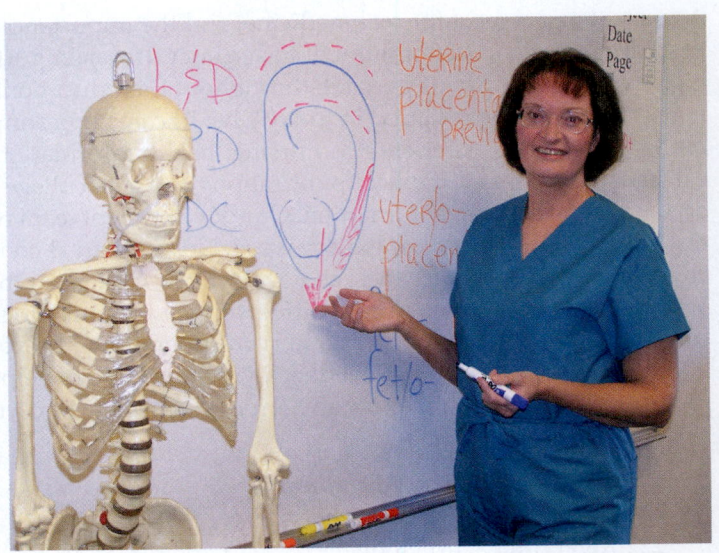

As a healthcare professional, Susan has worked in a variety of healthcare settings: acute care/ICU, long-term care, physicians' offices, and managed care. She has held positions as an intensive care nurse, plasmapheresis nurse, infection control officer, physician office auditor, medical transcriptionist, director of education, and director of quality management and corporate compliance for an HMO.

As an adjunct professor in the School of Health, Wellness, and Physical Education at Anne Arundel Community College in Arnold, Maryland, Susan taught courses in medical terminology, pathophysiology, pharmacology, and medical transcription. She was instrumental in gaining initial accreditation for the college's medical assisting program. Susan was a codeveloper of *The SUM Program for Medical Transcription Training* and reference books for Health Professions Institute. She developed the curricula for the bachelor, master's, and doctoral programs for the International Institute of Original Medicine. Susan has been a guest speaker at national seminars for accreditation of utilization management programs, medical transcription teacher training, and health information management certification examination review seminars.

Susan is also the author of the soon-to-be-released *Understanding Pharmacology for Health Professionals,* Sixth Edition (Pearson, 2021) and more than 40 articles published in medical transcription and health information management journals. With physician coauthors, she has written three nationally funded grants and two chapters in physicians' anesthesiology and ENT textbooks. Susan has also coauthored numerous abstracts and articles published in nationally known medical journals, and most recently she was the editor for an Opinion column that appeared in the *Journal of the American Medical Association.*

Susan holds a Master of Arts degree in adult education from Norwich University in Vermont, a Bachelor of Science degree in nursing from the Pennsylvania State University, and has state licensure as an RN. She is a member of and has national certification in medical transcription from the Association for Healthcare Documentation Integrity (AHDI) and is a member of and has national certification from the American Health Information Management Association (AHIMA).

About the Illustrator

The illustrations throughout this book are the result of a close collaborative effort between the author and medical illustrator. Every figure was custom developed specifically for this book and refined to be medically accurate, precise, unique, and fresh. From a pedagogical point of view, it was important that all of the art be consistent throughout, rather than presenting a conglomeration of styles and varying levels of detail. The illustrations for the fifth edition have been revised, clarified, and updated to reflect the highest degree of medical accuracy while retaining realism and ease of understanding for students.

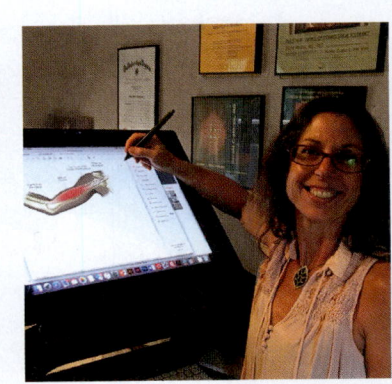

Anita Impagliazzo, **BA, MA, CMI,** is a medical and scientific illustrator in Charlottesville, Virginia. A graduate of the University of Virginia, she went on to complete the Biomedical Illustration Graduate Program at the University of Texas Southwestern Medical Center at Dallas. She was employed for several years by companies specializing in exhibits for medical malpractice litigation before starting her own business in 2001.

Anita's regular clients now include physicians and researchers at the University of Virginia, Tulane University, University of Pittsburgh, University of Florida, the Max Planck Institute, and the Royal College of London. She also provides pro bono work to St. Jude Children's Research Hospital. She has worked on multiple textbooks, including the popular Martini series of anatomy and physiology atlases and the revered Netter Collection of Medical Illustrations. Anita is a member of the Association of Medical Illustrators and the Society for Neuroscience. Her work has won several awards. She never tires of using medical language to learn and teach about the human body: how it works, how it fails, how it is fixed, and how the fixing fails.

About the Educational Consultant

James F. Allen, Jr., RN, MSN-Ed, MBA/HCM, JD, is an Adjunct Associate Professor at Lansing Community College in Lansing, Michigan. He earned his Master of Science in Nursing Education (MSN-Ed) at Western Governors University; his Master of Business Administration and Healthcare Management (MBA/HCM) at the University of Phoenix; and his Juris Doctorate (JD) from Thomas M. Cooley School of Law. Jim has taught courses both online and in the classroom in medical terminology, pathophysiology, pharmacology, and medical law and ethics. Since his college adopted the first edition, Jim has been an invaluable source of information and suggestions for improvement of *Medical Language*. Jim is the coauthor of *Medical Language STAT!* (Pearson, 2009) and the author of *Health Law and Medical Ethics for Healthcare Professionals* (Pearson, 2013).

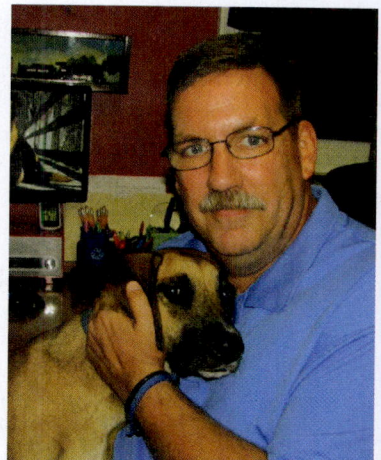

Consultants and Contributors

Each member of our development team has infused this book with ideas, vision, and a passion for medical language. Our team crafted the blueprints for this book and contributed to what has become a landmark educational tool. Their influence will continue to have an impact for decades to come as many students continue to study *Medical Language*. We are pleased to introduce the members of our team.

Physician Specialist Consultants

Stephen Caldwell, MD
Director of Hepatology
Digestive Health Center of Excellence
Charlottesville, Virginia

John H. Dirckx, MD
Former Medical Director,
University of Dayton
Student Health Center
Dayton, Ohio

Joseph Gibbons, MD
Internal Medicine Physician
Centennial Medical Group
Elkridge, Maryland

James Michelson, MD
Professor of Orthopedic Surgery
George Washington University School of Medicine
Washington, D.C.

Quality Assurance Editor

Garnet Tomich, BA
San Diego, California

Ancillary Content Providers

James F. Allen, Jr., RN, BSN, MBA/HCM, JD, MSN-Ed
Lansing Community College
Lansing, Michigan

Michael Battaglia, MS, EdD
Greenville Technical College
Greenville, South Carolina

Dale Brewer, BS, MEd, CMA, (AAMA)
Pensacola Junior College
Pensacola, Florida

Dean Chiarelli, MA, RD, HFS, CHES
Arizona State University
Phoenix, Arizona

Dianne Davis, BS, MS, ABD EdD
West Virginia University at Parkersburg
Parkersburg, West Virginia

Sarah E.W. Finch, PhD
Florida State College at Jacksonville
Jacksonville, Florida

Jean M. Krueger-Watson, PhD
Clark College
Vancouver, Washington

Angela Moderow, PT, MPT
Carolinas Rehabilitation
Charlotte, North Carolina

Janet Pandzik, MS, CMT, RMA
Good Careers Academy
San Antonio, Texas

Garnet Tomich, BA
San Diego, California

Katherine Twomey, MLS
Greenville Technical College
Greenville, South Carolina

Manuscript Reviewers for the Fifth Edition

Jana Allen, MT, ASCP
Volunteer State Community College
Gallatin, Tennessee

Peggy Anderson, DNP, MS, RN
Brigham Young University
Provo, Utah

Michelle Cooney, MA, MT(ASCP)
Moraine Valley Community College
Palos Hills, Illinois

Jeffrey Crisp, MS
Program Director, Allied Health Science
Spartanburg Community College
Spartanburg, South Carolina

Shelley Dennis, PhD, MD
Rio Salado Community College
Tempe, Arizona

Karalea Fisher, RHIT
Central New Mexico Community
College
Albuquerque, New Mexico

**Marie Hattabaugh, MAT, RT(R)(M),
CMA (AAMA)**
Pensacola State College
Pensacola, Florida

Rita Kealy, MM, MT(ASCP)
Moraine Valley Community College
Palos Hills, Illinois

LaShawn Lawrence, MS, RHIT, CCHP
Miami-Dade College
Miami, Florida

Jennifer Michael, MSRS, RT(R)
Northwestern State University
Natchitoches, Louisiana

Michele Miller, PhD, CMA(AAMA)
Lakeland Community College
Kirtland, Ohio

**B. Jeanine Newton-Riner, MHSA,
RRT, EMT-P**
Chattahoochee Technical College
Marietta, Georgia

Tammie Petersen, BSN, RNC-OB
Austin Community College
Austin, Texas

**Susan Stockmaster, OTR, CMAA
(AAMA)**
Trident Technical College
North Charleston, South Carolina

**Cheryl Travelstead, BS, AS, ASS,
RT(R)(BD)**
Tidewater Community College
Norfolk, Virginia

Deborah Uhlian, BS, AHI, RMA
Charles Stewart Mott Community
College
Flint, Michigan

**Brad Winterton, DVM, MPH,
DACVPM**
Weber State University
Ogden, Utah

Manuscript Reviewers for Earlier Editions

(*Reviewer conference attendee)

Denise M. Abrams, PT, MASS
SUNY Broome Community College
Appalachian, New York

Betsy Adams, AAS, BS, MSBE
Alamance Community College
Graham, North Carolina

Mercedes Alafriz-Gordon, BS
High Tech Institute
Phoenix, Arizona

Diana Alagna, RN, AHI, CPT
Branford Hall Career Institute
Southington, Connecticut

Jana Allen, BS, MT*
Volunteer State
Community College
Gallatin, Tennessee

Pam Anania, RN, APRN, MSN
Brookdale Community College
Lincroft, New Jersey

Ellen Anderson, RHIA
College of Lake County
Northfield, Illinois

Judy Anderson, MEd
Coastal Carolina Community College
Jacksonville, North Carolina

Wendy Anderson
MTI College
Sacramento, California

Lori Andreucci, MEd, CMT, CMA
Gateway Technical College
Racine, Wisconsin

Leah Beall, CST, BS
Fortis College
Westerville, Ohio

Debbie Bedford, CMA, AAS
North Seattle Community College
Seattle, Washington

Tricia Berry, OTR/L
Hamilton College
Urbandale, Iowa

Sue Biederman, MSHP, RHIA
Texas State University
San Marcos, Texas

Richard Boan, BS, MS, PhD
Midlands Technical College
Columbia, South Carolina

Jennifer Boles, MSN, RN, NCSN
Cincinnati State Technical and
Community College
Cincinnati, Ohio

Julie E. Boles, MS, RHIA
Ithaca College
Ithaca, New York

Annie M. Boster, PT
Bishop State Community College
Mobile, Alabama

Susan A. Boulden, RN
Mt. Hood Community College
Aloha, Oregon

Beth Braun, MA, PhD
Truman College
Chicago, Illinois

Shannon Bruley, BAS, AEMT-IC
Henry Ford Community College
Dearborn, Michigan

Juanita R. Bryant, CMA-A/C
Sierra College
Penn Valley, California

Thomas Bubar, BA, MS
Erie Community College
Williamsville, New York

Susan Buboltz, RN, MS, CMA
Madison Area Technical College
Madison, Wisconsin

**Patricia Bufalino, MA, MN, RN,
FNP**
Riverside Community College
Moreno Valley, California

Ginger Bushway
Mendocino College
Ukiah, California

Mary Butler, BS
Collin County Community College
McKinney, Texas

**Toni Cade, MBA, RHIA, CCS,
FAHIMA**
University of Louisiana at
Lafayette
Lafayette, Louisiana

**Cara L. Carreon, BS, RRT, CMA,
CPC**
Ivy Tech Community College
Lafayette, Indiana

Rafael Castilla, MD
Ho Ho Kus School
Ramsey, New Jersey

Julia I. Chapman, BS
Stark State College of Technology
North Canton, Ohio

**Dean Chiarelli, MA, RD, HFS,
CHES**
Arizona State University
Phoenix, Arizona

Kim Christmon, BS, RRT
Volunteer State Community
College
Gallatin, Tennessee

Paula-Beth Ciolek
National College of Business and
Technology
Richmond, Kentucky

Deresa Claybrook, MS, RHIT
Oklahoma City Community
College
Oklahoma City, Oklahoma

**Mike Cochran, BA, RT(R)(CT),
ARRT, VSRT, SWDSRT**
Southwest Virginia Community
College
Richlands, Virginia

Christine Cole, CCA
Williston State College
Williston, North Dakota

Ronald Coleman, EdD
Volunteer State Community
College
Gallatin, Tennessee

Bonnie Crist
Harrison College
Indianapolis, Indiana

Cathleen Currie, RN, BS
College of Southern Idaho
Twin Falls, Idaho

**Dianne Davis, BS, MS, ABD
EdD**
West Virginia University at
Parkersburg
Parkersburg, West Virginia

Mary Sayles, RN, MSN
Sierra College—Nevada County
Campus
Rocklin, California

Jody E. Scheller, MS, RHIA
Schoolcraft College
Garden City, Michigan

Patricia Schrull, MSN, MBA,
MEd, RN
Lorain County Community College
Elyria, Ohio

Theresa R. Schuldt, MEd, HT/HTL
(ASCP)
Rose State College
Midwest City, Oklahoma

Jan Sesser, BS, RMA (AMT), CMA
High Tech Institute
Phoenix, Arizona

Julie A. Shellenbarger, MBA, RHIA
University of Northwestern Ohio
Lima, Ohio

Donna Sue Shellman, MA, CPC
Gaston College
Dallas, North Carolina

Karin Sherrill, BSN
Mesa Community College
Gilbert, Arizona

Paula Silver, PharmD
ECPI University
Newport News, Virginia

Vicki Simpson, PhD, RN, CHES
Purdue University West Lafayette
West Lafayette, Indiana

Erin Sitterley
North Seattle Community College
Seattle, Washington

Tim J. Skaife, RT(R), MA
National Park Community College
Hot Springs, Arizona

Lynn G. Slack, CMA
ICM School of Business and
Medical Careers
Pittsburgh, Pennsylvania

Ellie Smith, RN, MSN
Cuesta College
San Luis Obispo, California

Sherman K. Sowby, PhD, CHES
California State University—Fresno
Fresno, California

Darla K. Sparacino, MEd, RHIA
Arkansas Tech University
Russelville, Arkansas

Carolyn Stariha, BS, RHIA
Houston Community College—
Coleman Campus
Houston, Texas

Kathy Stau, CPhT
Medix School
Smyrna, Georgia

Twila Sterling-Guillory, RN, MSN
McNeese State University
Lake Charles, Louisiana

Deb Stockberger, MSN, RN
North Iowa Community College
Mason City, Iowa

Paula L. Stoltz, CMT-F
Medical Transcription Education
Center
Fairlawn, Ohio

Diane Swift
State Fair Community College
Sedalia, Missouri

J. David Taylor, PhD, PT, CSCS
University of Central Arkansas
Conway, Arkansas

Sylvia Taylor, CMA, CPCA
Cleveland State Community
College
Cleveland, Tennessee

Jean Ternus, RN, MS
Kansas City Community College
Kansas City, Kansas

Cindy B. Thompson, BSRT, MA*
Alamance Community College
Graham, North Carolina

Lenette Thompson, CST
Piedmont Technical College
Greenwood, South Carolina

Margaret A. Tiemann, RN, BS
St. Charles Community College
Cottleville, Missouri

Mary Jane Tremethick, PhD, RN,
CHES
Northern Michigan University
Marquette, Michican

Valeria D. Truitt, BS, MAEd
Craven Community College
New Bern, North Carolina

Christine Tufts-Maher, MS, RHIA
Seminole Community College
Altamonte Springs, Florida

Pam Ventgen, CMA (AAMA),
CCS-P, CPC, CPC-I
University of Alaska—Anchorage
Anchorage, Alaska

Patricia Von Knorring
Tacoma Community College
Gig Harbor, Washington

Jane C. Walker, BBA, PhD, RN,
ASLNC-C, CPN, CNE
Walters State Community College
Morristown, Tennessee

Mary Warren-Oliver, BA
Gibbs College
Vienna, Virginia

Kristen Waterstram-Rich, MS,
CNMT
Rochester Institute of Technology
Rochester, New York

Kim Webb, RN, MN
Northern Oklahoma College
Tonkawa, Oklahoma

Richard Weidman, RHIA, CCS-P
Tacoma Community College
Tacoma, Washington

Bonnie Welniak, RN, MSN
Monroe County Community
College
Monroe, Michigan

Connie Werner, MS, RHIA
York College of Pennsylvania
York, Pennsylvania

Victoria Lee Wetle, RN, EdD
Chemeketa Community College
Salem, Oregon

David J. White, MA, MLIS
Baylor University
Waco, Texas

Jay W. Wilborn, MEd, MT(ASCP)
National Park Community College
Hot Springs, Arkansas

Tammy L. Wilder, RN, MSN,
CMSRN
Ivy Tech Community College
Evansville, Indiana

Antionette Woodall
Remington College—Cleveland
North Olmsted, Ohio

Scott Zimmer, MS
Metropolitan Community College
Omaha, Nebraska

Focus Group Participants

Kim Anthony Aaronson, BS, DC
Harry S. Truman College
Harold Washington College
Chicago, Illinois

Kendra J. Allen, LPN
Ohio Institute of Health Careers
Columbus, Ohio

Delena Kay Austin, BTIS, CMA
Macomb Community College
Clinton Township, Michigan

Molly Baxter
Baker College—Port Huron
Port Huron, Michigan

Joan Berry, RN, MSN, CNS
Lansing Community College
Lansing, Michigan

Kenneth Bretl, MA, RRT
College of DuPage
Glen Ellyn, Illinois

Carole Bretscher
Southwestern College
Bellrook, Ohio

Adrienne L. Carter, MEd, NRMA
Riverside Community College
Moreno Valley, California

Mary Dudash-White, MA, RHIA,
CCS
Sinclair Community College
Dayton, Ohio

Cathy Flite, MEd, RHIA
Temple University
Philadelphia, Pennsylvania

Sherry Gamble, RN, CNS, MSN,
CNOR
University of Akron
Akron, Ohio

Mary Garcia, BA, AD, RN
Northwestern Business College
Northeastern Illinois University
Truman College
Chicago, Illinois

Joyce Garozzo, MS, RHIA, CCS
Community College of
Philadelphia

Philadelphia, Pennsylvania

Patsy Gehring, PhD, RN, CS
Lakeland Community College
Kirkland, Ohio

Michelle Heller, CMA, RMA
Ohio Institute of Health Careers
Columbus, Ohio

Janet Hossli
Northwestern Business College
Chicago, Illinois

Trudi James-Parks, RT, BS
Lorain County Community College
Elyria, Ohio

Sherry L. Jones, RN, ASN
Western School of Health and
Business
Community College of Allegheny
County
Pittsburgh, Pennsylvania

Esther H. Kim
Chicago State University
Chicago, Illinois

Richelle S. Laipply, PhD, CMA
University of Akron
Akron, Ohio

Andrea M. Lane, CMA-C, BAS
RN, MS
Brookdale Community College
Lincroft, New Jersey

Mary Lou Liebal, BS, RTR, MA
Cuyahoga Community College
Cleveland, Ohio

Stacey Long, BS
Miami Jacobs Career College
Dayton, Ohio

Anne Loochtan, MEd
Columbus State Community
College
Cincinnati, Ohio

Anne M. Lunde, BS, CMT
Waubonsee Community College
Sugar Grove, Illinois

Janice Manning, MA, PCP
Baker College
Jackson, Michigan

Sandy Marks, RN, MS(HCA)
Cerritos College
Norwalk, California

Kathleen Masters, MS, RN
Monroe County Community
College
Monroe, Michigan

Mary Morgan, MS, CNMT
Columbus State Community
College
Columbus, Ohio

Andrew Muniz, OT, BBA, MBA
Baker College
Auburn Hills, Michigan

Michael Murphy, AAS, CMA,
CLP
Berdan Institute
Union, New Jersey

Stephen Nardozzi, BA
SUNY-Westchester Community
College
Valhalla, New York

Thank You

To the Pearson Development Team

My utmost thanks go to John Goucher, Courseware Portfolio Manager, Health Sciences, for bringing to completion the very successful most recent editions of *Medical Language*, as well as this new fifth edition. I also want to express my thanks to Melissa Bashe, Managing Producer, Health Sciences, who coordinated activities on the first edition and has now returned to expertly manage many facets of the fifth edition,

My gratitude and thanks go to Anita Impagliazzo, my medical illustrator. She embraced much more than her original role and quickly became a creative collaborator and advisor for all five editions. She is a wonderfully talented medical illustrator whose efforts made this book medically accurate, artistically unique, and without equal. By combining real-life photographs of people superimposed with medical illustrations, she created a never-before-seen level of medical realism, to the delight of the author and the awe of students and instructors alike.

My sincere thanks go to Laura S. Horowitz, York Content Development, my development editor. She expertly and seamlessly coordinated all aspects of the very complicated process of creating a new edition. Her professional expertise was a constant throughout the process, and all of the many steps and details involved would have been overwhelming and difficult to complete without her all-encompassing and timely editorial assistance and personal support.

My thanks go to Studio Montage for creating a beautiful, fresh, and inviting design and format for the fifth edition. My thanks go to all of members of the Pearson team from portfolio management assistants to project managers to marketing managers and sales representatives to the executive editors and the publisher!

My thanks go to the talented team at SPi Global, led by Patty Donovan, Project Management Team Lead/Nursing Science, Emily Tamburri, Editorial Project Manager, and Joanna Stein, Project Manager, who oversaw the extensive editing, layout, typesetting, and indexing of the fifth edition. In light of the complexity of the book, I especially appreciated their professionalism, flexibility, creative insights, and can-do approach.

My thanks go to the Pearson media team that designed and produced a spectacular array of learning applications to support my textbook.

To Students and Instructors

As the author, my thanks go to the many classes of students who motivated me to continually research and present medical language clearly and thoroughly. It was their warm response to my teaching methods and materials that encouraged me to keep improving in the classroom and throughout all five editions of the textbook.

My thanks go to the many reviewers, instructors, and practitioners—my colleagues—who have overwhelmingly validated my efforts to write about medical language with a uniquely interesting, lively, and fresh approach. Each and every person listed played an important role in the development of this book, and I hope they share my sense of pride and accomplishment in this fifth edition.

An Overview of *Medical Language*

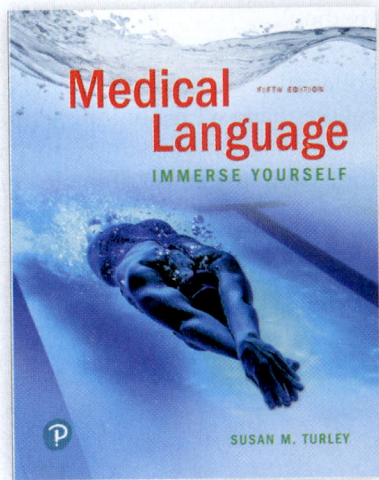

No new medical terminology book has touched the lives of so many people as profoundly as *Medical Language*. We credit the astounding success of the award-winning first edition and all subsequent editions to their special ability to meet the needs of students and instructors.

Students need to be immersed in the real world of medicine from the moment they begin to study medical terminology. That is why the chapters in *Medical Language* are named—not by body system (as is the case with anatomy textbooks and other medical terminology textbooks)—but by medical specialties, which reflects the practice of medicine in the real world. In addition, all of the text, illustrations, and photo images have been carefully revised and updated to reflect the most up-to-date medical information and the most realistic medical images available.

The emphasis on learning medical language as a language is reinforced by including see-and-say pronunciations for each bolded word in the text and providing a breakdown of each bolded word into its component word parts and their meanings.

The fifth edition builds on our commitment to excellence, and so we have once again challenged the author, our reviewers, and our development team to critique every feature, every page, every word—all to help enhance the learning and teaching process. The information in each section of a chapter is presented in a way that reflects the level of detail that the majority of instructors told us they need. The result of this feedback has been an intelligent reorganization as well as the integration of features that you, our customer, have asked for and will not find in any other medical terminology textbook.

Chapter Format

Each chapter follows a consistent organization designed for student success.

Chapter Overview, Learning Outcomes, and Medical Language Key

The first page of each chapter offers a brief chapter outline to help students see the scope of the chapter as well as its special features. Each section of the chapter is numbered, and this same numbering is consistently used throughout the chapter, including in all of the exercises. The overall learning outcome for the chapter can be fulfilled by students in a very practical way by successfully completing chapter exercises. Individual learning outcomes are listed under each numbered section. The first page ends with a Medical Language Key feature box that provides a word analysis of the medical specialty described in that chapter.

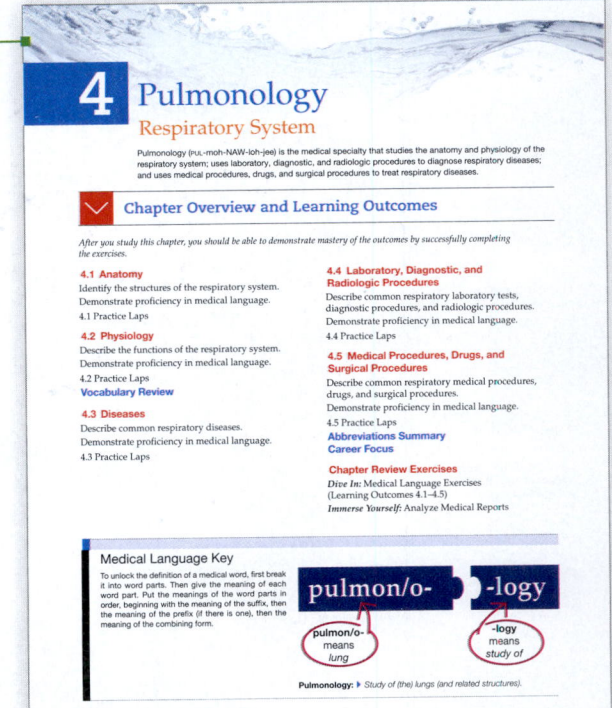

The following sections are included in most chapters. The material in these sections is comprehensive in its scope but is at a level that is appropriate for a terminology textbook as opposed to an anatomy, physiology, disease, laboratory, or surgical textbook. Each section is supplemented by a rich variety of medical illustrations and photographs as well as several different Special Features, as described later.

Anatomy
The first section in each chapter is a comprehensive presentation of the anatomy of the body system related to that chapter's medical specialty.

4.1 Anatomy

Upper Respiratory System

The upper respiratory system is in the head and neck. It includes the nose, nasal cavity, and pharynx (throat). *Note*: Some of these same structures—as well as others (the sinuses, adenoids, tonsils)—are part of the ears, nose, and throat (described in Chapter 15, Otolaryngology).

Practice Laps
The Anatomy section (and each subsequent numbered section) ends with a set of Practice Laps exercises that reinforce the material that has just been presented.

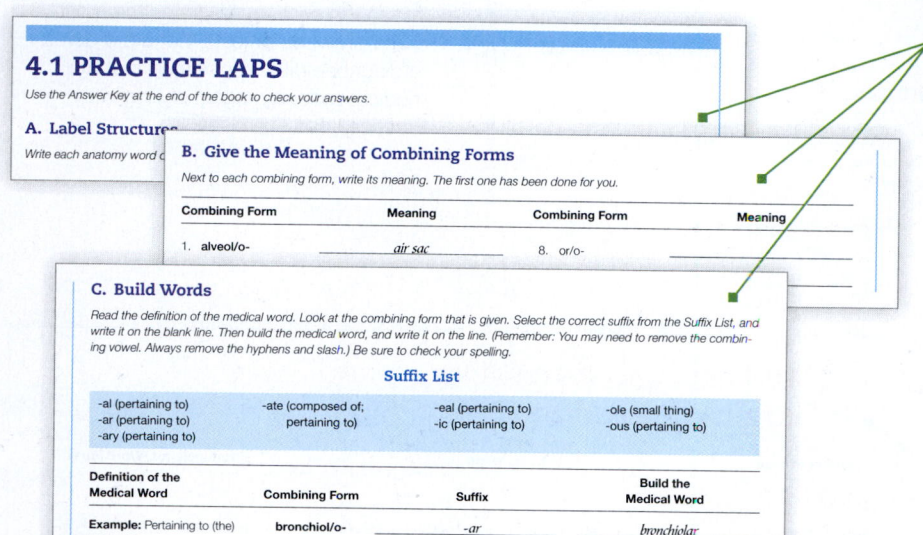

4.1 PRACTICE LAPS

Use the Answer Key at the end of the book to check your answers.

A. Label Structures

Write each anatomy word c...

B. Give the Meaning of Combining Forms

Next to each combining form, write its meaning. The first one has been done for you.

Combining Form	Meaning	Combining Form	Meaning
1. alveol/o-	*air sac*	8. or/o-	

C. Build Words

Read the definition of the medical word. Look at the combining form that is given. Select the correct suffix from the Suffix List, and write it on the blank line. Then build the medical word, and write it on the line. (Remember: You may need to remove the combining vowel. Always remove the hyphens and slash.) Be sure to check your spelling.

Suffix List

-al (pertaining to)	-ate (composed of;	-eal (pertaining to)	-ole (small thing)
-ar (pertaining to)	pertaining to)	-ic (pertaining to)	-ous (pertaining to)
-ary (pertaining to)			

Definition of the Medical Word	Combining Form	Suffix	Build the Medical Word
Example: Pertaining to (the) bronchiole	bronchiol/o-	*-ar*	*bronchiolar*

Physiology
This second section is a comprehensive presentation of the physiology of the body system related to that chapter's medical specialty.

4.2 Physiology

Breathing is normally an involuntary process that occurs without any conscious effort. **Respiratory control centers** in the brain regulate the depth and rate of respiration. Receptors in large arteries in the chest and neck send information to the brain about the level of oxygen in the blood, and receptors in the brain send information about the blood level of carbon dioxide. Based on this information, the respiratory control centers regulate the rate of respiration by sending nerve impulses to the **phrenic nerve**, causing the diaphragm to contract. You can voluntarily control your respiration (when you hold your breath), but eventually involuntary control takes over, forcing you to breathe.

Vocabulary Review

Word or Phrase	Description	Combining Forms
Overview		
cardiopulmonary	Pertaining to the heart and lungs	**cardi/o-** *heart* **pulmon/o-** *lung*
respiratory system	The structures of the upper respiratory system include the nose, nasal cavity, and pharynx (throat). The lower respiratory system includes the larynx (voice box), trachea (windpipe), bronchi, bronchioles, lungs, and thorax. Also known as the **respiratory tract**. The functions of the respiratory system are to bring oxygen into the body and expel carbon dioxide.	**spir/o-** *breathe; coil*
Anatomy of the Upper Respiratory System		
mucosa	**Mucous membrane** that lines most of the respiratory system. It warms and humidifies incoming air. It produces **mucus** to trap foreign particles and bacteria.	**muc/o-** *mucus*
nasal cavity	Hollow area inside the nose. The **nasal septum** divides the nasal cavity into right and left sides.	**nas/o-** *nose* **sept/o-** *dividing wall; septum*
pharynx	The throat. A shared passageway for both air and food. The **nasopharynx** is posterior to the nasal cavity, the **oropharynx** is posterior to the oral cavity, and the **laryngopharynx** is posterior to the larynx.	**pharyng/o-** *pharynx; throat* **nas/o-** *nose* **or/o-** *mouth* **laryng/o-** *larynx; voice box*
turbinates	Scroll-like projections of bone covered by mucous membrane on either side of the nasal cavity. They slow down and give moisture to inhaled air. Also known as **nasal conchae**.	**turbin/o-** *scroll-like structure*

Vocabulary Review
After the first two sections, a Vocabulary Review reinforces an understanding of anatomy and physiology with an at-a-glance review of each bolded word or phrase, its description, and related combining forms. Some chapters also contain an **Abbreviation Review** at this point.

4.3 Diseases

Note: Diseases of the nose, sinuses, pharynx, tonsils, adenoids, and larynx are described in Chapter 15, Otolaryngology.

Word or Phrase	Description	Pronunciation/Word Parts
Nose and Pharynx		
upper respiratory infection (URI)	Bacterial or viral infection of the nose and/or throat. Also known as a **common cold** or a **head cold** (see Figure 4-8 ■). Treatment: Antibiotic drug for a bacterial infection	**infection** (in-FEK-shun) **infect/o-** *disease within* **-ion** *action; condition*

4.4 Laboratory, Diagnostic, and Radiologic Procedures

Word or Phrase	Description	Pronunciation/Word Parts
Laboratory Tests and Diagnostic Procedures		
arterial blood gases (ABG)	Blood test to measure the partial pressure (p) of the gases oxygen (pO_2) and carbon dioxide (pCO_2) in the arterial blood. The pH (how acidic or alkaline the blood is) is also measured. The higher the level of carbon dioxide, the more acidic the blood and the lower the pH.	**arterial** (ar-TEER-ee-al) **arteri/o-** *artery* **-al** *pertaining to*

4.5 Medical Procedures, Drugs, and Surgical Procedures

Word or Phrase	Description	Pronunciation/Word Parts
Medical Procedures		
auscultation and percussion (A&P)	Auscultation uses a **stethoscope** to listen to breath sounds in all lobes of the lungs. Percussion uses the finger of one hand to tap over the finger of the other hand that is spread across the patient's back over a lobe of the lung. After a few taps, the hand is moved over another lobe. Auscultation and percussion tell the physician if the lung sounds are clear or if there is dullness because of the presence of fluid or a tumor (see Figure 4-24 ■).	**auscultation** (aws-kul-TAY-shun) **auscult/o-** *listening* **-ation** *being; having; process* **stethoscope** (STETH-oh-skohp) **steth/o-** *chest* **-scope** *instrument used to examine* **percussion** (per-KUH-shun) **percuss/o-** *tapping* **-ion** *action; condition*

Abbreviations Summary

A&P	auscultation and percussion	LUL	left upper lobe (of the lung)
ABG	arterial blood gases	MDI	metered-dose inhaler
AFB	acid-fast bacillus	MDR-TB	multidrug-resistant tuberculosis
AP	anteroposterior	MRI	magnetic resonance imaging
AQI	Air Quality Index	O_2	oxygen
ARDS	adult respiratory distress syndrome	PA	posteroanterior
BS	breath sounds	PCO_2, pCO_2	partial pressure of carbon dioxide
C&S	culture and sensitivity	PFT	pulmonary function test
CAT, CT	computerized axial tomography	PND	paroxysmal nocturnal dyspnea
CF	cystic fibrosis	PO_2, pO_2	partial pressure of oxygen
CO	carbon monoxide	PPD	packs per day (of cigarettes); purified protein derivative (TB test)
CO_2	carbon dioxide		
COPD	chronic obstructive pulmonary disease	RA	room air (no supplemental oxygen)
CPAP	continuous positive airway pressure (pronounced "SEE-pap")	RLL	right lower lobe (of the lung)
		RML	right middle lobe (of the lung)

Career Focus

Meet Susan, a respiratory therapist in a hospital

"I love my job. I've been doing it for 36 years. I probably could retire, but I choose not to. We treat neonates to geriatric patients. We treat asthma, COPD, and pulmonary fibrosis patients and give information to the patients' families. We also manage oxygen therapy, nebulizer therapy, and medication therapy. We do pulmonary function technology and blood gases. I feel that being a respiratory therapist allows me to feel respected and appreciated, not only by the medical staff, but by the patients because you are giving patient care. You are dealing with the patient directly, as well as the physician. You feel good at the end of the day when you leave."

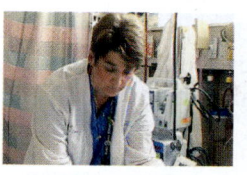

- **Respiratory therapists** are allied health professionals who perform pulmonary function tests and administer respiratory therapy with various types of equipment that provide oxygen or respiratory assistance to a patient.

- **Pulmonologists** are physicians who practice in the medical specialty of pulmonology. They diagnose and treat patients with respiratory problems. Physicians can take additional training and become board certified in the subspecialty of pediatric pulmonology.

- **Thoracic** (or cardiothoracic) **surgeons** perform pulmonary surgery, including surgery for cancer.

- **Oncologists** treat cancer of the lungs with drugs.

therapist (THAIR-ah-pist)
   therap/o- *treatment*
   -ist *person who specializes in*

pulmonologist (PUL-moh-NAW-loh-jist)
   pulmon/o- *lung*
   log/o- *study of; word*
   -ist *person who specializes in*

oncologist (ong-KAW-loh-jist)
   onc/o- *mass; tumor*
   log/o- *study of; word*
   -ist *person who specializes in*

Career Focus
This section orients students to a different healthcare career in each chapter.

Chapter Review Exercises
This section fortifies students with a fun and extensive variety of exercises. ***Dive In*** exercises are linked to each numbered section in the chapter and are designed for a range of learning styles. These exercises emphasize mastery of the medical information presented in each section as well as mastery of the language aspects of word parts and their meanings, building words, dividing words, singular and plural nouns, adjectives, spelling, and pronunciation. ***Immerse Yourself*** exercises emphasize the application of knowledge as students read real patient records and answer thought-provoking questions about their content.

Chapter Review Exercises

Dive In: Medical Language Exercises

Test your knowledge of the chapter by completing these review exercises. Use the Answer Key at the end of the book to check your answers. Note: Each of the numbered exercise headers corresponds to a numbered learning outcome at the beginning of the chapter.

4.1 Anatomy

MATCHING EXERCISE

Match each word or phrase to its description.

1. a
2. tu

Immerse Yourself: Analyze Medical Reports

Electronic Patient Record #1

This is an Office Visit in the SOAP note format. Read the note and answer the questions.

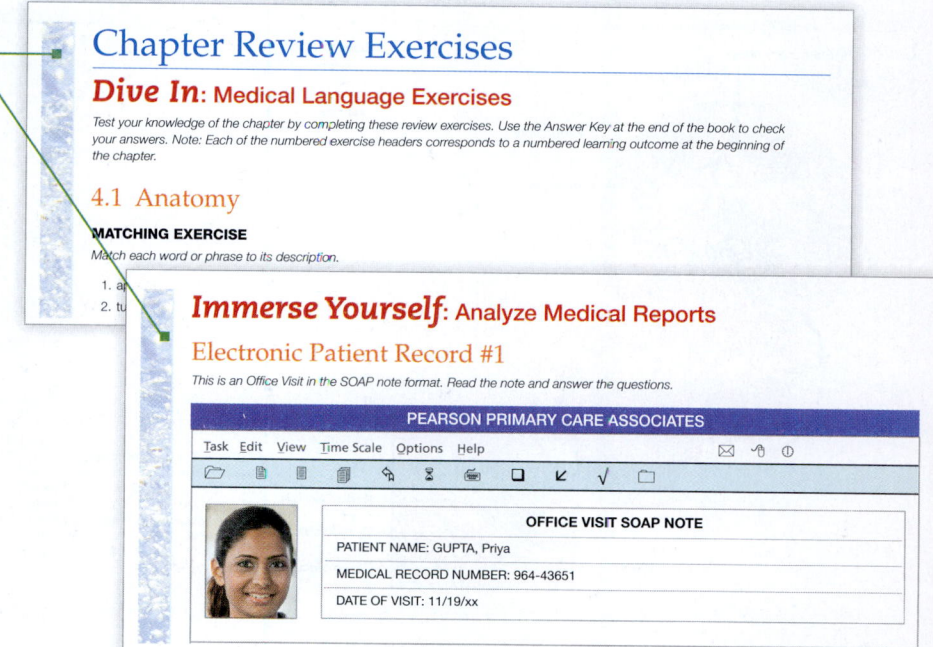

PEARSON PRIMARY CARE ASSOCIATES									

Task Edit View Time Scale Options Help

OFFICE VISIT SOAP NOTE

PATIENT NAME: GUPTA, Priya

MEDICAL RECORD NUMBER: 964-43651

DATE OF VISIT: 11/19/xx

My**Lab** Medical Terminology™

MyLab Medical Terminology is a premium online homework management system that includes a host of features to help you study. Registered users will find:

- A multitude of quizzes and activities built within the MyLab platform
- Powerful tools that track and analyze your results—allowing you to create a personalized learning experience
- Videos and audio pronunciations to help enrich your progress
- Streaming lesson presentations (guided lectures) and self-paced learning modules
- A space where you and your instructor can check your progress and manage your assignments

MyLab Medical Terminology Preview
This end-of-chapter reminder encourages students to make use of the rich variety of online interactive activities and games to further enhance their learning experience.

Special Features

"How would you describe the ideal medical terminology textbook?" That is the question we asked our development team of students and instructors. Their responses helped us craft an array of special features that make this book unique.

Vibrant Medical Illustrations and Photographs bring medical language to life and facilitate understanding, especially for visual learners.

Pronunciation/Word Parts are in the page margins (and within various tables), whenever a bolded word is introduced in the text. This feature gives students the tools to understand unfamiliar words on their own—a see-and-say pronunciation guide and the word parts and meanings of each bolded word—reinforcing that word building is an ongoing process.

Pronunciation/Word Parts

respiratory (RES-pih-rah-TOR-ee)
re- *again and again; backward; unable to*
spir/o- *breathe; coil*
-atory *pertaining to*
Respiratory: Pertaining to again and again (to) breathe

cardiopulmonary
(KAR-dee-oh-PUL-moh-NAIR-ee)
cardi/o- *heart*
pulmon/o- *lung*
-ary *pertaining to*

nose (NOHZ)

naris (NAY-rihs)

nares (NAY-reez)
Latin plural noun: Change the singular ending -is to -es.

nasal (NAY-zal)
nas/o- *nose*
-al *pertaining to*

cavity (KAV-ih-tee)
cav/o- *hollow space*
-ity *condition; state*

septum (SEP-tum)

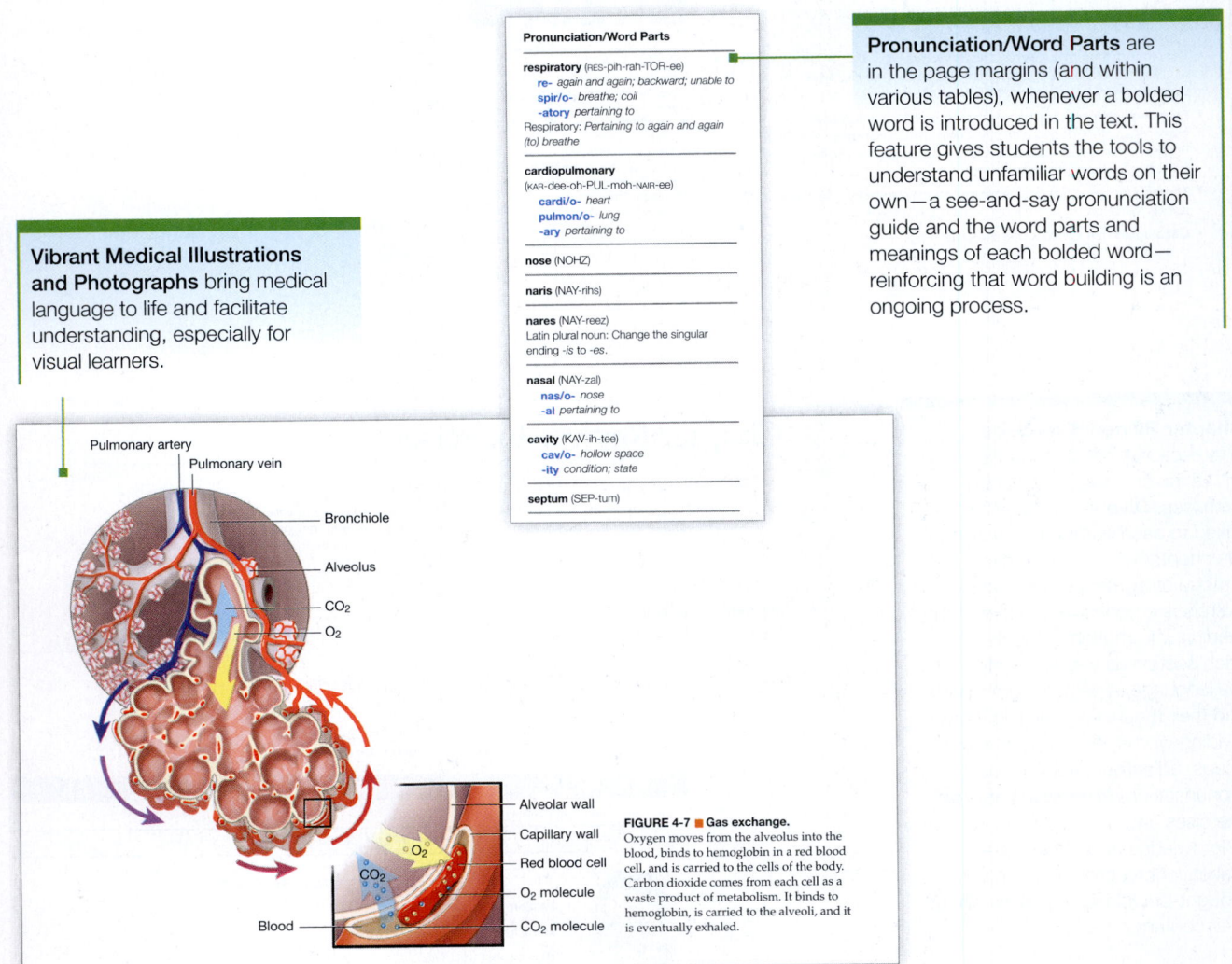

FIGURE 4-7 ■ **Gas exchange.**
Oxygen moves from the alveolus into the blood, binds to hemoglobin in a red blood cell, and is carried to the cells of the body. Carbon dioxide comes from each cell as a waste product of metabolism. It binds to hemoglobin, is carried to the alveoli, and it is eventually exhaled.

Labels: Pulmonary artery; Pulmonary vein; Bronchiole; Alveolus; CO_2; O_2; Alveolar wall; Capillary wall; Red blood cell; O_2 molecule; CO_2 molecule; Blood

Tables are used whenever appropriate to present the content in a visually organized way that students can more easily understand and study.

Table 5-3 Locations and Descriptions of the Veins

The veins are listed as they are encountered anatomically, beginning with the vena cava.

Veins	Location and Description	Pronunciation/Word Parts
superior vena cava	The **superior vena cava** brings deoxygenated blood from the head, neck, chest, and arms to the right atrium. The superior vena cava is named for its location, which is superior to the heart.	**vena cava** (VEE-nah KAY-vah) Latin plural noun: Change the singular ending -a to -ae. Example: The superior and inferior venae cavae
inferior vena cava	The **inferior vena cava** brings deoxygenated blood from the abdomen, pelvis, and legs to the right atrium. The inferior vena cava is named for its location, which is inferior to the heart. In the pelvic cavity in the area of the hip bones, the inferior vena cava ends as it divides to become the right and left iliac veins.	
jugular veins	The **jugular veins** bring deoxygenated blood from the head and neck to the superior vena cava. The jugular vein takes its name from a Latin word that means *neck*.	**jugular** (JUG-yoo-lar) **jugul/o-** *throat* **-ar** *pertaining to*
pulmonary veins	The **pulmonary veins** bring <u>oxygenated</u> blood from the lungs to the left atrium of the heart. Remember: The pulmonary veins are the exception because they are the only veins that carry <u>oxygenated</u> blood. The adjective for the lung is *pulmonary*.	**pulmonary** (PUL-moh-NAIR-ee) **pulmon/o-** *lung* **-ary** *pertaining to*
portal veins	The **portal veins** bring deoxygenated blood from the intestines and liver to the inferior vena cava. The portal vein is named for the porta hepatis, an opening (or portal) in the liver where blood vessels enter and exit.	**portal** (POR-tal) **port/o-** *point of entry* **-al** *pertaining to*
fibular veins	The **fibular veins** bring deoxygenated blood from the little toe side of the lower leg to the femoral veins. The fibular vein is named for the fibula bone in the lower leg.	**fibular** (FIH-byoo-lar) **fibul/o-** *fibula* **-ar** *pertaining to*
saphenous veins	The **saphenous veins** bring deoxygenated blood from the lower legs to the femoral veins. The saphenous vein takes its name from a Latin word that means *clearly visible*, as this vein often can be seen through the skin on the inside lower leg.	**saphenous** (SAF-eh-nuhs) **saphen/o-** *clearly visible* **-ous** *pertaining to*

Feature Boxes spark student interest with key details relating the material to the real world of medicine and include:

Across the Life Span brings an infusion of relevant information related to each stage of life from neonatalogy to pediatrics to geriatrics.

Across the Life Span

Pediatrics. In the uterus, the fetus does not breathe, and its lungs are collapsed. It receives oxygen from the mother's lungs via the placenta and umbilical cord. The lungs of the fetus do not function until the very first breath after birth. At that time, they must expand fully and stay expanded (which is helped by the presence of surfactant).

The normal respiratory rate for a newborn infant is 30–60 breaths per minute. The normal respiratory rate for an adult is 12–20 breaths per minute.

Geriatrics. As a person ages, the number of alveoli in the lungs decreases, and the remaining alveoli are less elastic. The thorax becomes stiff and is less able to expand on inhalation. In addition, a lifetime of exposure to air pollution, chemical fumes, and smoke causes damage to the lungs. These changes decrease pulmonary function in older adults.

Dive Deeper

The American College of Cardiology and the American Heart Association issued new guidelines for blood pressure and hypertension in 2017. Normal blood pressure is now anything *less than120/80.* The new guidelines are illustrated here.

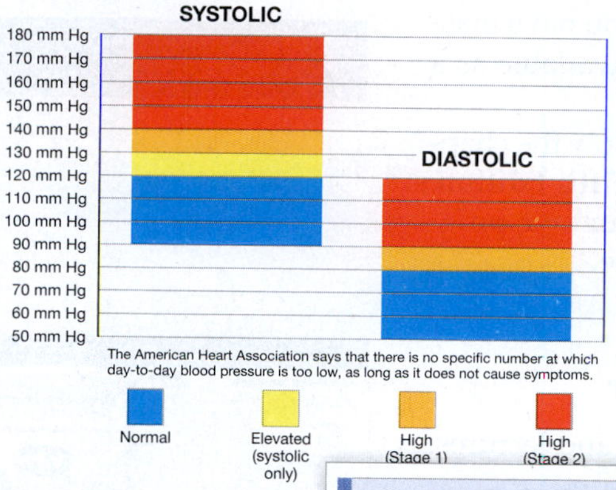

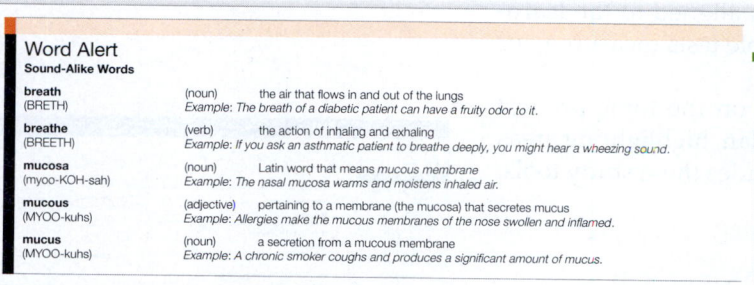

The American Heart Association says that there is no specific number at which day-to-day blood pressure is too low, as long as it does not cause symptoms.

Dive Deeper presents a quick, focused glance at pertinent additional in-depth details related to the material being covered.

Clinical Connections

Dietetics. The body produces its own supply of cholesterol to make bile, neurotransmitters, and male and female sex hormones. The diet contains additional cholesterol in foods from animal sources. An excessive amount of animal fat in the diet increases the cholesterol level in the blood. An excessive amount of sugar in the diet is converted by the body to triglycerides, and this causes an increased triglyceride level in the blood and increased storage as adipose tissue (fat). Fatty plaque deposits in the arteries grow more quickly in patients who eat high-fat diets or have uncontrolled diabetes mellitus.

Psychology. Some people have increased blood pressure readings just because they are nervous about being in a doctor's office. This is known as **white-coat hypertension**. This is not a true hypertension because, as soon as they leave the doctor's office, their blood pressure returns to normal.

Public Health. There are many factors that contribute to the development of coronary artery disease. These are known as **cardiac risk factors**. They include demographic factors (heredity, gender, age), medical factors (hypertension, hypercholesterolemia, diabetes mellitus, obesity), and lifestyle factors (smoking, lack of exercise, poor diet, stress, alcoholism).

Clinical Connections highlights the relationships between the chapter material and other medical specialties or presents snapshots of the ways technology is changing health care.

Word Alert
Sound-Alike Words

breath (BRETH)	(noun)	the air that flows in and out of the lungs *Example: The breath of a diabetic patient can have a fruity odor to it.*
breathe (BREETH)	(verb)	the action of inhaling and exhaling *Example: If you ask an asthmatic patient to breathe deeply, you might hear a wheezing sound.*
mucosa (myoo-KOH-sah)	(noun)	Latin word that means *mucous membrane* *Example: The nasal mucosa warms and moistens inhaled air.*
mucous (MYOO-kuhs)	(adjective)	pertaining to a membrane (the mucosa) that secretes mucus *Example: Allergies make the mucous membranes of the nose swollen and inflamed.*
mucus (MYOO-kuhs)	(noun)	a secretion from a mucous membrane *Example: A chronic smoker coughs and produces a significant amount of mucus.*

Word Alert presents important notes about the nuances, meanings, variations, and peculiarities of language and specific, selected bolded words in the chapter. Word Alert includes topics such as Abbreviations, Sound-Alike Words, and It's Greek to Me!, which gives useful reminders about how Greek and Latin combining forms remain part of medical language today.

Appendix A: Glossary of Medical Word Parts: Prefixes, Suffixes, and Combining Forms Appendix A gathers all medical word parts into one table to facilitate searching. Prefixes, suffixes, and combining forms and their meanings are indicated by color shading.

Appendix B: Glossary of Medical Abbreviations, Acronyms, and Short Forms gathers the shortened forms of medical language from the Abbreviations Summary feature within each chapter.

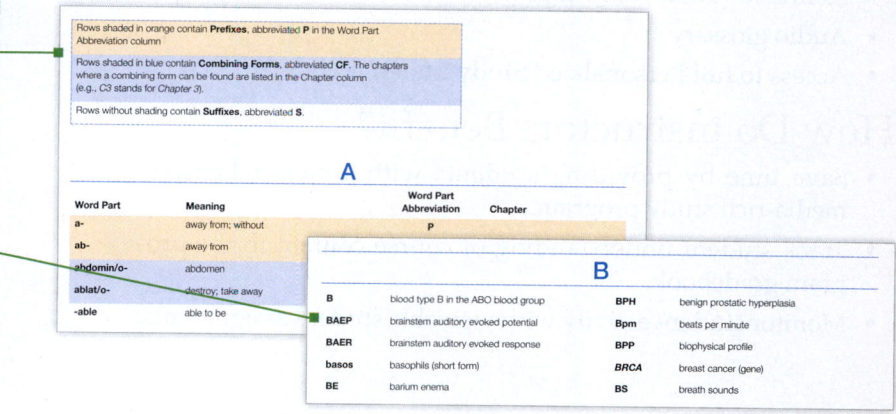

Rows shaded in orange contain **Prefixes**, abbreviated **P** in the Word Part Abbreviation column

Rows shaded in blue contain **Combining Forms**, abbreviated **CF**. The chapters where a combining form can be found are listed in the Chapter column (e.g., *C3* stands for *Chapter 3*).

Rows without shading contain **Suffixes**, abbreviated **S**.

A

Word Part	Meaning	Word Part Abbreviation	Chapter
a-	away from; without	P	
ab-	away from		
abdomin/o-	abdomen		
ablat/o-	destroy; take away		
-able	able to be		

B

B	blood type B in the ABO blood group	BPH	benign prostatic hyperplasia
BAEP	brainstem auditory evoked potential	Bpm	beats per minute
BAER	brainstem auditory evoked response	BPP	biophysical profile
basos	basophils (short form)	BRCA	breast cancer (gene)
BE	barium enema	BS	breath sounds

MyLab Medical Terminology™

What Is MyLab Medical Terminology?

MyLab Medical Terminology is a comprehensive online testing program that gives you, the student, the opportunity to test your understanding of information, concepts, and medical language to see how well you know the material. From the test results, MyLab Medical Terminology builds a self-paced, personalized study plan unique to your needs. Remediation in the form of etext pages, illustrations, exercises, audio segments, and video clips is provided for those areas in which you may need additional instruction, review, or reinforcement. You can then work through the program until your study plan is complete and you have mastered the content. MyLab Medical Terminology is available as a standalone program or with an embedded etext.

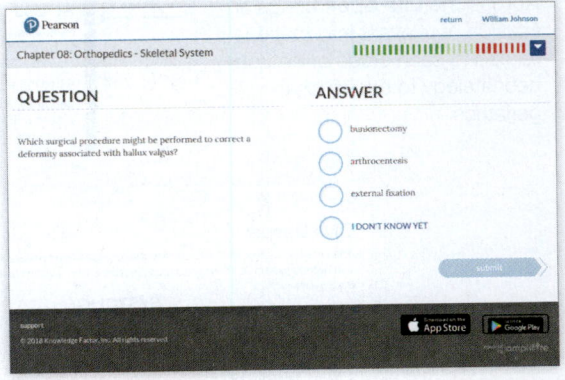

MyLab Medical Terminology is organized to follow the chapters and learning outcomes in *Medical Language*, **Fifth Edition**. With MyLab Medical Terminology, you can track your own progress through your entire medical terminology course.

How Do Students Benefit?

Here's how MyLab Medical Terminology helps you:

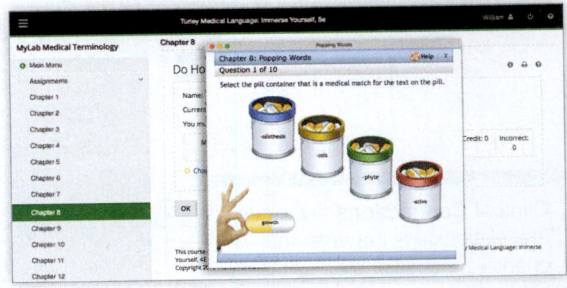

- Keep up with information presented in the text and lectures.
- Save time by focusing your study to review just the content you need.
- Increase your understanding of difficult concepts with study material that is appropriate for different learning styles.
- Remediate in areas in which you need additional review.

Key Features of MyLab Medical Terminology

Pre-Tests and Post-Tests. Using questions aligned to the learning outcomes in *Medical Language*, multiple tests measure your understanding of topics.

Personalized Study Material. Based on the topic pre-test results, you receive a personalized study plan, highlighting areas where you may need improvement. It includes these study tools:

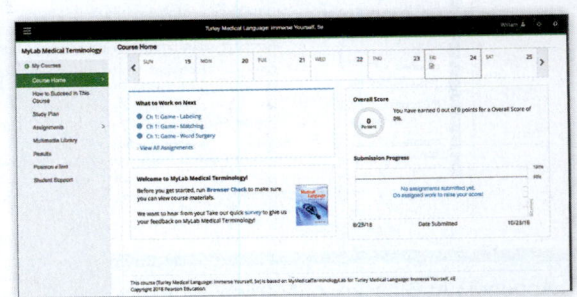

- Links to specific pages in the etext
- Images for review
- Interactive exercises
- Animations and video clips
- Audio glossary
- Access to full Personalized Study Material.

How Do Instructors Benefit?

- Save time by providing students with a comprehensive, media-rich study program.
- Track student understanding of course content in the program gradebook.
- Monitor student activity with viewable student assignments.

Contents

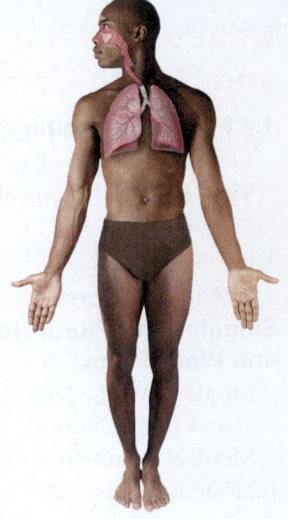

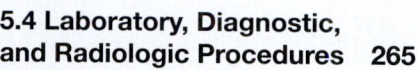
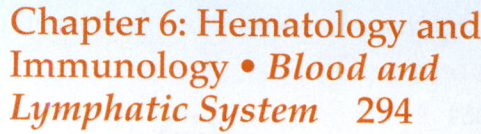

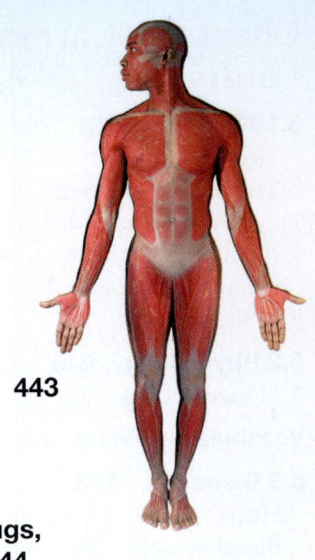

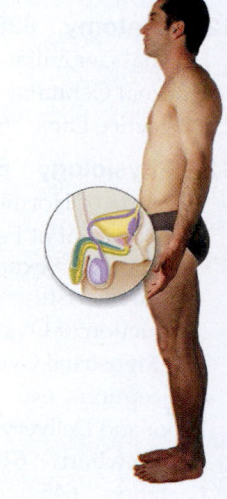

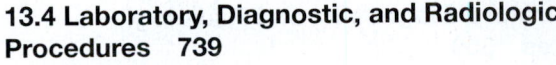

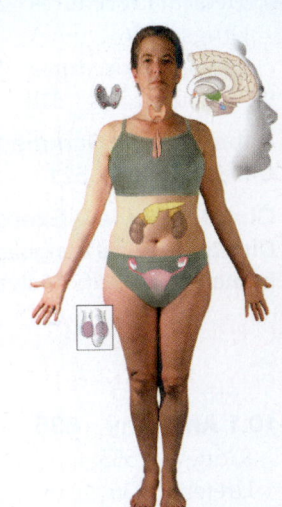

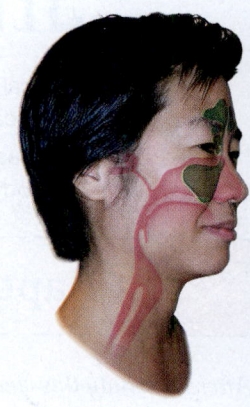

1 Medical Language and Health Care Today

Medical language (MED-ih-kal LANG-gwij) is the framework on which the practice of medicine is built. Healthcare professionals use medical language every day to communicate with each other.

Health care is the process by which trained and licensed professionals maintain or restore the health of the body and mind.

 ## Chapter Overview and Learning Outcomes

After you study this chapter, you should be able to demonstrate mastery of the outcomes by successfully completing the exercises.

1.1 Medical Language
Identify the five skills of medical language communication.
Describe the origins of medical language.
1.1 Practice Laps

1.2 Medical Words: Singular and Plural Nouns and Word Parts
Form the plural of common medical singular nouns.
Identify the characteristics of word parts (combining form, suffix, prefix).
Give the meaning of common medical word parts.
1.2 Practice Laps

1.3 Medical Words: Divide, Build, Spell, and Pronounce
Divide medical words into word parts.
Build medical words from word parts.
Spell and pronounce common medical words.
1.3 Practice Laps
Vocabulary Review

1.4 The Body in Health and Disease
Define *health* and *disease*.
Identify body planes, directions, and positions; body cavities; and body quadrants and regions.
Describe anatomy and physiology, body systems, and medical specialties.
Describe categories of diseases.
1.4 Practice Laps
Vocabulary Review

1.5 Health Care Today
Describe categories of healthcare professionals.
Describe the settings in which health care is provided.
Describe techniques used to perform a physical examination.
Describe the types and components of electronic health records.
1.5 Practice Laps
Vocabulary Review
Abbreviations Summary
Career Focus

Chapter Review Exercises
Dive In: Medical Language Exercises
(Learning Outcomes 1.1–1.5)
Immerse Yourself: Introduction to Medical Reports

Medical Language Key

To unlock the definition of a medical word, first break it into word parts. Then give the meaning of each word part. Put the meanings of the word parts in order, beginning with the meaning of the suffix, then the meaning of the prefix (if there is one), then the meaning of the combining form.

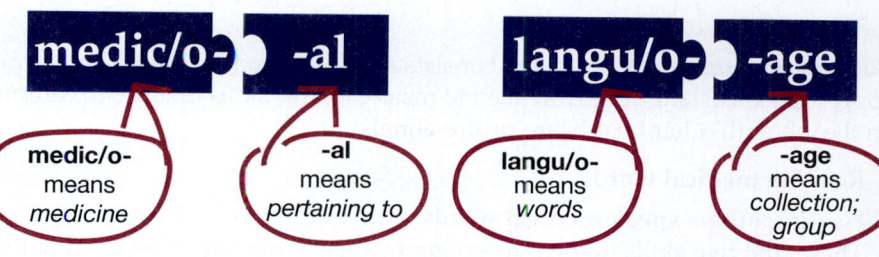

medic/o-) -al   langu/o-) -age

medic/o-
means
medicine

-al
means
pertaining to

langu/o-
means
words

-age
means
*collection;
group*

You are about to begin the study of medical language! Right now, medical words may seem complex, but, as you study, you will learn their meanings. Studying medical language involves time and effort, but healthcare professionals know that there is no substitute for a thorough, working knowledge of medical language. **Medical language** is the language of health care and medicine, and medical words are the "tools of the trade (see Figure 1-1 ■)." Learning medical language is the key to a successful career!

Dive Deeper

Medical Language versus Medical Terminology. There are many medical **terminology** textbooks on the market. These textbooks teach medical terms, but not medical language—the language that physicians, nurses, therapists, and other healthcare workers use. Medical terminology textbooks divide chapters by body systems, but *Medical Language* has chapters based on medical specialties, which reflects the practice of medicine in the real world. *Medical Language* reflects the way communication happens in medicine and health care today!

Pronunciation/Word Parts

medical (MED-ih-kal)
  medic/o- *medicine*
  -al *pertaining to*

language (LANG-gwij)
  langu/o- *words*
  -age *collection; group*

terminology (TER-mih-NAW-loh-jee)
  termin/o- *boundary; end; word*
  -logy *study of*

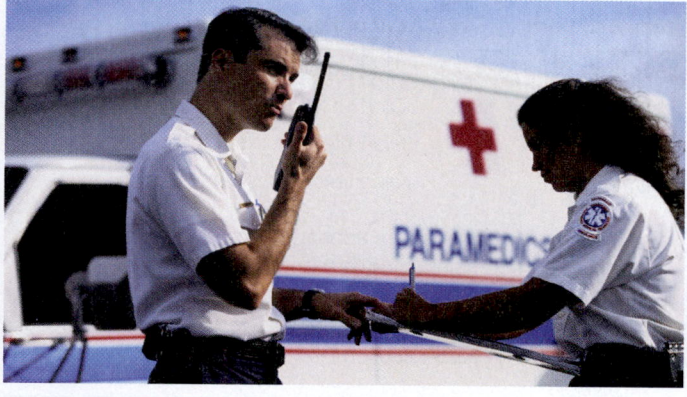

A.

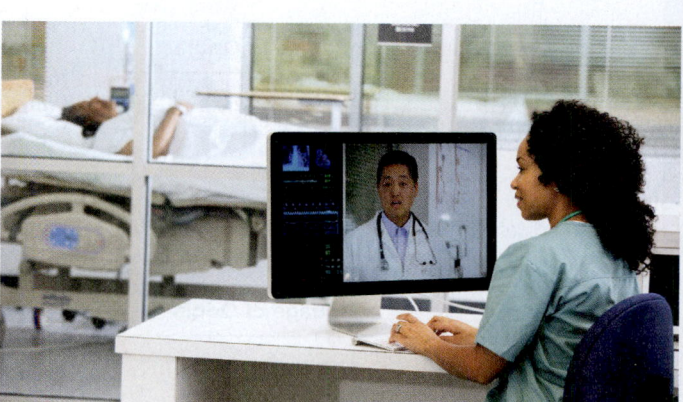

B.

FIGURE 1-1 ■ Medical language.
A. These paramedics are speaking and writing medical language as they describe the condition of the patient in the ambulance to healthcare professionals in the hospital's emergency department. **B.** This nurse is reading and analyzing a patient's electronic medical record as she speaks to the patient's physician who is listening to her report during a teleconference. How important do you think it is for each of these healthcare professionals to have a thorough, working knowledge of medical language?

1.1 Medical Language

Language Skills

Communication in any language consists of five language skills. These same skills apply to medical language. You need to master all five skills in order to communicate on the job with other healthcare professionals.

1. **Reading medical words**
2. **Hearing others speak medical words**
   These first two skills involve receiving medical language. This is similar to input coming into a computer.
3. **Thinking, analyzing, and understanding medical words**
   This three-part skill involves processing medical language. This is similar to the processing function of a computer.
4. **Writing (or typing) and spelling medical words**
5. **Speaking and pronouncing medical words**
   These two skills involve relaying medical language. This is similar to output coming from a computer.

   All of these skills are critical to the communication of medical language. This textbook, *Medical Language*, helps you develop all of these skills by giving you many opportunities to practice until you have mastered them.

The Origins of Medical Language

Let's start by looking at how medical language began. **Etymology** is the study of word origins. In medical language, many words came from other languages, particularly Greek and Latin. Why? Because in ancient times, both the Greeks and the Romans advanced the study and practice of medicine. They named anatomical structures, diseases, and treatments in their own languages, and many of these Greek and Latin words remain a part of medical language today. You'll be surprised to see how many of these words are familiar to you.

Pronunciation/Word Parts

communication (koh-MYOO-nih-KAY-shun)
communic/o- *impart; transmit*
-ation *being; having; process*

etymology (ET-ih-MAW-loh-jee)
etym/o- *word origin*
-logy *study of*

1. Reading
2. Hearing
3. Thinking, analyzing, and understanding
4. Writing (or typing) and spelling
5. Speaking and pronouncing

Word Alert

Word Origins. These medical words are identical to the original Greek and Latin words.

Medical Word	Language of Origin
pelvis	Latin *pelvis*
sinus	Latin *sinus*
thorax	Greek *thorax*

These medical words are similar to the original Greek and Latin words.

Medical Word	Language of Origin
artery	Latin *arteria*
muscle	Latin *musculus*
patient	Latin *patiens*
sperm	Greek *sperma*
urine	Latin *urina*
vein	Latin *vena*

These medical words are similar to words from Old English, French, or Dutch.

Medical Word	Language of Origin
bladder	Old English *blaedre*
drug	Old Dutch *droog*
heart	Old English *heorte*
physician	Old French *physicien*

It's Greek to Me! This feature appears at the end of each chapter. It lists common combining forms mentioned in that chapter, their language of origin (Greek or Latin), and how those combining forms were used in medical words in the chapter. (*Note:* You will learn about combining forms in a later section.)

Word	Greek	Latin	Medical Word Examples
intestine	enter/o-	intestin/o-	gastroenterology; gastrointestinal
nerve	neur/o-	nerv/o-	neurology; nervous system
skin	dermat/o-	integument/o-	dermatology; integumentary system

1.1 PRACTICE LAPS

Use the Answer Key at the end of the book to check your answers.

A. Matching Exercise

Match each word to its description.

1. bladder
2. drug
3. muscle
4. physician
5. sinus
6. sperm
7. thorax

_____ medical word that is similar to a Latin word

_____ medical word that is similar to an Old French word

_____ medical word that is similar to a Greek word

_____ medical word that is identical to a Latin word

_____ medical word that is identical to a Greek word

_____ medical word that is similar to an Old Dutch word

_____ medical word that is similar to an Old English word

B. True or False Exercise

Indicate whether each statement is true or false by writing **T** *or* **F** *on the line.*

1. _____ Studying medical language involves time and effort.
2. _____ Terminology is the study of word origins.
3. _____ In ancient times, both the Greeks and Romans named structures, diseases, and treatments in their own languages.
4. _____ All medical words originally came from the Latin language.
5. _____ The medical word *pelvis* and the Latin word *pelvis* are identical.
6. _____ Medical words are the "tools of the trade" for healthcare professionals.
7. _____ Communication in any language consists of five language skills.

C. Fill in the Blank Exercise

Name the five language skills.

1. _____
2. _____
3. _____
4. _____
5. _____

1.2 Medical Words: Singular and Plural Nouns and Word Parts

Medical Words: Singular and Plural Nouns

English Nouns

The rules for forming the plural of English words also apply to medical words. For most singular English nouns, form the plural by adding an *-s*.

> Examples: *gland* becomes *glands, hormone* becomes *hormones, intestine* becomes *intestines, kidney* becomes *kidneys, lung* becomes *lungs, nerve* becomes *nerves, rib* becomes *ribs,* and *tonsil* becomes *tonsils.*

For some singular English nouns that end in *-y*, form the plural by changing the *-y* to *-ies*.

Examples: *artery* becomes *arteries*, and *ovary* becomes *ovaries*.

Greek and Latin Nouns

The Greek and Latin languages are important sources of medical words. These languages had rules about how to form plural nouns, and those rules still apply today (see Table 1-1 ■). *Note*: When a Greek or Latin noun appears in a chapter, there will be a note there to remind you of those rules.

Table 1-1   Rules for Forming Greek and Latin Plural Nouns

Rule	Singular Noun	Plural Noun
Greek Singular and Plural Nouns		
1. When a Greek singular noun ends in *-is*, form the plural by changing *-is* to *-ides*.	iris	irides
2. When a Greek singular noun ends in *-nx*, form the plural by changing *-nx* to *-nges*.	phalanx	phalanges
3. When a Greek singular noun ends in *-oma*, form the plural by changing *-oma* to *-omata*.	carcinoma	carcinomata
4. When a Greek singular noun ends in *-on*, form the plural by changing *-on* to *-a*.	ganglion	ganglia
Latin Singular and Plural Nouns		
1. When a Latin singular noun ends in *-a*, form the plural by changing *-a* to *-ae*.	sclera vertebra	sclerae vertebrae
2. When a Latin singular noun ends in *-us*, form the plural by changing *-us* to *-i*.	bronchus thrombus	bronchi thrombi
3. When a Latin singular noun ends in *-um*, form the plural by changing *-um* to *–a*.	atrium bacterium	atria bacteria
4. When a Latin singular noun ends in *-is*, form the plural by changing *-is* to *-es*.	diagnosis testis	diagnoses testes
5. When a Latin singular noun ends in *-ex*, form the plural by changing *-ex* to *-ices*.	apex cortex	apices cortices

Medical Word Parts

Medical words contain word parts. Most medical words have two word parts, but even the longest medical word has only three different types of word parts: a prefix, combining form, and suffix.

Type of Word Part	Description
Prefix	An optional word beginning
Combining form	The foundation of a medical word
Suffix	A word ending

Dive Deeper

Learning medical language requires some memorization of word parts and their meanings.

If you know the meaning of a word part (especially a combining form), you can look at a medical word and already have an idea about its meaning because you know the meanings of its word parts.

Combining Forms

Because the combining form is the foundation of a medical word, let's begin our study of word parts by learning about combining forms. A combining form has the following characteristics:

- It is a word part that is the foundation of a medical word.
- It gives a medical word its main medical meaning.
- It has a root, a forward slash, a combining vowel, and a hyphen (see Figure 1-2 ■). Usually the combining vowel is an *o*, but occasionally it is an *a*, *e*, *i*, or *y*. The hyphen shows that a combining form is a word part, not a complete word.
- The majority of medical words contain a combining form. Some contain two combining forms, one right after the other. Example: *gastrointestinal* (the combining forms are **gastr/o-** and **intestin/o-**). Some medical words (such as *blood*, *health*, *heart*, or *nurse*), do not contain a combining form or any word parts at all.
- Two combining forms can have the same medical meaning because each is from a different language (see the feature *It's Greek to Me!* described previously.)

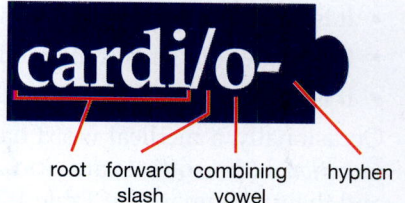

root forward combining hyphen
slash   vowel

FIGURE 1-2 ■ Combining form.
A combining form contains a root, forward slash, combining vowel, and hyphen. The hyphen shows that the combining form is a word part, not a complete word. The combining form **cardi/o-** means *heart*.

Dive Deeper

In *Medical Language*, each time a word part is mentioned, it is shown in **bold blue type** (see the paragraph above and Table 1-2 ■). This is to help you recognize that it is a word part. *Note*: Remember, word parts are not actual medical words because they contain forward slashes and hyphens that must be removed when a medical word is formed. Now let's look at some common combining forms and their meanings.

Table 1-2   Common Combining Forms and Their Meanings

Combining Form with a Nearly Identical Medical Meaning

Combining Form	Meaning	
abdomin/o-	abdomen	
arteri/o-	artery	
intestin/o-	intestine	
muscul/o-	muscle	
thyroid/o-	thyroid gland	
tonsill/o-	tonsil	
ven/o-	vein	

Combining Form Similar to a Common Medical Word

Combining Form	Meaning	Related Word
arthr/o-	joint	arthritis
cardi/o-	heart	cardiac
dermat/o-	skin	dermatologist
gastr/o-	stomach	gastric
mamm/o-	breast	mammogram
nas/o-	nose	nasal

Combining Form Not Similar to its Medical Meaning

Combining Form	Meaning	
cost/o-	rib	
cyan/o-	blue	
enter/o-	intestine	
hepat/o-	liver	
lapar/o-	abdomen	
leuk/o-	white	

Suffixes

Now let's turn our attention to another type of word part: suffixes. A suffix has the following characteristics:

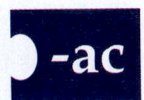

- It is a group of letters at the end of most medical words.
- It modifies or clarifies the medical meaning of the combining form.
- It is a word part that begins with a hyphen (see Figure 1-3 ■).

Occasionally, a medical word has two suffixes, one right after the other. Example: *nutritional* (the suffixes are **-ion** and **-al**). Now let's look at some common suffixes and their meanings (see Table 1-3 ■).

FIGURE 1-3 ■ Suffix.
A suffix begins with a hyphen to show that it is a word part, not a complete word. The suffix **-ac** means *pertaining to*.

Table 1-3   Common Suffixes and Their Meanings

Suffix	Meaning	Medical Word Example	Definition	Notes
Suffixes for an Adjective				
-ac	pertaining to	cardi**ac**	**pertaining to** (the) heart	Combining form **cardi/o-** means *heart*.
-al	pertaining to	intestin**al**	**pertaining to** (the) intestine	Combining form **intestin/o-** means *intestine*.
-ar	pertaining to	muscul**ar**	**pertaining to** (a) muscle	Combining form **muscul/o-** means *muscle*.
-ary	pertaining to	urin**ary**	**pertaining to** (the) urine	Combining form **urin/o-** means *urinary system; urine*.
-ic	pertaining to	pelv**ic**	**pertaining to** (the) pelvis	Combining form **pelv/o-** means *hip bone; pelvis; renal pelvis*.
-ine	pertaining to	uter**ine**	**pertaining to** (the) uterus	Combining form **uter/o-** means *uterus; womb*.
-ive	pertaining to	digest**ive**	**pertaining to** break down food	Combining form **digest/o-** means *break down food; digest*.
-ous	pertaining to	ven**ous**	**pertaining to** (a) vein	Combining form **ven/o-** means *vein*.
Suffixes for a Process				
-ation	being; having; process	urin**ation**	**process** (of making) urine	Combining form **urin/o-** means *urine; urinary system*.
-ion	action; condition	digest**ion**	**action** (to) break down food	Combining form **digest/o-** means *break down food; digest*.
Suffixes for a Disease				
-ia	condition; state; thing	pneumon**ia**	**condition** (of the) lung	Combining form **pneumon/o-** means *air; lung*.
-ism	disease from a specific cause; process	hypothyroid**ism**	**disease from a specific cause** (of) deficient thyroid gland (hormone)	Combining form **thyroid/o-** means *thyroid gland*.
-itis	infection of; inflammation of	tonsill**itis**	**infection of** (the) tonsil	Combining form **tonsill/o-** means *tonsil*.
-megaly	enlargement	cardio**megaly**	**enlargement** (of the) heart	Combining form **cardi/o-** means *heart*.
-oma	mass; tumor	neur**oma**	**tumor** (on a) nerve	Combining form **neur/o-** means *nerve*.
-osis	abnormal condition; process	vagin**osis**	**abnormal condition** (of the) vagina	Combining form **vagin/o-** means *vagina*.
-pathy	disease	arthro**pathy**	**disease** (of a) joint	Combining form **arthr/o-** means *joint*.
Suffixes for a Procedure				
-ectomy	surgical removal	tonsill**ectomy**	**surgical removal** (of the) tonsils	Combining form **tonsill/o-** means *tonsil*.
-gram	picture; record	mammo**gram** (see Figure 1-4 ■)	**picture** (of the) breast	Combining form **mamm/o-** means *breast*.
-graphy	process of recording	arterio**graphy**	**process of recording** (an) artery	Combining form **arteri/o-** means *artery*.
-metry	process of measuring	densito**metry**	**process of measuring** (the) density (of bone)	Combining form **densit/o-** means *density*.
-scope	instrument used to examine	colono**scope**	**instrument used to examine** (the) colon	Combining form **colon/o-** means *colon*.
-scopy	process of using an instrument to examine	gastro**scopy**	**process of using an instrument to examine** (the) stomach	Combining form **gastr/o-** means *stomach*.
-tomy	process of making an incision	laparo**tomy**	**process of making an incision** (in the) abdomen	Combining form **lapar/o-** means *abdomen*.

continued on next page

Table 1-3   Common Suffixes and Their Meanings

Suffix	Meaning	Medical Word Example	Definition	Notes
Suffixes for a Medical Specialty or Specialist				
-iatry	medical treatment	psych**iatry**	**medical treatment** (for the) mind	Combining form **psych/o-** means *mind*.
-ics	knowledge; practice	obstet**rics**	**knowledge and practice** (of) pregnancy and childbirth	Combining form **obstetr/o-** means *pregnancy and childbirth*.
-ist	person who specializes in; thing that specializes in	therap**ist** (see Figure 1-5 ■)	**person who specializes in** treatment	Combining form **therap/o-** means *treatment*.
-logy	study of	cardio**logy** (see Figure 1-6 ■)	**study of** (the) heart	Combining form **cardi/o-** means *heart*.

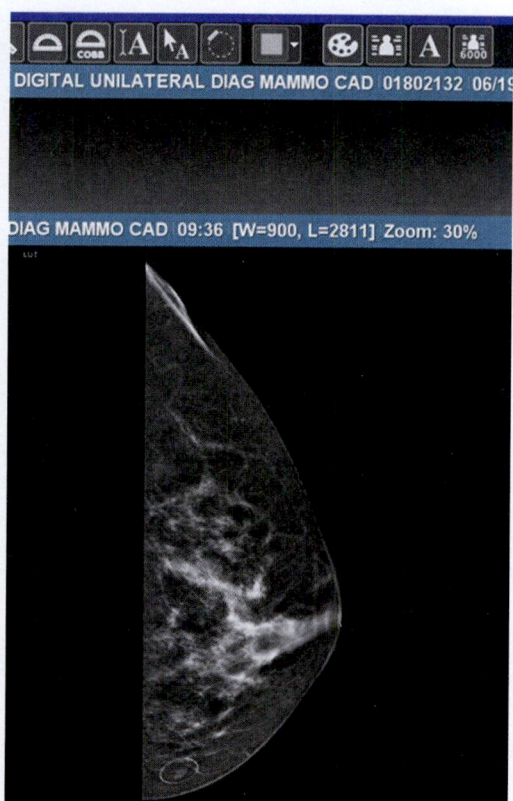

FIGURE 1-4 ■ **Mammogram.**
A mammogram is a picture of the breast that is created with x-rays. The suffix **-gram** means *picture; record.*

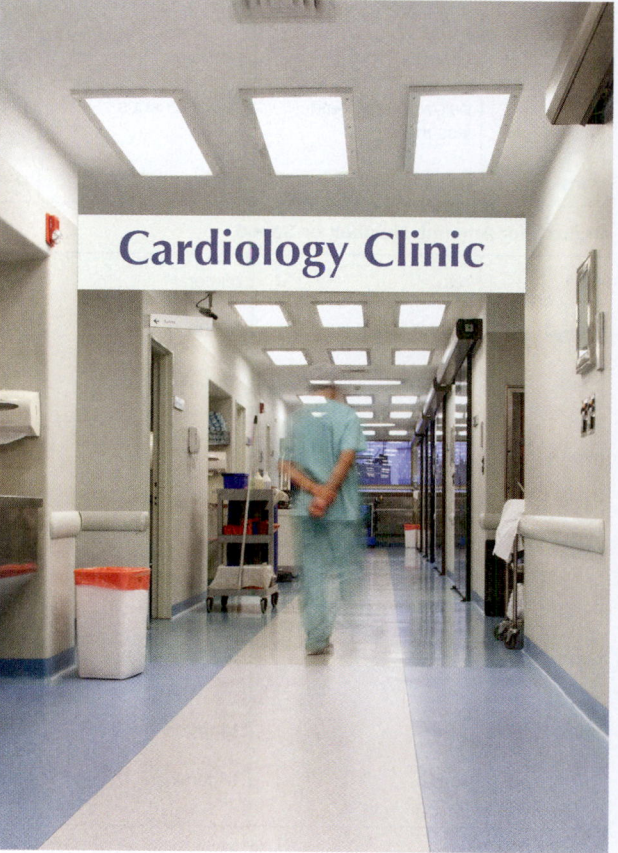

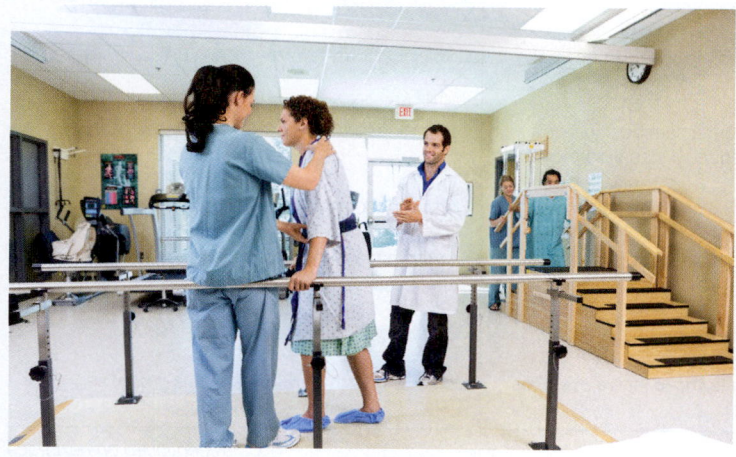

FIGURE 1-5 ■ **Therapist.**
This physical therapist is providing therapy to a patient. The suffix **-ist** means *person who specializes in.*

FIGURE 1-6 ■ **Cardiology clinic.**
There are many types of clinics located in a hospital or in other healthcare facilities.

Prefixes

Finally, let's look at the third type of word part: prefixes. A prefix has the following characteristics:

- It is a word part that, if present, is at the beginning of a word, but not every medical word contains a prefix.
- It modifies or clarifies the medical meaning of the combining form.
- It is a single letter or group of letters that ends with a hyphen (see Figure 1-7 ■).

Some common prefixes are shown in Table 1-4 ■. Take a moment to review them and learn their meanings so that you will be ready to use them in medical words.

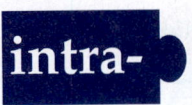

FIGURE 1-7 ■ Prefix.
A prefix ends with a hyphen to show that it is a word part, not a complete word. The prefix **intra-** means *within*.

Table 1-4   Common Prefixes and Their Meanings

Prefix	Meaning	Medical Word Example	Definition	Notes
Prefixes for Location or Direction				
epi-	above; upon	**epi**dermal	pertaining to **upon** (the) skin	Combining form **derm/o-** means *skin*.
inter-	between	**inter**costal	pertaining to **between** (the) ribs	Combining form **cost/o-** means *rib*.
intra-	within	**intra**venous (see Figure 1-8 ■)	pertaining to **within** (a) vein	Combining form **ven/o-** means *vein*.
peri-	around	**peri**cardial	pertaining to **around** (the) heart	Combining form **cardi/o-** means *heart*.
post-	after; behind	**post**nasal	pertaining to **behind** (the) nose	Combining form **nas/o-** means *nose*.
pre-	before; in front of	**pre**natal	pertaining to **before** (a) birth	Combining form **nat/o-** means *birth*.
sub-	below; underneath; less than	**sub**cutaneous	pertaining to **underneath** (the) skin	Combining form **cutane/o-** means *skin*.
trans-	across; through	**trans**vaginal	pertaining to **through** (the) vagina	Combining form **vagin/o-** means *vagina*.
Prefixes for Amount, Number, or Speed				
bi-	two	**bi**lateral	pertaining to **two** sides	Combining form **later/o-** means *side*.
brady-	slow	**brady**cardia	condition (of a) **slow** heart	Combining form **card/o-** means *heart*.
hemi-	one half	**hemi**plegia	condition (of) **one half** (of the body with a) paralysis	Combining form **pleg/o-** means *paralysis*.
hyper-	above; more than normal	**hyper**tension (see Figure 1-9 ■)	condition (of) **more than normal** pressure	Combining form **tens/o-** means *pressure; tension*.
hypo-	below; deficient	**hypo**thyroidism	disease from a specific cause (of) **deficient** thyroid gland (hormone)	Combining form **thyroid/o-** means *thyroid gland*.
poly-	many; much	**poly**neuritis	inflammation of **many** nerves	Combining form **neur/o-** means *nerve*.
quadri-	four	**quadri**plegia	condition (of) **four** (limbs with) paralysis	Combining form **pleg/o-** means *paralysis*.
tachy-	fast	**tachy**cardia	condition (of a) **fast** heart	Combining form **card/o-** means *heart*.
tri-	three	**tri**geminal	pertaining to **three** (nerve branches in a) group	Combining form **gemin/o-** means *group; set*.

continued on next page

Table 1-4   **Common Prefixes and Their Meanings**

Prefix	Meaning	Medical Word Example	Definition	Notes
Prefixes for Degree or Quality				
an-	not; without	**an**esthesia	condition (of being) **without** sensation	Combining form **esthes/o-** means *feeling; sensation*.
anti-	against	**anti**biotic	pertaining to (a drug that is) **against** living organisms	Combining form **bi/o-** means *living organism; living tissue*.
dys-	abnormal; difficult; painful	**dys**phagia	condition (of) **difficult** (or) **painful** eating (and) swallowing	Combining form **phag/o-** means *eating; swallowing*.
re-	again and again; backward; unable to	**re**spiration	process (of) **again and again** (to) breathe	Combining form **spir/o-** means *breathe; coil*.

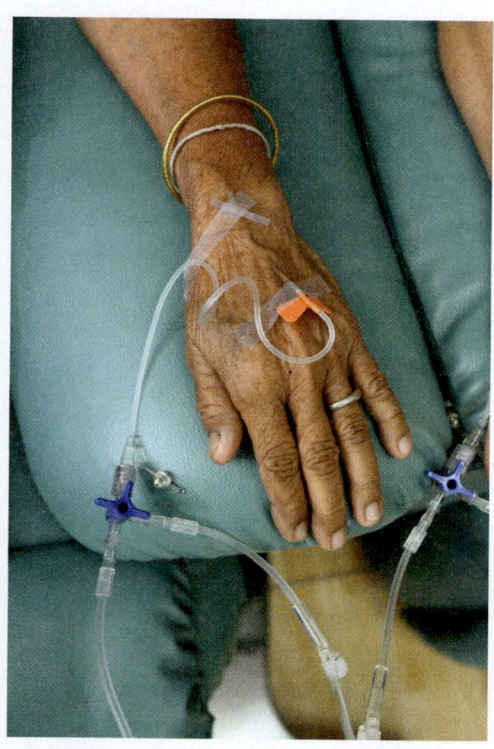

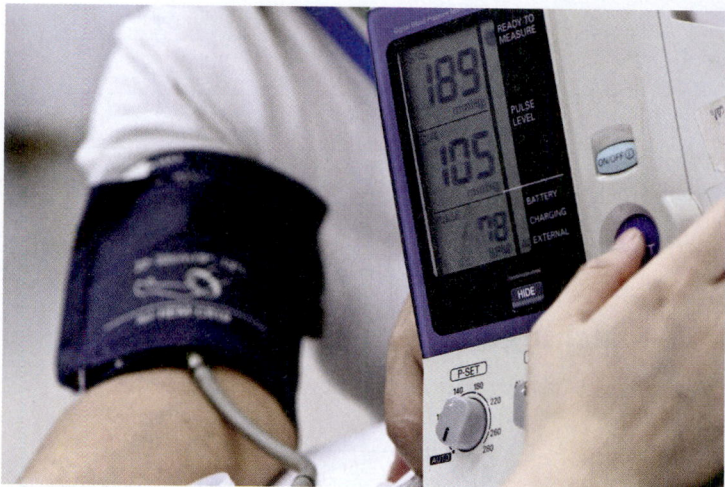

FIGURE 1-9 ■ Hypertension.
The numbers on this automated blood pressure machine are higher than a normal reading, which shows that the patient has hypertension. The prefix **hyper-** means *above; more than normal*.

FIGURE 1-8 ■ Intravenous.
The prefix **intra-** means *within*. The needle is placed within a vein to administer intravenous fluids.

1.2 PRACTICE LAPS

Use the Answer Key at the end of the book to check your answers.

A. Give the Meaning of Combining Forms

Next to each combining form, write its meaning. The first one has been done for you.

Combining Form	Meaning	Combining Form	Meaning
1. **spir/o-**	*breathe; coil*	4. arthr/o-	
2. abdomin/o-		5. bi/o-	
3. arteri/o-		6. colon/o-	

continued on next page

Combining Form	Meaning	Combining Form	Meaning
7. cost/o-	_____	21. nat/o-	_____
8. cutane/o-	_____	22. neur/o-	_____
9. dermat/o-	_____	23. obstetr/o-	_____
10. derm/o-	_____	24. pelv/o-	_____
11. digest/o-	_____	25. phag/o-	_____
12. enter/o-	_____	26. pleg/o-	_____
13. esthes/o-	_____	27. tens/o-	_____
14. gastr/o-	_____	28. therap/o-	_____
15. intestin/o-	_____	29. thyroid/o-	_____
16. lapar/o-	_____	30. tonsill/o-	_____
17. later/o-	_____	31. urin/o-	_____
18. leuk/o-	_____	32. uter/o-	_____
19. mamm/o-	_____	33. vagin/o-	_____
20. muscul/o-	_____	34. ven/o-	_____

B. Matching Exercise

Match each word part to its description.

1. anti-	_____ prefix meaning *fast*
2. brady-	_____ combining form meaning *liver*
3. cardi/o-	_____ suffix meaning *action; condition*
4. cyan/o-	_____ prefix meaning *around*
5. hepat/o-	_____ suffix meaning *mass; tumor*
6. -ion	_____ combining form meaning *nose*
7. -itis	_____ combining form meaning *heart*
8. nas/o-	_____ suffix meaning *pertaining to*
9. peri-	_____ prefix meaning *slow*
10. -oma	_____ combining form meaning *blue*
11. -ous	_____ suffix meaning *infection of; inflammation of*
12. tachy-	_____ prefix meaning *against*

C. True or False Exercise

*Indicate whether each statement is true or false by writing **T** or **F** on the line.*

1. _____ For most singular English words, form the plural by adding an -s.

2. _____ Greek and Latin languages had rules about how to form a plural noun, and those rules still apply today.

3. _____ By definition, a therapist is a person who specializes in treatment.

4. _____ The combining form **gastr/o-** means *rib*.

5. _____ The combining form **arthr/o-** means *joint*.

D. English Plural Noun Exercise

Write the plural form of each English singular noun. Be sure to check your spelling. The first one has been done for you.

1. **hormone**   *hormones*
2. kidney   _____
3. artery   _____

4. nerve   _____
5. ovary   _____

E. Greek Plural Noun Exercise

Write the plural form of each Greek singular noun. Be sure to check your spelling. The first one has been done for you.

1. **iris**   *irides*
2. phalanx   _____

3. carcinoma   _____
4. ganglion   _____

F. Latin Plural Noun Exercise

Write the plural form of each Latin singular noun. Be sure to check your spelling. The first one has been done for you.

1. **vertebra**   *vertebrae*
2. sclera   _____
3. bronchus   _____
4. alveolus   _____
5. thrombus   _____
6. atrium   _____

7. bacterium   _____
8. ovum   _____
9. diagnosis   _____
10. testis   _____
11. apex   _____

1.3 Divide and Build Medical Words

The third skill of medical language involves thinking, analyzing, and understanding. When you analyze something, you divide it into smaller pieces that are easier to understand. When you see or hear a medical word, you can analyze it by dividing it into its word parts. Or when you read the definition of a medical word, you can analyze it by selecting word parts to build the word itself. Here are the steps for dividing or building a medical word.

Divide Medical Words

Medical Word with a Combining Form and Suffix

Let's say you read or hear this medical word and want to know its definition.

cardiology

Step 1. Divide the medical word into its combining form and suffix.
(*Note*: At this point, you may not be able to look at a medical word and know that it contains a combining form and a suffix. However, as you memorize various word parts and their meanings, you will be able to do this.)

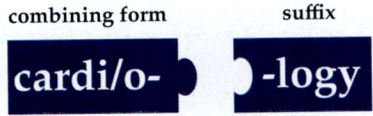

Step 2. Give the meaning of each word part.

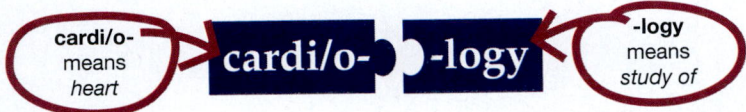

Step 3. Combine the meanings of the word parts; put the meaning of the suffix first, then the meaning of the combining form.

Step 4. Add small connecting words to make the definition.

suffix	**combining form**
study of	*heart*

Cardiology: *Study of (the) heart (and related structures)*

Medical Word with a Prefix, Combining Form, and Suffix

Let's say you read or hear this medical word and want to know its definition.

pericardial

Step 1. Divide the medical word into its prefix, combining form, and suffix.

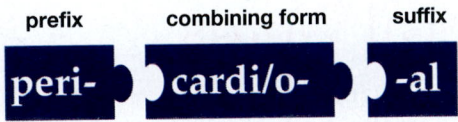

Step 2. Give the meaning of each word part.

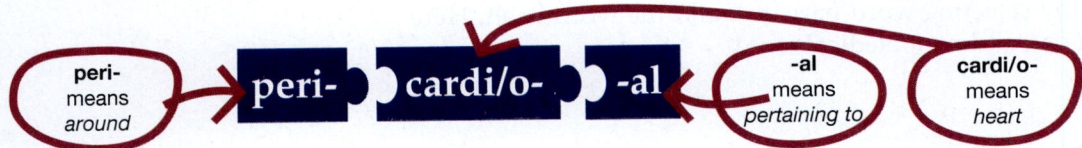

Step 3. Combine the meanings of the word parts; put the meaning of the suffix first, then the meaning of the prefix, then the meaning of the combining form.

Step 4. Add small connecting words to make the definition.

suffix	**prefix**	**combining form**
pertaining to	*around*	*heart*

Pericardial: *Pertaining to around (the) heart*

Build Medical Words

Medical words are like puzzles, and their word parts are the pieces of the puzzle. To build a medical word, begin with its definition. Select word parts that match that definition and put the word parts together (like puzzle pieces) in the correct way. Here are the steps for building a medical word.

Suffix that Begins with a Consonant

Let's say you want to build a medical word with this definition.

Study of the heart

Step 1. Select the suffix whose meaning matches the definition of that medical word. Then select the combining form whose meaning matches.

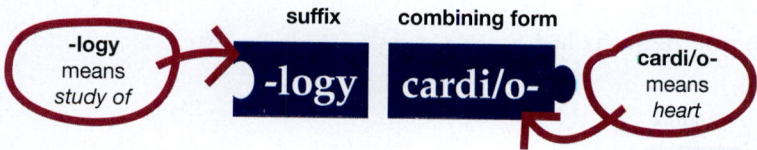

Step 2. Change the order of the word parts to put the suffix last.

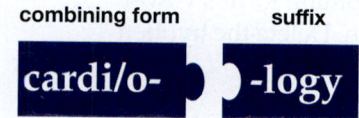

Step 3. Because the suffix begins with a consonant, keep the combining form's vowel, but delete the forward slash and hyphen. Delete the hyphen from the suffix. Then, join the two word parts.

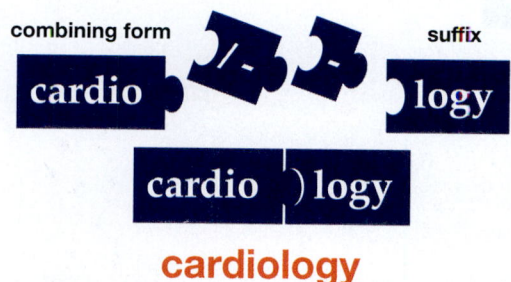

cardiology

Suffix that Begins with a Vowel

Let's say you want to build a medical word with this definition.

Pertaining to the heart

Step 1. Select the suffix whose meaning matches the definition of that medical word. Then select the combining form whose meaning matches.

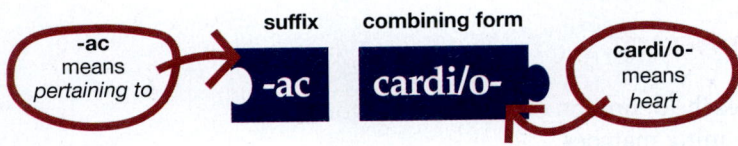

Step 2. Change the order of the word parts to put the suffix last.

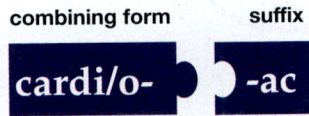

Step 3. Because the suffix begins with a vowel, delete the combining form's vowel. Also delete the combining form's forward slash and hyphen. Delete the hyphen from the suffix. Then, join the two word parts.

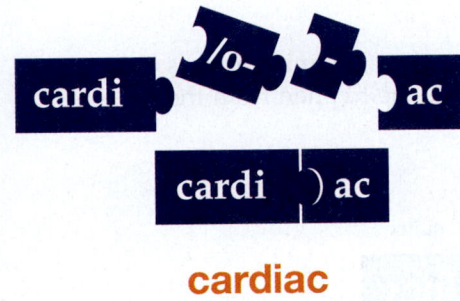

cardiac

Contains a Prefix

Let's say you want to build a medical word with this definition.

Pertaining to within the heart

Step 1. Select the suffix, prefix, and combining form whose meanings match the definition of the medical word.

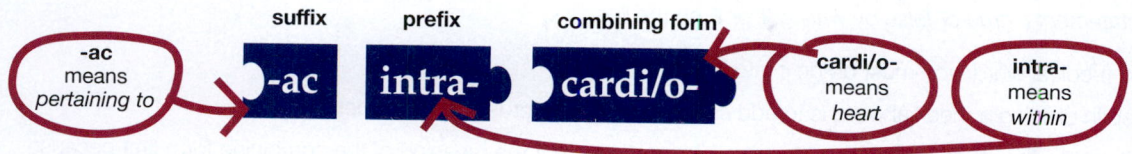

Step 2. Change the order of the word parts to put the suffix last, with the prefix first, followed by the combining form.

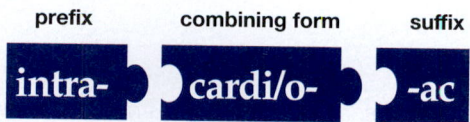

Step 3. Delete the hyphen from the prefix. Delete the forward slash, combining vowel, and hyphen from the combining form. Delete the hyphen from the suffix. Then, join the three word parts.

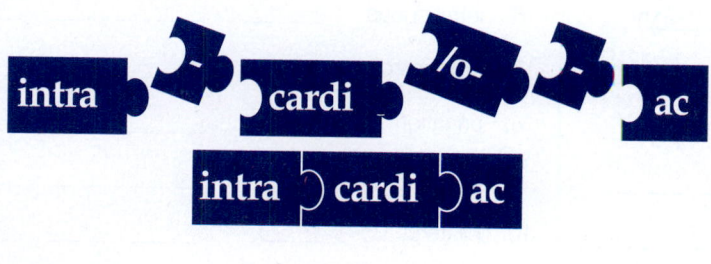

intracardiac

Write and Spell Medical Words

One of the five medical language skills is the spelling of medical words. Remembering the spelling of combining forms and other word parts and how to correctly build a medical word will also help you correctly spell the medical word. Writing and spelling medical words are emphasized in every chapter's exercises.

Speak and Pronounce Medical Words

One of the five medical language skills is the pronunciation of medical words. Knowing the definition of a medical word is important, but being able to pronounce the word correctly is equally important. In each chapter, as you read a medical word (in bold in the text), you will see an accompanying "see-and-say" pronunciation guide in the column next to the text (see Figure 1-10 ■). The syllables in the medical word are separated by hyphens. The primary (main) accented syllable is in all capital letters. The secondary accented syllable is in smaller capital letters. Use the pronunciation guide to say each syllable. In doing so, you are creating an accurate pronunciation memory for that medical word.

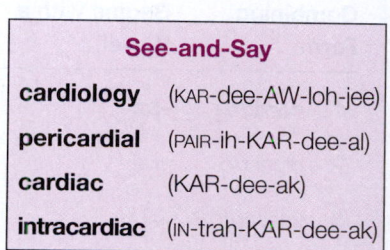

See-and-Say	
cardiology	(KAR-dee-AW-loh-jee)
pericardial	(PAIR-ih-KAR-dee-al)
cardiac	(KAR-dee-ak)
intracardiac	(IN-trah-KAR-dee-ak)

FIGURE 1-10 ■ Pronunciation.
Pronounce each syllable in the "see-and-say" pronunciation to hear the correct pronunciation of the medical word.

1.3 PRACTICE LAPS

Use the Answer Key at the end of the book to check your answers.

A. True or False Exercise

*Indicate whether each statement is true or false by writing **T** or **F** on the line.*

1. _____ To analyze a medical word, you must divide it into its word parts.

2. _____ The final step in dividing a medical word is to add small connecting words to make a definition.

3. _____ When you combine the meanings of the different word parts, you put the meaning of the combining form first because it is the most important.

4. _____ When a suffix begins with a consonant, keep the combining form's vowel when you build the medical word.

5. _____ To finish building a medical word, delete the hyphen from the combining form and the hyphen from the suffix.

6. _____ When a suffix begins with a vowel, delete the combining form's vowel when you build the medical word.

B. Dividing Medical Words Exercise

Separate these words into their component parts (prefix, combining form, suffix). Some words do not contain all three word parts. The first one has been done for you.

Medical Word	Prefix	Combining Form	Suffix
1. **cardiology**		*cardi/o-*	*-logy*
2. cardiac		_____	_____
3. intestinal		_____	_____
4. muscular		_____	_____
5. venous		_____	_____

Medical Word	Prefix	Combining Form	Suffix
6. intravenous	_____	_____	_____
7. bradycardia	_____	_____	_____
8. urination		_____	_____
9. tonsillitis		_____	_____
10. bilateral	_____	_____	_____

C. Build Medical Words Exercise

Practice building medical words by joining a combining form and a suffix. Write the medical word on the line. Be sure to check your spelling. The first one has been done for you.

Combining Form	Suffix that Begins with a Vowel	Medical Word
1. **cardi/o-**	**-ac**	*cardiac*
2. digest/o-	-ive	_____
3. intestin/o-	-al	_____
4. neur/o-	-oma	_____
5. therap/o-	-ist	_____
6. tonsill/o-	-itis	_____

Combining Form	Suffix that Begins with a Consonant	Medical Word
7. arthr/o-	-pathy	_____
8. cardi/o-	-logy	_____
9. cardi/o-	-megaly	_____
10. colon/o-	-scope	_____

D. Spell Medical Words Exercise

Look at each medical word and detect the spelling error. Then write the correct spelling on the line. The first one has been done for you.

Misspelled Medical Word	Correct Spelling
1. **sychiatry**	*psychiatry*
2. cardeac	
3. tonsilitis	
4. venus	
5. pelvik	
6. cardology	
7. hypertensin	
8. antebiotic	

E. Pronounce and Spell Exercise

Read the "see-and-say" pronunciation out loud. Practice pronouncing it several times. Write the medical word that it represents. Be sure to check your spelling. The first one has been done for you.

"See-and-Say" Pronunciation	Spell the Medical Word
1. **(ab-DAW-mih-nal)**	*abdominal*
2. (KAR-dee-ak)	
3. (KAR-dee-AW-loh-jee)	
4. (dy-JES-chun)	
5. (dy-JES-tiv)	
6. (in-TES-tih-nal)	
7. (MAM-oh-gram)	
8. (MUS-kyoo-lar)	
9. (sy-KY-ah-tree)	
10. (THAIR-ah-pist)	
11. (TAWN-sil-EK-toh-mee)	
12. (YOOR-ih-NAIR-ee)	
13. (PEL-vik)	
14. (VEE-nuhs)	

Vocabulary Review

Here are the word parts presented in the first part of this chapter. Take time to review them and learn their meanings so that you will be ready to use them when you see them in later chapters.

Combining Forms			
Combining Form	**Meaning**	**Combining Form**	**Meaning**
abdomin/o-	abdomen	**later/o-**	side
arteri/o-	artery	**leuk/o-**	white
arthr/o-	joint	**mamm/o-**	breast
bi/o-	living organism; living tissue	**medic/o-**	medicine
card/o-	heart	**muscul/o-**	muscle
cardi/o-	heart	**nas/o-**	nose
colon/o-	colon	**nat/o-**	birth
communic/o-	impart; transmit	**nerv/o-**	nerve
cost/o-	rib	**neur/o-**	nerve
cutane/o-	skin	**obstetr/o-**	pregnancy and childbirth
cyan/o-	blue	**pelv/o-**	hip bone; pelvis; renal pelvis
densit/o-	density	**phag/o-**	eating; swallowing
dermat/o-	skin	**pleg/o-**	paralysis
derm/o-	skin	**pneumon/o-**	air; lung
digest/o-	break down food; digest	**psych/o-**	mind
enter/o-	intestine	**spir/o-**	breathe; coil
esthes/o-	feeling; sensation	**tens/o-**	pressure; tension
etym/o-	word origin	**termin/o-**	boundary; end; word
gastr/o-	stomach	**therap/o-**	treatment
gemin/o-	group; set	**thyroid/o-**	thyroid gland
hepat/o-	liver	**tonsill/o-**	tonsil
intestin/o-	intestine	**urin/o-**	urinary system; urine
integument/o-	skin	**uter/o-**	uterus; womb
langu/o-	words	**vagin/o-**	vagina
lapar/o-	abdomen	**ven/o-**	vein

Suffixes

Suffix	Meaning	Suffix	Meaning
-ac	pertaining to	-ation	being; having; process
-al	pertaining to	-ectomy	surgical removal
-ar	pertaining to	-gram	picture; record
-ary	pertaining to	-graphy	process of recording
-ia	condition; state; thing	-logy	study of
-iatry	medical treatment	-megaly	enlargement
-ic	pertaining to	-metry	process of measuring
-ics	knowledge; practice	-oma	mass; tumor
-ine	pertaining to	-osis	abnormal condition; process
-ion	action; condition	-ous	pertaining to
-ism	disease from a specific cause; process	-pathy	disease
-ist	person who specializes in; thing that specializes in	-scope	instrument used to examine
-itis	infection of; inflammation of	-scopy	process of using an instrument to examine
-ive	pertaining to	-tomy	process of making an incision

Prefixes

Prefix	Meaning	Prefix	Meaning
an-	not; without	peri-	around
anti-	against	poly-	many; much
bi-	two	post-	after; behind
brady-	slow	pre-	before; in front of
dys-	abnormal; difficult; painful	quadri-	four
epi-	above; upon	re-	again and again; backward; unable to
hemi-	one half	sub-	below; underneath; less than
hyper-	above; more than normal	tachy-	fast
hypo-	below; deficient	trans-	across; through
inter-	between	tri-	three
intra-	within		

1.4 The Body in Health and Disease

Health

When the human body's countless parts function correctly, the body is in a state of **health**. The World Health Organization defines *health* as a state of complete physical, mental, and social well-being (and not just the absence of disease or infirmity). The healthy human body can be studied in several different ways. Each way approaches the body from a specific point of view and provides unique information, dividing or organizing the body in a logical way. These approaches include body planes, directions, and positions; body cavities; body quadrants and regions; anatomy and physiology; and body systems and medical specialties. It is important to understand the body in a state of health before learning about diseases of the body (described in a later section).

Body Planes, Directions, and Positions

As a reference point, the human body is studied in **anatomical position** (standing erect with the head up and eyes looking forward, arms by the sides with the palms facing forward, legs straight with the toes pointing forward). From that position, the body can be studied according to **body planes, directions, and positions**. A plane is an imaginary flat surface (like a plate of glass) that divides the body into two parts. There are three body planes: the sagittal plane, the coronal plane, and the transverse plane. Body directions represent movement away from or toward these planes.

Sagittal Plane: Body Directions and Positions

The **sagittal plane** is a vertical plane that divides the body in the midline into right and left sides (see Figure 1-11 ■). Moving from either side of the body toward the midline is moving in a **medial** direction, or medially. Moving from the midline toward either side of the body is moving in a **lateral** direction, or laterally (see Figure 1-12 ■). **Bilateral** is a position that indicates both sides of the body.

Pronunciation/Word Parts
health (HELTH)

anatomical (AN-ah-TAW-mih-kal)
  ana- *apart; excessive*
  tom/o- *cut; layer; slice*
  -ical *pertaining to*

sagittal (SAJ-ih-tal)
  sagitt/o- *front to back*
  -al *pertaining to*

medial (MEE-dee-al)
  medi/o- *middle*
  -al *pertaining to*

lateral (LAT-er-al)
  later/o- *side*
  -al *pertaining to*

bilateral (by-LAT-er-al)
  bi- *two*
  later/o- *side*
  -al *pertaining to*

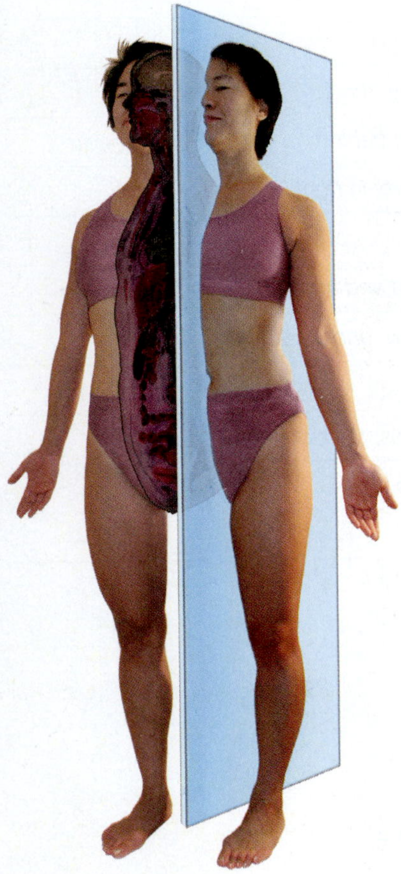

FIGURE 1-11 ■ Sagittal plane. The sagittal plane divides the body into right and left sections.

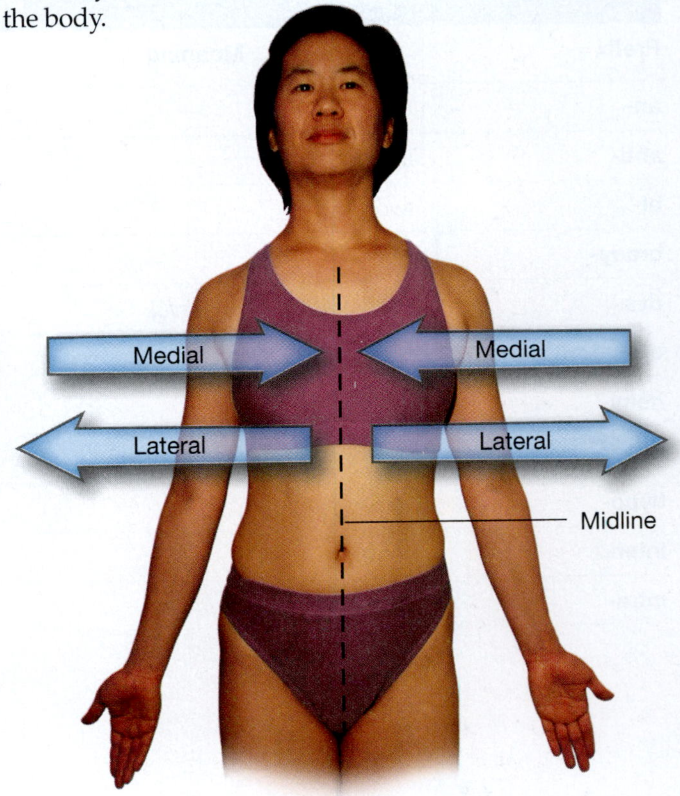

FIGURE 1-12 ■ Medial and lateral directions. Moving in a medial direction is moving toward the midline of the body. Moving in a lateral direction is moving away from the midline. Medial and lateral are opposite directions.

Clinical Connections

Surgery. Correctly identifying right and left is an important patient safety issue. Surgery can accidentally be performed on the wrong side if, prior to surgery, the surgeon did not mark the correct site of surgery or the anesthesiologist and surgical nurse did not ask the patient what was to be the site of the surgery.

Orthopedics. The sagittal and coronal planes are named for the sagittal and coronal sutures that join the bones of the cranium at the top of the head. Those body planes are oriented in the same directions as the sutures for which they are named.

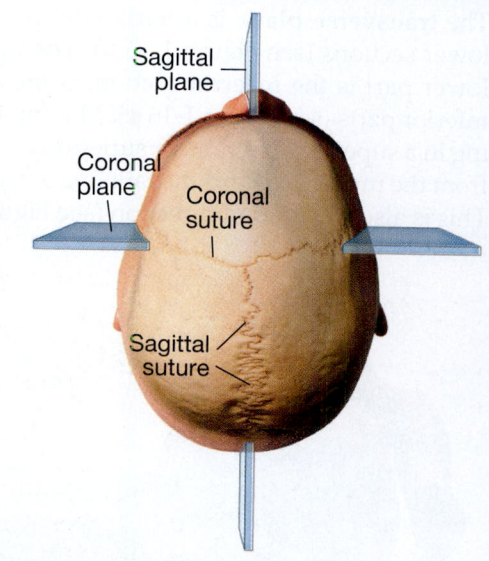

Coronal Plane: Body Directions and Positions

The **coronal plane** or **frontal plane** is a vertical plane that divides the body in the midline into front and back sections (see Figure 1-13 ■). The front of the body is the **anterior** or **ventral** section. Moving from the midline toward the front of the body is moving in an anterior direction, or anteriorly (see Figure 1-14 ■). The back of the body is the **posterior** or **dorsal** section. Moving from the midline toward the back of the body is moving in a posterior direction, or posteriorly. Lying face down is being in the **prone** position. Lying on the back is being in the **dorsal** or **dorsal supine** position.

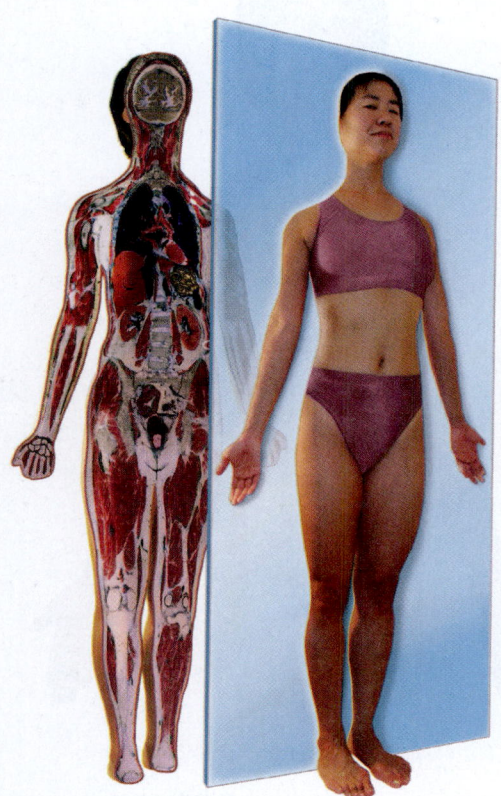

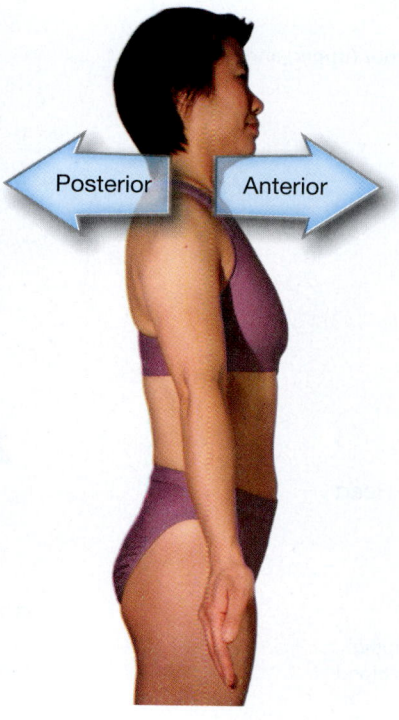

Posterior   Anterior

FIGURE 1-13 ■ Coronal plane.
The coronal plane or frontal plane divides the body into anterior (front) and posterior (back) sections.

Pronunciation/Word Parts

coronal (kor-OH-nal)
  coron/o- *structure that encircles like a crown*
  -al *pertaining to*

frontal (FRUN-tal)
  front/o- *front*
  -al *pertaining to*

anterior (an-TEER-ee-or)
  anter/o- *before; front part*
  -ior *pertaining to*

ventral (VEN-tral)
  ventr/o- *abdomen; front*
  -al *pertaining to*

posterior (pohs-TEER-ee-or)
  poster/o- *back part*
  -ior *pertaining to*

dorsal (DOR-sal)
  dors/o- *back; dorsum*
  -al *pertaining to*

prone (PROHN)

supine (soo-PINE)

FIGURE 1-14 ■ Anterior and posterior directions.
Moving in an anterior direction is moving toward the front of the body. Moving in a posterior direction is moving toward the back of the body. Anterior and posterior are opposite directions.

Transverse Plane: Body Directions

The **transverse plane** is a horizontal plane that divides the body into upper and lower sections (see Figure 1-15 ■). The upper part is the **superior** section, and the lower part is the **inferior** section. Some anatomical structures have superior and inferior parts (see Figure 1-16 ■). Moving from the midline toward the head is moving in a superior direction, or superiorly. This is also the **cephalad** direction. Moving from the midline toward the tailbone is moving in an inferior direction, or inferiorly. This is also the **caudad** direction (see Figure 1-17 ■).

Pronunciation/Word Parts

transverse (trans-VERS)
The prefix **trans-** means *across; through*, and the suffix **-verse** means *travel; turn*.

superior (soo-PEER-ee-or)
  super/o- *above*
  -ior *pertaining to*

inferior (in-FEER-ee-or)
  infer/o- *below*
  -ior *pertaining to*

cephalad (SEF-ah-lad)
  cephal/o- *head*
  -ad *in the direction of; toward*

caudad (KAW-dad)
  caud/o- *tailbone*
  -ad *in the direction of; toward*

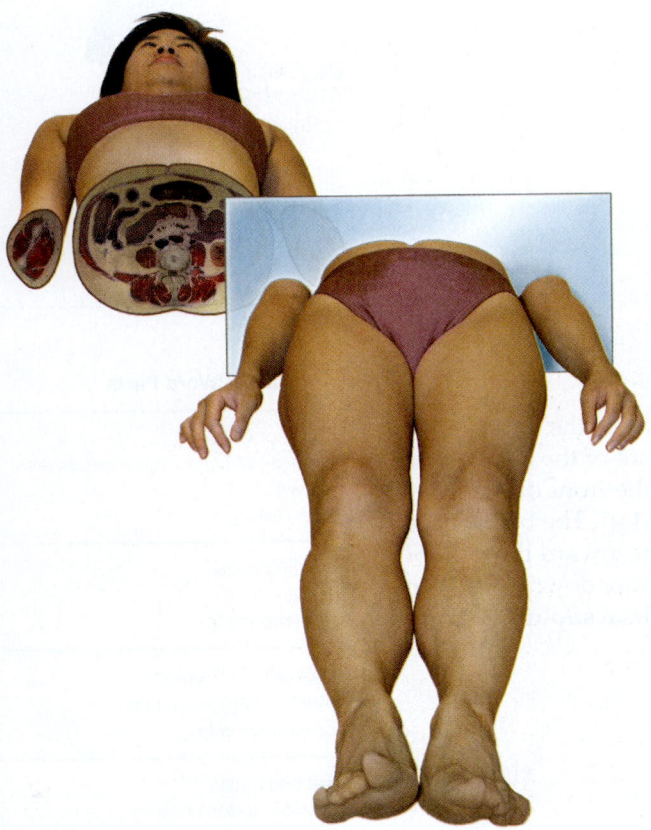

FIGURE 1-15 ■ Transverse plane.
The transverse plane divides the body into superior (upper) and inferior (lower) sections.

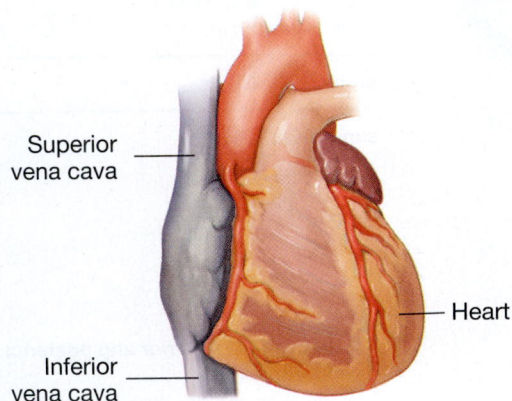

FIGURE 1-16 ■ Superior and inferior.
The superior vena cava brings blood from the upper body to the heart. The inferior vena cava brings blood from the lower body to the heart.

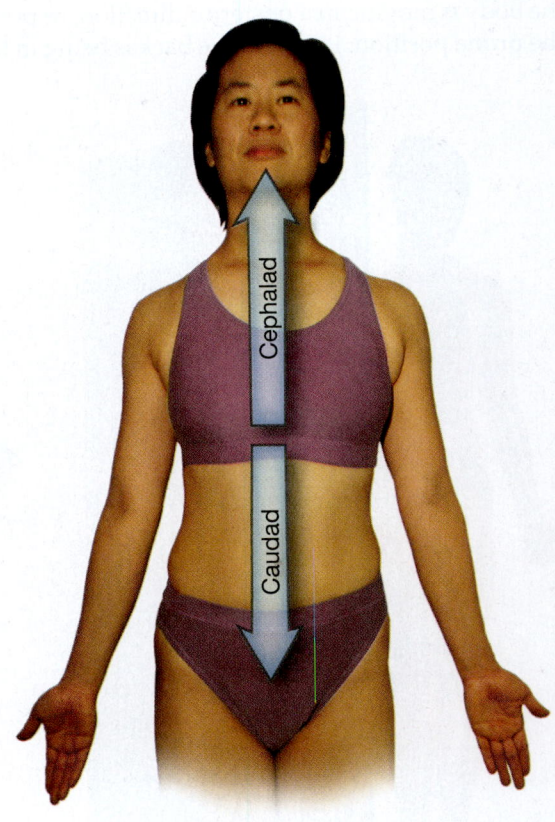

FIGURE 1-17 ■ Cephalad and caudad directions.
Moving in a cephalad direction is moving toward the head. Moving in a caudad direction is moving toward the tailbone. Cephalad and caudad are opposite directions.

Other Body Directions and Locations

Moving from the trunk of the body (and the point of attachment or origin of an arm or leg) toward the end of the arm or leg is moving in a **distal** direction, or distally. Moving from the end of an arm or leg toward its point of attachment (origin) on the trunk of the body is moving in a **proximal** direction, or proximally (see Figure 1-18 ■).

Structures on the surface of the body are superficial or **external**. Structures below the surface and inside the body are deep or **internal** (see Figure 1-19 ■).

Pronunciation/Word Parts

distal (DIS-tal)
   dist/o- *away from the center or point of origin*
   -al *pertaining to*

proximal (PRAWK-sih-mal)
   proxim/o- *near the center or point of origin*
   -al *pertaining to*

external (eks-TER-nal)
   extern/o- *outside*
   -al *pertaining to*

internal (in-TER-nal)
   intern/o- *inside*
   -al *pertaining to*

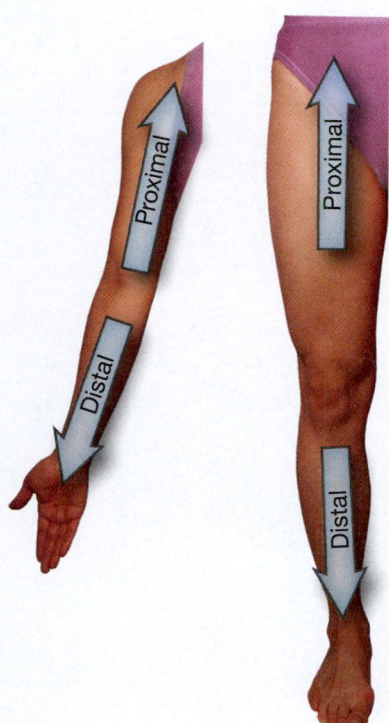

FIGURE 1-18 ■ Distal and proximal directions.
Moving in a distal direction is moving away from the trunk of the body toward the fingers or toes. Moving in a proximal direction is moving away from the fingers or toes toward the trunk. Distal and proximal are opposite directions.

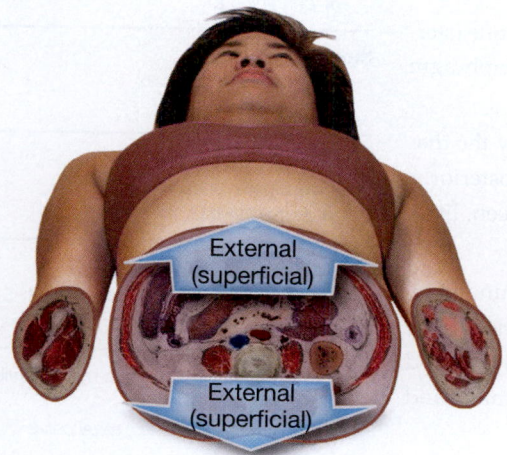
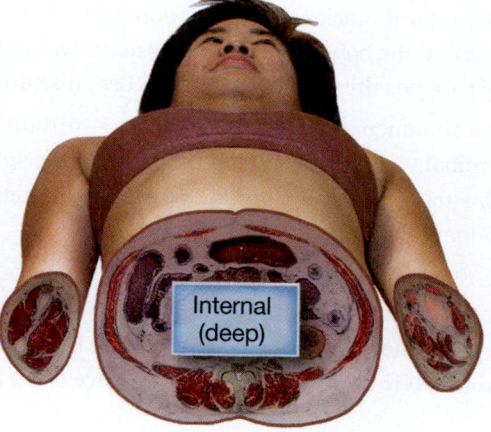

FIGURE 1-19 ■ External and internal.
External refers to the superficial or outer part of the body or an organ. Internal refers to deep inside the body or an organ. External and internal are opposite locations.

Body Cavities

The human body can also be studied according to its body cavities and their internal organs (see Figure 1-20 ■). A **cavity** is a hollow space. It is surrounded by bones or muscles that support and protect the organs and structures within the cavity. There are five body cavities.

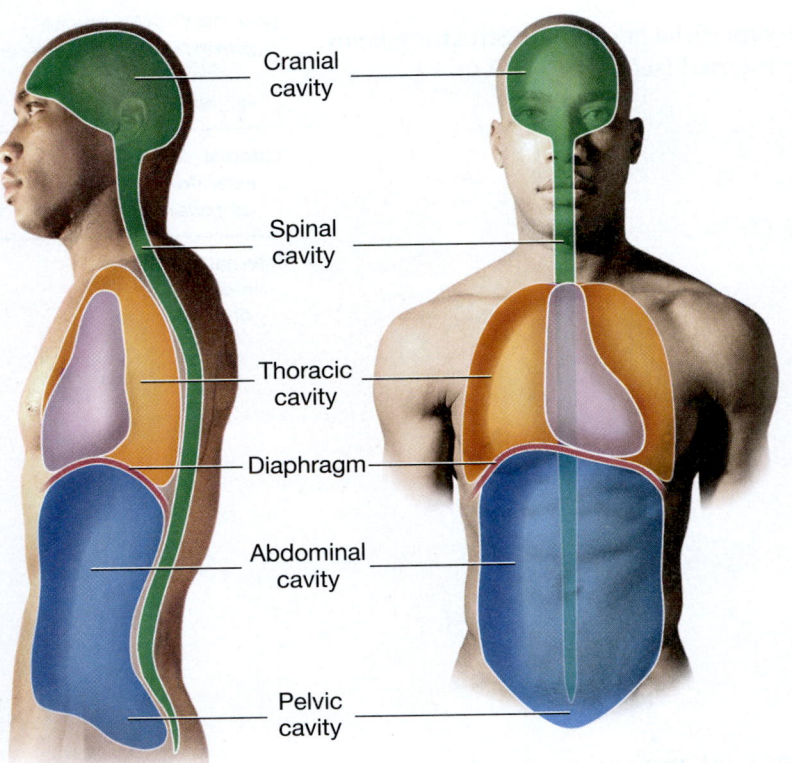

FIGURE 1-20 ■ **Body cavities.**
The cranial cavity becomes the spinal cavity along the back. The thoracic cavity is separated from the abdominal cavity by the diaphragm. The abdominal cavity is continuous with the pelvic cavity.

1. **Cranial cavity.** Within the bony cranium of the head; the cranial cavity contains the brain, cranial nerves, and related structures.

2. **Spinal cavity.** A continuation of the cranial cavity as it travels down the midline of the back; the spinal cavity is surrounded by the bones of the spine and contains the spinal cord, spinal nerves, and related structures. Also known as the *spinal canal.*

3. **Thoracic cavity.** Within the chest; the thoracic cavity is surrounded by the breastbone (sternum) anteriorly, the ribs bilaterally, the bones of the spine posteriorly, and the diaphragm inferiorly. The thoracic cavity contains the heart, lungs, and other structures.

4. **Abdominal cavity.** Within the abdomen; the abdominal cavity is surrounded by the diaphragm superiorly, the abdominal wall anteriorly, and the bones of the spine posteriorly. The abdominal cavity contains the stomach, small intestine, large intestine, spleen, liver, gallbladder, pancreas, and kidneys.

5. **Pelvic cavity.** A continuation of the abdominal cavity; the pelvic cavity is surrounded by the pelvic (hip) bones anteriorly and bilaterally and the bones of the spine posteriorly. The pelvic cavity contains the large intestine, uterus, bladder, some of the male genitalia, and other structures. The **abdominopelvic cavity** is the combined space of the abdominal and pelvic cavities.

Pronunciation/Word Parts

cavity (KAV-ih-tee)
  cav/o- *hollow space*
  -ity *condition; state*

cranial (KRAY-nee-al)
  crani/o- *cranium; top part of the skull*
  -al *pertaining to*

spinal (SPY-nal)
  spin/o- *backbone; spine*
  -al *pertaining to*

thoracic (thor-AS-ik)
  thorac/o- *chest; thorax*
  -ic *pertaining to*

abdominal (ab-DAW-mih-nal)
  abdomin/o- *abdomen*
  -al *pertaining to*

pelvic (PEL-vik)
  pelv/o- *hip bone; pelvis; renal pelvis*
  -ic *pertaining to*

abdominopelvic (ab-DAW-mih-noh-PEL-vik)
  abdomin/o- *abdomen*
  pelv/o- *hip bone; pelvis; renal pelvis*
  -ic *pertaining to*

Body Quadrants and Regions

The human body can be studied according to its quadrants and regions (see Figure 1-21 ▪). The anterior surface of the abdominopelvic area can be divided into four quadrants or nine regions, both of which are helpful as reference points during a physical examination of the internal organs.

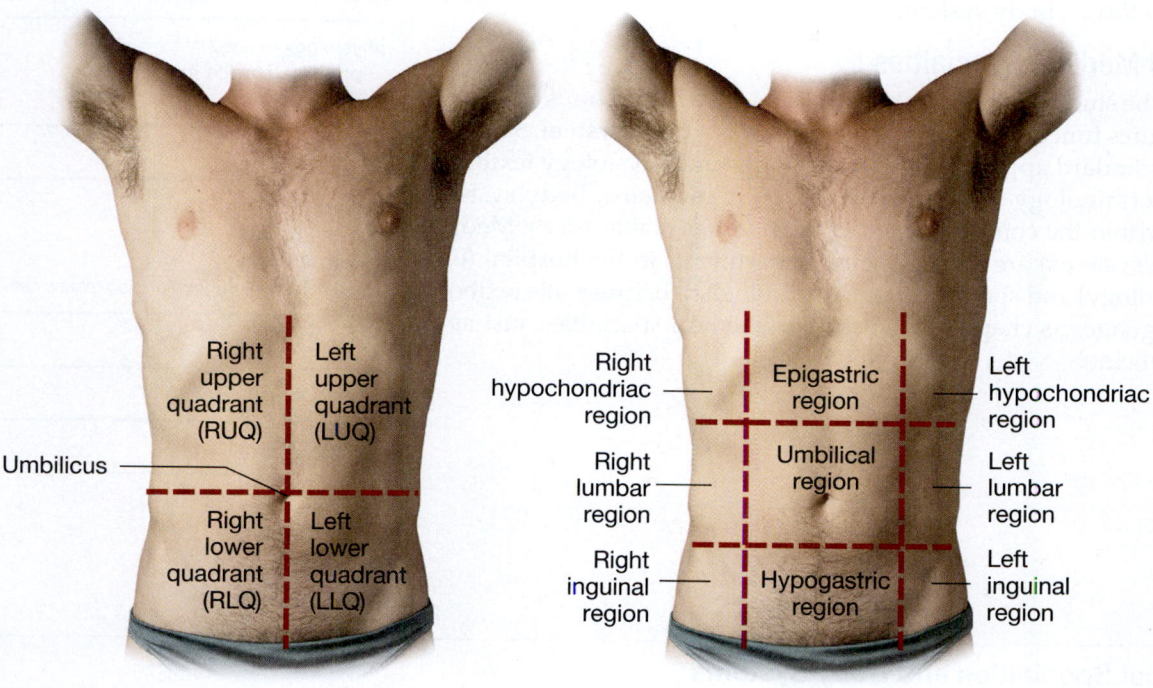

A.   B.

FIGURE 1-21 ▪ Body quadrants and regions.
A. Four quadrants are formed when a horizontal line and a vertical line cross at the umbilicus. The liver can be felt in the right upper quadrant and the stomach in the left upper quadrant. A patient with appendicitis has pain in the right lower quadrant. **B.** Nine regions are formed when two horizontal lines and two vertical lines form a square around the umbilicus.

The four **quadrants** include:

1. **Right upper quadrant (RUQ)**

2. **Left upper quadrant (LUQ)**

3. **Right lower quadrant (RLQ)**

4. **Left lower quadrant (LLQ)**.

The nine regions include the right and left **hypochondriac** regions, the **epigastric** region, the right and left **lumbar** regions, the **umbilical** region (centered around the umbilicus or navel), the right and left **inguinal** regions, and the **hypogastric** region.

Dive Deeper

The hypochondriac regions are on the right and left sides just below the cartilage that connects the ribs to the sternum. A hypochondriac is a person who is continually preoccupied with minor body sensations, often in the hypochondriac regions, and fears that these indicate disease. This is a psychiatric disorder. The lumbar regions of the abdominal area are so named because they are on the same level as the lumbar area of the lower back. Remember, when you are facing the patient (as in Figure 1-21), your right side corresponds to the patient's left side.

Pronunciation/Word Parts

quadrant (KWAH-drant)
  quadr/o- *four*
  -ant *pertaining to*

hypochondriac (HY-poh-CON-dree-ak)
  hypo- *below; deficient*
  chondr/o- *cartilage*
  -iac *pertaining to*
Hypochondriac: Pertaining to below (the) cartilage (of the ribs)

epigastric (EP-ih-GAS-trik)
  epi- *above; upon*
  gastr/o- *stomach*
  -ic *pertaining to*

lumbar (LUM-bar)
  lumb/o- *lower back*
  -ar *pertaining to*

umbilical (um-BIL-ih-kal)
  umbilic/o- *navel; umbilicus*
  -al *pertaining to*

inguinal (ING-gwih-nal)
  inguin/o- *groin*
  -al *pertaining to*

hypogastric (HY-poh-GAS-trik)
  hypo- *below; deficient*
  gastr/o- *stomach*
  -ic *pertaining to*

Anatomy and Physiology

Anatomy is the study of the structures of the human body. **Physiology** is the study of the functions of those structures. Anatomy begins with a **cell**, the smallest independently functioning structure in the body that can reproduce itself. Cells combine to form **tissues**, and tissues combine to form body **organs**. Several organs and related structures combine to form a body system.

Body Systems and Medical Specialties

The human body can be studied according to its various related structures (anatomy) and how those structures function together (physiology) as a **body system**. Studying body systems is the standard approach used in anatomy and physiology textbooks and many medical terminology textbooks. However, in medicine, body systems are always studied within the context of **medical specialties** (Table 1-5 ■). Medical specialties (not body systems) are used to name departments in the hospital (e.g., Department of Cardiology) and specialists (e.g., cardiologist). Because this textbook is about medical language, its chapters are based on medical specialties, just as in the real world of medicine!

Pronunciation/Word Parts

anatomy (ah-NAT-oh-mee)
The prefix **ana-** means *apart; excessive*, and the suffix **-tomy** means *process of cutting; process of making an incision*. Anatomy: *Process of cutting apart (the body)*

physiology (FIZ-ee-aw-loh-jee)
  physi/o- *physical function*
  -logy *study of*

cell (SEL)

cellular (SEL-yoo-lar)
  cellul/o- *cell*
  -ar *pertaining to*
The combining form **cyt/o-** also means *cell*.

tissue (TIH-shoo)

organ (OR-gan)

system (SIS-tem)

medical (MED-ih-kal)
  medic/o- *medicine*
  -al *pertaining to*

Table 1-5   Medical Specialties and Body Systems

Chapter	Medical Specialty/ Specialist	Body System/Anatomy and Physiology	Pronunciation/Word Parts
2	**Dermatology** dermatologist	**Integumentary system** Structures: Skin, hair, nails, subcutaneous tissue, and related structures Functions: Receives sensations, protects internal organs, synthesizes vitamin D, and regulates body temperature	**dermatology** (DER-mah-TAW-loh-jee) **dermat/o-** *skin* **-logy** *study of* **integumentary** (in-TEH-gyoo-MEN-tair-ee) **integument/o-** *skin* **-ary** *pertaining to*
3	**Gastroenterology** gastroenterologist	**Gastrointestinal system** Structures: Mouth, throat, esophagus, stomach, intestines, and related structures Functions: Digests food, absorbs nutrients, and removes undigested wastes. It sends sensory information to the brain for the sense of taste.	**gastroenterology** (GAS-troh-EN-ter-AW-loh-jee) **gastr/o-** *stomach* **enter/o-** *intestine* **-logy** *study of* **gastrointestinal** (GAS-troh-in-TES-tih-nal) **gastr/o-** *stomach* **intestin/o-** *intestine* **-al** *pertaining to*
4	**Pulmonology** pulmonologist	**Respiratory system** Structures: Nose, throat, larynx, trachea, bronchi, lungs, and related structures Functions: Brings oxygen into the body and expels carbon dioxide	**pulmonology** (PUL-moh-NAW-loh-jee) **pulmon/o-** *lung* **-logy** *study of* **respiratory** (RES-pih-rah-TOR-ee) **re-** *again and again; backward; unable to* **spir/o-** *breathe; coil* **-atory** *pertaining to*
5	**Cardiology** cardiologist	**Cardiovascular system** Structures: Heart, arteries, veins, capillaries, and related structures Function: Transports the blood throughout the body	**cardiology** (KAR-dee-AW-loh-jee) **cardi/o-** *heart* **-logy** *study of* **cardiovascular** (KAR-dee-oh-VAS-kyoo-lar) **cardi/o-** *heart* **vascul/o-** *blood vessel* **-ar** *pertaining to*

Chapter	Medical Specialty/ Specialist	Body System/Anatomy and Physiology	Pronunciation/Word Parts
6	**Hematology Immunology** hematologist immunologist	**Blood Lymphatic system** Structures: Blood cells, plasma; lymph glands, lymphoid tissues and organs, and related structures Functions: Transports blood cells, nutrients, oxygen, carbon dioxide, and waste products of cellular metabolism; the immune response destroys disease-causing organisms and abnormal cells.	**hematology** (HEE-mah-TAW-loh-jee) **hemat/o-** *blood* **-logy** *study of* **immunology** (IH-myoo-NAW-loh-jee) **immun/o-** *immune response* **-logy** *study of* **lymphatic** (lim-FAT-ik) **lymph/o-** *lymph; lymphatic system* **-atic** *pertaining to*
7	**Orthopedics** orthopedist	**Skeletal system** Structures: Bones, cartilage, ligaments, joints, and related structures Functions: Provides structural support and protection	**orthopedics** (OR-thoh-PEE-diks) **orth/o-** *straight* **ped/o-** *child* **-ics** *knowledge; practice* Orthopedics: *Knowledge and practice (of producing) straight(ness of the bones in a) child (or adult)* **skeletal** (SKEL-eh-tal) **skelet/o-** *skeleton* **-al** *pertaining to*
8	**Orthopedics** orthopedist	**Muscular system** Structures: Muscles, tendons, and related structures Functions: Produces movement of the body and maintains body posture	**orthopedics** (OR-thoh-PEE-diks) **orth/o-** *straight* **ped/o-** *child* **-ics** *knowledge; practice* **muscular** (MUS-kyoo-lar) **muscul/o-** *muscle* **-ar** *pertaining to*
9	**Neurology** neurologist	**Nervous system** Structures: Brain, cranial nerves, spinal cord, spinal nerves, other nerves, and related structures Functions: Receives and interprets sensory information and sends motor commands for body movement	**neurology** (nyoor-AW-loh-jee) **neur/o-** *nerve* **-logy** *study of* **nervous** (NER-vuhs) **nerv/o-** *nerve* **-ous** *pertaining to*
10	**Urology** urologist	**Urinary system** Structures: Kidneys, ureters, bladder, urethra, and related structures Functions: Removes waste products from the blood and excretes them in urine	**urology** (yoor-AW-loh-jee) **ur/o-** *urinary system; urine* **-logy** *study of* **urinary** (YOOR-ih-NAIR-ee) **urin/o-** *urinary system; urine* **-ary** *pertaining to*
11	**Male Reproductive Medicine**	**Male genitourinary system** Structures: Scrotum, testes, prostate gland, penile urethra, penis, and related structures Functions: Secretes the male hormone and produces and releases sperm	**reproductive** (REE-proh-DUK-tiv) **re-** *again and again; backward; unable to* **product/o-** *produce* **-ive** *pertaining to* **genital** (JEN-ih-tal) **genit/o-** *genitalia* **-al** *pertaining to*
12	**Gynecology Obstetrics** gynecologist obstetrician	**Female genital and reproductive system** Structures: Breasts, ovaries, uterus, vagina, and related structures Functions: Secretes the female hormone, produces ova, menstruates, conceives and bears babies, and produces milk to nourish babies	**gynecology** (GY-neh-KAW-loh-jee) **gynec/o-** *female; woman* **-logy** *study of* **obstetrics** (awb-STEH-triks) **obstetr/o-** *pregnancy and childbirth* **-ics** *knowledge; practice* Obstetrics: *Knowledge and practice (of treating women during) pregnancy and childbirth*

continued on next page

Table 1-5   Medical Specialties and Body Systems

Chapter	Medical Specialty/Specialist	Body System/Anatomy and Physiology	Pronunciation/Word Parts
13	**Endocrinology** endocrinologist	**Endocrine system** Structures: Hypothalamus, pituitary gland, pineal gland, thyroid gland, parathyroid glands, thymus, pancreas, adrenal glands, ovaries, and testes Functions: Secretes hormones and maintains body homeostasis	**endocrinology** (EN-doh-krih-NAW-loh-jee) **end/o-** *innermost; within* **crin/o-** *secrete* **-logy** *study of* Endocrinology: *Study of (glands) within (the body that) secrete (hormones into the blood)* **endocrine** (EN-doh-krin) **end/o-** *innermost; within* **-crine** *pertaining to secreting*
14	**Ophthalmology** ophthalmologist	**Eyes*** Structures: Eyes, lacrimal glands, and related structures Function: The sense of sight	**ophthalmology** (OFF-thal-MAW-loh-jee) **ophthalm/o-** *eye* **-logy** *study of*
15	**Otolaryngology** otolaryngologist	**Ears, nose, and throat*** Structures: Ears, nose, sinuses, throat, and larynx Functions: The sense of hearing and the sense of smell	**otolaryngology** (OH-toh-LAIR-ing-GAW-loh-jee) **ot/o-** *ear* **laryng/o-** *larynx; voice box* **-logy** *study of*

*The eyes, ears, and nose are sensory organs (not body systems); they are related to the special senses of vision, hearing, and smell.

There are additional medical specialties that focus on particular parts of the body, a specific disease or treatment, or selected populations (see Table 1-6 ■). Many of these medical specialties and their areas of interest are mentioned in Clinical Connections feature boxes in various chapters.

Table 1-6   Additional Medical Specialties

Medical Specialty/Specialist	Area of Interest	Pronunciation/Word Parts
Dentistry dentist	teeth	**dentistry** (DEN-tihs-tree) **dent/o-** *tooth* **-istry** *process related to a specialty*
Dietetics dietitian nutritionist	diet and nutrition	**dietetics** (DY-eh-TEH-tiks) **dietet/o-** *diet; foods* **-ics** *knowledge; practice*
Geriatrics geriatrician gerontologist	older persons	**geriatrics** (JAIR-ee-AT-riks) **ger/o-** *old age* **iatr/o-** *medical treatment; physician* **-ics** *knowledge; practice*
Neonatology neonatologist	newborn babies with medical problems	**neonatology** (NEE-oh-nay-TAW-loh-jee) **ne/o-** *new* **nat/o-** *birth* **-logy** *study of*
Oncology oncologist	cancer	**oncology** (ong-KAW-loh-jee) **onc/o-** *mass; tumor* **-logy** *study of*
Pediatrics pediatrician	children	**pediatrics** (PEE-dee-AT-riks) **ped/o-** *child* **iatr/o-** *medical treatment; physician* **-ics** *knowledge; practice*
Pharmacology pharmacist	drugs	**pharmacology** (FAR-mah-KAW-loh-jee) **pharmac/o-** *drug; medicine* **-logy** *study of*

Medical Specialty/ Specialist	Area of Interest	Pronunciation/Word Parts
Psychiatry psychiatrist, psychologist	mind and emotions	**psychiatry** (sy-KY-ah-tree) **psych/o-** mind **-iatry** medical treatment
Radiology radiologist	x-rays, sound waves, and other forms of radiation	**radiology** (RAY-dee-AW-loh-jee) **radi/o-** forearm bone; radius; x-rays **-logy** study of

Disease

Disease is any change in the normal structure or function of the body. This change might be slight and short-lived or severe and life-threatening. A **disorder** is a disturbance of action or function, most often applied to mental function and psychiatric conditions. The cause or origin of a disease is its **etiology**. In most cases, the cause of a disease is known or can be discovered through a physical examination and laboratory and diagnostic procedures. In some cases, however, the exact cause of a disease is never completely understood. **Preventive medicine** is health care that focuses on keeping a person healthy and preventing disease. But despite the best efforts of modern medicine, the human body does not always remain in a state of health. Much of medical language deals with diseases and how they are diagnosed and treated.

Disease Categories

Diseases can be divided into different categories based on their etiology (see Table 1-7 ■).

Pronunciation/Word Parts

disease (dih-ZEEZ)

etiology (EE-tee-AW-loh-jee)
eti/o- cause of disease
-logy study of

preventive (pree-VEN-tiv)
prevent/o- prevent
-ive pertaining to

medicine (MED-ih-sin)
medic/o- medicine
-ine pertaining to

Table 1-7   Disease Categories

Disease Type	Etiology	Pronunciation/Word Parts
Congenital	Caused by an abnormality in the fetus as it develops or caused by an abnormal process that occurs during gestation or birth Examples: Cleft lip and palate, cerebral palsy	**congenital** (con-JEN-ih-tal) **congenit/o-** present at birth **-al** pertaining to
Degenerative	Caused by the progressive destruction of cells due to disease or the aging process Examples: Multiple sclerosis, loss of hearing, arthritis	**degenerative** (dee-JEN-er-ah-TIV) **de-** reversal of; without **gener/o-** creation; production **-ative** pertaining to
Environmental	Caused by exposure to substances in the environment Examples: Breathing problems from smoking, allergies to pollen, skin cancer from the sun	**environmental** (en-VY-rawn-MEN-tal)
Genetic	Caused by a mutation in a person's genes and chromosomes during fetal development Example: Down syndrome	**genetic** (jeh-NEH-tik) **gene/o-** gene **-tic** pertaining to
Hereditary	Caused by an inherited recessive defective gene passed to a child from a parent who carries the defective gene but does not have the disease Examples: Cystic fibrosis, hemophilia, sickle cell disease	**hereditary** (heh-RED-ih-TAIR-ee) **heredit/o-** genetic inheritance **-ary** pertaining to
Hospital-acquired infection	Caused by exposure to a disease-causing agent while in the hospital environment. Previously known as a **nosocomial infection**. Example: Wound infection after surgery	**nosocomial** (NOH-soh-KOH-mee-al) **nosocomi/o-** hospital **-al** pertaining to
Iatrogenic	Caused by medicine or treatment that was given to the patient Examples: Wrong drug given to a patient, surgery performed on the wrong body part, an incompatible blood type given as a blood transfusion, side effect of a drug	**iatrogenic** (eye-AT-roh-JEN-ik) **iatr/o-** medical treatment; physician **gen/o-** arising from; produced by **-ic** pertaining to

continued on next page

Table 1-7 Disease Categories

Disease Type	Etiology	Pronunciation/Word Parts

Idiopathic	Having no identifiable or confirmed cause
	Example: Idiopathic thrombocytopenia (a blood disease)
		idiopathic (ID-ee-oh-PATH-ik)
		  idi/o- *individual; unknown*
		  path/o- *disease*
		  -ic *pertaining to*

Infectious	Caused by a **pathogen** (a disease-causing microorganism such as a bacterium, virus, fungus, etc.). A **communicable** disease is an infectious disease that is transmitted by direct or indirect contact with an infected person, animal, or insect.
	Examples: Gonorrhea (a sexually transmitted disease), rabies (from an animal bite), tuberculosis (from being near a person with tuberculosis who is coughing)
		infectious (in-FEK-shuhs)
		  infect/o- *disease within*
		  -ious *pertaining to*
		Infectious: *Pertaining to disease(-causing organisms) within (the body)*
		
		pathogen (PATH-oh-jen)
		  path/o- *disease*
		  -gen *that which produces*
		
		communicable (koh-MYOO-nih-kah-BUL)
		  communic/o- *impart; transmit*
		  -able *able to be*

Neoplastic	Caused by the growth of either a benign (not cancerous) or malignant (cancerous) mass or tumor
	Examples: Benign cyst, cancerous tumor of the skin
		neoplastic (NEE-oh-PLAS-tik)
		  ne/o- *new*
		  plast/o- *formation; growth*
		  -ic *pertaining to*

Nutritional	Caused by a lack of nutritious food, insufficient amounts of food, or an inability to utilize the nutrients in food
	Examples: Malnutrition, pernicious anemia
		nutritional (noo-TRIH-shun-al)
		  nutrit/o- *nourishment*
		  -ion *action; condition*
		  -al *pertaining to*

Onset, Course, and Outcome of Disease

Onset of a Disease

The beginning or onset of disease is often noticed because of the appearance of symptoms or signs. A **symptom** is any deviation from health that is experienced or felt by the patient. When a symptom can be seen or detected by others, it is known as a **sign**. An elevated temperature, coughing, tremors, paleness, vomiting, or a lump that can be seen or felt would all be signs of disease. Symptoms and signs may be **acute** (sudden in nature and severe in intensity), **subacute** (less severe in intensity), or **chronic** (continuing for 3 months or more). An **exacerbation** is a sudden worsening in the severity of the symptoms or signs. A **remission** is a temporary improvement in the symptoms or signs of a disease without the underlying disease being cured. A **relapse** or recurrence is a return of the original symptoms or signs of the disease. A **sequela** is a complication that is caused by the original disease and remains after the original disease has resolved. **Symptomatology** is the clinical picture of all of the patient's symptoms and signs. Patients who are **asymptomatic** (showing no symptoms or signs) can still have a disease, but one that can only be detected by laboratory and diagnostic procedures. A **syndrome** is a set of symptoms and signs associated with and characteristic of a particular disease.

Course and Outcome of a Disease

The course of a disease includes all events from the onset of the disease until the final outcome. The course and outcome of a disease can be affected by treatment when the physician prescribes drugs or orders therapy for the patient. If the treatment is **therapeutic**, the symptoms or signs of the disease disappear. A disease that is **refractory** (resistant) does not respond to treatment. Certain diseases that cannot be treated with drugs or therapy may require **surgery**.

Pronunciation/Word Parts

symptom (SIMP-tum)

acute (ah-KYOOT)

subacute (SUB-ah-KYOOT)

chronic (KRAW-nik)
  chron/o- *time*
  -ic *pertaining to*

exacerbation (eg-ZAS-er-BAY-shun)
  exacerb/o- *increase; provoke*
  -ation *being; having; process*

remission (ree-MIH-shun)
  remiss/o- *send back*
  -ion *action; condition*

sequela (see-KWEL-ah)

symptomatology (SIMP-toh-mah-TAW-loh-jee)
  symptomat/o- *collection of symptoms*
  -logy *study of*

asymptomatic (AA-simp-toh-MAT-ik)
  a- *away from; without*
  symptomat/o- *collection of symptoms*
  -ic *pertaining to*

syndrome (SIN-drohm)
  The prefix **syn-** means *together*, and the suffix **-drome** means *a running*.

therapeutic (THAIR-ah-PYOO-tik)
  therapeut/o- *therapy; treatment*
  -ic *pertaining to*

refractory (ree-FRAK-tor-ee)
  re- *again and again; backward; unable to*
  fract/o- *bend; break up*
  -ory *having the function of*
Refractory: *Having the function of (a disease that treatment is) unable to break up (or cure)*

surgery (SER-jer-ee)
  surg/o- *operative procedure*
  -ery *process*

The **prognosis** is the predicted outcome of a disease. The natures of many diseases are so well-known that the physician can predict with a great deal of accuracy what the patient's course and outcome will be.

The course of a disease ends in one of the following outcomes. **Recuperation** or recovery is a return to a normal state of health. When recuperation is not complete, a residual chronic disease or disability remains. A **disability** is a permanent loss of the ability to perform certain activities or to function in a given way. A **terminal illness** is one from which the patient cannot recover, and one that eventually results in death.

Pronunciation/Word Parts

prognosis (prawg-NOH-sihs)
  pro- *before*
  gnos/o- *knowledge*
  -osis *abnormal condition; process*

recuperation (ree-KOO-per-AA-shun)
  recuper/o- *recover*
  -ation *being; having; process*

disability (DIS-ah-BIL-ah-tee)

terminal (TER-mih-nal)
  termin/o- *boundary; end; word*
  -al *pertaining to*

1.4 PRACTICE LAPS

Use the Answer Key at the end of the book to check your answers.

A. Label Structures

Write each anatomy word or phrase in the correct numbered box. Be sure to check your spelling.

| anterior (ventral) | lateral | posterior (dorsal) |
| distal | medial | proximal |

1.

2.

3.

4.

5.

6.

abdominal cavity   diaphragm   spinal cavity
cranial cavity   pelvic cavity   thoracic cavity

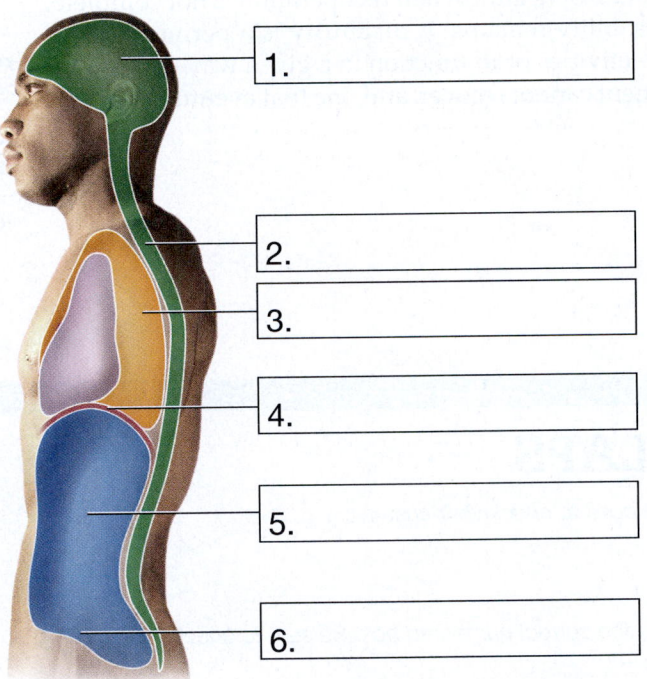

1. _____

2. _____

3. _____

4. _____

5. _____

6. _____

epigastric region   left inguinal region   right inguinal region
hypogastric region   left lumbar region   right lumbar region
left hypochondriac region right hypochondriac region umbilical region

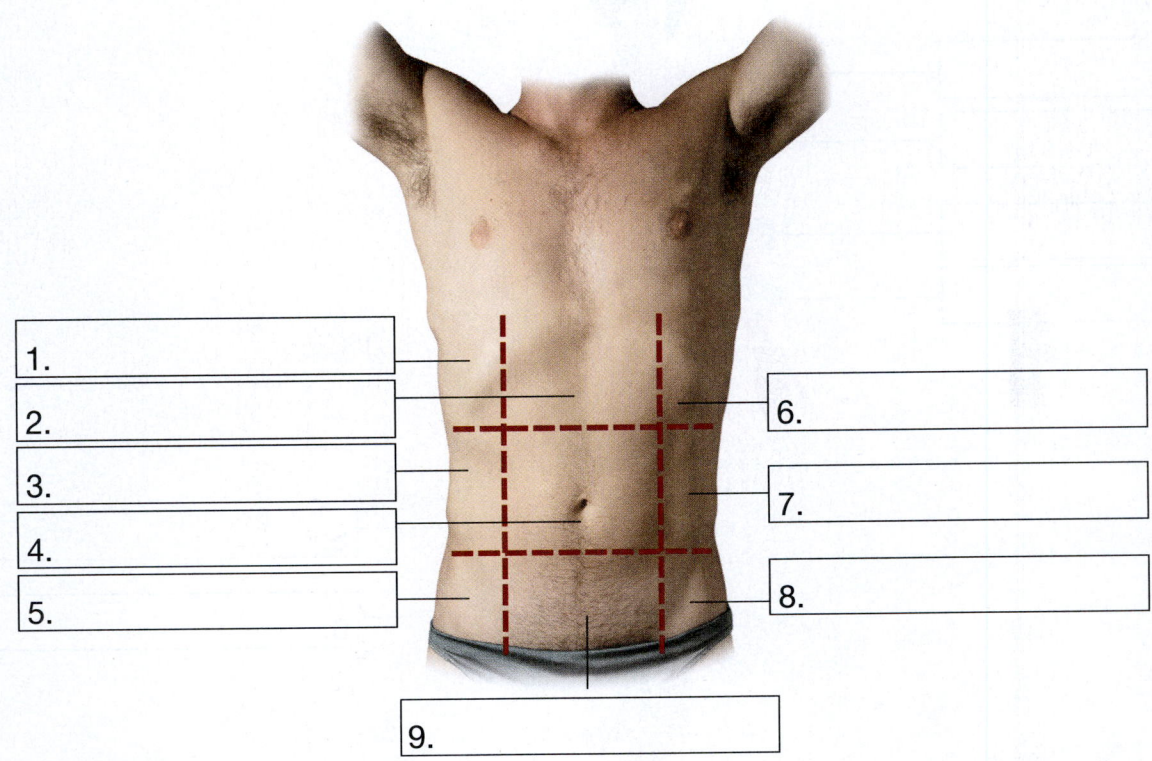

1. _____

2. _____

3. _____

4. _____

5. _____

6. _____

7. _____

8. _____

9. _____

B. Give the Meaning of Combining Forms

Next to each combining form, write its meaning. The first one has been done for you.

Combining Form	Meaning	Combining Form	Meaning
1. dors/o-	*back; dorsum*	31. gen/o-	
2. abdomin/o-		32. ger/o-	
3. anter/o-		33. gnos/o-	
4. cardi/o-		34. gynec/o-	
5. caud/o-		35. hemat/o-	
6. cav/o-		36. heredit/o-	
7. cellul/o-		37. iatr/o-	
8. cephal/o-		38. idi/o-	
9. chondr/o-		39. immun/o-	
10. chron/o-		40. infect/o-	
11. communic/o-		41. infer/o-	
12. congenit/o-		42. inguin/o-	
13. coron/o-		43. integument/o-	
14. crani/o-		44. intern/o-	
15. crin/o-		45. intestin/o-	
16. cyt/o-		46. laryng/o-	
17. dent/o-		47. later/o-	
18. dermat/o-		48. lumb/o-	
19. dietet/o-		49. lymph/o-	
20. dist/o-		50. medic/o-	
21. end/o-		51. medi/o-	
22. enter/o-		52. muscul/o-	
23. eti/o-		53. nat/o-	
24. exacerb/o-		54. ne/o-	
25. extern/o-		55. nerv/o-	
26. fract/o-		56. neur/o-	
27. front/o-		57. nosocomi/o-	
28. gastr/o-		58. nutrit/o-	
29. gener/o-		59. obstetr/o-	
30. genit/o-		60. onc/o-	

continued on next page

Combining Form	Meaning	Combining Form	Meaning
61. ophthalm/o-		79. remiss/o-	
62. orth/o-		80. sagitt/o-	
63. ot/o-		81. skelet/o-	
64. path/o-		82. spin/o-	
65. ped/o-		83. spir/o-	
66. pelv/o-		84. super/o-	
67. pharmac/o-		85. surg/o-	
68. physi/o-		86. symptomat/o-	
69. plas/o-		87. termin/o-	
70. poster/o-		88. therapeut/o-	
71. prevent/o-		89. thorac/o-	
72. product/o-		90. tom/o-	
73. proxim/o-		91. umbilic/o-	
74. psych/o-		92. urin/o-	
75. pulmon/o-		93. ur/o-	
76. quadr/o-		94. vascul/o-	
77. radi/o-		95. ventr/o-	
78. recuper/o-			

Vocabulary Review

Word or Phrase	Description	Combining Forms
Health		
abdominal cavity	Body cavity that is surrounded by the diaphragm superiorly, the abdominal wall anteriorly, and the bones of the spine posteriorly. It contains the stomach, small intestine, large intestine, spleen, liver, gallbladder, pancreas, and kidneys.	**abdomin/o-** *abdomen*
abdominopelvic cavity	Body cavity formed by the combined abdominal and pelvic cavities	**abdomin/o-** *abdomen* **pelv/o-** *hip bone; pelvis; renal pelvis*
anatomical position	Standard position of the body for the purpose of study. The body is erect, head up and eyes looking forward, arms by the sides with palms facing forward, and legs straight with the toes pointing forward.	**tom/o-** *cut; layer; slice*
anatomy	Study of the structures of the human body	**tom/o-** *cut; layer; slice*
anterior	Body position on the front of the body or an organ. Also known as *ventral*. Body direction of moving from the midline toward the front of the body.	**anter/o-** *before; front part*

Word or Phrase	Description	Combining Forms
blood	Body system of blood cells and plasma. It transports blood cells, nutrients, oxygen, carbon dioxide, and waste products of cellular metabolism.	**hemat/o-** *blood*
body cavity	Hollow space surrounded by bones or muscles that support and protect organs and structures within the cavity. There are five body cavities.	**cav/o-** *hollow space*
body plane	An imaginary flat surface that divides the body into two parts. There are three planes: the sagittal plane, coronal plane, and transverse plane.	
body quadrants	Four divisions on the anterior surface of the abdominopelvic area: left upper quadrant (LUQ), right upper quadrant (RUQ), left lower quadrant (LLQ), and right lower quadrant (RLQ)	**quadr/o-** *four*
body regions	Nine divisions on the anterior surface of the abdominopelvic area: hypochondriac regions (2), epigastric region, lumbar regions (2), umbilical region, inguinal regions (2), and the hypogastric region	
body system	Several organs and related structures that function together	
cardiology	Medical specialty related to the cardiovascular system. The physician specialist is a cardiologist.	**cardi/o-** *heart*
cardiovascular system	Body system that includes the heart, arteries, veins, capillaries, and related structures. It transports the blood throughout the body.	**cardi/o-** *heart* **vascul/o-** *blood vessel*
caudad	Body direction of moving from the midline toward the tailbone	**caud/o-** *tailbone*
cell	Smallest, independently functioning structure in the body that can reproduce itself	**cellul/o-** *cell* **cyt/o-** *cell*
cephalad	Body direction of moving away from the midline toward the head	**cephal/o-** *head*
coronal plane	Vertical plane that divides the body in the midline into front (anterior) and back (posterior) sections. Also known as the *frontal plane*.	**coron/o-** *structure that encircles like a crown* **front/o-** *front*
cranial cavity	Body cavity within the bony cranium of the head; it contains the brain, cranial nerves, and related structures	**crani/o-** *cranium; top part of the skull*
dentistry	Medical specialty related to the teeth. The medical specialist is a dentist.	**dent/o-** *tooth*
dermatology	Medical specialty related to the integumentary system. The physician specialist is a dermatologist.	**dermat/o-** *skin*
dietetics	Medical specialty related to diet and nutrition. The healthcare specialists are dietitians and nutritionists.	**dietet/o-** *diet; foods*
disease	Any change in the normal structure or function of the body	
distal	Body direction of moving from the trunk of the body (and the point of attachment or origin of an arm or leg) toward the end of the arm or leg	**dist/o-** *away from the center or point of origin*
dorsal	Body position of lying on the back. Also known as the *dorsal supine position*.	**dors/o-** *back; dorsum*
ears, nose, and throat	Related structures in the head and neck. The ears and nose are sensory organs that function in the special senses of hearing, balance, and smell	

Word or Phrase	Description	Combining Forms
endocrine system	Body system that includes the hypothalamus, pituitary gland, pineal gland, thyroid gland, parathyroid glands, thymus, pancreas, adrenal glands, ovaries, and testes. It secretes hormones and maintains body homeostasis.	**end/o-** *innermost; within* **crin/o-** *secrete*
endocrinology	Medical specialty related to the endocrine system. The physician specialist is an endocrinologist.	**end/o-** *innermost; within* **crin/o-** *secrete*
epigastric region	Region on the anterior surface of the abdominopelvic area, superior to the umbilical region	**gastr/o-** *stomach*
etiology	Cause or origin of a disease	**eti/o-** *cause of disease*
external	Body position on the outer, superficial surface of the body or an organ	**extern/o-** *outside*
eyes	Sensory organs that function in the special sense of sight	
female genital and reproductive system	Body system that includes the breasts, ovaries, uterus, vagina, and related structures. It secretes the female hormone, produces ova, menstruates, conceives and bears children, and produces milk to nourish babies.	**genit/o-** *genitalia* **product/o-** *produce*
gastroenterology	Medical specialty related to the gastrointestinal system. The physician specialist is a gastroenterologist.	**gastr/o-** *stomach* **enter/o-** *intestine*
gastrointestinal system	Body system that includes the mouth, throat, esophagus, stomach, intestines, and related structures. It digests food, absorbs nutrients, and removes undigested wastes. It sends sensory information to the brain for the sense of taste.	**gastr/o-** *stomach* **intestin/o-** *intestine*
geriatrics	Medical specialty related to older adults. The physician specialist is a geriatrician or gerontologist.	**ger/o-** *old age* **iatr/o-** *medical treatment; physician*
gynecology	Medical specialty related to the female genital system. The physician specialist is a gynecologist.	**gynec/o-** *female; woman*
health	State of complete physical, mental, and social well-being	
hematology	Medical specialty related to the blood. The physician specialist is a hematologist.	**hemat/o-** *blood*
hypochondriac regions	Right and left regions on the anterior surface of the abdominopelvic area, just below the cartilage of the ribs	**chondr/o-** *cartilage*
hypogastric region	Region on the anterior surface of the abdominopelvic area. It is inferior to the umbilical region.	**gastr/o-** *stomach*
immunology	Medical specialty related to the lymphatic system and the immune response. The physician specialist is an immunologist.	**immun/o-** *immune response*
inferior	Body position on the lower part of the body or an organ	**infer/o-** *below*
inguinal regions	Right and left regions on the anterior surface of the abdominopelvic area. They are lateral to the hypogastric region.	**inguin/o-** *groin*
integumentary system	Body system that includes the skin, hair, nails, subcutaneous tissue, and related structures. It receives sensations, protects internal organs, synthesizes vitamin D, and regulates body temperature.	**integument/o-** *skin*
internal	Body position on the inside of the body or an organ	**intern/o-** *inside*

Word or Phrase	Description	Combining Forms
lateral	Body direction of moving from the midline toward either side of the body. Bilateral is a position that indicates both sides.	**later/o-** *side*
lumbar regions	Right and left regions on the anterior surface of the abdominopelvic area. They are lateral to the umbilical region.	**lumb/o-** *lower back*
lymphatic system	Body system that includes the lymphatic glands, lymphoid tissues, and organs. It recognizes and destroys disease-causing organisms and abnormal cells.	**lymph/o-** *lymph; lymphatic system*
male genitourinary system	Body system in the male that includes the scrotum, testes, prostate gland, penile urethra, penis, and related structures. It secretes the male hormone and produces and releases sperm.	**genit/o-** *genitalia* **product/o-** *produce*
male reproductive medicine	Medical specialty related to the male genitourinary system	**product/o-** *produce*
medial	Body direction of moving from either side of the body toward the midline	**medi/o-** *middle*
medical specialty	Basis of the practice of medicine	**medic/o-** *medicine*
muscular system	Body system that includes the muscles, tendons, and related structures. It produces body movement and maintains body posture.	**muscul/o-** *muscle*
neonatology	Medical specialty related to newborn babies with medical problems. The physician specialist is a neonatologist.	**ne/o-** *new* **nat/o-** *birth*
nervous system	Body system that includes the brain, cranial nerves, spinal cord, spinal nerves, other nerves, and related structures. It receives and interprets sensory information and sends motor commands for body movement.	**nerv/o-** *nerve*
neurology	Medical specialty related to the nervous system. The physician specialist is a neurologist.	**neur/o-** *nerve*
obstetrics	Medical specialty related to the female reproductive system during pregnancy and childbirth. The physician specialist is an obstetrician.	**obstetr/o-** *pregnancy and childbirth*
oncology	Medical specialty related to cancer. The physician specialist is an oncologist.	**onc/o-** *mass; tumor*
ophthalmology	Medical specialty related to the eyes. The physician specialist is an ophthalmologist.	**ophthalm/o-** *eye*
organ	Body structure composed of tissues	
orthopedics	Medical specialty related to the skeletal system and muscular system. The physician specialist is an orthopedist.	**orth/o-** *straight* **ped/o-** *child*
otolaryngology	Medical specialty related to the ears, nose, and throat. The physician specialist is an otolaryngologist.	**ot/o-** *ear* **laryng/o-** *larynx; voice box*
pediatrics	Medical specialty related to children. The physician specialist is a pediatrician.	**ped/o-** *child* **iatr/o-** *medical treatment; physician*
pelvic cavity	Body cavity that is continuous with the abdominal cavity. It is surrounded by the pelvic bones anteriorly and bilaterally and bones of the spine posteriorly. It contains the large intestine, uterus, bladder, some of the male genitalia, and related structures.	**pelv/o-** *hip bone; pelvis; renal pelvis*
pharmacology	Medical specialty related to drugs. The medical specialist is a pharmacist.	**pharmac/o-** *drug; medicine*

Word or Phrase	Description	Combining Forms
physiology	Study of the functions of the human body	**physi/o-** *physical function*
posterior	Body position on the back of the body or an organ. Body direction of moving from the midline toward the back of the body.	**poster/o-** *back part*
preventive medicine	Health care that focuses on keeping a person healthy and preventing disease	**prevent/o-** *prevent*
prone	Body position of lying face down on the anterior surface of the body	
proximal	Body direction of moving from the end of an arm or leg toward its point of attachment (origin) on the trunk of the body	**proxim/o-** *near the center; near the point of origin*
psychiatry	Medical specialty related to the mind and emotions. The medical specialists are psychiatrists and psychologists.	**psych/o-** *mind*
pulmonology	Medical specialty related to the respiratory system. The physician specialist is a pulmonologist.	**pulmon/o-** *lung*
radiology	Medical specialty related to x-rays, sound waves, and other forms of radiation and energy to create images. The physician specialist is a radiologist.	**radi/o-** *forearm bone; radius; x-rays*
respiratory system	Body system that includes the nose, throat, larynx, trachea, bronchi, lungs, and related structures. It brings oxygen into the body and expels carbon dioxide.	**spir/o-** *breathe; coil*
sagittal plane	Vertical plane that divides the body in the midline into right and left sections	**sagitt/o-** *front to back*
skeletal system	Body system that includes the bones, cartilage, ligaments, joints, and related structures. It supports and protects the body.	**skelet/o-** *skeleton*
spinal cavity	Body cavity surrounded by the bones of the spine. It contains the spinal cord, spinal nerves, and related structures. Also known as the *spinal canal*.	**spin/o-** *backbone; spine*
superior	Body position on the upper part of the body or an organ. Body direction of moving from the midline toward the head.	**super/o-** *above*
thoracic cavity	Body cavity that is surrounded by the breastbone (sternum) anteriorly, ribs bilaterally, bones of the spine posteriorly, and the diaphragm inferiorly. It contains the heart, lungs, and other structures.	**thorac/o-** *chest; thorax*
tissue	Body structure formed of cells	
transverse plane	Horizontal plane that divides the body in the midline into upper (superior) and lower (inferior) parts	**vers/o-** *travel; turn*
umbilical region	Region on the anterior surface of the abdominopelvic area. It is centered around the umbilicus.	**umbilic/o-** *navel; umbilicus*
urinary system	Body system that includes the kidneys, ureters, bladder, urethra, and related structures. It removes waste products from the blood and excretes them in the urine.	**urin/o-** *urinary system; urine*
urology	Medical specialty related to the urinary system. The physician specialist is a urologist.	**ur/o-** *urinary system; urine*
ventral	Body position on the front of the body	**ventr/o-** *abdomen; front*

Word or Phrase	Description	Combining Forms
Disease		
acute	Symptoms and signs of diseases that are sudden in nature and severe in intensity	
asymptomatic	Showing no symptoms or signs of disease	**symptomat/o-** *collection of symptoms*
chronic	Symptoms and signs of disease that continue for 3 months or longer	**chron/o-** *time*
congenital disease	Caused by an abnormality in fetal development or an abnormal process that occurs during gestation or birth	**congenit/o-** *present at birth*
degenerative disease	Caused by progressive destruction of cells due to disease or the aging process	**gener/o-** *creation; production*
disability	Permanent loss of the ability to perform certain activities or function in a given way	
disease	Any change in the normal structure or function of the body	
environmental disease	Caused by exposure to substances in the environment	
etiology	The cause or origin of a disease	**eti/o-** *cause of disease*
exacerbation	Sudden worsening in the severity of symptoms or signs	**exacerb/o-** *increase; provoke*
genetic disease	Caused by a mutation in a person's genes or chromosomes during fetal development	**gene/o-** *gene*
hereditary disease	Caused by an inherited recessive defective gene, passed to a child from a parent who carries the defective gene but does not have the disease	**heredit/o-** *genetic inheritance*
hospital-acquired infection	Caused by exposure to a disease-causing agent while in the hospital. Previously known as a *nosocomial infection*.	**nosocomi/o-** *hospital*
iatrogenic disease	Caused by medicine or treatment given to the patient	**iatr/o-** *medical treatment; physician* **gen/o-** *arising from; produced by*
idiopathic disease	Having no identifiable or confirmed cause	**idi/o-** *individual; unknown* **path/o-** *disease*
infectious disease	Caused by a pathogen. A *communicable disease* is an infectious disease that is transmitted by direct or indirect contact with an infected person, animal, or insect.	**infect/o-** *disease within* **communic/o-** *impart; transmit*
neoplastic disease	Caused by the growth of a benign (not cancerous) or a malignant (cancerous) tumor or mass	**ne/o-** *new* **plast/o-** *formation; growth*
nutritional disease	Caused by lack of nutritious food, too little food, or an inability to utilize the food that is eaten	**nutrit/o-** *nourishment*
pathogen	Disease-causing microorganism, such as a bacterium, virus, fungus, etc.	**path/o-** *disease*
prognosis	Predicted course and outcome of a disease	**gnos/o-** *knowledge*
recuperation	Process of recovery and return to a normal state of health	**recuper/o-** *recover*
refractory	Pertaining to a disease that does not respond well to treatment	**fract/o-** *bend; break up*

Word or Phrase	Description	Combining Forms
remission	Temporary improvement in the symptoms or signs of a disease without the underlying disease being cured	**remiss/o-** *send back*
sequela	Complication that is caused by the original disease and remains after the original disease has resolved	
sign	Symptom that can be seen or detected by others	
surgery	Operative procedure to treat a disease that cannot be treated with drugs or therapy	**surg/o-** *operative procedure*
symptom	Any deviation from health that is experienced and felt by the patient	
symptomatology	Clinical picture of all the patient's symptoms and signs	**symptomat/o-** *collection of symptoms*
syndrome	Set of symptoms and signs associated with and characteristic of a specific disease	
subacute	Symptoms and signs that are less severe in intensity than acute symptoms	
terminal illness	Disease from which there is no hope of recovery and one that will eventually result in the patient's death	**termin/o-** *boundary; end; word*
therapeutic	Treatment that makes the symptoms and signs of a disease disappear	**therapeut/o-** *therapy; treatment*

1.5 Health Care Today

Healthcare Professionals

Physicians

A **physician** or **doctor** leads the members of the healthcare team and directs their activities. The physician examines the patient, orders tests (if necessary), diagnoses diseases, and treats diseases by prescribing medicines or therapy. Physicians who graduate from medical school receive a Doctor of Medicine (M.D.) degree. Physicians who graduate from a school of osteopathy receive a Doctor of Osteopathy (D.O.) degree. After medical school, physicians complete residency training and select a specialized area for their medical practice (e.g., family practice, pediatrics, psychiatry, etc.). **Surgeons** are physicians who complete additional training in surgical techniques.

Primary care physicians (PCPs) are physicians who specialize in family practice or pediatrics. They see the majority of patients on a day-to-day basis in their offices. A physician or doctor who is on the medical staff of a hospital and admits a patient to the hospital, directs their care, and discharges them is known as the **attending physician**.

Other doctors graduate from schools that focus their training on just one part of the body or one aspect of medicine. Chiropractors have a Doctor of Chiropracty (D.C.) degree and only treat the alignment of the bones, muscles, and nerves. Optometrists have a Doctor of Optometry (O.D.) degree and only treat the eyes. Podiatrists have a Doctor of Podiatric Medicine (D.P.M.) degree and only treat the feet. Dentists have a Doctor of Dental Surgery (D.D.S.) degree and only treat the teeth. Pharmacists have a Doctor of Pharmacy (Pharm.D.) degree. They fill prescriptions for medicines as well as consult with physicians and patients.

Pronunciation/Word Parts

physician (fih-ZIH-shun)
  physi/o- *physical function*
  -ician *skilled expert; skilled professional*
Note: The duplicated letter *i* is deleted when the word is formed.

surgeon (SER-jun)
  surg/o- *operative procedure*
  -eon *person who performs*

Physician Extenders

Physician extenders are healthcare professionals who perform some of the duties of a physician. They examine, diagnose, and treat patients and some of them can prescribe medicines. Most work under the supervision of a physician or doctor (MD or DO).

Physician extenders include physician's assistants (PAs), nurse practitioners (NPs), certified nurse midwives (CNMs), and certified registered nurse anesthetists (CRNAs).

Allied Health Professionals

Allied health professionals support the physician and perform specific services ordered by the physician. **Nurses**, such as a registered nurse (RN), licensed practical nurse (LPN), or licensed vocational nurse (LVN), examine patients, make nursing diagnoses, and administer treatments or medicines ordered by the physician. Nurses give hands-on care and focus on the physical and emotional needs of the patient and the family (see Figure 1-22 ■).

Other allied health professionals include **technologists**, **technicians**, and **therapists**, as well as dietitians, medical assistants, phlebotomists, dental hygienists, and audiologists.

Healthcare Settings

Health care is provided in many different settings, depending on the healthcare needs of the patient and which setting can medically and cost effectively meet those needs.

Hospital

A **hospital** is a healthcare facility that is the traditional setting for providing care for patients who are acutely ill and require medical or surgical care for longer than 24 hours. Each hospital stay begins with an admission and ends with a discharge from the hospital. The attending physician must write an order in the patient's electronic medical record to admit or discharge the patient. The attending physician also monitors the patient's care and orders diagnostic tests, treatments, therapies, medicines, and surgeries, as needed. A patient in the hospital is an **inpatient**.

A hospital is divided into floors or nursing units that provide care for specific types of patients. There are also specialty care units such as the **intensive care unit (ICU)**. **Ancillary** departments in the hospital provide additional types of services and include the radiology department, **physical therapy (PT)** department, dietary department, **emergency department (ED)** or **emergency room (ER)**, clinical laboratory, and pharmacy. Nonmedical departments provide other services such as health information management (medical records), finances and billing, housekeeping, and so on.

Pronunciation/Word Parts

technologist (tek-NAW-loh-jist)
  techn/o- technical skill
  log/o- study of; word
  -ist person who specializes in; thing that specializes in

technician (tek-NIH-shun)
  techn/o- technical skill
  -ician skilled expert; skilled professional

therapist (THAIR-ah-pist)
  therap/o- treatment
  -ist person who specializes in; thing that specializes in

hospital (HAWS-pih-tal)

inpatient (IN-pay-shent)

ancillary (AN-sih-LAIR-ee)
  ancill/o- accessory; servant
  -ary pertaining to

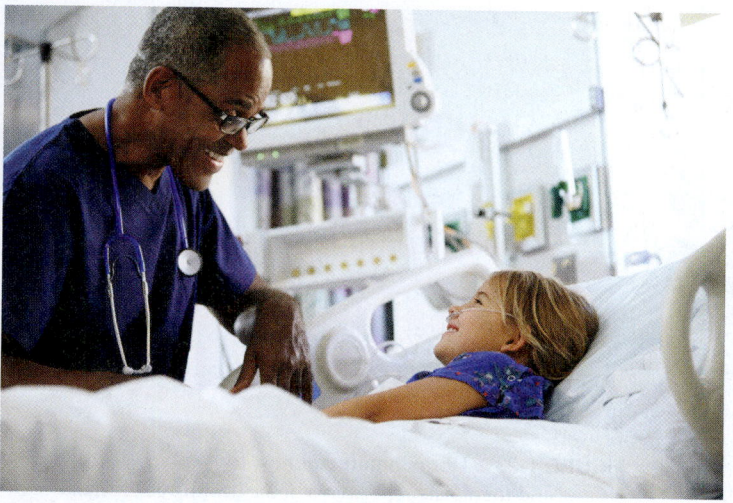

FIGURE 1-22 ■ Nurse in the intensive care unit.
Nurses give hands-on care and focus on the physical and emotional needs of the patient and family.

Physician's Office

The physician's office is one of the most frequently used healthcare settings. A single physician (or a group of physicians in a group practice) maintains an office where patients are seen, diagnosed, treated, and counseled. Some offices have their own laboratory and x-ray equipment for performing diagnostic tests. Seriously ill patients who cannot be quickly diagnosed or adequately treated in the office are sent to a hospital.

Clinic

Some **clinics** provide healthcare services similar to that of a physician's office but for just one type of patient or one type of disease. For example, a well-baby clinic provides care to newborn infants, and a methadone clinic treats recovering drug addicts. Outpatient clinics are located in a hospital or in a separate facility. Their patients are known as **outpatients** because they are not admitted to the clinic and do not stay overnight. **Walk-in clinics**, often located in or near pharmacies, provide services such as treating minor injuries or illnesses, giving immunizations, and performing sports physicals. They are typically staffed by a nurse practitioner. **Urgent care clinics** are similar to walk-in clinics, but they have additional capabilities and have a physician on staff. They can treat patients with more serious illnesses and injuries, but not life-threatening ones, and are often open on weekends when primary care offices are closed.

Ambulatory Surgery Center

An **ambulatory surgery center (ASC)** is a facility where minor surgery is performed, and the patient does not stay overnight.

Long-Term Care Facility

A **long-term care facility**, previously known as a *nursing home*, is primarily a residential facility for older adults or those with disabilities who are unable to care for themselves. Long-term care facilities provide 24-hour nursing care. Persons in long-term care facilities are referred to as **residents** rather than *patients* because the facility is considered their home or residence. **Skilled nursing facilities (SNFs)** are long-term care facilities with a special nursing unit that provides the higher level of medical and nursing care that is needed for patients who have recently been discharged from the hospital. Many long-term care facilities also provide **rehabilitation** services to prepare a patient to live independently at home.

Home Health Agency

A **home health agency** provides a range of healthcare services to persons (who are known as **clients**) in their homes. These services are particularly useful for those who are unable to come to a physician's office or clinic and do not want to live in a long-term care facility (see Figure 1-23 ■).

Pronunciation/Word Parts

clinic (KLIN-ik)

outpatient (OUT-pay-shent)

ambulatory (AM-byoo-lah-TOR-ee)
  ambulat/o- *walking*
  -ory *having the function of*

rehabilitation (REE-hah-BIL-ih-TAY-shun)
  re- *again and again; backward; unable to*
  habilit/o- *give ability*
  -ation *being; having; process*
Rehabilitation: *Process (to) again and again give ability*

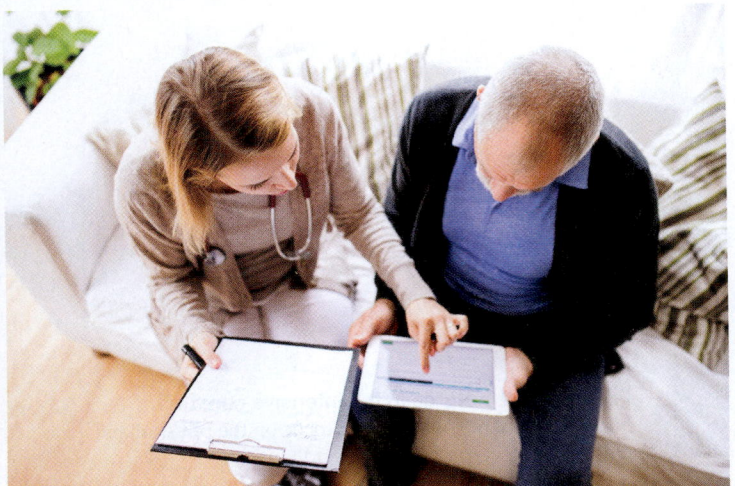

FIGURE 1-23 ■ Home health agency.
Nurses and therapists sent from a home health agency make regularly scheduled visits to assess patients in their homes.

Hospice

A **hospice** is an inpatient facility for patients who are dying from a terminal illness, and their physicians have certified that they have less than 6 months to live. Hospice services include **palliative** care (supportive medical and nursing care to keep the patient comfortable but does not provide a cure), pain management, counseling, and emotional support for the patient and family. Hospice care can also be provided in the patient's home.

Pronunciation/Word Parts

hospice (HAWS-pihs)

palliative (PAL-ee-ah-TIV)
   palliat/o- *reduce the severity*
   -ive *pertaining to*

Across the Life Span

Most people think of the healthcare settings of a long-term care facility and hospice as only pertaining to older adults. In fact, some chronically ill or severely handicapped children and young adults are cared for in long-term care facilities. All ages of patients who are terminally ill can receive hospice care in a hospice facility or at home.

History and Physical Examination

To fully understand the patient's symptoms and signs, the physician takes the patient's history and performs a physical examination. For the history of the present illness, the physician asks the patient in detail about the location, onset, duration, and severity of the symptoms. The physician also asks about the patient's past medical history, past surgical history, family history, social history, and history of allergies to drugs and other substances. Then the physician performs a physical examination to look for signs of disease. The physician uses the techniques shown in Table 1-8 ■ (as needed) during the physical examination.

Table 1-8 Physical Examination Techniques

Technique	Pronunciation/Word Parts

Inspection
Using the eyes or an instrument to examine the external surfaces or internal cavities of the body
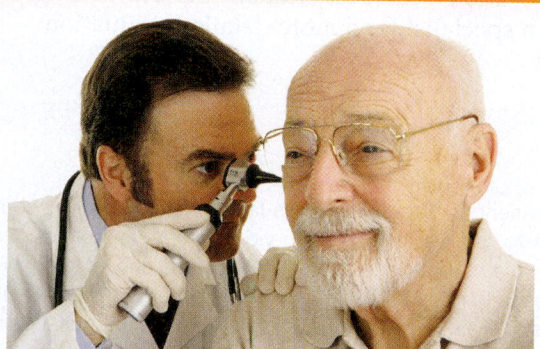
	inspection (in-SPEK-shun)
	  inspect/o- *looking at*
	  -ion *action; condition*

Palpation
Using the fingers to feel masses or enlarged organs or to detect tenderness or pain
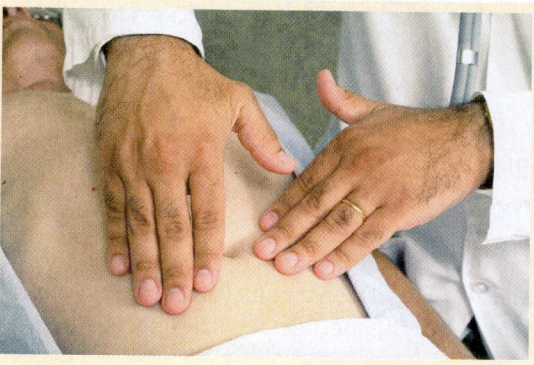
	palpation (pal-PAY-shun)
	  palpat/o- *feeling; touching*
	  -ion *action; condition*

continued on next page

Table 1-8   Physical Examination Techniques

Technique		Pronunciation/Word Parts
Auscultation Using a stethoscope to listen to the sounds of the heart, lungs, or intestines	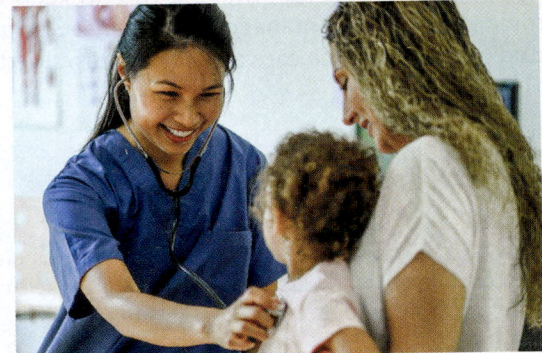	**auscultation** (AWS-kul-TAY-shun) **auscult/o-** *listening* **-ation** *being; having; process*
Percussion Using the finger of one hand to tap on the finger of the other hand that is spread over a body cavity and listening to the sound that is produced	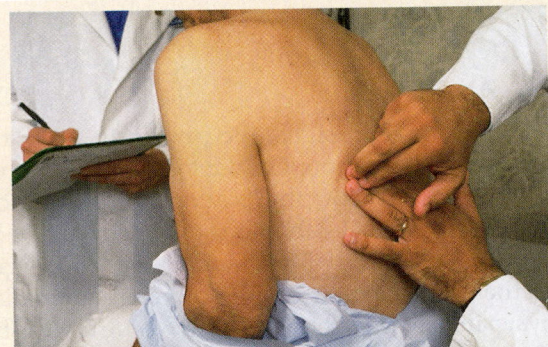	**percussion** (per-KUH-shun) **percuss/o-** *tapping* **-ion** *action; condition*

Based on the patient's history and the results of the physical examination, the physician can **rule out (R/O)** most diseases and make a **diagnosis** that identifies the nature and cause of the disease. If it is not possible to make a diagnosis, the physician makes a tentative or working diagnosis and orders laboratory tests and/or diagnostic procedures or refers the patient to a specialist for a more detailed evaluation.

Pronunciation/Word Parts

diagnosis (DY-ag-NOH-sihs)

Clinical Connections

Telehealth. In the past, physician–patient contact was always face to face. Now, telecommunication advances allow patients to receive care through videoconferencing sessions, remote monitoring of vital signs, and so on. Physicians also use videoconferencing to consult with specialists (e-consulting). Surgeons in one part of the world do telesurgery with on-site and remote robots and three-dimensional visualization to operate on a patient thousands of miles away.

Electronic Health Records

Many of the medical language skills discussed in the first part of this chapter are used when dealing with medical records. Let's briefly look at some of the more common types of medical records.

The **medical record** is where healthcare professionals document all care provided to a patient. In the past, the medical record was mainly used to document diseases, treatments, surgeries, and so on. Now, the medical record reflects an emphasis on keeping the patient in good health and preventing disease. Most physicians' office medical records include a checklist that documents preventive care given to the patient (immunizations, routine physical exams, etc.), as well as things the patient should do (limit sun exposure and apply sunscreen, have smoke detectors in the home, use seat belts, do monthly self-examination of the breasts or testicles, secure firearms kept in the home, etc.).

The paper medical record has been the traditional form of medical record. Its disadvantages are that only one healthcare professional can access it at a time, it can be lost or damaged, and it can take hours or even days to retrieve a patient's past medical records that are stored off-site. This delay can compromise the delivery of quality care.

Most physicians' offices, hospitals, and other healthcare facilities have converted some or all of their paper medical records to **electronic health records (EHRs)**.

Clinical Connections

Health information management. The electronic health record (EHR), **electronic medical record (EMR)**, or **electronic patient record (EPR)** provides seamless, immediate, and simultaneous access by several healthcare professionals to all parts of a patient's record regardless of where those parts were created or stored. The federal government's goal is to have the electronic health record and electronic prescribing of drugs (e-prescribing) available everywhere. These electronic records go beyond storing a patient's medical information. They also alert physicians to potential errors, suggest additional diagnostic tests, spot trends in the patient's condition, and warn about prescribing the wrong drug.

Types of Documents in the Electronic Health Record

The format and content of an electronic health record varies from one setting to the next. Short narrative notes and checklists are used in many physicians' offices and clinics. These notes usually contain a brief history of the present illness, pertinent past medical or surgical history, a physical examination, a diagnosis, treatments, and a follow-up plan.

Hospitals have more extensive documentation than physicians' offices. Common documents for a hospitalized patient include the admission **History and Physical Examination (H&P)**, **Operative Report**, and **Discharge Summary (DS)**. These documents include standard headings, as described below.

Standard Headings in Healthcare Documents

- **Chief Complaint (CC)**
- **History of Present Illness (HPI)**
- **Past Medical (and Surgical) History (PMH)**
- **Social History (SH)** and **Family History (FH)**
- **Review of Systems (ROS)**
- **Physical Examination (PE)**
- **Laboratory and X-ray Data**
- **Diagnosis (Dx)**
- **Disposition**

In addition, physicians write orders and progress notes, nurses write nurses' notes, and other departments contribute notes or use preprinted forms to record information.

Dive Deeper

The electronic health record is a medicolegal record. This means that it not only contains medical documents but that those are also legal documents that can be used in a court of law. Before patients can be treated at any type of healthcare facility, they must sign a **consent to treatment** form that gives physicians and other healthcare professionals the right to treat them. Treatment without consent is against the law and could constitute battery (touching another person without his or her consent or causing harm). For a patient who is a minor, the parent or legal guardian signs the consent to treatment form. In an emergency situation, implied consent allows care to be provided until the patient is awake and able to consent or until a legally appropriate person is able to consent for the patient. Prior to a surgery, the physician describes the purpose of the surgery and informs the patient of alternatives, risks, and possible outcomes or complications. Then the patient signs a consent to surgery form.

A patient must also sign a form that allows the facility to contact the insurance company to obtain payment for any health care that is provided. Under the federal regulations of **HIPAA** (**Health Insurance Portability and Accountability Act** of 1996), all healthcare settings must provide patients with a statement verifying that their medical record information is secure and is released only to authorized healthcare providers, insurance companies, or healthcare quality monitoring organizations.

1.5 PRACTICE LAPS

Use the Answer Key at the end of the book to check your answers.

A. Give the Meaning of Combining Forms

Next to each combining form, write its meaning. The first one has been done for you.

Combining Form	Meaning	Combining Form	Meaning
1. **therap/o-**	*treatment*	5. palliat/o-	
2. ambulat/o-		6. physi/o-	
3. ancill/o-		7. surg/o-	
4. habilit/o-		8. techn/o-	

B. Define Abbreviations

1. Dx		4. H&P	
2. ED		5. PCP	
3. EHR		6. SNF	

Vocabulary Review

Word or Phrase	Description	Combining Forms
Health Care Today		
allied health professionals	Healthcare professionals who support the work of physicians and perform specific services ordered by the physician. Allied health professionals include nurses, technologists, technicians, therapists, and others.	
ambulatory surgery center (ASC)	Facility where minor surgical procedures are performed. The patient is an **outpatient** who does not stay overnight.	**ambulat/o-** *walking* **surg/o-** *operative procedure*
ancillary department	Department in the hospital that provides services to support the medical and surgical care being given in a hospital. Examples: Radiology department, physical therapy department, dietary department, emergency department, clinical laboratory, and pharmacy	**ancill/o-** *accessory; servant*
attending physician	Physician on the medical staff of a hospital who admits patients, directs their care, and discharges them	**physi/o-** *physical function*
auscultation	Using a stethoscope to listen to the sounds of the heart, lungs, or intestines	**auscult/o-** *listening*
clinic	An ambulatory facility that provides healthcare services, often for just one type of patient or one type of disease Examples: Well-baby clinic for newborns, walk-in clinics, urgent care clinics. Clinic patients are known as **outpatients** and the facility is an outpatient clinic.	
consent to treatment	Form that must be signed that gives a physician and others the right to treat the patient	
diagnosis	A determination based on knowledge about the cause of the patient's symptoms and signs	**gnos/o-** *knowledge*
discharge	Release from the hospital of a patient who no longer needs hospital-level care. The patient can be discharged to home or transferred to another healthcare facility.	
electronic health record (EHR)	Paperless medical record that provides seamless, immediate, and simultaneous access by several healthcare professionals regardless of where the parts of the record were created or stored. Also known as the **electronic medical record (EMR)** or **electronic patient record (EPR)**.	
HIPAA	The Health Insurance Portability and Accountability Act states that all healthcare facilities must provide the patient with a statement that his or her medical record information is secure and only released to authorized organizations.	
home health agency	Agency that provides a range of healthcare services to patients in their homes. These patients are known as **clients**.	
hospice	Facility for patients who have a terminal illness and require **palliative** care, pain management, counseling, and emotional support for the patient and the family. Hospice care can also be provided in the patient's home.	**palliat/o-** *reduce the severity*
hospital	Healthcare facility that provides care for acutely ill medical and surgical patients for longer than 24 hours. The patient being treated is an **inpatient**. The patient is admitted, occupies a bed in the hospital, and is discharged.	

Word or Phrase	Description	Combining Forms
inpatient	A patient in a hospital	
inspection	Using the eyes or an instrument to examine the body	**inspect/o-** *looking at*
intensive care unit (ICU)	Specialty care unit within a hospital	
long-term care facility	Residential facility for persons who are unable to care for themselves. A long-term care facility, previously known as a *nursing home*, provides 24-hour nursing care, and some provide **rehabilitation** services. Persons in this facility are known as **residents**.	**habilit/o-** *give ability*
nurse	Allied health professional who examines patients, makes nursing diagnoses, and gives medicines and treatment ordered by a physician	
palliative care	Supportive medical and nursing care that keeps the patient comfortable but does not cure the disease	**palliat/o-** *reduce the severity*
palpation	Using the fingers to press on a body part to feel a mass, an enlarged organ, tenderness, or pain	**palpat/o-** *feeling; touching*
percussion	Tapping one finger on another finger of a hand that is spread across the chest, abdomen, or back to listen for differences in sound in a body cavity	**percuss/o-** *tapping*
physician	Healthcare professional—Doctor of Medicine (MD) or Doctor of Osteopathy (DO)—who directs the activities of the healthcare team. The physician examines the patient, orders tests, diagnoses, and treats diseases. Other healthcare professionals graduate from schools that focus their training on just one part of the body or one aspect of medicine—Doctor of Chiropracty (DC), Doctor of Optometry (OD), Doctor of Podiatric Medicine (DPM), Doctor of Dental Surgery (DDS), or Doctor of Pharmacy (PharmD). A primary care physician (PCP) is a general practitioner who specializes in family practice or pediatrics.	**physi/o-** *physical function*
physician extender	Healthcare professionals who perform some of the duties of physicians or doctors and work under their supervision. They examine, diagnose, and treat patients. Some can prescribe medicines. Physician extenders include physician's assistants, nurse practitioners, certified nurse midwives, and certified registered nurse anesthetists.	
physician's office	Facility where a physician (or a group of physicians in a group practice) maintains an office. The ambulatory patients here are outpatients and are seen for a short period of time to diagnose and prescribe treatment for diseases that do not require hospitalization.	
skilled nursing facility (SNF)	Long-term care facility with a special nursing unit that admits patients from the hospital and provides a higher level of medical and nursing care. Persons in this facility are known as **residents**.	
surgeon	Physician or doctor who performs surgery	**surg/o-** *operative procedure*
technician	Allied health professional who has technical skill in a particular field of medicine	**techn/o-** *technical skill*
technologist	Allied health professional who specializes in a technical area of a field of medicine and performs technical tests	**techn/o-** *technical skill* **log/o-** *study of; word*
therapist	Allied health professional who performs therapy on patients to treat a specific disease or condition	**therap/o-** *treatment*

Abbreviations Summary

ASC	ambulatory surgery center		**LLQ**	left lower quadrant
CC	Chief Complaint		**LPN**	licensed practical nurse
CNM	certified nurse midwife		**LUQ**	left upper quadrant
CRNA	certified registered nurse anesthetist		**LVN**	licensed vocational nurse
D.C.	Doctor of Chiropracty		**M.D.**	Doctor of Medicine
D.D.S.	Doctor of Dental Surgery		**NP**	nurse practitioner
D.O.	Doctor of Osteopathy		**O.D.**	Doctor of Optometry
D.P.M.	Doctor of Podiatric Medicine		**PA**	physician's assistant
DS	Discharge Summary		**PE**	Physical Examination
Dx	diagnosis		**PCP**	primary care physician
ED	Emergency Department		**Pharm.D.**	Doctor of Pharmacy
EHR	electronic health record		**PMH**	Past Medical History
EMR	electronic medical record		**PT**	physical therapy
EPR	electronic patient record		**RLQ**	right lower quadrant
ER	Emergency Room		**RN**	registered nurse
FH	Family History		**R/O**	rule out
H&P	History and Physical		**ROS**	Review of Systems
HIPAA	Health Insurance Portability and Accountability Act		**RUQ**	right upper quadrant
HPI	History of Present Illness		**SH**	Social History
ICU	intensive care unit		**SNF**	skilled nursing facility

Word Alert

Abbreviations. Abbreviations are commonly used in all types of medical documents; however, they can mean different things to different people and their meanings can be misinterpreted. Always verify the meaning of an abbreviation.

CC means *chief complaint*, but it also means *cubic centimeter* (a measure of volume).

H&P means *history and physical* (*examination*), but the sound-alike abbreviation *HNP* stands for *herniated nucleus pulposus*.

PA means *physician's assistant*, but it also means *posteroanterior*.

PE means *physical examination*, but it also means *pressure-equalizing (tube)* and *pulmonary embolus*.

It's Greek to Me! Some words are related to two different combining forms. Why? In ancient times, the Greeks and the Romans independently advanced the study and practice of medicine, naming things in their own languages. Combining forms from both Greek and Latin remain a part of medical language today.

Word	Greek	Latin	Medical Word Examples
intestine	enter/o-	intestin/o-	gastroenterology; gastrointestinal
nerve	neur/o-	nerv/o-	neurology; nervous system
skin	dermat/o-	integument/o-	dermatology; integumentary system

Career Focus

Meet Erica, a paramedic

"I was always interested in health care. EMTs give basic life support. They can do things such as backboarding a patient, splinting, giving oxygen, taking vital signs, and transporting patients to the hospital. Paramedics also give advanced life support. We can start intravenous lines and give medications. We can defibrillate, give electrocardiotherapy. It's hard to describe a typical day because no day is like any other. We give care to patients with chest pain, shortness of breath, diabetes, seizures, and trauma (obviously auto accidents, but also industrial accidents) and transport them to the hospital. I use medical terminology when I'm writing my run reports. Those reports are medical and legal documents. They can be looked at by lawyers in the future. I always want my reports to look professional and be medically correct."

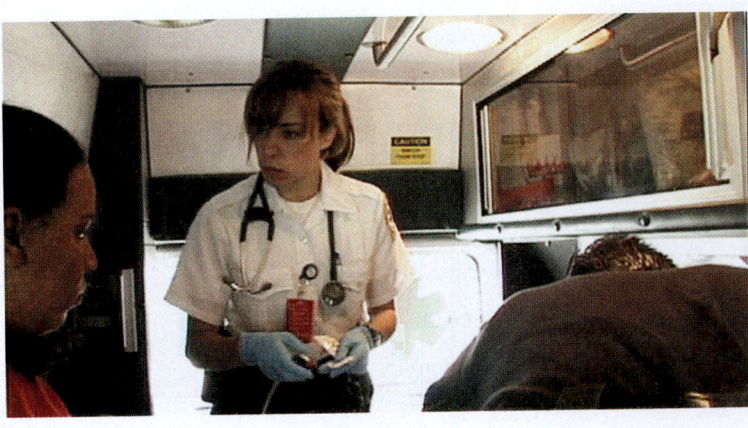

- **Paramedics** are allied health professionals who respond to emergency calls from the community, treat patients in ambulances, and transport them to the emergency department of the hospital. The paramedic provides medical care in a setting that is apart from a hospital or physician's office.

paramedic (PAIR-ah-MED-ik)
Paramedic contains the prefix **para-**, which means *apart from,* and **medic** (a shortened form of *medical*). A paramedic works apart from the healthcare professionals who are in the hospital.

Chapter Review Exercises

Dive In: Medical Language Exercises

Test your knowledge of the chapter by completing these review exercises. Use the Answer Key at the end of the book to check your answers. Note: Each of the numbered exercise headers corresponds to a numbered learning outcome at the beginning of the chapter.

1.1 Medical Language

CIRCLE EXERCISE

Circle the correct answer from the choices given.

1. Language skills consist of all of the following *except* (**listening, spelling, terminology**).
2. Etymology is the study of (**Greek, languages, word origins**).
3. Medical words come from all of these sources *except* (**Arabic, Latin, Old Dutch, Old French**).

TRUE OR FALSE EXERCISE

*Indicate whether each statement is true or false by writing **T** or **F** on the line.*

1. _____ Terminology is the study of word origins.
2. _____ Medical words are the "tools of the trade" for healthcare professionals.
3. _____ Reading medical words and hearing medical words is similar to input coming into a computer.
4. _____ Speaking and pronouncing are skills needed to relay medical language.

RELATED COMBINING FORMS EXERCISE

Write the combining forms on the lines provided. (Hint: See the It's Greek to Me! feature box.)

1. Two combining forms that mean *intestine*.   _____   _____

2. Two combining forms that mean *nerve*.   _____   _____

3. Two combining forms that mean *skin*.   _____   _____

1.2 Medical Words: Singular and Plural Nouns and Word Parts

MATCHING EXERCISE

Match each word or phrase to its description. A word or phrase can have more than one description.

1. combining form
2. suffix
3. prefix

_____ begins with a hyphen

_____ contains the main meaning of the medical word

_____ ends with a combining vowel

_____ always is positioned at the end of a medical word

_____ if present, is always at the beginning of a medical word

_____ an optional word part

_____ when there is no prefix, this is the first word part

MATCHING EXERCISE

Match each word part to its meaning.

1. anti-
2. arteri/o-
3. arthr/o-
4. cardi/o-
5. cost/o-
6. cyan/o-
7. -gram
8. -graphy
9. hepat/o-
10. inter-
11. lapar/o-
12. -logy
13. mamm/o-
14. -megaly
15. muscul/o-
16. nas/o-
17. -oma
18. -pathy
19. poly-
20. sub-

_____ against
_____ between
_____ rib
_____ heart
_____ mass; tumor
_____ liver
_____ study of
_____ muscle
_____ picture; record
_____ blue
_____ nose
_____ below; underneath; less than
_____ enlargement
_____ joint
_____ many; much
_____ disease
_____ artery
_____ process of recording
_____ breast
_____ abdomen

CIRCLE EXERCISE

Circle the correct answer from the choices given.

1. When a Latin singular noun ends in -*a*, form the plural as (**-ae, -es, -ices**).
2. The main medical meaning of a word comes from its (**combining form, prefix, suffix**).
3. The combining form *enter/o-* means (**heart, intestine, rib**).
4. When a Latin singular noun ends in -*us*, form the plural as (**-a, -i, -y**).
5. Daniel Fields broke his left middle (**phalanges, phalanx**) while playing baseball.
6. Baby Phong Nyugen's mother took him to the doctor when she noticed that his left (**testes, testis**) was not present in the scrotum.
7. On the x-ray, Leona Calvin's spine showed fractures of several (**vertebra, vertebrae**).
8. The laboratory identified several (**bacteria, bacterium**) that were causing the infection.
9. There are many (**alveolus, alveoli**) or air sacs in the lungs.
10. When a woman ovulates, her ovary releases an egg or (**ovum, ova**).

TRUE OR FALSE EXERCISE

*Indicate whether each statement is true or false by writing **T** or **F** on the line.*

1. _____ The three word parts in medical language are spelling, reading, and Greek.
2. _____ Every medical word contains a prefix.
3. _____ The suffix is the foundation of a medical word.
4. _____ A root and a combining vowel together form a medical word.
5. _____ The suffixes -*al* and -*ic* both mean *pertaining to*.

PLURAL NOUN EXERCISE

Read the singular noun and write its plural form on the line. Be sure to check your spelling. The first one has been done for you.

Singular Noun	Plural Noun	Singular Noun	Plural Noun
1. **iris**	*irides*	8. bacterium	
2. diagnosis		9. ganglion	
3. ovum		10. vertebra	
4. phalanx		11. artery	
5. ovary		12. thrombus	
6. hormone		13. testis	
7. bronchus		14. ovary	

1.3 Divide and Build Medical Words

DIVIDING WORDS EXERCISE

Separate these words into their component parts (prefix, combining form, suffix). Some words do not contain all three word parts. The first one has been done for you.

Medical Word	Prefix	Combining Form	Suffix
1. **language**		*langu/o-*	*-age*
2. medical			
3. etymology			
4. bilateral			
5. cardiac			
6. intestinal			
7. muscular			
8. uterine			
9. urinary			
10. digestive			
11. pericardial			
12. hypertension			
13. antibiotic			
14. cardiomegaly			
15. tonsillectomy			

BUILDING WORDS EXERCISE

Practice building medical words by joining a combining form and a suffix. Write the medical word on the line. Be sure to check your spelling. The first one has been done for you.

Suffix List

-ation (being; having; process)   -ive (pertaining to)   -pathy (disease)

-ics (knowledge; practice)   -logy (study of)   -scopy (process of using an
                                                                   instrument to examine)
-itis (inflammation of; infection of) -ous (pertaining to)

Definition of the Medical Word	Combining Form	Suffix	Build the Medical Word
Example: Study of (the) heart	**cardi/o-**	*-logy*	*cardiology*

[*You think* study of (-logy) + heart (cardi/o-). *You change the order of the word parts to put the suffix last. You write* cardiology.]

1. Pertaining to break down food	digest/o-	_____	_____
2. Pertaining to (a) vein	ven/o-	_____	_____
3. Knowledge (and) practice (of) pregnancy and childbirth	obstetr/o-	_____	_____
4. Process (of making) urine	urin/o-	_____	_____
5. Infection of (the) tonsils	tonsill/o-	_____	_____
6. Disease (of a) joint	arthr/o-	_____	_____
7. Process of using an instrument to examine (the) stomach	gastr/o-	_____	_____

SPELLING EXERCISE

Look at each medical word and detect the spelling error. Then write the correct spelling of the word on the line.

Misspelled Medical Word	Correct Spelling	Misspelled Medical Word	Correct Spelling
1. cardeac	_____	5. tonsilitis	_____
2. subcutayneous	_____	6. urinashun	_____
3. mamografee	_____	7. venus	_____
4. takicardia	_____		

SPELLING EXERCISE

Read each medical word pronunciation and write the medical word that it represents. Be sure to check your spelling. The first one has been done for you.

1. **(KAR-dee-ak)**	*cardiac*	4. (nyoor-AW-loh-jee)	_____
2. (YOOR-ih-NAY-shun)	_____	5. (TAWN-sil-EYE-tihs)	_____
3. (IN-trah-VEE-nuhs)	_____	6. (SUB-kyoo-TAY-nee-uhs)	_____

1.4 The Body in Health and Disease

MATCHING EXERCISE

Match each word to its description.

1. cavity	_____ increased symptoms
2. dietetics	_____ knowledge and practice of foods
3. distal	_____ pregnancy and childbirth
4. exacerbation	_____ opposite of prone
5. genetic	_____ pertaining to genes and chromosomes
6. geriatrics	_____ hollow space
7. obstetrics	_____ opposite of proximal
8. plane	_____ end of life
9. supine	_____ having no identifiable cause
10. terminal	_____ specialty for older adults
11. idiopathic	_____ imaginary surface

CIRCLE EXERCISE

Circle the correct answer from the choices given.

1. The cause of a disease is the (**etiology, sequela, syndrome**).
2. A disease that does not respond well to treatment is said to be (**acute, refractory, therapeutic**).
3. A/An (**exacerbation, remission, sequela**) is a temporary improvement in the symptoms and signs of a disease.
4. When a disease involves a recessive gene that is inherited from one's parents, the disease is (**congenital, hereditary, nutritional**).
5. Dr. James Gibbons treated Al Smith's (**gastric, gastroscopy**) ulcer by prescribing medication.
6. The physical examination at the walk-in clinic revealed that Jose Rodriguez had (**tonsillectomy, tonsillitis**).
7. Alan Witherspoon underwent a (**cardiac, cardiomegaly**) stress test to evaluate his heart.
8. Alicyn Smart experienced severe abdominal pain, and the emergency department physician scheduled her to have an (**appendectomy, appendicitis**).
9. Dr. Matthew Cohen decided to specialize in treating the (**tonsillectomy, urinary**) system.
10. When Briana Wright began feeling depressed, she made an appointment with a (**psychotherapy, psychiatrist**).

TRUE OR FALSE EXERCISE

*Indicate whether each statement is true or false by writing **T** or **F** on the line.*

1. _____ The sagittal plane divides the body into superior and inferior sections.
2. _____ Cephalad is the opposite direction of caudad.
3. _____ The cranial cavity is continuous with the spinal cavity.
4. _____ Dermatology studies the integumentary system.
5. _____ The respiratory system is related to the medical specialty of pulmonology.
6. _____ An iatrogenic disease is caused by the physician or the treatment.
7. _____ An exacerbation is a complication caused by the original disease.

DIVIDING WORDS EXERCISE

Separate these words into their component parts (prefix, combining form, suffix). Some words do not contain all three word parts. The first one has been done for you.

Medical Word	Prefix	Combining Form	Suffix	Medical Word	Prefix	Combining Form	Suffix
1. **anatomical**	*ana-*	*tom/o-*	*-ical*	7. asymptomatic	___	___	___
2. nosocomial		___	___	8. posterior		___	___
3. cephalad		___	___	9. reproductive	___	___	___
4. gynecology		___	___	10. thoracic		___	___
5. degenerative	___	___	___	11. urinary		___	___
6. ophthalmology		___	___				

BUILDING WORDS EXERCISE

Practice building medical words by joining a combining form and a suffix. Write the medical word on the line. Be sure to check your spelling. The first one has been done for you.

Suffix List

-al (pertaining to)	-ery (process)	-ics (knowledge; practice)
-ant (pertaining to)	-gen (that which produces)	-ious (pertaining to)
-ary (pertaining to)	-ic (pertaining to)	-logy (study of)

Definition of the Medical Word	Combining Form	Suffix	Build the Medical Word
Example: Study of (the) heart	**cardi/o-**	*-logy*	*cardiology*

[*You think* study of (-logy) + heart (cardi/o-). *You change the order of the word parts to put the suffix last. You write cardiology.*]

Definition of the Medical Word	Combining Form	Suffix	Build the Medical Word
1. Pertaining to (being) present at birth	congenit/o-	___	___
2. That which produces disease	path/o-	___	___
3. Study of (a) collection of symptoms	symptomat/o-	___	___
4. Pertaining to therapy (or) treatment	therapeut/o-	___	___
5. Process (of an) operative procedure	surg/o-	___	___
6. Study of (the) cause of disease	eti/o-	___	___
7. Pertaining to (the) skin	integument/o-	___	___
8. Pertaining to four	quadr/o-	___	___
9. Knowledge (and) practice (of) pregnancy and childbirth	obstetr/o-	___	___
10. Pertaining to disease within	infect/o-	___	___
11. Pertaining to genetic inheritance	heredit/o-	___	___

SPELLING EXERCISE

Look at each medical word and detect the spelling error. Then write the correct spelling of the medical word on the line. The first one has been done for you.

Misspelled Medical Word	Correct Spelling	Misspelled Medical Word	Correct Spelling
1. **cardeac**	*cardiac*	5. takicardia	
2. subcutayneous		6. tonsilitis	
3. mamografee		7. urinashun	
4. sychiatry		8. venus	

SPELLING EXERCISE

You hear someone speaking the medical words given below. Read each pronunciation and then write the medical word it represents. Be sure to check your spelling. The first one has been done for you.

1. **(KAR-dee-ak)**	*cardiac*	6. (noo-MOHN-yah)	
2. (nyoor-AW-loh-jee)		7. (heh-PAT-ik)	
3. (TAWN-sil-EYE-tihs)		8. (mam-AW-grah-fee)	
4. (YOO-ter-in)		9. (ah-NAT-oh-mee)	
5. (SUB-kyoo-TAY-nee-uhs)		10. (PEE-dee-AT-riks)	

1.5 Health Care Today

MATCHING EXERCISE

Match each abbreviation to its description.

1. MD   _____ minor outpatient surgery is performed here
2. NP   _____ physician extender who delivers babies
3. SNF   _____ doctor who treats the feet
4. ASC   _____ physician who graduated from a medical school
5. CNM   _____ registered nurse
6. DPM   _____ acts as a physician extender
7. RN   _____ patients here are known as *residents*
8. DDS   _____ ancillary department within a hospital
9. ED   _____ doctor who treats the teeth

TRUE OR FALSE EXERCISE

*Indicate whether each statement is true or false by writing **T** or **F** on the line.*

1. _____ The medical record is where healthcare professionals document care provided to a patient.
2. _____ The medical record of today is mainly used to document diseases, treatments, and surgeries.
3. _____ The medical record is a medicolegal document.
4. _____ By law, the format of a medical record must be the same in all healthcare facilities.
5. _____ A consent to treat form signed by the patient allows the healthcare facility to contact HIPAA for payment for any medical care provided.
6. _____ Doctors and therapists form the core of the healthcare team.
7. _____ A hospital stay begins with the physician's order to admit the patient.
8. _____ A nurse orders therapy for a patient.
9. _____ A Doctor of Chiropractic treats only the eyes.
10. _____ A dietitian is an example of a technologist.

FILL IN THE BLANK EXERCISE

Describe three advantages of the electronic health record versus a paper medical record.

1. _____

2. _____

3. _____

DIVIDING WORDS EXERCISE

Separate these words into their component parts (prefix, combining form, suffix). Some words do not contain all three word parts. The first one has been done for you.

Medical Word	Prefix	Combining Form	Suffix
1. **palliative**		*palliat/o-*	*-ive*
2. rehabilitation	_____	_____	_____
3. ambulatory		_____	_____
4. physician		_____	_____
5. technician		_____	_____

BUILDING WORDS EXERCISE

Read the definition of the medical word. Look at the combining form that is given. Select the correct suffix from the Suffix List, and write it on the blank line. Then build the medical word, and write it on the line. (Remember: You may need to remove the combining vowel. Always remove the hyphens and slash.) Be sure to check your spelling.

Suffix List

-ation (being; having; process)	-ician (skilled expert; skilled professional)	-ist (person who specializes in)
-eon (person who performs)	-ion (action; condition)	-ive (pertaining to)

Definition of the Medical Word	Combining Form	Suffix	Build the Medical Word
Example: Action (of) looking at (the body)	**inspect/o-**	*-ion*	*inspection*

[*You think* action (-ion) + looking at (inspect/o-). You change the order of the word parts to put the suffix last. You write inspection.]

1. Person who specializes in treatment	therap/o-	_____	_____
2. Person who performs (an) operative procedure	surg/o-	_____	_____
3. Pertaining to reducing the severity	palliat/o-	_____	_____
4. Skilled professional (with) technical skill	techn/o-	_____	_____
5. Action (of) feeling (or) touching	palpat/o-	_____	_____
6. Process (of) listening	auscult/o-	_____	_____
7. Action (of) tapping	percuss/o-	_____	_____

DEFINE ABBREVIATIONS

Write the definition for each abbreviation on the line provided.

1. EPR _____

2. DS _____

3. CC _____

4. H&P _____

5. Dx _____

6. ROS _____

Immerse Yourself: Introduction to Medical Reports

You Write the Medical Report

Complete each sentence with the correct medical specialty. Be sure to check your spelling. The first one has been done for you.

1. Diseases of the female genital system are studied in the medical specialty of __*gynecology*__.

2. Mrs. Claire English is 4 months' pregnant. She is under the care of a physician who specializes in _____.

3. Bobby McCollum seems to constantly have a runny nose, a sore throat, and repeated ear infections. His regular physician referred him to a specialist in the medical specialty of _____ for possible surgery on his ears.

4. _____ is the medical specialty that helps patients who have diseases of the nervous system.

5. County road worker Jeremy Walker accidentally touched poison ivy while clearing some brush. He has severe itching and redness on the skin of his hands and arms. He has an appointment this afternoon in the _____ clinic.

6. Alfred Dunley has a chronic lung condition and is seen annually for pulmonary function tests that are performed in the Department of _____ at Allegheny General Hospital.

7. Sarah Gibbs was born 4 weeks prematurely, but is going home today after being cared for by the nurses and doctors who specialize in _____.

8. When Chris Sutton fell down the steps, she went to the emergency room and a physician from the medical specialty of _____ read her x-rays and found she had fractured her little toe.

9. The team physician for the Baltimore Ravens football team is a specialist in the field of _____ because team members have so many bone and muscle injuries during the season.

MyLab Medical Terminology™

MyLab Medical Terminology is a premium online homework management system that includes a host of features to help you study. Registered users will find:

- A multitude of activities and assignments built within the MyLab platform

- Powerful tools that track and analyze your results—allowing you to create a personalized learning experience

- Videos and audio pronunciations to help enrich your progress

- Streaming lesson presentations (guided lectures) and self-paced learning modules

- A space where you and your instructor can check your progress and manage your assignments

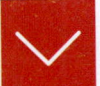

2 Dermatology
Integumentary System

Dermatology (DER-mah-TAW-loh-jee) is the medical specialty that studies the anatomy and physiology of the integumentary system; uses laboratory and diagnostic procedures to diagnose integumentary diseases; and uses medical procedures, drugs, and surgical procedures to treat integumentary diseases.

∨ Chapter Overview and Learning Outcomes

After you study this chapter, you should be able to demonstrate mastery of the outcomes by successfully completing the exercises.

2.1 Anatomy
Identify the structures of the integumentary system.
Demonstrate proficiency in medical language.
2.1 Practice Laps

2.2 Physiology
Describe the functions of the integumentary system.
Demonstrate proficiency in medical language.
2.2 Practice Laps
Vocabulary Review

2.3 Diseases
Describe common integumentary diseases.
Demonstrate proficiency in medical language.
2.3 Practice Laps

2.4 Laboratory and Diagnostic Procedures
Describe common integumentary laboratory tests and diagnostic procedures.
Demonstrate proficiency in medical language.
2.4 Practice Laps

2.5 Medical Procedures, Drugs, and Surgical Procedures
Describe common integumentary medical procedures, drugs, and surgical procedures.
Demonstrate proficiency in medical language.
2.5 Practice Laps
Abbreviations Summary
Career Focus

Chapter Review Exercises
Dive In: Medical Language Exercises
(Learning Outcomes 2.1–2.5)

Immerse Yourself: Analyze Medical Reports

Medical Language Key

To unlock the definition of a medical word, first break it into word parts. Then give the meaning of each word part. Put the meanings of the word parts in order, beginning with the meaning of the suffix, then the meaning of the prefix (if there is one), then the meaning of the combining form.

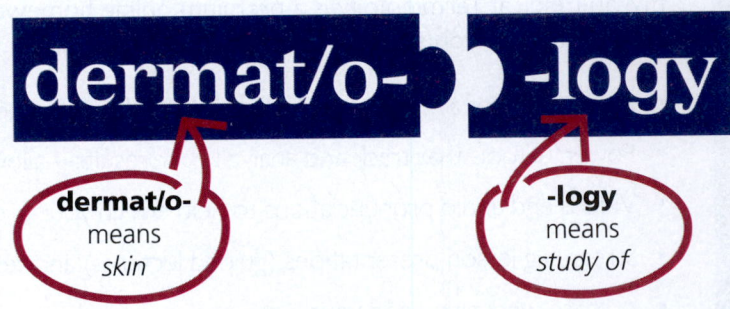

dermat/o- means *skin*

-logy means *study of*

Dermatology: ▶ *Study of (the) skin (and related structures).*

The **integumentary system** (see Figure 2-1 ■) is a large, flexible body system that covers most of the surface of the body. The structures of the integumentary system include the skin, the nails, and the subcutaneous tissue. The structures of the skin itself include the epidermis and the dermis with its glands, hair, and hair follicles. The subcutaneous tissue lies beneath the dermis.

The functions of the integumentary system include protection, repair, sensation, synthesis of vitamin D, and thermoregulation. In addition, the integumentary system has many functions that relate to the body as a whole and provide information about how well the body is maintaining homeostasis.

2.1 Anatomy

Skin

The skin consists of two different layers—the epidermis and the dermis—as well as glands and hair follicles within the dermis. Another adjective for the skin is **cutaneous**.

Epidermis

The **epidermis** is the thin, outermost layer of the skin (see Figure 2-2 ■), and it is categorized as **epithelium** that is made up of **epithelial tissue**. The superficial or **squamous layer** of the epidermis contains some living cells, but its surface cells are dead cells that are filled with **keratin**, a hard, fibrous protein. These dead cells form a protective layer, but they are constantly being shed in a process known as **exfoliation**. In contrast, the deepest or **basal layer** of the epidermis is composed of living cells that are constantly dividing and moving to the surface. The epidermis does contain **melanocytes**, pigment cells that produce **melanin**, a dark brown or black pigment. The epidermis does not contain any blood vessels. It receives nutrients and oxygen from blood vessels in the dermis beneath it.

Dermis

The **dermis** is a thicker layer beneath the epidermis (see Figure 2-2), and it is categorized as connective tissue. The dermis contains **collagen** (white protein fibers) that make it firm. It also contains **elastin** (yellow elastin fibers) that make it flexible. The dermis contains a number of different structures: arteries, veins, and nerves, as well as sebaceous glands, sudoriferous glands, and hair follicles.

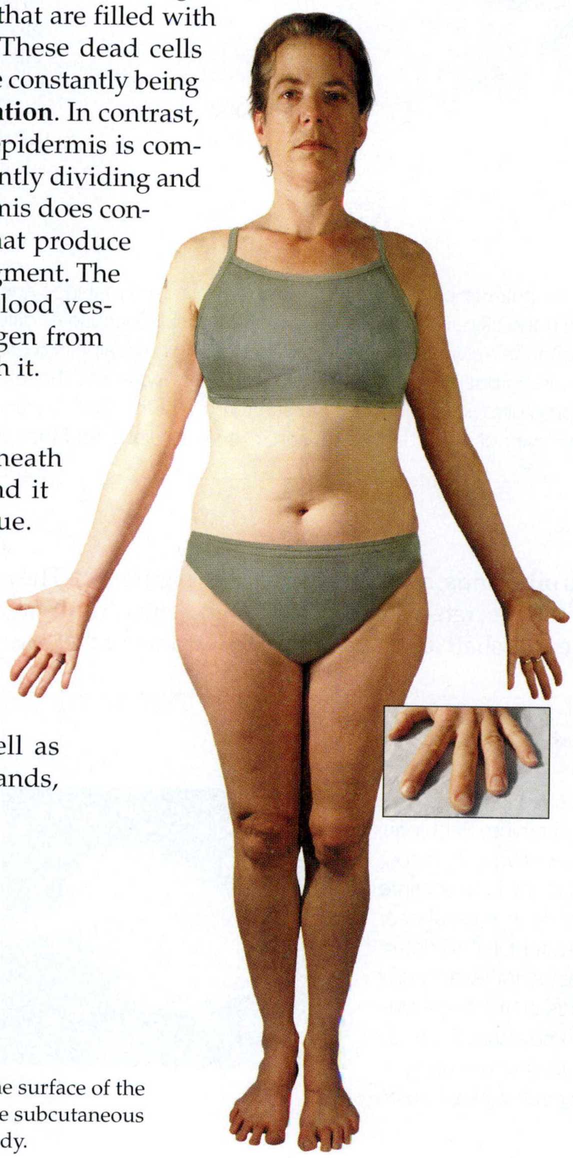

FIGURE 2-1 ■ Integumentary system.
The integumentary system covers most of the surface of the body. It consists of the skin, the nails, and the subcutaneous tissue. The skin is the largest organ in the body.

Pronunciation/Word Parts

integumentary (in-TEH-gyoo-MEN-tair-ee)
  integument/o- *skin*
  -ary *pertaining to*

cutaneous (kyoo-TAY-nee-uhs)
  cutane/o- *skin*
  -ous *pertaining to*
Cutaneous is another adjective for *skin*. The combining forms **cut/i-, derm/a-, dermat/o-,** and **derm/o-** also mean *skin*.

epidermis (EP-ih-DER-mihs)

epidermal (EP-ih-DER-mal)
  epi- *above; upon*
  derm/o- *skin*
  -al *pertaining to*

epithelium (EP-ih-THEE-lee-um)
  epi- *above; upon*
  theli/o- *cellular layer*
  -um *period of time; structure*

epithelial (EP-ih-THEE-lee-al)
  epi- *above; upon*
  theli/o- *cellular layer*
  -al *pertaining to*

squamous (SKWAY-muhs)
  squam/o- *scale-like cell*
  -ous *pertaining to*

keratin (KAIR-ah-tin)
  kerat/o- *cornea; hard, fibrous protein*
  -in *substance*

exfoliation (eks-FOH-lee-AA-shun)
  ex- *away from; out*
  foli/o- *leaf*
  -ation *being; having; process*
Exfoliation: *Process (of a skin cell moving) away from (the body like a) leaf (falling off a tree)*

basal (BAY-sal)
  bas/o- *alkaline; base of a structure*
  -al *pertaining to*

melanocyte (meh-LAN-oh-SITE)
  melan/o- *black*
  -cyte *cell*
Melanocyte: *Cell (in the skin that produces a dark brown or) black (pigment)*

melanin (MEL-ah-nin)
  melan/o- *black*
  -in *substance*

dermis (DER-mihs)

dermal (DER-mal)
  derm/o- *skin*
  -al *pertaining to*

collagen (KAW-lah-jen)
  coll/a- *fibers that hold together*
  -gen *that which produces*

elastin (ee-LAS-tin)
  elast/o- *flexing; stretching*
  -in *substance*

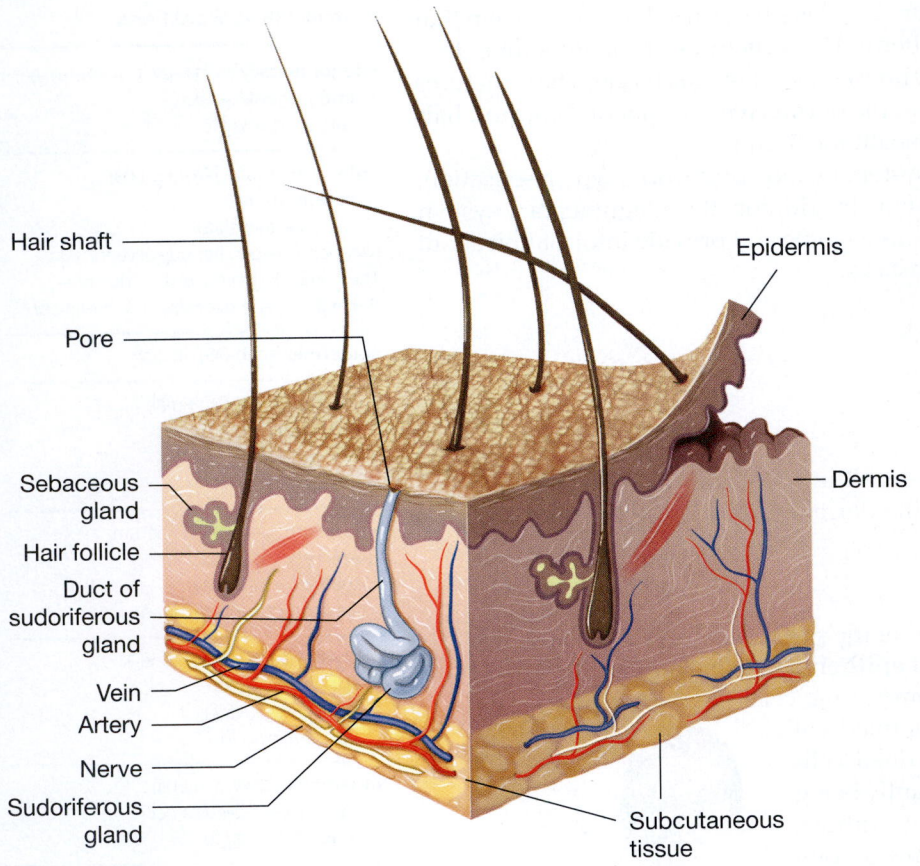

Hair shaft

Pore

Sebaceous gland

Hair follicle

Duct of sudoriferous gland

Vein

Artery

Nerve

Sudoriferous gland

Epidermis

Dermis

Subcutaneous tissue

Pronunciation/Word Parts

sebaceous (seh-BAY-shus)
   sebace/o- *oil; sebum*
   -ous *pertaining to*
The combining form **seb/o-** also means *oil; sebum.*

exocrine (EKS-oh-krin)
   ex/o- *away from; external; outward*
   -crine *pertaining to secreting*

sebum (SEE-bum)

FIGURE 2-2 ■ Skin and subcutaneous tissue. The skin is composed of the epidermis and the dermis. The epidermis contains dead protective cells at its surface and living, actively dividing cells at its base. The dermis contains sebaceous glands, sudoriferous glands, and hair follicles. The subcutaneous tissue, a type of connective tissue, lies beneath the dermis.

Dive Deeper

Melanocyte-stimulating hormone from the anterior pituitary gland in the brain causes melanocytes to produce melanin. All races of people have the same number of melanocytes in the skin. Differences in skin color occur because of differing levels of melanin production. Dark-skinned people produce more melanin than fair-skinned people. Individuals who have albinism have a normal number of melanocytes, but the cells produce insufficient or no melanin. Exposure to the sun's ultraviolet rays increases the rate of melanin production, which produces a suntan. Melanin in the epidermis absorbs ultraviolet light from the sun to protect the DNA in skin cells from undergoing genetic mutation. During prolonged sun exposure, melanin cannot absorb all of the sun's ultraviolet light, and the result is a sunburn.

Sebaceous Glands

The **sebaceous glands**, also known as **oil glands**, are in the dermis (see Figure 2-2). They are a type of **exocrine gland** because they secrete a substance through a duct. That substance is **sebum** (oil). Sebum coats the hair shaft and moisturizes the surface of the skin.

Clinical Connections

Forensic Science. Oil from the sebaceous glands leaves a fingerprint when a person touches something. Each person's fingerprint is a unique combination of whorls, loops, or arches. Detectives can scan a fingerprint from a crime scene and match it to fingerprints on file in a database. Cells from a hair follicle can be analyzed for DNA to determine a person's identity. Hair can be tested for evidence of toxins or poisons. White horizontal bands on the fingernails indicate arsenic poisoning. Detectives know that if a body was buried in moist dirt, its adipose (fatty) tissue decomposes and forms a characteristic waxy substance known as **adipocere** (grave wax).

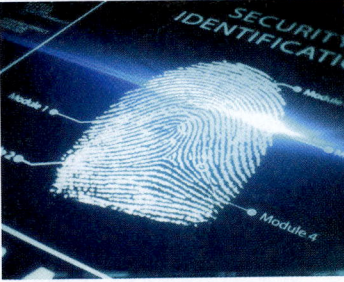

adipocere (AD-ih-poh-SEER)
   adip/o- *fat*
   -cere *waxy substance*

Sudoriferous Glands

The **sudoriferous glands**, also known as **sweat glands**, are in the dermis (see Figure 2-2). They are also a type of exocrine gland. They secrete sweat through a duct that ends at a pore on the surface of the skin. Sweat contains water, sodium, and small amounts of body wastes (ammonia, creatinine, urea). It is the sodium that gives sweat its salty taste. Although sweat is odorless, bacteria on the surface of the skin digest sweat, and their waste products produce the odor associated with sweat. The process of producing sweat is **diaphoresis**, and the sweat itself is **perspiration**.

Hair

Each hair forms within a hair **follicle** in the dermis (see Figure 2-2). Hair cells are filled with keratin, which makes the hair shaft strong. Usually, hairs lie flat against the surface of the skin, but, when the skin is cold (or when a person experiences a strong emotion), the hairs stand up; this is known as **piloerection**. Just as melanin from melanocytes colors the skin, it also colors the hair. Dark hair contains melanin, but blond hair and red hair contain a variant of melanin that contains more sulfur, and so the hair appears more yellow or red. Hair covers most of the body, although its consistency and color vary from one part of the body to the next and from one person to another. During adolescence, under the influence of hormones, additional hair grows in facial, axillary, and pubic areas to show the onset of sexual maturity.

Pronunciation/Word Parts

sudoriferous (SOO-doh-RIF-er-uhs)
  sudor/i- *sweat*
  fer/o- *bear*
  -ous *pertaining to*
The combining form **hidr/o-** also means *sweat*.

diaphoresis (DY-ah-for-EE-sihs)
  dia- *complete; through*
  phor/o- *bear; carry; range*
  -esis *abnormal condition; process*

perspiration (PER-spih-RAY-shun)
  per- *through; throughout*
  spir/o- *breathe; coil*
  -ation *being; having; process*

hair (HAIR)
The combining form **trich/o-** means *hair*. The word *schizotrichia* means *condition of split hairs*.

follicle (FAW-lih-kul)
  folli/o- *sac-like structure*
  -cle *small thing*

Across the Life Span

Pediatrics. In the mother's uterus, a fetus begins to develop hair at 10 weeks of age. The first hair, which is very fine, covers the entire body and is called **lanugo**. This is still present on babies who are born prematurely. Scalp hair usually develops later, but some babies are born with a full head of hair, whereas others are bald!

Geriatrics. As a person ages, melanocytes stop producing melanin, and the hair appears gray or white.

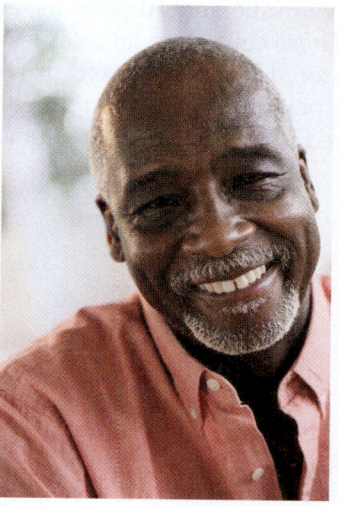

lanugo (lah-NOO-goh)

ungual (UNG-gwal)
  ungu/o- *fingernail; toenail*
  -al *pertaining to*
Ungual is the adjective for *nail*. The combining form **onych/o-** also means *fingernail; toenail*.

Nails

The nails cover and protect the distal ends of the fingers and toes because those areas are easily injured. Each nail consists of several parts (see Figure 2-3 ■). The outer layer—the hard, translucent **nail plate**—is composed of dead cells that contain keratin. The **nail root** is located beneath the skin on the upper surface of the finger and toe. It produces the cells of the nail plate, first the **lunula** (the visible white, half-moon) that then becomes the hard, top nail plate. The **cuticle**, a layer of dead cells, lies along the proximal base of the nail. Beneath the top nail plate is the **nail bed** or *quick*, which contains nerves and blood vessels. Blood vessels in the nail bed give the nail plate its color—normally this is pink, but it can become bluish-purple if the person's oxygen level in the blood is decreased.

follicular (foh-LIH-kyoo-lar)
  follicul/o- *follicle*
  -ar *pertaining to*

piloerection (PY-loh-eh-REK-shun)
  pil/o- *hair*
  erect/o- *stand up*
  -ion *action; condition*

lunula (LOO-nyoo-lah)
  lun/o- *moon*
  -ula *small thing*

cuticle (KYOO-tih-kul)
  cut/i- *skin*
  -cle *small thing*

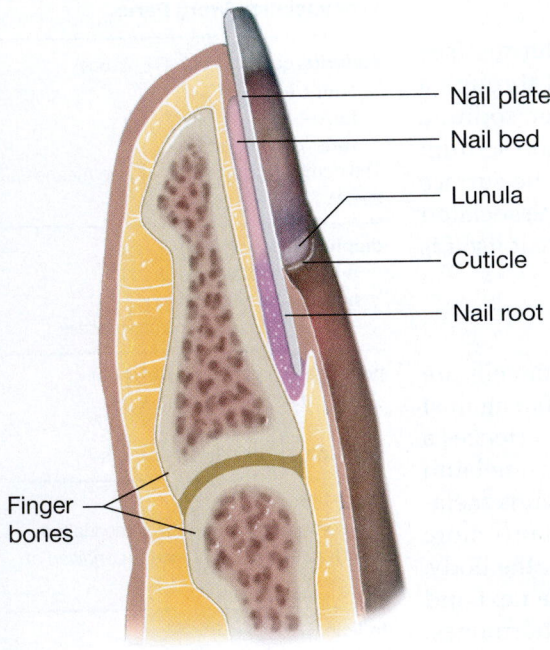

Nail plate
Nail bed
Lunula
Cuticle
Nail root
Finger bones

FIGURE 2-3 ■ **Nail.**
The nail is composed of both living and dead cells. The nail root produces keratin-containing cells that form the lunula. As those cells grow from the lunula, they die and harden to form the nail plate, the protective covering on the distal end of the finger or toe.

Subcutaneous Tissue

The **subcutaneous tissue** (SQ, subcu, subQ) (see Figure 2-2) is directly beneath the dermis. It is composed of connective tissue and **adipose tissue** (fatty tissue). The adipose tissue contains **lipocytes**. These cells store fat as an energy reserve for the body. However, the amount of fat stored usually far exceeds any energy needs the body might have! Depending on a person's metabolism, dietary intake of sugars and fats, and the amount of fat stored in the lipocytes, the subcutaneous tissue can be thin or several inches thick.

Pronunciation/Word Parts

subcutaneous (SUB-kyoo-TAY-nee-uhs)
sub- *below; underneath; less than*
cutane/o- *skin*
-ous *pertaining to*

adipose (AD-ih-pohs)
adip/o- *fat*
-ose *full of*

lipocyte (LIP-oh-site)
lip/o- *fat; lipid*
-cyte *cell*

Across the Life Span

Pediatrics. The skin of an infant is smooth and very flexible. It has no wrinkles because of elastin (elastic fibers) in the dermis and the thick layer of fat in the subcutaneous tissue. This fat layer conserves body heat and protects the internal organs as the infant learns to walk.

Geriatrics. In older adults, the amount of elastin decreases, and the skin develops sags and wrinkles. The fat in the subcutaneous layer thins, the skin appears translucent, and arteries and veins—especially in the hands—become obvious. There is a simultaneous underproduction and overproduction of melanin that gives the skin a mottled, irregular appearance with age spots. In persons who smoke, the nicotine in cigarettes decreases oxygen levels in the skin and destroys the collagen. This causes deep wrinkles and gives a leathery quality to the skin.

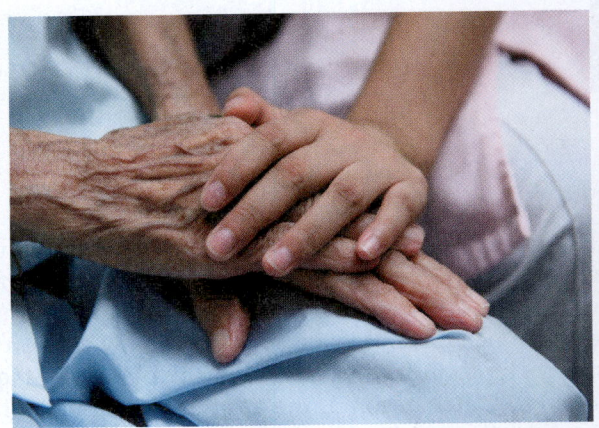

2.1 PRACTICE LAPS

Use the Answer Key at the end of the book to check your answers.

A. Label Structures

Write each anatomy word or phrase in the correct numbered box. Be sure to check your spelling.

artery	epidermis	nerve	subcutaneous tissue
dermis	hair follicle	pore	sudoriferous gland
duct of sudoriferous gland	hair shaft	sebaceous gland	vein

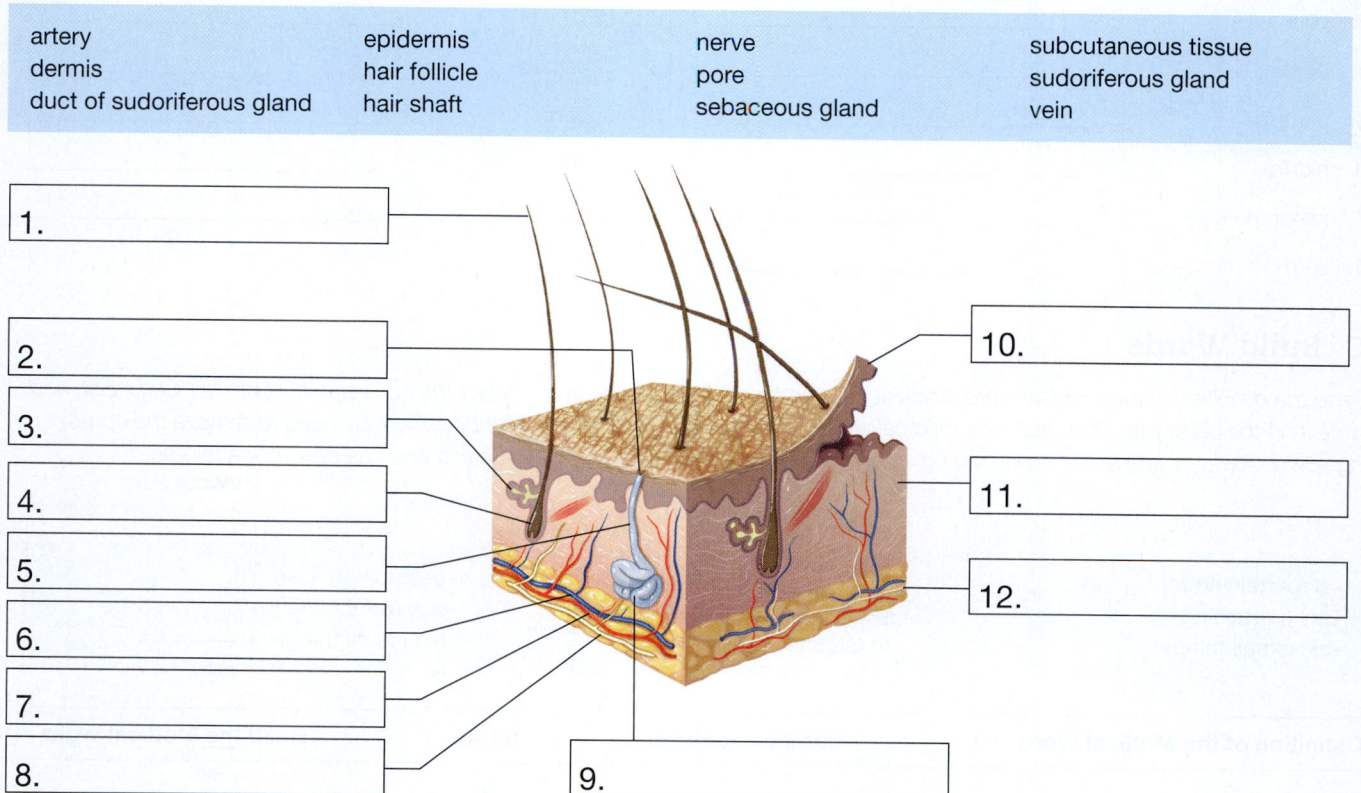

1.

2.

3.

4.

5.

6.

7.

8.

9.

10.

11.

12.

Write each anatomy word or phrase in the correct numbered box. Be sure to check your spelling.

cuticle	lunula	nail plate
finger bone	nail bed	nail root

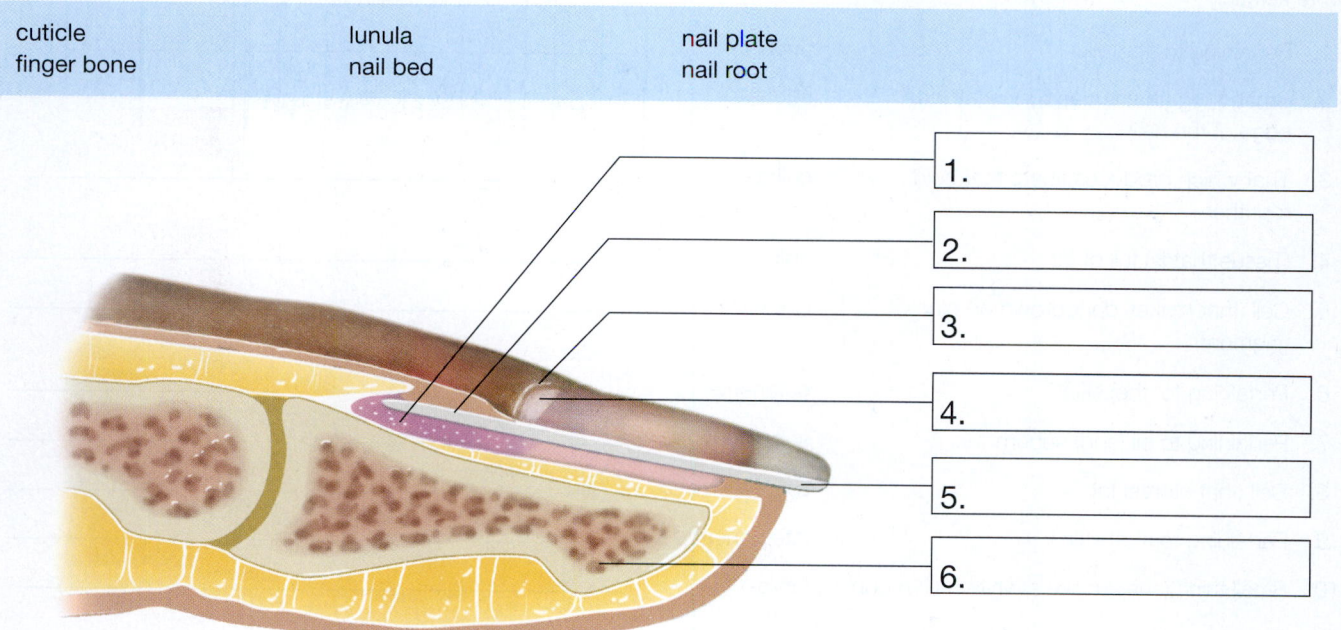

1.

2.

3.

4.

5.

6.

B. Give the Meaning of Combining Forms

Next to each combining form, write its meaning. The first one has been done for you.

Combining Form	Meaning	Combining Form	Meaning
1. **follicul/o-**	*follicle*	9. melan/o-	
2. adip/o-		10. onych/o-	
3. cutane/o-		11. pil/o-	
4. dermat/o-		12. sebace/o-	
5. derm/o-		13. sudor/i-	
6. hidr/o-		14. theli/o-	
7. integument/o-		15. trich/o-	
8. lip/o-			

C. Build Words

Read the definition of the medical word. Look at the combining form that is given. Select the correct suffix from the Suffix List, and write it on the blank line. Then build the medical word, and write it on the line. (Remember: You may need to remove the combining vowel. Always remove the hyphens and slash.) Be sure to check your spelling. The first one has been done for you.

Suffix List

-al (pertaining to)	-cyte (cell)	-ose (full of)
-ary (pertaining to)	-gen (that which produces)	-ous (pertaining to)
-cle (small thing)	-in (substance)	-ula (small thing)

Definition of the Medical Word	Combining Form	Suffix	Build the Medical Word
Example: Substance (of) hard, fibrous protein	**kerat/o-**	*-in*	*keratin*

[*You think* substance (-in) + hard, fibrous protein (kerat/o-). *You change the order of the word parts to put the suffix last. You write* keratin.]

Definition of the Medical Word	Combining Form	Suffix	Build the Medical Word
1. Pertaining to (the) nail	ungu/o-		
2. Small thing (that is dead) skin (at the edge of the nail)	cut/i-		
3. That which produces fibers that hold together	coll/a-		
4. (Tissue that is) full of fat	adip/o-		
5. Cell (that makes dark brown or) black (pigment)	melan/o-		
6. Pertaining to (the) skin	cutane/o-		
7. Pertaining to oil (and) sebum	sebace/o-		
8. Cell (that stores) fat	lip/o-		
9. Pertaining to (the) skin	integument/o-		
10. Small thing (shaped like a white half) moon	lun/o-		
11. Substance (that produces) black	melan/o-		

2.2 Physiology

The integumentary system has many functions, including those that relate to the body as a whole, as well as to other individual body systems.

Pronunciation/Word Parts

protection (proh-TEK-shun)
 protect/o- *defend; protect*
 -ion *action; condition*

flora (FLOOR-ah)

nosocomial (NOH-soh-KOH-mee-al)
 nosocomi/o- *hospital*
 -al *pertaining to*

1. **Protection.** The integumentary system is the body's first line of defense and protection against injury and infection. Each component of the integumentary system has a specific protective function.

   The dead cells on the surface of the epidermis create a dry and slightly acidic environment that discourages the growth of microorganisms. The keratin in these cells also makes the skin waterproof. The constant shedding of epidermal cells prevents microorganisms from multiplying and entering the skin to cause infection. Sweat and sebum (oil) secreted by the skin contain antibodies and enzymes that kill bacteria. **Normal skin flora** (bacteria that live on the skin and thrive under these conditions) never cause infection; in fact, normal skin flora actually inhibit the growth of disease-causing microorganisms by competing for space and nutrients.

   The hair on the head protects the skin from the ultraviolet rays of the sun. The nails protect the distal ends of the fingers and toes from injury. The cuticle is adherent to the nail plate to prevent microorganisms from entering and causing infection in the tissues of the fingers and toes. The subcutaneous layer acts as a cushion to protect the bones and internal organs from injury.

2. **Repair.** When a small injury to the skin does occur, the skin is able to repair itself. Cells in the basal layer of the epidermis move upward and cover the wound. When there is a deeper wound, a blood clot forms and many cells come together to form a scab. The scab eventually falls off as new cells from the dermis and basal layer of the epidermis fill in the wound. The integumentary system's role as an external barrier complements the work of the immune system (described in Chapter 6, Hematology and Immunology) as it fights infection within the body.

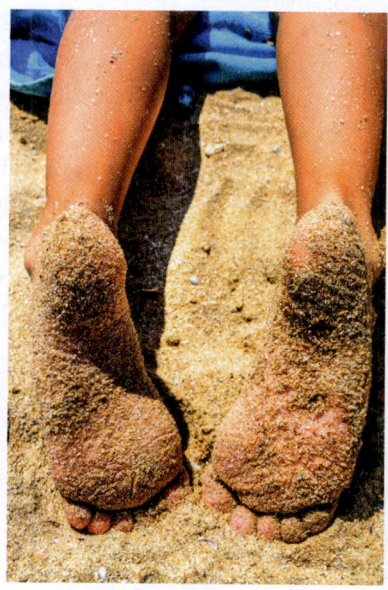

Clinical Connections

Public Health. The integumentary system is the body's first line of defense against infection. And yet, ironically, bacteria and viruses on the skin can be a source of infection to others. In 1847, it was discovered that the simple act of handwashing prevented the spread of disease. In hospitals and other healthcare facilities, caregivers wash their hands before caring for each patient. This is to prevent **healthcare–associated infections (HAIs)**, previously known as **nosocomial infections**.

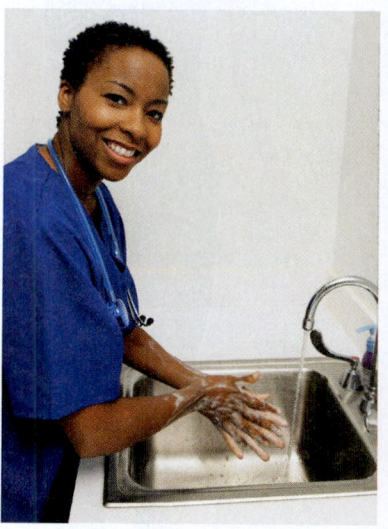

3. **Sensation.** The integumentary system contains sensory receptors in the dermis that respond to light touch, pressure, vibration, pain, or temperature. The integumentary system complements the work of the nervous system, as the nervous system relays and interprets skin sensations. When you touch something hot, the sensation from the skin travels on a nerve to the spinal cord. The spinal cord immediately sends a motor command to a muscle to pull your hand away from the heat. After your hand has moved, your brain receives the sensory information and thinks "That was hot!" A **dermatome** is a specific area on the skin that sends sensory information through a spinal nerve to the spinal cord (see Figure 2-4 ■).

4. **Vitamin D synthesis. Synthesis** is the process of putting separate components together to make a new substance. In the integumentary system, synthesis occurs as the sun's ultraviolet rays convert cholesterol in the epidermis into vitamin D. The amount of vitamin D produced depends on the amount of sunlight (time of day, season of the year). About 20–45 minutes of sunlight per week produces sufficient amounts of vitamin D to meet the body's needs. Vitamin D is stored in lipocytes in the subcutaneous tissue. Vitamin D helps the body absorb and use calcium from foods and also protects the entire body against some types of cancer. The integumentary system's role in storing vitamin D complements the function of the skeletal system that uses the absorbed calcium for bone growth and complements the function of the muscular system that uses calcium for muscle contractions.

Pronunciation/Word Parts

sensation (sen-SAY-shun)
 sens/o- *feeling*
 -ation *being; having; process*

dermatome (DER-mah-tohm)
 derm/a- *skin*
 -tome *area with distinct edges; instrument used to cut*

synthesis (SIN-theh-sihs)
 synth/o- *put together*
 -esis *abnormal condition; process*

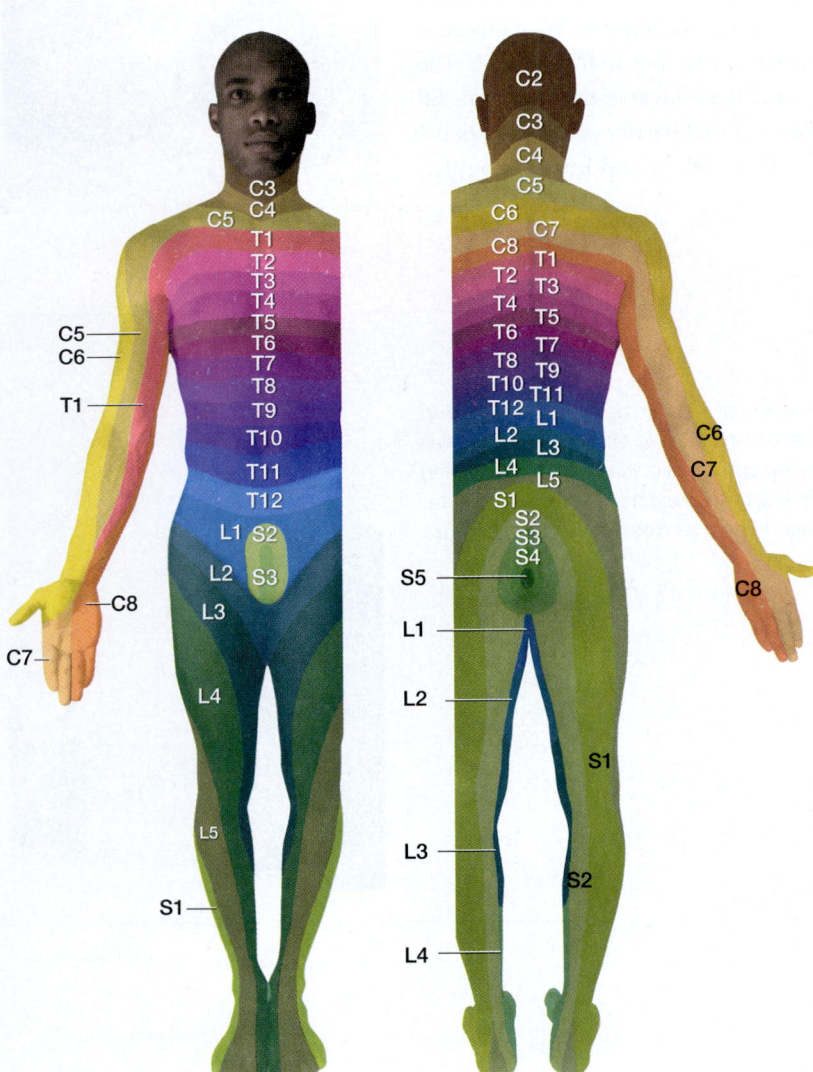

FIGURE 2-4 ■ Dermatomes of the body.
One of the functions of the skin is the sense of touch. A dermatome is a specific area of the skin that sends sensory information from the skin through a spinal nerve to the spinal cord. Each dermatome is named according to the level at which the spinal nerve enters the spinal cord. *C* stands for the spinal cord at the level of the neck (*cervic/o-* means *neck*). *T* stands for the spinal cord at the level of the thorax. *L* stands for the spinal cord at the level of the lumbar area (lower back). *S* stands for the spinal cord at the level of the sacrum (the last bones in the spine). The skin of the face sends sensory information through the cranial nerves that go directly to the brain.

5. **Thermoregulation. Thermoregulation** is the process of controlling and adjusting the body's temperature. The integumentary system assists in thermoregulation in the following ways. The subcutaneous tissue is a stored layer of fat that conserves internal body heat. In a cool environment, small muscles at the base of each hair follicle contract. This creates raised areas on the skin (goosebumps) and the hairs become erect (piloerection), both of which create some heat on the skin's surface. When the body is hot, temperature receptors in the skin send impulses to the hypothalamus in the brain, which then signals the sudoriferous glands to secrete sweat. Water in the sweat evaporates from the skin and cools the surface of the body. Also, blood vessels in the dermis dilate, and heat from the blood is radiated out from the body.

6. **Homeostasis. Homeostasis** is the process of maintaining the balance, equilibrium, and stability of all body systems and their functions. Thermoregulation, as described before, is one aspect of the larger picture of homeostasis. The integumentary system provides a window into the inner workings of different body systems to help maintain homeostasis. When facial, axillary, and pubic hair fail to appear during adolescence, this indicates hormone failure from the endocrine system. A yellowish discoloration of the skin indicates liver disease. When the nails and the skin around the mouth take on a bluish-purple color, this indicates that the entire body needs more oxygen.

Pronunciation/Word Parts

thermoregulation
(THER-moh-REH-gyoo-LAY-shun)
   therm/o- heat
   regulat/o- control
   -ion action; condition

homeostasis (HOH-mee-oh-STAY-sihs)
   home/o- same
   -stasis standing still; staying in one place

Clinical Connection

Forensic Science. When a person drowns or suffocates, there is a high level of carbon dioxide (CO_2) in the blood, and the skin shows the bluish color of cyanosis. However, when a person dies in a fire or from inhaling the fumes from car exhaust or a faulty space heater, there is a high level of carbon monoxide (CO) in the blood. Carbon monoxide poisoning causes a characteristic cherry-red skin color.

2.2 PRACTICE LAPS

Use the Answer Key at the end of the book to check your answers.

A. Give the Meaning of Combining Forms

Next to each combining form, write its meaning. The first one has been done for you.

Combining Form	Meaning	Combining Form	Meaning
1. **protect/o-**	*defend; protect*	5. regulat/o-	
2. derm/a-		6. sens/o-	
3. home/o-		7. therm/o-	
4. nosocomi/o-			

continued on next page

B. Build Words

Read the definition of the medical word. Look at the combining form that is given. Select the correct suffix from the Suffix List, and write it on the blank line. Then build the medical word, and write it on the line. (Remember: You may need to remove the combining vowel. Always remove the hyphens and slash.) Be sure to check your spelling. The first one has been done for you.

Suffix List

-al (pertaining to)
-ation (being; having; process)
-ion (action; condition)

-stasis (standing still; staying in one place)
-tome (area with distinct edges; instrument used to cut)

Definition of the Medical Word	Combining Form	Suffix	Build the Medical Word
Example: Action (to) defend (or) protect	**protect/o-**	*-ion*	*protection*

[*You think* action *(-ion)* + defend; protect *(protect/o-).* You change the order of the word parts to put the suffix last. *You write* protection.]

1. Pertaining to (a) hospital	nosocomi/o-	_____	_____
2. Process (of) having feeling	sens/o-	_____	_____
3. Area (on the skin) with distinct edges	derm/a-	_____	_____
4. (Body functions are) staying in one place (and remaining the) same	home/o-	_____	_____

Vocabulary Review

Word or Phrase	Description	Combining Forms
Overview		
integumentary system	The structures of the integumentary system consist of the skin (and its structures and glands), the nails, and the subcutaneous tissue. This body system covers most of the surface of the body and is the body's first line of defense against injury and infection. Functions of the integumentary system include protection, repair, sensation, vitamin D synthesis, thermoregulation, and homeostasis.	**integument/o-** *skin*
Anatomy of the Integumentary System		
adipose tissue	Fatty tissue that is part of the subcutaneous tissue. It contains lipocytes that store fat as an energy reserve.	**adip/o-** *fat*
collagen	Firm, white protein fibers in the dermis	**coll/a-** *fibers that hold together*
cutaneous	Pertaining to the skin	**cutane/o-** *skin*
cuticle	Layer of dead cells that lie along the proximal edge of the nail. The cuticle keeps microorganisms from entering the deeper tissues.	**cut/i-** *skin*

Word or Phrase	Description	Combining Forms
dermis	Layer of skin beneath the epidermis. It contains collagen and elastin fibers. It also contains arteries, veins, and nerves, as well as sebaceous glands, sudoriferous glands, and hair follicles.	**derm/o-** *skin*
diaphoresis	The process of sweating. The sweat itself is **perspiration**. Sweat is secreted by the sudoriferous glands. Bacteria on the skin that digest sweat produce its characteristic odor.	**phor/o-** *bear; carry; range* **spir/o-** *breathe; coil*
elastin	Yellow elastic fibers in the dermis	**elast/o-** *flexing; stretching*
epidermis	Thin, outermost layer of the skin. The most superficial part or **squamous layer** of the epidermis consists of dead cells filled with keratin. The deepest part or **basal layer** contains constantly dividing cells that are moving toward the surface.	**derm/o-** *skin* **squam/o-** *scale-like cell* **bas/o-** *alkaline; base of a structure*
epithelium	Type of tissue that includes the epidermis, as well as mucous membranes that line internal cavities that connect to the outside of the body. Also known as **epithelial tissue**.	**theli/o-** *cellular layer*
exfoliation	Normal process of the constant shedding of dead cells from the most superficial part of the epidermis	**foli/o-** *leaf*
exocrine gland	Type of gland that secretes substances through a duct. The sebaceous (oil) glands and sudoriferous (sweat) glands in the dermis are both exocrine glands.	**ex/o-** *away from; external; outward*
follicle	Structure in the dermis in which each hair forms	**folli/o-** *sac-like structure* **follicul/o-** *follicle*
hair	Structure that grows as a shaft from a follicle in the dermis. Hair cells are filled with keratin.	**pil/o-** *hair* **trich/o-** *hair*
keratin	Hard, fibrous protein in the outermost cells of the epidermis. Keratin is also in the hair and nails.	**kerat/o-** *cornea; hard, fibrous protein*
lipocyte	Cell in the adipose tissue of the subcutaneous tissue; it stores fat as an energy reserve.	**lip/o-** *fat; lipid*
lunula	Whitish half-moon shape that is the visible part of the nail root	**lun/o-** *moon*
melanin	Dark brown or black pigment that gives color to the skin and hair	**melan/o-** *black*
melanocyte	Pigment cell in the epidermis. Melanocyte-stimulating hormone in the anterior pituitary gland in the brain causes melanocytes to produce melanin.	**melan/o-** *black*
nail bed	Layer of living tissue beneath the nail plate. It contains nerves and blood vessels. Also known as the *quick*.	
nail plate	Hard, translucent protective covering over the distal end of each finger and toe. It is composed of dead cells that contain keratin. Also known as the *nail*.	**onych/o-** *fingernail; toenail* **ungu/o-** *fingernail; toenail*
nail root	Located beneath the skin of the finger or toe. It produces cells that form the lunula and nail plate.	

Word or Phrase	Description	Combining Forms
piloerection	Process in which body hairs become erect when the skin is cold.	**pil/o-** *hair* **erect/o-** *stand up*
sebaceous gland	Exocrine gland in the dermis that secretes **sebum** (oil) through a duct. Sebum coats the hair and moisturizes the skin. Also known as an **oil gland**.	**sebace/o-** *oil; sebum* **seb/o-** *oil; sebum*
skin	The skin is a major part of the integumentary system. The skin consists of two layers—the epidermis and the dermis.	**cutane/o-** *skin* **cut/i-** *skin* **derm/a-** *skin* **dermat/o-** *skin* **derm/o-** *skin* **integument/o-** *skin*
subcutaneous tissue	Tissue layer beneath the dermis. It is composed of connective tissue and adipose tissue.	**cutane/o-** *skin*
sudoriferous gland	Exocrine gland in the dermis. It secretes sweat through a duct that ends at a pore on the surface of the skin. Also known as a **sweat gland**.	**sudor/i-** *sweat* **fer/o-** *bear* **hidr/o-** *sweat*

Physiology of the Integumentary System

Word or Phrase	Description	Combining Forms
dermatome	Area of the skin that sends sensory information through a nerve to the spinal cord	**derm/a-** *skin*
healthcare–associated infection (HAI)	Infection that occurs in hospitals and other healthcare facilities when caregivers do not wash their hands. Previously known as a **nosocomial infection.**	**nosocomi/o-** *hospital*
homeostasis	Balance, equilibrium, and stability of all body systems and functions	**home/o-** *same*
normal skin flora	Bacteria that live on the skin and inhibit the growth of disease-causing microorganisms	
protection	The integumentary system is the body's first line of defense and protection against injury and infection.	**protect/o-** *defend; protect*
sensation	Sensory receptors in the dermis respond to light touch, pressure, vibration, pain, or temperature. The nervous system then relays and interprets skin sensations.	**sens/o-** *feeling*
synthesis	Process of putting together sunlight and the skin to create vitamin D	**synth/o-** *put together*
thermoregulation	Actions of the integumentary system to help control body temperature: the subcutaneous layer conserves body heat, the skin creates heat with goosebumps and piloerection, and the sudoriferous glands secrete sweat to evaporate and cool the body.	**therm/o-** *heat* **regulat/o-** *control*

Abbreviation Review

CO	carbon monoxide		**HAI**	healthcare–associated infection
CO_2	carbon dioxide			

2.3 Diseases

Word or Phrase	Description	Pronunciation/Word Parts

General

| dermatitis | Infection or inflammation of the skin. This can be due to injury to the skin itself or to a disease within the body that manifests itself on the skin. Treatment: Correct the underlying cause. | **dermatitis** (DER-mah-TY-tihs) **dermat/o-** *skin* **-itis** *infection of; inflammation of* |
| edema | Excessive amounts of fluid move from the blood into the dermis or subcutaneous tissue and cause swelling (see Figure 2-5 ■). Local areas of edema on the skin can be caused by inflammation, an allergic reaction, or an infection. Large areas of edema on the skin are associated with diseases of the cardiovascular or urinary systems. Treatment: Correct the underlying cause. | **edema** (eh-DEE-mah) |

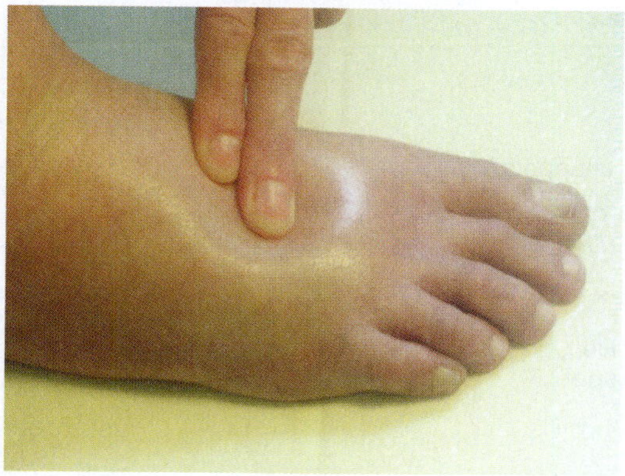

FIGURE 2-5 ■ Skin edema.
Fingertip pressure on an area of severe edema displaces the tissue fluid and produces a deep indentation in the tissue. This is known as *pitting edema.*

| hemorrhage | An injury to the blood vessels releases blood into the skin; this process is known as **extravasation**. • **Petechiae** are pinpoint areas of blood caused by small ruptured blood vessels. • **Contusion** is a hemorrhage of a larger amount of blood into the skin. An **ecchymosis** is a hemorrhage that is 3 cm in diameter or larger. A contusion or an ecchymosis is commonly known as a **bruise**. • **Hematoma** is an elevated, localized collection of blood under the skin. Treatment: None, except in cases of extensive skin trauma with hemorrhaging. | **hemorrhage** (HEM-oh-rij) **hem/o-** *blood* **-rrhage** *excessive discharge; excessive flow* **extravasation** (eks-TRAV-ah-SAY-shun) **extra-** *outside* **vas/o-** *blood vessel; vas deferens* **-ation** *being; having; process* **petechiae** (peh-TEE-kee-ee) **contusion** (con-TOO-shun) **contus/o-** *bruising* **-ion** *action; condition* **ecchymosis** (EK-ih-MOH-sihs) **ecchym/o-** *blood in the tissue* **-osis** *abnormal condition; process* **ecchymoses** (EK-ih-MOH-seez) Greek plural noun: Change the singular ending *-is* to *-es*. **hematoma** (HEE-mah-TOH-mah) **hemat/o-** *blood* **-oma** *mass; tumor* |

Word or Phrase	Description	Pronunciation/Word Parts
lesion	Any visible damage or variation from normal skin, whether from disease or injury (see Figure 2-6 ■). Treatment: Correct the underlying cause.	**lesion** (LEE-shun)

LESION	DESCRIPTION	COLOR	CONTENTS	EXAMPLE
Cyst	Elevated circular mound	Skin color or erythema	Semisolid or partly fluid filled	Acne sebaceous cyst
Fissure	Small, cracklike crevice	Erythema	None; some fluid exudate	Dry, chapped skin
Macule	Flat circle	Pigmented brown or black	None	Freckle, age spot
Papule	Elevated	Skin color or erythema	Solid	Acne pimple
Pustule	Elevated	White top	Pus	Acne whitehead
Scale	Flat to slightly elevated, thin flake	White	None	Dandruff, psoriasis
Vesicle	Elevated with pointed top	Erythema with a transparent top	Clear fluid	Herpes, chickenpox, shingles
Wheal	Elevated with broad, flat top	Erythema with a pale top	Clear fluid	Insect bites, urticaria

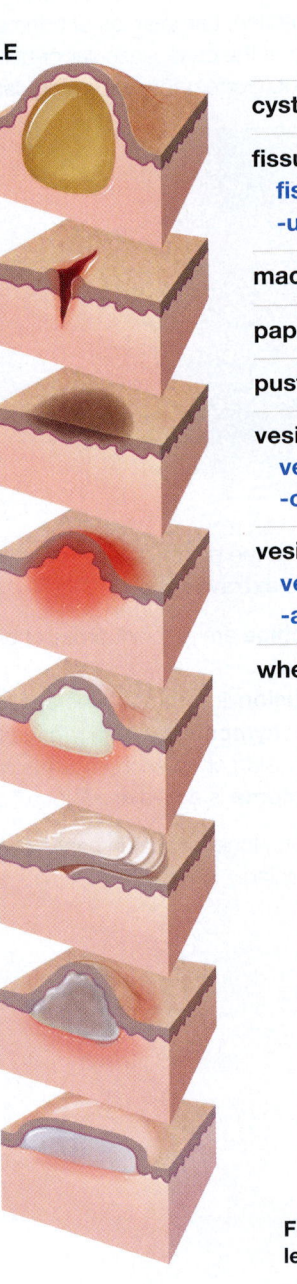

cyst (SIST)

fissure (FIH-shur)
  fiss/o- *splitting*
  -ure *result of; system*

macule (MAK-yool)

papule (PAP-yool)

pustule (PUS-tyool)

vesicle (VES-ih-kul)
  vesic/o- *bladder; fluid-filled sac*
  -cle *small thing*

vesicular (veh-SIH-kyoo-lar)
  vesicul/o- *fluid-filled sac*
  -ar *pertaining to*

wheal (HWEEL)

FIGURE 2-6 ■ Types of skin lesions.

Word or Phrase	Description	Pronunciation/Word Parts

neoplasm	Any new growth that occurs on the skin. A neoplasm can be **benign** (not cancerous) or **malignant** (cancerous). *Note:* Malignant neoplasms are described later in the chapter.
	Treatment: Excision of a benign neoplasm, if necessary
		neoplasm (NEE-oh-plazm)
		  ne/o- *new*
		  -plasm *formed substance; growth*
		
		benign (bee-NINE)
		
		malignant (mah-LIG-nant)
		  malign/o- *cancer*
		  -ant *pertaining to*

pruritus	Pruritus is caused by the release of histamine as part of an allergic reaction of the skin. Also known as *itching*.
	Treatment: Topical or oral antihistamine drug or corticosteroid drug
		pruritus (proo-RY-tuhs)
		
		pruritic (proo-RIH-tik)
		  prurit/o- *itching*
		  -ic *pertaining to*

rash	Any type of skin lesion that is pink to red, flat or raised, itchy or not itchy. Certain diseases (chickenpox, measles) have characteristic rashes. Treatment: Topical or oral antihistamine drug or corticosteroid drug	

xeroderma	Excessive dryness of the skin. It is caused by aging, cold weather with low humidity, vitamin A deficiency, or dehydration.
	Treatment: Correct the underlying cause.
		xeroderma (ZEER-oh-DER-mah)
		  xer/o- *dry*
		  -derma *skin*

Skin Color Conditions

albinism	Genetic mutation that causes a lack of pigment in the skin, hair, and iris of the eye. There is a normal number of melanocytes, but they produce insufficient or no melanin.
	Treatment: None
		albinism (AL-by-NIZ-em)
		  albin/o- *white*
		  -ism *disease from a specific cause; process*

cyanosis	Bluish-purple discoloration of the skin and nails due to a decreased level of oxygen in the blood (see Figure 2-7 ■). It is caused by cardiac or respiratory disease. The patient is said to be **cyanotic**. In healthy persons, areas of skin exposed to the cold can temporarily exhibit cyanosis.
	Treatment: Correct the underlying cause.
		cyanosis (SY-ah-NOH-sihs)
		  cyan/o- *blue*
		  -osis *abnormal condition; process*
		
		cyanotic (SY-ah-NAW-tik)
		  cyan/o- *blue*
		  -tic *pertaining to*

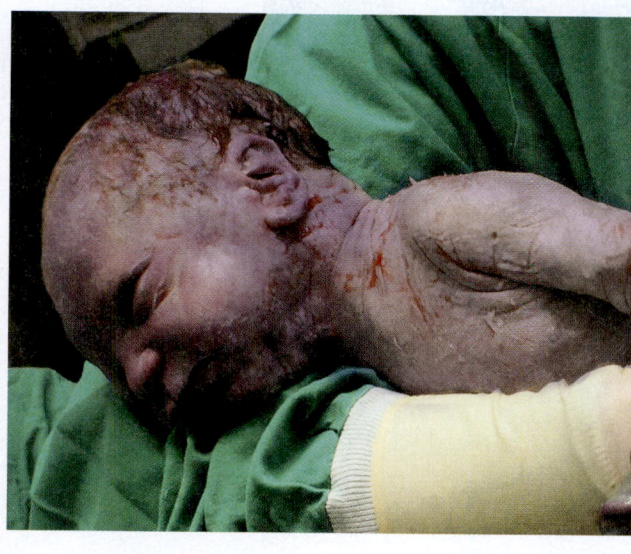

FIGURE 2-7 ■ Cyanosis.
This newborn baby shows cyanosis of the head and face. This is a normal finding at birth. The cyanosis gradually disappears as the newborn breathes and cries.

Word or Phrase	Description	Pronunciation/Word Parts
erythema	Reddish discoloration of the skin. It can be confined to a local area of infection or inflammation, or it can affect large areas of the skin, as in sunburn. The area is said to be **erythematous**. Treatment: Correct the underlying cause.	**erythema** (AIR-ih-THEE-mah) **erythematous** (AIR-ih-THEM-eh-tuhs) 　**erythemat/o-** *redness* 　**-ous** *pertaining to*
jaundice	Yellowish discoloration of the skin and mucous membranes, as well as the whites of the eyes (see Figure 3-22 in Chapter 3). It is associated with liver disease. The patient's diseased liver cannot process (conjugate) bilirubin, and so unconjugated bilirubin in the blood moves into the tissues and colors the skin yellow. The patient is said to be *jaundiced*. A patient without any sign of jaundice is said to be **anicteric**. *Note: Icterus* is an older word for jaundice. Treatment: Correct the underlying cause.	**jaundice** (JAWN-dihs) 　**jaund/o-** *yellow* 　**-ice** *quality; state* **anicteric** (AN-ik-TAIR-ik) 　**an-** *not; without* 　**icter/o-** *jaundice* 　**-ic** *pertaining to*
necrosis	Gray-to-black discoloration of the skin in areas where the tissue has died (see Figure 2-8 ■). **Necrotic** tissue can develop in a burn, pressure injury, wound, or any tissue with a poor blood supply. Necrosis with subsequent bacterial invasion and infection is **gangrene**, and the area is said to be **gangrenous**. Treatment: Removal of the necrotic tissue or body part	**necrosis** (neh-KROH-sihs) 　**necr/o-** *dead body; dead tissue* 　**-osis** *abnormal condition; process* **necrotic** (neh-KRAW-tik) 　**necr/o-** *dead body; dead tissue* 　**-tic** *pertaining to* **gangrene** (GANG-green) **gangrenous** (GANG-greh-nuhs) 　**gangren/o-** *gangrene* 　**-ous** *pertaining to*

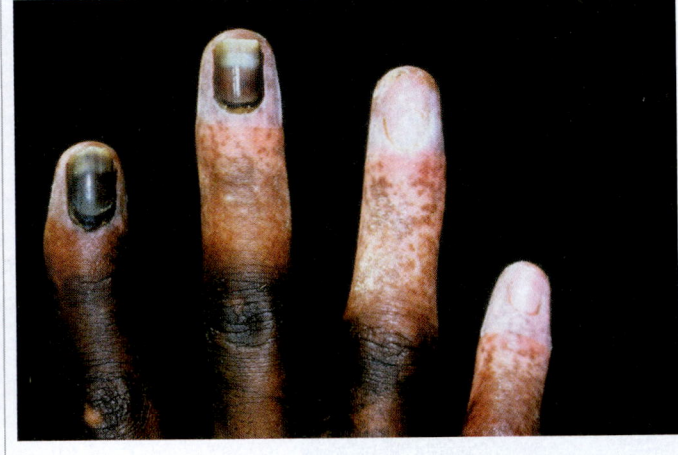

FIGURE 2-8 ■ Necrosis.
This patient's right hand shows necrosis of the skin due to severe frostbite. The index and middle fingers may need to be amputated. The third and fourth fingers show pallor (paleness), indicating poor blood flow, which may eventually progress to tissue death and necrosis.

Word or Phrase	Description	Pronunciation/Word Parts
vitiligo	Autoimmune disorder in which melanocytes are slowly destroyed. There are white patches of **depigmentation** interspersed with areas of normally pigmented skin (see Figure 2-9 ■). Treatment: Ultraviolet phototherapy or an oral repigmentation drug	**vitiligo** (VIT-ih-LY-goh) **depigmentation** (dee-PIG-men-TAY-shun) **de-** *reversal of; without* **pigment/o-** *pigment* **-ation** *being; having; process*

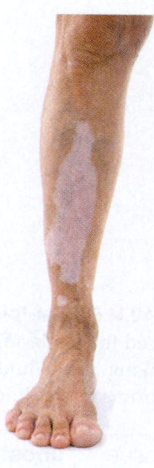 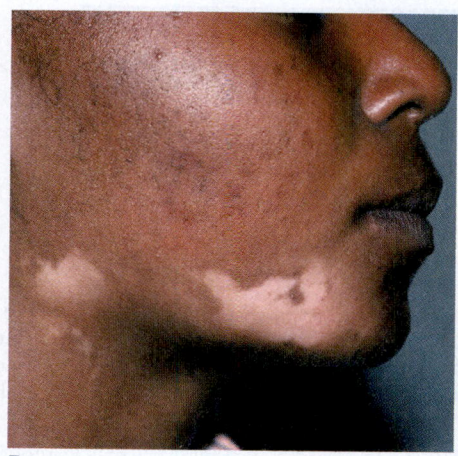

A.   B.

FIGURE 2-9 ■ Vitiligo.
A. This patient has an area of depigmentation on the right leg, due to vitiligo. **B.** Vitiligo occurs as irregular, ever-expanding areas because it is a progressive autoimmune disorder.

Clinical Connections

Obstetrics. Melanocyte-stimulating hormone (from the anterior pituitary gland in the brain) can become overactive during pregnancy, causing melanocytes to produce too much melanin. This results in dark, hyperpigmented areas on the face (**chloasma** or the "mask of pregnancy") and/or a vertical dark line on the skin of the abdomen from the umbilicus downward (**linea nigra**).

chloasma (kloh-AZ-mah)

linea nigra (LIN-ee-ah NY-grah)

Skin Injuries

abrasion	A sliding or scraping injury that mechanically removes the epidermis. Also known as a **brush burn**. Treatment: Apply a protective covering until it is healed.	**abrasion** (ah-BRAY-shun) **abras/o-** *scrape off* **-ion** *action; condition*
blister	Fluid-filled sac with a thin, transparent covering of epidermal cells. It occurs when a repetitive rubbing injury separates the epidermis from the dermis, releasing tissue fluid and creating a fluid-filled sac. Blisters often form on the heel from walking in poorly fitting shoes or on the hand from constant rubbing against an object such as a tool. Treatment: Apply a protective covering before the activity.	**blister** (BLIS-ter)
burns	Heat (fire, hot objects, steam, boiling water), electrical current (lightning, electrical outlets or cords), chemicals, and radiation or x-rays (sunshine or prescribed radiation therapy) can create a burn of the epidermis or dermis.	
superficial burn	Involves only the epidermis. There is erythema, pain, and swelling, but not blisters. Also known as a **first-degree burn**. Treatment: Topical anti-infective drug to prevent infection	

Word or Phrase	Description	Pronunciation/Word Parts
partial-thickness burn	Involves the epidermis and the upper part of the dermis. There is erythema, pain, and swelling, but also a blister or a larger **bulla** that forms as the epidermis detaches from the dermis and the space between fills with tissue fluid (see Figure 2-10 ■). Also known as a **second-degree burn**. Treatment: Second-degree burns that cover a large area require debridement and skin grafting.	**bulla** (BUL-ah) **bullae** (BUL-ee) Latin plural noun: Change the singular ending -a to -ae.

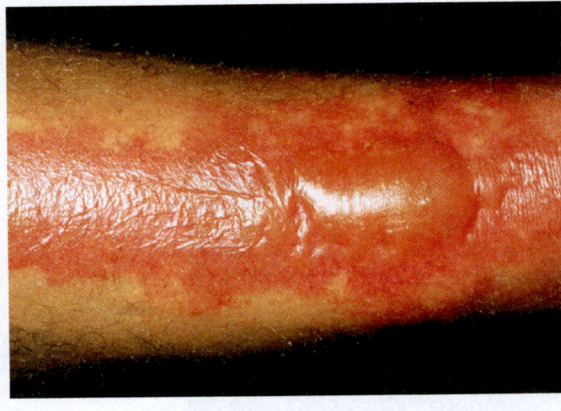

FIGURE 2-10 ■ Partial-thickness burn of the leg.
A burn caused the epidermis to separate from the dermis. Leaking tissue fluid caused the epidermis to swell and form a large, fluid-filled bulla.

Word or Phrase	Description	Pronunciation/Word Parts
full-thickness burn	Involves the epidermis, dermis, and sometimes the subcutaneous tissue and muscle layer beneath it. If nerves in the dermis are destroyed, there is local **anesthesia** with loss of sensation of pain. Also known as a **third-degree burn**. **Eschar** is a thick scar of necrotic tissue that forms on a full-thickness burn. Eschar must be removed because it traps fluid, delays healing, and can become infected. Treatment: Third-degree burns require debridement and skin grafting.	**anesthesia** (AN-es-THEE-zha) **an-** not; without **esthes/o-** feeling; sensation **-ia** condition; state; thing **eschar** (ES-kar)
callus	Repetitive rubbing injury that causes the epidermis to gradually thicken into a wide, elevated pad. A **corn** is a callus with a hard central area with a pointed tip that causes pain. Treatment: Removal	**callus** (KAL-uhs)
cicatrix	Fibrous tissue composed of collagen; it forms as an injury heals. Also known as a **scar**.	**cicatrix** (SIK-ah-triks)
excoriation	Superficial injury with a sharp object (such as a fingernail, animal claw, or thorn) that creates a linear **scratch** on the skin. Treatment: Topical antibiotic drug to prevent infection	**excoriation** (eks-KOR-ee-AA-shun) **excori/o-** take out skin **-ation** being; having; process
keloid	A very firm, abnormally large scar. It grows larger than the original injury because of an overproduction of collagen as the injury heals (see Figure 2-11 ■). Unlike a scar, a keloid does not decrease in size over time. Treatment: Surgical removal, although a keloid often grows back	**keloid** (KEE-loyd) **kel/o-** tumor **-oid** resembling

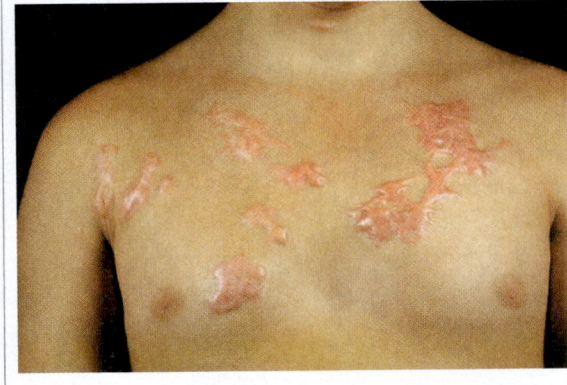

FIGURE 2-11 ■ Keloid.
A keloid is a scar that continues to grow until it is larger than the original injury. Depending on its location and size, a keloid can be cosmetically unacceptable.

Word or Phrase	Description	Pronunciation/Word Parts
laceration	Linear penetrating wound. It can have clean-cut or torn, ragged skin edges (see Figure 2-12 ■). Treatment: Close with sutures, or use surgical glue for a small laceration. 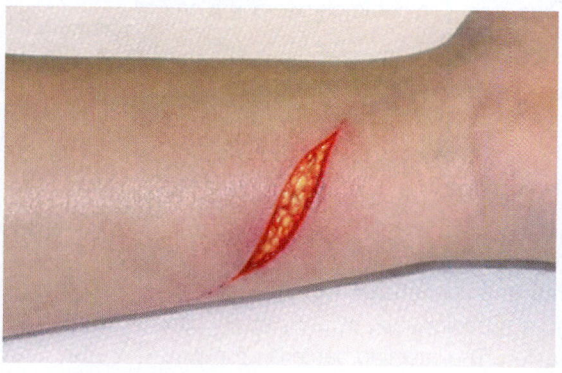 **FIGURE 2-12 ■ Laceration.** This deep laceration of the forearm was caused by a piece of glass that penetrated through the epidermis and dermis to expose the adipose tissue in the subcutaneous layer.	**laceration** (LAS-er-AA-shun) **lacer/o-** *tearing* **-ation** *being; having; process*
pressure injury	Epidermis and dermis break down, resulting in a shallow or deep ulcer (see Figure 2-13 ■). This occurs because constant pressure on the skin decreases blood flow to that area. Also known as a **pressure ulcer**, **bedsore**, or **decubitus ulcer**. Treatment: Frequent repositioning; increased protein intake to rebuild tissue; and debridement of any necrotic tissue to promote healing 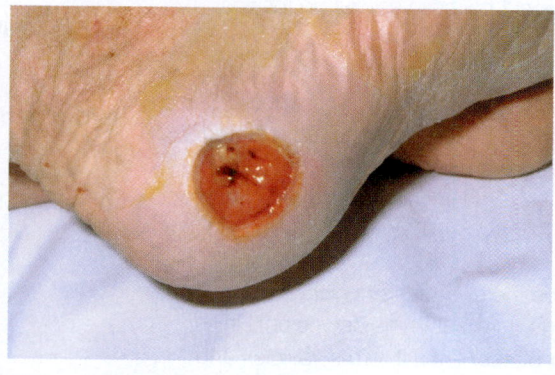 **FIGURE 2-13 ■ Pressure injury.** This pressure injury was caused by continuous pressure on the heel when the patient remained lying on his back for a prolonged period of time.	**decubitus** (dee-KYOO-bih-tuhs) **ulcer** (UL-ser) *Decubitus* is a Latin word meaning *lying down*.

Across the Life Span

Geriatrics. Pressure injuries are common in patients in nursing homes. They often occur at pressure points overlying bony prominences such as the hip, sacrum, or heel. Confinement to bed or a wheelchair, decreased fat in the subcutaneous tissue, poor nutrition, uncontrolled diabetes mellitus, or circulatory problems predispose older patients to developing pressure injuries. Frequent repositioning and keeping the skin dry helps prevent pressure injuries. A normal level of protein (albumin) in the blood indicates that the patient can build tissues and heal an existing pressure injury. A low level of albumin is treated nutritionally by offering the patient high-protein snacks.

Obstetrics. Stretch marks (**striae**) in the skin of the abdomen and buttocks are the result of small tears in the dermis as the skin stretches to accommodate the pregnant uterus. These are irregular, reddened lines that later become lighter and shiny as they heal as scar tissue.

striae (STRY-ee)

Word or Phrase	Description	Pronunciation/Word Parts

Skin Infections

abscess	Localized, pus-containing pocket under the skin from a bacterial infection. It is usually caused by *Staphylococcus aureus*, a common bacterium on the skin. • **Furuncle.** Localized, elevated abscess around a hair follicle. Also known as a **boil**. • **Carbuncle.** Several furuncles connected by channels through the subcutaneous tissue or to the skin surface. Treatment: Incision and drainage of the pus; antibiotic drug	**abscess** (AB-sehs) **furuncle** (FYOOR-ung-kul) **carbuncle** (KAR-bung-kul)

cellulitis	Infection and inflammation that spreads through the skin, subcutaneous tissue, and muscle. It develops from a superficial cut, scratch, insect bite, blister, or splinter that becomes infected. The infecting bacteria produce enzymes that allow the infection to spread between the tissue layers. There is erythema (often as a red streak), warmth, and pain.
	Treatment: Antibiotic drug
		cellulitis (SEL-yoo-LY-tihs)
		  cellul/o- *cell*
		  -itis *infection of; inflammation of*

herpes	Infection caused by the herpes virus. There are clusters of vesicles, erythema, edema, and pain. The vesicles rupture, releasing clear fluid that forms crusts. • **Herpes simplex virus (HSV) type 1** causes vesicles on the lips. These tend to recur during illness and stress. Also known as **cold sores** or **fever blisters**. • **Herpes simplex virus (HSV) type 2** is a sexually transmitted disease that causes vesicles in the genital area. These tend to recur during illness and stress. Also known as **genital herpes**. • **Herpes whitlow** is infection at the distal fingernail because of contact with either herpes simplex type 1 or type 2. The virus enters through a small tear in the cuticle. • **Herpes varicella-zoster** causes the skin rash of chickenpox during childhood. The virus then remains dormant in the nerves until it is activated in later life by illness or stress. Then it forms vesicles and crusts along a dermatome and is very painful. Also known as **shingles** (see Figure 2-14 ■). Treatment: Topical or oral antiviral drug	**herpes** (HER-peez) **herpes simplex** (HER-peez SIM-pleks) **herpes whitlow** (HER-peez WHIT-loh) **herpes varicella-zoster** (HER-peez VAIR-ih-SEH-lah ZAW-ster) **shingles** (SHING-gulz)

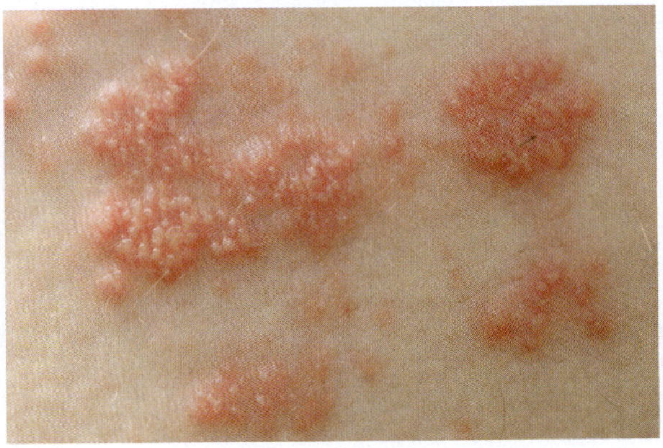

FIGURE 2-14 ■ Shingles.
The vesicles and crusts of shingles. The lesions occur along a dermatome (an area of skin associated with a specific spinal nerve that goes to the spinal cord).

Word or Phrase	Description	Pronunciation/Word Parts
tinea	Skin infection caused by a fungus that feeds on epidermal cells. There is severe itching and burning with red, scaly lesions. Because some lesions are round, it was thought to be caused by a worm, and so it was (and still is) called **ringworm**. Tinea is named according to where it occurs on the body. • **Tinea capitis** occurs on the scalp and causes hair loss (see Figure 2-15 ■). • **Tinea corporis** occurs on the trunk and extremities. • **Tinea cruris** occurs in the groin and genital areas. Also known as **jock itch**. • **Tinea pedis** occurs on the feet. Also known as **athlete's foot**. Treatment: Topical antifungal drug 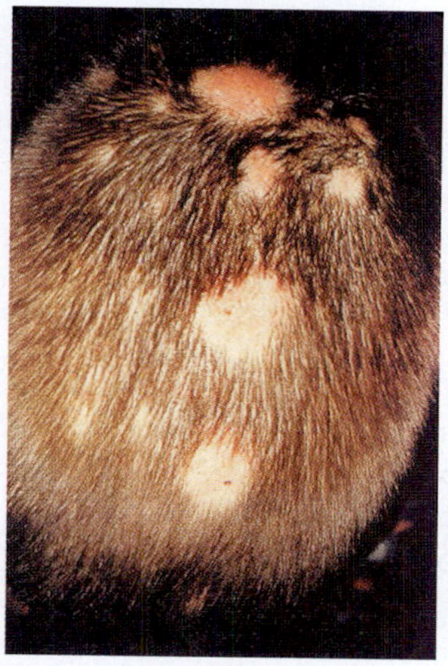 **FIGURE 2-15 ■ Tinea capitis.** This fungal infection, known as *ringworm*, occurs on the scalp and causes itching and hair loss. Because the skin lesions are often round, it was thought to be caused by a worm.	**tinea** (TIN-ee-ah) Originally, it was thought to be caused by an insect (*tinea* in Latin). **capitis** (KAP-ih-tihs) Latin word meaning *of the head*. **corporis** (KOR-por-ihs) Latin word meaning *of the body*. **cruris** (KROOR-ihs) Latin word meaning *of the leg*. **pedis** (PEE-dihs) Latin word meaning *of the foot*.
verruca	Irregular, rough skin lesion caused by the human papillomavirus. It usually occurs on the hands, fingers, or the soles of the feet (plantar wart). Also known as a **wart**. Treatment: Topical drug to break down the wart; cryosurgery or electro-surgery to destroy the wart	**verruca** (veh-ROO-kah)

Skin Infestations

pediculosis	Infestation of parasitic lice and their eggs (nits) in the scalp, hair, eyelashes, or genital hair. Lice are easily transmitted from one person to another by combs or hats.
	Treatment: Shampoo and skin lotion to kill lice
		pediculosis
		(peh-DIH-kyoo-LOH-sihs)
		  pedicul/o- *lice*
		  -osis *abnormal condition; process*

scabies	Infestation of parasitic mites that tunnel under the skin and produce vesicles that are itchy. Treatment: Shampoo and skin lotion to kill mites	**scabies** (SKAY-beez)

Word or Phrase	Description	Pronunciation/Word Parts

Allergic Skin Conditions

contact dermatitis	Local reaction from contact with a substance that is an allergen or irritant. Examples: Chemicals (deodorant, soap, detergent, makeup, urine), metals, synthetic products (latex gloves, Spandex bathing suit or girdle), plants (poison ivy), or animals (see Figure 2-16 ■). The skin becomes inflamed and irritated. Treatment: Topical or oral antihistamine drug or corticosteroid drug	**dermatitis** (DER-mah-TY-tihs) **dermat/o-** *skin* **-itis** *infection of; inflammation of*

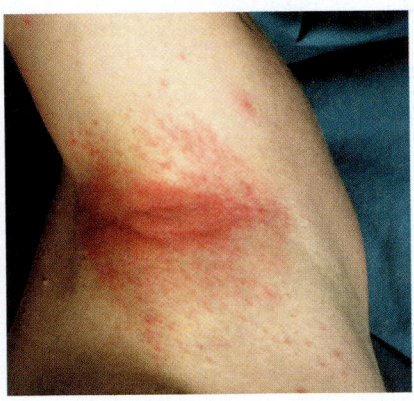

FIGURE 2-16 ■ Severe contact dermatitis. This skin reaction was caused by the application of a new deodorant containing chemical ingredients that caused irritation.

urticaria	Local allergic reaction due to food, plants, animals, insect bites, or drugs. There are raised areas of redness and edema that appear suddenly. Itching causes the areas to enlarge. Also known as **hives**. Each individual area is known as a **wheal**. A large wheal is a **welt**. Treatment: Topical or oral antihistamine drug or corticosteroid drug	**urticaria** (ER-tih-KAIR-ee-ah) **wheal** (HWEEL)

Clinical Connections

Occupational Health. According to the Occupational Safety and Health Administration (OSHA), 8 to 12 percent of healthcare workers are sensitive or allergic to latex. This occurs because of constant exposure to latex medical products, particularly the gloves used in medical examinations and surgeries. This allergy causes skin rashes, hives, itching, and asthma. Nonlatex gloves can be used instead to protect workers while still preventing the spread of infection.

Benign Neoplasms of the Skin

actinic keratosis	**Benign** (not cancerous) **neoplasm**. This raised, irregular, rough area of skin is dry and feels like sandpaper. It develops in middle-aged persons in areas exposed to the sun. The area can become cancerous. Also known as **solar keratosis**. Treatment: Avoid sun exposure.	**actinic** (ak-TIN-ik) **actin/o-** *rays of the sun* **-ic** *pertaining to* **keratosis** (KAIR-ah-TOH-sihs) **kerat/o-** *cornea; hard, fibrous protein* **-osis** *abnormal condition; process* **benign** (bee-NINE) **neoplasm** (NEE-oh-plasm) **ne/o-** *new* **-plasm** *formed substance; growth* **solar** (SOH-lar) **sol/o-** *sun* **-ar** *pertaining to*

Word or Phrase	Description	Pronunciation/Word Parts
hemangioma	Benign mass of superficial, dilated blood vessels that is present at birth (see Figure 2-17 ■). Most disappear without treatment by age 3. **FIGURE 2-17 ■ Hemangioma.** The bright red color of this skin lesion is because of the large number of dilated blood vessels it contains.	**hemangioma** (hee-MAN-jee-OH-mah) **hem/o-** *blood* **angi/o-** *blood vessel; lymphatic vessel* **-oma** *mass; tumor*
lipoma	Benign growth of adipose tissue in the subcutaneous layer. It makes a soft, rounded, fatty elevation in the skin. Treatment: Removal, if desired	**lipoma** (ly-POH-mah) **lip/o-** *fat; lipid* **-oma** *mass; tumor*
nevus	Benign skin lesion that is present at birth and has a variety of colors and shapes (see Figure 2-18 ■). • **Mole.** A raised and round nevus. • **Port-wine stain.** A flat, red-to-purple, and irregularly shaped nevus. It can be over a large area, often on the head and neck. Also known as a **birthmark**. Treatment: Excision of a mole if clothing irritates it; laser treatment to remove a port-wine stain nevus A. B. **FIGURE 2-18 ■ Nevus.** A. This mole is a pigmented nevus that has a round top. Other moles are flatter, darker in color, and can contain a hair. B. The shape and color of a port-wine stain nevus resembles a puddle of spilled red wine.	**nevus** (NEE-vuhs)
papilloma	Soft, flesh-colored growth that protrudes outwardly from the skin as a flap or a polyp on a stalk. Also known as a **skin tag**. Treatment: Removal by cryotherapy, electrocautery, or surgical excision, if desired	**papilloma** (PAP-ih-LOH-mah) **papill/o-** *elevated structure* **-oma** *mass; tumor*

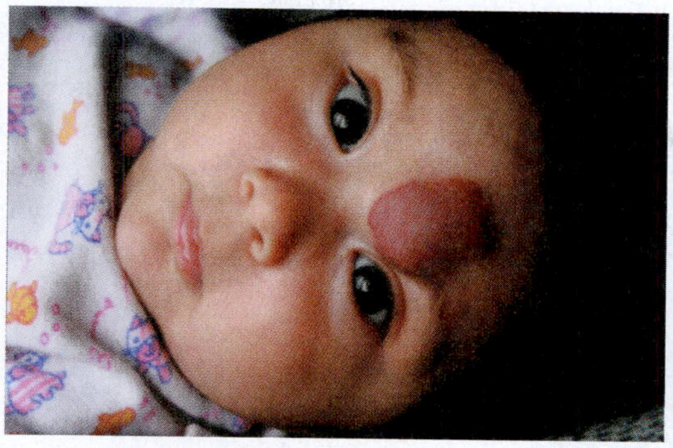

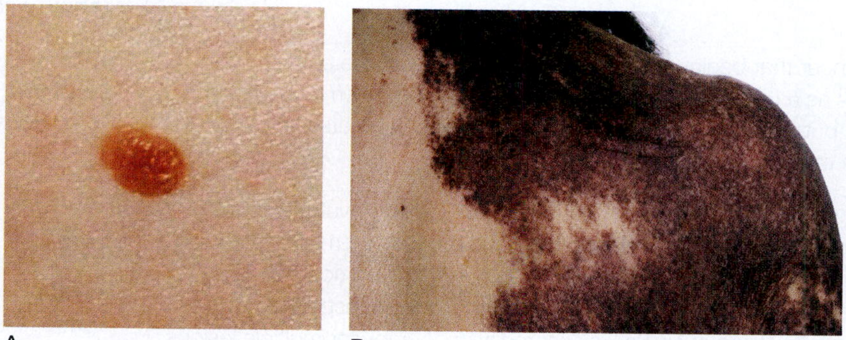

Across the Life Span

Geriatrics. Senile lentigo are light-to-dark brown, flat macules on the hands and face of older adults; they occur in areas chronically exposed to the sun. Also known as *liver spots* or *age spots*.

Treatment: None

senile (SEE-nile)
sen/o- *old age*
-ile *pertaining to*

lentigo (len-TY-goh)

Word or Phrase	Description	Pronunciation/Word Parts
syndactyly	Congenital abnormality in which the skin and soft tissues are joined between the fingers or toes (see Figure 2-19 ■). In some cases, the nails are also joined. **Polydactyly** is a congenital abnormality in which there are extra fingers or toes. Treatment: Surgical correction, if desired	**syndactyly** (sin-DAK-tih-lee) The prefix **syn-** means *together.* Syndactyly: *Condition of the fingers or toes (being) together* **polydactyly** (PAW-lee-DAK-tih-lee) The prefix **poly-** means *many; much.* Polydactyly: *Condition of the fingers or toes (with) many (more than normal)*

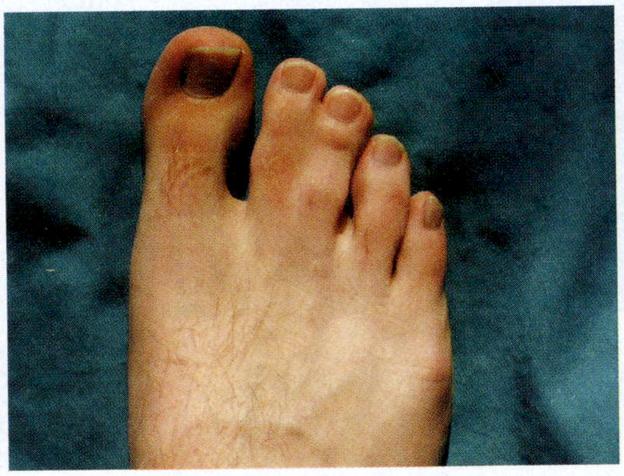

FIGURE 2-19 ■ Syndactyly.
The skin and soft tissues of the second and third toes are fused together in this patient with syndactyly.

Malignant Neoplasms of the Skin

cancer of the skin	A **cancerous** lesion or **malignancy** in areas of the skin that are chronically exposed to ultraviolet light radiation from the sun. Skin cancer is more common in older adults (because of a lifetime of sun exposure) and in fair-skinned persons (because there is less melanin to absorb radiation).
	Treatment: Mohs surgery to remove the cancer; chemotherapy drugs; photodynamic therapy
		cancer (KAN-ser)
		
		cancerous (KAN-ser-uhs)
		  cancer/o- *cancer*
		  -ous *pertaining to*
		
		malignancy (mah-LIG-nan-see)
		  malign/o- *cancer*
		  -ancy *state*

basal cell carcinoma	Skin cancer that begins in the basal (bottom) layer of the epidermis. It appears as a raised, pearly bump. It is the most common type of skin cancer, but it is a slow-growing cancer that does not metastasize to other parts of the body.	**carcinoma** (KAR-sih-NOH-mah)
		  carcin/o- *cancer*
		  -oma *mass; tumor*

Kaposi sarcoma	Cancer of the skin and subcutaneous tissue. It is an elevated, irregular, dark reddish-blue tumor. It also involves the mucous membranes and internal organs. This previously rare cancer is now commonly seen in patients with AIDS because of their impaired immune response.
	Treatment: Excision of single lesions; radiation therapy for multiple lesions
		Kaposi (kah-POH-see)
		
		sarcoma (sar-KOH-mah)
		  sarc/o- *connective tissue*
		  -oma *mass; tumor*

malignant melanoma	Skin cancer of the melanocytes in the epidermis (see Figure 2-20 ■). It grows quickly and can spread (metastasize) to other parts of the body (see the Clinical Connections box on the next page).	**malignant** (mah-LIG-nant)
		  malign/o- *cancer*
		  -ant *pertaining to*
		
		melanoma (MEL-ah-NOH-mah)
		  melan/o- *black*
		  -oma *mass; tumor*
		Melanoma: *Tumor (whose color varies from brown to) black*

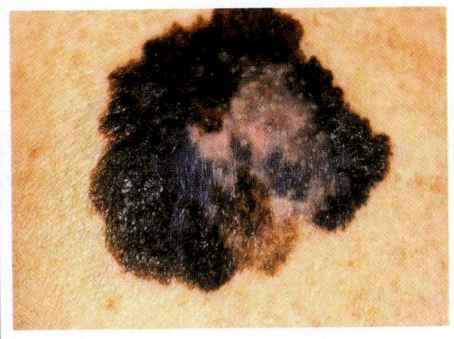

FIGURE 2-20 ■ Malignant melanoma.
This lesion reveals four of the five typical characteristics of a malignant melanoma: asymmetry, irregular edges, varying shades of color, and a size greater than ¼ inch. The fifth characteristic—an increase in size (evolving)— would be seen over time.

Word or Phrase	Description	Pronunciation/Word Parts

Clinical Connections

Oncology. Depletion of the earth's ozone layer has led to many cases of malignant melanoma. Using sunscreen and avoiding prolonged sun exposure, particularly during midday, helps to decrease this risk. Self-examination of the skin should be done frequently. Irregular or changing skin lesions should be examined by a dermatologist. The American Cancer Society suggests using the **ABCDE** rule to identify the warning signs of malignant melanoma.

Asymmetry: One side has a different shape than the other side.
Border: Irregular or ragged.
Color: Varies from black to brown with patches of pink, red, or white within the same lesion.
Diameter: Greater than 6 mm (¼ inch).
Evolving: Changing in size, shape, or color over time.

Word or Phrase	Description	Pronunciation/Word Parts
squamous cell carcinoma	Skin cancer that begins in the superficial (squamous cell) layer of the epidermis. It appears as a red bump or an ulcer. It often develops from an actinic keratosis. It is the second most common type of skin cancer, but it grows slowly.	**squamous** (SKWAY-muhs) **squam/o-** scale-like cell **-ous** pertaining to

Autoimmune Disorders of the Skin

Word or Phrase	Description	Pronunciation/Word Parts
psoriasis	Autoimmune disorder that produces an excessive number of abnormal epidermal cells. The skin is itchy, red, and covered with silvery scales and plaques on the scalp, elbows, hands, and knees (see Figure 2-21 ■). Illness and stress can cause a flareup, and psoriasis has a hereditary component. Treatment: Topical coal tar drug, vitamin A drug, vitamin D drug, and corticosteroid drug; light therapy with a psoralen drug and ultraviolet light A (PUVA) or ultraviolet light B (UVB)	**psoriasis** (sor-EYE-ah-sihs) **psor/o-** itching **-iasis** abnormal condition; process

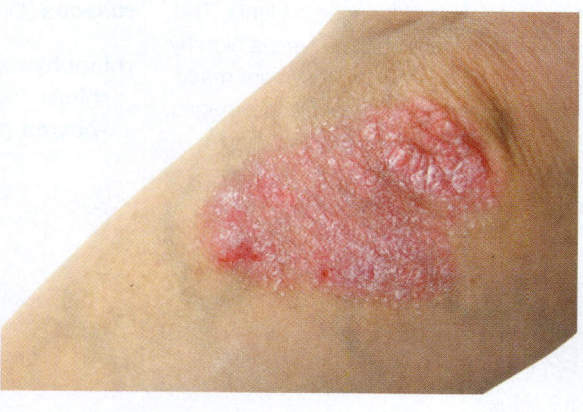

FIGURE 2-21 ■ Psoriasis.
Psoriasis produces characteristic elevated, erythematous lesions that are topped by silvery scales and plaques. The elbows and the knees are common sites of psoriasis.

Word or Phrase	Description	Pronunciation/Word Parts
scleroderma	Autoimmune disorder that causes the skin and internal organs to harden over time due to abnormal deposits of collagen. Treatment: Corticosteroid drug	**scleroderma** (SKLAIR-oh-DER-mah) **scler/o-** hard; sclera **-derma** skin
systemic lupus erythematosus (SLE)	Autoimmune disorder in which collagen in the skin and connective tissue deteriorates. There is joint pain, sensitivity to sunlight, and fatigue. Often there is a characteristic butterfly-shaped, erythematous rash over the nose and cheeks and a red rash on other body parts. Treatment: Corticosteroid drug	**systemic** (sis-TEM-ik) **system/o-** body as a whole **-ic** pertaining to **lupus erythematosus** (LOO-puhs AIR-eh-THEM-ah-TOH-suhs)

Clinical Connections

Immunology. Autoimmune disorders are disorders of the immune system in which the body makes antibodies against its own tissues, causing pain, changes in the tissues, and loss of function. In addition to the three autoimmune disorders of the skin described above, vitiligo (described previously; see Figure 2-9) is also an autoimmune disorder.

Word or Phrase	Description	Pronunciation/Word Parts

Diseases of the Sebaceous Glands

acne vulgaris — Chronic skin condition of the face, shoulders, and back during adolescence. The sebaceous glands secrete excessive amounts of sebum. Excess sebum enlarges the pores and turns black as the oil is exposed to the air; this becomes a **blackhead**. Alternatively, excess sebum blocks the pore and causes a red, raised **papule**. As bacteria feed on the sebum, it produces inflammation and infection; this draws white blood cells to the area and forms **pustules** or **whiteheads** (see Figure 2-22 ■ and Table 2-1). The blackheads, papules, and whiteheads of acne vulgaris are collectively known as **comedos**. In severe cystic acne, the papules enlarge to form deep, pus-filled cysts.
Treatment: Oil-removing topical cleanser; topical or oral antibiotic drug to kill skin bacteria; oral vitamin A–type drug for severe cystic acne

acne vulgaris (AK-nee vul-GAIR-ihs)

papule (PAP-yool)

pustule (PUS-tyool)

comedo (KOH-meh-doh)

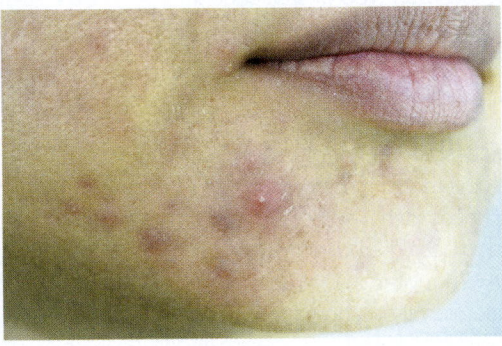

FIGURE 2-22 ■ Acne vulgaris.
This adolescent girl has acne vulgaris with small and large papules and a pustule. Increased secretions of the sebaceous glands during puberty trigger the onset of acne vulgaris.

rosacea — Chronic skin condition of the face and neck in middle-aged patients. The sebaceous glands secrete excessive amounts of sebum. There is blotchy erythema (redness) and dilated superficial blood vessels; these are made worse by heat, cold, stress, emotions, certain foods, alcoholic beverages, or sunlight (see Figure 2-23 ■). Men can develop **rhinophyma**, an erythematous, irregular enlargement of the nose.
Treatment: Topical antibacterial drug; laser surgery to destroy small, superficial blood vessels

rosacea (roh-ZAY-shee-ah)

rhinophyma (RY-noh-FY-mah)
  rhin/o- *nose*
  -phyma *growth; tumor*

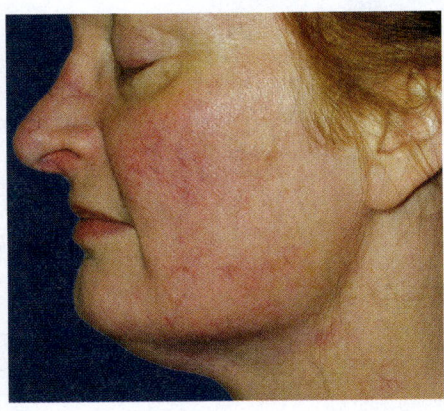

FIGURE 2-23 ■ Rosacea.
This patient's face shows the blotchy, rose-colored erythema and dilated superficial blood vessels of rosacea. Even the eyelids and neck are affected.

Table 2-1   Comparison of Acne Vulgaris and Rosacea

	Site	Comedos	Pustules and Papules	Dilated Blood Vessels	Age
Acne vulgaris	face, shoulders, back	yes	yes	no	adolescence
Rosacea	face, neck	no	no	yes	middle age

Word or Phrase	Description	Pronunciation/Word Parts
seborrhea	Overproduction of sebum that occurs at a time other than adolescence. Oily areas alternate with dry, scaly skin and dandruff. There can also be erythema and crusty, yellow deposits from leaking tissue fluids. In adults, it often occurs after illness or stress. It can also be caused by allergies. In infants, it is called **cradle cap**. In children or adults, it is called **eczema**. Treatment: Topical corticosteroid drug; medicated shampoo	**seborrhea** (SEB-oh-REE-ah) **seb/o-** *oil; sebum* **-rrhea** *discharge; flow* **eczema** (EK-zeh-mah)

Diseases of the Sudoriferous Glands

anhidrosis	Congenital absence of the sudoriferous glands and inability to sweat and tolerate heat. Treatment: Avoid overheating.	**anhidrosis** (AN-hy-DROH-sihs) **an-** *not; without* **hidr/o-** *sweat* **-osis** *abnormal condition; process*
diaphoresis	Diaphoresis is the normal process of sweating. Excessive sweating can point to an underlying serious condition, such as a myocardial infarction, hyperthyroidism, hypoglycemia, or withdrawal from narcotic drugs. The patient is said to be **diaphoretic**. Treatment: Correct the underlying cause.	**diaphoresis** (DY-ah-foh-REE-sihs) **dia-** *complete; through* **phor/o-** *bear; carry; range* **-esis** *abnormal condition; process* Diaphoresis: *Process through (the skin to) carry (sweat)* **diaphoretic** (DY-ah-foh-RET-ik) **dia-** *complete; through* **phor/o-** *bear; carry; range* **-etic** *pertaining to*

Diseases of the Hair

alopecia	Loss of hair from the scalp. Skin diseases such as tinea capitis can cause hair loss. Alopecia can also be caused by chemotherapy drugs that kill rapidly dividing cancer cells, but also kill rapidly dividing hair cells. Chronic hair loss usually begins in middle age. In men, a decreased level of testosterone in the blood and decreased blood flow to the scalp cause the hair follicles to shrink. The hair on the top of the scalp thins; this is known as **male pattern baldness**. In women, menopause causes a decreased level of estradiol in the blood; the estradiol level is lower than the level of male hormone, and this hormonal change causes the woman's hair to thin. Treatment: Topical drug to dilate the arteries and increase blood flow to the scalp; oral drug to block the effect of DHT (substance that is increased in the balding scalp); estradiol drug for women; hair transplantation (moving small areas of scalp hair to areas of baldness)	**alopecia** (AL-oh-PEE-sha) **alopec/o-** *bald* **-ia** *condition; state; thing*
hirsutism	Excessive, dark hair on the forearms and upper lip of a woman. It is caused by an increased level of male hormone, which is produced by a tumor in the woman's adrenal gland cortex. Treatment: Correct the underlying cause.	**hirsutism** (HER-soo-tizm) **hirsut/o-** *hairy* **-ism** *disease from a specific cause; process*

Word or Phrase	Description	Pronunciation/Word Parts
Diseases of the Nails		
clubbing and cyanosis	Abnormal downward curved and bluish fingernails and stunted growth of the fingers associated with a chronic lack of oxygen in patients with cystic fibrosis (see Figure 4-11). Treatment: Treat the underlying cause.	
onychomycosis	Fungal infection of the fingernails or toenails. It infects the nail root and deforms the nail as it grows (see Figure 2-24 ■). Treatment: Topical or oral antifungal drug; treatment with a laser 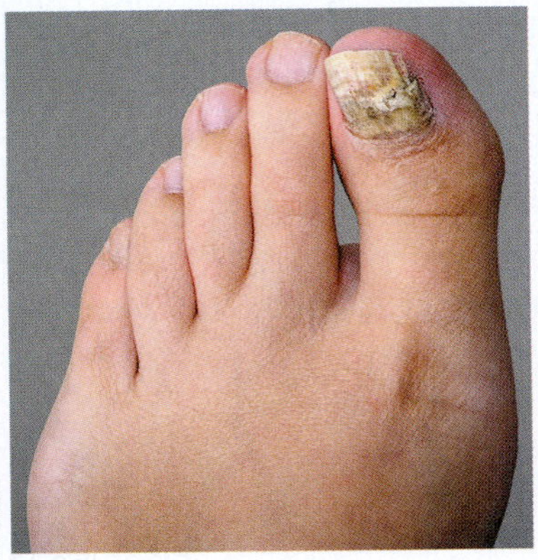	**onychomycosis** (ON-ih-KOH-my-KOH-sihs) **onych/o-** *fingernail; toenail* **myc/o-** *fungus* **-osis** *abnormal condition; process*

FIGURE 2-24 ■ Onychomycosis.
A fungal infection can involve one or all of the nails of the hands or feet. The nails become discolored, misshapen, thickened, and raised up from the nail bed.

2.3 PRACTICE LAPS

Use the Answer Key at the end of the book to check your answers.

A. Give the Meaning of Combining Forms

Next to each combining form, write its meaning. The first one has been done for you.

Combining Form	Meaning	Combining Form	Meaning
1. actin/o-	*rays of the sun*	10. lip/o-	
2. albin/o-		11. malign/o-	
3. contus/o-		12. necr/o-	
4. cyan/o-		13. onych/o-	
5. dermat/o-		14. pedicul/o-	
6. erythemat/o-		15. prurit/o-	
7. hem/o-		16. psor/o-	
8. kel/o-		17. xer/o-	
9. lacer/o-			

B. Build Words

Read the definition of the medical word. Look at the combining form that is given. Select the correct suffix from the Suffix List, and write it on the blank line. Then build the medical word, and write it on the line. (Remember: You may need to remove the combining vowel. Always remove the hyphens and slash.) Be sure to check your spelling.

Suffix List

-cle (small thing)
-derma (skin)
-ia (condition; state; thing)
-iasis (abnormal condition;
    process)

-ism (disease from a specific cause;
    process)
-itis (infection of;
    inflammation of)
-oma (mass; tumor)

-osis (abnormal condition; process)
-ous (pertaining to)
-plasm (formed substance; growth)
-rrhage (excessive discharge;
    excessive flow)

Definition of the Medical Word	Combining Form	Suffix	Build the Medical Word
Example: Pertaining to cancer	**cancer/o-**	*-ous*	*cancerous*

[*You think* pertaining to (-ous) + cancer (cancer/o-). You change the order of the word parts to put the suffix last. You write cancerous.]

	Definition	Combining Form	Suffix	Build the Medical Word
1.	Abnormal condition (of) itching	psor/o-		
2.	Abnormal condition (of) lice	pedicul/o-		
3.	Infection of (or) inflammation of (the) skin	dermat/o-		
4.	Tumor (composed of) fat	lip/o-		
5.	Abnormal condition (of) dead tissue	necr/o-		
6.	Condition (of being) bald	alopec/o-		
7.	Formed substance (or) growth (on the skin that is) new	ne/o-		
8.	Tumor (of variable colors and) black	melan/o-		
9.	Small thing (on the skin that is a) fluid-filled sac	vesic/o-		
10.	Abnormal condition (of the skin being) blue	cyan/o-		
11.	Excessive flow (of) blood	hem/o-		
12.	Disease from a specific cause (of being) hairy	hirsut/o-		
13.	Pertaining to redness	erythemat/o-		
14.	Skin (that is) dry	xer/o-		

C. Define Abbreviations

1. HSV _____

2. SLE _____

2.4 Laboratory and Diagnostic Procedures

Word or Phrase	Description	Pronunciation/Word Parts

Laboratory Tests and Diagnostic Procedures

Word or Phrase	Description	Pronunciation/Word Parts
allergy skin testing	Skin test in which **allergens** (animal dander, foods, plants, pollen, etc.) in a liquid form are given by **intradermal** injections into the skin. If the patient is allergic to a particular allergen, a wheal will form at the site of that injection (see Figure 2-25 ■). Alternately, the allergen is scratched into the skin, and the procedure is known as a **scratch test**. 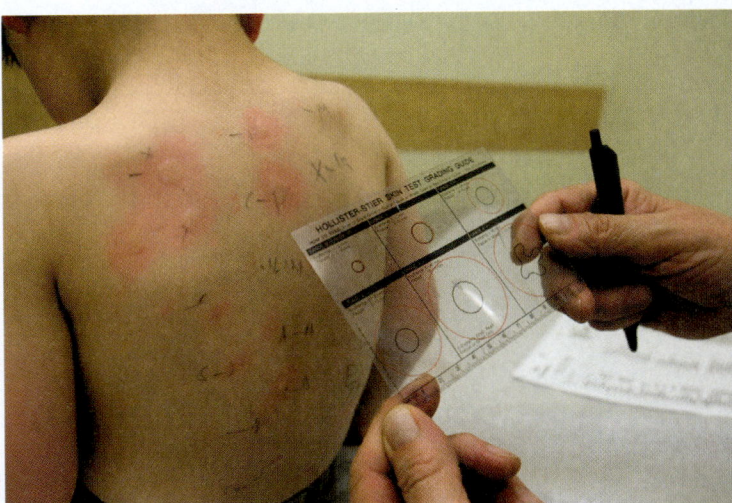 FIGURE 2-25 ■ **Allergy skin testing.** This patient's back shows a number of wheals where the body's immune response was triggered by the injected allergens. The size of the wheal corresponds to the degree of allergy to that allergen. No wheal formation means that the patient is not allergic to that allergen.	**allergen** (AL-er-jen) Allergen: *That which produces an allergy* **intradermal** (IN-trah-DER-mal) **intra-** *within* **derm/o-** *skin* **-al** *pertaining to*
culture and sensitivity (C&S)	Laboratory test in which a specimen of the **exudate** (oozing fluid or pus) from an ulcer, wound, burn, laceration, or skin infection is tested to identify the bacterium present and its sensitivity to specific antibiotic drugs (see the Clinical Connections box on the next page).	**sensitivity** (SEN-sih-TIV-ih-tee) **sensitiv/o-** *affected by; sensitive to* **-ity** *condition; state* **exudate** (EKS-yoo-dayt) **exud/o-** *oozing fluid* **-ate** *composed of; pertaining to*

Word or Phrase	Description	Pronunciation/Word Parts

Clinical Connections

Microbiology and Pharmacology. This culture plate contains a culture medium that can grow bacteria. A sample of pus from a patient's skin wound has been swabbed across it. Disks containing various antibiotic drugs are placed on the culture medium. If the bacterium in the pus is resistant to the antibiotic drug, there will only be a narrow clear ring of no growth around the disk. If the bacterium is sensitive to the antibiotic drug, there will be a wide clear ring of no growth around the antibiotic disk. This is the antibiotic drug the physician will prescribe to treat the patient's wound infection.

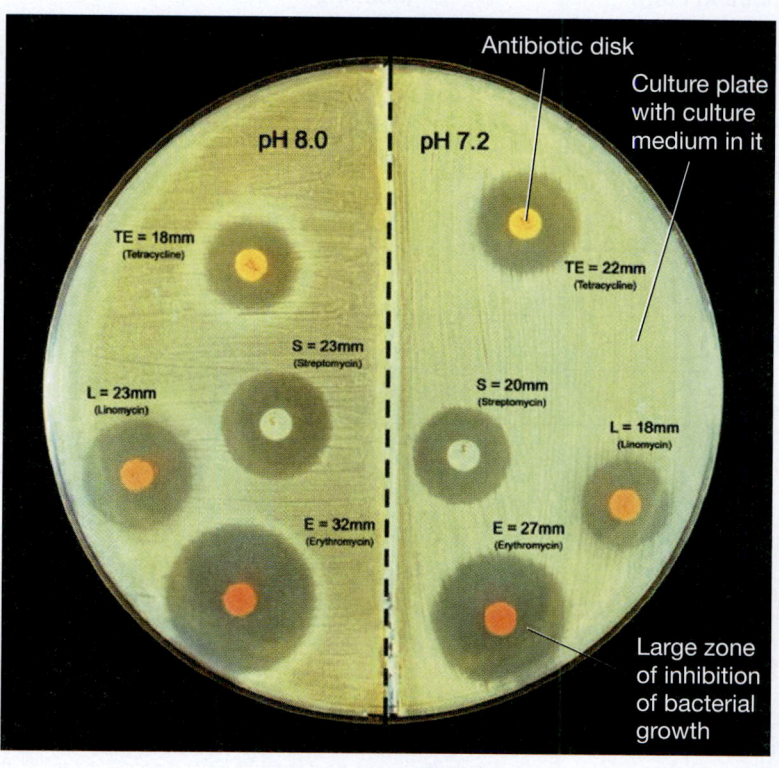

Word or Phrase	Description	Pronunciation/Word Parts
RAST	Blood test that measures the amount of immunoglobulin E (IgE) that is produced when the patient's blood is mixed with a specific allergen. IgE is active during allergic reactions in the body. The test produces a computerized printout that shows which allergens the patient is allergic to and how severe the allergy is. RAST stands for *radioallergosorbent test*. A more sensitive test is the ImmunoCAP Specific IgE test.	
skin scraping	Skin test in which a skin scraping is done with the edge of a scalpel to obtain cells from a skin lesion. The cells are examined under a microscope to make a diagnosis. Often used to diagnose tinea capitis (ringworm).	
Tzanck test	Skin test in which a skin scraping is done to obtain fluid from a vesicle. The fluid is smeared on a slide, stained, and examined under a microscope. Herpes virus infections and shingles show characteristic giant cells with herpes viruses in them.	**Tzanck** (TSANGK)
Wood lamp or light	Skin test that uses ultraviolet light to highlight areas of abnormal skin. In a darkened room, ultraviolet light makes vitiligo appear bright white and tinea capitis (ringworm) appear blue-green because the fungus fluoresces (glows).	

2.4 PRACTICE LAPS

Use the Answer Key at the end of the book to check your answers.

A. Give the Meaning of Combining Forms

Next to each combining form, write its meaning. The first one has been done for you.

Combining Form	Meaning
1. derm/o-	*skin*
2. exud/o-	
3. sensitiv/o-	

B. Define Abbreviations

1. C&S _____

2. IgE _____

3. RAST _____

2.5 Medical Procedures, Drugs, and Surgical Procedures

Word or Phrase	Description	Pronunciation/Word Parts

Medical Procedures

| Botox injections | Procedure in which the drug Botox is injected into the muscle to release deep wrinkle lines on the face (see Figure 2-26 ■). The drug keeps the muscle from contracting and creating wrinkles. This treatment is only effective for several months. | **Botox** (BOH-tawks) |

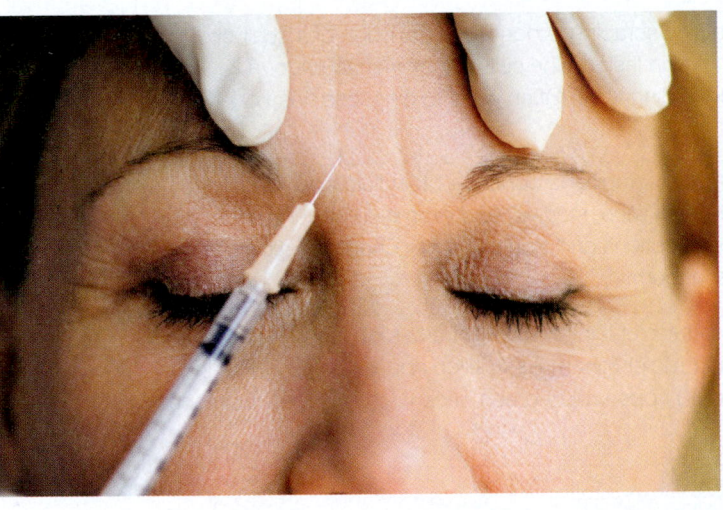

FIGURE 2-26 ■ Botox injection.
The drug Botox is actually a diluted version of the neurotoxin from the bacterium *Clostridium botulinum* type A that is known to cause food poisoning (botulism) and is present in canned goods with bulging ends.

Word or Phrase	Description	Pronunciation/Word Parts
collagen injections	Procedure in which a liquid that contains collagen is injected into wrinkles or acne scars. This plumps the skin and decreases the depth of the wrinkle or scar.	
cryolipolysis	Procedure (popularly known as CoolSculpting®) that is noninvasive and uses a device that is placed on the skin. The device is cold, and it targets and freezes fat cells, causing them to crystalize and die. It does not freeze skin cells or cause frostbite, as skin cells contain more water and freeze at a lower temperature than fat cells. In a few weeks, the body naturally eliminates the dead fat cells, causing a reduction in unwanted fat deposits.	**cryolipolysis** (KRY-oh-lih-POH-lih-sihs) **cry/o-** cold **lip/o-** fat **-lysis** process to break down or destroy
cryosurgery	Procedure in which liquid nitrogen is sprayed or painted onto a wart, mole, or other benign lesion or onto a small malignant lesion. The liquid nitrogen freezes and destroys the lesion.	**cryosurgery** (KRY-oh-SER-jer-ee) **cry/o-** cold **surg/o-** operative procedure **-ery** process
curettage	Procedure that uses a **curet** to scrape off a superficial skin lesion. A curet is a metal instrument that ends in a small ring with a sharp edge. Curettage is often combined with electrodesiccation for complete removal of a lesion.	**curettage** (kyoor-eh-TAWZH) **curet** (kyoor-ET)
debridement	Procedure in which necrotic tissue is removed (debrided) from a burn, wound, or ulcer. This is done to prevent infection from developing, to determine the depth of the wound, or to create a clean, raw surface that is ready to heal or receive a skin graft. • Mechanical debridement consists of putting on a wet dressing, letting it dry, removing the dressing, and pulling off necrotic tissue with it. • Topical debridement uses enzyme drugs to debride by chemically dissolving necrotic tissue. Medically sterilized maggots are used to eat necrotic tissue and the bacteria in it. • Surgical debridement of a large area is done under anesthesia using a scalpel or a curet.	**debridement** (deh-BREED-maw) *Note:* The pronunciation reflects the French origin of this word.
electrosurgery	Procedure that uses an electrical current to remove a nevus, wart, skin tag, or small malignant lesion. The electrical current passes through an electrode and evaporates the lesion. • **Fulguration.** The electrode is held away from the skin and transmits the electrical current to the skin lesion as a spark. • **Electrodesiccation.** The electrode is touched or inserted into the skin lesion to deliver the electrical current. • **Electrosection.** A special electrode is used that can cut and remove the lesion.	**electrosurgery** (ee-LEK-troh-SER-jer-ee) **electr/o-** electricity **surg/o-** operative procedure **-ery** process **fulguration** (FUL-gyoor-AA-shun) **fulgur/o-** spark of electricity **-ation** being; having; process **electrodesiccation** (ee-LEK-troh-DES-ih-KAY-shun) **electr/o-** electricity **desicc/o-** dry up **-ation** being; having; process **electrosection** (ee-LEK-troh-SEK-shun) **electr/o-** electricity **sect/o-** cut **-ion** action; condition

Word or Phrase	Description	Pronunciation/Word Parts
incision and drainage (I&D)	Procedure to remove fluid or pus from a cyst or abscess. A scalpel is used to make an incision. Most of the fluid or pus is manually expressed (pushed out with gloved hands), and the remainder is allowed to drain out.	**incision** (in-SIH-shun) **in-** *in; not; within* **cis/o-** *cut* **-ion** *action; condition*
laser surgery	Procedure that uses pulses of laser light to remove birthmarks, tattoos, enlarged superficial blood vessels (rosacea), wrinkles, scars, or unwanted hair. A tunable laser has a specific wavelength of light that only reacts with certain colors (the red of a birthmark, the black pigment of a tattoo, etc.) to break up that color and the tissue around it. Surrounding tissue of a different color is unharmed.	**laser** (LAY-zer) *Laser* is an acronym, a word made from the first letters of the phrase *light amplification by stimulated emission of radiation.*
skin examination	Procedure to examine the patient's skin or just one skin lesion, rash, or tumor. The dermatologist uses a lens to magnify the area (see Figure 2-27 ■).	

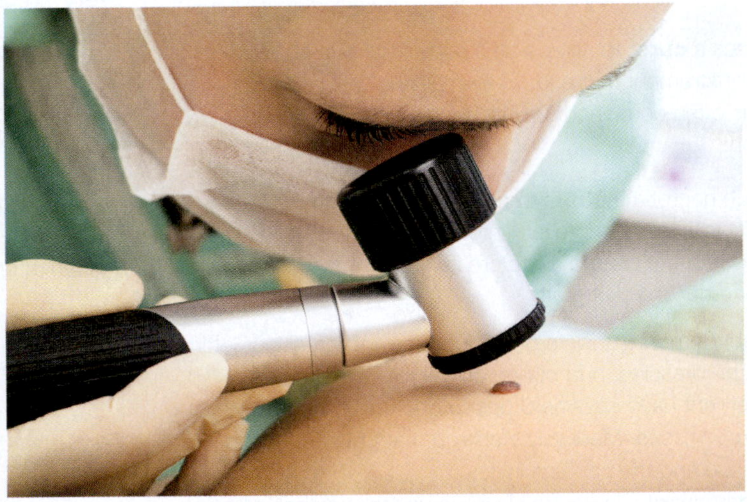

FIGURE 2-27 ■ Skin examination. The dermatologist is using a magnifying lens to examine a lesion on this patient's skin. The area may need to be biopsied to obtain a diagnosis.

Word or Phrase	Description	Pronunciation/Word Parts
skin resurfacing	Procedure that removes the epidermis. It is used to treat acne scars and skin tone irregularities, remove tattoos, and promote the regrowth of smoother skin. • **Chemical peel** uses a liquid acid to remove the epidermis. • **Dermabrasion** uses a rapidly spinning wire brush or diamond surface to mechanically scrape away (abrade) the epidermis. • **Laser skin resurfacing** uses a computer-controlled laser to vaporize the epidermis. Also known as a **laser peel**. • **Microdermabrasion** uses aluminium oxide crystals to abrade and remove the epidermis.	**dermabrasion** (DER-mah-BRAY-shun) **derm/o-** *skin* **abras/o-** *scrape off* **-ion** *action; condition* **microdermabrasion** (MY-kroh-DER-mah-BRAY-shun) **micr/o-** *one millionth; small* **derm/o-** *skin* **abras/o-** *scrape off* **-ion** *action; condition*
skin turgor assessment	Healthcare professionals assess a patient's level of hydration by testing the **skin turgor**. A fold of skin pinched between the thumb and fingertips of the healthcare professional should flatten out immediately when released. Dehydration causes the fold of skin to remain elevated ("tenting" of the skin) or to flatten out very slowly.	**turgor** (TER-ger)

Across the Life Span

Geriatrics. Older people often fail to drink enough fluids. This may be due to (1) a lack of activity and a decreased feeling of thirst or (2) avoiding the inconvenience or difficulty of frequent trips to the bathroom. This leads to dehydration.

Word or Phrase	Description	Pronunciation/Word Parts
suturing	Procedure that uses sutures to bring the edges of the skin together and close a wound after a laceration, injury, or at the end of a surgical procedure (see Figure 2-28 ■)	**suturing** (SOO-chur-ing)

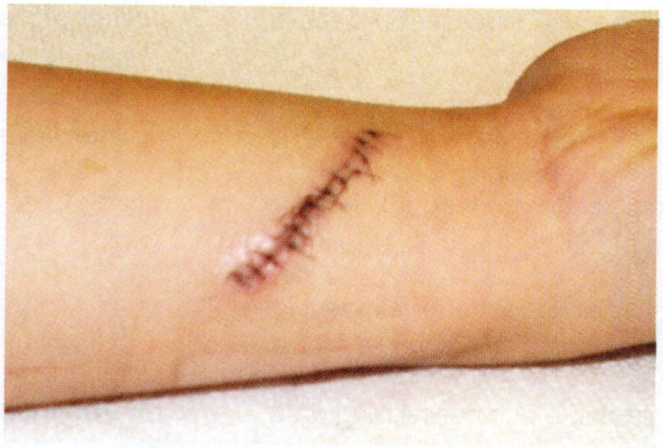

A. 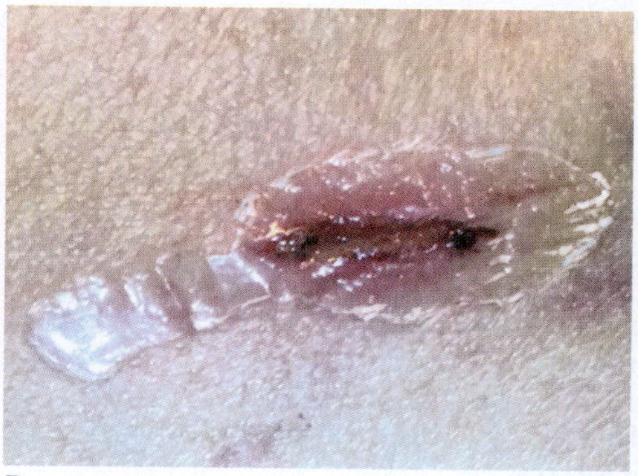   B.

FIGURE 2-28 ■ Wound closure.
A. After an anesthetic drug was given to numb the area, this laceration in the forearm was sewn closed with two layers of sutures, the first in the deeper tissues and the second to close the skin edges. After a week, the skin sutures were removed. The deeper sutures, which were made of a material that was absorbed by the body, did not need to be removed. **B.** Surgical glue applied topically is an alternative to suturing a small wound.

Word or Phrase	Description	Pronunciation/Word Parts
Ultherapy®	Procedure that uses ultrasound waves directed to the dermis and subcutaneous tissues. It stimulates the production of new collagen to lift and tighten the skin of the face and neck.	

Category	Indication	Pronunciation/Word Parts

Drugs

Category	Indication	Pronunciation/Word Parts
anesthetic drug	Provides temporary numbness of the skin while injuries and skin diseases are treated or skin lesions are removed. Applied topically or injected.	**anesthetic** (AN-es-THEH-tik) **an-** *not; without* **esthet/o-** *feeling; sensation* **-ic** *pertaining to*
antibiotic drug	Treats bacterial infections of the skin or acne vulgaris. Applied topically or given orally.	**antibiotic** (AN-tee-by-AW-tik) **anti-** *against* **bi/o-** *living organism; living tissue* **-tic** *pertaining to*
antifungal drug	Treats ringworm (tinea) when applied topically. Treats a fungal infection of the nail when applied topically or given orally.	**antifungal** (AN-tee-FUN-gal) **anti-** *against* **fung/o-** *fungus* **-al** *pertaining to*
antipruritic drug	Decreases itching. Applied topically or given orally.	**antipruritic** (AN-tee-proo-RIH-tik) **anti-** *against* **prurit/o-** *itching* **-ic** *pertaining to*
antiviral drug	Treats herpes simplex virus infections. Applied topically or given orally.	**antiviral** (AN-tee-VY-ral) **anti-** *against* **vir/o-** *virus* **-al** *pertaining to*

Category	Indication	Pronunciation/Word Parts
coal tar drug	Treats psoriasis. Causes epidermal cells to multiply more slowly to decrease itching. Coal tar is a by-product of the processing of bituminous coal. It contains more than 10,000 different chemicals. Applied topically.	
corticosteroid drug	Treats skin inflammation associated with many different skin diseases. Applied topically or given orally.	**corticosteroid** (KOR-tih-koh-STAIR-oyd) **cortic/o-** cortex; outer region **-steroid** steroid
drug for alopecia	Improves blood flow to the skin to increase hair growth. Applied topically or given orally to block the production of DHT.	
drug for infestations	Treats scabies (mites) and pediculosis (lice). Applied topically as a lotion and shampoo.	
photodynamic therapy (PDT)	Treats cancer of the skin with laser light and a photosensitizing drug.	**photodynamic** (FOH-toh-dy-NAM-ik) **phot/o-** light **dynam/o-** movement; power **-ic** pertaining to
psoralen drug	Treats psoriasis. Psoralen sensitizes the skin to the ultraviolet light therapy, damages cellular DNA, and decreases the rate of cell division. This combination is known as PUVA (psoralen drug and ultraviolet A light)	**psoralen** (SOR-ah-len)
vitamin A–type drug	Treats acne vulgaris or severe cystic acne. Causes epidermal cells to multiply rapidly to keep the pores from becoming clogged. Applied topically or given orally.	

Clinical Connections

Pharmacology. The administration of drugs often involves the skin. **Topical** drugs such as creams, lotions, and ointments are applied to the surface of the skin and are absorbed into the skin for a local drug effect. **Transdermal** drug patches are applied to the surface of the skin and release small amounts of a drug over time; the drug is absorbed through the skin, but it has an effect throughout the entire body (a systemic effect). The **intradermal** route of drug administration uses a needle to inject a liquid drug just beneath the epidermis. This is used for the Mantoux tuberculosis test and allergy testing. The **hypodermic** route of drug administration uses a needle to inject a liquid drug into the subcutaneous tissue (see Figure 2-29 ■).

topical (TOP-ih-kal)
  topic/o- specific area
  -al pertaining to

transdermal (trans-DER-mal)
  trans- across; through
  derm/o- skin
  -al pertaining to

intradermal (IN-trah-DER-mal)
  intra- within
  derm/o- skin
  -al pertaining to

hypodermic (HY-poh-DER-mik)
  hypo- below; deficient
  derm/o- skin
  -ic pertaining to

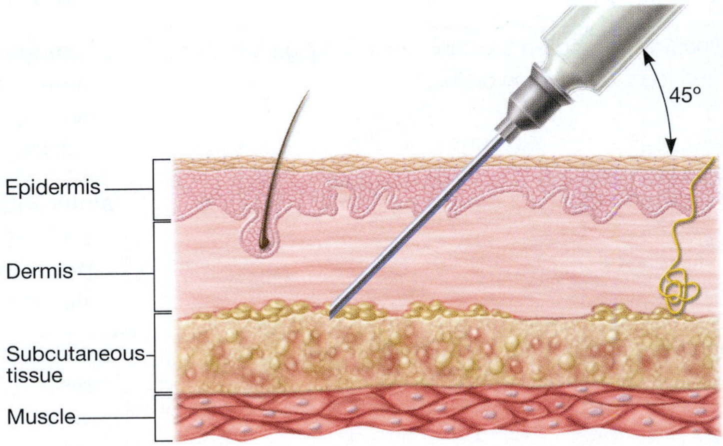

Epidermis
Dermis
Subcutaneous tissue
Muscle
45°

FIGURE 2-29 ■ Hypodermic injection.

Word or Phrase	Description	Pronunciation/Word Parts

Surgical Procedures

biopsy (Bx)	Procedure done to remove all or part of a skin lesion or tumor. The biopsy specimen is sent to the pathology department of the hospital for examination under a microscope to obtain a diagnosis.
	
	• **Excisional biopsy** uses a scalpel to remove the entire skin lesion or tumor.
	• **Incisional biopsy** uses a scalpel to make an incision to remove just a portion of the skin lesion or tumor.
	• **Punch biopsy** uses a circular metal cutter to remove a core of tissue from the skin lesion or tumor (see Figure 2-30 ■).
	• **Shave biopsy** uses a scalpel to shave off a superficial skin lesion in the epidermis.
		biopsy (BY-awp-see)
		  bi/o- *living organism; living tissue*
		  -opsy *process of viewing*
		
		excisional (ek-SIH-shun-al)
		  ex- *away from*
		  cis/o- *cut*
		  -ion *action; condition*
		  -al *pertaining to*
		
		incisional (in-SIH-shun-al)
		  in- *in; not; within*
		  cis/o- *cut*
		  -ion *action; condition*
		  -al *pertaining to*

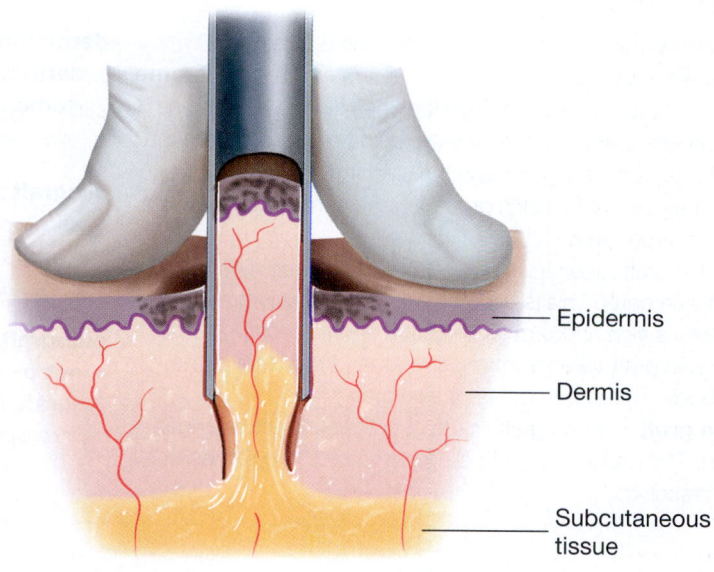

Epidermis

Dermis

Subcutaneous tissue

FIGURE 2-30 ■ Punch biopsy.
A punch biopsy uses a circular metal cutter to remove a plug-shaped core that includes the epidermis, dermis, and subcutaneous tissue.

dermatoplasty	Procedure of any type that involves plastic surgery to the skin, such as skin grafting, removal of a keloid, facelift, etc.	**dermatoplasty** (DER-mah-toh-PLAS-tee)
		  dermat/o- *skin*
		  -plasty *process of reshaping by surgery*

liposuction	Procedure to remove excessive adipose tissue deposits from the breasts, abdomen, hips, legs, or buttocks. A cannula inserted through a small incision is used to suction out the subcutaneous tissue (see Figure 2-31 ■). Ultrasonic-assisted liposuction uses ultrasonic waves to break up the fatty tissue before it is removed. Also known as **suction-assisted lipectomy**.	**liposuction** (LIP-oh-SUK-shun)
		  lip/o- *fat; lipid*
		  suct/o- *suck*
		  -ion *action; condition*
		
		lipectomy (ly-PEK-toh-mee)
		  lip/o- *fat; lipid*
		  -ectomy *surgical removal*

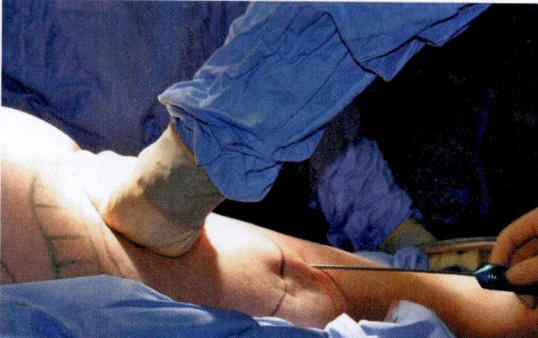

FIGURE 2-31 ■ Liposuction.
This plastic surgeon is performing liposuction to remove fat from the patient's thigh and hip. Lines drawn on the skin show the areas of greatest fat deposit that are to be removed. Both legs will be done to achieve a symmetrical result.

Word or Phrase	Description	Pronunciation/Word Parts
Mohs surgery	Procedure to remove skin cancer, particularly tumors with irregular shapes and depths. An operating microscope is used during the surgery to examine each layer of excised tissue. If it still shows cancerous cells, more tissue is removed until no cancer cells are seen.	**Mohs** (MOHZ)
rhytidectomy	Procedure to remove wrinkles and tighten loose, aging skin on the face and neck. Also known as a **facelift**. A **blepharoplasty**, the removal of fat and drooping skin from around the eyelids, is often done at the same time.	**rhytidectomy** (RIH-tih-DEK-toh-mee) **rhytid/o-** wrinkle **-ectomy** surgical removal **blepharoplasty** (BLEF-ah-roh-PLAS-tee) **blephar/o-** eyelid **-plasty** process of reshaping by surgery
skin grafting	Procedure that uses human or artificial skin to provide a temporary covering or permanent layer of skin over a burn or wound. A **dermatome** makes a shallow, continuous cut to remove (harvest) skin to be used as a graft. A split-thickness skin graft contains the epidermis and part of the dermis. A full-thickness skin graft contains the epidermis and all of the dermis. Tiny holes can be cut in a skin graft to create a mesh that can be stretched to cover a larger area. • **Allograft** is a skin graft taken from a dead body (cadaver). It is frozen and stored in a skin bank. This is used as a temporary skin graft to protect the patient's skin and prevent infection and fluid loss. • **Autograft** is a skin graft taken from another area (donor site) of the patient's own body. This is a permanent skin graft. • **Synthetic skin graft** is a skin graft made of collagen fibers arranged in a lattice pattern. The patient's own healing skin grows into this as the graft gradually dissolves.	**dermatome** (DER-mah-tohm) **derm/a-** skin **-tome** area with distinct edges; instrument used to cut **allograft** (AL-oh-graft) **all/o-** other; strange **-graft** tissue for implant or transplant **autograft** (AW-toh-graft) **aut/o-** self **-graft** tissue for implant or transplant

2.5 PRACTICE LAPS

Use the Answer Key at the end of the book to check your answers.

A. Give the Meaning of Combining Forms

Next to each combining form, write its meaning. The first one has been done for you.

Combining Form	Meaning	Combining Form	Meaning
1. abras/o-	*scrape off*	8. fulgur/o-	
2. aut/o-		9. fung/o-	
3. bi/o-		10. lip/o-	
4. cis/o-		11. phot/o-	
5. cry/o-		12. rhytid/o-	
6. dermat/o-		13. surg/o-	
7. esthet/o-			

B. Build Words

Read the definition of the medical word. Look at the combining form that is given. Select the correct suffix from the Suffix List, and write it on the blank line. Then build the medical word, and write it on the line. (Remember: You may need to remove the combining vowel. Always remove the hyphens and slash.) Be sure to check your spelling.

Suffix List

-ation (being; having; process)
-ectomy (surgical removal)
-graft (tissue for implant or transplant)

-opsy (process of viewing)
-plasty (process of reshaping by surgery)
-tome (instrument used to cut)

Definition of the Medical Word	Combining Form	Suffix	Build the Medical Word
Example: Process of reshaping by surgery (on the) eyelid	**blephar/o**	*-plasty*	*blepharoplasty*
1. Process of viewing (a sample of) living tissue	bi/o-		
2. Process of reshaping by surgery (on the) skin	dermat/o-		
3. Surgical removal (of) fat	lip/o-		
4. Having (a) spark of electricity (go to the skin)	fulgur/o-		
5. Tissue for transplant (from a person's own) self	aut/o-		
6. Surgical removal (of) wrinkles	rhytid/o-		
7. Instrument used to cut (the) skin	derm/a-		

C. Define Abbreviations

1. Bx _____

2. I&D _____

3. PDT _____

4. PUVA _____

Abbreviations Summary

Bx	biopsy		**PDT**	photodynamic therapy
C&S	culture and sensitivity		**PUVA**	psoralen (drug and) ultraviolet A (light therapy)
Derm	dermatology (short form)		**SLE**	systemic lupus erythematosus
HAI	healthcare–associated infection		**SQ**	subcutaneous
HSV	herpes simplex virus		**subcu**	subcutaneous (short form)
I&D	incision and drainage		**subQ**	subcutaneous (short form)
IgE	immunoglobulin E		**UVB**	ultraviolet light B

Word Alert

Homonyms. These words are spelled alike and pronounced alike, but have different meanings.

dermatome   (noun)   a specific area of the skin that sends sensory information through a spinal nerve to the spinal cord
Example: The patient had shingles on the chest and back along the T6 dermatome.

dermatome   (noun)   a surgical instrument used to make a shallow, continuous cut to form a skin graft
Example: After the patient's donor site was prepped and draped, a dermatome was used to obtain a split-thickness skin graft.

It's Greek to Me! Did you notice that some words have two different combining forms? Combining forms from both Greek and Latin remain a part of medical language today.

Word	Greek	Latin	Medical Word Examples
fat	lip/o-	adip/o-	lipocyte; adipose tissue
hair or hairy	trich/o-	hirsut/o-, pil/o-	schizotrichia; hirsutism, piloerection
itching	psor/o-	prurit/o-	psoriasis; pruritic
nail	onych/o-	ungu/o-	onychomycosis; ungual
skin	derm/a-, derm/o-, dermat/o-	cutane/o-, cut/i-, integument/o-	dermatome, intradermal, dermatologist; subcutaneous, cuticle, integumentary

Career Focus

Meet Toral, a physician's assistant in a cosmetic surgeon's office

"Growing up, I always knew I would be in medicine. At first, I entertained the idea of becoming a nurse. Then I entertained the idea of becoming a physician. Being a physician's assistant allows me to see my own patients, treat and diagnose, write prescriptions, care for patients, and advise them. I also assist in laser procedures and all surgical procedures. Our everyday language is medical terminology—from talking to the physician, to talking to my coworkers, to typing in the medical records. With so many patients being Internet-savvy, they come in talking in medical terminology!"

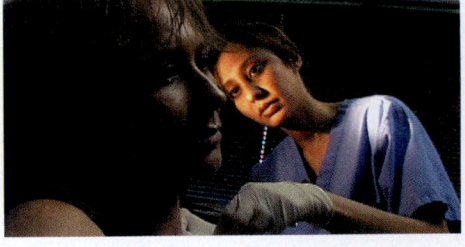

- **Physician's assistants** are physician extenders who are licensed to perform basic medical care under the supervision of a physician. They perform physical examinations, diagnose, prescribe drugs, and perform minor surgery. They can assist the physician during more extensive surgery. They work in physicians' offices, clinics, and hospitals.

- **Dermatologists** are physicians who practice in the medical specialty of dermatology. They diagnose and treat patients with diseases of the skin. Physicians can take additional training and become board certified in the subspecialty of pediatric dermatology. Malignancies of the skin are treated medically by an oncologist or surgically by a dermatologist, a general surgeon, or a plastic surgeon.

- **Plastic surgeons** are physicians who perform plastic and reconstructive surgery to reshape the body. They remove lesions and scars and perform liposuction and other procedures that reshape the skin and subcutaneous tissue.

- **Oncologists** are physicians who specialize in treating cancer with chemotherapy drugs. Surgeons perform surgery to remove cancerous tumors.

dermatologist (DER-mah-TAW-loh-jist)
  dermat/o- *skin*
  log/o- *study of; word*
  -ist *person who specializes in; thing that specializes in*

plastic (PLAS-tik)
  plast/o- *formation; growth*
  -ic *pertaining to*

surgeon (SER-jun)
  surg/o- *operative procedure*
  -eon *person who performs*

oncologist (ong-KAW-loh-jist)
  onc/o- *mass; tumor*
  log/o- *study of; word*
  -ist *person who specializes in; thing that specializes in*

Chapter Review Exercises

Dive In: Medical Language Exercises

Test your knowledge of the chapter by completing these review exercises. Use the Answer Key at the end of the book to check your answers. Note: Each of the numbered exercise headers corresponds to a numbered learning outcome at the beginning of the chapter.

2.1 Anatomy

MATCHING EXERCISE

Match each word or phrase to its description.

1. basal layer
2. cutaneous
3. dermis
4. epidermis
5. exfoliation
6. lipocytes
7. lunula
8. melanocytes
9. sudoriferous glands

_____ shedding of dead cells from the epidermis
_____ outermost layer of skin
_____ another name for *sweat glands*
_____ white half-moon on the nail plate
_____ cells that are in the adipose tissue
_____ cells that produce brown or black pigment
_____ deepest part of the epidermis
_____ contains sebaceous glands and sweat glands
_____ pertaining to the skin

CIRCLE EXERCISE

Circle the correct answer from the choices given.

1. The (**lunula, nail bed, nail plate**) is also known as the *quick*.
2. (**Collagen, Keratin, Melanin**) is a hard, fibrous protein found in the most superficial cells of the epidermis.
3. Piloerection involves contraction of the muscle around a (**dermatome, hair, lipocyte**).
4. (**Exfoliation, Perspiration, Sudoriferous**) is the normal shedding of skin cells.
5. *Ungual* is the adjective form for (**hair, nail, skin**).

TRUE OR FALSE EXERCISE

*Indicate whether each statement is true or false by writing **T** or **F** on the line.*

1. _____ The integumentary system consists of the nails, hair, and dermis.
2. _____ The epithelium is the outermost layer of the skin.
3. _____ Sebaceous glands are exocrine glands.
4. _____ Melanin is produced by melanocytes in the subcutaneous tissue.

DIVIDING WORDS EXERCISE

Separate these words into their component parts (prefix, combining form, suffix). Some words do not contain all three word parts. The first one has been done for you.

Medical Word	Prefix	Combining Form	Suffix	Medical Word	Prefix	Combining Form	Suffix
1. **diaphoresis**	*dia-*	*phor/o-*	*-esis*	6. collagen		_____	_____
2. integumentary		_____	_____	7. cuticle		_____	_____
3. melanocyte		_____	_____	8. adipose		_____	_____
4. dermal		_____	_____	9. subcutaneous	_____	_____	_____
5. exfoliation	_____	_____	_____	10. lipocyte		_____	_____

SPELLING EXERCISE

Read each medical word pronunciation and write the medical word that it represents. Be sure to check your spelling. The first one has been done for you.

1. **(kyoo-TAY-nee-uhs)**   *cutaneous*
2. (EP-ih-DERM-mal)   _____
3. (meh-LAN-oh-SITE)   _____
4. (seh-BAY-shus)   _____
5. (DY-ah-for-EE-sihs)   _____

6. (UNG-gwal)   _____
7. (SUB-kyoo-TAY-nee-uhs)   _____
8. (AD-ih-pohs)   _____
9. (LIP-oh-site)   _____

2.2 Physiology

MATCHING EXERCISE

Match each word or phrase to its description.

1. subcutaneous fat
2. homeostasis
3. nosocomial
4. vitamin D synthesis
5. dermatome
6. integumentary system

_____ occurs in the dermis

_____ sends skin sensations to a spinal nerve

_____ body's first line of defense

_____ helps with thermoregulation

_____ balance and equilibrium of all body systems

_____ healthcare–associated infection

TRUE OR FALSE EXERCISE

*Indicate whether each statement is true or false by writing **T** or **F** on the line.*

1. _____ Sunlight on the skin helps produce vitamin D.
2. _____ Normal skin flora are bacteria that can cause infection.
3. _____ Goosebumps are one way the skin creates heat.
4. _____ When a person dies in a fire, the high level of carbon monoxide makes the skin cherry red.
5. _____ A dermatome is associated with healthcare-associated infections.
6. _____ The skin repairs itself with cells from the basal layer of the epidermis that move upward.

DIVIDING WORDS EXERCISE

Separate these words into their component parts (prefix, combining form, suffix). Some words do not contain all three word parts. The first one has been done for you.

Medical Word	Prefix	Combining Form	Suffix
1. **sensation**		*sens/o-*	*-ation*
2. dermatome		_____	_____
3. homeostasis		_____	_____
4. nosocomial		_____	_____

SPELLING EXERCISE

Read each medical word pronunciation and write the medical word that it represents. Be sure to check your spelling. The first one has been done for you.

1. **(proh-TEK-shun)**   *protection*
2. (NOH-soh-KOH-mee-al)   _____
3. (THER-moh-REH-gyoo-LAY-shun)   _____
4. (HOH-mee-oh-STAY-sihs)   _____

2.3 Diseases

MATCHING EXERCISE

Match each word or phrase to its description.

1. abscess	_____ infection or inflammation of the skin
2. alopecia	_____ yellowish coloration of the skin
3. bullae	_____ localized collection of pus
4. callus	_____ often seen in patients with aids
5. pressure injury	_____ autoimmune disorder with depigmentation patches
6. dermatitis	_____ thickened, firm pad on the epidermis
7. skin cancer	_____ fungal infection of the nails
8. hematoma	_____ present in partial-thickness burns
9. jaundice	_____ frequent repositioning avoids this
10. Kaposi sarcoma	_____ baldness
11. onychomycosis	_____ collection of blood under the skin
12. vitiligo	_____ malignant melanoma

CIRCLE EXERCISE

Circle the correct answer from the choices given.

1. This skin lesion is a (**cyst, fissure, papule, wheal**).

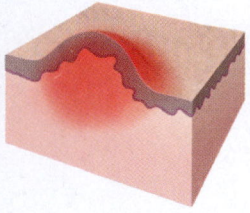

2. This skin lesion is a (**cyst, laceration, macule, vesicle**).

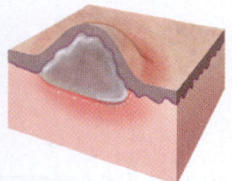

3. This skin lesion is a (**cyst, macule, scale, wheal**).

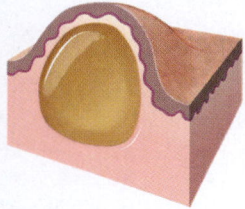

4. All of the following are changes that occur in the skin during pregnancy *except* (**dermatome, linea nigra, striae**).
5. A macule is a/an (**crevice, elevated, flat**) lesion.
6. An acne whitehead is also called a (**cyst, pustule, wheal**).
7. The thick, black crust over a full-thickness burn is known as a/an (**cicatrix, eschar, keloid**).
8. Tinea pedis occurs on the skin of the (**feet, groin, trunk of the body**).
9. A yellow color of the skin is known as (**cyanosis, jaundice, scleroderma**).
10. Fungal infection of the toenail is known as (**onychomycosis, ringworm, verruca**).

TRUE OR FALSE EXERCISE

*Indicate whether each statement is true or false by writing **T** or **F** on the line.*

1. _____ A neoplasm is always a malignant growth of the skin.

2. _____ Bluish discoloration of the skin from a lack of oxygen is known as a *bruise*.

3. _____ An abnormally enlarged scar is known as a *keloid*.

4. _____ Actinic keratoses are rough, raised areas due to long-term sun exposure.

5. _____ Rhinophyma is a complication of severe acne vulgaris of the nose.

6. _____ Hirsutism is a lack of hair due to aging.

7. _____ Psoriasis is treated with coal tar drugs and PUVA.

PLURAL NOUN AND ADJECTIVE EXERCISE

Read the noun and write its plural form and/or adjective form on the line. Be sure to check your spelling. The first one has been done for you.

Singular Noun	Plural Noun	Adjective
1. **cancer**		*cancerous* or *malignant*
2. cyanosis		_____
3. diaphoresis		_____
4. gangrene		_____
5. necrosis		_____
6. pruritus		_____
7. vesicle	_____	_____

DIVIDING WORDS EXERCISE

Separate these words into their component parts (prefix, combining form, suffix). Some words do not contain all three word parts. The first one has been done for you.

Medical Word	Prefix	Combining Form	Suffix
1. **diaphoresis**	*dia-*	*phor/o-*	*-esis*
2. anesthesia	_____	_____	_____
3. anhidrosis	_____	_____	_____
4. depigmentation	_____	_____	_____
5. extravasation	_____	_____	_____

SPELLING EXERCISE

Read each medical word pronunciation and write the medical word that it represents. Be sure to check your spelling. The first one has been done for you.

1. (las-er-AA-shun)   *laceration*

2. (SIK-ah-triks) _____

3. (AIR-ih-THEM-eh-tuhs) _____

4. (hee-MAN-jee-OH-mah) _____

5. (NEE-oh-plazm) _____

6. (ON-ih-KOH-my-KOH-sihs) _____

7. (PAW-lee-DAK-tih-lee) _____

8. (proo-RY-tuhs) _____

9. (sor-EYE-ah-sihs) _____

10. (VIT-ih-LY-goh) _____

ENGLISH AND MEDICAL WORD EQUIVALENTS

For each English word or phrase, write its equivalent medical word. Be sure to check your spelling. The first one has been done for you.

English Word	Medical Word	English Word	Medical Word
1. age spots or liver spots	*senile lentigo*	7. fungal infection of the nail	
2. baldness		8. infestation with lice	
3. bedsore		9. infestation with mites	
4. blackhead		10. port-wine stain	
5. brush burn		11. ringworm on the scalp	
6. cradle cap		12. wart	

2.4 Laboratory and Diagnostic Procedures

MATCHING EXERCISE

Match each word or phrase to its description.

1. allergy skin testing   _____ fluid from an ulcer, wound, or burn
2. culture and sensitivity   _____ done to diagnose herpes
3. exudate   _____ done to determine what bacterium is causing an infection
4. skin scraping   _____ done to diagnose ringworm
5. antibiotic disks   _____ scratch test is one example
6. Tzanck test   _____ placed on a culture plate

SPELLING EXERCISE

Read each medical word pronunciation and write the medical word that it represents. Be sure to check your spelling. The first one has been done for you.

1. **(TSANGK)**   *Tzanck*
2. (EKS-yoo-dayt)
3. (SEN-sih-TIV-ih-tee)
4. (IN-trah-DERM-mal)

2.5 Medical Procedures, Drugs, and Surgical Procedures

MATCHING EXERCISE

Match each word or phrase to its description.

1. Botox   _____ uses liquid nitrogen to remove a small malignant skin lesion
2. cryosurgery   _____ topical drug patch that acts systemically
3. dermatome   _____ freezes fat cells to remove unwanted fat
4. incision and drainage _____ can remove tattoos
5. laser surgery   _____ creates a skin graft for burn patients
6. transdermal   _____ used to treat an abscess that contains pus
7. cryolipolysis   _____ injection that relaxes deep wrinkles
8. fulguration   _____ uses electricity to remove a wart or skin tag

CIRCLE EXERCISE

Circle the correct answer from the choices given.

1. Electrosurgery includes all of the following *except* (**debridement, fulguration, electrodesiccation**).
2. Surgical debridement is done with a (**curet, electrode, transdermal patch**).
3. Allergy skin testing uses (**hypodermic, intradermal, transdermal**) injection of an allergen.
4. A surgical procedure to remove wrinkles from the face is a/an (**autograft, Botox injection, rhytidectomy**).
5. A/an (**dermatoplasty, excisional biopsy, incisional biopsy**) removes just a piece of a large skin lesion.
6. Each of the following is a skin resurfacing technique *except* (**chemical peel, dermabrasion, incision and drainage**).
7. Each of the following drugs is used to treat psoriasis *except* (**antifungal drugs, coal tar drugs, psoralen**).
8. Suturing takes place following a/an (**abrasion, collagen injection, laceration**).

TRUE OR FALSE EXERCISE

*Indicate whether each statement is true or false by writing **T** or **F** on the line.*

1. _____ Lipectomy is the surgical removal of fat by using suction through an incision.
2. _____ Vitamin A–type drugs are used to treat alopecia.
3. _____ An antiviral cream is an example of a topical drug.
4. _____ Drugs for vitiligo cause depigmentation of the skin.
5. _____ A dermatome is used to harvest a skin graft.
6. _____ Mohs surgery is used to remove skin cancers that have irregular shapes and depths.

DIVIDING WORDS EXERCISE

Separate these words into their component parts (prefix, combining form, suffix). Some words do not contain all three word parts. The first one has been done for you.

Medical Word	Prefix	Combining Form	Suffix
1. **fulguration**		*fulgur/o-*	*-ation*
2. incision			
3. antifungal			
4. biopsy			
5. dermatoplasty			
6. allograft			
7. rhytidectomy			
8. transdermal			

SPELLING EXERCISE

Read each medical word pronunciation and write the medical word that it represents. Be sure to check your spelling. The first one has been done for you.

1. (**IN-trah-DER-mal**) _intradermal_
2. (AN-tee-proo-RIH-tik) _____
3. (KRY-oh-SER-jer-ee) _____
4. (kyoor-eh-TAWZH) _____
5. (DER-mah-BRAY-shun) _____
6. (BY-awp-see) _____
7. (trans-DER-mal) _____
8. (DER-mah-TAW-loh-jist) _____

Immerse Yourself: Analyze Medical Reports

Electronic Patient Record

This is an Office Visit Note. Read the note and answer the questions.

PEARSON PRIMARY CARE ASSOCIATES

Task Edit View Time Scale Options Help

OFFICE VISIT NOTE

PATIENT NAME:	GUNDERSON, Denise
PATIENT NUMBER:	191-46-3985
DATE OF VISIT:	November 19, 20xx

HISTORY

The patient developed erythema nodosum, which is an unusual adverse reaction in the skin following an untreated strep throat. She had swelling and edema in her right foot, but it then spread to her right leg and to areas on her chest, left knee, and left foot. These areas were extremely painful and erythematous; her right knee developed a large, painful nodule under the skin. Her right foot was so painful and edematous that it was nearly impossible for her to walk. When the dorsum of her right foot developed cellulitis, she finally came to our office last week, and she was placed on the antibiotic drug azithromycin. She had just taken her last scheduled dose of azithromycin when she describes suddenly having a very itchy scalp. When she scratched her scalp, she could feel multiple raised areas. About 20 minutes later, there were twice as many raised areas on her scalp, and now she could see wheals on her cheeks and on her chest. When the wheals became large welts, she became concerned about not being able to breathe and took two antihistamine tablets. After that, the welts and itching began to subside. Although she was feeling better, she decided to come to the office today to be examined.

PHYSICAL EXAMINATION

Integumentary system: There are a few small, scattered hives still visible on her trunk and arms. The welts on her scalp and face have completely disappeared. The cellulitis of her right foot has cleared up and the nodules from the erythema nodosum have disappeared.

ASSESSMENT

1. Severe urticaria, secondary to a systemic allergic drug reaction to azithromycin.
2. Right foot cellulitis, resolved.
3. Resolving erythema nodosum following an untreated strep throat.

PLAN

A note has been made in the patient's medical record that she is allergic to azithromycin. The acute phase of this allergic reaction has passed. The patient has been instructed to never take that antibiotic drug again. Follow up as needed for her resolving erythema nodosum.

Bonita R. Grant, M.D.

Bonita R. Grant, M.D.

BRG: smt
D: 11/19/xx
T: 11/19/xx

1. Divide *cellulitis* into word parts and give the meaning of each word part.

   Word Part   **Meaning**

   _____   _____

   _____   _____

2. The patient has erythema on her legs. If you wanted to use the adjective form of *erythema*, you would say, "She has _____ areas on her legs."

3. What is the medical word for *itching*? _____

4. Circle the word that means reddened: (**edematous, erythematous, flare-up**)

5. Which are larger—welts or wheals? _____

6. The patient's urticaria was due to a (**cellulitis, drug reaction, strep throat**).

7. What unusual skin condition did the patient develop after having an untreated strep throat? _____

You Create The Electronic Health Record

Read the patient's words. Then read the partial sentence in the electronic health record and fill in the blank with the correct medical word.

1. Patient's words: "I had chickenpox when I was a child. Now, I have this painful skin thing of crusting and raised red areas along my left back and side. It really hurts."

   You type: "The elderly patient has a past history of infection with the _____ _____-_____ virus as a child. She now presents with the vesicles and crusts of _____ along the T6 _____ on the left side."

2. Patient's words: "When I looked in the mirror, I noticed some round areas on my head where I don't have any hair."

   You type: "Examination of the scalp reveals the characteristic round skin lesions caused by the fungus _____ _____. I prescribed a topical _____ drug to treat the ringworm."

3. Patient's words: "I cut myself on a piece of broken glass."

   You type: Examination of the right forearm reveals a long skin _____, but the bleeding has stopped. After a topical _____ drug was placed on the skin to numb the area, the edges of the wound were brought together and _____ were placed to close the wound."

4. Patient's words: "I noticed a strange-looking thing on my skin. It is black and brown with some pink in it, and it seems to be getting bigger."

   You type: "Examination reveals an irregularly shaped lesion of several colors. It has been growing larger. Tentative diagnosis: Malignant _____. The patient was given a consultation for a plastic surgeon to perform a skin _____ to examine the cells and provide a diagnosis."

Research Medical Words

On the job, you will encounter new medical words. Practice your medical language research skills by looking up the medical words in this Office Chart Note and writing their definitions on the lines.

OFFICE CHART NOTE

ASSESSMENT:
This 14-year-old female was brought in by her mother. The mother states that the patient continually bites her fingernails despite all attempts to discourage her. Her fingernails are always bitten to the quick, and the skin around them is frequently bloody. The patient states she is unable to stop. When the mother stepped out of the examination room, the patient became tearful as she related pressure at school and an impending divorce between her parents.

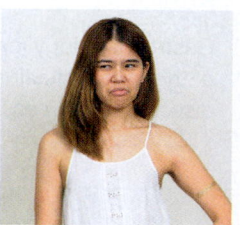

On examination, the fingernails show evidence of chronic biting, right hand greater than left. The patient is right-handed. Examination of the feet also shows evidence of nail biting. There is erythema and swelling of the tissue along the medial nail groove of her right great toe where the nail was bitten away and is growing back but is ingrown. The skin on the lower arms bilaterally shows aggressive scratching of small, isolated insect bites. The scalp shows some small, patchy areas where there is an absence of hair. The patient admits to some hair-pulling, but her greatest concern is that her hair "can never look pretty because I have split ends."

DIAGNOSES:

1. Onychophagia

2. Onychocryptosis

3. Trichotillomania

4. Schizotrichia

PLAN:
The medial side of the nail on the right great toe was trimmed with clippers. The patient was given a prescription for a 7-day course of an antibiotic drug. The patient will get a haircut and use moisturizing shampoo and conditioner. The patient's mother was also given a referral for the patient to see a child psychologist for counseling.

Research and define the following medical words.

1. onychophagia _____

2. onychocryptosis _____

3. trichotillomania _____

4. schizotrichia _____

MyLab Medical Terminology™

MyLab Medical Terminology is a premium online homework management system that includes a host of features to help you study. Registered users will find:

- A multitude of quizzes and activities built within the MyLab platform

- Powerful tools that track and analyze your results—allowing you to create a personalized learning experience

- Videos and audio pronunciations to help enrich your progress

- Streaming lesson presentations (guided lectures) and self-paced learning modules

- A space where you and your instructor can check your progress and manage your assignments

3 Gastroenterology

Gastrointestinal System

Gastroenterology (GAS-troh-EN-ter-AW-loh-jee) is the medical specialty that studies the anatomy and physiology of the gastrointestinal system, uses laboratory, diagnostic, and radiologic procedures to diagnose gastrointestinal diseases, and uses medical procedures, drugs, and surgical procedures to treat gastrointestinal diseases.

∨ Chapter Overview and Learning Outcomes

After you study this chapter, you should be able to demonstrate mastery of the outcomes by successfully completing the exercises.

3.1 Anatomy
Identify the structures of the gastrointestinal system.
Demonstrate proficiency in medical language.
3.1 Practice Laps

3.2 Physiology
Describe the functions of the gastrointestinal system.
Demonstrate proficiency in medical language.
3.2 Practice Laps
Vocabulary Review

3.3 Diseases
Describe common gastrointestinal diseases.
Demonstrate proficiency in medical language.
3.3 Practice Laps

3.4 Laboratory, Diagnostic, and Radiologic Procedures
Describe common gastrointestinal laboratory tests, diagnostic procedures, and radiologic procedures.
Demonstrate proficiency in medical language.
3.4 Practice Laps

3.5 Medical Procedures, Drugs, and Surgical Procedures
Describe common gastrointestinal medical procedures, drugs, and surgical procedures.
Demonstrate proficiency in medical language.
3.5 Practice Laps
Abbreviations Summary
Career Focus

Chapter Review Exercises
Dive In: Medical Language Exercises (Learning Outcomes 3.1–3.5)

Immerse Yourself: Analyze Medical Reports

Medical Language Key

To unlock the definition of a medical word, first break it into word parts. Then give the meaning of each word part. Put the meanings of the word parts in order, beginning with the meaning of the suffix, then the meaning of the prefix (if there is one), then the meaning of the combining form.

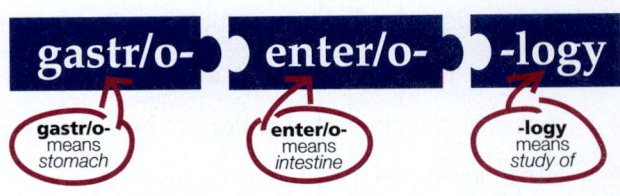

Gastroenterology: ▶ *Study of (the) stomach (and) intestine(s) (and related structures).*

The **gastrointestinal (GI) system** is an elongated body system that begins at the mouth, continues through the thoracic cavity, fills much of the abdominopelvic cavity, and ends on the surface of the lower body (see Figure 3-1 ■). The upper gastrointestinal system extends from the mouth to the stomach. The lower gastrointestinal system extends from the small intestine to the anus. The gastrointestinal system is also known as the **gastrointestinal tract** or **alimentary canal**, as a tract is a continuing pathway and a canal is a tubular channel.

The functions of the gastrointestinal system are to digest food, absorb nutrients, and remove waste materials from the body. The gastrointestinal system is also known as the **digestive system** or **digestive tract**.

3.1 Anatomy

Oral Cavity and Pharynx

The gastrointestinal system begins in the mouth or **oral cavity** (see Figure 3-2 ■). The oral cavity (and the entire gastrointestinal system) is lined with **mucosa**, a mucous membrane that produces thin mucus. The oral cavity contains the teeth, gums, tongue, hard palate, and soft palate.

The teeth bring pieces of food into the oral cavity. The **tongue** is a large muscle that fills the oral cavity and assists with eating and talking, as it mixes food particles with saliva. The sense of taste is also associated with the tongue. Receptors on the tongue perceive taste and send this sensory information to the **gustatory cortex** in the brain.

The sight, smell, and taste of food cause the **salivary glands** to release saliva into the oral cavity. There are three pairs of salivary glands on either side of the head: the **parotid glands**, **sublingual glands**, and **submandibular glands** (see Figure 3-3 ■). **Saliva** is a lubricant that moistens the food particles as they are chewed. Saliva contains the digestive enzyme amylase.

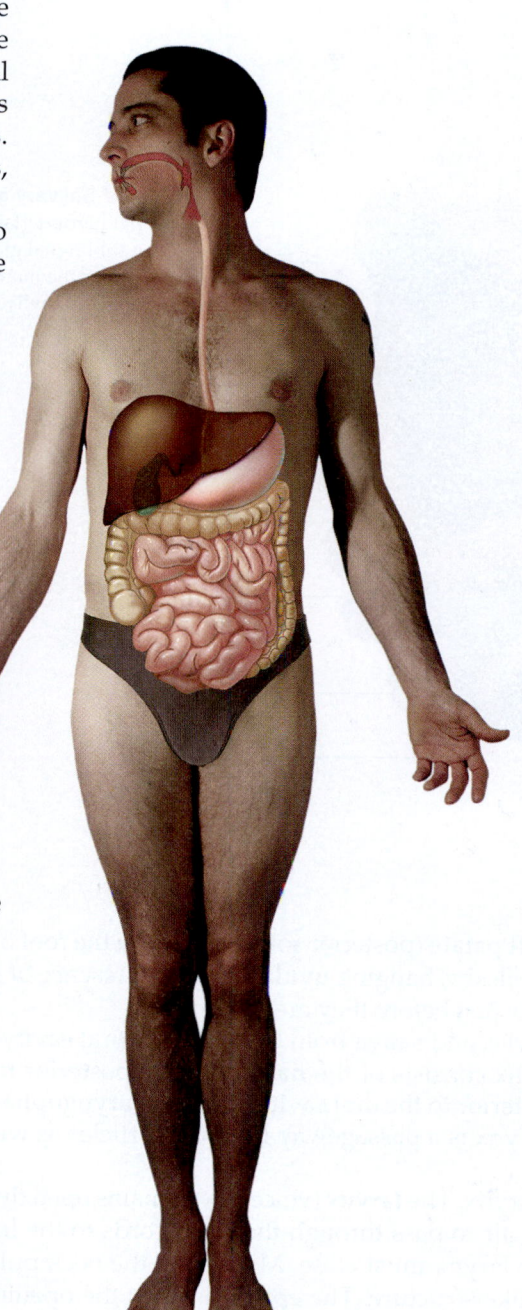

FIGURE 3-1 ■ Gastrointestinal system.
The gastrointestinal system consists of organs and glands connected in a pathway. Food enters the body, is digested, nutrients are absorbed into the blood, and undigested wastes are eliminated from the body.

Pronunciation/Word Parts

gastrointestinal (GAS-troh-in-TES-tih-nal)
  gastr/o- *stomach*
  intestin/o- *intestine*
  -al *pertaining to*

system (SIHS-tem)

tract (TRAKT)

alimentary (AL-ih-MEN-tair-ee)
  aliment/o- *food; nourishment*
  -ary *pertaining to*

canal (kah-NAL)

digestive (dy-JES-tiv)
  digest/o- *break down food; digest*
  -ive *pertaining to*

oral (OR-al)
  or/o- *mouth*
  -al *pertaining to*
Oral is the adjective for *mouth*. The combining form **stomat/o-** also means *mouth*.

cavity (KAV-ih-tee)

mucosa (myoo-KOH-sah)

mucosal (myoo-KOH-sal)
  mucos/o- *mucous membrane*
  -al *pertaining to*

tongue (TUNG)
Tongue is from an Old English word meaning *organ of speech*. The combining form **gloss/o-** means *tongue*.

lingual (LING-gwal)
  lingu/o- *tongue*
  -al *pertaining to*
Lingual is the adjective for *tongue*.

gustatory (GUS-tah-TOR-ee)
  gustat/o- *sense of taste*
  -ory *having the function of*

salivary (SAL-ih-VAIR-ee)
  saliv/o- *saliva*
  -ary *pertaining to*
The combining form **sial/o-** means *saliva; salivary gland*.

parotid (pah-RAW-tid)
  par- *beside*
  ot/o- *ear*
  -id *origin; resembling; source*

sublingual (sub-LING-gwal)
  sub- *below; underneath*
  lingu/o- *tongue*
  -al *pertaining to*

submandibular (SUB-man-DIH-byoo-lar)
  sub- *below; underneath*
  mandibul/o- *lower jaw; mandible*
  -ar *pertaining to*

saliva (sah-LY-vah)

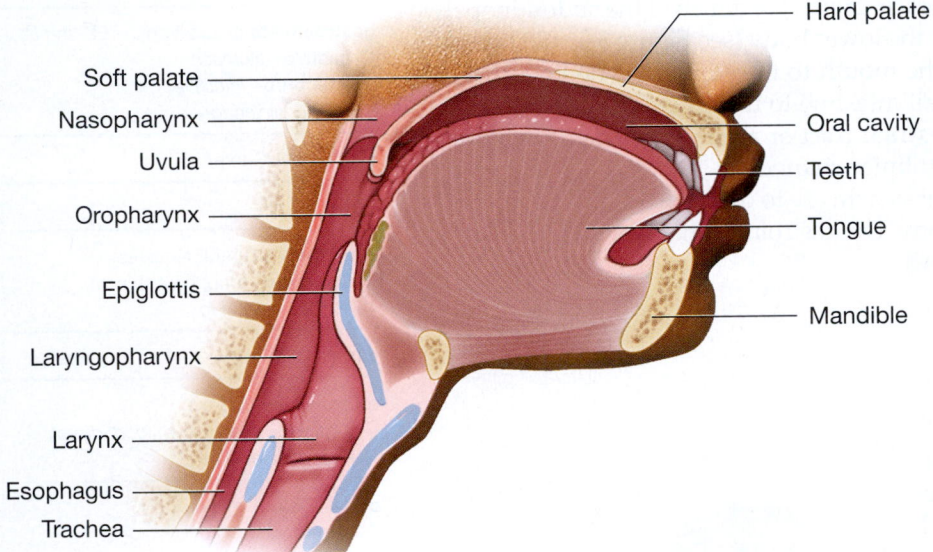

Hard palate

Soft palate

Nasopharynx

Uvula

Oropharynx

Epiglottis

Laryngopharynx

Larynx

Esophagus

Trachea

Oral cavity

Teeth

Tongue

Mandible

FIGURE 3-2 ■ **Oral cavity and pharynx.**
The oral cavity contains the teeth, tongue, and the hard and soft palates. Food passes from the oral cavity into the pharynx (throat) and then into the esophagus.

FIGURE 3-3 ■ **Salivary glands.**
The large, flat parotid glands are on either side of the head in front of the ear. The sublingual glands are under the tongue. The submandibular glands are under the mandible (lower jaw). Ducts from these glands bring saliva into the oral cavity.

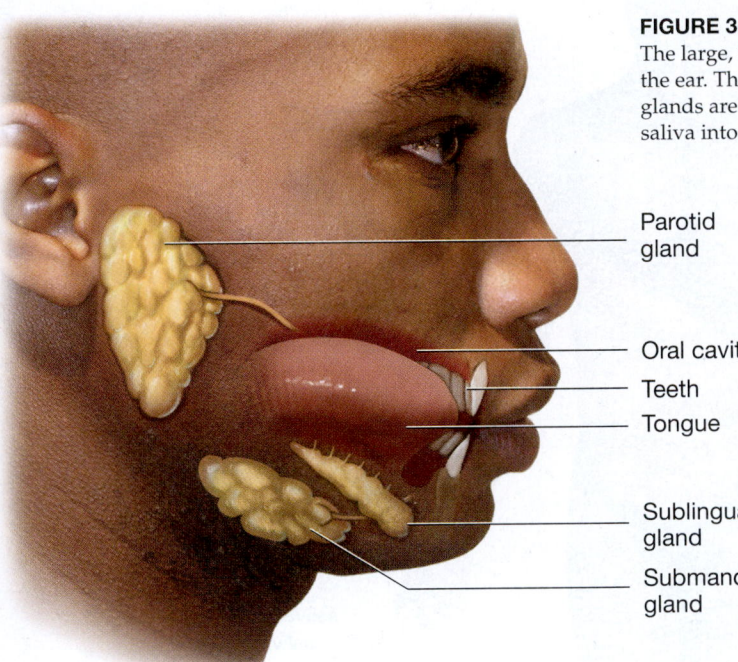

Parotid gland

Oral cavity

Teeth

Tongue

Sublingual gland

Submandibular gland

Pronunciation/Word Parts

palate (PAL-at)

uvula (YOO-vyoo-lah)

pharynx (FAIR-ingks)
Pharynx is a Greek word that means *throat.*

pharyngeal (fah-RIN-jee-al)
  pharyng/o- *pharynx; throat*
  -eal *pertaining to*

nasopharynx (NAY-soh-FAIR-ingks)
  nas/o- *nose*
  -pharynx *pharynx; throat*

oropharynx (OR-oh-FAIR-ingks)
  or/o- *mouth*
  -pharynx *pharynx; throat*

laryngopharynx (lah-RING-goh-FAIR-ingks)
  laryng/o- *larynx; voice box*
  -pharynx *pharynx; throat*

larynx (LAIR-ingks)

laryngeal (lah-RIN-jee-al)
  laryng/o- *larynx; voice box*
  -eal *pertaining to*

epiglottis (EP-ih-GLAW-tihs)
The combining form **glott/o-** means *glottis of the larynx.*

The **hard palate** (bone) and **soft palate** (posterior soft tissue) form the roof of the oral cavity. The soft palate and the fleshy, hanging **uvula** sense the presence of food particles in the posterior oral cavity just before they are swallowed.

Swallowing moves food particles and saliva from the posterior oral cavity into the **pharynx** or throat. The pharynx consists of the **nasopharynx** (posterior to the nasal cavity), the **oropharynx** (posterior to the oral cavity), and the **laryngopharynx** (posterior to the larynx). The pharynx is a passageway for food particles as well as for inhaled and exhaled air.

Inferior to the pharynx is the larynx. The **larynx** (voice box) remains open during breathing and speaking, allowing air to pass through the vocal cords to the lungs. However, during swallowing, the larynx must close. Muscles in the neck pull the larynx up to the **epiglottis**, a lid-like structure. The epiglottis seals the opening to the larynx so that swallowed food particles are diverted and go into the esophagus to the stomach, not into the trachea to the lungs.

Across the Life Span

Pediatrics. The first food for many babies is colostrum from the mother's breast. Colostrum is rich in nutrients and contains maternal antibodies. For the first few days of life, the newborn's intestinal tract is permeable and allows these antibodies to be absorbed from the intestine into the blood, where they provide the baby with passive immunity to common infectious diseases that the mother has had.

Geriatrics. Older adults often complain that food is not as tasty as when they were young. The aging process causes a very real decline in the ability to smell and taste food as the number of receptors in the nose and tongue decreases.

Esophagus

From the pharynx, swallowed food particles move into the **esophagus** (see Figure 3-2), a flexible tube approximately 10 inches in length that is between the pharynx and the stomach. The upper part of the esophagus is located in the neck; the lower part is in the thoracic cavity. The esophagus is lined with mucosa that produces thin mucus. With coordinated muscle contractions of its wall (known as **peristalsis**), the esophagus moves food particles toward the stomach.

Stomach

The **stomach** (see Figure 3-4 ■) is a large, elongated sac in the upper abdominal cavity. It receives food particles from the esophagus. The stomach is divided into four regions: the cardia, fundus, body, and pylorus. The **cardia** is the first part of the stomach where it joins the esophagus. The **fundus** is the rounded, top part of the stomach. The body is the main part of the stomach. The **pylorus** is the narrowed, last part of the stomach where it joins the duodenum. The gastric mucosa is arranged in thick, deep folds, or **rugae** that expand as the stomach fills. The stomach produces hydrochloric acid and the digestive enzymes of pepsinogen and gastrin. The gastric mucosa produces thin mucus that protects the lining of the stomach from the hydrochloric acid.

Chyme is a semisolid mixture of food particles, saliva, and digestive enzymes. Two sphincters (muscular rings) keep chyme in the stomach. The **lower esophageal sphincter** is located at the distal end of the esophagus. This sphincter prevents chyme from flowing back into the esophagus. The **pyloric sphincter** is located at the distal end of the stomach. It keeps chyme in the stomach for an hour or so after eating until it opens, and the chyme moves into the small intestine.

Pronunciation/Word Parts

esophagus (eh-SAW-fah-guhs)

esophageal (eh-SAW-fah-JEE-al)
  esophag/o- *esophagus*
  -eal *pertaining to*

peristalsis (PAIR-ih-STAL-sihs)
The prefix **peri-** means *around*.
The suffix **-stalsis** means *process of contraction*.

stomach (STUM-ak)

gastric (GAS-trik)
  gastr/o- *stomach*
  -ic *pertaining to*
Gastric is the adjective for *stomach*.

cardia (KAR-dee-ah)

fundus (FUN-duhs)

pylorus (py-LOR-uhs)

pyloric (py-LOR-ik)
  pylor/o- *pylorus*
  -ic *pertaining to*

rugae (ROO-jee)
Rugae is a Latin plural noun. Because there are so many rugae in the stomach, the singular form (*ruga*) is not used.

chyme (KIME)

sphincter (SFINGK-ter)
  sphinct/o- *close tightly*
  -er *person who does or produces; thing that does or produces*

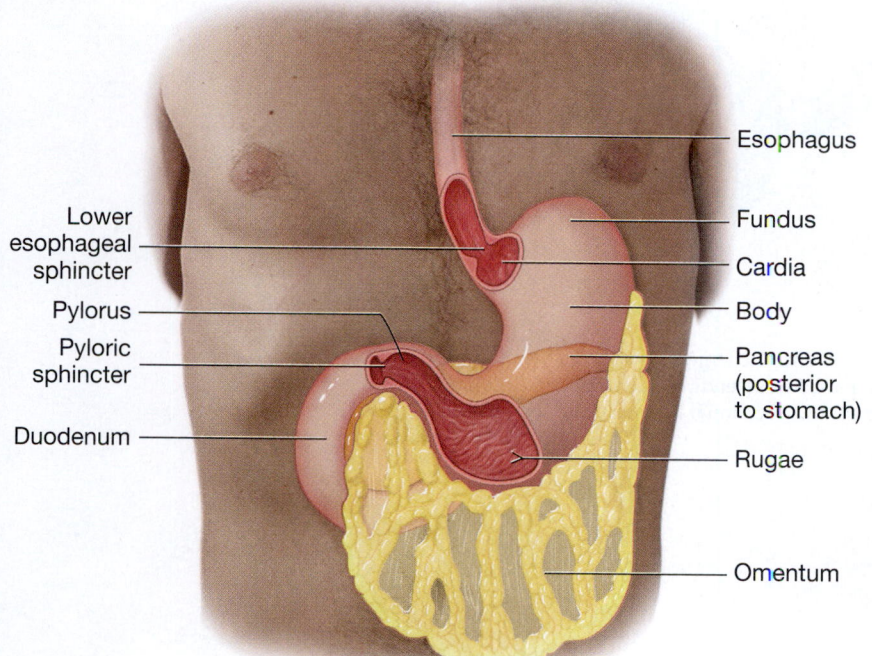

FIGURE 3-4 ■ **Stomach.**
The stomach has four regions. The cardia is a small area where the esophagus joins the stomach. The fundus is the rounded top of the stomach. The body is the large, curved part of the stomach. The pylorus is where the stomach narrows to join the first part of the small intestine.

Small Intestine

The **small intestine** or **small bowel** is located in the abdominopelvic cavity. It is a long tubular structure between the stomach and the large intestine. The small intestine receives chyme from the stomach. The small intestine consists of the duodenum, jejunum, and ileum (see Figure 3-5 ■).

The **duodenum** is an approximately 10-inch, C-shaped segment of small intestine that begins at the stomach and ends at the jejunum. The **jejunum**, the second part of the small intestine, is an 8-foot coiled segment. The **ileum** is 12 feet in length and is the final part of the small intestine.

The small intestine produces digestive enzymes, and other digestive enzymes from the gallbladder and pancreas (described in the next section) flow through ducts into the duodenum. The small intestine contains thousands of **villi**, which are microscopic, thin structures that project into the **lumen** (central, open area). Villi increase the amount of surface area to maximize the absorption of digested nutrients and water from the small intestine into the blood. Peristalsis slowly moves food through the small intestine as it is being digested, and then the remaining waste material and water move into the large intestine.

Pronunciation/Word Parts

intestine (in-TES-tin)

intestinal (in-TES-tih-nal)
  intestin/o- *intestine*
  -al *pertaining to*
The combining form **enter/o-** also means *intestine.*

duodenum (DOO-oh-DEE-num)

duodenal (DOO-oh-DEE-nal)
  duoden/o- *duodenum*
  -al *pertaining to*
Duodenum comes from a Latin word meaning *twelve.* Roman physicians found that the duodenum was always 12 fingerbreadths (10 inches) in length.

jejunum (jeh-JOO-num)

jejunal (jeh-JOO-nal)
  jejun/o- *jejunum*
  -al *pertaining to*

ileum (IL-ee-um)

ileal (IL-ee-al)
  ile/o- *ileum*
  -al *pertaining to*

villi (VIL-eye)
Villi is a Latin plural noun. Because there are so many villi, the singular form (*villus*) is not used.

lumen (LOO-men)

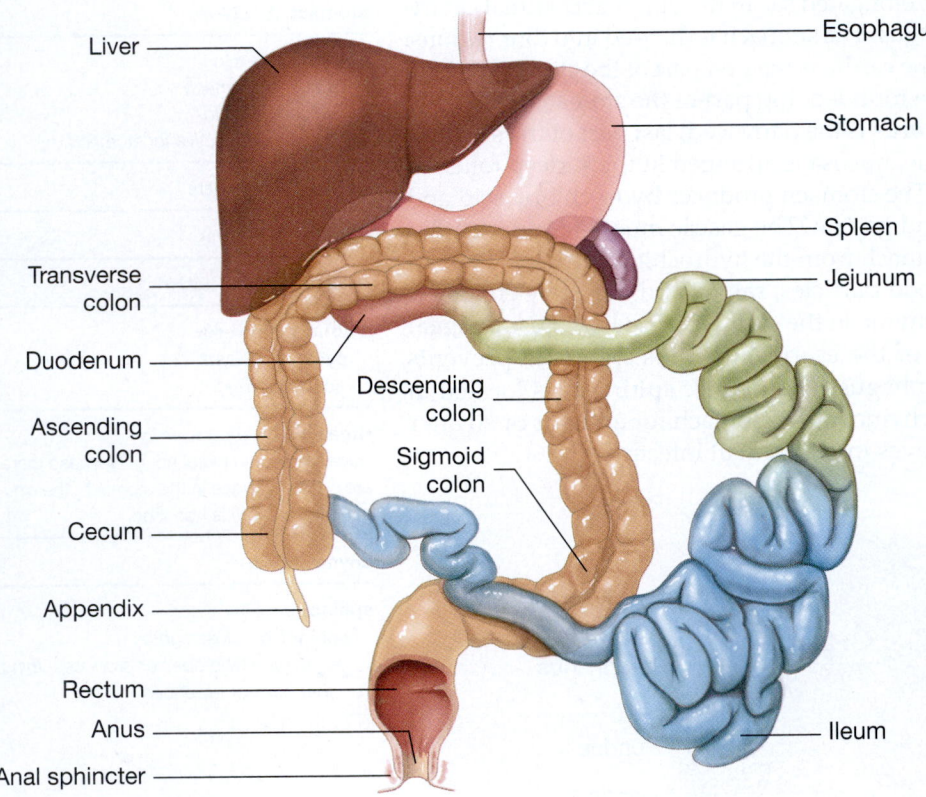

FIGURE 3-5 ■ Small and large intestines.
The small intestine consists of the duodenum, jejunum, and ileum. The large intestine consists of the cecum, colon, rectum, and anus. The colon is divided into parts: the ascending colon, transverse colon, descending colon, and sigmoid colon. Each part is named for the direction it is going or for its shape.

Pronunciation/Word Parts

Word Alert
Sound-Alike Words

ileum	(noun)	the final part of the small intestine
		Example: The ileum is the segment of small intestine just before the large intestine begins.
ilium	(noun)	the most superior part of the hip bone
		Example: The ilium contains the cup-shaped socket of the hip joint.

Large Intestine

The **large intestine** or **large bowel** is approximately 5 feet in length and is located in the abdominopelvic cavity. The walls of the large intestine contain **haustra** (puckered pouches) that can expand to receive large amounts of waste material and water from the ileum. This waste material and water move slowly through the parts of the large intestine, which include the cecum, colon, rectum, and anus (see Figure 3-5).

The first part of the large intestine, the **cecum**, is a short sac. The **ileocecal valve** keeps the waste material and water from flowing back into the ileum. Hanging from the external wall of the cecum is the **appendix**, a thin pouch that is usually 4 inches long but can be up to 8 inches long! The appendix is not part of the gastrointestinal system; it contains lymphoid tissue that is active in an immune response (described in Chapter 6, Hematology and Immunology).

The **colon** is the second and longest part of the large intestine. The parts of the colon include the **ascending colon**, **transverse colon**, **descending colon**, and **sigmoid colon**. The colon travels through all four quadrants of the abdominopelvic cavity. From the cecum, the ascending colon travels upward, the transverse colon travels across, and the descending colon travels downward. Then the sigmoid colon bends toward the midline in an S-shaped curve that joins the rectum.

The **rectum** is a short, straight final segment of the large intestine, and it connects to the outside of the body. The **anus**, the external opening of the rectum, is located between the buttocks. The **anal sphincter** is a muscular ring whose opening and closing is under conscious, voluntary control.

Abdominopelvic Cavity

The anterior **abdominal wall** is divided into four quadrants or nine regions (described in Chapter 1, Medical Language and Health Care Today).

The **abdominopelvic cavity** is a continuous cavity within the abdomen and pelvis, and it contains the largest organs of the gastrointestinal system. The abdominopelvic cavity is lined with **peritoneum**, a double-layered serous membrane. One layer lines the walls of the abdominopelvic cavity. The other layer surrounds the gastrointestinal organs. The peritoneum secretes **peritoneal fluid**, a watery fluid that fills the spaces between the gastrointestinal organs and allows them to slide past each other during the movements of digestion.

---

haustra (HAW-strah)
Haustra is a Latin plural noun. Because there are so many haustra, the singular form (*haustrum*) is not used.

cecum (SEE-kum)

cecal (SEE-kal)
  cec/o- cecum
  -al *pertaining to*

ileocecal (IL-ee-oh-SEE-kal)
  ile/o- *ileum*
  cec/o- *cecum*
  -al *pertaining to*

appendix (ah-PEN-diks)
  append/o- *small structure hanging from a larger structure*
  -ix *thing*

appendiceal (AP-en-DIH-see-al)
  appendic/o- *appendix*
  -eal *pertaining to*

colon (KOH-lon)

colonic (koh-LAW-nik)
  colon/o- *colon*
  -ic *pertaining to*
The combining form **col/o-** also means *colon*.

sigmoid (SIG-moyd)
Sigmoid is a combination of the S-shaped Greek letter *sigma* Σ and the suffix **-oid** (resembling). The combining form **sigmoid/o-** means *sigmoid colon*.

rectum (REK-tum)

rectal (REK-tal)
  rect/o- *rectum*
  -al *pertaining to*
The combining form **proct/o-** means *rectum and anus*.

anus (AA-nuhs)

anal (AA-nal)
  an/o- *anus*
  -al *pertaining to*

abdominal (ab-DAW-mih-nal)
  abdomin/o- *abdomen*
  -al *pertaining to*
The combining forms **celi/o-** and **lapar/o-** also mean *abdomen*.

abdominopelvic (ab-DAW-mih-noh-PEL-vik)
  abdomin/o- *abdomen*
  pelv/o- *hip bone; pelvis; renal pelvis*
  -ic *pertaining to*

cavity (KAV-ih-tee)

peritoneum (PAIR-ih-toh-NEE-um)

peritoneal (PAIR-ih-toh-NEE-al)
  peritone/o- *peritoneum*
  -al *pertaining to*
The combining form **periton/o-** also means *peritoneum*.

One part of the peritoneum in the center of the abdominopelvic cavity becomes the **omentum** (see Figure 3-4). The omentum supports the stomach and hangs down as a broad, fatty covering to protect the small intestine. The other part of the peritoneum becomes the **mesentery**, a thick, fan-shaped sheet that supports loops of the jejunum and ileum (see Figure 3-18).

Accessory Organs

The liver, gallbladder, and pancreas are accessory organs of the gastrointestinal system. They contribute to the process of digestion, but food does not actually pass through them.

The **liver**, a large, dark red-brown organ, is located in the right upper quadrant (RUQ) of the abdominal cavity (see Figure 3-6 ■). Liver cells (**hepatocytes**) produce the digestive enzyme **bile**, which is a thick, yellow-green fluid. Bile contains bile acids, the yellow pigment **bilirubin**, and the green pigment **biliverdin**. Bile produced by the liver flows through the common hepatic duct and into the common bile duct (CBD). When that duct is full, bile fills the cystic duct of the gallbladder and then the gallbladder itself. All of the **bile ducts** are collectively known as the **biliary tree**.

The **gallbladder** is a teardrop-shaped, dark green sac posterior to the liver (see Figure 3-6). It concentrates and stores bile from the liver. Fatty chyme in the duodenum causes the gallbladder to contract and release bile into the duodenum.

The **pancreas** is a yellow, elongated, triangular organ that is posterior to the stomach (see Figure 3-6). The pancreas secretes several digestive enzymes through the pancreatic duct and into the duodenum. The **pancreas** is a gland of both the gastrointestinal system and the endocrine system (described in Chapter 13, Endocrinology).

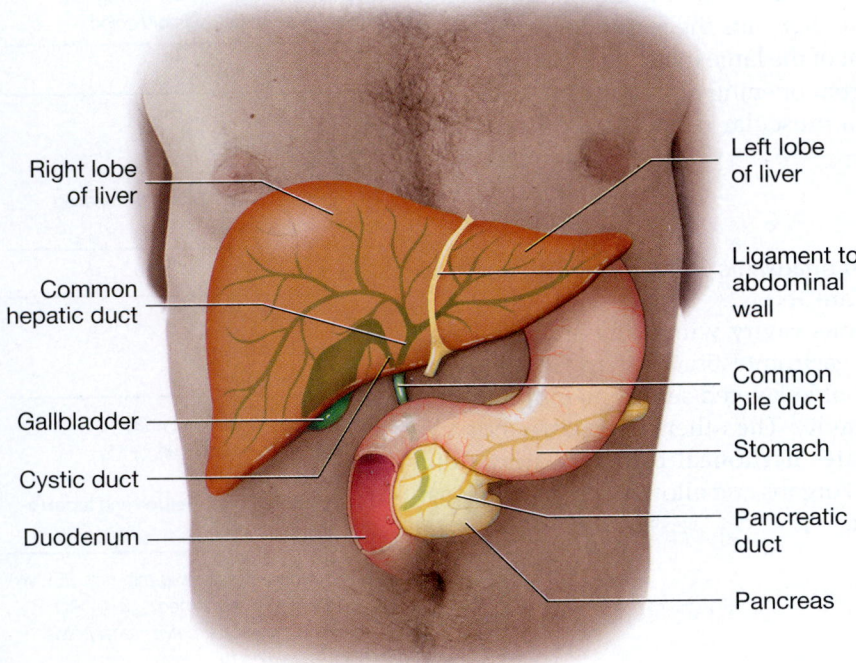

Right lobe of liver

Common hepatic duct

Gallbladder

Cystic duct

Duodenum

Left lobe of liver

Ligament to abdominal wall

Common bile duct

Stomach

Pancreatic duct

Pancreas

FIGURE 3-6 ■ Biliary tree.
Bile flows through hepatic ducts in the liver that merge to form the common hepatic duct. It joins the cystic duct from the gallbladder and becomes the common bile duct. Because of their branched appearance, these ducts are known as the *biliary tree.* The pancreatic duct joins the common bile duct just before it enters the duodenum.

Pronunciation/Word Parts

omentum (oh-MEN-tum)

mesentery (MEZ-en-TAIR-ee)

mesenteric (MEZ-en-TAIR-ik)
  mesenter/o- *middle thing between the intestines*
  -ic *pertaining to*

liver (LIV-er)

hepatic (heh-PAT-ik)
  hepat/o- *liver*
  -ic *pertaining to*
Hepatic is the adjective for *liver.*

hepatocyte (HEP-ah-toh-SITE)
  hepat/o- *liver*
  -cyte *cell*

bile (BILE)
The combining forms **bil/i-, bili/o-,** and **chol/e-** mean *bile; gall.*

bilirubin (BIL-ih-ROO-bin)
  bil/i- *bile; gall*
  rub/o- *red*
  -in *substance*
Rub/o- refers to red blood cells that are used by the liver to make bilirubin.

biliverdin (BIL-ih-VER-din)
Verd/o- means *green.*

bile duct (BILE DUKT)
The combining form **cholangi/o-** means *bile duct,* and **choledoch/o-** means *common bile duct.*

biliary (BIL-ee-AIR-ee)
  bili/o- *bile; gall*
  -ary *pertaining to*
Gall is an older name for *bile.*

gallbladder (GAWL-blad-er)
The combining form **cholecyst/o-** means *gallbladder.*

pancreas (PAN-kree-as)

pancreatic (PAN-kree-AT-ik)
  pancreat/o- *pancreas*
  -ic *pertaining to*

3.1 PRACTICE LAPS

Use the Answer Key at the end of the book to check your answers.

A. Label Structures

Write each anatomy word or phrase in the correct numbered box. Be sure to check your spelling.

| esophagus | parotid gland | sublingual gland | teeth |
| oral cavity | pharynx | submandibular gland | tongue |

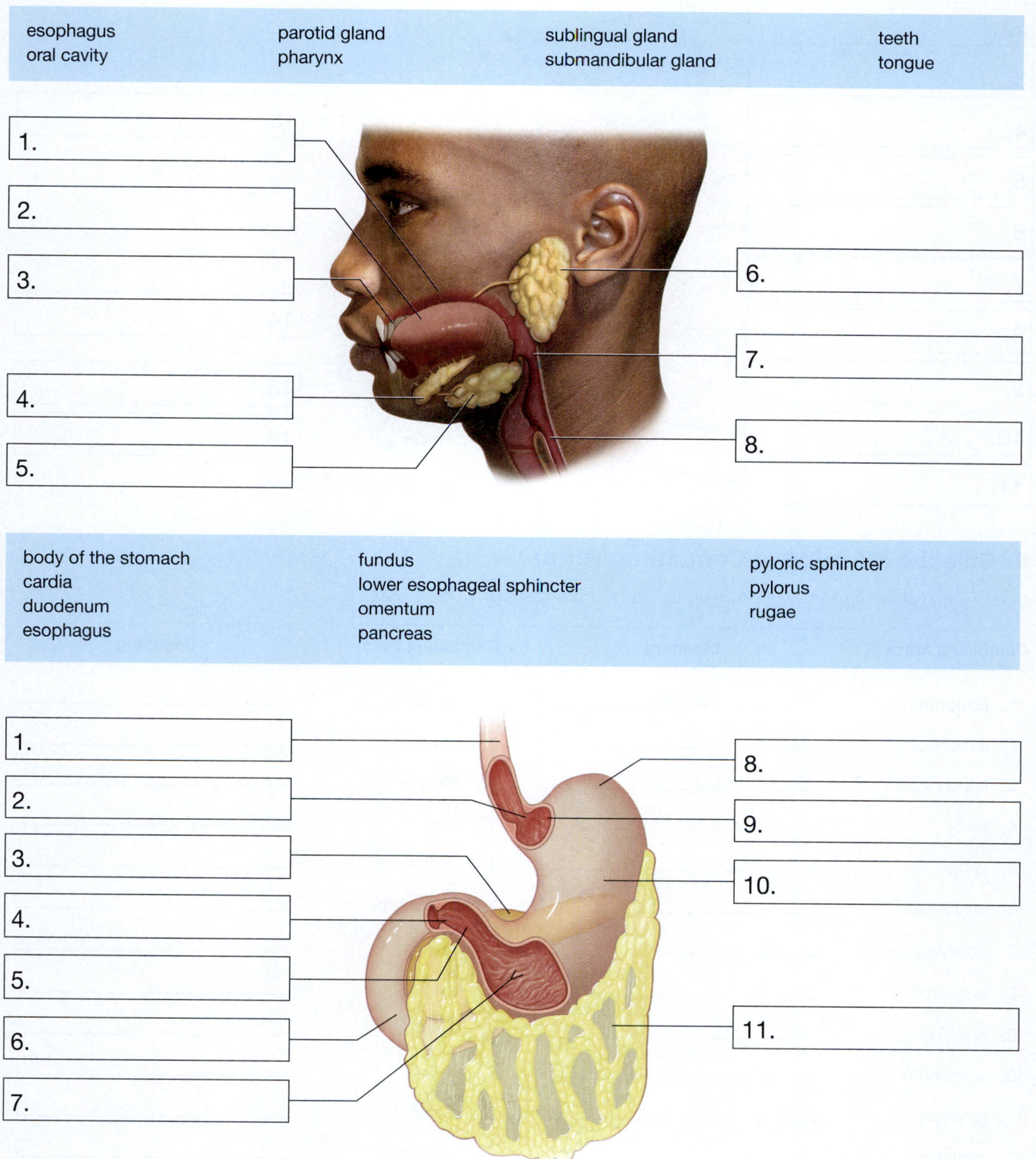

1.
2.
3.
4.
5.
6.
7.
8.

body of the stomach	fundus	pyloric sphincter
cardia	lower esophageal sphincter	pylorus
duodenum	omentum	rugae
esophagus	pancreas	

1.
2.
3.
4.
5.
6.
7.
8.
9.
10.
11.

anal sphincter	cecum	ileum	rectum
anus	descending colon	jejunum	sigmoid colon
appendix	duodenum	liver	stomach
ascending colon	gallbladder	pancreas	transverse colon

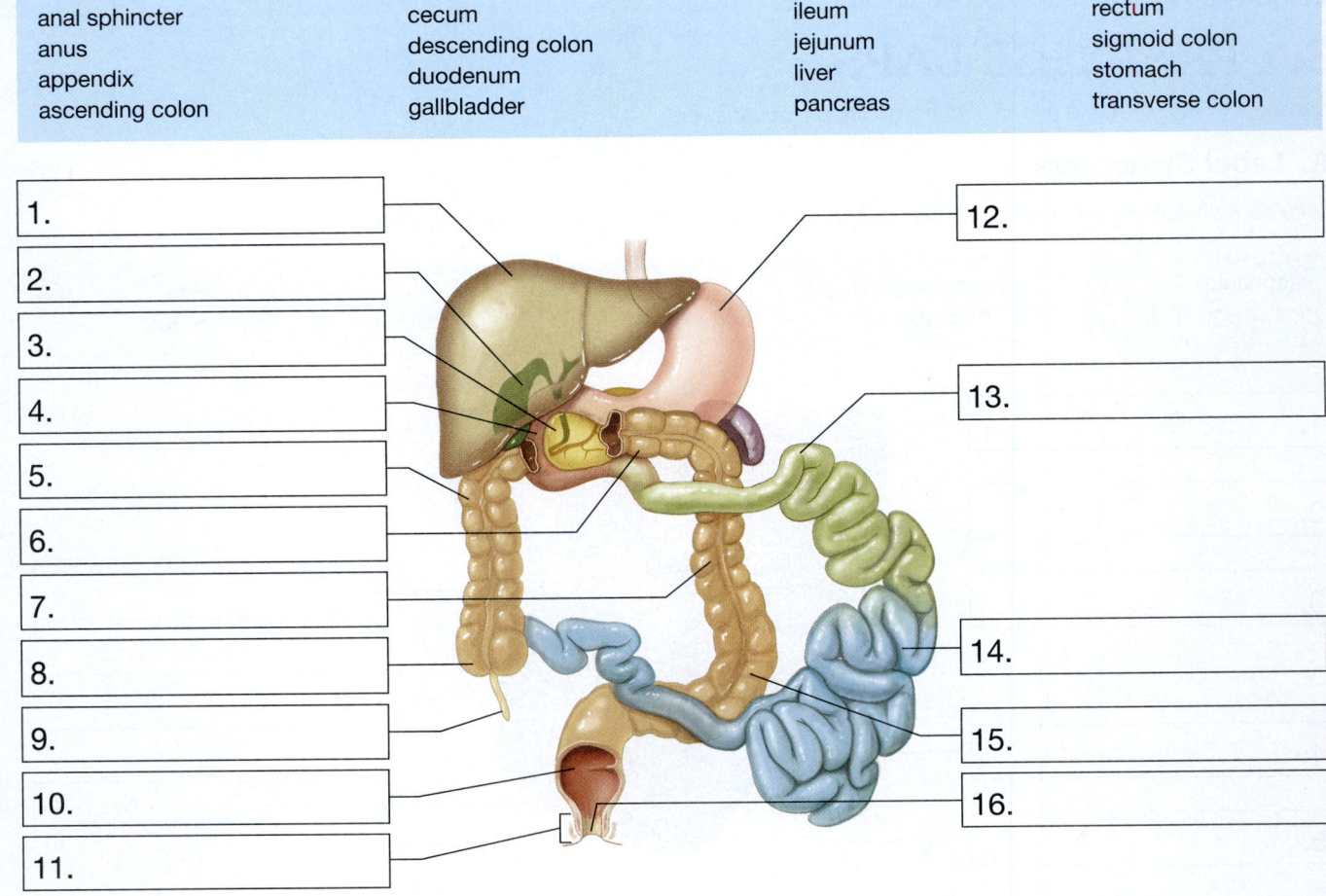

1. _____

2. _____

3. _____

4. _____

5. _____

6. _____

7. _____

8. _____

9. _____

10. _____

11. _____

12. _____

13. _____

14. _____

15. _____

16. _____

B. Give the Meaning of Combining Forms

Next to each combining form, write its meaning. The first one has been done for you.

Combining Form	Meaning	Combining Form	Meaning
1. **abdomin/o-**	*abdomen*	14. intestin/o-	_____
2. aliment/o-	_____	15. jejun/o-	_____
3. appendic/o-	_____	16. lingu/o-	_____
4. bili/o-	_____	17. or/o-	_____
5. cec/o-	_____	18. peritone/o-	_____
6. cholecyst/o-	_____	19. pharyng/o-	_____
7. colon/o-	_____	20. proct/o-	_____
8. duoden/o-	_____	21. pylor/o-	_____
9. enter/o-	_____	22. rect/o-	_____
10. esophag/o-	_____	23. saliv/o-	_____
11. gastr/o-	_____	24. sigmoid/o-	_____
12. gustat/o-	_____	25. stomat/o-	_____
13. hepat/o-	_____		

C. Build Words

Read the definition of the medical word. Look at the combining form that is given. Select the correct suffix from the Suffix List, and write it on the blank line. Then build the medical word, and write it on the line. (Remember: You may need to remove the combining vowel. Always remove the hyphens and slash.) Be sure to check your spelling.

Suffix List

-al (pertaining to) -ary (pertaining to)	-cyte (cell) -eal (pertaining to)	-er (thing that does or produces) -ic (pertaining to)	-ix (thing) -ory (having the function of)

Definition of the Medical Word	Combining Form	Suffix	Build the Medical Word
Example: Pertaining to (the) ileum	*ile/o-*	*-al*	*ileal*

[*You think* pertaining to (-al) + ileum (ile/o-). You change the order of the word parts to put the suffix last. You combine the word parts and write ileal.]

	Definition of the Medical Word	Combining Form	Suffix	Build the Medical Word
1.	Pertaining to (the) appendix	appendic/o-	_____	_____
2.	Pertaining to (the) colon	colon/o-	_____	_____
3.	Cell (that is in the) liver	hepat/o-	_____	_____
4.	Pertaining to (the) bile	bili/o-	_____	_____
5.	Pertaining to food (and) nourishment	aliment/o-	_____	_____
6.	Pertaining to (the) mouth	or/o-	_____	_____
7.	Having the function of (the) sense of taste	gustat/o-	_____	_____
8.	Pertaining to (the) stomach	gastr/o-	_____	_____
9.	Pertaining to (the) saliva	saliv/o-	_____	_____
10.	Thing (that is a) small structure hanging from a larger structure	append/o-	_____	_____
11.	Pertaining to (the) intestine	intestin/o-	_____	_____
12.	Pertaining to (the) liver	hepat/o-	_____	_____
13.	Thing that does close tightly	sphinct/o-	_____	_____
14.	Pertaining to (the) esophagus	esophag/o-	_____	_____

3.2 Physiology

The functions of the gastrointestinal system are to digest food, absorb nutrients, and remove waste products from the body. This involves the processes of digestion, absorption, and elimination.

Digestion

The process of digestion begins in the oral cavity and continues throughout the small intestine (see Figure 3-7 ■). Digestion consists of two processes: mechanical digestion and chemical digestion.

Mechanical digestion involves some type of physical force and movement, and it has three steps: mastication, deglutition, and peristalsis. **Mastication** involves the

Pronunciation/Word Parts

digestion (dy-JES-chun)
  digest/o- *break down food; digest*
  -ion *action; condition*

mechanical (meh-KAN-ih-kal)
  mechanic/o- *physical force; tool*
  -al *pertaining to*

mastication (MAS-tih-KAY-shun)
  mastic/o- *chewing*
  -ation *being; having; process*

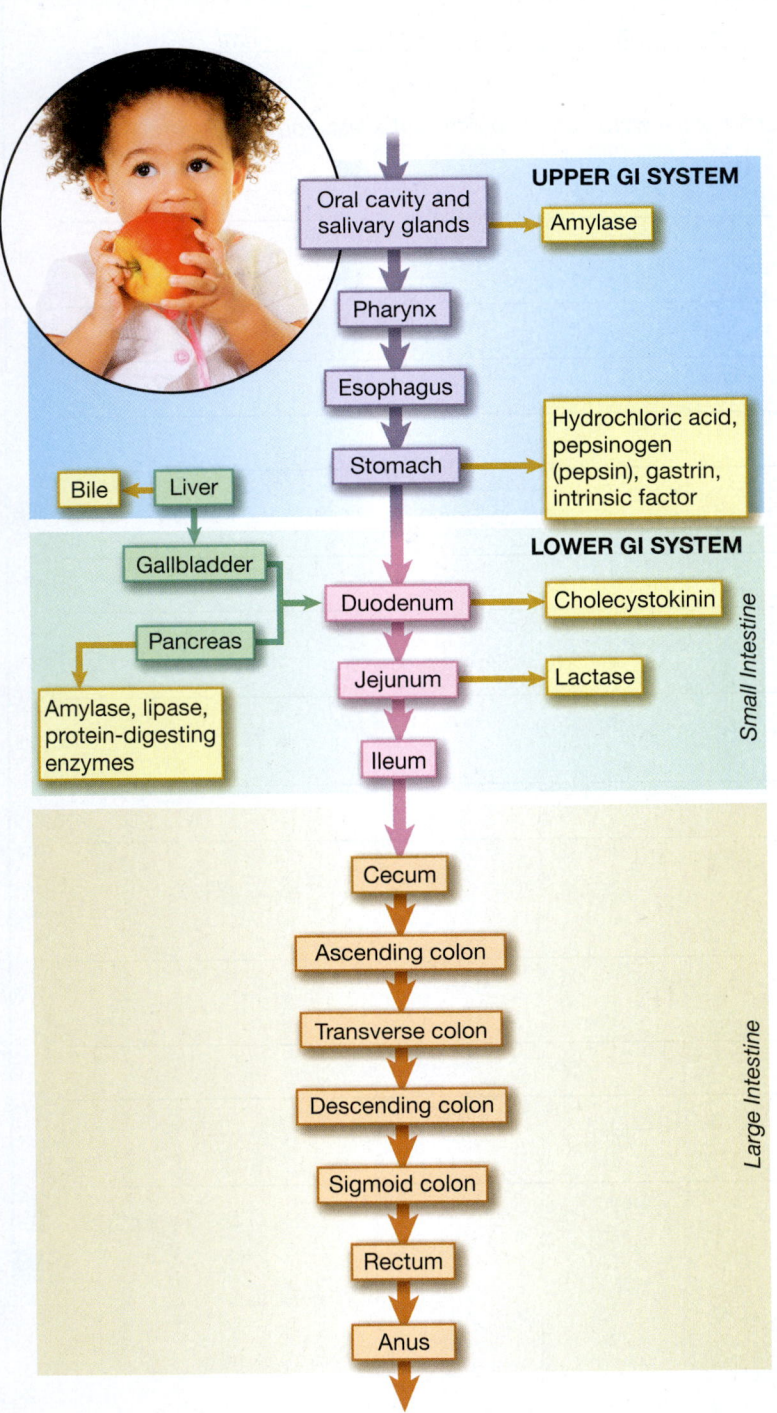

UPPER GI SYSTEM

Oral cavity and salivary glands → Amylase

Pharynx

Esophagus

Stomach → Hydrochloric acid, pepsinogen (pepsin), gastrin, intrinsic factor

Bile ← Liver

LOWER GI SYSTEM

Gallbladder

Pancreas

Amylase, lipase, protein-digesting enzymes

Duodenum → Cholecystokinin

Jejunum → Lactase

Ileum

Small Intestine

Cecum

Ascending colon

Transverse colon

Descending colon

Sigmoid colon

Rectum

Anus

Large Intestine

FIGURE 3-7 ■ **Gastrointestinal system.**
Everyone enjoys eating! The gastrointestinal system helps you taste and enjoy the food you eat and then uses mechanical and chemical digestion processes to break down that food into nutrients that nourish your body.

teeth as they tear, chew, and grind food in the oral cavity, as well as the tongue as it moves food particles around in the mouth and mixes them with saliva. **Deglutition** is the process of swallowing that occurs when food particles in the oral cavity are swallowed and move into the pharynx. It is important to realize that, during swallowing, the epiglottis closes off the entrance to the larynx (voice box), so that food particles in the pharynx do not enter the larynx and go into the lungs. If the larynx is not yet closed, this initiates the gag reflex. Deglutition moves food particles from the pharynx and into the esophagus. In the esophagus, the mechanical digestion process of peristalsis begins. **Peristalsis** involves coordinated waves of contractions of smooth muscle in the walls of the esophagus, stomach, and intestines to move food particles, then chyme, and finally waste materials and water through the digestive system.

Chemical digestion uses digestive enzymes, acids, and other substances to chemically break down food into its component parts. **Enzymes** are substances that speed up chemical reactions. Chemical digestion begins in the oral cavity. The enzyme **amylase** in saliva begins to break down carbohydrate foods.

Chemical digestion continues in the stomach, as the stomach secretes the following substances.

- **Hydrochloric acid**. This strong acid breaks down food fibers and converts pepsinogen to the digestive enzyme pepsin. Hydrochloric acid also destroys microorganisms in foods and liquids that have been eaten.
- **Pepsinogen**. This inactive substance is converted to **pepsin**, a digestive enzyme that breaks down protein foods.
- **Gastrin**. This hormone stimulates the release of more hydrochloric acid and pepsinogen.
- **Intrinsic factor**. This substance helps the stomach absorb vitamin B_{12}.

Chemical digestion continues in the small intestine. In order to digest the sugars in foods, the small intestine produces lactase and other sugar-digesting enzymes. **Lactase** breaks down complex sugar molecules and the sugar in milk to become the simple sugar **glucose**, which is the only source of energy that body cells can use. In order to digest the fats in food, the duodenum releases **cholecystokinin**, a hormone that stimulates the gallbladder to release bile into the duodenum when there is fatty chyme in the duodenum. **Bile** breaks down fats in the chyme into small fat globules. This chemical process is known as **emulsification**. Cholecystokinin also stimulates the pancreas to secrete its digestive enzymes into the duodenum. The pancreatic digestive enzymes include the following.

- **Amylase**. This pancreatic digestive enzyme continues the digestion of carbohydrates that began in the oral cavity. Amylase further breaks down complex sugar molecules into glucose and into food fibers to be eliminated.
- **Lipase**. This pancreatic digestive enzyme breaks down small fat globules into fatty acids.
- Protein-digesting enzymes break down protein molecules into amino acids, the building blocks of cells and tissues.

Absorption

The process of absorption occurs as substances move into the blood that is in blood vessels that surround the gastrointestinal system. In the oral cavity, water and some of the fluids in foods and drinks are absorbed into the blood that is in blood vessels under the tongue. In the stomach, water and some liquid/dissolved drugs are absorbed into the blood. However, partially digested food particles as chyme in the stomach are not yet absorbed into the blood. It is only when digestion is complete that water and food nutrients are absorbed from the small intestine. The majority of absorption of food nutrients and water takes place in the ileum. Absorption of any remaining water takes place in the large intestine.

Pronunciation/Word Parts

deglutition (DEE-gloo-TIH-shun)
  deglutit/o- *swallowing*
  -ion *action; condition*

peristalsis (PAIR-ih-STAL-sihs)
The prefix **peri-** means *around*. The suffix **-stalsis** means *process of contraction*.

chemical (KEM-ih-kal)
  chem/o- *chemical; drug*
  -ical *pertaining to*

enzyme (EN-zime)
The suffix **-ase** is associated with enzymes.

amylase (AM-ih-lays)
  amyl/o- *carbohydrate; starch*
  -ase *enzyme*

hydrochloric acid (HY-droh-KLOR-ik AS-id)
  hydr/o- *fluid; water*
  chlor/o- *chloride*
  -ic *pertaining to*

pepsinogen (pep-SIN-oh-jen)
  pepsin/o- *pepsin*
  -gen *that which produces*

pepsin (PEP-sin)
  peps/o- *digestion*
  -in *substance*

gastrin (GAS-trin)
  gastr/o- *stomach*
  -in *substance*

lactase (LAK-tays)
  lact/o- *milk*
  -ase *enzyme*

glucose (GLOO-kohs)
  gluc/o- *glucose; sugar*
  -ose *full of*

cholecystokinin (KOH-lee-SIHS-toh-KY-nin)
  cholecyst/o- *gallbladder*
  kin/o- *movement*
  -in *substance*

bile (BILE)
The combining forms **bil/i-**, **bili/o-**, and **chol/e-** mean *bile; gall*.

emulsification (ee-MUL-sih-fih-KAY-shun)
  emulsific/o- *liquid with suspended particles*
  -ation *being; having; process*

amylase (AM-ih-lays)
  amyl/o- *carbohydrate; starch*
  -ase *enzyme*

lipase (LIH-pays)
  lip/o- *fat; lipid*
  -ase *enzyme*
The combining form **steat/o-** means *fat*.

absorption (ab-SORP-shun)
  absorpt/o- *absorb; take in*
  -ion *action; condition*

Elimination

The process of elimination occurs when undigested food fibers, waste material, and the remaining water are eliminated from the body in a solid waste form known as a **bowel movement (BM)** or **feces** or **stool**. The process of elimination is **defecation**. Some gas, known as **flatus**, may also be passed at that time.

Pronunciation/Word Parts

elimination (ee-LIM-ih-NAY-shun)
  elimin/o- *remove from the body*
  -ation *being; having; process*

feces (FEE-seez)

fecal (FEE-kal)
  fec/o- *feces; stool*
  -al *pertaining to*
The combining form **fec/a-** also means *feces; stool.*

stool (STOOL)

defecation (DEF-eh-KAY-shun)
  de- *reversal of; without*
  fec/o- *feces; stool*
  -ation *being; having; process*
The combining form **chez/o-** means *pass feces.*

flatus (FLAY-tuhs)
The combining form **flatul/o-** means *flatus; gas.*

Clinical Connections

Dietetics. The liver plays an important role in regulating nutrients such as glucose and amino acids. Excess glucose in the blood is stored in the liver as glycogen and is released when the blood glucose level is low. The liver uses amino acids from protein foods to build plasma proteins and clotting factors for the blood.

Individuals whose small intestine does not produce enough of the digestive enzyme lactase experience bloating and pass excessive amounts of gas (flatus) when they drink milk or eat dairy products. This is caused by undigested lactose. Beans contain a particular sugar that cannot be completely broken down in the small intestine; eating beans can also cause gas. For some people, eating the gluten in certain grains (wheat, barley, rye, or oats) causes celiac disease (described in a later section).

Hematology. The stomach plays an indirect role in the production of red blood cells. It secretes intrinsic factor that allows vitamin B_{12} (a building block of red blood cells) to be absorbed from the intestine into the blood. When the stomach does not produce enough intrinsic factor, vitamin B_{12} is not absorbed; the red blood cells that are formed are very large, fragile, and die prematurely; this is the disease of pernicious anemia (described in Chapter 6, Hematology and Immunology).

Immunology. Some parts of the gastrointestinal system are also part of the body's immune response (described in Chapter 6 Hematology and Immunology). Saliva contains antibodies that kill microorganisms in the food we eat. Hydrochloric acid in the stomach kills microorganisms. Small masses of lymphatic tissue (Peyer's patches) on the walls of the small intestine also kill microorganisms. The appendix, which contains lymphoid tissue and is a structure of the lymphatic system, also participates in the immune response to kill microorganisms. However, if large numbers of microorganisms are present in the food, they can still cause a gastrointestinal illness.

Microbiology. The large intestine is inhabited by millions of beneficial bacteria that produce vitamin K to supplement the vitamin K in the diet. These beneficial bacteria feed on any undigested material; they also change the yellow-green color of bile to the characteristic brown color of the feces.

Radiology. As the ascending colon nears the liver, it bends at a right angle known as the hepatic flexure. As the transverse colon nears the spleen, it bends at a right angle known as the splenic flexure. These bends (flexures) in the colon are landmarks that are mentioned in radiology reports of the abdomen.

3.2 PRACTICE LAPS

Use the Answer Key at the end of the book to check your answers.

A. Give the Meaning of Combining Forms

Next to each combining form, write its meaning. The first one has been done for you.

Combining Form	Meaning	Combining Form	Meaning
1. **absorpt/o-**	*absorb; take in*	8. fec/o-	
2. amyl/o-		9. gastr/o-	
3. chez/o-		10. lact/o-	
4. deglutit/o-		11. lip/o-	
5. digest/o-		12. mastic/o-	
6. elimin/o-		13. pepsin/o-	
7. emulsific/o-		14. peps/o-	

B. Build Words

Read the definition of the medical word. Look at the combining form that is given. Select the correct suffix from the Suffix List, and write it on the blank line. Then build the medical word, and write it on the line. (Remember: You may need to remove the combining vowel. Always remove the hyphens and slash.) Be sure to check your spelling.

Suffix List

-al (pertaining to) -ase (enzyme)	-ation (being; having; process)	-gen (thing that produces) -in (substance)	-ion (action; condition)

Definition of the Medical Word	Combining Form	Suffix	Build the Medical Word
Example: Enzyme (that breaks apart) carbohydrates	**amyl/o-**	*-ase*	*amylase*

[*You think* enzyme *(-ase)* + carbohydrate *(amyl/o-)*. *You change the order of the word parts to put the suffix last. You write* amylase.]

1. Action (of) swallowing	deglutit/o-	_____	_____
2. Action (to) absorb (or) take in	absorpt/o-	_____	_____
3. Process (to) remove from the body	elimin/o-	_____	_____
4. Pertaining to feces (or) stool	fec/o-	_____	_____
5. Substance (that stimulates) the stomach	gastr/o-	_____	_____
6. Enzyme (that breaks apart) milk	lact/o-	_____	_____
7. Thing that produces pepsin	pepsin/o-	_____	_____
8. Process (of) chewing	mastic/o-	_____	_____
9. Enzyme (that breaks apart) fat (or) lipid	lip/o-	_____	_____

Vocabulary Review

Word or Phrase	Description	Combining Forms
Overview		
alimentary canal	Another name for the gastrointestinal sysztem	**aliment/o-** *food; nourishment*
digestive system	Another name for the gastrointestinal system. Also known as the **digestive tract**.	**digest/o-** *break down food; digest*
gastrointestinal (GI) system	The structures of the gastrointestinal system include the oral cavity (teeth, gums, tongue, hard palate, soft palate), salivary glands (parotid, sublingual, submandibular), pharynx, esophagus, stomach, small and large intestines, rectum, anus, and the accessory organs (liver, gallbladder, pancreas). The functions of the gastrointestinal system are to digest food, absorb nutrients, and remove waste materials. Also known as the **gastrointestinal tract**.	**gastr/o-** *stomach* **intestin/o-** *intestine*
Anatomy of the Oral Cavity, Pharynx, and Larynx		
larynx	Structure below the pharynx. It is closed during swallowing when muscles in the neck pull it up to the **epiglottis**, a lid-like structure, so that swallowed food particles go into the esophagus and stomach.	**laryng/o-** *larynx; voice box* **glott/o-** *glottis of the larynx*

Word or Phrase	Description	Combining Forms
mucosa	Mucous membrane that produces thin mucus. It lines the oral cavity and the entire gastrointestinal system.	**mucos/o-** *mucous membrane*
oral cavity	Mouth. Hollow area that contains the teeth, gums, tongue, hard palate, and soft palate.	**or/o-** *mouth* **stomat/o-** *mouth*
palate	Hard palate (bone) and soft palate (posterior soft tissue) form the roof of the oral cavity. The soft palate ends in the fleshy, hanging **uvula**. The soft palate and uvula sense the presence of food particles in the posterior oral cavity just before they are swallowed.	
pharynx	Throat. A passageway for food particles and air. It is between the oral cavity and the esophagus. The pharynx includes the **nasopharynx** (posterior to the nasal cavity), the **oropharynx** (posterior to the oral cavity) and the **laryngopharynx** (posterior to the larynx).	**pharyng/o-** *pharynx; throat* **nas/o-** *nose* **or/o-** *mouth* **laryng/o-** *larynx; voice box*
salivary glands	Three pairs of glands (**parotid**, **sublingual**, and **submandibular**) on either side of the head; they release saliva into the oral cavity. **Saliva** moistens food particles and contains the digestive enzyme amylase.	**saliv/o-** *saliva* **sial/o-** *saliva; salivary gland* **ot/o-** *ear* **lingu/o-** *tongue* **mandibul/o-** *lower jaw; mandible*
tongue	Large muscle that fills the oral cavity and assists with eating and talking. It contains receptors for the sense of taste. The **gustatory cortex** in the brain receives sensory information about taste from receptors on the tongue.	**gloss/o-** *tongue* **lingu/o-** *tongue* **gustat/o-** *sense of taste*

Anatomy of the Esophagus and Stomach

Word or Phrase	Description	Combining Forms
cardia	First part of the stomach where the stomach joins the esophagus	
chyme	Semisolid mixture of food particles, saliva, and digestive enzymes in the stomach and small intesine	
esophagus	Flexible tube approximately 10 inches in length that connects the pharynx to the stomach. It contains the lower esophageal sphincter.	**esophag/o-** *esophagus*
fundus	Rounded, top part of the stomach	
lower esophageal sphincter	Muscular ring at the distal end of the esophagus. It keeps chyme in the stomach from flowing back into the esophagus.	**esophag/o-** *esophagus* **sphinct/o-** *close tightly*
pyloric sphincter	Muscular ring at the distal end of the stomach. It closes to keep chyme in the stomach or opens to let chyme flow into the duodenum.	**pylor/o-** *pylorus* **sphinct/o-** *close tightly*
pylorus	Narrowed, last part of the stomach where it joins the duodenum. It contains the pyloric sphincter.	**pylor/o-** *pylorus*
rugae	Thick, deep folds in the gastric mucosa that expand to accommodate a large amount of swallowed food particles	
stomach	Large, elongated sac in the upper abdominal cavity. It is between the esophagus and the small intestine. Regions of the stomach: cardia, fundus, body, and pylorus. Rugae are thick, deep folds in the mucosa that allow the stomach to expand.	**gastr/o-** *stomach*

Anatomy of the Small and Large Intestines

Word or Phrase	Description	Combining Forms
anus	External opening of the rectum. The **anal sphincter** is under voluntary control.	**an/o-** *anus* **sphinct/o-** *close tightly*

Word or Phrase	Description	Combining Forms
appendix	Long, thin pouch on the exterior wall of the cecum. It contains lymphoid tissue and is part of the immune response; it does not play a role in digestion.	**appendic/o-** *appendix* **append/o-** *small structure hanging from a larger structure*
cecum	Short sac that is the first part of the large intestine. It contains the **ileocecal valve** that keeps waste materials and water from flowing back into the ileum from the large intestine. The appendix is attached to the cecum's external wall.	**cec/o-** *cecum* **ile/o-** *ileum*
colon	Second and longest part of the large intestine. It includes the **ascending colon**, **transverse colon**, **descending colon**, and S-shaped **sigmoid colon**.	**col/o-** *colon* **colon/o-** *colon* **sigmoid/o-** *sigmoid colon*
duodenum	The 10-inch, C-shaped, first part of the small intestine. It is between the stomach and the jejunum.	**duoden/o-** *duodenum*
ileum	Third and final part of the small intestine. It is 12 feet long and is located between the jejunum and the cecum of the large intestine.	**ile/o-** *ileum*
jejunum	Second part of the small intestine. It is an 8-foot coiled segment between the duodenum and the ileum.	**jejun/o-** *jejunum*
haustra	Puckered pouches in the intestinal wall that expand to receive large amounts of waste materials.	
large intestine	Large, tubular structure in the abdominopelvic cavity. It is about 5 feet in length and is located between the small intestine and the anus. The large intestine includes the cecum, colon, rectum, and anus. Also known as the **large bowel**.	**intestin/o-** *intestine* **enter/o-** *intestine*
lumen	Central, open area inside a tubular structure such as the esophagus, small intestine, and large intestine	
rectum	Short, straight segment that is the last part of the large intestine. It is between the sigmoid colon and the outside of the body.	**rect/o-** *rectum* **proct/o-** *rectum and anus*
small intestine	Long, tubular structure in the abdominopelvic cavity. It is between the stomach and the large intestine. It receives chyme from the stomach. The small intestine includes the duodenum, jejunum, and ileum. It produces lactase and other sugar-digesting enzymes. Also known as the **small bowel**.	**intestin/o-** *intestine* **enter/o-** *intestine*
villi	Thousands of microscopic, thin structures in the mucosa that project into the lumen of the small intestine. They increase the surface area to maximize absorption of digested nutrients and water from the small intestine.	

Abdominopelvic Cavity and Accessory Organs

abdominopelvic cavity	Continuous cavity within the abdomen and pelvis. It contains the largest organs of the gastrointestinal system. It is lined with peritoneum.	**abdomin/o-** *abdomen* **pelv/o-** *hip bone; pelvis; renal pelvis* **celi/o-** *abdomen* **lapar/o-** *abdomen*
bile	Thick, yellow-green digestive enzyme produced by the liver; it flows through the bile ducts and is stored in the gallbladder. It contains bile acids, the yellow pigment **bilirubin**, and the green pigment **biliverdin**.	**bil/i-** *bile; gall* **bili/o-** *bile; gall* **chol/e-** *bile; gall* **rub/o-** *red* **verd/o-** *green*

Word or Phrase	Description	Combining Forms
bile ducts	Bile from the liver flows through the common hepatic duct into the common bile duct (CBD). When that duct is full, bile fills the cystic duct and then the gallbladder. The bile ducts are also known as the **biliary tree**.	**bili/o-** *bile; gall* **cholangi/o-** *bile duct* **choledoch/o-** *common bile duct*
gallbladder	An accessory organ of the gastrointestinal system. The gallbladder is a teardrop-shaped, dark green sac posterior to the liver. It stores and concentrates bile. Fatty chyme in the duodenum causes the gallbladder to contract and release bile into the duodenum.	**cholecyst/o-** *gallbladder*
liver	An accessory organ of the gastrointestinal system. The liver is a large, dark red-brown organ in the right upper quadrant (RUQ) of the abdominal cavity. It contains **hepatocytes** that produce bile.	**hepat/o-** *liver*
mesentery	Thick, fan-shaped sheet of peritoneum that supports loops of the jejunum and ileum	**mesenter/o-** *middle thing between the intestines*
omentum	Broad, fatty covering of peritoneum that supports the stomach and protects the small intestine	
pancreas	An accessory organ of the gastrointestinal system. The pancreas is a yellow, elongated, triangular organ posterior to the stomach. It secretes amylase, lipase, and protein-digesting enzymes through the pancreatic duct into the duodenum. The pancreas is also a gland of the endocrine system.	**pancreat/o-** *pancreas*
peritoneum	Double-layered serous membrane that lines the abdominopelvic cavity and surrounds the gastrointestinal organs. It secretes **peritoneal fluid**, a watery fluid that fills the spaces between the gastrointestinal organs.	**peritone/o-** *peritoneum* **periton/o-** *peritoneum*

Physiology of Digestion

Word or Phrase	Description	Combining Forms
absorption	Process by which water and fluids in the oral cavity move into the blood that is in blood vessels under the tongue. Also, in the stomach, water and some liquid/dissolved drugs are absorbed. The majority of absorption of food nutrients and water takes place in the ileum. Any remaining water is absorbed into the blood from the large intestine.	**absorpt/o-** *absorb; take in*
amylase	Digestive enzyme in saliva that begins the digestion of carbohydrates in the oral cavity. Amylase is also secreted by the pancreas, and it further breaks down complex sugar molecules into glucose.	**amyl/o-** *carbohydrate; starch*
bile	Digestive enzyme released by the gallbladder. Bile breaks down fats in the chyme into small fat globules.	
chemical digestion	Digestive process that involves digestive enzymes, acids, and other substances to chemically break down food. It includes emulsification.	**chem/o-** *chemical; drug*
cholecystokinin	Hormone produced by the duodenum when it receives fatty chyme from the stomach. Cholecystokinin stimulates the gallbladder to release bile, and it also stimulates the pancreas to secrete its digestive enzymes into the duodenum.	**cholecyst/o-** *gallbladder* **kin/o-** *movement*
chyme	Semisolid mixture of food particles, saliva, and digestive enzymes in the stomach and small intestine	

Word or Phrase	Description	Combining Forms
defecation	Process by which undigested food fibers, waste materials, and water are eliminated from the body as a **bowel movement** or **feces** or **stool**. The passage of **flatus** (gas) may also occur.	**fec/o-** *feces; stool* **fec/a-** *feces; stool* **chez/o-** *pass feces* **flatul/o-** *flatus; gas*
deglutition	Process of swallowing food particles and moving them into the pharynx. This is part of mechanical digestion.	**deglutit/o-** *swallowing*
digestion	Process of breaking down food into nutrients that can be used by the body. Digestion begins in the oral cavity and continues throughout the small intestine. It includes mechanical digestion and chemical digestion.	**digest/o-** *break down food; digest* **mechanic/o-** *physical force; tool* **chem/o-** *chemical; drug*
elimination	Process in which food fibers, waste materials, and water are eliminated from the body in a solid form. Also known as *defecation*.	**elimin/o-** *remove from the body*
emulsification	Process in which bile breaks down fats in the chyme into small fat globules. This is part of chemical digestion.	**emulsific/o-** *liquid with suspended particles*
enzymes	Substances that speed up chemical reactions. Enzymes are produced by the salivary glands, stomach, small intestine, and pancreas. An enzyme name usually ends in *-ase*.	
gastrin	Hormone produced by the stomach. It stimulates the release of hydrochloric acid and pepsinogen.	**gastr/o-** *stomach*
glucose	Simple sugar that is the only source of energy that body cells can use	**gluc/o-** *glucose; sugar*
hydrochloric acid	Strong acid produced by the stomach. It breaks down food fibers and converts pepsinogen to pepsin.	**hydr/o-** *fluid; water* **chlor/o-** *chloride*
intrinsic factor	Substance produced by the stomach. It helps the stomach absorb vitamin B_{12} from foods.	
lactase	Digestive enzyme produced by the small intestine. It breaks down complex sugar molecules and the sugar in milk to the simple sugar **glucose**.	**lact/o-** *milk*
lipase	Digestive enzyme secreted by the pancreas. It breaks down small fat globules into fatty acids.	**lip/o-** *fat; lipid*
mastication	The teeth tear, chew, and grind food in the oral cavity. The tongue moves food particles and mixes them with saliva. This is part of mechanical digestion.	**mastic/o-** *chewing*
mechanical digestion	Digestive process that involves some type of physical force and movement. It includes mastication, deglutition, and peristalsis.	**mechanic/o-** *physical force; tool*
pepsin	Digestive enzyme in the stomach that breaks down protein foods	**peps/o-** *digestion*
pepsinogen	Inactive substance produced by the stomach. It is converted by hydrochloric acid to the digestive enzyme pepsin.	**pepsin/o-** *pepsin*
peristalsis	Coordinated waves of smooth muscle contractions of the esophagus, stomach, and intestines. Peristalsis moves food particles, chyme, waste materials, and water through the gastrointestinal system. Peristalsis is part of mechanical digestion.	

3.3 Diseases

Word or Phrase	Description	Pronunciation/Word Parts

Eating

anorexia	Decreased appetite because of disease or the gastrointestinal side effect of a drug. The patient is said to be **anorexic**. Treatment: Correct the underlying cause.	**anorexia** (AN-oh-REK-see-ah) **an-** *not; without* **orex/o-** *appetite* **-ia** *condition; state; thing* **anorexic** (AN-oh-REK-sik)

Clinical Connections

Psychiatry. Anorexia nervosa is a psychiatric disorder in which a person has an extreme fear of being fat and feels an obsessive desire to be thinner (see Figure 3-8 ■). The person decreases his or her food intake to the point of starvation but tries to keep this from family and friends by making excuses for not eating and by wearing clothes that conceal the extreme weight loss.

Bulimia is a psychiatric disorder in which a person gorges him- or herself on excessive amounts of food (**binge eating**) and then, for fear of gaining weight, rids (**purges**) him- or herself of food by using laxative drugs or with self-induced vomiting. There is a continuous cycle of binging and purging.

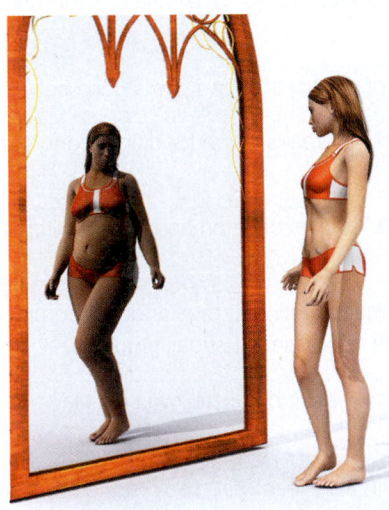

FIGURE 3-8 ■ **Anorexia nervosa.**
A person with anorexia nervosa denies being too thin and appears to herself as being fat when she looks in a mirror.

dysphagia	Painful eating or difficulty swallowing. Painful eating can be caused by an infection in the mouth, poorly fitting dentures, or radiation therapy to the mouth for cancer. Difficulty swallowing can be caused by a tumor or by a stroke that makes it difficult to coordinate the muscles for swallowing. Treatment: Soft foods for painful eating. Antibiotic drug for a bacterial infection. Thickened liquids for difficult swallowing. Removal of a tumor.	**dysphagia** (dis-FAY-jee-ah) **dys-** *abnormal; difficult; painful* **phag/o-** *eating; swallowing* **-ia** *condition; state; thing*
polyphagia	Excessive overeating due to an overactive thyroid gland, diabetes mellitus, or a psychiatric illness. Treatment: Correct the underlying cause.	**polyphagia** (PAW-lee-FAY-jee-ah) **poly-** *many; much* **phag/o-** *eating; swallowing* **-ia** *condition; state; thing*

Word or Phrase	Description	Pronunciation/Word Parts

Oral Cavity and Salivary Glands

Word or Phrase	Description	Pronunciation/Word Parts
glossitis	Infection or inflammation of the tongue. This can be caused by a bacterial or viral infection, food allergies, abrasive or spicy foods, or a vitamin B deficiency. Treatment: Correct the underlying cause.	**glossitis** (GLAW-SY-tihs) **gloss/o-** *tongue* **-itis** *infection of; inflammation of*
sialolithiasis	A stone (**sialolith**) forms in the salivary gland and becomes lodged in the duct, blocking the flow of saliva. The salivary gland, oral cavity, and face become swollen. When the salivary gland contracts to release saliva, the stone blocks the flow of saliva, and the duct spasms, causing pain. Treatment: Surgical removal of the stone	**sialolithiasis** (sy-AL-oh-lith-EYE-ah-sihs) **sial/o-** *saliva; salivary gland* **lith/o-** *stone* **-iasis** *abnormal condition; process* **sialolith** (sy-AL-oh-lith) **sial/o-** *saliva; salivary gland* **-lith** *stone*
stomatitis	Inflammation of the mucosa in the oral cavity. Stomatitis can be caused by poorly fitting dentures or by an infection. Treatment: Correct the underlying cause.	**stomatitis** (STOH-mah-TY-tihs) **stomat/o-** *mouth* **-itis** *infection of; inflammation of* Do not confuse the sound-alike words *stomatitis* and *stomach*.

Esophagus and Stomach

Word or Phrase	Description	Pronunciation/Word Parts
dyspepsia	Mild, temporary **epigastric** pain, sometimes with gas or nausea (see Figure 3-9 ■). Also known as **indigestion**. Treatment: Antacid drug; avoid spicy foods, fatty foods, alcohol and things that cause dyspepsia. Correct underlying diseases such as gastroesophageal reflux, peptic ulcer, etc.	**dyspepsia** (dis-PEP-see-ah) **dys-** *abnormal; difficult; painful* **peps/o-** *digestion* **-ia** *condition; state; thing* **epigastric** (EP-ih-GAS-trik) **epi-** *above; upon* **gastr/o-** *stomach* **-ic** *pertaining to* **indigestion** (IN-dy-JES-chun) **in-** *in; not; within* **digest/o-** *break down food; digest* **-ion** *action; condition*

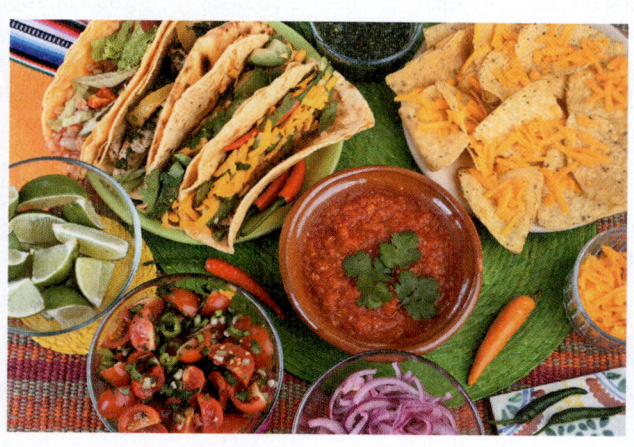

FIGURE 3-9 ■ Dyspepsia.
Dyspepsia can be caused by excess stomach acid, reflux of stomach acid into the esophagus, overeating, eating spicy foods, or stress.

Word or Phrase	Description	Pronunciation/Word Parts
esophageal varix	Swollen, protruding vein in the mucosa of the esophagus (see Figure 3-10 ■). Liver disease causes blood to back up in the large vein from the intestines to the liver, so the blood takes an alternate route through smaller veins in the esophagus, but eventually these veins become engorged. Esophageal varices are easily irritated by swallowed food. They can hemorrhage suddenly, causing death. Treatment: Correct the underlying liver disease. Surgery: A drug is injected into the varix to harden it.	**varix** (VAIR-iks) **varices** (VAIR-ih-seez) Latin plural noun: Change the singular ending -ix to -ices.

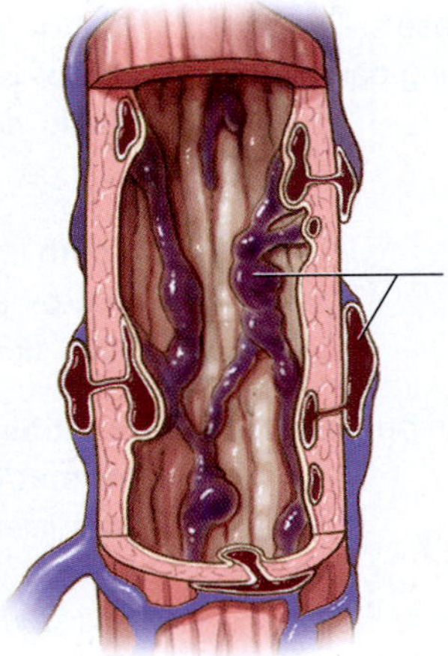

Esophageal varices

FIGURE 3-10 ■ **Esophageal varices.**
A varix is a dilated, swollen vein in the mucosa. There can be bleeding as swallowed food irritates a varix. Esophageal varices can be seen when an endoscope with a light is passed through the mouth and into the esophagus.

Word or Phrase	Description	Pronunciation/Word Parts

gastritis	Acute or chronic infection or inflammation of the stomach due to a bacterial infection, spicy foods, alcohol, or excess acid production.
	Treatment: Antacid drug; antibiotic drug for a bacterial infection; H_2 blocker and proton pump inhibitor drugs to decrease the production of acid; avoid spicy foods and alcohol.
		gastritis (gas-TRY-tihs)
		  gastr/o- stomach
		  -itis infection of; inflammation of

gastroenteritis	Acute infection or inflammation of the stomach and intestines. There is abdominal pain, nausea and vomiting, and diarrhea. It is caused by a virus (from the flu) or a bacterium (from contaminated food).
	Treatment: Antiemetic drug (to prevent vomiting); antidiarrheal drug; antibiotic drug for a bacterial infection
		gastroenteritis (GAS-troh-EN-ter-EYE-tihs)
		  gastr/o- stomach
		  enter/o- intestine
		  -itis infection of; inflammation of

gastroesophageal reflux disease (GERD)	Chronic inflammation and irritation due to **reflux** of stomach acid back into the esophagus because the lower esophageal sphincter does not close tightly. This causes a sore throat, belching, and **esophagitis** with chronic inflammation. It can lead to esophageal ulcers or cancer of the esophagus.
	Treatment: Eat small, frequent meals. Elevate the head of the bed while sleeping. Avoid alcohol and foods that stimulate stomach acid production. Antacid drug to neutralize acid; H_2 blocker or proton pump inhibitor drugs to decrease the production of acid. Surgery to repair the sphincter.
		gastroesophageal (GAS-troh-eh-SAW-fah-JEE-al)
		  gastr/o- stomach
		  esophag/o- esophagus
		  -eal pertaining to
		
		reflux (REE-fluks)
		
		esophagitis (eh-SAW-fah-JY-tihs)
		  esophag/o- esophagus
		  -itis infection of; inflammation of

heartburn	Temporary, mild inflammation of the esophagus due to reflux of stomach acid back into the esophagus. Also known as **pyrosis**.
	Treatment: Antacid drug
		pyrosis (py-ROH-sihs)
		  pyr/o- burning; fire
		  -osis abnormal condition; process

hematemesis	Vomiting (emesis) of blood caused by bleeding in the stomach or esophagus. This can be due to an esophageal or gastric ulcer or esophageal varices. Coffee-grounds emesis contains old, dark blood that has been partially digested by the stomach.
	Treatment: Correct the underlying cause.
		hematemesis (HEE-mah-TEM-eh-sihs)
		  hemat/o- blood
		  -emesis abnormal condition of vomiting
		The combining form **emet/o-** means vomiting.

Word or Phrase	Description	Pronunciation/Word Parts

nausea and vomiting (N&V)	Nausea is an unpleasant, queasy feeling in the stomach. It is caused by infection or inflammation of the stomach or by motion sickness that affects the inner ear. Vomiting or **emesis** is the expelling of chyme from the stomach through the mouth. It is triggered when impulses from the stomach or inner ear stimulate the vomiting center in the brain. **Vomitus** is the expelled chyme. Retching (dry heaves) is continual vomiting when there is no longer anything in the stomach. **Regurgitation** is the reflux of small amounts of chyme and acid coming back into the mouth, but without vomiting.
	Treatment: Antiemetic drug; correct the underlying cause.
		nausea (NAW-see-ah)
		
		emesis (EM-eh-sihs)
		
		vomitus (VAW-mih-tuhs)
		
		regurgitation
		(ree-GER-jih-TAY-shun)
		  regurgit/o- backward flow
		  -ation being; having; process

Clinical Connections

Obstetrics. Morning sickness is the vomiting associated with early pregnancy. **Hyperemesis gravidarum** is excessive vomiting during the first months of pregnancy. These conditions are thought to be due to changes in hormone levels in the pregnant woman's body (described in Chapter 12, Gynecology and Obstetrics).

hyperemesis (HY-per-EM-eh-sihs)

gravidarum (GRAV-ih-DAIR-um)
Gravidarum is a Latin word that means *of pregnancy.*

Word or Phrase	Description	Pronunciation/Word Parts

peptic ulcer disease (PUD)	Chronic irritation, burning pain, and erosion of the mucosa with the formation of an ulcer. An esophageal ulcer, a gastric ulcer in the stomach, and a duodenal ulcer are all peptic ulcers. A **gastric ulcer** (see Figure 3-11 ■) is most commonly caused by the bacterium *Helicobacter pylori*, which has also been linked to cancer of the stomach. Ulcers can also be caused by excessive hydrochloric acid, stress, and drugs (such as aspirin) that irritate the mucosa.
	Treatment: Antacid drug to neutralize acid; H_2 blocker or proton pump inhibitor drugs to decrease the production of acid. Antibiotic drug to treat *H. pylori* infection. Avoid spicy foods, smoking, alcohol, caffeine, and aspirin-containing drugs.
		peptic (PEP-tik)
		  pept/o- digestion
		  -ic pertaining to
		
		ulcer (UL-ser)
		
		gastric (GAS-trik)
		  gastr/o- stomach
		  -ic pertaining to

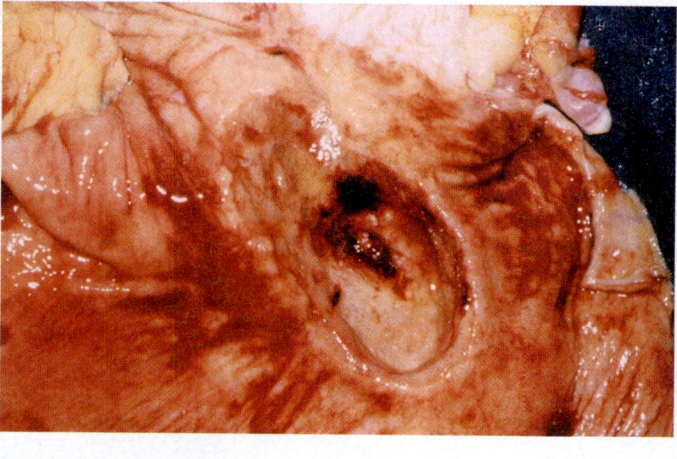

FIGURE 3-11 ■ Gastric ulcer.
This gastric mucosa is raw and irritated with a large central ulcer crater. The bright red blood indicates a recent episode of bleeding from the ulcer.

Word or Phrase	Description	Pronunciation/Word Parts

stomach cancer	Cancerous tumor of the stomach that begins in glands in the gastric mucosa, and so it is categorized as an **adenocarcinoma**. It is caused by chronic irritation from a *Helicobacter pylori* infection.
	Treatment: Surgery to remove the cancer and part of the stomach (gastrectomy)
		cancer (KAN-ser)
		
		cancerous (KAN-ser-uhs)
		  cancer/o- cancer
		  -ous pertaining to
		
		adenocarcinoma
		(AD-eh-noh-KAR-sih-NOH-mah)
		  aden/o- gland
		  carcin/o- cancer
		  -oma mass; tumor

Word or Phrase	Description	Pronunciation/Word Parts

Duodenum, Jejunum, Ileum

ileus	Absence of normal peristalsis in the small and large intestines. Obstipation, a tumor, or a hernia can cause an obstruction that slows peristalsis. Intestinal infection or trauma or the use of narcotic drugs for pain can slow peristalsis. **Postoperative ileus** occurs after the intestines are manipulated during abdominal surgery.
	Treatment: Intravenous fluids for temporary nutritional support; surgery (bowel resection and anastomosis) may be needed.
		ileus (IL-ee-uhs)
		Note: Do not confuse *ileus* with the anatomic structure of the *ileum*.
		
		postoperative
		(post-AW-per-ah-TIV)
		  post- *after; behind*
		  operat/o- *perform a procedure; surgery*
		  -ive *pertaining to*

intussusception	Telescoping of one segment of intestine inside the lumen of the next segment (see Figure 3-12A ■). There is vomiting and abdominal pain. The cause is unknown.
	Treatment: Surgery (bowel resection and anastomosis)
		intussusception
		(IN-tuh-suh-SEP-shun)
		  intussuscept/o- *receive within*
		  -ion *action; condition*

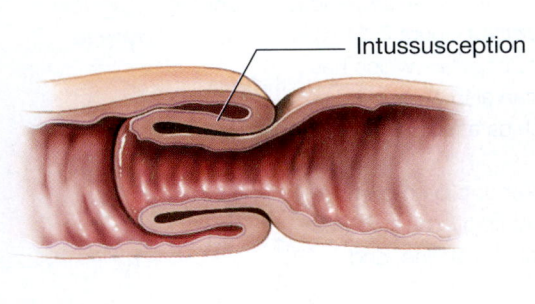
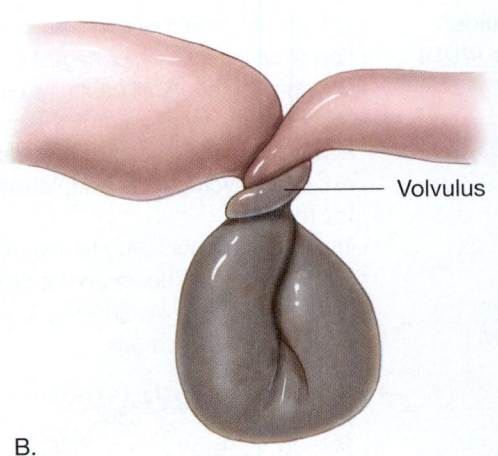

FIGURE 3-12 ■ Intussusception and volvulus of the intestine.
A. In an intussusception, the intestine folds back on itself in the same way that one part of a telescope slides into the other. **B.** In a volvulus, the intestine becomes twisted. Both of these conditions stop peristalsis and decrease blood flow to the intestine.

volvulus	Twisting of the intestine around itself (see Figure 3-12B). There is vomiting and abdominal pain. Also known as **malrotation**. Causes include poor support of the intestine with twisting of the mesentery or the formation of abdominal **adhesions** between the loops of intestine.
	Treatment: Surgery of an exploratory laparotomy and lysis of adhesions; bowel resection and anastomosis, if needed
		volvulus (VAWL-vyoo-luhs)
		
		malrotation (MAL-roh-TAY-shun)
		  mal- *bad; inadequate*
		  rotat/o- *rotate*
		  -ion *action; condition*
		
		adhesion (ad-HEE-zhun)

Cecum and Colon

appendicitis	Infection and inflammation of the appendix as waste materials become trapped in the lumen of the appendix. The abdominal pain increases and then localizes to the right lower quadrant (RLQ). If the physician presses on that area and then quickly removes the hand to release the pressure, the abdominal wall rebounds to its original position, and the patient complains of severe **rebound pain**. An infected appendix can rupture (burst), spilling infection into the abdominopelvic cavity and causing peritonitis.
	Treatment: Surgery to remove the appendix (appendectomy)
		appendicitis (ah-PEN-dih-SY-tihs)
		  appendic/o- *appendix*
		  -itis *infection of; inflammation of*

Word or Phrase	Description	Pronunciation/Word Parts
colon cancer	Cancerous tumor of the colon. It occurs when colonic polyps or ulcerative colitis become cancerous. It is also linked to a high-fat diet. There can be blood in the feces. Treatment: Preventive surgery to remove polyps before they become cancerous; surgery to remove the cancer and the affected intestine (bowel resection) and reroute the colon to a new opening in the abdominal wall (colostomy)	

diverticulum	Weakness in the wall of the colon where the mucosa forms an abnormal pouch or tube-shaped sac that opens into the lumen of the colon. Diverticula can be caused by eating a low-fiber diet that forms small, compact feces. Then, increased intra-abdominal pressure and straining to pass feces eventually creates diverticula. **Diverticulosis** is the condition of multiple diverticula (see Figure 3-13 ■). If feces become trapped inside a diverticulum, this causes inflammation, infection, abdominal pain, and fever, a condition known as **diverticulitis** (see Figure 3-14 ■).
	Prevention: High-fiber diet
	Treatment: Antibiotic drug to treat diverticulitis; surgery (bowel resection and anastomosis) to remove the affected segment of the colon
		diverticulum
		(DY-ver-TIH-kyoo-lum)
		
		diverticula (DY-ver-TIH-kyoo-lah)
		Latin plural noun: Change the singular ending -*um* to -*a*.
		
		diverticulosis
		(DY-ver-TIH-kyoo-LOH-sihs)
		  diverticul/o- *diverticulum*
		  -osis *abnormal condition; process*
		
		diverticulitis
		(DY-ver-TIH-kyoo-LY-tihs)
		  diverticul/o- *diverticulum*
		  -itis *infection of; inflammation of*

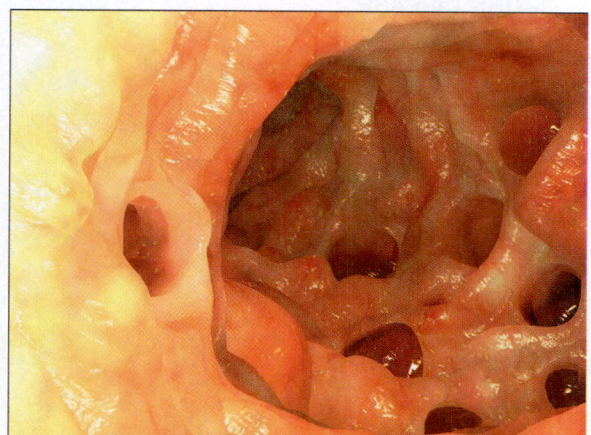

FIGURE 3-13 ■ Diverticula.
These pouches in the wall of the colon are diverticular sacs where feces can become trapped.

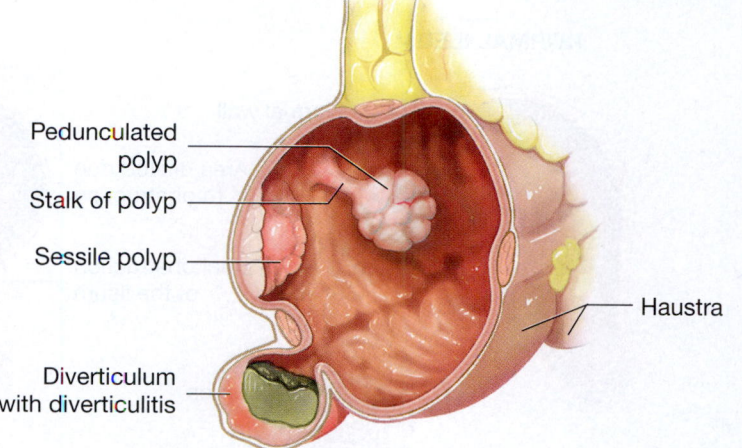

FIGURE 3-14 ■ Diverticulitis and polyposis.
This diverticulum has become infected from trapped feces. These polyps (described later in this section) can be irritated by the passage of feces and can become cancerous.

Clinical Connections

Dietetics. Diverticular disease was unknown until the early 1900s, when refined flour began to replace whole wheat flour. Diverticular disease is common in countries where people eat a low-fiber diet, but it remains uncommon in third-world countries where there is a high-fiber diet. Fiber creates bulk and holds water to keep the feces soft.

Word or Phrase	Description	Pronunciation/Word Parts

gluten sensitivity enteropathy	Autoimmune disorder and toxic reaction to the gluten found in certain grains (wheat, barley, rye, oats). The small intestine is damaged by the inflammatory response. Also known as **celiac disease**.
	Treatment: Avoid eating foods and food products that contain gluten.
		gluten (GLOO-ten)
		
		enteropathy (EN-ter-AW-pah-thee)
		  enter/o- *intestine*
		  -pathy *disease*
		
		celiac (SEE-lee-ak)
		  celi/o- *abdomen*
		  -ac *pertaining to*

inflammatory bowel disease (IBD)	Chronic inflammation of various parts of the small and large intestines. There is diarrhea, bloody feces, abdominal cramps, and fever. The cause is not known. There are two types of inflammatory bowel disease:
	• **Crohn disease** (or **regional enteritis**) affects regions of the ileum and colon (see Figure 3-15 ■). There are areas of normal mucosa ("skip areas") and then inflammation. There are ulcers and thickening of the intestinal wall that can cause a partial obstruction in the intestine.
	• **Ulcerative colitis** affects the colon and rectum and causes inflammation and ulcers.
	Treatment: Corticosteroid drug to decrease inflammation; surgery (bowel resection) to remove the affected intestine and reroute the intestine through a new opening in the abdominal wall (ileostomy, colostomy)
		Crohn (KROHN)
		
		enteritis (EN-ter-EYE-tihs)
		  enter/o- *intestine*
		  -itis *infection of; inflammation of*
		
		ulcerative (UL-ser-ah-TIV)
		  ulcerat/o- *ulcer*
		  -ive *pertaining to*
		
		colitis (KOH-LY-tihs)
		  col/o- *colon*
		  -itis *infection of; inflammation of*

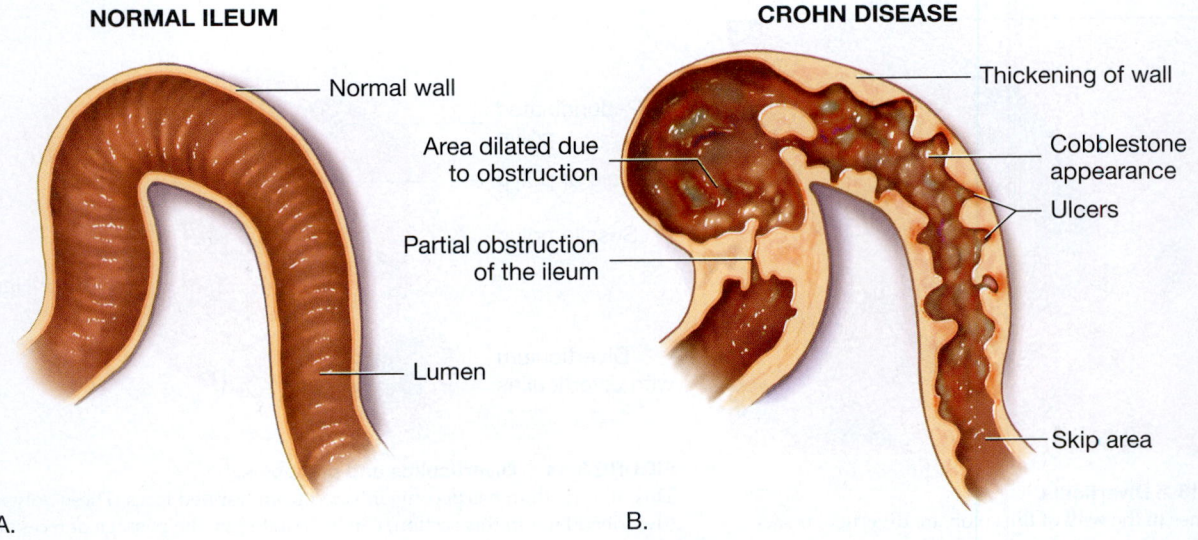

NORMAL ILEUM

— Normal wall

— Lumen

CROHN DISEASE

— Thickening of wall

— Cobblestone appearance

— Ulcers

— Skip area

Area dilated due to obstruction

Partial obstruction of the ileum

A.

B.

FIGURE 3-15 ■ Crohn disease.
A. This segment of normal intestine shows an open lumen throughout and an intestinal wall without thickening or ulcers. **B.** Crohn disease shows thickening of the intestinal wall and ulcers. There is also a partial obstruction.

Word or Phrase	Description	Pronunciation/Word Parts

irritable bowel syndrome (IBS)	Disorder of the function of the colon, although the mucosa of the colon never shows any visible signs of inflammation. There is cramping, abdominal pain, bloating, diarrhea alternating with constipation, and excessive mucus. The cause is not known but may be related to lactose intolerance or emotional stress. Also known as **spastic colon** or **mucous colitis**. Treatment: Antidiarrheal, antispasmodic, and antianxiety drugs; high-fiber diet and laxative drugs to prevent constipation; avoidance of foods that contain lactose	**spastic** (SPAS-tik)
		  spast/o- *spasm*
		  -ic *pertaining to*
		
		colitis (koh-LY-tihs)
		  col/o- *colon*
		  -itis *infection of; inflammation of*

polyposis	Condition of numerous polyps. **Polyps** are small, fleshy, benign or precancerous growths in the mucosa of the colon. A **pedunculated polyp** has a thin stalk that supports an irregular, ball-shaped top. A **sessile polyp** is a mound with a broad base (see Figure 3-14 and Figure 3-16 ■). Although polyps are benign, they can become cancerous.
	Treatment: Surgery to remove the polyps (polypectomy)
		polyposis (PAW-lih-POH-sihs)
		  polyp/o- *polyp*
		  -osis *abnormal condition; process*
		
		polyp (PAW-lip)
		
		pedunculated
		(peh-DUNG-kyoo-LAY-ted)
		
		sessile (SES-il)

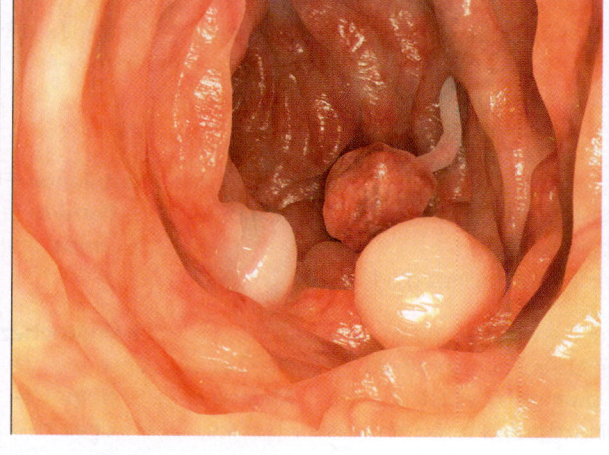

FIGURE 3-16 ■ Colonic polyps.
This patient has two sessile polyps (in the front) and one pedunculated polyp on a stalk (in the rear) in the mucosal folds in the wall of the colon.

Rectum and Anus

hemorrhoids	Swollen, protruding veins in the rectum (internal hemorrhoids) or on the skin around the anus (external hemorrhoids). They are caused by increased intra-abdominal pressure from straining to pass feces. Also known as **piles**. A hemorrhoid is irritated by feces, and its surface bleeds easily.
	Treatment: Topical corticosteroid drug to decrease irritation; surgery to remove the hemorrhoids (hemorrhoidectomy)
		hemorrhoid (HEM-oh-royd)
		  hemorrh/o- *flowing of blood*
		  -oid *resembling*

proctitis	Inflammation of the rectum due to radiation therapy done to treat cancer. It can also be caused by ulcers or infection.
	Treatment: Correct the underlying cause.
		proctitis (prawk-TY-tihs)
		  proct/o- *rectum and anus*
		  -itis *infection of; inflammation of*

rectocele	The wall of the rectum protrudes into the adjacent vaginal wall, causing it to collapse inwardly and block the vaginal canal in a female. This is a type of hernia. A rectocele can also protrude to the outside of the body.
	Treatment: Surgery to repair the defect
		rectocele (REK-toh-seel)
		  rect/o- *rectum*
		  -cele *hernia*

Word or Phrase	Description	Pronunciation/Word Parts

Defecation and Feces

Word or Phrase	Description	Pronunciation/Word Parts
constipation	Failure to have regular, soft bowel movements. This can be due to decreased peristalsis, lack of dietary fiber, inadequate water intake, lack of exercise, or the side effect of a drug. **Obstipation** is severe, unrelieved constipation that can cause a bowel obstruction. A **fecalith** is hardened feces that becomes a stone-like mass. This can form in the appendix or in a diverticulum. Treatment: Laxative drug; a high-fiber diet; increased water intake; enemas	**constipation** (CON-stih-PAY-shun) **constip/o-** *compacted feces* **-ation** *being; having; process* **obstipation** (AWB-stih-PAY-shun) **obstip/o-** *severe constipation* **-ation** *being; having; process* **fecalith** (FEE-kah-lith) **fec/a-** *feces; stool* **-lith** *stone*
diarrhea	Abnormally frequent, loose, and sometimes watery feces. It is caused by an infection (bacteria, viruses), irritable bowel syndrome, ulcerative colitis, lactose intolerance, or the side effect of a drug. There is increased peristalsis, and the feces move through the large intestine before the water can be absorbed. Treatment: Antidiarrheal drug; lactase enzyme supplement; antibiotic drug to treat a bacterial infection	**diarrhea** (DY-ah-REE-ah) The prefix **dia-** means *complete; through*. The suffix **-rrhea** means *discharge; flow*.
flatulence	Presence of excessive amounts of flatus (gas) in the stomach or intestines. It can be caused by milk (lactose intolerance), indigestion, or incomplete digestion of carbohydrates such as beans. Treatment: Lactase enzyme supplement; antigas drug	**flatulence** (FLAT-yoo-lens) **flatul/o-** *flatus; gas* **-ence** *state*
hematochezia	Blood in the feces. The source of bleeding can be an ulcer, cancer, Crohn disease, or a polyp, diverticulum, or hemorrhoid. Bright red blood indicates active bleeding in the lower gastrointestinal system. **Melena** is a dark, tar-like feces that contains digested blood from bleeding in the esophagus or stomach. Treatment: Correct the underlying cause of bleeding.	**hematochezia** (hee-MAH-toh-KEE-zha) **hemat/o-** *blood* **chez/o-** *pass feces* **-ia** *condition; state; thing* **melena** (meh-LEE-nah) The combining form **melan/o-** means *black*.
steatorrhea	Greasy, frothy, foul-smelling feces that contain undigested fats. There is a deficiency of the enzyme lipase, which digests fats, because of pancreatic disease, cancer, or cystic fibrosis. Treatment: Correct the underlying cause.	**steatorrhea** (stee-AT-oh-REE-ah) **steat/o-** *fat* **-rrhea** *discharge; flow*

Across the Life Span

Pediatrics. Feces forms in the intestine while the fetus is in the uterus. Swallowed amniotic fluid and sloughed-off fetal skin cells mix with mucus and bile to form **meconium**, a thick, sticky, green-to-black stool that is passed after birth. In the newborn nursery, the nurse checks to see that the anus and rectum are **patent** (open). **Colic** is common in babies, causing crampy abdominal pain after feeding. It can be due to overfeeding, feeding too quickly, inadequate burping, or a food allergy to milk.

Geriatrics. Constipation is a common complaint in older adults. A diet of refined foods with low fiber, lack of water intake, and inactivity contribute to the formation of small, hard feces. Narcotic drugs used to treat chronic, severe pain can cause constipation and that can develop into a bowel obstruction in older adults. Some older patients have **incontinence**, which is an inability to voluntarily control the anal sphincter and the passage of feces; this can be due to paralysis or dementia.

meconium (meh-KOH-nee-um)

colic (KAW-lik)
col/o- *colon*
-ic *pertaining to*

incontinence (in-CON-tih-nens)
in- *in; not; within*
contin/o- *hold together*
-ence *state*
Incontinence: *State (of) not (being able to) hold together (feces in the colon)*

Word or Phrase	Description	Pronunciation/Word Parts

Abdominal Wall and Abdominopelvic Cavity

hernia

Defect and weakness in the muscle of the diaphragm or the abdominal wall. The defect allows the intestine and the peritoneum around it to bulge through (hernia sac), causing swelling and pain. There is an inherited tendency to hernias, but hernias can also be caused by pregnancy, obesity, or heavy lifting. Hernias are named in two different ways.

- Hernias are named according to how easily the intestine can move back into its normal position. **A sliding or reducible hernia** has the intestine move back and forth between the hernia sac and the abdominopelvic cavity (see Figure 3-17 ■). In an **incarcerated hernia**, the intestine swells within the hernia sac, becomes trapped, and can no longer go back into the abdominopelvic cavity. A **strangulated hernia** is an incarcerated hernia sac whose blood supply has been cut off (see Figure 3-17). This leads to tissue death (necrosis).
- Hernias are named according to their location. A **hiatal hernia** occurs when the stomach bulges into the opening where the esophagus passes through the diaphragm. A **ventral hernia** occurs anywhere on the anterior abdominal wall (except at the umbilicus). An **umbilical hernia** occurs at the umbilicus (navel). An **omphalocele** is an umbilical hernia that is present at birth, and it has no covering of skin, only a hernia sac of peritoneum (see Figure 3-17). An **inguinal hernia** is in the groin. An **incisional hernia** is along the suture line of a prior abdominal surgical incision.

Treatment: Surgery to correct the hernia (herniorrhaphy)

hernia (HER-nee-ah)
The combining form **herni/o-** means *hernia; protruding part.*

incarcerated (in-KAR-ser-AA-ted)
  incarcer/o- *imprison*
  -ated *composed of; pertaining to a condition*

hiatal (hy-AA-tal)
  hiat/o- *gap; opening*
  -al *pertaining to*

ventral (VEN-tral)
  ventr/o- *abdomen; front*
  -al *pertaining to*

umbilical (um-BIL-ih-kal)
  umbilic/o- *navel; umbilicus*
  -al *pertaining to*

omphalocele (OM-fal-oh-SEEL)
  omphal/o- *navel; umbilicus*
  -cele *hernia*

inguinal (ING-gwih-nal)
  inguin/o- *groin*
  -al *pertaining to*

incisional (in-SIH-zhun-al)
  in- *in; not; within*
  cis/o- *cut*
  -ion *action; condition*
  -al *pertaining to*

SLIDING HERNIA

Loop of intestine in hernia sac

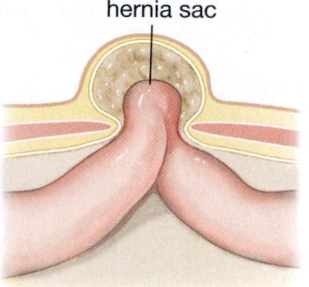

A.

STRANGULATED HERNIA

Entrapped, necrotic loop of intestine

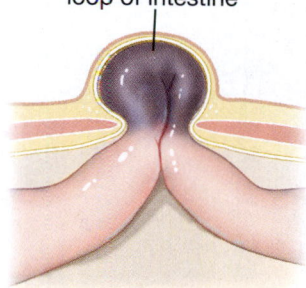

B.

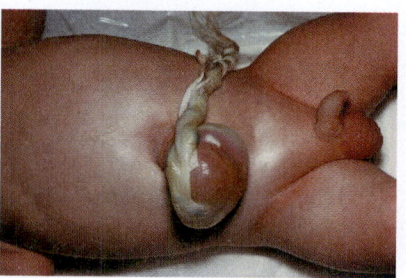

C.

FIGURE 3-17 ■ Hernia.
A. In a sliding hernia, the intestine and peritoneum move in and out of the hernia sac. **B.** In a strangulated hernia, the intestine is trapped in the hernia sac and its tissues begin to die. **C.** This baby was born with an omphalocele, a hernia at the umbilicus. The hernia sac is only a layer of peritoneum with the intestine inside. This baby needs to have immediate surgery to correct the omphalocele and repair the abdominal wall defect.

Clinical Connections

Neonatology. In a male before birth, the testes (male sex glands) normally move through the inguinal canal (an opening in the abdominal wall muscle) and into the scrotum. If the inguinal canal fails to close (around 2 years of age), a loop of intestine can pass through the canal, go into the scrotum, and create an inguinal hernia.

Word or Phrase	Description	Pronunciation/Word Parts
peritonitis	Infection and inflammation of the peritoneum (see Figure 3-18 ■). It occurs when an ulcer, diverticulum, or cancerous tumor breaks through the wall of the stomach or intestine or when an infected appendix ruptures. Stomach or intestinal contents and bacteria spill into the abdominopelvic cavity. Treatment: Surgery (exploratory laparotomy) to cleanse the abdominal cavity of infected fluids and tissues; correct the underlying cause; antibiotic drug for bacterial infection 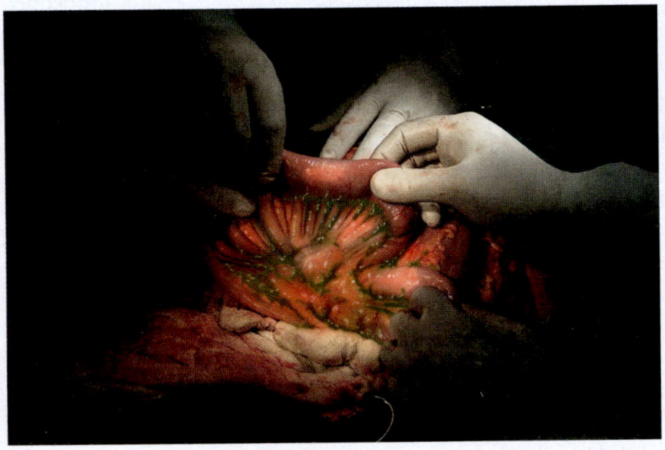 **FIGURE 3-18 ■ Peritonitis.** The surgeon is holding a loop of duodenum, showing the mesentery attached to the small intestine. This patient developed peritonitis when a duodenal ulcer perforated the intestinal wall and green bile from the gallbladder and chyme from the stomach spilled into the abdominal cavity. The areas of white are white blood cells (pus) that are fighting this infection.	**peritonitis** (PAIR-ih-toh-NY-tihs) **periton/o-** *peritoneum* **-itis** *infection of; inflammation of*

Word or Phrase	Description	Pronunciation/Word Parts

Liver

ascites	Accumulation of **ascitic** fluid in the abdominopelvic cavity (see Figure 3-19 ■). Liver disease causes a backup of blood and increased blood pressure in the veins of the abdomen. This pressure pushes fluid out of the blood into the abdominopelvic cavity and grossly distends the abdomen. Treatment: Removal of ascitic fluid from the abdomen using a needle (abdominocentesis) or permanent drainage of excess fluid via an implanted tube (shunt), if needed	**ascites** (ah-SY-teez) **ascitic** (ah-SIT-ik) **ascit/o-** *ascites* **-ic** *pertaining to*

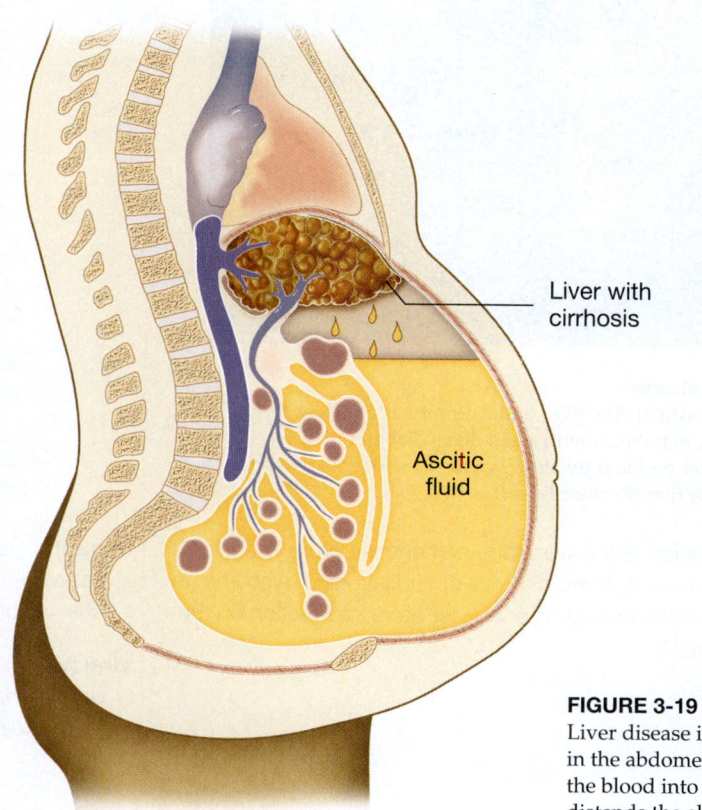

Liver with cirrhosis

Ascitic fluid

FIGURE 3-19 ■ Ascites.
Liver disease increases the blood pressure in veins in the abdomen. The pressure pushes fluid from the blood into the abdominopelvic cavity, and this distends the abdomen.

Word Alert
Sound-Alike Words

acidic (ah-SID-ik)	(adjective)	pertaining to an acid, having a low pH *Example: Hydrochloric acid creates an acidic (low pH) environment in the stomach.*
ascitic (ah-SIT-ik)	(adjective)	pertaining to ascites *Example: Ascitic fluid can accumulate in the abdominopelvic cavity.*

Word or Phrase	Description	Pronunciation/Word Parts
cirrhosis	Chronic, progressive inflammation and finally irreversible degeneration of the liver, with enlargement, nodules, and scarring (see Figure 3-20 ■). Liver function is severely impaired. There is nausea and vomiting, weakness, and jaundice. Cirrhosis is caused by alcoholism, viral hepatitis, or chronic obstruction of the bile ducts. Treatment: Correct the underlying cause. 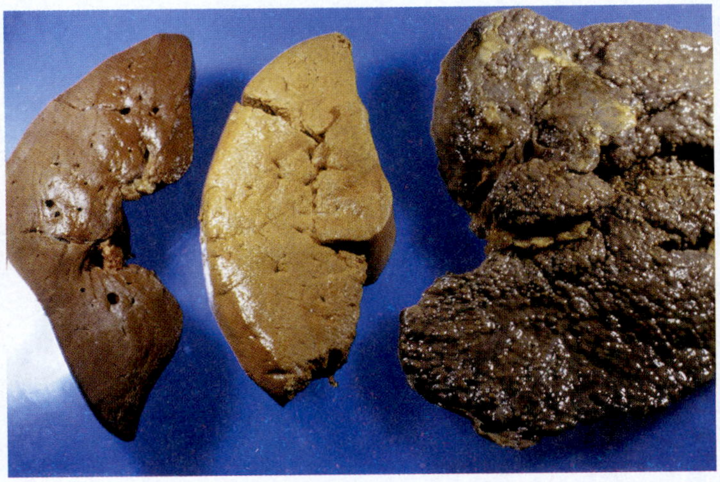 **FIGURE 3-20** ■ **Liver disease.** The liver on the left is normal. The liver in the center has a yellow, fatty appearance that occurs in patients with alcoholism, diabetes mellitus, or lipid disorders. The liver on the right shows cirrhosis with enlargement, nodules, and scar tissue that decrease liver function.	**cirrhosis** (sih-ROH-sihs) **cirrh/o-** *yellow* **-osis** *abnormal condition; process*
hepatitis	Infection and inflammation of the liver from the hepatitis virus. There is weakness, anorexia, nausea, fever, dark urine, and jaundice. Also known as **viral hepatitis**. See the Dive Deeper box for more information on the various types of hepatitis.	**hepatitis** (HEP-ah-TY-tihs) **hepat/o-** *liver* **-itis** *infection of; inflammation of* **viral** (VY-ral) **vir/o-** *virus* **-al** *pertaining to*

Word or Phrase	Description	Pronunciation/Word Parts

Dive Deeper

Hepatitis is the most common chronic liver disease. There are four types of hepatitis. Each is caused by a different virus.

- **Hepatitis A** is caused by the hepatitis A virus (HAV). It produces an acute but short-lived infection; most people recover completely. It is caused by water or food that is contaminated with feces from a person who is already infected with HAV. Also known as **infectious hepatitis**.

  Prevention: Vaccination
  Treatment: None needed because most people recover completely

- **Hepatitis B** is caused by the hepatitis B virus (HBV). It produces an acute infection, but most people recover completely. However, it can continue as a chronic infection for months. During that time, the infected person is a carrier and can infect others. It is caused by exposure to the blood of a person who is already infected with HBV (see Figure 3-21 ■). It is also spread during sexual activity by contact with saliva and vaginal secretions. An infected mother can pass hepatitis B to her fetus before birth or when breastfeeding. Also known as **serum hepatitis**.

  Prevention: Vaccination; healthcare workers are vaccinated because of their constant exposure to patients' blood and body fluids.

- **Hepatitis C** is caused by the hepatitis C virus (HCV). It produces an acute infection that continues as a chronic infection. It is caused by exposure to contaminated needles or to the blood of a person who is already infected with HCV. Hepatitis C is not easily transmitted during sexual activity or from a mother to her fetus. Chronic hepatitis C is the main cause of chronic liver disease, cirrhosis, and liver cancer.

  Treatment: Antiviral drugs specifically for HCV can achieve a nearly 100% cure rate.

- **Hepatitis D** is a secondary infection caused by a mutated (changed) hepatitis virus. It develops only in patients who already have hepatitis B. Also known as **delta hepatitis**.

infectious (in-FEK-shus)
infect/o- *disease within*
-ious *pertaining to*

serum (SEER-um)
Serum is the fluid portion of the blood (without the cells and clotting factors).

delta (DEL-tah)
The Greek word *delta* means *change.*

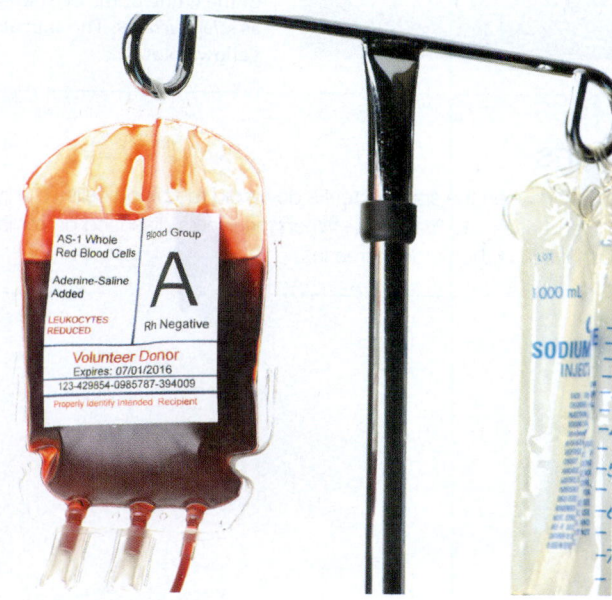

FIGURE 3-21 ■ Blood transfusion.
Receiving infected blood during a blood transfusion, coming in contact with blood-contaminated instruments, or the sharing of needles by drug addicts can result in hepatitis B or hepatitis C.

Word or Phrase	Description	Pronunciation/Word Parts
hepatomegaly	Enlargement of the liver due to cirrhosis, hepatitis, or cancer (see Figure 3-20). The enlarged liver can be felt on palpation of the abdomen. The degree of enlargement is measured as the number of fingerbreadths from the lower edge of the right rib cage to the lower edge of the liver. **Hepatosplenomegaly** is enlargement of both the liver and the spleen. Treatment: Correct the underlying cause.	**hepatomegaly** (HEP-ah-toh-MEG-ah-lee) **hepat/o-** *liver* **-megaly** *enlargement* **hepatosplenomegaly** (HEP-ah-toh-SPLEN-oh-MEG-ah-lee) **hepat/o-** *liver* **splen/o-** *spleen* **-megaly** *enlargement*
jaundice	Yellowish discoloration of the skin and whites of the eyes (scleral icterus) (see Figure 3-22 ■). There is an increased level of unconjugated bilirubin in the blood that enters the tissues, giving them a yellow color. The patient is said to be *jaundiced*. If a patient does not have jaundice, he or she is **nonicteric**. Jaundice occurs for these reasons: • If the liver is too diseased or is too immature (in premature newborn infants) to conjugate bilirubin. • If there is too much unconjugated bilirubin in the blood because of the destruction of large numbers of red blood cells. • If a gallstone is obstructing the flow of bile in the bile ducts (**obstructive jaundice**). Treatment: Correct the underlying cause.	**jaundice** (JAWN-dihs) **jaund/o-** *yellow* **-ice** *quality; state* **nonicteric** (NON-ik-TAIR-ik) **non-** *not* **icter/o-** *jaundice* **-ic** *pertaining to* **obstructive** (awb-STRUK-tiv) **obstruct/o-** *blocked by a barrier* **-ive** *pertaining to*

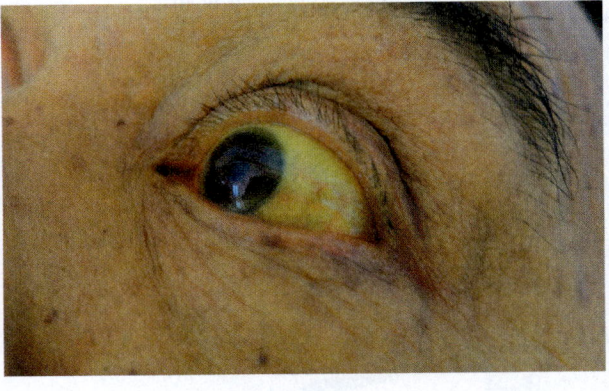

FIGURE 3-22 ■ Jaundice.
Jaundice can be seen as a yellow discoloration of the white of the eye (sclera). This is known as *scleral icterus*. The skin also has a slight yellow color.

Clinical Connections

Hematology. Bilirubin is produced when the spleen breaks down old red blood cells. The liver joins (conjugates) this bilirubin to another substance and uses it to make bile. When the liver is diseased or immature and cannot do this, the amount of unconjugated bilirubin in the blood increases.

Word or Phrase	Description	Pronunciation/Word Parts

liver cancer	Cancerous tumor of the liver (see Figure 3-23 ■). This is usually a secondary cancer that began in another part of the body and spread (metastasized) to the liver. Also known as a **hepatoma** or **hepatocellular carcinoma**.
	Treatment: Surgery to remove the tumor; chemotherapy drugs
		hepatoma (HEP-ah-TOH-mah)
		  hepat/o- *liver*
		  -oma *mass; tumor*
		
		hepatocellular
		(HEP-ah-toh-SEL-yoo-lar)
		  hepat/o- *liver*
		  cellul/o- *cell*
		  -ar *pertaining to*
		
		carcinoma (KAR-sih-NOH-mah)
		  carcin/o- *cancer*
		  -oma *mass; tumor*

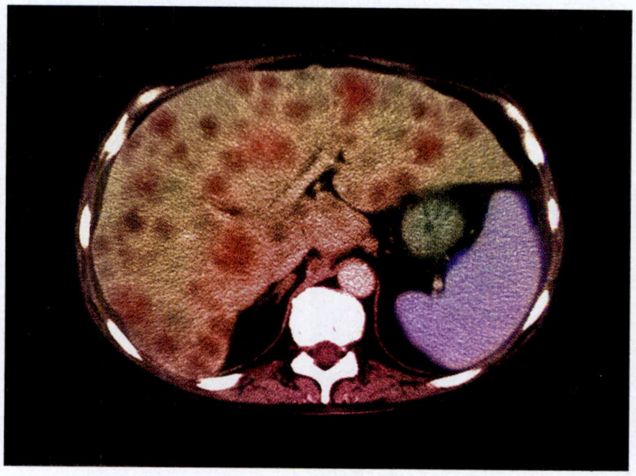

FIGURE 3-23 ■ **Liver cancer.**
This colorized computerized tomography (CT scan) of the abdomen shows an enlarged (tan) liver, nearly filling the abdominal cavity, with many red-brown areas of cancer. A CT scan is read as if you were standing at the patient's feet, looking up. The white area in the center bottom is a vertebra of the spine, and the white areas around the edges are ribs.

Gallbladder and Bile Ducts

Word or Phrase	Description	Pronunciation/Word Parts

gallbladder cancer	Cancerous tumor in the ducts of the gallbladder. Also known as a **cholangiocarcinoma**.
	Treatment: Surgery to remove the cancerous gallbladder (cholecystectomy); radiation therapy and chemotherapy drugs
		cholangiocarcinoma
		(koh-LAN-jee-oh-KAR-sih-NOH-mah)
		  cholangi/o- *bile duct*
		  carcin/o- *cancer*
		  -oma *mass; tumor*

cholangitis	Acute or chronic inflammation of the bile ducts because of cirrhosis or gallstones.
	Treatment: Correct the underlying cause.
		cholangitis (KOH-lan-JY-tihs)
		  cholangi/o- *bile duct*
		  -itis *infection of; inflammation of*
		Note: The duplicated letter *i* is deleted.

cholecystitis	Acute cholecystitis occurs when a gallstone blocks the cystic duct of the gallbladder. As the gallbladder contracts, the duct spasms, causing severe pain (**biliary colic**). Chronic cholecystitis occurs when a gallstone partially blocks the cystic duct, causing backup of bile and thickening of the gallbladder wall.
	Prevention: Avoid fatty foods that cause the gallbladder to contract.
	Treatment: Drug to dissolve the gallstone; surgery to remove the gallbladder (cholecystectomy)
		cholecystitis
		(KOH-lee-sihs-TY-tihs)
		  cholecyst/o- *gallbladder*
		  -itis *infection of; inflammation of*

Word or Phrase	Description	Pronunciation/Word Parts

cholelithiasis	The presence of gallstones in the gallbladder (see Figure 3-24 ■). When the bile is too concentrated, it forms a thick sediment (sludge) that becomes small gallstones (gravel) and then larger gallstones. Cramping symptoms can be mild, or there can be severe biliary colic when there are many gallstones and the gallbladder contracts or when a gallstone becomes lodged in a bile duct. **Choledocholithiasis** is a gallstone that is lodged in the common bile duct (see Figure 3-25 ■).
	Prevention: Avoid fatty foods that cause the gallbladder to contract.
	Treatmeant: Drug to dissolve the gallstone; surgery to remove the gallbladder (cholecystectomy) or to remove a gallstone from the common bile duct (choledocholithotomy)
		cholelithiasis
		(KOH-lee-lith-EYE-ah-sihs)
		   chol/e- *bile; gall*
		   lith/o- *stone*
		   -iasis *abnormal condition; process*
		
		 choledocholithiasis
		(koh-LED-oh-KOH-lith-EYE-ah-sihs)
		   choledoch/o- *common bile duct*
		   lith/o- *stone*
		   -iasis *abnormal condition; process*

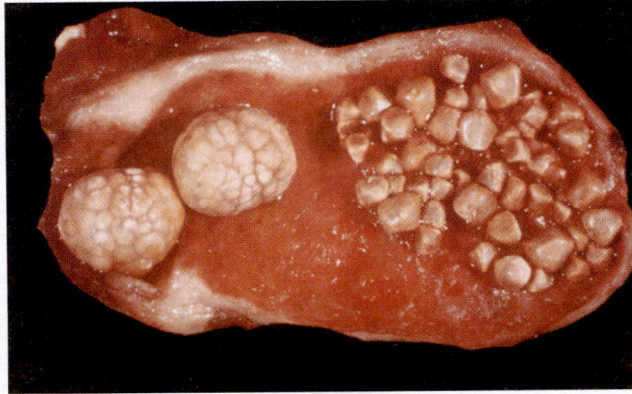

FIGURE 3-24 ■ Cholelithiasis.
This patient's gallbladder was removed during surgery. It contained numerous small and large gallstones.

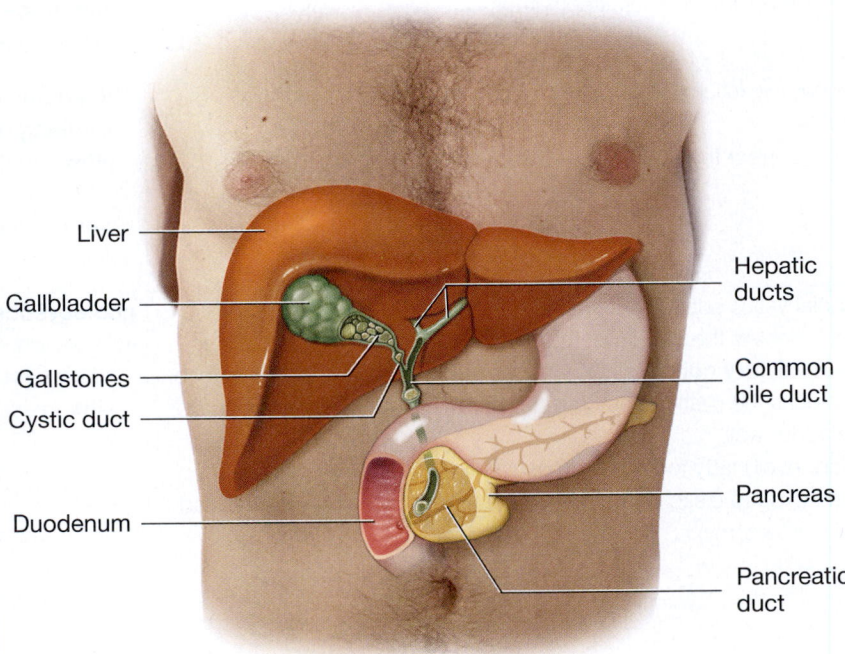

FIGURE 3-25 ■ Gallstones in the biliary and pancreatic ducts.
A gallstone in the cystic duct causes bile to back up into the gallbladder. A gallstone in the upper common bile duct causes bile to back up into the gallbladder and liver. A gallstone in the lower common bile duct keeps pancreatic digestive enzymes from entering the duodenum.

Word or Phrase	Description	Pronunciation/Word Parts
Pancreas		
pancreatic cancer	Cancerous tumor (**adenocarcinoma**) of the pancreas. The pancreas is a gland that secretes its digestive enzymes through a duct, and so this cancer is also known as **ductal cell carcinoma**. Most patients are in the advanced stage when they are diagnosed, and so survival is usually less than 1 year. Treatment: Chemotherapy drugs; surgery to remove the tumor	**adenocarcinoma** (AD-eh-noh-KAR-sih-NOH-mah) **aden/o-** *gland* **carcin/o-** *cancer* **-oma** *mass; tumor*
pancreatitis	Infection or inflammation of the pancreas. There is abdominal pain and nausea and vomiting. Inflammation occurs when a gallstone blocks the common bile duct and the pancreatic duct and pancreatic enzymes back up into the pancreas. Inflammation can also be due to chronic alcoholism. Infection of the pancreas is caused by bacteria or viruses. Treatment: Stop drinking alcohol; antibiotic drug to treat a bacterial infection; surgery to remove the gallstone (choledocholithotomy)	**pancreatitis** (PAN-kree-ah-TY-tihs) **pancreat/o-** *pancreas* **-itis** *infection of; inflammation of*

3.3 PRACTICE LAPS

Use the Answer Key at the end of the book to check your answers.

A. Give the Meaning of Combining Forms

Next to each combining form, write its meaning. The first one has been done for you.

Combining Form	Meaning	Combining Form	Meaning
1. **appendic/o-**	*appendix*	12. herni/o-	
2. carcin/o-		13. jaund/o-	
3. celi/o-		14. obstip/o-	
4. cholangi/o-		15. omphal/o-	
5. cholecyst/o-		16. orex/o-	
6. choledoch/o-		17. phag/o-	
7. fec/a-		18. polyp/o-	
8. gastr/o-		19. regurgit/o-	
9. gloss/o-		20. sial/o-	
10. hemat/o-		21. steat/o-	
11. hemorrh/o-			

B. Build Words

Read the definition of the medical word. Look at the combining form that is given. Select the correct suffix from the Suffix List, and write it on the blank line. Then build the medical word, and write it on the line. (Remember: You may need to remove the combining vowel. Always remove the hyphens and slash.) Be sure to check your spelling.

Suffix List

-al (pertaining to)
-ation (being; having; process)
-cele (hernia)
-emesis (abnormal condition of vomiting)

-ion (action; condition)
-itis (infection of; inflammation of)
-ive (pertaining to)
-lith (stone)
-megaly (enlargement)

-oma (mass; tumor)
-osis (abnormal condition; process)
-pathy (disease)
-rrhea (discharge; flow)

Definition of the Medical Word	Combining Form	Suffix	Build the Medical Word
Example: Infection of (or) inflammation of (the) pancreas	**pancreat/o-**	*-itis*	*pancreatitis*

[*You think* infection of (or) inflammation of (-itis) + pancreas (pancreat/o-). You change the order of the word parts to put the suffix last. You write pancreatitis.]

1. Mass (or) tumor (that is a) cancer	carcin/o-		
2. Action (of part of intestine to) receive within	intussuscept/o-		
3. Abnormal condition of vomiting blood	hemat/o-		
4. Abnormal condition (of having a) diverticulum	diverticul/o-		
5. Pertaining to (an) ulcer	ulcerat/o-		
6. Infection of (or) inflammation of (the) appendix	appendic/o-		
7. Hernia (of the) rectum	rect/o-		
8. Pertaining to (the) navel	umbilic/o-		
9. Having compacted feces	constip/o-		
10. Abnormal condition (of) yellow	cirrh/o-		
11. Disease (of the) intestine	enter/o-		
12. Stone (made of) feces	fec/a-		
13. Infection of (or) inflammation of (the) gallbladder	cholecyst/o-		
14. Enlargement (of the) liver	hepat/o-		
15. Abnormal condition (of) polyps	polyp/o-		
16. Infection of (or) inflammation of (the) rectum and anus	proct/o-		

Definition of the Medical Word	Combining Form	Suffix	Build the Medical Word
17. Tumor (of the) liver	hepat/o-	_____	_____
18. Infection of (or) inflammation (of the) stomach	gastr/o-	_____	_____
19. Stone (in the) salivary gland	sial/o-	_____	_____
20. Discharge (of) fat	steat/o-	_____	_____

C. Define Abbreviations

1. GERD _____

2. HAV _____

3. IBD _____

4. IBS _____

5. N&V _____

6. PUD _____

3.4 Laboratory, Diagnostic, and Radiologic Procedures

Word or Phrase	Description	Pronunciation/Word Parts

Laboratory Tests and Diagnostic Procedures

Word or Phrase	Description	Pronunciation/Word Parts
albumin	Blood test for albumin, the major protein molecule in the blood. It is part of the panel of blood tests known as *liver function tests* (described later in this section). Because albumin is produced by the liver, liver disease results in a low level of albumin in the blood. The albumin level is also low in patients with malnutrition from poor protein intake.	**albumin** (al-BYOO-min)
CLO test	Gastric mucosa rapid screening test to detect the presence of the bacterium *Helicobacter pylori*. A biopsy of the patient's gastric mucosa is placed on a test pad that contains urea. If *H. pylori* bacteria are present, they metabolize the urea to ammonia, which changes the color of the test pad.	**CLO** (KLOH) *CLO* stands for *Campylobacter-like organism* (because *H. pylori* used to be categorized with the genus *Campylobacter*).
culture and sensitivity (C&S)	Fecal test in which a sample of the patient's feces is swabbed onto a culture dish that contains a nutrient medium for growing bacteria. After the bacterium grows, it can be identified by the appearance of the colonies. Then disks of different antibiotic drugs are placed in the culture dish. If the bacteria are resistant to that antibiotic drug, there will only be a small zone of inhibition (no growth) around it. If the bacteria are sensitive to that antibiotic drug, there will be a medium or large zone of inhibition around that disk.	**sensitivity** (SEN-sih-TIV-ih-tee) **sensitiv/o-** *affected by; sensitive to* **-ity** *condition; state*
fecal occult blood test	Fecal test for occult (hidden) blood in the feces. The feces are tested with the chemical reagent guaiac. Also known as a **stool guaiac test**. If blood is present, the guaiac will turn blue (guaiac-positive). The result of the test can only tell that blood is present. It cannot tell how much blood or where the bleeding is coming from.	**occult** (oh-KULT) **guaiac** (GWY-ak)

Word or Phrase	Description	Pronunciation/Word Parts
gastric analysis	Stomach test to determine the amount of hydrochloric acid in the stomach. A nasogastric (NG) tube is inserted, and gastric fluid is collected. Then a drug is given to stimulate acid production, and another sample is collected.	

liver function tests (LFTs)	Panel of individual blood tests performed at the same time to give a comprehensive picture of the function of the liver. LFTs include these blood tests:
	• **Albumin** (See previous description.)
	• **Bilirubin**. An elevated blood level occurs with liver disease or gallstones.
	• **ALP (alkaline phosphatase)**. An enzyme that is found in both liver cells and bone cells. An elevated blood level occurs with liver disease or bone disease.
	• **ALT (alanine transaminase)** and **AST (aspartate transaminase)**. Enzymes that are mainly found in the liver. Elevated blood levels occur when damaged liver cells release these enzymes.
	• **GGT** or **GGTP (gamma-glutamyl transpeptidase)**. An enzyme that is mainly found in the liver. An elevated blood level occurs when damaged liver cells release this enzyme into the blood.
	• **Prothrombin time**. Prothrombin is a blood clotting factor produced by the liver (described in Chapter 6, Hematology and Immunology).
		albumin (al-BYOO-min)
		
		bilirubin (BIL-ih-ROO-bin)
		  bil/i- *bile; gall*
		  rub/o- *red*
		  -in *substance*
		
		alkaline phosphatase (AL-kah-lin FAWS-fah-tays)
		
		prothrombin (proh-THRAWM-bin)

ova and parasites (O&P)	Fecal test to determine if there is a parasitic infection in the gastrointestinal system. Ova are the eggs of parasitic worms. They can be seen in the feces or by examining a fecal sample under a microscope.	**ova** (OH-vah) Latin plural noun: Change the singular ending *-um* to *-a*. **parasite** (PAIR-ah-site)

Radiologic and Nuclear Medicine Procedures

| **barium enema (BE)** | Radiologic procedure that uses a liquid contrast medium (barium) inserted into the rectum (see Figure 3-26 ■). Barium outlines and coats the walls of the colon and rectum, and then an x-ray is taken. This test is used to identify polyps, diverticula, or tumors. | **barium** (BAIR-ee-um)

enema (EN-eh-mah) |

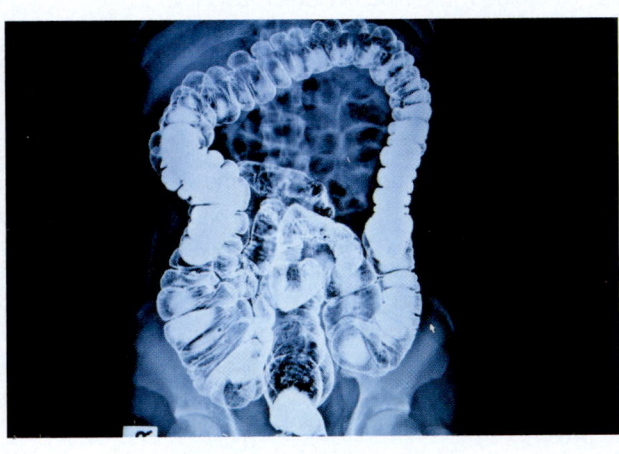

FIGURE 3-26 ■ **Barium enema.**
Barium contrast medium inserted through the rectum fills the sigmoid colon, descending colon, transverse colon, ascending colon, and cecum on this x-ray.

Word or Phrase	Description	Pronunciation/Word Parts

cholangiography	Radiologic procedure that uses an iodinated contrast dye to outline the bile ducts. Then an x-ray is taken to show gallstones in the gallbladder and bile ducts or thickening of the gallbladder wall. The x-ray image is a **cholangiogram**.
	
	• **Intravenous cholangiography**. The iodinated contrast dye is injected intravenously, travels through the blood to the liver, and is excreted with bile into the gallbladder.
	• **Percutaneous transhepatic cholangiography**. A needle is passed through the skin of the abdomen, and the iodinated contrast dye is injected into the liver.
	• **Endoscopic retrograde cholangiopancreatography (ERCP)**. An endoscope and a catheter are used to inject iodinated contrast dye to visualize the common bile duct and pancreatic duct (see Figure 3-27 ■).
		cholangiography
		(koh-LAN-jee-AW-grah-fee)
		  cholangi/o- *bile duct*
		  -graphy *process of recording*
		
		cholangiogram
		(koh-LAN-jee-oh-GRAM)
		  cholangi/o- *bile duct*
		  -gram *picture; record*
		
		intravenous (IN-trah-VEE-nuhs)
		  intra- *within*
		  ven/o- *vein*
		  -ous *pertaining to*
		
		percutaneous
		(PER-kyoo-TAY-nee-uhs)
		  per- *through; throughout*
		  cutane/o- *skin*
		  -ous *pertaining to*
		
		transhepatic (TRANS-heh-PAT-ik)
		  trans- *across; through*
		  hepat/o- *liver*
		  -ic *pertaining to*
		
		endoscopic (EN-doh-SKAW-pik)
		  end/o- *innermost; within*
		  scop/o- *examine with an instrument*
		  -ic *pertaining to*
		
		retrograde (REH-troh-grayd)
		
		cholangiopancreatography
		(koh-LAN-jee-oh-PAN-kree-ah-TAW-grah-fee)
		  cholangi/o- *bile duct*
		  pancreat/o- *pancreas*
		  -graphy *process of recording*

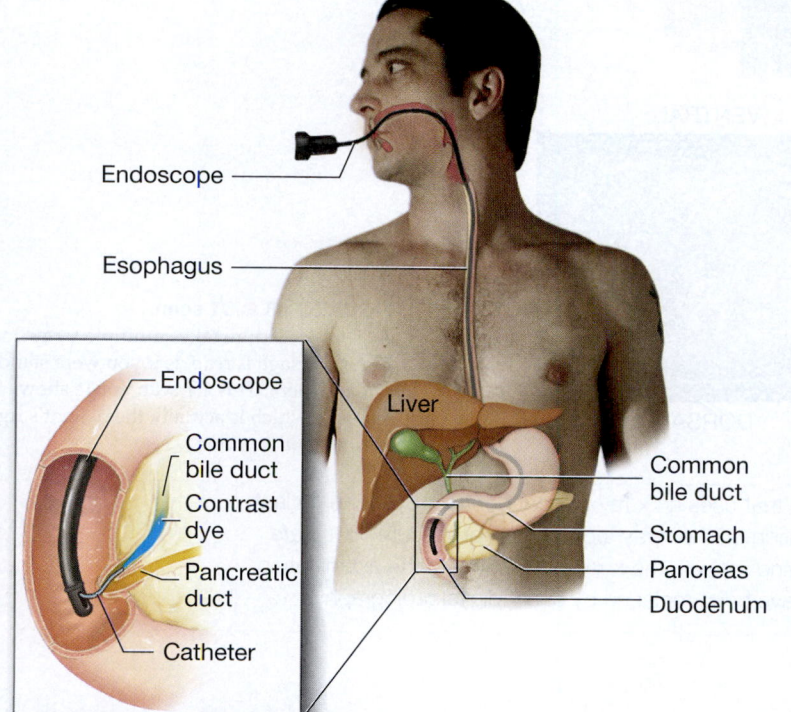

FIGURE 3-27 ■ Endoscopic retrograde cholangiopancreatography.
An endoscope is passed through the mouth, esophagus, stomach, and into the duodenum. A catheter is passed through the endoscope, and then contrast dye is injected to visualize the common bile duct and pancreatic duct. *Retrograde* means the contrast dye is injected in the opposite direction of the normal flow of bile.

Word or Phrase	Description	Pronunciation/Word Parts
cholescintigraphy	Nuclear medicine procedure that uses a radioactive drug given intravenously to detect areas of decreased uptake related to an obstruction in the cystic duct. Also known as a **HIDA scan** (abbreviation for the chemical name of the radioactive drug).	**cholescintigraphy** (KOH-lee-sin-TIH-grah-fee) **chol/e-** *bile; gall* **scint/i-** *point of light* **-graphy** *process of recording*
computerized axial tomography (CAT, CT scan)	Radiologic procedure that uses x-rays to create images of abdominal organs and structures in many thin, successive "slices" (see Figure 3-28 ■).	**tomography** (toh-MAW-grah-fee) **tom/o-** *cut; layer; slice* **-graphy** *process of recording*

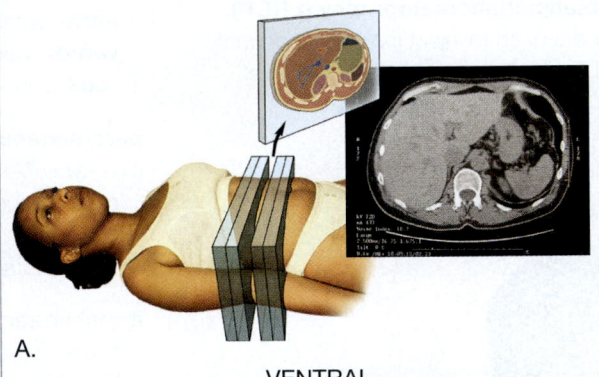

A.

VENTRAL

Liver
Ribs
R
Stomach
Spleen
Left kidney
R
DORSAL   Vertebra

B.

FIGURE 3-28 ■ CT scan.
A. This procedure takes multiple x-ray images in slices.
B. A CT image is read as if you were standing at the feet of the patient. This CT scan image shows the liver on the left side, which is actually the patient's right side when viewed from her feet.

| flat plate of the abdomen | Radiologic procedure that uses an x-ray without contrast dye. The patient lies in the supine position on the x-ray table for this procedure. *Flat plate* refers to the patient lying flat with the x-ray plate beneath the examination table. X-rays plates have been replaced by direct digital radiography. | |

Word or Phrase	Description	Pronunciation/Word Parts

gallbladder ultrasound	Radiologic procedure that uses ultra high-frequency sound waves (not x-rays) to create images of the gallbladder. It is used to identify gallstones and thickening of the gallbladder wall. The image is a **gallbladder sonogram**.	**ultrasound** (UL-trah-sound)
		
		sonogram (SAW-noh-gram)
		  son/o- *sound*
		  -gram *picture; record*

magnetic resonance imaging (MRI)	Radiologic procedure that uses a strong magnetic field to align protons in the atoms of the patient's body. The protons emit signals to form very detailed images of abdominal organs and structures in thin, successive "slices."	**magnetic** (mag-NET-ik)
		  magnet/o- *magnet*
		  -ic *pertaining to*

oral cholecystography (OCG)	Radiologic procedure that uses tablets of iodinated contrast dye taken orally. The tablets dissolve in the small intestine. The contrast dye is absorbed into the blood, travels to the liver, and is excreted with bile into the gallbladder. An x-ray is taken to identify stones in the gallbladder and biliary ducts or thickening of the gallbladder wall. The x-ray image is an **oral cholecystogram**.	**cholecystography**
		(KOH-lee-sihs-TAW-grah-fee)
		  cholecyst/o- *gallbladder*
		  -graphy *process of recording*
		
		cholecystogram
		(KOH-lee-SIHS-toh-gram)
		  cholecyst/o- *gallbladder*
		  -gram *picture; record*

upper gastrointestinal series (UGI)	Radiologic procedure that uses a liquid contrast medium (barium) that is swallowed (a barium meal). Barium coats and outlines the walls of the esophagus, stomach, and duodenum. Also known as a **barium swallow**. Fluoroscopy (a continuously moving x-ray image on a monitor) is used to follow the barium through the small intestine (see Figure 3-29 ■). This is a **small bowel follow-through**. Individual x-rays are taken at specific times throughout the procedure. This test identifies ulcers, tumors, or obstruction in the esophagus, stomach, and small intestine.	

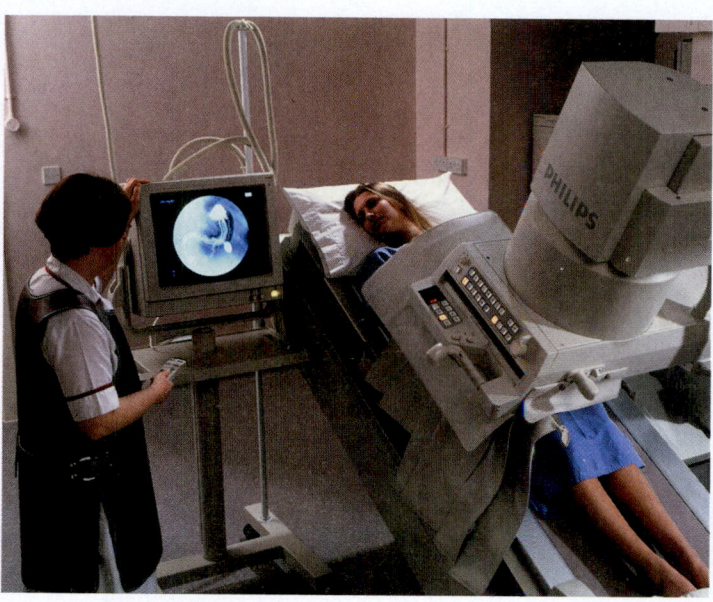

FIGURE 3-29 ■ Upper gastrointestinal series with fluoroscopy.
This patient swallowed the contrast medium barium. The tilted table allows the barium to flow with gravity and coat her stomach and intestines, outlining them to make them visible on the monitor that is showing a continuously moving x-ray image. The radiologist is wearing a lead apron to protect her from exposure to the x-rays.

3.4 PRACTICE LAPS

Use the Answer Key at the end of the book to check your answers.

A. Give the Meaning of Combining Forms

Next to each combining form, write its meaning. The first one has been done for you.

Combining Form	Meaning	Combining Form	Meaning
1. **bil/i-**	*bile; gall*	7. sensitiv/o-	
2. cholangi/o-		8. scop/o-	
3. chol/e-		9. son/o-	
4. cholecyst/o-		10. tom/o-	
5. cutane/o-		11. ven/o-	
6. pancreat/o-			

B. Build Words

Read the definition of the medical word. Look at the combining form that is given. Select the correct suffix from the Suffix List, and write it on the blank line. Then build the medical word, and write it on the line. (Remember: You may need to remove the combining vowel. Always remove the hyphens and slash.) Be sure to check your spelling.

Suffix List

-gram (picture; record)	-graphy (process of recording)	-ity (condition; state)

Definition of the Medical Word	Combining Form	Suffix	Build the Medical Word
Example: Process of recording (the) bile duct	**cholangi/o-**	*-graphy*	*cholangiography*

[You think process of recording (-graphy) + bile duct (cholangi/o-). You change the order of the word parts to put the suffix last. You write cholangiography.]

Definition of the Medical Word	Combining Form	Suffix	Build the Medical Word
1. Process of recording (images as a) cut, layer (or) slice	tom/o-		
2. State (of being) sensitive to	sensitiv/o-		
3. Picture (or) record (of the) gallbladder	cholecyst/o-		
4. Process of recording (the) gallbladder	cholecyst/o-		
5. Picture (or) record (of the) bile duct	cholangi/o-		

C. Define Abbreviations

1. BE _____

2. C&S _____

3. LFTs _____

4. O&P _____

5. UGI _____

3.5 Medical Procedures, Drugs, and Surgical Procedures

Word or Phrase	Description	Pronunciation/Word Parts

Medical Procedures

insertion of nasogastric (NG) tube	Procedure to insert a long, flexible **nasogastric tube** through the nose into the stomach. It is used to drain secretions from the stomach, take a sample of gastric acid, or give feedings or drugs to a patient on a temporary basis (see Figure 3-30 ■).	**nasogastric** (NAY-zoh-GAS-trik) **nas/o-** *nose* **gastr/o-** *stomach* **-ic** *pertaining to*

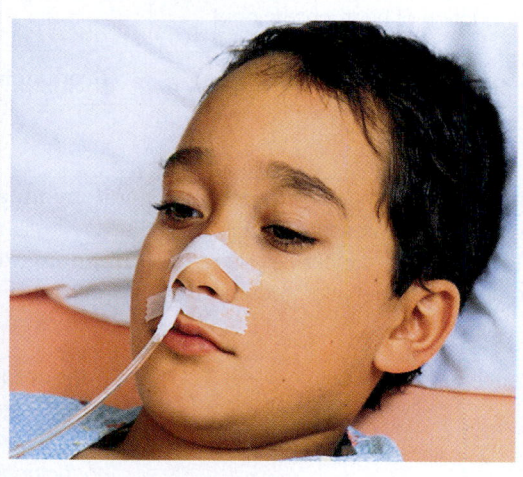

FIGURE 3-30 ■ Nasogastric tube.
This patient has a nasogastric (NG) tube. It was inserted into the nose and, as he swallowed, it was advanced through the esophagus and into the stomach and then taped to the skin to hold it in position. Only liquid feedings or liquid drugs can be given through an NG tube.

enema	Procedure to insert water into the rectum to stimulate a bowel movement and relieve constipation	**enema** (EN-eh-mah)

Category	Indication	Pronunciation/Word Parts

Drugs

antacid drug	Treats heartburn by neutralizing acid in the stomach	**antacid** (ant-AS-id) The prefix **anti-** means *against*.
antibiotic drug	Treats gastrointestinal infections caused by bacteria. Antibiotic drugs are not effective against viral gastrointestinal infections.	**antibiotic** (AN-tee-by-AW-tik) **anti-** *against* **bi/o-** *living organism; living tissue* **-tic** *pertaining to*
antidiarrheal drug	Treats diarrhea by slowing down peristalsis, which increases water absorption from feces	**antidiarrheal** (AN-tee-DY-ah-REE-al) **anti-** *against* **dia-** *complete; through* **rrhe/o-** *discharge; flow* **-al** *pertaining to*
antiemetic drug	Treats nausea and vomiting and motion sickness	**antiemetic** (AN-tee-eh-MET-ik) **anti-** *against* **emet/o-** *vomiting* **-ic** *pertaining to*
drug for gallstones	Dissolves gallstones (instead of surgical removal)	

Category	Indication	Pronunciation/Word Parts
H₂ blocker drug	Treats gastroesophageal reflux disease (GERD) and peptic ulcer disease (PUD) by blocking H₂ (histamine 2) receptors in the stomach that trigger the release of hydrochloric acid	

laxative drug	Treats constipation by softening the feces or by adding dietary fiber. A **suppository** directly stimulates peristalsis by its presence in the rectum.	**laxative** (LAK-sah-tiv)
		
		suppository
		(soo-PAW-zih-TOR-ee)
		   supposit/o- *placed beneath*
		   -ory *having the function of*

proton pump inhibitor drug	Treats gastroesophageal reflux disease (GERD) and peptic ulcer disease (PUD) by blocking the final step in the production of hydrochloric acid	

Word or Phrase	Description	Pronunciation/Word Parts

Surgical Procedures

abdominocentesis	Procedure to remove fluid from the abdomen using a needle inserted into the abdominal cavity. It is done to relieve abdominal pressure from fluid associated with ascites. It is also done to identify any cancer cells in the peritoneal fluid or to identify blood in the peritoneal fluid after abdominal trauma.	**abdominocentesis**
		(ab-DAW-mih-NOH-sen-TEE-sihs)
		   abdomin/o- *abdomen*
		   -centesis *procedure to puncture*

appendectomy	Procedure to remove the appendix because of appendicitis	**appendectomy**
		(AP-en-DEK-toh-mee)
		   append/o- *small structure hanging from a larger structure*
		   -ectomy *surgical removal*

bariatric surgery	Procedure to treat severe obesity. It limits food intake and nutrient absorption by decreasing the size of the stomach. Also known as **weight loss surgery**.
	• A **gastric balloon** is swallowed uninflated and then inflated once it is in the stomach.
	• An **adjustable gastric band** is placed across the upper part of the stomach to decrease its total size.
	• A **gastric sleeve** removes 80% of the stomach. This is also known as a **gastroplasty**.
		bariatric (BAIR-ee-AT-rik)
		   bar/o- *weight*
		   iatr/o- *medical treatment; physician*
		   -ic *pertaining to*
		
		surgery (SIR-jer-ee)
		   surg/o- *operative procedure*
		   -ery *process*
		
		gastroplasty (GAS-troh-PLAS-tee)
		   gastr/o- *stomach*
		   -plasty *process of reshaping by surgery*

biopsy	Procedure to remove a small piece of tissue from an ulcer, polyp, mass, or tumor. It is examined under a microscope to look for abnormal or cancerous cells.	**biopsy** (BY-awp-see)
		   bi/o- *living organism; living tissue*
		   -opsy *process of viewing*

Word or Phrase	Description	Pronunciation/Word Parts
bowel resection and anastomosis	Procedure to remove a section of diseased intestine and rejoin the intestine. An end-to-end anastomosis joins the two cut ends of the intestine together. An end-to-side anastomosis joins one end to the side of another part of the intestine.	**resection** (ree-SEK-shun) **resect/o-** *cut out; remove* **-ion** *action; condition* **anastomosis** (ah-NAS-toh-MOH-sihs) **anastom/o-** *create an opening between two structures* **-osis** *abnormal condition; process*
cholecystectomy	Procedure to remove the gallbladder. This is done as a minimally invasive **laparoscopic cholecystectomy** that uses a **laparoscope** that is inserted through tiny incisions in the abdominal wall (see Figure 3-31 ■).	**cholecystectomy** (KOH-lee-sihs-TEK-toh-mee) **cholecyst/o-** *gallbladder* **-ectomy** *surgical removal* **laparoscopic** (LAP-ar-oh-SKAW-pik) **lapar/o-** *abdomen* **scop/o-** *examine with an instrument* **-ic** *pertaining to* **laparoscope** (LAP-ar-oh-SKOHP) **lapar/o-** *abdomen* **-scope** *instrument used to examine*

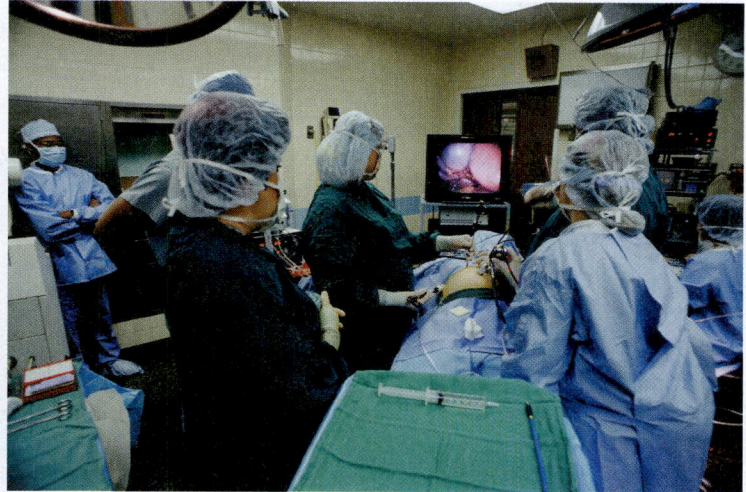

FIGURE 3-31 ■ Laparoscopic cholecystectomy.
Carbon dioxide gas is used to inflate the abdominal cavity and separate the organs. A laparoscope is inserted through one of several small incisions; it is used to visualize the gallbladder (on the computer screen), while other instruments grasp and remove the gallbladder.

Dive Deeper

Robotic surgery was first performed during a laparoscopic cholecystectomy. Now robots are used routinely for many different types of surgery. As the laparoscope provides a 3-D image of the operative site, the surgeon sits at a console and manipulates the robotic arms that hold various surgical instruments.

Word or Phrase	Description	Pronunciation/Word Parts
choledocholi-thotomy	Procedure to make an incision in the common bile duct to remove a gallstone	**choledocholithotomy** (koh-LED-oh-KOH-lith-AW-toh-mee) **choledoch/o-** *common bile duct* **lith/o-** *stone* **-tomy** *process of cutting; process of making an incision*
colostomy	Procedure to remove the diseased part of the colon and create a new opening in the abdominal wall where feces can leave the body (see Figure 3-32 ■). The cut end of the colon is brought out through the abdominal wall. The edges of the colon are rolled to make a mouth-like opening (**stoma**), and this is sutured to the abdominal wall. The patient wears a plastic disposable pouch that adheres to the abdominal wall to collect feces. If part of the ileum and colon are removed and a stoma created, the procedure is known as an **ileostomy**.	**colostomy** (koh-LAW-stoh-mee) **col/o-** *colon* **-stomy** *surgically created opening* **stoma** (STOH-mah) **ileostomy** (IL-ee-AW-stoh-mee) **ile/o-** *ileum* **-stomy** *surgically created opening*

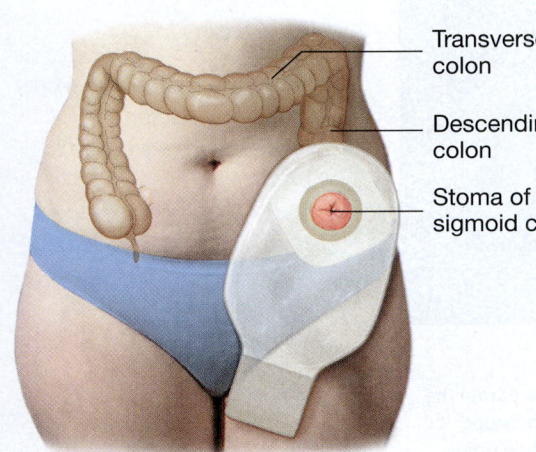

Transverse colon

Descending colon

Stoma of the sigmoid colon

A.

B.

FIGURE 3-32 ■ Colostomy and stoma.
A. This colostomy is performed on the sigmoid colon. The red mucosa of the cut end of the sigmoid colon was rolled back on itself to create a stoma, which is sutured to the abdominal wall. **B.** The patient wears a plastic disposable colostomy bag that adheres to the skin and collects feces.

Word or Phrase	Description	Pronunciation/Word Parts
endoscopy	Procedure that uses an **endoscope** (a flexible, fiberoptic scope with a magnifying lens and a light source) to internally examine the gastrointestinal system. An endoscopic procedure can be coupled with another procedure such as a biopsy or removal of a polyp.	**endoscopy** (en-DAW-skoh-pee) **end/o-** *innermost; within* **-scopy** *process of using an instrument to examine* **endoscope** (EN-doh-skohp) **end/o-** *innermost; within* **-scope** *instrument used to examine*

Word or Phrase	Description	Pronunciation/Word Parts

Dive Deeper

These procedures use an endoscope inserted through the nose or mouth.

- **Esophagoscopy**: Visualization and examination of the esophagus
- **Gastroscopy**: Visualization and examination of the stomach (after the endoscope first passes through the esophagus)
- **Esophagogastroduodenoscopy (EGD)**: Visualization and examination of the esophagus first, followed by the stomach, and then the duodenum

These procedures use an endoscope inserted through the rectum.

- **Sigmoidoscopy**: Visualization and examination of the rectum and sigmoid colon using a sigmoidoscope
- **Colonoscopy**: Visualization and examination of the entire colon using a **colonoscope** (see Figure 3-33 ■)

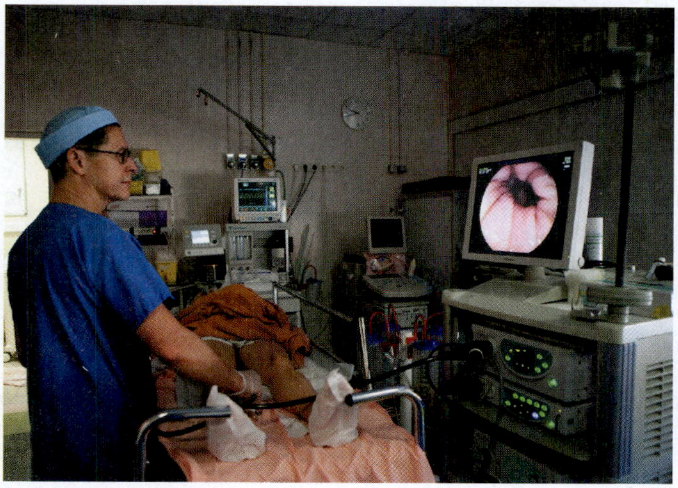

FIGURE 3-33 ■ Colonoscopy.
A colonoscope with a camera is passed through the patient's anus to examine the rectum and colon. The images are transmitted to a computer screen for viewing and are also recorded for the patient's electronic medical record.

esophagoscopy
(eh-SAW-fah-GAW-skoh-pee)
　esophag/o- *esophagus*
　-scopy *process of using an instrument to examine*

gastroscopy
(gas-TRAW-skoh-pee)
　gastr/o- *stomach*
　-scopy *process of using an instrument to examine*

esophagogastroduodenoscopy
(eh-SAW-fah-goh-GAS-troh-DOO-oh-den-AW-skoh-pee)
　esophag/o- *esophagus*
　gastr/o- *stomach*
　duoden/o- *duodenum*
　-scopy *process of using an instrument to examine*

sigmoidoscopy
(SIG-moyd-AW-skoh-pee)
　sigmoid/o- *sigmoid colon*
　-scopy *process of using an instrument to examine*

colonoscopy
(KOH-lon-AW-skoh-pee)
　colon/o- *colon*
　-scopy *process of using an instrument to examine*

colonoscope
(koh-LAW-noh-skohp)
　colon/o- *colon*
　-scope *instrument used to examine*

Word or Phrase	Description	Pronunciation/Word Parts
exploratory laparotomy	Procedure that uses a long abdominal incision to open the abdominopelvic cavity widely so that it can be explored for evidence of trauma or disease of any of the gastrointestinal organs.	**laparotomy** (LAP-ar-AW-toh-mee) **lapar/o-** *abdomen* **-tomy** *process of cutting; process of making an incision*
gastrectomy	Procedure to remove all or part of the stomach because of a cancerous or benign tumor	**gastrectomy** (gas-TREK-toh-mee) **gastr/o-** *stomach* **-ectomy** *surgical removal*

Word or Phrase	Description	Pronunciation/Word Parts

gastrostomy	Procedure to create a temporary or permanent opening from the abdominal wall into the stomach to insert a gastrostomy feeding tube. This is done for patients who have had an NG tube for some time but still cannot eat on their own.
	
	For a **percutaneous endoscopic gastrostomy (PEG)**, a permanent PEG feeding tube is inserted through the abdominal wall. Then, under visual guidance from an endoscope that was previously passed through the mouth, the PEG tube is positioned in the stomach (see Figure 3-34 ■).
		gastrostomy
		(gas-TRAW-stoh-mee)
		  gastr/o- *stomach*
		  -stomy *surgically created opening*
		percutaneous
		(PER-kyoo-TAY-nee-uhs)
		  per- *through; throughout*
		  cutane/o- *skin*
		  -ous *pertaining to*
		endoscopic (EN-doh-SKAW-pik)
		  end/o- *innermost; within*
		  scop/o- *examine with an instrument*
		  -ic *pertaining to*

Abdominal wall
Skin
PEG tube
Stomach

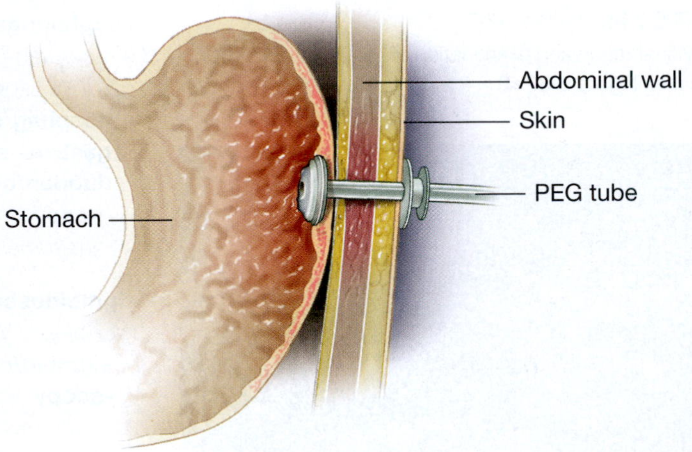

FIGURE 3-34 ■ PEG tube.
This permanent feeding tube was inserted during a percutaneous endoscopic gastrostomy.

Word or Phrase	Description	Pronunciation/Word Parts

hemorrhoid-ectomy	Procedure to remove hemorrhoids from the rectum or from around the anus	**hemorrhoidectomy**
		(HEM-oh-royd-EK-toh-mee)
		  hemorrhoid/o- *hemorrhoid*
		  -ectomy *surgical removal*

herniorrhaphy	Procedure that uses sutures or surgical mesh to close a defect in the abdominal muscle wall where there is a hernia	**herniorrhaphy**
		(HER-nee-OR-ah-fee)
		  herni/o- *hernia; protruding part*
		  -rrhaphy *procedure of suturing*

jejunostomy	Procedure to create a temporary or permanent opening from the abdominal wall into the jejunum to insert a jejunostomy feeding tube.
	For a **percutaneous endoscopic jejunostomy (PEJ)**, a PEJ tube is inserted through the abdominal wall. Then, under visual guidance from an endoscope that was previously passed through the mouth, the PEJ tube is positioned in the jejunum.
		jejunostomy
		(JEH-joo-NAW-stoh-mee)
		  jejun/o- *jejunum*
		  -stomy *surgically created opening*

Word or Phrase	Description	Pronunciation/Word Parts
liver transplantation	Procedure to remove a severely damaged liver from a patient with end-stage liver disease and insert a new liver from a donor. The patient (the recipient) is matched by blood type and tissue type to the donor. Liver transplant patients must take immunosuppressant drugs for the rest of their lives to keep their bodies from rejecting the foreign tissue that is their new liver.	**transplantation** (TRANS-plan-TAY-shun) **transplant/o-** *move and put in another place* **-ation** *being; having; process*
polypectomy	Procedure to remove one or more polyps from the colon using forceps for a sessile polyp or a wire snare positioned around the thin stalk of a pedunculated polyp.	**polypectomy** (PAW-lih-PEK-toh-mee) **polyp/o-** *polyp* **-ectomy** *surgical removal*

3.5 PRACTICE LAPS

Use the Answer Key at the end of the book to check your answers.

A. Give the Meaning of Combining Forms

Next to each combining form, write its meaning. The first one has been done for you.

Combining Form	Meaning	Combining Form	Meaning
1. **anastom/o-**	*create an opening between two structures*	11. lapar/o-	
2. append/o-		12. lith/o-	
3. bar/o-		13. nas/o-	
4. cholecyst/o-		14. polyp/o-	
5. choledoch/o-		15. resect/o-	
6. col/o-		16. rrhe/o-	
7. gastr/o-		17. supposit/o-	
8. hemorrhoid/o-		18. surg/o-	
9. herni/o-		19. transplant/o-	
10. iatr/o-			

B. Build Words

Read the definition of the medical word. Look at the combining form that is given. Select the correct suffix from the Suffix List, and write it on the blank line. Then build the medical word, and write it on the line. (Remember: You may need to remove the combining vowel. Always remove the hyphens and slash.) Be sure to check your spelling.

Suffix List

-ation (being; having; process)	-opsy (process of viewing)	-rrhaphy (procedure of suturing)
-centesis (procedure to puncture)	-ory (having the function of)	-scope (instrument used to examine)
-ectomy (surgical removal)	-osis (abnormal condition; process)	-stomy (surgically created opening)
-ery (process)	-plasty (process of reshaping by	-tomy (process of cutting; process
-ion (action; condition)	surgery)	of making an incision)

Definition of the Medical Word	Combining Form	Suffix	Build the Medical Word
Example: Action (to) cut out (and) remove	**resect/o-**	*-ion*	*resection*

[*You think* action *(-ion)* + cut out (and) remove *(resect/o-)*. *You change the order of the word parts to put the suffix last. You write* resection.]

1. Surgical removal (of the) stomach	gastr/o-	_____	_____
2. Instrument used to examine (the) abdomen	lapar/o-	_____	_____
3. Process of making an incision (to remove a) stone	lith/o-	_____	_____
4. Procedure of suturing (a) hernia	herni/o-	_____	_____
5. Surgical removal (of a) polyp	polyp/o-	_____	_____
6. Process (of an) operative procedure	surg/o-	_____	_____
7. Process (to) move and put in another place	transplant/o-	_____	_____
8. Procedure to puncture (the) abdomen	abdomin/o-	_____	_____
9. Surgical removal (of) small thing hanging from larger structure	append/o-	_____	_____
10. Process of viewing living tissue	bi/o-	_____	_____
11. Surgical removal (of the) gallbladder	cholecyst/o-	_____	_____
12. Surgically created opening (in the) colon	col/o-	_____	_____
13. Process of reshaping by surgery (on the) stomach	gastr/o-	_____	_____
14. Process (to) create an opening	anastom/o-	_____	_____
15. Surgical removal (of a) hemorrhoid	hemorrhoid/o-	_____	_____
16. Having the function of (something) placed beneath	supposit/o-	_____	_____

C. Define Abbreviations

1. EGD _____   3. PEG _____

2. NG _____

Abbreviations Summary

ABD, abd	abdomen	**HAV**	hepatitis A virus
ALP	alkaline phosphatase	**HBV**	hepatitis B virus
ALT	alanine aminotransferase; alanine transaminase	**HCV**	hepatitis C virus
AST	aspartate aminotransferase; aspartate transaminase	**IBD**	inflammatory bowel disease
		IBS	irritable bowel syndrome
BE	barium enema	**LFTs**	liver function tests
BM	bowel movement	**MRI**	magnetic resonance imaging
C&S	culture and sensitivity	**N&V**	nausea and vomiting
CAT, CT	computerized axial tomography	**NG**	nasogastric
CBD	common bile duct	**O&P**	ova and parasites
CLO	*Campylobacter*-like organism	**OCG**	oral cholecystogram; oral cholecystography
EGD	esophagogastroduodenoscopy	**PEG**	percutaneous endoscopic gastrostomy
ERCP	endoscopic retrograde cholangiopancreatography	**PEJ**	percutaneous endoscopic jejunostomy
		PUD	peptic ulcer disease
GERD	gastroesophageal reflux disease	**RLQ**	right lower quadrant (of the abdomen)
GGTP, GGT	gamma-glutamyl transpeptidase	**RUQ**	right upper quadrant (of the abdomen)
GI	gastrointestinal	**UGI**	upper gastrointestinal (series)

Word Alert

It's Greek to Me! Did you notice that some words have two different combining forms? Combining forms from both Greek and Latin remain a part of medical language today.

Word	Greek	Latin	Medical Word Examples
abdomen	celi/o-	abdomin/o-	celiac disease; abdominal
	lapar/o-	ventr/o-	laparoscopy; ventral
break down food; digest		digest/o-	digestive
digestion	peps/o-, pept/o-		pepsin, peptic
fat	steat/o-	lip/o-	steatorrhea; lipase
intestine	enter/o-	intestin/o-	gastroenteritis; gastrointestinal
mouth	stomat/o-	or/o-	stomatitis; oral
navel; umbilicus	omphal/o-	umbilic/o-	omphalocele; umbilical
rectum	proct/o-	rect/o-	proctitis; rectal
saliva	sial/o-	saliv/o-	sialolith; salivary
tongue	gloss/o-	lingu/o-	glossitis; sublingual
yellow	icter/o-	jaund/o-	nonicteric; jaundice

Career Focus
Meet Patricia, a medical assistant

"The best part of my job as a medical assistant is dealing with the patients. I love coming to work and doing it every day. It's just very fulfilling to me. I love helping people. I love talking to them. I love learning about their families, and that's what you find in this kind of practice. This is a huge clinic. It has internal medicine, pediatrics, OB/GYN, and plastic surgery. We have a specialty department with ears, nose, and throat doctors. We have optometry; we have physical therapy. I work with patients. I bring them in, I weigh them, take their blood pressure, find out what their problem is, write down their problem, and go to the physician and tell why the patient is here. I definitely think medical assistants are the first line of defense for the doctor. I bring everything to the doctor. We work as a team. We have a great rapport together and with our patients."

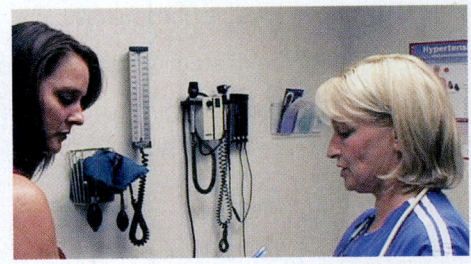

- **Medical assistants** are allied health professionals who perform and document a variety of clinical and laboratory procedures and assist the physician during medical procedures in the office or clinic.

- **Gastroenterologists** are physicians who practice in the medical specialty of gastroenterology. They diagnose and treat patients with diseases of the gastrointestinal system. Physicians can take additional training and become board certified in the subspecialty of pediatric gastroenterology. Cancerous tumors of the gastrointestinal system are treated medically by an **oncologist** or surgically by a general **surgeon**.

---

gastroenterologist
(GAS-troh-EN-ter-AW-loh-jist)
  gastr/o- *stomach*
  enter/o- *intestine*
  log/o- *study of; word*
  -ist *person who specializes in*

---

oncologist (ong-KAW-loh-jist)
  onc/o- *mass; tumor*
  log/o- *study of; word*
  -ist *person who specializes in*

---

surgeon (SER-jun)
  surg/o- *operative procedure*
  -eon *person who performs*

Chapter Review Exercises

Dive In: Medical Language Exercises

Test your knowledge of the chapter by completing these review exercises. Use the Answer Key at the end of the book to check your answers. Note: Each of the numbered exercise headers corresponds to a numbered learning outcome at the beginning of the chapter.

3.1 Anatomy

MATCHING EXERCISE

Match each word or phrase to its description.

1. biliary tree
2. colostrum
3. esophagus
4. gustatory cortex
5. jejunum
6. omentum
7. oral cavity
8. pharynx
9. sublingual gland
10. villi

_____ throat

_____ absorb nutrients in the small intestine

_____ one of the salivary glands

_____ also known as the *mouth*

_____ first food for a baby

_____ collectively all of the bile ducts

_____ fatty covering over the small intestine

_____ between the pharynx and stomach

_____ receives sensory information from tongue's taste receptors

_____ second part of the small bowel

CIRCLE EXERCISE

Circle the correct answer from the choices given.

1. All of the following are salivary glands *except* (**fundus, parotid, sublingual**).
2. (**Bile, Cardia, Peritoneal fluid**) is a thick, yellow-green fluid.
3. The (**anus, duodenum, haustra**) is a 10-inch, C-shaped segment of small intestine.
4. Chyme contains all of the following *except* (**food particles, digestive enzymes, rugae**).
5. The (**cecum, hard palate, gallbladder**) is a dark green sac posterior to the liver.
6. The (**ileum, parotid gland, pylorus**) is the last of the four regions of the stomach.

TRUE OR FALSE EXERCISE

*Indicate whether each statement is true or false by writing **T** or **F** on the line.*

1. _____ The mesentery provides support to the colon and rectum.
2. _____ Hepatocytes are liver cells that produce bile.
3. _____ The uvula hangs from the sigmoid colon.
4. _____ The lumen is the central, open area of the intestines.

PLURAL NOUN AND ADJECTIVE EXERCISE

Read the noun and write its plural form and/or adjective form on the line. Only write in the plural noun or adjective if there is a blank line there for it. Be sure to check your spelling. The first one has been done for you.

Singular Noun	Plural Noun	Adjective	Singular Noun	Plural Noun	Adjective
1. **mucosa**		*mucosal*	10. liver		_____
2. abdomen		_____	11. pancreas		_____
3. anus		_____	12. pharynx		_____
4. appendix		_____	13. pylorus		_____
5. cecum		_____	14. rectum		_____
6. duodenum		_____	15. saliva		_____
7. esophagus		_____	16. stomach		_____
8. ileum		_____	17. tongue		_____
9. intestine	_____	_____			

DIVIDING WORDS EXERCISE

Separate these words into their component parts (prefix, combining form, suffix). Some words do not contain all three word parts. The first one has been done for you.

Medical Word	Prefix	Combining Form	Suffix	Medical Word	Prefix	Combining Form	Suffix
1. **oral**		*or/o-*	*-al*	7. hepatic		_____	_____
2. abdominal		_____	_____	8. parotid	_____	_____	_____
3. biliary		_____	_____	9. pharyngeal		_____	_____
4. digestive		_____	_____	10. salivary		_____	_____
5. gastric		_____	_____	11. sphincter		_____	_____
6. gustatory		_____	_____	12. sublingual	_____	_____	_____

SPELLING EXERCISE

Read each medical word pronunciation and write the medical word that it represents. Be sure to check your spelling. The first one has been done for you.

1. **(ab-DAW-mih-nal)** *abdominal*
2. (PAN-kree-AT-ik) _____
3. (myoo-KOH-sah) _____
4. (sub-LING-gwal) _____
5. (YOO-vyoo-lah) _____
6. (fah-RIN-jee-al) _____
7. (jeh-JOO-num) _____
8. (SIG-moyd) _____
9. (heh-PAT-ik) _____
10. (BIL-ee-AIR-ee) _____

3.2 Physiology

MATCHING EXERCISE

Match each word or phrase to its description.

1. amylase
2. deglutition
3. elimination
4. emulsification
5. gastrin
6. glucose
7. hydrochloric acid
8. intrinsic factor

_____ stimulates the release of hydrochloric acid and pepsinogen
_____ produced by the stomach
_____ a simple sugar
_____ also known as *defecation*
_____ digestive enzyme
_____ chemical process of breaking down fats
_____ swallowing
_____ helps the stomach absorb vitamin B_{12}

CIRCLE EXERCISE

Circle the correct answer from the choices given.

1. Amylase digests all of the following *except* (**carbohydrates, fats, starches**).
2. (**Deglutition, Emulsification, Mastication**) is the medical name for chewing.
3. A bowel movement is known as all of the following *except* (**feces, flatus, stool**).
4. Lactase breaks down (**amylase, fat, sugar**).
5. Mechanical digestion includes (**absorption, deglutition, elimination**).

TRUE OR FALSE EXERCISE

*Indicate whether each statement is true or false by writing **T** or **F** on the line.*

1. _____ Amylase is produced by the salivary glands and by the pancreas.
2. _____ Pepsinogen is an inactive substance until it is converted to pepsin.
3. _____ The gallbladder releases bile into the stomach.
4. _____ Digestion begins in the oral cavity and continues throughout the small intestine.
5. _____ Partially digested foods in the stomach can be absorbed into blood vessels around the stomach.

DIVIDING WORDS EXERCISE

Separate these words into their component parts (prefix, combining form, suffix). Some words do not contain all three word parts. The first one has been done for you.

Medical Word	Prefix	Combining Form	Suffix	Medical Word	Prefix	Combining Form	Suffix
1. **absorption**		*absorpt/o-*	*-ion*	6. gastrin		_____	_____
2. amylase		_____	_____	7. lactose		_____	_____
3. defecation	_____	_____	_____	8. mastication		_____	_____
4. deglutition		_____	_____	9. pepsinogen		_____	_____
5. digestion		_____	_____				

SPELLING EXERCISE

Read each medical word pronunciation and write the medical word that it represents. Be sure to check your spelling. The first one has been done for you.

1. **(meh-KAN-ih-kal)** _____*mechanical*_____
2. (dy-JES-chun) _____
3. (PAIR-ih-STAL-sihs) _____
4. (EN-zime) _____
5. (GLOO-kohs) _____

3.3 Diseases

MATCHING EXERCISE

Match each word or phrase to its description.

1. anorexia	_____ caused by a ruptured appendix
2. appendicitis	_____ rebound pain in the right lower quadrant
3. Crohn disease	_____ baby's first stool
4. dyspepsia	_____ indigestion
5. gastroenteritis	_____ severe constipation
6. hepatoma	_____ "skip areas" in the mucosa
7. jaundice	_____ liver cancer
8. meconium	_____ stone in the salivary gland
9. obstipation	_____ decreased appetite
10. pedunculated polyp	_____ expelled chyme
11. peritonitis	_____ thin stalk with ball-shaped top
12. sialolithiasis	_____ caused by a bacterium or a virus
13. volvulus	_____ malrotation of the intestine
14. vomitus	_____ yellow eyes and skin

CIRCLE EXERCISE

Circle the correct answer from the choices given.

1. Glossitis is infection or inflammation of the (**colon, esophagus, tongue**).
2. GERD is treated in all of the following ways *except* (**avoid alcohol, elevate the head of the bed while sleeping, take an antibiotic drug**).
3. Telescoping of one segment of intestine inside the next segment is (**intussusception, irritable bowel syndrome, proctitis**).
4. Diverticula can be caused by (**a bacterial infection, eating a low-fiber diet, hepatitis**).
5. (**Celiac disease, Diarrhea, Polyps**) is an autoimmune disorder with sensitivity to certain grains.
6. A swollen, protruding vein in the rectum is a (**hemorrhoid, rectocele, varix**).
7. A hernia can be caused by all of the following *except* (**heavy lifting, jaundice, obesity**).
8. Liver disease with fluid in the abdominopelvic cavity is (**ascites, cirrhosis, hepatomegaly**).

TRUE OR FALSE EXERCISE

*Indicate whether each statement is true or false by writing **T** or **F** on the line.*

1. _____ Anorexia is the shortened name for anorexia nervosa.
2. _____ Hematemesis is the vomiting of blood.
3. _____ Gastric ulcers are commonly caused by *Helicobacter pylori*.
4. _____ Postoperative ileus can occur after abdominal surgery.
5. _____ Melena is a dark, tar-like feces of digested blood.
6. _____ An inguinal hernia occurs in the groin.
7. _____ Hepatomegaly is enlargement of the gallbladder.
8. _____ Polyphagia is painful eating or difficulty swallowing.
9. _____ A polyp in the colon can become cancerous.
10. _____ Crohn disease is a type of gluten sensitivity enteropathy.

DIVIDING WORDS

Separate these words into their component parts (prefix, combining form, suffix). Some words do not contain all three word parts. The first one has been done for you.

Medical Word	Prefix	Combining Form	Suffix	Medical Word	Prefix	Combining Form	Suffix
1. **carcinoma**		*carcin/o-*	*-oma*	11. hematemesis		_____	_____
2. anorexia	____	_____	____	12. hemorrhoid		_____	_____
3. appendicitis		_____	____	13. hepatomegaly		_____	_____
4. cirrhosis		_____	____	14. malrotation	____	_____	____
5. diverticulosis		_____	____	15. polyphagia	____	_____	____
6. dysphagia	____	_____	____	16. polyposis		_____	____
7. enteropathy		_____	____	17. postoperative	____	_____	____
8. epigastric	____	_____	____	18. rectocele		_____	____
9. fecalith		_____	____	19. sialolith		_____	____
10. glossitis		_____	____	20. steatorrhea		_____	____

SPELLING EXERCISE

Read each medical word pronunciation and write the medical word that it represents. Be sure to check your spelling. The first one has been done for you.

1. **(HER-nee-ah)** _____ *hernia* _____
2. (AN-oh-REK-see-ah) _____
3. (KOH-lee-sihs-TY-tihs) _____
4. (sih-ROH-sihs) _____
5. (DY-ver-TIH-kyoo-LOH-sihs) _____
6. (dis-FAY-jee-ah) _____
7. (GAS-troh-EN-ter-EYE-tihs) _____
8. (HEE-mah-TEM-eh-sihs) _____
9. (HEM-oh-royd) _____
10. (IL-ee-uhs) _____
11. (JAWN-dihs) _____
12. (PAIR-ih-toh-NY-tihs) _____
13. (PAW-lip) _____
14. (HEP-ah-TY-tihs) _____

3.4 Laboratory, Diagnostic, and Radiologic Procedures

MATCHING EXERCISE

Match each word or phrase to its description.

1. albumin
2. barium
3. barium swallow
4. cholangiography
5. CLO test
6. HIDA scan
7. occult
8. sonogram

_____ also known as *cholescintigraphy*

_____ major protein molecule in the blood

_____ radiologic procedure to outline the bile ducts

_____ picture of sound waves

_____ hidden

_____ detects *Helicobacter pylori*

_____ liquid contrast medium

_____ part of an upper GI series

TRUE OR FALSE EXERCISE

*Indicate whether each statement is true or false by writing **T** or **F** on the line.*

1. _____ A CT scan creates thin, successive slices of abdominal organs.
2. _____ An elevated blood alkaline phosphatase is due to liver disease or bone disease.
3. _____ Albumin is a digestive enzyme found in the blood.
4. _____ Blood tests can be done for direct, indirect, and total bilirubin.
5. _____ The fecal occult blood test is also known as the *stool guaiac test*.
6. _____ The O&P test can show parasites in the gastrointestinal system.
7. _____ Barium can be taken by mouth or given as an enema.

DIVIDING WORDS EXERCISE

Separate these words into their component parts (prefix, combining form, suffix). Some words do not contain all three word parts. The first one has been done for you.

Medical Word	Prefix	Combining Form	Suffix	Medical Word	Prefix	Combining Form	Suffix
1. **sensitivity**		*sensitiv/o-*	*-ity*	5. sonogram		_____	_____
2. cholangiogram		_____	_____	6. tomography		_____	_____
3. intravenous	_____	_____	_____	7. transhepatic	_____	_____	_____
4. percutaneous	_____	_____	_____				

SPELLING EXERCISE

Read each medical word pronunciation and write the medical word that it represents. Be sure to check your spelling. The first one has been done for you.

1. **(al-BYOO-min)** _____*albumin*_____
2. (BIL-ih-ROO-bin) _____
3. (oh-KULT) _____
4. (koh-LAN-jee-AW-grah-fee) _____
5. (EN-doh-SKAW-pik) _____
6. (toh-MAW-grah-fee) _____
7. (KOH-lee-SIHS-toh-gram) _____

3.5 Medical Procedures, Drugs, and Surgical Procedures

MATCHING EXERCISE

Match each word or phrase to its description.

1. abdominocentesis
2. antacid
3. antiemetic
4. biopsy
5. gastric balloon
6. herniorrhaphy
7. laparoscope
8. suppository
9. stoma
10. wire snare

_____ type of bariatric surgery
_____ uses surgical mesh
_____ used during a cholecystectomy
_____ used to do a polypectomy
_____ drug to treat vomiting
_____ uses a needle to treat ascites
_____ placed in the rectum
_____ tissue examined under a microscope
_____ surgically created mouth-like opening of intestine
_____ drug to neutralize stomach acid

CIRCLE EXERCISE

Circle the correct answer from the choices given.

1. An H$_2$ blocker drug is used to treat all of the following *except* (**GERD, O&P, PUD**).
2. The combining form *bar/o-* means (**barium, bowel, weight**).
3. An endoscope has all of the following *except* (**a light, a magnifying lens, a surgical mesh**).
4. A (**gastrectomy, gastroscopy, gastrostomy**) is a permanent opening created in the stomach to insert a feeding tube.
5. A percutaneous tube is inserted through the (**mouth, skin, stomach**).

TRUE OR FALSE EXERCISE

*Indicate whether each statement is true or false by writing **T** or **F** on the line.*

1. _____ An NG tube is used to feed a patient on a temporary basis.
2. _____ An antiemetic drug slows peristalsis and stops diarrhea.
3. _____ Bariatric surgery is also known as *weight loss surgery*.
4. _____ Choledocholithotomy removes a stone from the colon.
5. _____ An exploratory laparotomy uses a long incision to open up the abdomen.

DIVIDING WORDS EXERCISE

Separate these words into their component parts (prefix, combining form, suffix). Some words do not contain all three word parts. The first one has been done for you.

Medical Word	Prefix	Combining Form	Suffix	Medical Word	Prefix	Combining Form	Suffix
1. **antibiotic**	*anti-*	*bi/o-*	*-tic*	8. herniorrhaphy		_____	_____
2. anastomosis		_____	_____	9. laparoscope		_____	_____
3. antiemetic	_____	_____	_____	10. laparotomy		_____	_____
4. appendectomy		_____	_____	11. percutaneous	_____	_____	_____
5. biopsy		_____	_____	12. polypectomy		_____	_____
6. cholecystectomy		_____	_____	13. suppository		_____	_____
7. colostomy		_____	_____				

SPELLING EXERCISE

Read each medical word pronunciation and write the medical word that it represents. Be sure to check your spelling. The first one has been done for you.

1. **(ant-AS-id)** ___antacid___
2. (ab-DAW-mih-NOH-sen-TEE-sihs) _____
3. (AN-tee-eh-MET-ik) _____
4. (BAIR-ee-AT-rik) _____
5. (BY-awp-see) _____

6. (KOH-lee-sihs-TEK-toh-mee) _____
7. (koh-LAW-stoh-mee) _____
8. (en-DAW-skoh-pee) _____
9. (HER-nee-OR-ah-fee) _____
10. (NAY-zoh-GAS-trik) _____

Immerse Yourself: Analyze Medical Reports

Electronic Patient Record #1

This report is an Office Visit SOAP Note. Read the note and answer the questions.

PEARSON PEDIATRIC ASSOCIATES

Task   Edit   View   Time Scale   Options   Help

OFFICE VISIT SOAP NOTE

PATIENT NAME: NGUYEN, Thi

PATIENT NUMBER: 6824-97

DATE OF VISIT: 11/19/20xx

SUBJECTIVE: The mother reports that this 5-year-old female was well until 2 days ago, when she was at a county fair and ate food from a food truck. Later that evening, she was anorexic. The next morning, she had N&V, mild dyspepsia, and then later diarrhea.

OBJECTIVE: Temperature 101, heart rate 160, respiratory rate 38, blood pressure 115/80. The child is flushed and sweaty and appears lethargic and slightly dehydrated. She complains of abdominal pain.

ASSESSMENT: Gastroenteritis.

PLAN: Increased fluid intake. Tylenol for fever. Call the office if not improved in 24 hours.

---

1. Divide these words into their word parts. Give the meanings of the word parts.

   a. anorexic

Word Part	Meaning
_____	_____
_____	_____
_____	_____

   b. dyspepsia

Word Part	Meaning
_____	_____
_____	_____
_____	_____

c. gastroenteritis

Word Part	Meaning
_____	_____
_____	_____

2. What is the meaning of the abbreviation *N&V*? _____

3. What is the probable cause of the patient's gastroenteritis? _____

4. Research the meaning of these words.

lethargic _____

dehydrated _____

Electronic Patient Record #2

This is an Admission History and Physical Examination. Read the report and answer the questions.

PEARSON GENERAL HOSPITAL

Task   Edit   View   Time Scale   Options   Help

ADMISSION HISTORY AND PHYSICAL EXAMINATION

PATIENT NAME: MARTINEZ, Javier

HOSPITAL NUMBER: 138-524-7193

DATE OF ADMISSION: November 19, 20xx

HISTORY OF PRESENT ILLNESS

This is a 20-year-old Hispanic male who experienced severe abdominal pain beginning on the morning of admission. He was awakened at 6:00 A.M. by sharp pains in the stomach. Drinking a glass of milk, which usually helps this type of pain, was not effective. He also took his customary antacid, but with no relief. He went to class and ate lunch at the college, then developed nausea and vomiting. An hour later, he developed watery diarrhea with approximately three to four bowel movements over the next few hours. He denies any history of ulcerative colitis or Crohn disease. By this evening, his pain was so severe that he came to the emergency room to be seen.

PHYSICAL EXAMINATION

Temperature 100.2, pulse 84, respiratory rate 30, blood pressure 132/88. He is alert and oriented, lying uncomfortably in bed. Abdominal examination: Abdomen is soft. There is rebound tenderness in the RLQ.

LABORATORY DATA

Labs drawn in the emergency room showed an elevated white blood cell count of 14.6. Bilirubin and amylase were within normal limits. Urinalysis was unremarkable.

IMPRESSION

Acute appendicitis.

DISCUSSION

A detailed discussion was carried out with the patient and his parents. The dangers of waiting and observing his condition were described as well as the indications, possible risks, complications, and alternatives to an appendectomy. They agree with the plan to perform an appendectomy, and the patient will be taken to the operating room shortly.

James R. Rodgers, M.D.

James R. Rodgers, M.D.
JRR/bjg

D: 11/19/xx
T: 11/19/xx

1. The patient had sharp pains in his stomach. If you wanted to use the adjective form of *stomach*, you would say, "He had sharp _____ pains."

2. Divide *appendicitis* into its two word parts and give the meaning of each word part.

Word Part   **Meaning**

_____   _____

_____   _____

3. What does the abbreviation *RLQ* mean? _____

4. What is the abbreviation for *nausea and vomiting*? _____

5. What is the category of drug that neutralizes acid in the stomach?

_____

6. What is another medical name for *vomiting*?

_____

7. What is the medical word that means *surgical removal of the appendix*?

_____

8. The patient has taken milk and an antacid in the past for his stomach pains. This suggests he has a previous history of what disease condition? Circle the correct answer.

   pyrosis   **colon cancer**   **flatulence**   **hemorrhoids**

9. An elevated white blood cell count is associated with an infection. Where was the site of this patient's infection?

_____

10. The danger in waiting and observing the patient's condition was that he could develop a ruptured appendix that would lead to what condition? Circle the correct answer.

   peritonitis   **gastritis**   **cholecystitis**

11. The patient had a finding of "rebound tenderness" on the physical examination. Describe what a physician would do to check for rebound tenderness.

_____

12. The patient's bilirubin was within normal limits. This tells you that he is not having any problems with which of these organs?

   stomach   **liver**   **pancreas**

13. The patient's amylase was within normal limits. This tells you that he is not having any problems with which of these organs?

   pancreas   **colon**   **esophagus**

You Create the Electronic Health Record

Read the patient's words. Then read the partial sentence in the electronic health record and fill in the blank with the correct medical word. The first one has been done for you.

1. The patient says, "I can't explain it. I just don't seem to have any appetite for the past few weeks, and that's not like me at all."

   You write: The patient is complaining of _____*anorexia*_____ that has been present for the past few weeks.

2. The patient says, "I had cancer of the colon in 2018 and they took out my colon and made this new opening in my abdomen."

   You write: The patient had cancer of the colon in 2018, the colon was removed, and a _____ was created with a permanent stoma.

3. The patient says, "Oh that bug was going around, and I caught it from my kids—you know that intestinal virus with nausea, vomiting, and diarrhea. I had it for 4 days."

   You write: The patient developed viral _____ with symptoms of nausea, vomiting, and diarrhea for 4 days.

4. The patient says, "I strain most times when I try to pass a stool, but it never gets really bad."

   You write: The patient reports that she has frequent episodes of _____, but denies having any

   _____.

5. The patient says, "I don't want to but I know I am supposed to have one of those procedures where they use an instrument to look into your bowel, so I guess it's time to go."

   You write: The patient is apprehensive about having a _____ performed, but is agreeable to my referring her for this procedure.

6. The patient says, "I went to see that doctor at the hospital who specializes in treating the GI system, and he said I have an ulcer."

   You write: The patient was seen by a _____ at the hospital, who diagnosed her as having an ulcer.

7. The patient says, "This is an emergency. I have an old ulcer in my esophagus, but today I just started vomiting up blood. I know I am an alcoholic, and my liver has disease and my abdomen is all swollen up with fluid, too."

   You write: The patient has a history of an _____ ulcer and today had an episode of _____. He has a past history of alcoholism with a diagnosis of _____, and now has an enlarged abdomen with _____.

8. The patient says, "I have an acidy, irritated stomach with gas when I eat spicy foods."

   You write: The patient complains of _____ with _____ after eating spicy foods.

9. The patient says, "You know I have had these stones in my gallbladder that keep giving me trouble, so is it time for me to have them taken out?"

   You write: The patient has _____ and is now considering the surgical option of having a _____ done.

10. The patient says, "You know that stroke that I had last year. Well, I still have difficulty eating from that. I also lost weight and now my dentures don't fit right and they hurt when I eat."

    You write: The patient is complaining of _____ due to impairment from a past stroke. She also notes weight loss that resulted in poorly fitting dentures that cause _____ in the oral cavity.

My**Lab** Medical Terminology™

MyLab Medical Terminology is a premium online homework management system that includes a host of features to help you study. Registered users will find:

- A multitude of quizzes and activities built within the MyLab platform

- Powerful tools that track and analyze your results—allowing you to create a personalized learning experience

- Videos and audio pronunciations to help enrich your progress

- Streaming lesson presentations (guided lectures) and self-paced learning modules

- A space where you and your instructor can check your progress and manage your assignments

4 Pulmonology
Respiratory System

Pulmonology (PUL-moh-NAW-loh-jee) is the medical specialty that studies the anatomy and physiology of the respiratory system; uses laboratory, diagnostic, and radiologic procedures to diagnose respiratory diseases; and uses medical procedures, drugs, and surgical procedures to treat respiratory diseases.

∨ Chapter Overview and Learning Outcomes

After you study this chapter, you should be able to demonstrate mastery of the outcomes by successfully completing the exercises.

4.1 Anatomy
Identify the structures of the respiratory system.
Demonstrate proficiency in medical language.
4.1 Practice Laps

4.2 Physiology
Describe the functions of the respiratory system.
Demonstrate proficiency in medical language.
4.2 Practice Laps
Vocabulary Review

4.3 Diseases
Describe common respiratory diseases.
Demonstrate proficiency in medical language.
4.3 Practice Laps

4.4 Laboratory, Diagnostic, and Radiologic Procedures
Describe common respiratory laboratory tests, diagnostic procedures, and radiologic procedures.
Demonstrate proficiency in medical language.
4.4 Practice Laps

4.5 Medical Procedures, Drugs, and Surgical Procedures
Describe common respiratory medical procedures, drugs, and surgical procedures.
Demonstrate proficiency in medical language.
4.5 Practice Laps
Abbreviations Summary
Career Focus

Chapter Review Exercises
Dive In: Medical Language Exercises
(Learning Outcomes 4.1–4.5)
Immerse Yourself: Analyze Medical Reports

Medical Language Key

To unlock the definition of a medical word, first break it into word parts. Then give the meaning of each word part. Put the meanings of the word parts in order, beginning with the meaning of the suffix, then the meaning of the prefix (if there is one), then the meaning of the combining form.

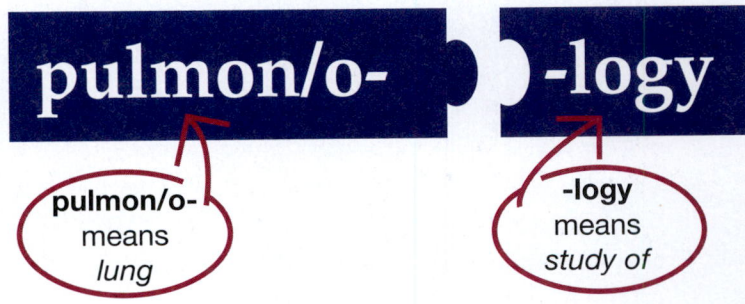

pulmon/o-
means
lung

-logy
means
study of

Pulmonology: ▶ *Study of (the) lungs (and related structures).*

The **respiratory system** consists of a pathway of air passages that begins at the nose and ends in the lungs (see Figure 4-1 ■). The respiratory system is also known as the **respiratory tract** because a tract is a pathway. The respiratory system is divided into upper and lower parts. The structures of the upper respiratory system include the nose, nasal cavity, and pharynx. The structures of the lower respiratory system include the larynx, trachea, bronchi, bronchioles, lungs, and thorax.

The functions of the respiratory system are to bring oxygen into the body and expel the waste product of carbon dioxide. The respiratory system works in conjunction with the cardiovascular system and **cardiopulmonary** reflects that close connection. Without the action of the heart, oxygen brought into the lungs would never reach the body's cells, and carbon dioxide produced by the body's cells would never reach the lungs to be exhaled.

4.1 Anatomy

Upper Respiratory System

The upper respiratory system is in the head and neck. It includes the nose, nasal cavity, and pharynx (throat). *Note*: Some of these same structures—as well as others (the sinuses, adenoids, tonsils)—are part of the ears, nose, and throat (described in Chapter 15, Otolaryngology).

Nose and Nasal Cavity

The **nose** has two external openings known as the **nares** (nostrils), and it contains the **nasal cavity** (see Figure 4-2 ■). The cavity is divided in the center by the **nasal septum**, a wall of cartilage and bone. On each side of the nasal cavity are three scroll-like projections of bone covered with mucous membrane; these are the **turbinates** or **nasal conchae**. These projections slow down inhaled air. The nasal cavity and turbinates are lined with **mucosa**, a **mucous membrane** that warms and moisturizes the air and produces **mucus**. Mucus and hairs in the nose trap inhaled particles of dust, pollen, smoke, and bacteria and keep them from entering the lungs.

Pharynx

The nasal cavity merges with the **pharynx** (throat) (see Figure 4-3 ■). The pharynx is a passageway for both air and food. The pharynx has three parts: the **nasopharynx** that is posterior to the nasal cavity, the **oropharynx** that is posterior to the oral cavity, and the **laryngopharynx** that is posterior to the larynx (voice box). The laryngopharynx leads into either the esophagus or the larynx.

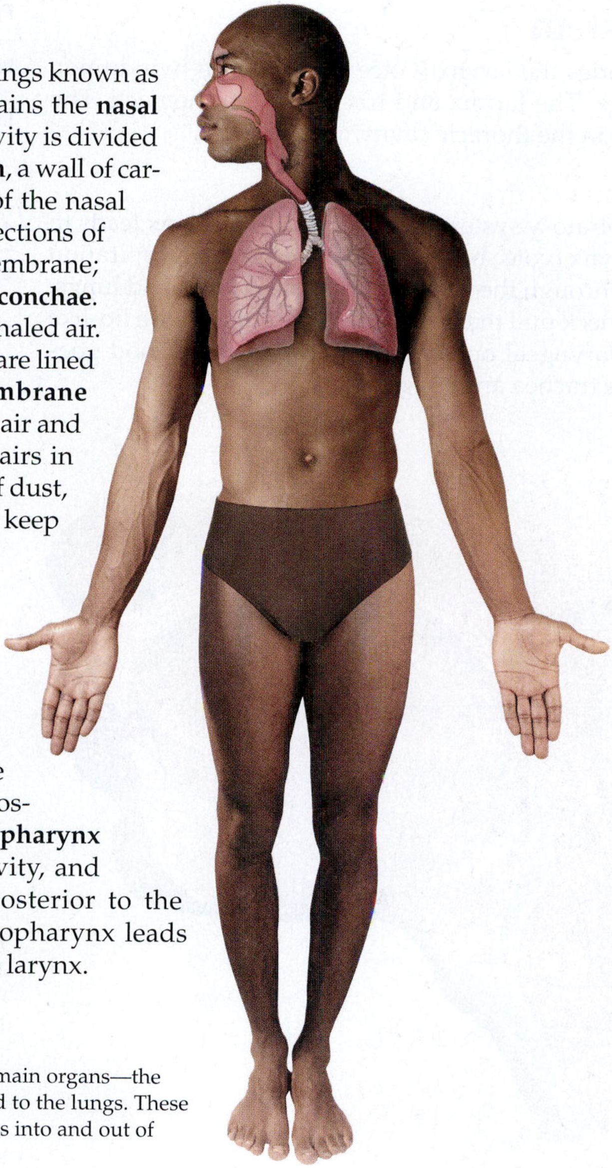

FIGURE 4-1 ■ Respiratory system.
The respiratory system consists of two main organs—the lungs—and related structures connected to the lungs. These form a pathway through which air flows into and out of the body.

Pronunciation/Word Parts

respiratory (RES-pih-rah-TOR-ee)
   re- again and again; backward; unable to
   spir/o- breathe; coil
   -atory pertaining to
Respiratory: *Pertaining to again and again (to) breathe*

cardiopulmonary
(KAR-dee-oh-PUL-moh-NAIR-ee)
   cardi/o- heart
   pulmon/o- lung
   -ary pertaining to

nose (NOHZ)

naris (NAY-rihs)

nares (NAY-reez)
Latin plural noun: Change the singular ending *-is* to *-es*.

nasal (NAY-zal)
   nas/o- nose
   -al pertaining to

cavity (KAV-ih-tee)
   cav/o- hollow space
   -ity condition; state

septum (SEP-tum)

septal (SEP-tal)
   sept/o- dividing wall; septum
   -al pertaining to

turbinate (TER-bih-nayt)
   turbin/o- scroll-like structure
   -ate composed of; pertaining to

conchae (CON-kee)

mucosa (myoo-KOH-sah)

mucous (MYOO-kuhs)
   muc/o- mucus
   -ous pertaining to

mucus (MYOO-kuhs)

pharynx (FAIR-ingks)

pharyngeal (fah-RIN-jee-al)
   pharyng/o- pharynx; throat
   -eal pertaining to

nasopharynx (NAY-soh-FAIR-ingks)
   nas/o- nose
   -pharynx pharynx; throat

oropharynx (OR-oh-FAIR-ingks)
   or/o- mouth
   -pharynx pharynx; throat

laryngopharynx (lah-RING-goh-FAIR-ingks)
   laryng/o- larynx; voice box
   -pharynx pharynx; throat

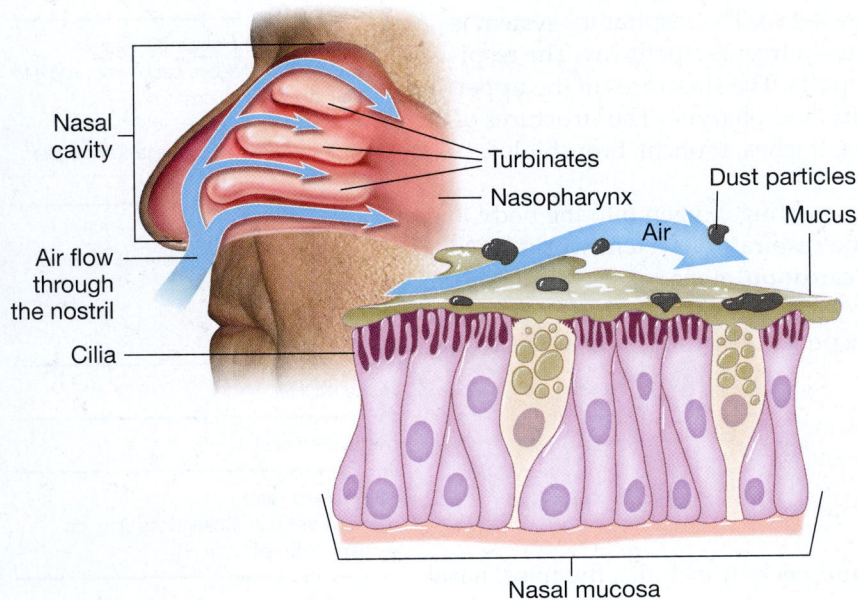

FIGURE 4-2 ■ **Nasal cavity.**
Air entering the nasal cavity swirls around the turbinates, allowing the mucosa to warm and moisten the air before it goes to the lungs. This helps the body maintain its core temperature. The mucosa also produces mucus to trap inhaled particles and bacteria before they enter the lungs. The cilia move in waves to clear away mucus and debris.

Lower Respiratory System

The lower respiratory system includes the larynx (voice box), trachea (windpipe), bronchi, bronchioles, and the lungs. The larynx and trachea are in the neck. The bronchi, bronchioles, and lungs are in the thoracic cavity.

Larynx

The first structure of the lower respiratory system is the larynx. The larynx leads to the trachea (see Figure 4-3). The **larynx** (voice box) remains open during respiration and speaking, allowing air to pass through the vocal cords to the trachea and lungs. During swallowing, muscles in the neck pull the larynx up to the **epiglottis**, a lid-like structure. The epiglottis seals the laryngeal opening so that swallowed food goes into the esophagus and not into the trachea and lungs.

Pronunciation/Word Parts

larynx (LAIR-ingks)

laryngeal (lah-RIN-jee-al)
   laryng/o- *larynx; voice box*
   -eal *pertaining to*

epiglottis (EP-ih-GLAW-tihs)

epiglottic (EP-ih-GLAW-tik)
   epi- *above; upon*
   glott/o- *glottis of the larynx*
   -ic *pertaining to*

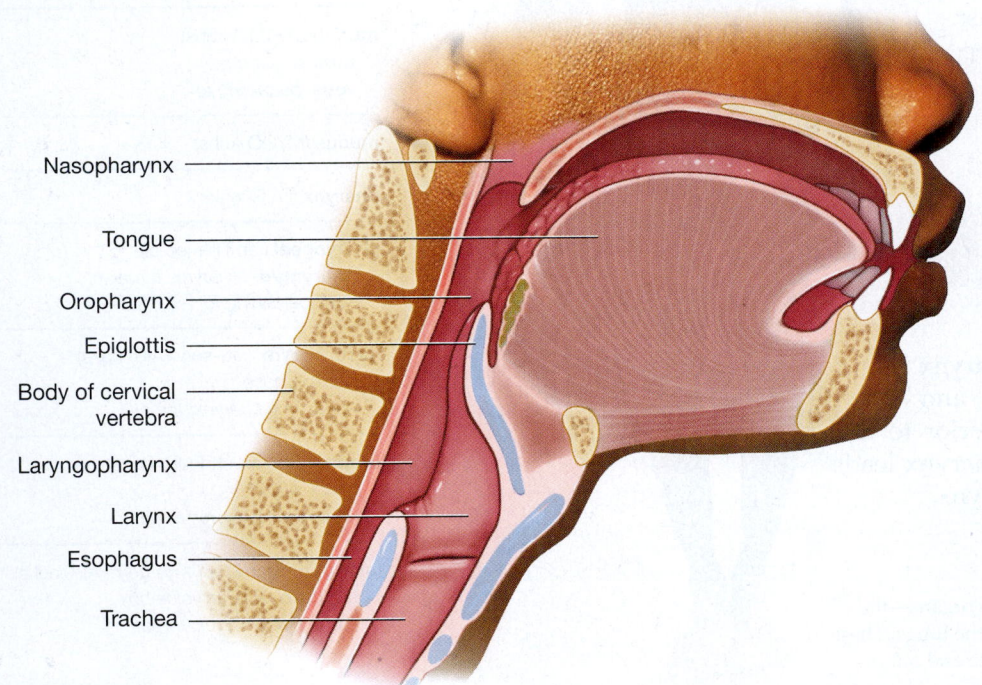

FIGURE 4-3 ■ **Pharynx and larynx.**
The pharynx (throat) has three parts: nasopharynx, oropharynx, and laryngopharynx. The larynx is open during breathing. During swallowing, muscles in the neck pull the larynx up to meet the epiglottis, and the epiglottis covers the larynx so that swallowed food cannot enter the lungs.

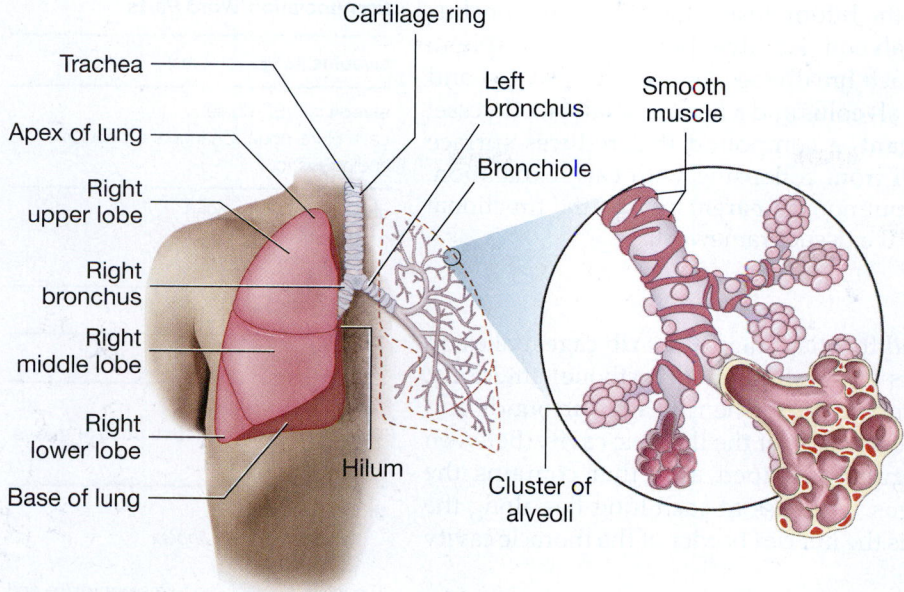

Cartilage ring
Trachea
Apex of lung
Right upper lobe
Right bronchus
Right middle lobe
Right lower lobe
Base of lung
Left bronchus
Smooth muscle
Bronchiole
Hilum
Cluster of alveoli

FIGURE 4-4 ■ **Trachea, bronchi, bronchioles, lungs, and alveoli.**
The trachea divides into the right and left bronchi. A bronchus enters the lung at its hilum and then divides into bronchioles. At the end of each bronchiole are alveoli, which are clusters of microscopic air sacs where oxygen and carbon dioxide gases are exchanged.

Trachea

Below the vocal cords, the larynx merges into the trachea. The **trachea** (windpipe) is approximately 1 inch in diameter and 4 inches in length (see Figure 4-4 ■). The central opening within the trachea is the **lumen**. C-shaped rings of cartilage support the trachea, but the posterior surface of the trachea has no cartilage. This allows the esophagus to expand when a large amount of food is swallowed and moves past the posterior surface of the trachea.

Bronchi and Bronchioles

The trachea divides into the right and left **bronchi** (see Figure 4-4). Rings of cartilage support the bronchi. Each **bronchus** enters a lung and branches into smaller **bronchioles**. The smallest bronchioles have walls of smooth muscle, but no cartilage. The lumen is the central opening within the bronchi and bronchioles. **Bronchopulmonary** refers to the bronchi and the lungs.

The trachea, bronchi, and bronchioles look like the trunk and branches of an upside-down tree, and they are called the **bronchial tree**. The bronchial tree is lined with **cilia**, small hairs that move in waves to carry mucus and foreign particles toward the throat where they can be swallowed or expelled by coughing.

Clinical Connections

Public Health. Smoking immobilizes and eventually destroys the cilia. Without the action of the cilia, smoke particles enter the lung and are deposited there, and mucus accumulates, causing a constant "smoker's cough."

Lungs

The **lungs** are spongy, air-filled structures. Each lung contains **lobes**, large divisions that are visible on the lung's outer surface (see Figure 4-4). The larger right lung has three lobes: right upper lobe (RUL), right middle lobe (RML), and right lower lobe (RLL). The left lung has two lobes: left upper lobe (LUL) and left lower lobe (LLL).

The **apex** is the rounded top of each lung. A bronchus enters each lung at the **hilum** (an indentation in the lung). The pulmonary arteries and pulmonary veins

Pronunciation/Word Parts

trachea (TRAY-kee-ah)

tracheal (TRAY-kee-al)
  trache/o- *trachea; windpipe*
  -al *pertaining to*

lumen (LOO-men)

bronchus (BRONG-kuhs)

bronchi (BRONG-ki)
Latin plural noun: Change the singular ending *-us* to *-i*.

bronchial (BRONG-kee-al)
  bronchi/o- *bronchus*
  -al *pertaining to*

bronchiole (BRONG-kee-ohl)
  bronchi/o- *bronchus*
  -ole *small thing*

bronchiolar (BRONG-kee-OH-lar)
  bronchiol/o- *bronchiole*
  -ar *pertaining to*

bronchopulmonary
(BRONG-koh-PUL-moh-NAIR-ee)
  bronch/o- *bronchus*
  pulmon/o- *lung*
  -ary *pertaining to*

cilia (SIL-ee-ah)

lung (LUNG)

pulmonary (PUL-moh-NAIR-ee)
  pulmon/o- *lung*
  -ary *pertaining to*
The related combining forms **pneum/o-** and **pneumon/o-** mean *air; lung*.

lobe (LOHB)

lobar (LOH-bar)
  lob/o- *lobe of an organ*
  -ar *pertaining to*

apex (AA-peks)

hilum (HY-lum)

hilar (HY-lar)
  hil/o- *indentation*
  -ar *pertaining to*

for each of the lobes also enter and exit at the hilum. Inside the lung, the bronchus branches into bronchioles, which end in alveoli. An **alveolus** is a hollow sphere of cells that expands and contracts with each breath (see Figure 4-4). Oxygen and carbon dioxide are exchanged between the alveolus and a nearby small blood vessel (capillary). The alveolus secretes **surfactant**, a compound that reduces surface tension and keeps the walls of the alveoli from collapsing with each exhalation. Collectively, the alveoli are known as the pulmonary **parenchyma**—the functional part of the lung—as opposed to its connective tissue framework.

Thorax

The **thorax** is the area between the neck and the diaphragm. The **rib cage** makes up the bony wall of the thorax, and it consists of the sternum (breastbone) anteriorly, the ribs laterally, and bones of the spine posteriorly. The rib cage surrounds and protects the **thoracic cavity**. The lungs take up most of the thoracic cavity. Between the lungs is the **mediastinum**, an irregularly shaped area that contains the trachea, as well as the heart and esophagus. The base of each lung lies along the **diaphragm**, a sheet of skeletal muscle that is the inferior border of the thoracic cavity (see Figure 4-5 ■).

Each lung is located within a pleural cavity that is lined by the **pleurae**, a double-layered serous membrane. The pleura that is next to the lung's surface is the **visceral pleura**; the pleura next to the wall of the thoracic cavity is the **parietal pleura** (see Figure 4-5). The pleurae secrete **pleural fluid** into the **pleural space**, the narrow space between the two layers of pleurae. Pleural fluid is a slippery, watery fluid that allows the visceral pleura and parietal pleura to slide smoothly past each other as the lungs expand and contract during inspiration and expiration.

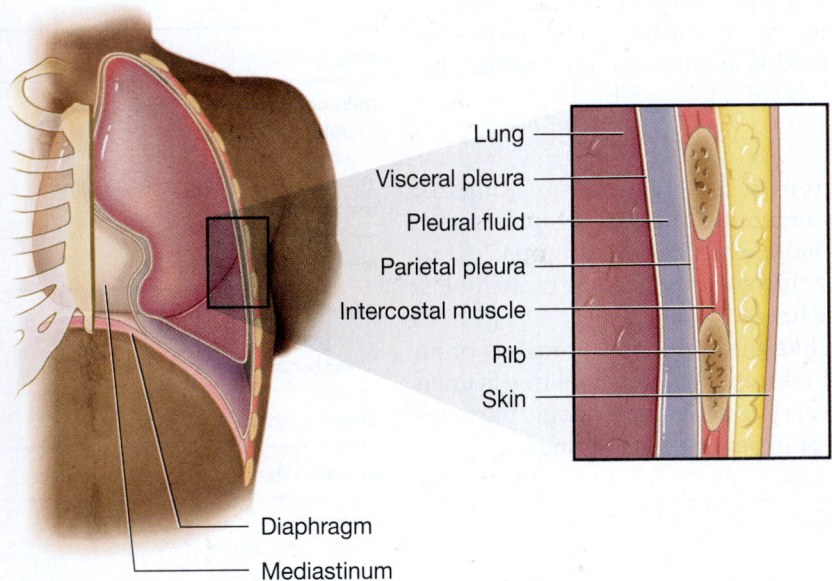

Lung
Visceral pleura
Pleural fluid
Parietal pleura
Intercostal muscle
Rib
Skin

Diaphragm

Mediastinum

FIGURE 4-5 ■ Diaphragm and pleurae.
The diaphragm is the inferior border of the thoracic cavity. The visceral pleura is next to the surface of the lung. The parietal pleura is next to the wall of the thoracic cavity. The pleurae secrete pleural fluid.

Pronunciation/Word Parts

alveolus (al-VEE-oh-luhs)

alveoli (al-VEE-oh-lie)
Latin plural noun: Change the singular ending -us to -i.

alveolar (al-VEE-oh-lar)
   alveol/o- air sac
   -ar pertaining to

surfactant (ser-FAK-tant)

parenchyma (pah-RENG-kih-mah)

thorax (THOR-aks)
The related combining form **cost/o-** means rib.

thoracic (thor-AS-ik)
   thorac/o- chest; thorax
   -ic pertaining to
The related combining forms **pector/o-** and **steth/o-** mean chest.

cavity (KAV-ih-tee)
   cav/o- hollow space
   -ity condition; state

mediastinum (MEE-dee-ah-STY-num)

diaphragm (DY-ah-fram)

diaphragmatic (DY-ah-frag-MAT-ik)
   diaphragmat/o- diaphragm
   -ic pertaining to

pleura (PLOOR-ah)

pleurae (PLOOR-ee)
Latin plural noun: Change the singular ending -a to -ae.

pleural (PLOOR-al)
   pleur/o- lung membrane
   -al pertaining to

visceral (VIS-eh-ral)
   viscer/o- large internal organs
   -al pertaining to

parietal (pah-RY-eh-tal)
   pariet/o- wall of a cavity
   -al pertaining to

4.1 PRACTICE LAPS

Use the Answer Key at the end of the book to check your answers.

A. Label Structures

Write each anatomy word or phrase in the correct numbered box. Be sure to check your spelling.

apex of lung	cluster of alveoli	lower lobe of lung	rib
bronchioles	diaphragm	nasal cavity	sternum
bronchus	larynx	pharynx	trachea

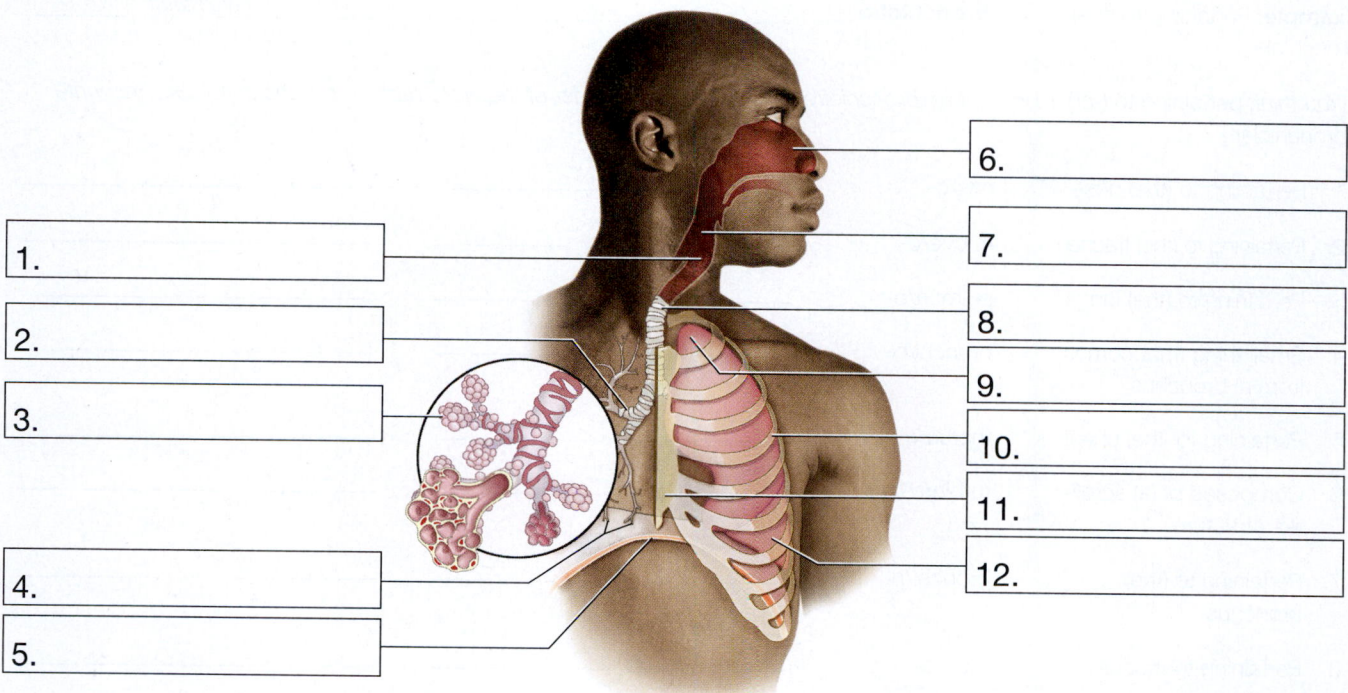

1.
2.
3.
4.
5.
6.
7.
8.
9.
10.
11.
12.

B. Give the Meaning of Combining Forms

Next to each combining form, write its meaning. The first one has been done for you.

Combining Form	Meaning	Combining Form	Meaning
1. **alveol/o-**	*air sac*	8. or/o-	
2. bronchi/o-		9. pharyng/o-	
3. bronchiol/o-		10. pleur/o-	
4. bronch/o-		11. pulmon/o-	
5. diaphragmat/o-		12. sept/o-	
6. laryng/o-		13. thorac/o-	
7. nas/o-		14. trache/o-	

C. Build Words

Read the definition of the medical word. Look at the combining form that is given. Select the correct suffix from the Suffix List, and write it on the blank line. Then build the medical word, and write it on the line. (Remember: You may need to remove the combining vowel. Always remove the hyphens and slash.) Be sure to check your spelling.

Suffix List

-al (pertaining to)	-ate (composed of;	-eal (pertaining to)	-ole (small thing)
-ar (pertaining to)	pertaining to)	-ic (pertaining to)	-ous (pertaining to)
-ary (pertaining to)			

Definition of the Medical Word	Combining Form	Suffix	Build the Medical Word
Example: Pertaining to (the) bronchiole	**bronchiol/o-**	*-ar*	*bronchiolar*

[*You think* pertaining to (-ar) + bronchiole (*bronchiol/o-*). You change the order of the word parts to put the suffix last. You write bronchiolar.]

1. Pertaining to (the) nose	nas/o-		
2. Pertaining to (the) trachea	trache/o-		
3. Pertaining to (the) lungs	pulmon/o-		
4. Small thing (that comes from a) bronchus	bronchi/o-		
5. Pertaining to (the) chest	thorac/o-		
6. Composed of (a) scroll-like structure	turbin/o-		
7. Pertaining to (the) bronchus	bronchi/o-		
8. Pertaining to mucus	muc/o-		
9. Pertaining to (the) larynx	laryng/o-		
10. Pertaining to (the) diaphragm	diaphragmat/o-		
11. Pertaining to (the) alveolus	alveol/o-		

4.2 Physiology

Breathing is normally an involuntary process that occurs without any conscious effort. **Respiratory control centers** in the brain regulate the depth and rate of respiration. Receptors in large arteries in the chest and neck send information to the brain about the level of oxygen in the blood, and receptors in the brain send information about the blood level of carbon dioxide. Based on this information, the respiratory control centers regulate the rate of respiration by sending nerve impulses to the **phrenic nerve**, causing the diaphragm to contract. You can voluntarily control your respiration (when you hold your breath), but eventually involuntary control takes over, forcing you to breathe.

Pronunciation/Word Parts

respiratory (RES-pih-rah-TOR-ee)
  re- *again and again; backward; unable to*
  spir/o- *breathe; coil*
  -atory *pertaining to*

phrenic (FREN-ik)
  phren/o- *diaphragm; mind*
  -ic *pertaining to*

Respiration consists of breathing in and breathing out. Breathing in is **inhalation** or **inspiration**. Breathing out is **exhalation** or **expiration**. One inhalation and one exhalation are counted as one respiration.

During inhalation, the diaphragm contracts and moves downward, and the **intercostal muscles** between the ribs pull the ribs up and out. This enlarges the thoracic cavity and creates negative internal pressure that causes air to flow into the lungs. During exhalation, the diaphragm and intercostal muscles relax, the thoracic cavity returns to its previous size, and air flows slowly out of the nose. Having a normal depth and rate of respiration is known as **eupnea**. For forceful expiration, a different set of intercostal muscles—as well as the abdominal muscles—contract strongly (see Figure 4-6 ■). This quickly decreases the size of the thoracic cavity and expels a large volume of air in just a few seconds.

Processes of Respiration

Respiration involves five separate processes:

1. **Ventilation.** Movement of air in and out of the lungs. The respiratory system performs this process.

2. **External respiration.** Movement of **oxygen** (O_2) gas molecules from inhaled air into the alveoli and then into the blood. External respiration also involves the movement of **carbon dioxide** (CO_2) gas molecules from the blood into the alveoli and then into exhaled air (see Figure 4-7 ■). External respiration is the exchange of these two gases within the alveoli. The respiratory system and the blood perform this process together.

3. **Gas transport.** Transport of oxygen and carbon dioxide gas molecules in the blood. Oxygen gas molecules in the blood are transported by hemoglobin in red blood cells, and this forms the compound **oxyhemoglobin**. Then this **oxygenated** blood travels from the lungs to the heart, where it is pumped throughout the body to reach every cell. Carbon dioxide gas molecules also bind to hemoglobin in the red blood cells and travel from body cells back to the lungs. The cardiovascular system and the blood perform this process.

4. **Internal respiration.** Movement of oxygen gas molecules from the blood into the cells of the body. Also, the movement of carbon dioxide gas molecules from the cells into the blood. Internal respiration is the exchange of those two gases between the blood and each cell. The blood and individual cells perform this process.

5. **Cellular respiration.** Oxygen is used by every cell to produce energy during the process of **metabolism**. Carbon dioxide is a waste product of cellular metabolism. This process is performed by every cell.

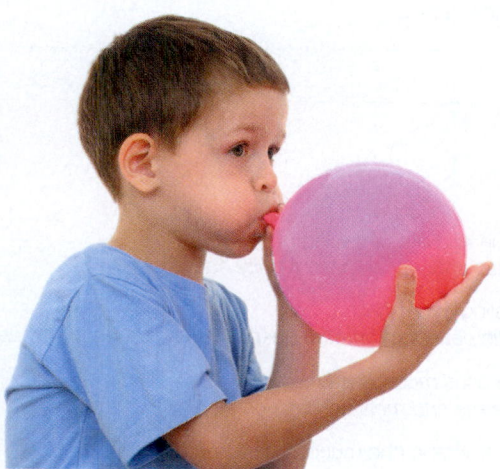

FIGURE 4-6 ■ Forceful exhalation.
When you want to forcefully exhale air, your intercostal muscles and abdominal muscles contract. This quickly decreases the size of the thoracic cavity and expels a large volume of air in just a few seconds—perfect for blowing up a balloon, blowing bubbles, or whistling.

Pronunciation/Word Parts

respiration (RES-pih-RAY-shun)
  re- *again and again; backward; unable to*
  spir/o- *breathe; coil*
  -ation *being; having; process*

inhalation (IN-hah-LAY-shun)
  in- *in; not; within*
  hal/o- *breathe*
  -ation *being; having; process*

inspiration (IN-spih-RAY-shun)
  in- *in; not; within*
  spir/o- *breathe; coil*
  -ation *being; having; process*

exhalation (EKS-hah-LAY-shun)
  ex- *away from; out*
  hal/o- *breathe*
  -ation *being; having; process*

expiration (EKS-pih-RAY-shun)
  ex- *away from; out*
  spir/o- *breathe; coil*
  -ation *being; having; process*
The letter *s* in **spir/o-** is deleted because the prefix **ex-** already has an *s* sound.

intercostal (IN-ter-KAW-stal)
  inter- *between*
  cost/o- *rib*
  -al *pertaining to*

eupnea (YOOP-nee-ah)
The prefix **eu-** means *good; normal.*
Eupnea: *Breathing (that is) normal*
The combining form **pne/o-** means *breathing.*

ventilation (VEN-tih-LAY-shun)
  ventil/o- *air movement*
  -ation *being; having; process*

oxygen (AWK-seh-jen)
The combining forms **ox/i-** and **ox/o-** mean *oxygen.* The combining form **ox/y-** means *oxygen; quick.*

carbon dioxide (KAR-bun dy-AWK-side)
The combining form **capn/o-** means *carbon dioxide.*

oxyhemoglobin
(AWK-see-HEE-moh-GLOH-bin)
  ox/y- *oxygen; quick*
  hem/o- *blood*
  glob/o- *comprehensive; shaped like a globe*
  -in *substance*

oxygenated (AWK-seh-jen-AA-ted)
  ox/y- *oxygen; quick*
  gen/o- *arising from; produced by*
  -ated *composed of; pertaining to a condition*

cellular (SEL-yoo-lar)
  cellul/o- *cell*
  -ar *pertaining to*

metabolism (meh-TAB-oh-lizm)
  metabol/o- *transformation*
  -ism *disease from a specific cause; process*

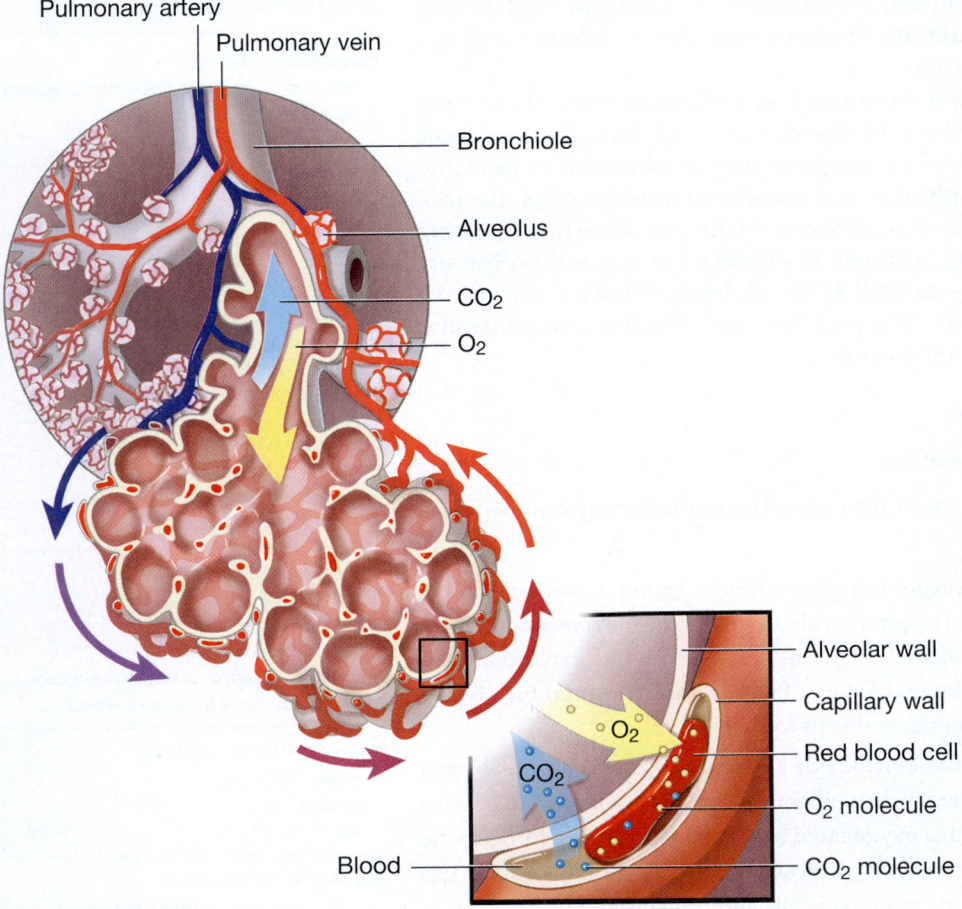

FIGURE 4-7 ■ **Gas exchange.**
Oxygen moves from the alveolus into the blood, binds to hemoglobin in a red blood cell, and is carried to the cells of the body. Carbon dioxide comes from each cell as a waste product of metabolism. It binds to hemoglobin, is carried to the alveoli, and it is eventually exhaled.

Across the Life Span

Pediatrics. In the uterus, the fetus does not breathe, and its lungs are collapsed. It receives oxygen from the mother's lungs via the placenta and umbilical cord. The lungs of the fetus do not function until the very first breath after birth. At that time, they must expand fully and stay expanded (which is helped by the presence of surfactant).

The normal respiratory rate for a newborn infant is 30–60 breaths per minute. The normal respiratory rate for an adult is 12–20 breaths per minute.

Geriatrics. As a person ages, the number of alveoli in the lungs decreases, and the remaining alveoli are less elastic. The thorax becomes stiff and is less able to expand on inhalation. In addition, a lifetime of exposure to air pollution, chemical fumes, and smoke causes damage to the lungs. These changes decrease pulmonary function in older adults.

Word Alert
Sound-Alike Words

breath (BRETH)	(noun)	the air that flows in and out of the lungs *Example: The breath of a diabetic patient can have a fruity odor to it.*
breathe (BREETH)	(verb)	the action of inhaling and exhaling *Example: If you ask an asthmatic patient to breathe deeply, you might hear a wheezing sound.*
mucosa (myoo-KOH-sah)	(noun)	Latin word that means *mucous membrane* *Example: The nasal mucosa warms and moistens inhaled air.*
mucous (MYOO-kuhs)	(adjective)	pertaining to a membrane (the mucosa) that secretes mucus *Example: Allergies make the mucous membranes of the nose swollen and inflamed.*
mucus (MYOO-kuhs)	(noun)	a secretion from a mucous membrane *Example: A chronic smoker coughs and produces a significant amount of mucus.*

4.2 PRACTICE LAPS

Use the Answer Key at the end of the book to check your answers.

A. Label Functions

Write each physiology word or phrase in the correct numbered box. Be sure to check your spelling.

bronchiole	carbon dioxide gas molecules	oxygen gas molecules
capillary wall	cluster of alveoli	red blood cell

1.

2.

3.

4.

5.

6.

B. Give the Meaning of Combining Forms

Next to each combining form, write its meaning. The first one has been done for you.

Combining Form	Meaning	Combining Form	Meaning
1. **capn/o-**	*carbon dioxide*	6. ox/o-	
2. cost/o-		7. ox/y-	
3. hal/o-		8. phren/o-	
4. metabol/o-		9. spir/o-	
5. ox/i-		10. ventil/o-	

C. Build Words

Read the definition of the medical word. Look at the combining form that is given. Select the correct suffix from the Suffix List, and write it on the blank line. Then build the medical word, and write it on the line. (Remember: You may need to remove the combining vowel. Always remove the hyphens and slash.) Be sure to check your spelling.

Suffix List

-ar (pertaining to)	-ic (pertaining to)
-ation (being; having; process)	-ism (disease from a specific cause; process)

Definition of the Medical Word	Combining Form	Suffix	Build the Medical Word
Example: Pertaining to (a) cell	**cellul/o-**	*-ar*	*cellular*

[*You think* pertaining to (*-ar*) + cell (*cellul/o-*). *You change the order of the word parts to put the suffix last. You write* cellular.]

1. Pertaining to (the nerve for the) diaphragm	phren/o-	_____	_____
2. Process (of) air movement	ventil/o-	_____	_____
3. Process (of) transformation (that happens within a cell)	metabol/o-	_____	_____

Vocabulary Review

Word or Phrase	Description	Combining Forms
Overview		
cardiopulmonary	Pertaining to the heart and lungs	**cardi/o-** *heart* **pulmon/o-** *lung*
respiratory system	The structures of the upper respiratory system include the nose, nasal cavity, and pharynx (throat). The lower respiratory system includes the larynx (voice box), trachea (windpipe), bronchi, bronchioles, lungs, and thorax. Also known as the **respiratory tract**. The functions of the respiratory system are to bring oxygen into the body and expel carbon dioxide.	**spir/o-** *breathe; coil*
Anatomy of the Upper Respiratory System		
mucosa	**Mucous membrane** that lines most of the respiratory system. It warms and humidifies incoming air. It produces **mucus** to trap foreign particles and bacteria.	**muc/o-** *mucus*
nasal cavity	Hollow area inside the nose. The **nasal septum** divides the nasal cavity into right and left sides.	**nas/o-** *nose* **sept/o-** *dividing wall; septum*
pharynx	The throat. A shared passageway for both air and food. The **nasopharynx** is posterior to the nasal cavity, the **oropharynx** is posterior to the oral cavity, and the **laryngopharynx** is posterior to the larynx.	**pharyng/o-** *pharynx; throat* **nas/o-** *nose* **or/o-** *mouth* **laryng/o-** *larynx; voice box*
turbinates	Scroll-like projections of bone covered by mucous membrane on either side of the nasal cavity. They slow down and give moisture to inhaled air. Also known as **nasal conchae**.	**turbin/o-** *scroll-like structure*

Word or Phrase	Description	Combining Forms
Anatomy of the Lower Respiratory System		
alveolus	Hollow sphere of cells in the lungs where oxygen and carbon dioxide gas molecules are exchanged	**alveol/o-** *air sac*
apex	Rounded top of each lung	
bronchiole	Small tubular air passageway that branches off from a bronchus and then branches into several alveoli. Its wall contains smooth muscle.	**bronchiol/o-** *bronchiole*
bronchus	Tubular air passageway supported by cartilage rings. Each bronchus enters a lung and branches into bronchioles. The **bronchial tree** includes the trachea, bronchi, and bronchioles. **Bronchopulmonary** refers to the bronchi and the lungs.	**bronchi/o-** *bronchus* **bronch/o-** *bronchus* **pulmon/o-** *lung*
cilia	Small hairs that move in waves to take mucus and foreign particles toward the throat to be expelled by coughing or to be swallowed	
epiglottis	Lid-like structure that seals off the opening to the larynx, so that swallowed food goes into the esophagus, not into the trachea	**glott/o-** *glottis of the larynx*
hilum	Indentation on the medial side of each lung where the bronchus, pulmonary arteries, and pulmonary veins enter and exit the lung	**hil/o-** *indentation*
larynx	Structure that contains the vocal cords and is a passageway for inhaled and exhaled air. Also known as the **voice box**.	**laryng/o-** *larynx; voice box*
lobe	Large division of a lung, whose dividing line is visible on the lung's outer surface	**lob/o-** *lobe of an organ*
lumen	Central opening through which air flows inside the trachea, bronchus, or bronchiole	
lung	Spongy, air-filled structures that contain alveoli	**pneum/o-** *air; lung* **pneumon/o-** *air; lung* **pulmon/o-** *lung*
parenchyma	Functional part of the lung (i.e., the alveoli) as opposed to the connective tissue framework	
surfactant	Compound that reduces surface tension and keeps the walls of the alveoli from collapsing with each exhalation	
trachea	Tube supported by C-shaped rings of cartilage. It is an air passageway between the larynx and the bronchi. Also known as the **windpipe**.	**trache/o-** *trachea; windpipe*
Anatomy of the Thorax		
diaphragm	Sheet of skeletal muscle that divides the thoracic cavity from the abdominal cavity. It is active in breathing.	**diaphragmat/o-** *diaphragm*
intercostal muscles	Sets of muscles between the ribs that contract to pull the ribs up and out during inhalation or down and in during forceful exhalation	**cost/o-** *rib*
mediastinum	Irregularly shaped area within the thoracic cavity. It contains the trachea (and heart and esophagus).	
phrenic nerve	Nerve that, when stimulated by the respiratory control centers, causes the diaphragm to contract and move downward; this expands the thoracic cavity and causes inspiration.	**phren/o-** *diaphragm; mind*
pleurae	Double-layered membrane that lines each pleural cavity and secretes pleural fluid. The **visceral pleura** is next to the lung's surface. The **parietal pleura** is next to the wall of the thoracic cavity. The space in between is filled with **pleural fluid**.	**pleur/o-** *lung membrane* **viscer/o-** *large internal organs* **pariet/o-** *wall of a cavity*

Word or Phrase	Description	Combining Forms
pleural cavity	Area surrounded by pleura. Each pleural cavity contains a lung.	**pleur/o-** *lung membrane*
pleural space	Narrow space between the two layers of pleurae. It is filled with pleural fluid.	**pleur/o-** *lung membrane*
rib cage	Bony wall that surrounds and protects the thoracic cavity. It consists of the sternum (breastbone), ribs, and bones of the spine.	**cost/o-** *rib*
thoracic cavity	Hollow space surrounded by the rib cage. It contains the lungs and structures in the mediastinum.	**thorac/o-** *chest; thorax* **cav/o-** *hollow space*
thorax	Area between the neck and the diaphragm	**thorac/o-** *chest; thorax* **pector/o-** *chest* **steth/o-** *chest*

Physiology of Respiration		
carbon dioxide	Exhaled gas that is a waste product of cellular metabolism. It is carried by the hemoglobin in red blood cells.	**capn/o-** *carbon dioxide*
eupnea	Normal depth and rate of respiration	
exhalation	Breathing out. Also known as **expiration**.	**hal/o-** *breathe* **spir/o-** *breathe; coil*
inhalation	Breathing in. Also known as **inspiration**.	**hal/o-** *breathe* **spir/o-** *breathe; coil*
metabolism	Process that uses oxygen to produce energy within body cells and produces carbon dioxide as a waste product	**metabol/o-** *transformation*
oxygen	Inhaled gas that is used by each cell to produce energy in the process of metabolism. Oxygen is carried by the hemoglobin in red blood cells. Blood that contains oxygen is **oxygenated**.	**ox/y-** *oxygen; quick* **ox/i-** *oxygen* **ox/o-** *oxygen* **gen/o-** *arising from; produced by*
oxyhemoglobin	Compound formed when oxygen combines with the hemoglobin in red blood cells	**ox/y-** *oxygen; quick* **hem/o-** *blood* **glob/o-** *comprehensive; shaped like a globe*
respiration	Consists of five processes: **ventilation** (movement of air in and out of the lungs), **external respiration** (exchange of oxygen and carbon dioxide gas molecules between the alveoli and the blood), **gas transport** of oxygen and carbon dioxide through the blood, **internal respiration** (exchange of oxygen and carbon dioxide between the blood and the cells), and **cellular respiration** (use of oxygen to produce energy in the cell while producing carbon dioxide as a waste product of metabolism).	**spir/o-** *breathe; coil* **ventil/o-** *air movement* **cellul/o-** *cell*
respiratory control centers	Centers in the brain that control the rate of respiration	**spir/o-** *breathe; coil*

Abbreviation Review

CO₂	carbon dioxide		**RLL**	right lower lobe (of the lung)
LLL	left lower lobe (of the lung)		**RML**	right middle lobe (of the lung)
LUL	left upper lobe (of the lung)		**RUL**	right upper lobe (of the lung)
O₂	oxygen			

4.3 Diseases

Note: Diseases of the nose, sinuses, pharynx, tonsils, adenoids, and larynx are described in Chapter 15, Otolaryngology.

Word or Phrase	Description	Pronunciation/Word Parts

Nose and Pharynx

Word or Phrase	Description	Pronunciation/Word Parts
upper respiratory infection (URI)	Bacterial or viral infection of the nose and/or throat. Also known as a **common cold** or a **head cold** (see Figure 4-8 ◼). Treatment: Antibiotic drug for a bacterial infection 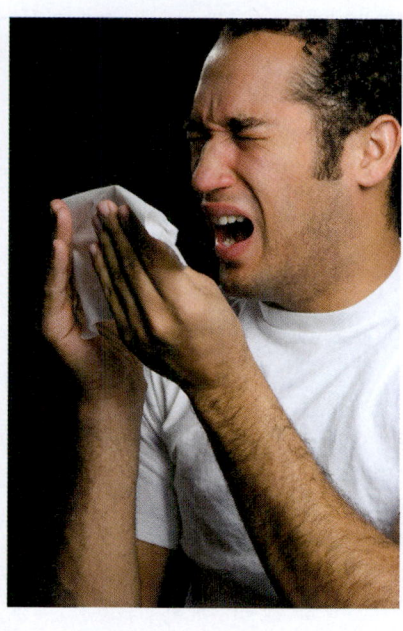 **FIGURE 4-8** ◼ **Upper respiratory infection.** An upper respiratory infection is caused by a bacterium or virus. It spreads easily to others on unwashed hands or by droplets of mucus and saliva that are expelled into the air during sneezing and coughing.	**infection** (in-FEK-shun) **infect/o-** *disease within* **-ion** *action; condition*

Trachea, Bronchi, and Bronchioles

Word or Phrase	Description	Pronunciation/Word Parts
asthma	Hyperreactivity of the bronchi and bronchioles. Inflammation and swelling of the mucosa, excessive mucus production. **Bronchospasm** (contraction of the smooth muscle) narrows the lumens of the bronchi and bronchioles, causing shortness of breath, coughing, wheezing from narrowing of the lumen and bronchospasm, and difficulty exhaling. Attacks are triggered by exposure to allergens, dust, mold, smoke, inhaled chemicals, exercise, cold air, or emotional stress. Patients with asthma are said to be **asthmatic**. Asthma is a type of reactive airway disease. **Status asthmaticus** is a prolonged, extremely severe, life-threatening asthma attack. Prevention: Avoid things that trigger asthma attacks. Prevent attacks by daily use of a corticosteroid drug, bronchodilator drug, or leukotriene receptor blocker drug. Treatment: Inhaled bronchodilator drug during attacks; oxygen for severe attacks	**asthma** (AZ-mah) **bronchospasm** (BRONG-koh-spazm) **bronch/o-** *bronchus* **-spasm** *sudden, involuntary muscle contraction* **asthmatic** (az-MAT-ik) **asthm/o-** *asthma* **-atic** *pertaining to* **status asthmaticus** (STAT-uhs az-MAT-ih-kuhs)

Across the Life Span

Pediatrics. Asthma is prevalent in children living in substandard housing in high-congregate areas. Researchers found that exposure to cockroaches appears to be a strong asthma trigger. Extermination of live cockroaches does not eliminate the problem because cockroach droppings and carcasses remain behind the walls.

Geriatrics. Older patients can find that their asthma is more difficult to control because of age-related changes in their lungs and in the muscles of respiration.

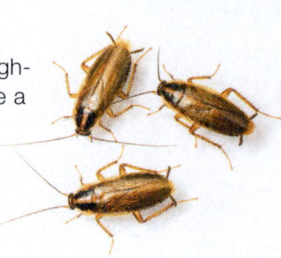

Word or Phrase	Description	Pronunciation/Word Parts
bronchitis	Acute or chronic infection or inflammation of the bronchi. Acute bronchitis with infection is due to bacteria or viruses. There is mucus production, coughing of mucus (sputum) out of the mouth, wheezing, and a fever. Chronic bronchitis is due to air pollution or smoking. There is a constant cough, mucus production, and wheezing. Treatment: Bronchodilator drug; corticosteroid drug for inflammation; antibiotic drug for a bacterial infection	**bronchitis** (brong-KY-tihs) **bronch/o-** *bronchus* **-itis** *infection of; inflammation of* **sputum** (SPYOO-tum)
bronchiectasis	Chronic, permanent enlargement and loss of elasticity of the bronchioles. Chronic inflammation destroys the smooth muscle and allows secretions to accumulate. There is a large amount of mucus with coughing. Often seen in patients with cystic fibrosis. Treatment: Bronchodilator drug; oxygen therapy	**bronchiectasis** (BRONG-kee-EK-tah-sihs) **bronchi/o-** *bronchus* **-ectasis** *condition of dilation*
reactive airway disease	Group of conditions that all show reversible narrowing of the airway lumens with wheezing, caused by an external factor. Includes asthma, chronic obstructive pulmonary disease, and upper respiratory infections.	

Lungs

abnormal breath sounds	Normal respirations sound like a soft wind rushing through a tunnel. These are examples of abnormal breath sounds. Treatment: Correct the underlying cause. • **Pleural friction rub:** Creaking, grating, or rubbing sound. Caused by inflamed layers of pleurae rubbing against each other. • **Rales:** Irregular crackling or bubbling sounds. Wet rales are caused by fluid or infection in the alveoli. Dry rales are caused by chronic irritation or fibrosis. Also known as *crackles*. • **Rhonchi:** Humming, whistling, or snoring sounds. Caused by swelling, mucus, or a foreign body that partially obstructs the bronchi. • **Stridor:** High-pitched, harsh, crowing sound. Caused by edema or an obstruction in the trachea or larynx. • **Wheezes:** High-pitched whistling or squeaking sounds. It is caused by narrowing of the lumen due to bronchospasm from asthma, a lung infection, an allergic reaction, or a foreign body obstructing the airways.	**rales** (RAWLZ) **rhonchi** (RONG-ki) **stridor** (STRY-dor) **wheezes** (WHEE-zehs)

Word or Phrase	Description	Pronunciation/Word Parts
acute respiratory distress syndrome (ARDS)	Condition in which many alveoli are damaged and become filled with fluid. The alveoli do not make surfactant, and so they collapse after each breath (see Figure 4-9 ■). Caused by a severe infection, extensive burns, or injury to the lungs (aspiration of vomit or inhalation of chemical fumes). Treatment: Oxygen therapy; use of a respirator; surfactant drug given through an endotracheal tube. Correct the underlying cause.	

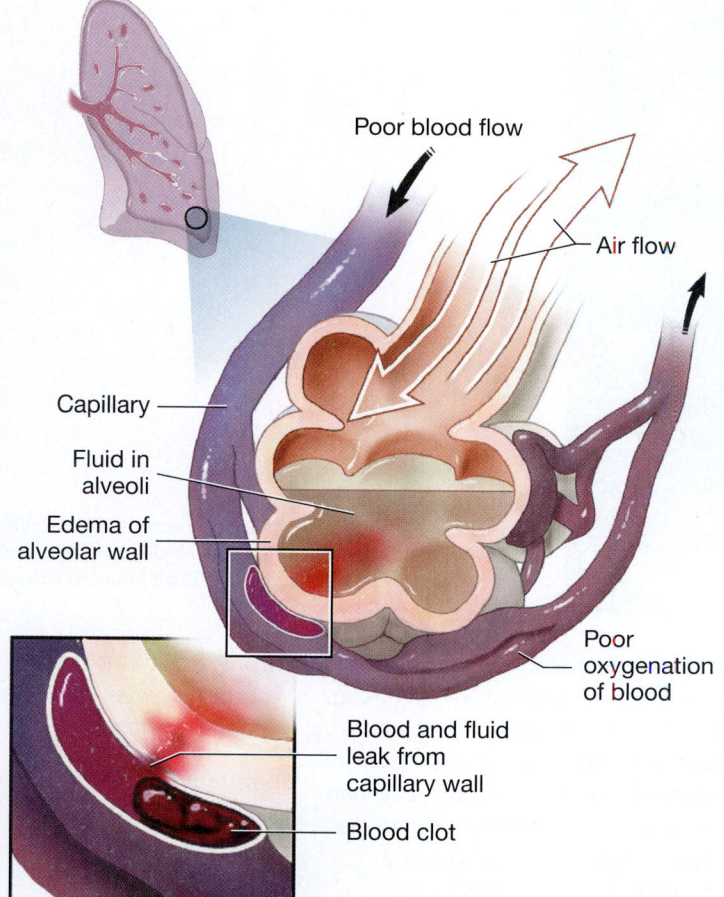

Poor blood flow

Air flow

Capillary

Fluid in alveoli

Edema of alveolar wall

Poor oxygenation of blood

Blood and fluid leak from capillary wall

Blood clot

FIGURE 4-9 ■ Acute respiratory distress syndrome. The alveolus is edematous and filled with fluid. There is poor blood flow in the capillary around the alveolus with some blood clots. The capillary walls leak fluid and blood into the alveolus. Blood coming back to the heart (and going to the rest of the body) does not contain enough oxygen.

Dive Deeper

Infant respiratory distress syndrome (IRDS) develops in premature infants who produce too little surfactant because their lungs are not fully mature. There is nasal flaring (the nostrils flare with each breath to draw in more air) and grunting (the larynx closes against the epiglottis to maintain pressure in the lungs to keep the alveoli from collapsing). The flexible sternum (breastbone) is pulled inward with each inspiration (sternal **retraction**).

Treatment: Oxygen and the use of a respirator, if needed; surfactant drug given by endotracheal tube

retraction (ree-TRAK-shun)
  re- *again and again; backward; unable to*
  tract/o- *pulling*
  -ion *action; condition*
Retraction: *Action (of) backward pulling (of the sternum)*

Word or Phrase	Description	Pronunciation/Word Parts
atelectasis	Incomplete expansion of part or all of a lung. Caused by mucus, a tumor, trauma, or a foreign body that blocks the bronchus (see Figure 4-10 ■). Also known as **collapsed lung**. This can develop postoperatively in patients who have shallow breathing and no cough reflex. Treatment: Correct the underlying cause. Insert a chest tube to reinflate the lung. 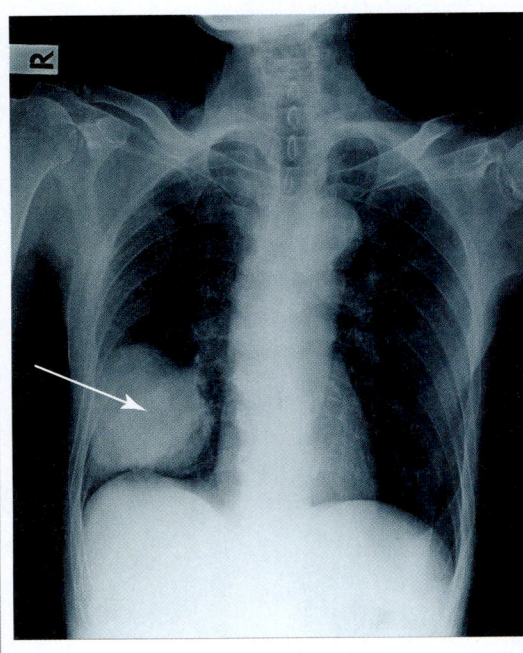 **FIGURE 4-10** ■ **Atelectasis.** This chest x-ray shows an area of atelectasis–a hazy, white patch–where the patient's right lower lobe has collapsed. Remember, the patient's right lung is on your left side when you look at the x-ray.	**atelectasis** (AT-eh-LEK-tah-sihs) **atel/o-** *incomplete* **-ectasis** *condition of dilation*
chronic obstructive pulmonary disease (COPD)	Any type of chronic obstructive lung disease, including chronic bronchitis or **emphysema**. Caused by chronic exposure to air pollution or smoking. There is inflammation of the bronchi with severe coughing, shortness of breath (dyspnea), and sputum production. Emphysema causes the alveoli to hyperinflate and rupture, creating large air pockets in the lungs. Air can be inhaled but not exhaled. Chronic overexpansion of the lungs deforms the thorax (barrel chest). COPD is a type of reactive airway disease. Treatment: Bronchodilator drug; corticosteroid drug; oxygen therapy	**chronic** (KRAW-nik) **chron/o-** *time* **-ic** *pertaining to* **obstructive** (awb-STRUK-tiv) **obstruct/o-** *blocked by a barrier* **-ive** *pertaining to* **emphysema** (EM-fih-SEE-mah) **em-** *in* **phys/o-** *distend; grow; inflate* **-ema** *condition* Emphysema: *Condition in (the lungs of being) distend(ed and) inflate(d)*

Word or Phrase	Description	Pronunciation/Word Parts

cystic fibrosis (CF)	Hereditary, eventually fatal disease caused by a recessive gene. Cystic fibrosis affects exocrine cells that secrete mucus, digestive enzymes, or sweat. The mucus is abnormally viscous (thick) and blocks the alveoli, causing dyspnea. Constant coughing causes bronchiectasis. There are frequent bacterial infections in the lungs. A chronic lack of oxygen causes cyanosis of the skin and clubbing of the fingertips (see Figure 4-11 ■). Mucus blocks pancreatic ducts and pancreatic enzymes, so fats are not digested properly. The patient has diarrhea and is undernourished. The pancreas develops fibrous cysts, hence the name *cystic fibrosis*. The sweat glands are overactive, producing too much sweat, and the patient loses large amounts of sodium.
	Treatment: Daily postural drainage (gravity helps drain the thick mucus) and chest percussion therapy to loosen mucus; bronchodilator drug; corticosteroid drug; digestive enzymes; high-salt diet
		cystic (SIS-tik)
		  cyst/o- *bladder; fluid-filled sac; semisolid cyst*
		  -ic *pertaining to*
		Cystic: *Pertaining to semisolid cysts (that are in the pancreas, not the lungs)*
		
		fibrosis (fy-BROH-sihs)
		  fibr/o- *fiber*
		  -osis *abnormal condition; process*

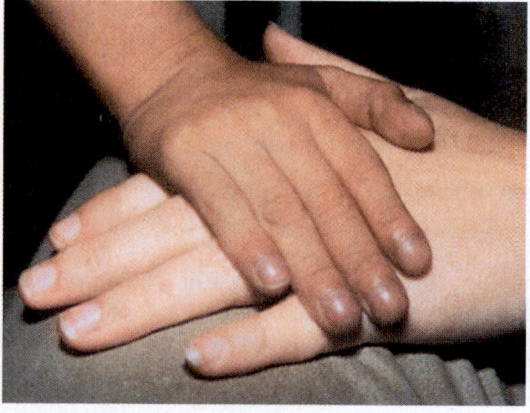

FIGURE 4-11 ■ Cystic fibrosis.
The hand of a child with cystic fibrosis compared to a normal adult hand (beneath). Cyanosis of the skin and clubbing of the fingertips are common in patients with cystic fibrosis. A low level of oxygen causes blood in the arteries to be bluish rather than bright red, and the skin color is cyanotic. The chronic lack of oxygen causes the fingertips and fingernails to grow abnormally.

Word or Phrase	Description	Pronunciation/Word Parts

empyema	Localized collection of **purulent** material (pus) in the thoracic cavity. Caused by a lung infection. Also known as **pyothorax**.
	Treatment: Antibiotic drug; surgery to drain the pus
		empyema (EM-py-EE-mah)
		  em- *in*
		  py/o- *pus*
		  -ema *condition*
		Empyema: *Condition in (the lungs of) pus*
		
		purulent (PYOOR-yoo-lent)
		  purul/o- *pus*
		  -ent *pertaining to*
		
		pyothorax (PY-oh-THOR-aks)
		  py/o- *pus*
		  -thorax *chest; thorax*

Word Alert
Sound-Alike Words

emphysema (noun) chronic, irreversibly damaged alveoli that are enlarged and trap air in the lungs
Example: Emphysema caused this patient to have a barrel chest.

empyema (noun) localized collection of pus in the thoracic cavity
Example: She will be started immediately on an intravenous antibiotic drug for her empyema.

Word or Phrase	Description	Pronunciation/Word Parts
influenza	Acute viral infection of the upper and lower respiratory system. Symptoms include nasal mucus, sneezing, fever, severe muscle aches, and a cough. Also known as the **flu**. It occurs most often in the fall and winter months. Influenza plus a secondary bacterial infection can cause pneumonia and death in older adults. Prevention: Annual flu vaccination Treatment: Analgesic drug; antiviral drug	**influenza** (IN-floo-EN-zah)

Clinical Connections

Public Health. The analgesic drug aspirin should not be used to treat symptoms of the flu. It can cause **Reye syndrome**, mainly in children and teenagers. It produces a high level of ammonia in the blood and brain, with vomiting, seizures, and liver failure. Instead, acetaminophen should be used to treat the symptoms of any viral infection.

Reye (RYE)

syndrome (SIN-drohm)

Word or Phrase	Description	Pronunciation/Word Parts
legionnaires' disease	Severe, sometimes fatal, bacterial infection. There are flu-like symptoms, body aches, and fever, followed by severe pneumonia with liver and kidney degeneration. Treatment: Antibiotic drug that is effective against this bacterium	**legionnaire** (LEE-jen-AIR)

Dive Deeper

Legionnaires' disease was first identified in 1976 when many people at an American Legion convention in Philadelphia became sick. Physicians and epidemiologists from the Centers for Disease Control and Prevention (CDC) found that the building's air conditioning system was contaminated with **Legionella pneumophila**, a bacterium that is attracted to the lungs. The bacterium was named for the site (American Legion) and its attraction (phil/o-) to the lungs (pneum/o-).

Legionella pneumophila (LEE-jeh-NEL-ah noo-MAW-fih-lah) The combining form **pneum/o-** means *air; lung.* The combining form **phil/o-** means *attraction to; fondness for.*

Word or Phrase	Description	Pronunciation/Word Parts

lung cancer	Cancerous tumor of the lungs that is more common in smokers. Years of smoking leave tar deposits in the lungs (see Figure 4-12 ■). Even nonsmokers who frequently breathe secondhand smoke have these deposits. These areas can become **cancerous** tumors. Lung cancer destroys normal tissue as it spreads (see Figure 4-13 ■). Lung cancers are named according to the location or the characteristics of the original **malignant** cell. **Adenocarcinoma** is the most common type of lung cancer, and it begins in the mucus-producing glands in the bronchi. **Bronchogenic carcinoma** begins in the epithelial cells that line the inner wall of the bronchi. **Large cell carcinoma** is cancer of the lung's tissue, as is **small cell carcinoma** (also known as **oat cell carcinoma** because of the shape of the cancerous cell).
	Prevention: Quitting smoking can reduce the risk of developing lung cancer.
	Treatment: Surgery to remove a lobe of the lung (lobectomy) or the entire lung (pneumonectomy); chemotherapy drug and/or radiation therapy
		cancer (KAN-ser)
		
		cancerous (KAN-ser-uhs)
		  cancer/o- *cancer*
		  -ous *pertaining to*
		
		malignant (mah-LIG-nant)
		  malign/o- *cancer*
		  -ant *pertaining to*
		
		adenocarcinoma
		(AD-eh-noh-KAR-sih-NOH-mah)
		  aden/o- *gland*
		  carcin/o- *cancer*
		  -oma *mass; tumor*
		
		bronchogenic
		(BRONG-koh-JEN-ik)
		  bronch/o- *bronchus*
		  gen/o- *arising from; produced by*
		  -ic *pertaining to*

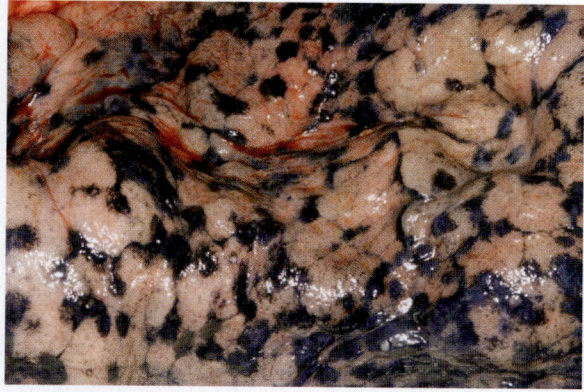

FIGURE 4-12 ■ Tar deposits in the lung.
This section of lung tissue shows hundreds of large and small deposits of black tar from years of smoking. Cigarette tar also contains carcinogens that can cause cancer.

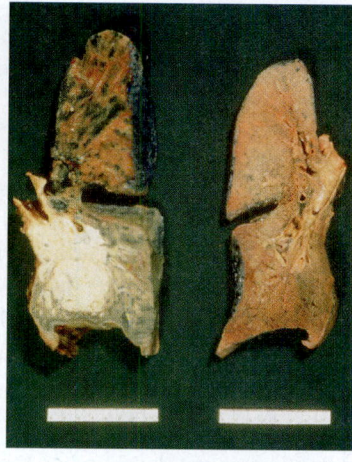

FIGURE 4-13 ■ Lung cancer.
These are two autopsy specimens of lungs. The lung on the left shows a large, white cancerous tumor that has nearly destroyed the base of the lung. There are also darkened areas in the upper lung that are tar deposits due to heavy smoking. The lung on the right is normal. It has a mostly pink color with some small darkened areas due to air pollution or light smoking.

Clinical Connections

Public Health. According to the American Lung Association, the average smoker smokes 15 cigarettes a day. **Packs per day (PPD)** of cigarettes is a standardized way to measure smoking. **Pack-years** equals the number of packs per day times the number of years of smoking. Scientific research studies first linked smoking to cancer in 1950. It was not until 1965 that Congress required a warning label on cigarettes that said that smoking was hazardous to your health.

Word or Phrase	Description	Pronunciation/Word Parts

occupational lung diseases	Group of diseases that are all caused by long-term exposure to inhaled irritants or particles that cause pulmonary fibrosis, and the alveoli lose their elasticity.
	
	• **Anthracosis** (coal miner's lung or black lung disease) is caused by coal dust.
	• **Asbestosis** is caused by asbestos fibers.
	• **Pneumoconiosis** is a general word for any occupational lung disease caused by inhaling some type of dust or particle.
	
	Prevention: Wear a filter mask to prevent inhalation of particles.
	Treatment: Bronchodilator drug; corticosteroid drug
		anthracosis (AN-thrah-KOH-sihs)
		  anthrac/o- *coal*
		  -osis *abnormal condition; process*
		Anthracosis: *Abnormal condition (of the lungs caused by inhaling) coal (dust)*
		
		asbestosis (AS-bes-TOH-sihs)
		  asbest/o- *asbestos*
		  -osis *abnormal condition; process*
		
		pneumoconiosis
		(NOO-moh-KOH-nee-OH-sihs)
		  pneum/o- *air; lung*
		  coni/o- *dust*
		  -osis *abnormal condition; process*

Clinical Connections

Public Health. Sick building syndrome is caused by inadequate ventilation coupled with indoor air pollutants and fumes released by carpeting, adhesives, paint that contains volatile organic compounds (VOCs), copy machines, cleaning agents, etc. It causes symptoms of headache; eye, nose, and throat irritation; cough; dizziness; difficulty concentrating; and fatigue.
Treatment: The symptoms subside or disappear when the person leaves the building.

Word or Phrase	Description	Pronunciation/Word Parts

pneumonia	Infection of some or all of the lobes of the lungs (see Figure 4-14 ■). Fluid, microorganisms, and white blood cells fill the alveoli and air passages. There is difficulty breathing, with coughing and mucus production. Inflammation of the pleurae causes pain on inspiration. Pneumonia is named according to the cause or the part of the lung that is affected.
	
	• **Bacterial pneumonia** is caused by a bacterium.
	• **Viral pneumonia** is caused by a virus.
	• **Double pneumonia** involves both lungs.
	
	Additional types of pneumonia are described on the next page.
	
	Treatment: Antibiotic drug for bacterial pneumonia; antiviral drug for viral pneumonia; oxygen therapy and use of a respirator, if needed
		pneumonia (noo-MOHN-yah)
		  pneumon/o- *air; lung*
		  -ia *condition; state; thing*

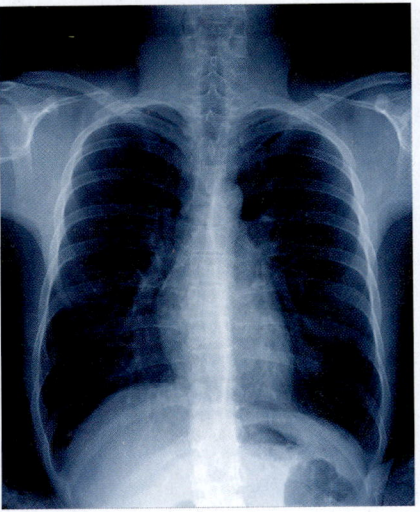

A.

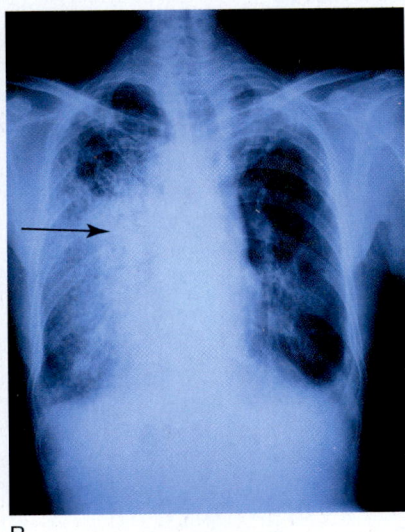

B.

FIGURE 4-14 ■ Pneumonia.
A. Normal chest x-ray. **B.** The chest x-ray shows a dense gray-white area of pneumonia in the patient's right lung. Remember, the patient's right lung is on your left side when you look at the x-ray.

Word or Phrase	Description	Pronunciation/Word Parts
aspiration pneumonia	Caused by foreign matter (chemicals, vomit, etc.) that is inhaled into the lungs	**aspiration** (AS-pih-RAY-shun) **aspir/o-** *breathe in; suck in* **-ation** *being; having; process*
broncho-pneumonia	Affects the bronchi, bronchioles, and alveoli in the lung	**bronchopneumonia** (BRONG-koh-noo-MOHN-yah) **bronch/o-** *bronchus* **pneumon/o-** *air; lung* **-ia** *condition; state; thing*
lobar pneumonia	Affects one lobe of the lung. **Panlobar** pneumonia affects all the lobes of one lung.	**lobar** (LOH-bar) **panlobar** (pan-LOH-bar) **pan-** *all* **lob/o-** *lobe of an organ* **-ar** *pertaining to*
pneumococcal pneumonia	Caused by the bacterium *Streptococcus pneumoniae*. Prevention: Pneumococcal vaccination of at-risk patients (infants, older adults)	**pneumococcal** (NOO-moh-KAW-kal) **pneum/o-** *air; lung* **cocc/o-** *spherical bacterium* **-al** *pertaining to*
Pneumocystis jiroveci pneumonia	Caused by the fungus *Pneumocystis jiroveci*. This fungus infects many people during childhood, causing a mild infection; then it lies dormant in the lungs within small cysts (*Pneumocystis*). In patients with AIDS and other immunosuppressant diseases, it emerges from the cysts and causes severe pneumonia. This is a type of **opportunistic infection** because it waits for an opportunity to cause disease in a person whose immune system is weakened. Treatment: Antifungal drug	***Pneumocystis jiroveci*** (NOO-moh-SIS-tihs YEE-roh-VET-zee) **opportunistic** (AW-por-too-NIS-tik) **opportun/o-** *taking advantage of an opportunity; well timed* **-ist** *person who specializes in; thing that specializes in* **-ic** *pertaining to*
walking pneumonia	Caused by the bacterium *Mycoplasma pneumoniae*. This is mild pneumonia; the patient does not feel well but can continue daily activities.	
pulmonary edema	Edema (fluid) collects in the alveoli. It is most commonly caused by failure of the left side of the heart to pump blood; this creates a backup of blood in the pulmonary circulation. Also can be caused by chest wall trauma or pneumonia, as fluid leaves the blood and enters the alveoli. Symptoms include dyspnea and orthopnea. Treatment: Correct the underlying heart failure; oxygen therapy	**edema** (eh-DEE-mah)

Word or Phrase	Description	Pronunciation/Word Parts
pulmonary embolism	Blockage of a pulmonary artery or one of its branches by an **embolus** (see Figure 4-15 ■). An embolus can develop if a patient is on prolonged bedrest, or from an injury that creates a blood clot in the leg (deep vein thrombosis), or from a fractured bone that releases a fat globule. The embolus (blood clot or fat globule) travels through the blood to a pulmonary artery where it acts as a plug and occludes (blocks) blood flow. There is a decreased level of oxygen in the blood, and the patient has shortness of breath. A large pulmonary embolus can be fatal. Treatment: Oxygen therapy; drugs to dissolve a blood clot (and prevent more blood clots from forming)	**embolism** (EM-boh-lizm) **embol/o-** *embolus; occluding plug* **-ism** *disease from a specific cause; process* **embolus** (EM-boh-luhs)

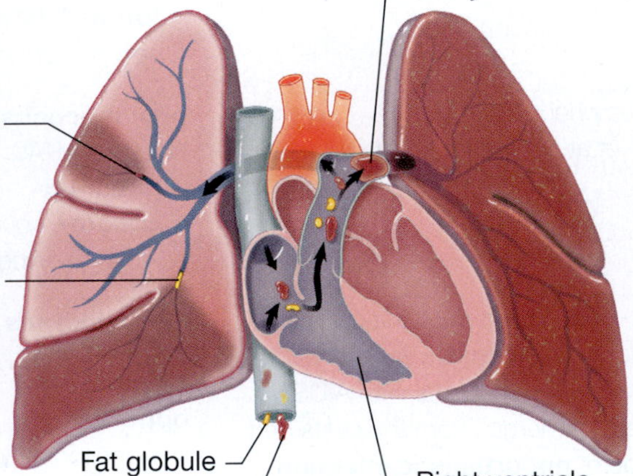

Large blood clot in left pulmonary artery

Small blood clot in branch of right pulmonary artery

Fat globule in branch of right pulmonary artery

Fat globule

Blood clot

Right ventricle of heart

FIGURE 4-15 ■ **Pulmonary embolus.**
An embolus (blood clot or fat globule) originates from veins anywhere in the body and travels to the heart. It easily goes through the large right ventricle of the heart, but it becomes trapped when it leaves the heart and goes into the smaller branches of the pulmonary arteries. Once the embolus becomes trapped, it blocks the flow of blood to the lung. The blood never reaches the alveoli to pick up oxygen. This lowers the overall oxygen content of the blood in the body. The alveoli collapse in that area of the lung.

Word or Phrase	Description	Pronunciation/Word Parts
severe acute respiratory syndrome (SARS)	Severe viral infection that can be fatal. There is a history of travel in an airplane or close contact with another person with SARS. Symptoms include fever, dyspnea, and cough. Treatment: Oxygen therapy and use of a respirator.	
tuberculosis (TB)	Infection caused by the bacterium *Mycobacterium tuberculosis* (see Figure 4-16 ■) and spread by airborne droplets and coughing. If the patient's immune system is strong, the bacteria cause no symptoms; this is known as a **latent tuberculosis infection (LTBI)**. Otherwise, the bacteria multiply, producing **tubercles** (soft nodules of necrosis) in the lungs, as well as symptoms of fever, cough, weight loss, night sweats, and hemoptysis (coughing up blood). Treatment: Antibiotic drugs used to treat bacterial infections are not effective against this bacterium. The patient must be treated with several antitubercular drugs for 9 months. **Multidrug-resistant tuberculosis (MDR-TB)** is resistant to at least two of the common antitubercular drugs.	**tuberculosis** (too-BER-kyoo-LOH-sihs) **tubercul/o-** *nodule* **-osis** *abnormal condition; process* **latent** (LAY-tent) **lat/o-** *dormant; hidden* **-ent** *pertaining to* **tubercle** (TOO-ber-kul) **tuber/o-** *nodule* **-cle** *small thing*

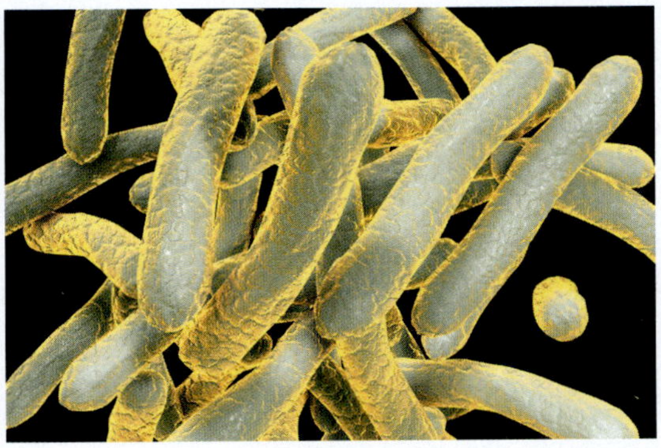

FIGURE 4-16 ■ *Mycobacterium tuberculosis.*
This bacterium causes tuberculosis. A rod-shaped bacterium like this is also known as a *bacillus*. It has an unusual waxy, external coating that makes it resistant to treatment with just one drug.

Word or Phrase	Description	Pronunciation/Word Parts

Thorax

hemothorax	Presence of blood in the thoracic cavity, usually from trauma.
	Treatment: Thoracentesis and insertion of a chest tube to remove blood and fluid
		hemothorax
		(HEE-moh-THOR-aks)
		  hem/o- *blood*
		  -thorax *chest; thorax*

pleural effusion	Accumulation of excessive fluid in the space between the visceral and parietal pleurae. Caused by infection or inflammation of the pleurae and lungs.
	Treatment: Antibiotic drug for infection; thoracentesis to remove the fluid
		effusion (ee-FYOO-shun)
		  effus/o- *pouring out*
		  -ion *action; condition*

pleurisy	Infection or inflammation of the pleurae due to pneumonia, trauma, or a tumor. Also known as **pleuritis**. The visceral and parietal pleurae rub against each other, causing pain on inspiration. This rubbing sound, as heard through a stethoscope, is a pleural friction rub.
	Treatment: Correct the underlying cause.
		pleurisy (PLOOR-ih-see)
		  pleur/o- *lung membrane*
		  -isy *condition of infection; condition of inflammation*
		
		pleuritis (ploor-EYE-tihs)
		  pleur/o- *lung membrane*
		  -itis *infection of; inflammation of*

pneumothorax	A large volume of air in the pleural space. A pneumothorax is a fully collapsed lung. This is usually caused by a penetrating injury to the chest, but a spontaneous pneumothorax can occur when alveoli rupture from lung disease. Air spreads apart the visceral and parietal pleurae and collapses the lung. *Note:* Air within the lung is normal; air between the visceral and parietal pleurae is abnormal.
	Treatment: Thoracentesis and insertion of a chest tube to remove the air
		pneumothorax
		(NOO-moh-THOR-aks)
		  pneum/o- *air; lung*
		  -thorax *chest; thorax*

Respiration

apnea	Absence of spontaneous respirations due to respiratory failure or respiratory arrest. Patients having an episode of apnea are said to be **apneic**. In premature infants, the immature central nervous system fails to maintain a consistent respiratory rate, and there are long pauses between breaths. Middle-aged, obese patients who snore excessively have **obstructive sleep apnea**. They stop breathing many times during the night as the airway is obstructed (by the soft palate or by obesity of the neck); then they take a gasping breath that often awakens them. This causes sleep deprivation, fatigue, and difficulty concentrating during the day.
	Treatment: Home apnea monitor for infants. Sleep apnea study to determine the cause in adults. Continuous positive airway pressure (CPAP) apparatus on the nose at night to provide positive pressure to keep the airway open.
		apnea (AP-nee-ah)
		
		apneic (AP-nee-ik)
		  a- *away from; without*
		  pne/o- *breathing*
		  -ic *pertaining to*
		
		obstructive (awb-STRUK-tiv)
		  obstruct/o- *blocked by a barrier*
		  -ive *pertaining to*

Dive Deeper

Sudden infant death syndrome (SIDS) is an acute event in which an apparently healthy infant under 1 year of age suddenly dies. This was previously known as *crib death*. The cause is unknown; it may be due to respiratory arrest from vomiting and aspirating stomach contents, from asphyxiation with soft bedding blocking the nose, from sleep apnea, or from an imbalance of neurotransmitters in the brain. Parents are cautioned to position babies on their backs to sleep. The national campaign for the prevention of SIDS is called "Safe to Sleep."

bradypnea	Abnormally slow rate of breathing (less than 10 breaths per minute in adults). Caused by a chemical imbalance in the blood or by brain damage that affects the respiratory control centers of the brain. Treatment: Correct the underlying cause.	**bradypnea** (BRAD-ip-NEE-ah) The prefix **brady-** means *slow*.

Word or Phrase	Description	Pronunciation/Word Parts
cough	Protective mechanism to forcefully expel accidentally inhaled food, irritating particles (smoke, dust), or internally produced mucus. A cough can be productive (sputum is expelled) or it can be nonproductive. **Expectoration** is coughing up sputum from the lungs. **Hemoptysis** is coughing up blood-tinged sputum. Treatment: Expectorant drug for a productive cough; antitussive drug for a nonproductive cough. Correct the underlying cause.	**expectoration** (eks-PEK-toh-RAY-shun) **ex-** *away from; out* **pector/o-** *chest* **-ation** *being; having; process* Expectoration: *Process (of expelling sputum) out (of the) chest* **hemoptysis** (hee-MAWP-tih-sihs) **hem/o-** *blood* **-ptysis** *condition of coughing up*
dyspnea	Difficult, labored, or painful respirations. Patients are said to be **dyspneic**. Also known as **shortness of breath (SOB)**. **Dyspnea on exertion (DOE)** occurs after brief activity in patients with severe chronic obstructive pulmonary disease (COPD). **Paroxysmal nocturnal dyspnea (PND)** is a sudden attack of shortness of breath that occurs at night (nocturnal) when fluid builds up in the lungs because the patient is lying supine. Treatment: Sleeping propped up on pillows or in a chair; oxygen therapy. Correct the underlying cause.	**dyspnea** (DISP-nee-ah) **dyspneic** (DISP-nee-ik) **dys-** *abnormal; difficult; painful* **pne/o-** *breathing* **-ic** *pertaining to* **paroxysmal** (PAIR-awk-SIZ-mal)
orthopnea	Difficulty breathing when lying supine. The patient can breathe and sleep comfortably only when in an upright or semi-upright position. Dyspnea and congestion occur if the patient lies down. The severity of orthopnea is expressed as the number of pillows that are needed (e.g., two-pillow orthopnea). Treatment: Oxygen therapy. Correct the underlying cause.	**orthopnea** (or-THAWP-nee-ah) The combining form **orth/o-** means *straight.* Orthopnea: *Breathing (that is only comfortable in a) straight (up position)*
tachypnea	Abnormally rapid rate of breathing (see Figure 4-17 ■). The patient is said to be **tachypneic**. Treatment: Oxygen therapy. Correct the underlying cause.	**tachypnea** (TAK-ip-NEE-ah) **tachypneic** (TAK-ip-NEE-ik) **tachy-** *fast* **pne/o-** *breathing* **-ic** *pertaining to*

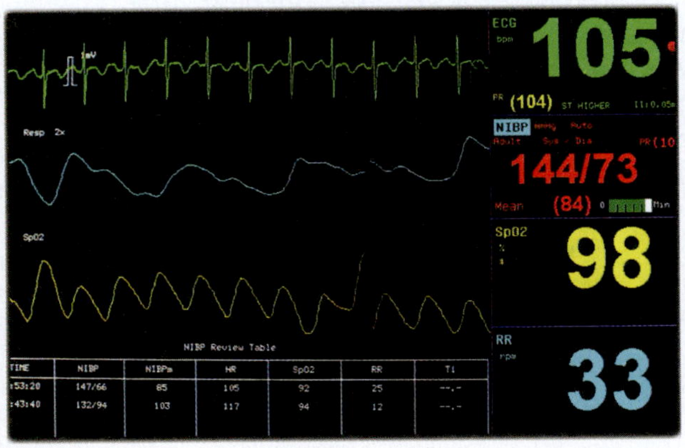

FIGURE 4-17 ■ Tachypnea.
This monitor screen shows the patient's heart rate in green (105 beats per minute), blood pressure in red (144/73), saturated partial oxygen (SpO2) in yellow (98), and respiratory rate in blue (33 respirations per minute). The normal respiratory rate for an adult is 12–20 breaths per minute, and so this patient is tachypneic. The increased respiratory rate could be due to lung disease or to pain.

Oxygen and Carbon Dioxide

anoxia	Complete lack (or a severely decreased level) of oxygen in the arterial blood and body tissues. Caused by a lack of oxygen in the inhaled air or by an obstruction that prevents oxygen from reaching the lungs. Treatment: Oxygen therapy. Correct the underlying cause.	**anoxia** (an-AWK-see-ah) **an-** *not; without* **ox/o-** *oxygen* **-ia** *condition; state; thing*

Word or Phrase	Description	Pronunciation/Word Parts
asphyxia	An abnormally high level of carbon dioxide with an abnormally low level of oxygen in the blood that produces a decreased heart rate and blueness of the skin. Caused by choking, drowning, suffocating, or a **foreign body object (FBO).** Treatment: Correct the underlying cause. May need cardiopulmonary resuscitation.	**asphyxia** (as-FIK-see-ah)

Clinical Connections

Obstetrics. Birth asphyxia occurs when the fetus in the uterus does not get enough oxygen through the umbilical cord and placenta before or during birth. This can be caused by premature separation of the placenta from the uterine wall, an umbilical cord that is wrapped tightly around the fetus's neck, or an umbilical cord that is compressed by the weight of the fetus during delivery.

Word or Phrase	Description	Pronunciation/Word Parts
cyanosis	Bluish discoloration of the skin and nail beds because of a low level of oxygen and a high level of carbon dioxide in the blood and tissues. **Circumoral cyanosis** occurs around the mouth (see Figure 4-18 ■). The patient is said to be **cyanotic**. Treatment: Oxygen therapy. Correct the underlying cause.	**cyanosis** (SY-ah-NOH-sihs) **cyan/o-** *blue* **-osis** *abnormal condition; process* **cyanotic** (SY-ah-NAW-tik) **cyan/o-** *blue* **-tic** *pertaining to* **circumoral** (SIR-kum-OR-al) **circum-** *around* **or/o-** *mouth* **-al** *pertaining to*

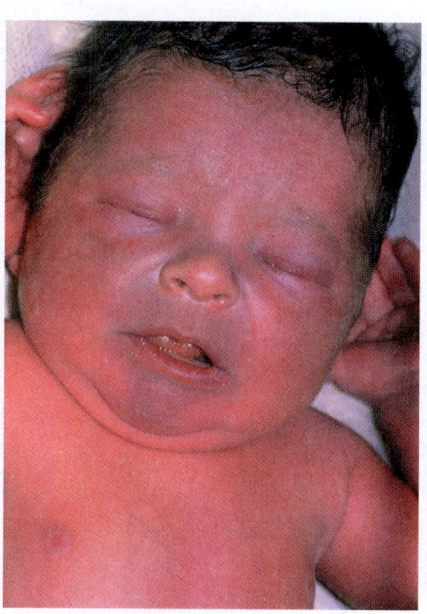

FIGURE 4-18 ■ Cyanosis.
This newborn infant shows cyanosis of his face. He has a structural defect of his heart and, each time his heart beats, it pumps deoxygenated blood (instead of oxygenated blood) to the cells of his body.

Clinical Connections

Environmental Health. One new car in 1960 generated as much air pollution as 20 new cars today. The **Air Quality Index (AQI)** is a scale that rates the quality of the air daily. An AQI of 0–50 is good; over 100 is unhealthy for sensitive people, and over 300 is hazardous for everyone. Scientists feel that air pollution is a factor in global warming.

Public Health. In children, exposure to secondhand smoke is linked to asthma, respiratory infections, and middle ear infections. Many states ban smoking in public places such as restaurants and bars because even secondhand smoke is a carcinogen, according to the Environmental Protection Agency.

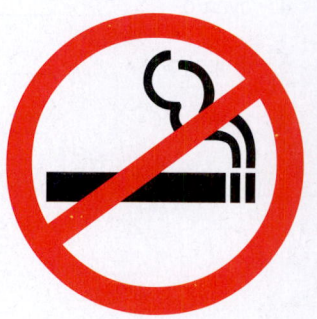

Word or Phrase	Description	Pronunciation/Word Parts
hypercapnia	Very high level of carbon dioxide (CO_2) in the arterial blood. Treatment: Oxygen therapy. Correct the underlying cause.	**hypercapnia** (HY-per-KAP-nee-ah) **hyper-** *above; more than normal* **capn/o-** *carbon dioxide* **-ia** *condition; state; thing*
hypoxemia	Very low level of oxygen in the arterial blood. **Hypoxia** is a very low level of oxygen in the cells. Treatment: Oxygen therapy. Correct the underlying cause.	**hypoxemia** (HY-pawk-SEE-mee-ah) **hypo-** *below; deficient* **ox/o-** *oxygen* **-emia** *condition of the blood; substance in the blood* **hypoxia** (hy-PAWK-see-ah) **hypo-** *below; deficient* **ox/o-** *oxygen* **-ia** *condition; state; thing*

4.3 PRACTICE LAPS

Use the Answer Key at the end of the book to check your answers.

A. Give the Meaning of Combining Forms

Next to each combining form, write its meaning. The first one has been done for you.

Combining Form	Meaning	Combining Form	Meaning
1. **anthrac/o-**	*coal*	7. malign/o-	
2. asthm/o-		8. obstruct/o-	
3. carcin/o-		9. pneum/o-	
4. cyan/o-		10. pneumon/o-	
5. embol/o-		11. py/o-	
6. hem/o-		12. tubercul/o-	

B. Build Words

Read the definition of the medical word. Look at the combining form that is given. Select the correct suffix from the Suffix List, and write it on the blank line. Then build the medical word, and write it on the line. (Remember: You may need to remove the combining vowel. Always remove the hyphens and slash.) Be sure to check your spelling.

Suffix List

-ar (pertaining to)	-ism (disease from a specific	-ptysis (condition of coughing up)
-atic (pertaining to)	cause; process)	-spasm (sudden, involuntary muscle
-cle (small thing)	-itis (infection of; inflammation of)	contraction)
-ectasis (condition of dilation)	-osis (abnormal condition; process)	-thorax (chest; thorax)

Definition of the Medical Word	Combining Form	Suffix	Build the Medical Word
Example: Pertaining to (a) lobe of an organ	**lob/o-**	*-ar*	*lobar*

[*You think* pertaining to *(-ar)* + lobe *(lob/o-)*. You change the order of the word parts to put the suffix last. You write lobar.]

1. Abnormal condition (of being) blue	cyan/o-	_____	_____
2. Small thing (that is a) nodule	tuber/o-	_____	_____
3. Condition of coughing up blood	hem/o-	_____	_____
4. Sudden, involuntary muscle contraction (around the) bronchus	bronch/o-	_____	_____
5. Pertaining to asthma	asthm/o-	_____	_____
6. Infection (or) inflammation of (the) bronchus	bronch/o-	_____	_____
7. Condition of dilation (of the lung that is) incomplete	atel/o-	_____	_____
8. Chest (that contains) pus	py/o-	_____	_____
9. Disease from a specific cause (of an) occluding plug	embol/o-	_____	_____
10. Chest (that contains) blood	hem/o-	_____	_____

C. Define Abbreviations

1. CF   _____
2. COPD _____
3. DOE   _____
4. ARDS _____

5. LTBI _____
6. SIDS _____
7. TB   _____
8. URI   _____

4.4 Laboratory, Diagnostic, and Radiologic Procedures

Word or Phrase	Description	Pronunciation/Word Parts

Laboratory Tests and Diagnostic Procedures

Word or Phrase	Description	Pronunciation/Word Parts
arterial blood gases (ABG)	Blood test to measure the partial pressure (p) of the gases oxygen (pO_2) and carbon dioxide (pCO_2) in the arterial blood. The pH (how acidic or alkaline the blood is) is also measured. The higher the level of carbon dioxide, the more acidic the blood and the lower the pH.	**arterial** (ar-TEER-ee-al) **arteri/o-** *artery* **-al** *pertaining to*
carboxyhemo-globin	Blood test to measure the level of carbon monoxide (CO) in the blood. An increased level is caused by exposure to fire, smoke, or fumes in a closed, unventilated space. Carbon monoxide is carried by hemoglobin as carboxyhemoglobin. A blood level above 50% is fatal.	**carboxyhemoglobin** (kar-BAWK-see-HEE-moh-GLOH-bin) **carbox/y-** *carbon monoxide* **hem/o-** *blood* **glob/o-** *comprehensive; shaped like a globe* **-in** *substance*
oximetry	Procedure to measure the degree of hemoglobin saturation of the blood. An **oximeter**, a small, noninvasive clip device, is placed on the patient's index finger or earlobe. It emits light waves that penetrate the skin and are absorbed or reflected by saturated hemoglobin in red blood cells (that is bound to oxygen) versus unsaturated hemoglobin (not bound to oxygen). The oximeter displays the oxygen saturation level of the blood but not the carbon dioxide level. A **pulse oximeter** measures the pulse rate as well (see Figure 4-19 ■).	**oximetry** (awk-SIM-eh-tree) **ox/i-** *oxygen* **-metry** *process of measuring* **oximeter** (awk-SIM-eh-ter) **ox/i-** *oxygen* **-meter** *instrument used to measure*

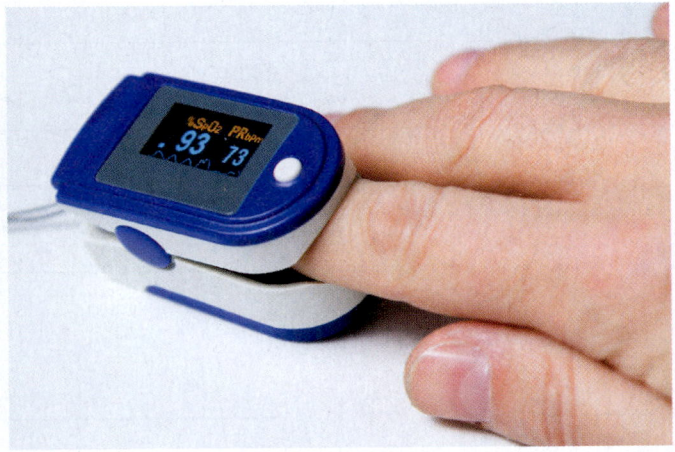

FIGURE 4-19 ■ Pulse oximeter.
This device is used in ambulances and in hospitals (at the patient's bedside) to provide a quick and accurate measurement of the percentage of the patient's hemoglobin that is saturated with oxygen, 93 percent, and the pulse rate (PR), 73. Here, both of this patient's readings are within normal limits.

Word or Phrase	Description	Pronunciation/Word Parts
pulmonary function test (PFT)	Procedure to measure the capacity of the lungs and the volume of air during inhalation and exhalation (see Figure 4-20 ■). The forced vital capacity (FVC) measures the amount of air that can be forcefully exhaled from the lungs after inhaling fully. The forced expiratory volume (FEV_1) measures the volume of air that can be forcefully exhaled in 1 second. The FVC and FEV_1 results are displayed on a computer.	

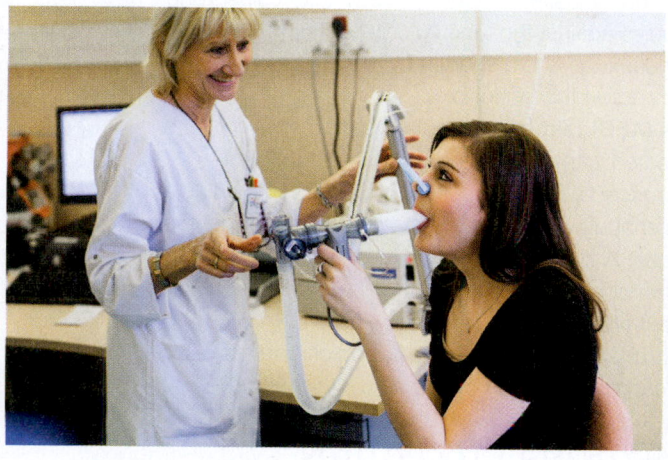

FIGURE 4-20 ■ Pulmonary function test.
This young woman who has cystic fibrosis has to have periodic pulmonary function tests. The blue clip on her nose ensures that air only flows in and out of her mouth to her lungs, so that the volume of air in her lungs can be accurately measured.

Word or Phrase	Description	Pronunciation/Word Parts
sleep study	Procedure to determine whether a patient has obstructive sleep apnea. Sensors record the patient's brain waves, eye movements, heart rate, breathing rate, blood pressure, movements of the extremities, and the oxygen level in the blood (see Figure 4-21 ■). Also known as **polysomnography**.	**polysomnography** (PAW-lee-sawm-NAW-grah-fee) **poly-** *many; much* **somn/o-** *sleep* **-graphy** *process of recording*

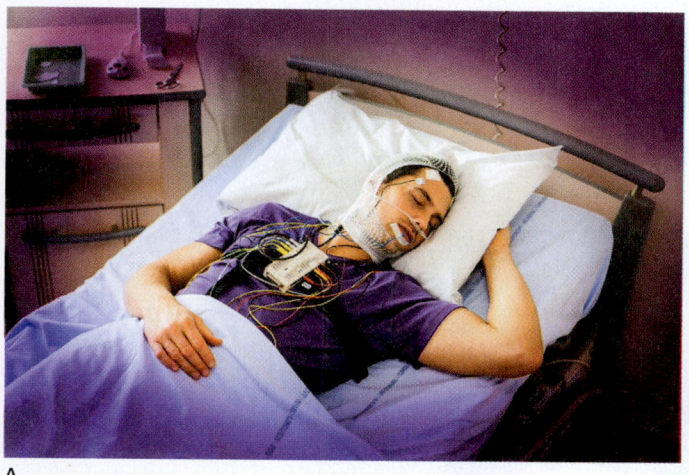
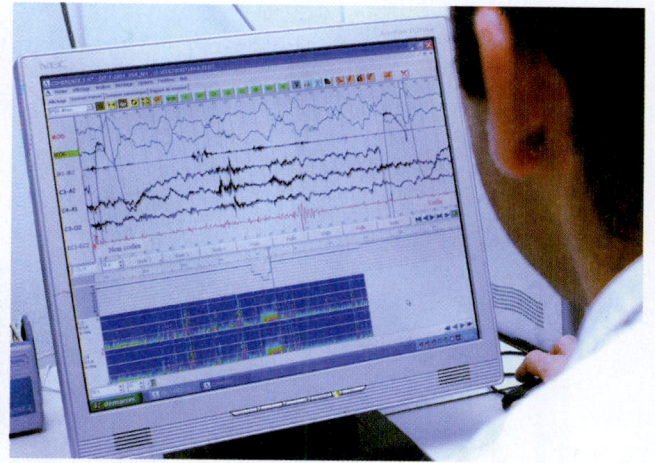

A.   B.

FIGURE 4-21 ■ Sleep study.
A. This patient is being electronically monitored while he sleeps. Sensors record his brain waves, eye movements, heart rate, respiratory rate, blood pressure, and the oxygen level in his blood. **B.** A physician continuously monitors each of the sensor recordings.

Word or Phrase	Description	Pronunciation/Word Parts
sputum culture and sensitivity (C&S)	Laboratory test to identify the bacterium causing a pulmonary infection. A specimen of the patient's sputum is placed in a culture dish with disks of antibiotic drugs to see which drug the bacterium is sensitive to; this will be the antibiotic drug prescribed.	

Word or Phrase	Description	Pronunciation/Word Parts
tuberculosis tests	Tests to determine whether a patient has been exposed to tuberculosis. • The **tine test** is a screening test that uses a four-pronged device (similar to the tines on a fork) to puncture the skin and introduce **PPD (purified protein derivative)**, which is a part of the bacterium *Mycobacterium tuberculosis*. • The **Mantoux test** uses an intradermal injection of PPD. For both tests, a raised skin reaction of a certain size within 48–72 hours after the test is a positive test result and indicates prior exposure to tuberculosis and the presence of antibodies against the tuberculosis bacterium. A positive test is followed by a chest x-ray and a sputum culture to determine whether the patient has active tuberculosis. • An **acid-fast bacillus (AFB) test** uses a sputum specimen that is smeared on a slide, treated with a stain, and then washed. When examined under a microscope, the tuberculosis bacterium (known as a *bacillus* because of its shape) will hold fast to the acid stain's color, even when the slide is washed. A culture of the sputum is then performed to confirm the diagnosis of tuberculosis. • The **Xpert sputum test** (the "while-you-wait" test) uses DNA technology, takes 100 minutes, is more accurate, and can detect tuberculosis that is already resistant to drugs.	**Mantoux** (man-TOO)

Radiologic and Nuclear Medicine Procedures

chest radiography	Radiologic procedure that uses x-rays to create a digital image of the lungs. Also known as a **chest x-ray (CXR)**. • **Anteroposterior (AP) chest x-ray**: the x-rays enter through the patient's anterior chest and exit through the posterior chest. • **Posteroanterior (PA) chest x-ray**: the x-rays enter through the patient's posterior chest and exit through the anterior chest (see Figure 4-22 ■). • **Lateral chest x-ray**: the x-rays enter through the patient's side and exit through the other side.	**radiography** (RAY-dee-AW-grah-fee) **radi/o-** *forearm bone; radius; x-rays* **-graphy** *process of recording*

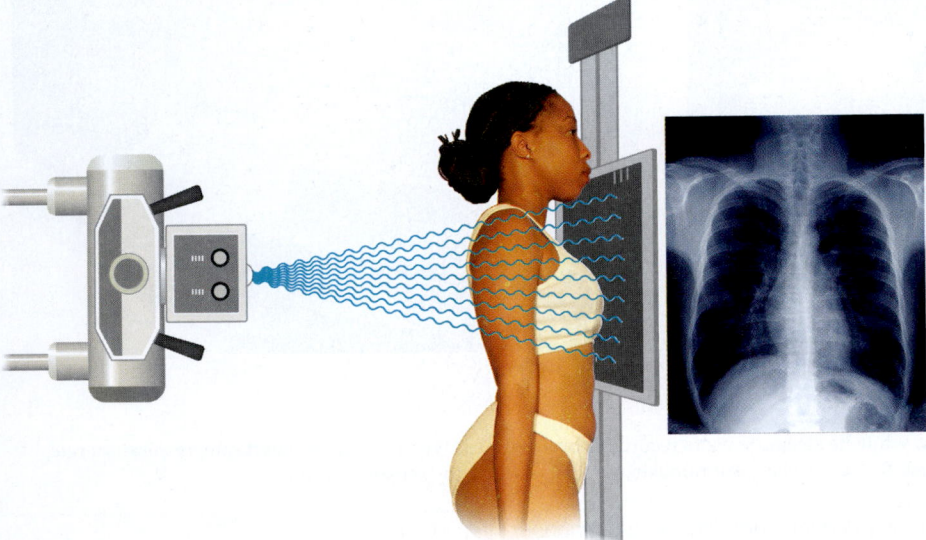

FIGURE 4-22 ■ PA Chest x-ray.
This patient is having a PA (posteroanterior) chest x-ray. The x-ray machine projects a set of crossed lines onto the patient's back to help the radiologic technologist center the x-ray beam. The patient is asked to remain still so that the image will not show motion artifact (blurring). The x-rays penetrate the patient's posterior chest and exit through the patient's anterior chest to create a digital image.

Clinical Connections

Radiology. X-rays were discovered in 1895 by Wilhelm Roentgen; he took the first x-ray, which was of his wife's hand! A roentgen is the international unit of x-ray radiation. X-ray film has been replaced by digital x-ray images. Chest x-rays are the most common diagnostic radiologic procedure; 150 million are performed each year.

Word or Phrase	Description	Pronunciation/Word Parts
computerized axial tomography (CAT, CT)	Radiologic procedure that uses x-rays to create multiple digital cross-sectional images by scanning one narrow slice of tissue at a time (see Figure 4-23 ■).	**tomography** (toh-MAW-grah-fee) **tom/o-** *cut; layer; slice* **-graphy** *process of recording*

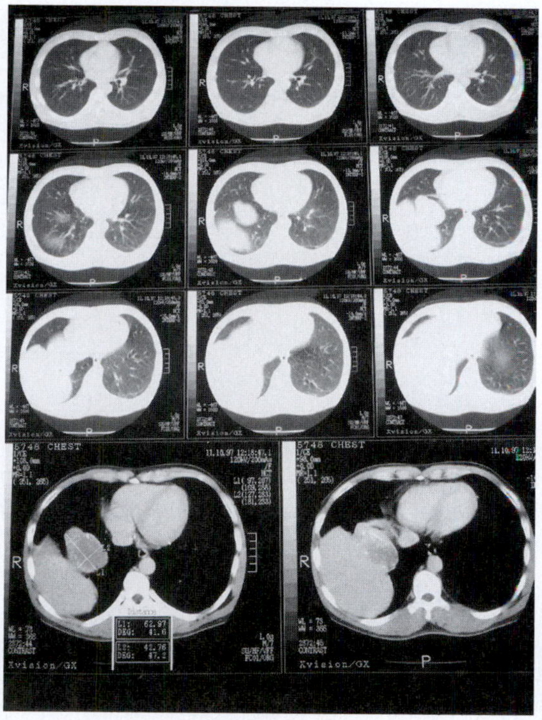

FIGURE 4-23 ■ CT scan of the chest.
The radiologist is able to see details of structures and detect subtle changes from one CT "slice" image to the next.

Word or Phrase	Description	Pronunciation/Word Parts
lung scan	Nuclear medicine procedure that uses an inhaled radioactive gas to evaluate ventilation (air flow) in the lungs as well as an intravenous radioactive drug to evaluate perfusion (blood flow to the lungs). Areas of decreased uptake ("cold spots") indicate pneumonia, atelectasis, or pleural effusion. Also known as a **ventilation-perfusion (V/Q) scan**. The *Q* stands for *quotient*.	**ventilation** (VEN-tih-LAY-shun) **ventil/o-** *air movement* **-ation** *being; having; process* **perfusion** (per-FYOO-shun) **per-** *through; throughout* **fus/o-** *pouring* **-ion** *action; condition*
magnetic resonance imaging (MRI)	Radiologic procedure that uses a magnet and radio waves to produce a magnetic field that affects the rotational axis of protons in atoms in the body's tissues. The MRI machine scans one narrow slice of tissue at a time to create multiple images. This procedure does not expose the patient to any radiation or x-rays, which is preferred in pediatric patients and patients who are pregnant.	

4.4 PRACTICE LAPS

Use the Answer Key at the end of the book to check your answers.

A. Give the Meaning of Combining Forms

Next to each combining form, write its meaning. The first one has been done for you.

Combining Form	Meaning	Combining Form	Meaning
1. **arteri/o-**	*artery*	5. radi/o-	
2. carbox/y-		6. somn/o-	
3. hem/o-		7. tom/o-	
4. ox/i-		8. ventil/o-	

B. Build Words

Read the definition of the medical word. Look at the combining form that is given. Select the correct suffix from the Suffix List, and write it on the blank line. Then build the medical word, and write it on the line. (Remember: You may need to remove the combining vowel. Always remove the hyphens and slash.) Be sure to check your spelling.

Suffix List

-ation (being; having; process)	-graphy (process of recording)	-meter (instrument used to measure)	-metry (process of measuring)

Definition of the Medical Word	Combining Form	Suffix	Build the Medical Word
Example: Process of measuring (the level of) oxygen	**ox/i-**	*-metry*	*oximetry*

[*You think* process of measuring *(-metry)* + oxygen *(ox/i-).* You change the order of the word parts to put the suffix last. *You write* oximetry.]

1. Instrument used to measure (the level of) oxygen	ox/i-		
2. Process of recording x-rays	radi/o-		
3. Process (of) air movement	ventil/o-		
4. Process of measuring (to) breathe	spir/o-		

C. Define Abbreviations

1. ABG	4. FVC
2. C&S	5. pCO_2
3. CXR	6. PFT

4.5 Medical Procedures, Drugs, and Surgical Procedures

Word or Phrase	Description	Pronunciation/Word Parts

Medical Procedures

auscultation and percussion (A&P)	Auscultation uses a **stethoscope** to listen to breath sounds in all lobes of the lungs. Percussion uses the finger of one hand to tap over the finger of the other hand that is spread across the patient's back over a lobe of the lung. After a few taps, the hand is moved over another lobe. Auscultation and percussion tell the physician if the lung sounds are clear or if there is dullness because of the presence of fluid or a tumor (see Figure 4-24 ■).	**auscultation** (AWS-kul-TAY-shun)
		  auscult/o- *listening*
		  -ation *being; having; process*
		
		stethoscope (STETH-oh-skohp)
		  steth/o- *chest*
		  -scope *instrument used to examine*
		
		percussion (per-KUH-shun)
		  percuss/o- *tapping*
		  -ion *action; condition*

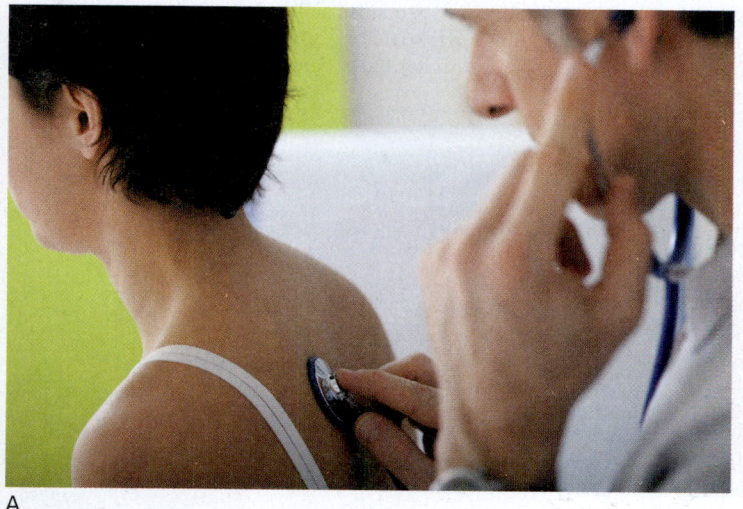 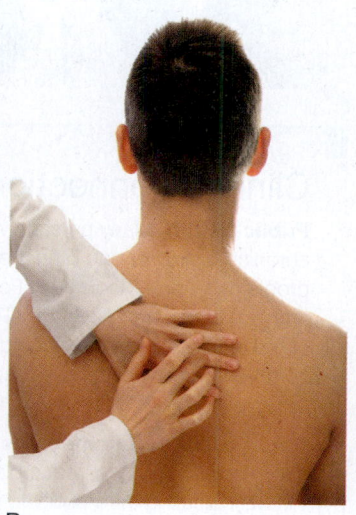

A.   B.

FIGURE 4-24 ■ Auscultation and percussion.
A. The physician asks the patient to take a deep breath as he listens through a stethoscope to the breath sounds in each of the lobes of the lungs. **B.** During percussion, the examiner uses her hands to identify sounds of dullness in the lungs.

cardiopulmonary resuscitation (CPR)	Procedure to provide air to the lungs and circulate the blood when a patient stops breathing and the heart stops beating. Mouth-to-mouth resuscitation involves forcing air into the patient's lungs while chest compressions pump blood through the heart. Current American Heart Association CPR guidelines allow a layperson to perform only chest compressions because there is a sufficient amount of oxygen in the blood if the blood is circulated by the chest compressions.	**cardiopulmonary** (KAR-dee-oh-PUL-moh-NAIR-ee)
		  cardi/o- *heart*
		  pulmon/o- *lung*
		  -ary *pertaining to*
		
		resuscitation (ree-SUS-ih-TAY-shun)
		  resuscit/o- *raise up again; revive*
		  -ation *being; having; process*

Word or Phrase	Description	Pronunciation/Word Parts
chest percussion therapy	For patients with severe lung disease and mucus production or for patients with cystic fibrosis and thick mucus, the respiratory therapist uses cupped hands, hitting (percussion) against the patient's back to loosen the mucus, or uses a vibrating device to loosen the mucus (see Figure 4-25 ■). The patient can then cough up the mucus.	

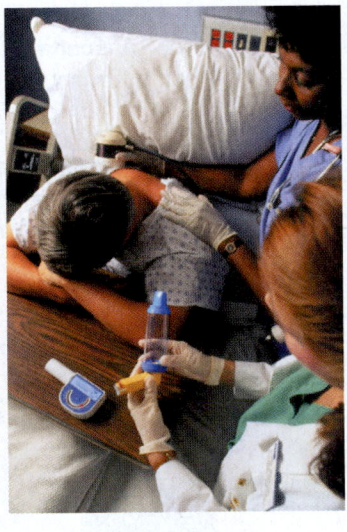

FIGURE 4-25 ■ Chest percussion therapy.
This young man has been hospitalized. The respiratory therapist is using a vibrating device on his back to shake loose the thick mucus in his lungs so that he can cough it up. The nurse is preparing a drug for the patient to inhale.

Clinical Connections

Public Health. Many persons with chronic respiratory and other health problems wear a Medic Alert Foundation emblem bracelet or necklace. The back of the emblem describes their disease so that this information is available in an emergency even if they are unconscious.

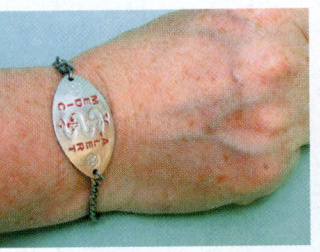

Emergency Medicine. The universal sign of choking is two hands placed at the throat, indicating the inability to speak or breath. **Abdominal thrusts** (formerly the **Heimlich maneuver**) is a procedure to assist a choking victim with an airway obstruction. The rescuer stands behind the victim and places a fist on the victim's abdominal wall just below the diaphragm and, with both hands, gives a sudden push inward and upward. This generates an exhaled burst of air that pushes the obstruction into the mouth where it can be coughed out or removed.

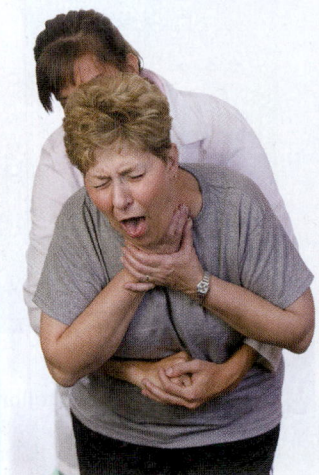

Heimlich (HYM-lik)

Word or Phrase	Description	Pronunciation/Word Parts
endotracheal intubation	Procedure in which an **endotracheal tube (ETT)** is inserted into the trachea. A lighted **laryngoscope** helps visualize the vocal cords (see Figure 4-26 ■). The tube goes through the oral cavity and pharynx, between the vocal cords of the larynx, and into the trachea. This establishes an airway for a patient who is not breathing or needs a respirator. This procedure is performed by paramedics in an ambulance, by physicians or respiratory therapists in the emergency department, or by anesthesiologists in the operating room prior to surgical procedures. Alternatively, a **nasotracheal tube** can be inserted through the nasopharynx to reach the trachea.	**endotracheal** (EN-doh-TRAY-kee-al) **end/o-** _innermost; within_ **trache/o-** _trachea; windpipe_ **-al** _pertaining to_ **intubation** (IN-too-BAY-shun) **in-** _in; not; within_ **tub/o-** _tube_ **-ation** _being; having; process_ **laryngoscope** (lah-RING-goh-skohp) **laryng/o-** _larynx; voice box_ **-scope** _instrument used to examine_ **nasotracheal** (NAY-soh-TRAY-kee-al) **nas/o-** _nose_ **trache/o-** _trachea; windpipe_ **-al** _pertaining to_

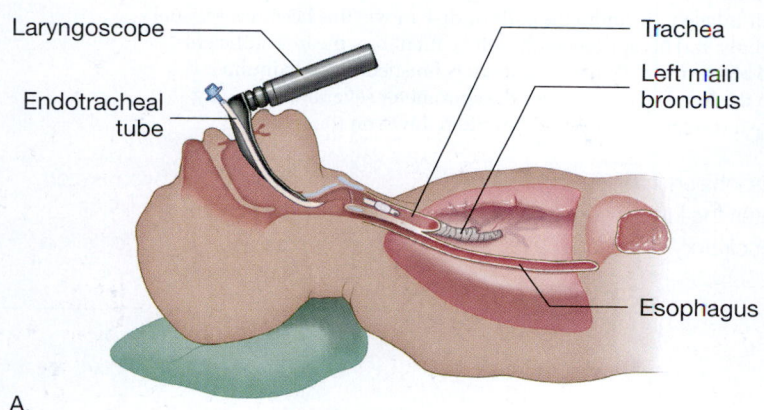

A.

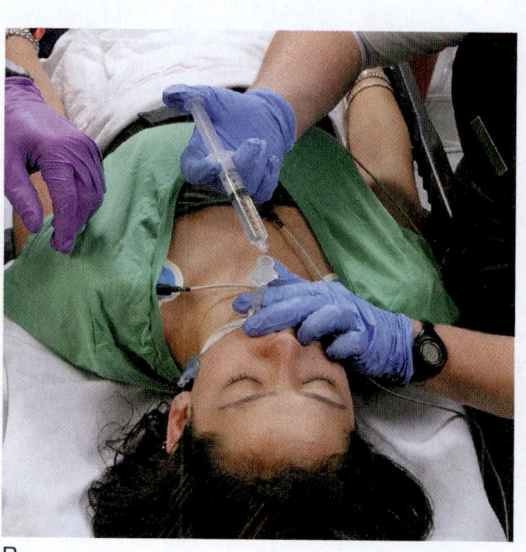

B.

FIGURE 4-26 ■ Endotracheal intubation.
A. A laryngoscope is used to visualize the vocal cords prior to insertion of an endotracheal tube. The endotracheal tube is positioned in the trachea, with the tip of the tube just above the bronchi. A small balloon at the tip of the tube is inflated to hold the tube in place, and the external part of the tube is taped to the patient's cheek. **B.** An endotracheal tube can be connected to a respirator that breathes for the patient; it can also be used to deliver certain drugs to the lungs in an emergency.

Word or Phrase	Description	Pronunciation/Word Parts
incentive spirometry	Procedure that uses the medical device of a **spirometer** to encourage patients (give them an incentive) to breathe deeply to prevent atelectasis (see Figure 4-27 ■). It is the most common type of pulmonary function test.	**spirometry** (spih-RAW-meh-tree) **spir/o-** *breathe; coil* **-metry** *process of measuring* **spirometer** (spih-RAW-meh-ter) **spir/o-** *breathe; coil* **-meter** *instrument used to measure*

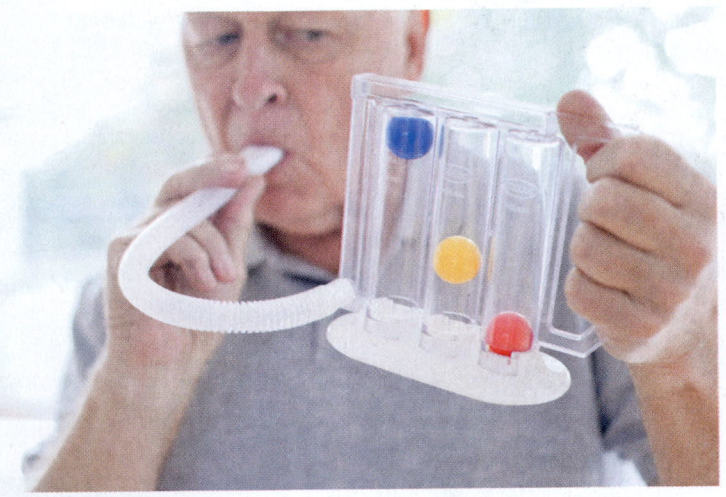
A.

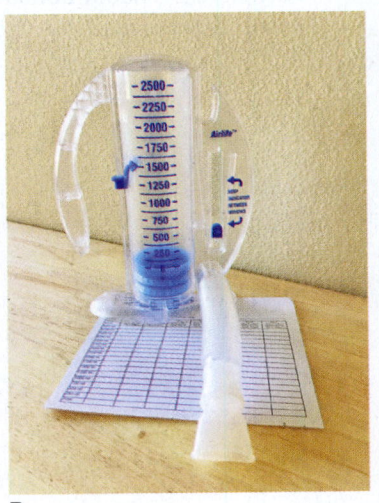
B.

FIGURE 4-27 ■ Incentive spirometers.
A. A spirometer is a portable plastic device with a mouthpiece. The patient inhales through the device's mouthpiece, which causes balls or a disk to move. The greater the volume of air inhaled, the more the balls or disk move; this becomes a visual incentive to encourage the patient to breathe even more deeply. **B.** This spirometer has the patient breathe in a sufficient volume to keep the blue indicator on the right between the blue arrows. When the patient is finished, the maximum volume that was inhaled is marked with the blue arrow on the left. The patient uses the spirometer several times a day, each time striving to inhale a greater volume, as marked by the arrow on the left and written down on the record.

Word or Phrase	Description	Pronunciation/Word Parts
nebulizer treatment	Device that creates a fine mist that is inhaled into the lungs. The mist contains a drug that deeply penetrates the lung tissue. Used to treat asthma, cystic fibrosis, and other respiratory diseases.	**nebulizer** (NEH-byoo-LY-zer) **nebul/o-** *mist* **-izer** *thing that affects in a particular way*

Word or Phrase	Description	Pronunciation/Word Parts
oxygen therapy	Procedure to provide additional oxygen to patients with pulmonary disease. **Room air (RA)** contains 21% oxygen. A patient can need percentages of oxygen ranging from 22% to 100%. Oxygen can be delivered to the patient via a **nasal cannula** (see Figure 4-28 ■) or a face mask. An infant can receive oxygen through a rigid plastic hood placed over the head or by being in an oxygen tent. Oxygen is drying, and so patients who need a high flow of oxygen or prolonged oxygen therapy receive humidified oxygen (bubbled through water). A patient who requires respiratory assistance as well as oxygen is placed on a **respirator (ventilator)**, a mechanical device that breathes for the patient or assists with some breaths (see Figure 4-29 ■). Respirators can provide up to 100% oxygen, as well as pressure to keep the alveoli from collapsing. A **resuscitator bag (Ambu bag)** is a handheld device that is squeezed to temporarily breathe for a patient through a face mask or endotracheal tube.	**cannula** (KAN-yoo-lah) **respirator** (RES-pih-RAY-tor) **re-** *again and again; backward; unable to* **spir/o-** *breathe; coil* **-ator** *person who does or produces; thing that does or produces* **ventilator** (VEN-tih-LAY-tor) **ventil/o-** *air movement* **-ator** *person who does or produces; thing that does or produces* **resuscitator** (ree-SUS-ih-TAY-tor) **resuscit/o-** *raise up again; revive* **-ator** *person who does or produces; thing that does or produces* **Ambu** (AM-boo)

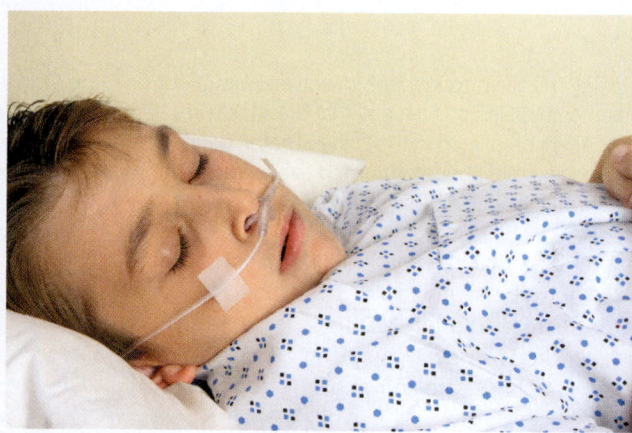

FIGURE 4-28 ■ Nasal cannula.
This patient is receiving oxygen therapy through a nasal cannula, a plastic tube with two short, flexible prongs that rest just inside the nostrils. A nasal cannula can provide an oxygen concentration up to 40 percent. The fraction of inspired (inhaled) oxygen is the FiO$_2$.

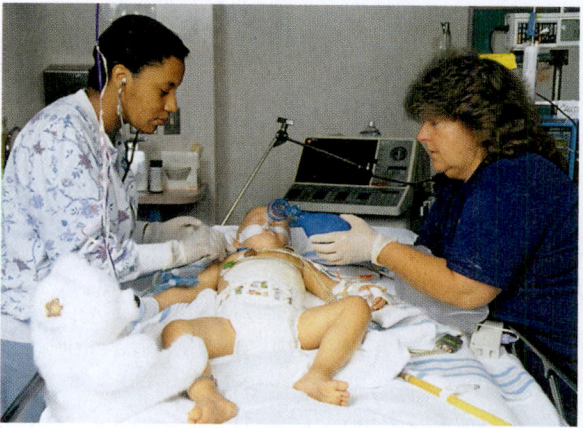

FIGURE 4-29 ■ Oxygen therapy with a respirator.
This infant in the pediatric intensive care unit has an endotracheal tube to assist with breathing. The nurse on the left is using a stethoscope to auscultate breath sounds in the infant's right lung. The nurse on the right is squeezing a blue Ambu bag to breathe for the infant until the endotracheal tube is reconnected to the respirator. The infant's pink skin color shows that the level of oxygen in the blood is adequate because of treatment with the respirator and oxygen.

Category	Indication	Pronunciation/Word Parts

Drugs

antibiotic drug	Treats respiratory infections caused by bacteria	**antibiotic** (AN-tee-by-AW-tik)
		  anti- *against*
		  bi/o- *living organism; living tissue*
		  -tic *pertaining to*

antitubercular drug	Treats tuberculosis. More than one antitubercular drug must be used in combination for 9 months to be effective.	**antitubercular**
		(AN-tee-too-BER-kyoo-lar)
		  anti- *against*
		  tubercul/o- *nodule*
		  -ar *pertaining to*

antitussive drug	Suppresses the cough center in the brain. Used to treat chronic bronchitis and nonproductive coughs. Some are narcotic drugs.	**antitussive** (AN-tee-TUH-siv)
		  anti- *against*
		  tuss/o- *cough*
		  -ive *pertaining to*

antiviral drug	Treats influenza virus infection, particularly in at-risk patients with asthma or lung disease. Also used to treat viral pneumonia.	**antiviral** (AN-tee-VY-ral)
		  anti- *against*
		  vir/o- *virus*
		  -al *pertaining to*

Clinical Connections

Public Health. Influenza vaccinations (flu shots) are given to prevent influenza. Each February, the Centers for Disease Control and Prevention (CDC) selects those strains of influenza that are most prevalent in Asia and other parts of the world to include in the flu vaccine that will be offered in the United States before the start of flu season. Flu viruses mutate constantly, so the influenza vaccine must be reformulated every year. Persons who get flu shots can still get the flu from other strains of influenza not included in the flu vaccine.

bronchodilator drug	Dilates constricted airways by relaxing the smooth muscles that surround the bronchioles. Used to treat asthma, COPD, emphysema, and cystic fibrosis. Given orally or inhaled through a **metered-dose inhaler (MDI)** (see Figure 4-30 ■). When a strong bronchodilator drug is given through an inhaler to treat the symptoms of an acute asthma attack, it is known as a *rescue inhaler*.	**bronchodilator**
		(BRONG-koh-DY-lay-tor)
		  bronch/o- *bronchus*
		  dilat/o- *dilate; widen*
		  -or *person who does or produces; thing that does or produces*

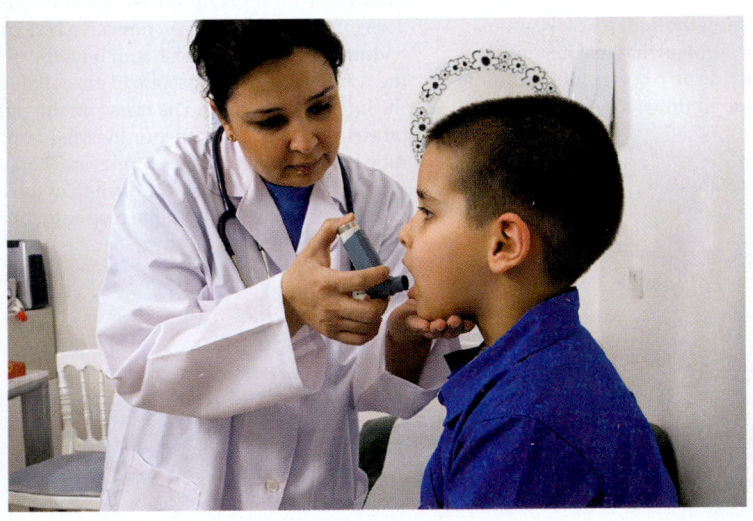

FIGURE 4-30 ■ Metered-dose inhaler.
A metered-dose inhaler (MDI) automatically delivers a premeasured dose of a bronchodilator drug or corticosteroid drug into the lungs as the patient inhales through the mouth. The dose is prescribed as the number of metered sprays or puffs. This healthcare professional is using a metered-dose inhaler device to administer a bronchodilator drug to this pediatric patient who has asthma symptoms.

Category	Indication	Pronunciation/Word Parts
corticosteroid drug	Blocks the immune system from causing inflammation in the lungs. Used to treat asthma and COPD. Given by a metered-dose inhaler, orally, or intravenously.	**corticosteroid** (KOR-tih-koh-STAIR-oyd) **cortic/o-** *cortex; outer region* **-steroid** *steroid*
expectorant drug	Reduces the thickness of sputum so that it can be coughed up. Used to treat a productive cough.	**expectorant** (eks-PEK-toh-rant) **ex-** *away from; out* **pector/o-** *chest* **-ant** *pertaining to*
leukotriene receptor blocker drug	Blocks leukotriene, which causes inflammation and edema. Used to treat asthma.	**leukotriene** (LOO-koh-TRY-een)
mast cell stabilizer drug	Stabilizes mast cells and prevents them from releasing histamine that causes bronchospasm during an allergic reaction. Used to treat asthma.	
pneumococcal vaccination	Used to prevent pneumococcal pneumonia.	
smoking cessation drug	Binds to nicotine receptors and prevents them from being activated if the patient smokes. Used to stop smoking (see Figure 4-31 ■).	

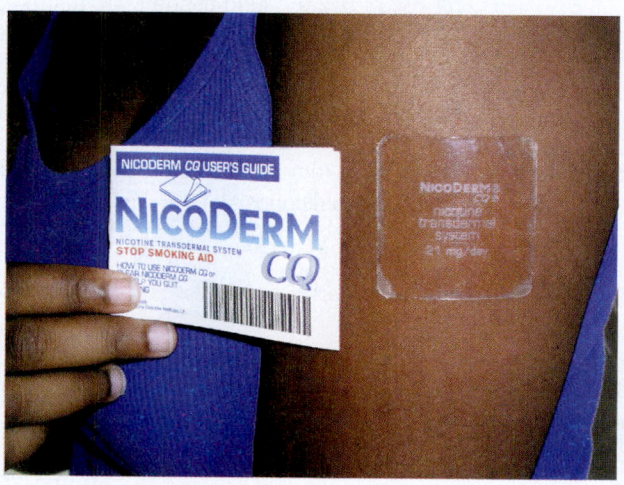

FIGURE 4-31 ■ Smoking cessation drug.
This over-the-counter drug comes as a skin patch. It supplies nicotine in a gradually decreasing dose until the patient no longer needs nicotine and can stop smoking.

Word or Phrase	Description	Pronunciation/Word Parts

Surgical Procedures

Word or Phrase	Description	Pronunciation/Word Parts
bronchoscopy	Procedure that uses a lighted **bronchoscope** inserted through the mouth and larynx to examine the trachea and bronchi. Attachments on the bronchoscope can remove foreign bodies, suction thick mucus, or perform a biopsy.	**bronchoscopy** (brong-KAW-skoh-pee) **bronch/o-** *bronchus* **-scopy** *process of using an instrument to examine* **bronchoscope** (BRONG-koh-skohp) **bronch/o-** *bronchus* **-scope** *instrument used to examine*
chest tube insertion	Procedure that inserts a plastic tube into the thoracic cavity to remove accumulated air, fluid, pus, or blood due to trauma or infection. The tube is connected to a container (to measure the drainage) and to a suction device. Used to treat a pneumothorax or a hemothorax.	

Word or Phrase	Description	Pronunciation/Word Parts
lung resection	Procedure to remove part of or the entire lung. A wedge resection removes a small wedge-shaped piece of lung tissue. A segmental resection removes a large piece or a segment of a lobe. A **lobectomy** removes an entire lobe (see Figure 4-32 ■). A **pneumonectomy** removes an entire lung. A lung resection is done as a biopsy procedure to look for cancer or to treat severe emphysema or lung cancer.	**resection** (ree-SEK-shun) **resect/o-** *cut out; remove* **-ion** *action; condition* **lobectomy** (loh-BEK-toh-mee) **lob/o-** *lobe of an organ* **-ectomy** *surgical removal* **pneumonectomy** (NOO-moh-NEK-toh-mee) **pneumon/o-** *air; lung* **-ectomy** *surgical removal*

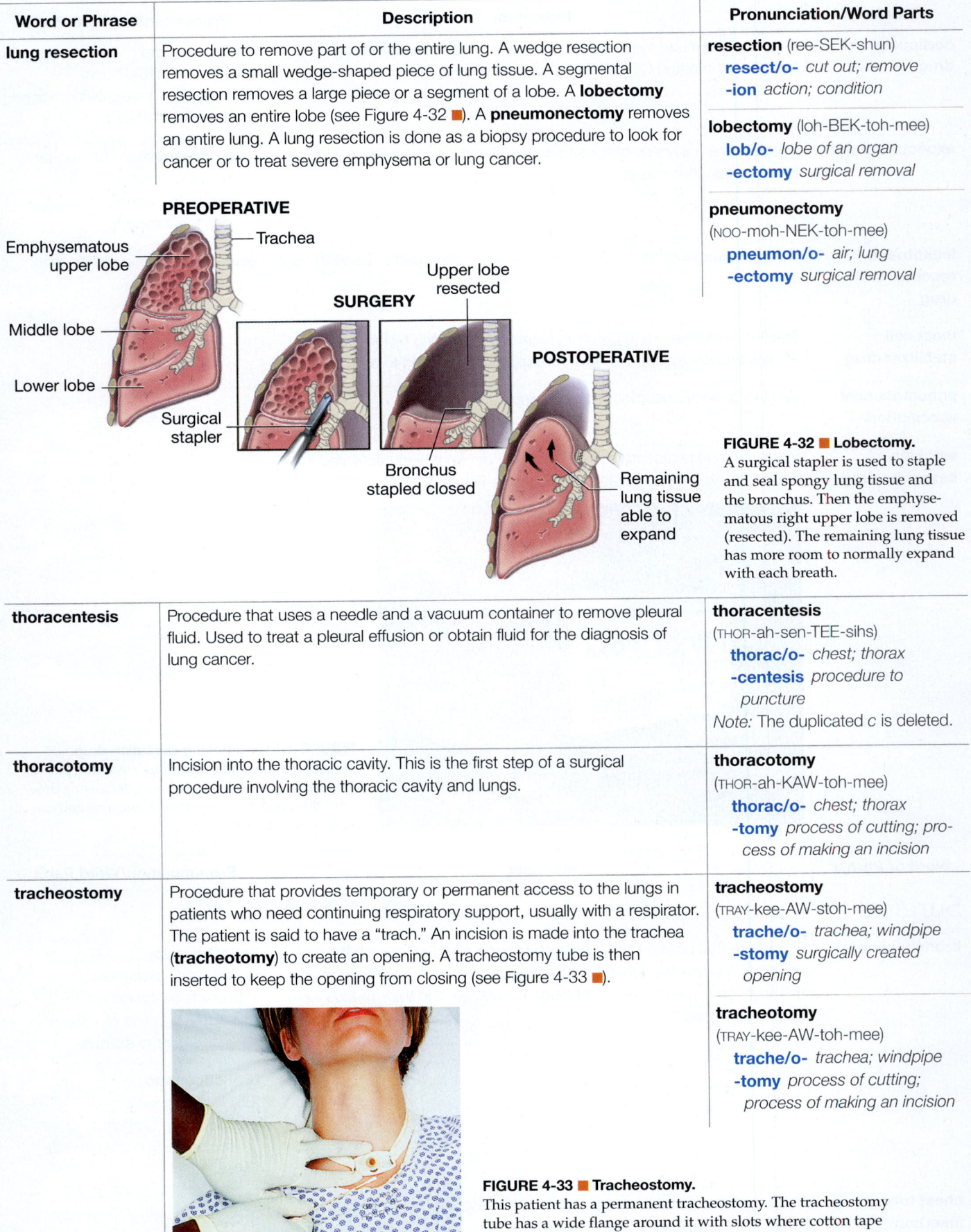

FIGURE 4-32 ■ Lobectomy.
A surgical stapler is used to staple and seal spongy lung tissue and the bronchus. Then the emphysematous right upper lobe is removed (resected). The remaining lung tissue has more room to normally expand with each breath.

Word or Phrase	Description	Pronunciation/Word Parts
thoracentesis	Procedure that uses a needle and a vacuum container to remove pleural fluid. Used to treat a pleural effusion or obtain fluid for the diagnosis of lung cancer.	**thoracentesis** (THOR-ah-sen-TEE-sihs) **thorac/o-** *chest; thorax* **-centesis** *procedure to puncture* *Note:* The duplicated *c* is deleted.
thoracotomy	Incision into the thoracic cavity. This is the first step of a surgical procedure involving the thoracic cavity and lungs.	**thoracotomy** (THOR-ah-KAW-toh-mee) **thorac/o-** *chest; thorax* **-tomy** *process of cutting; process of making an incision*
tracheostomy	Procedure that provides temporary or permanent access to the lungs in patients who need continuing respiratory support, usually with a respirator. The patient is said to have a "trach." An incision is made into the trachea (**tracheotomy**) to create an opening. A tracheostomy tube is then inserted to keep the opening from closing (see Figure 4-33 ■).	**tracheostomy** (TRAY-kee-AW-stoh-mee) **trache/o-** *trachea; windpipe* **-stomy** *surgically created opening* **tracheotomy** (TRAY-kee-AW-toh-mee) **trache/o-** *trachea; windpipe* **-tomy** *process of cutting; process of making an incision*

FIGURE 4-33 ■ Tracheostomy.
This patient has a permanent tracheostomy. The tracheostomy tube has a wide flange around it with slots where cotton tape can be inserted and tied around the patient's neck to secure the tube within the trachea. The nurse is cleansing the area to remove mucus.

4.5 PRACTICE LAPS

Use the Answer Key at the end of the book to check your answers.

A. Give the Meaning of Combining Forms

Next to each combining form, write its meaning. The first one has been done for you.

Combining Form	Meaning	Combining Form	Meaning
1. **auscult/o-**	*listening*	8. resect/o-	
2. bronch/o-		9. resuscit/o-	
3. laryng/o-		10. spir/o-	
4. lob/o-		11. steth/o-	
5. nebul/o-		12. thorac/o-	
6. percuss/o-		13. trache/o-	
7. pneumon/o-			

B. Build Words

Read the definition of the medical word. Look at the combining form that is given. Select the correct suffix from the Suffix List, and write it on the blank line. Then build the medical word, and write it on the line. (Remember: You may need to remove the combining vowel. Always remove the hyphens and slash.) Be sure to check your spelling.

Suffix List

-ation (being; having; process)
-ator (thing that does or produces)
-ectomy (surgical removal)
-meter (instrument used to measure)

-scope (instrument used to examine)
-scopy (process of using an instrument to examine)

-stomy (surgically created opening)
-tomy (process of cutting; process of making an incision)

Definition of the Medical Word	Combining Form	Suffix	Build the Medical Word
Example: Process (used to) revive	**resuscit/o-**	*-ation*	*resuscitation*

[You think process (-ation) + raise up; revive (resuscit/o-). You change the order of the word parts to put the suffix last. You write resuscitation.]

Definition of the Medical Word	Combining Form	Suffix	Build the Medical Word
1. Instrument used to examine (the) larynx	laryng/o-		
2. Process (of) listening	auscult/o-		
3. Process of making an incision (into the) chest	thorac/o-		
4. Instrument used to measure (the) breath	spir/o-		
5. Thing that produces movement of air	ventil/o-		
6. Surgical removal (of a) lobe of an organ (the lung)	lob/o-		
7. Surgically created opening (in the) trachea	trache/o-		
8. Process of using an instrument to examine (the) bronchus	bronch/o-		

C. Define Abbreviations

1. A&P _____

2. CPR _____

3. ETT _____

4. MDI _____

5. RA _____

Abbreviations Summary

A&P	auscultation and percussion		**LUL**	left upper lobe (of the lung)
ABG	arterial blood gases		**MDI**	metered-dose inhaler
AFB	acid-fast bacillus		**MDR-TB**	multidrug-resistant tuberculosis
AP	anteroposterior		**MRI**	magnetic resonance imaging
AQI	Air Quality Index		**O_2**	oxygen
ARDS	acute respiratory distress syndrome		**PA**	posteroanterior
BS	breath sounds		**PCO_2, pCO_2**	partial pressure of carbon dioxide
C&S	culture and sensitivity		**PFT**	pulmonary function test
CAT, CT	computerized axial tomography		**PND**	paroxysmal nocturnal dyspnea
CF	cystic fibrosis		**PO_2, pO_2**	partial pressure of oxygen
CO	carbon monoxide		**PPD**	packs per day (of cigarettes); purified protein derivative (TB test)
CO_2	carbon dioxide			
COPD	chronic obstructive pulmonary disease		**RA**	room air (no supplemental oxygen)
CPAP	continuous positive airway pressure (pronounced "SEE-pap")		**RLL**	right lower lobe (of the lung)
			RML	right middle lobe (of the lung)
CPR	cardiopulmonary resuscitation		**RRT**	registered respiratory therapist
CXR	chest x-ray		**RUL**	right upper lobe (of the lung)
DOE	dyspnea on exertion		**SARS**	severe acute respiratory syndrome
ETT	endotracheal tube		**SIDS**	sudden infant death syndrome
FBO	foreign body object		**SOB****	shortness of breath
FEV_1	forced expiratory volume (in 1 second)		**SpO_2**	saturated partial oxygen
FiO_2	fraction (percentage) of inspired oxygen		**TB**	tuberculosis
FVC	forced vital capacity		**URI**	upper respiratory infection
IRDS	infant respiratory distress syndrome		**V/Q**	ventilation-perfusion (scan)
LLL	left lower lobe (of the lung)			
LTBI	latent tuberculosis infection			

**This abbreviation is still in use, but many hospitals have removed it from their official list of abbreviations because it also has an undesirable meaning that is unrelated to the respiratory system.

Word Alert

Abbreviations. Abbreviations are commonly used in all types of medical documents; however, they can mean different things to different people and their meanings can be misinterpreted. Always verify the meaning of an abbreviation.

- *A&P* means *auscultation and percussion*, but it also means *anatomy and physiology*.
- *BS* means *breath sounds*, but it also means *bowel sounds*.
- *C&S* means *culture and sensitivity*, but it can be confused with the sound-alike abbreviation *CNS* (central nervous system).
- *PND* means *paroxysmal nocturnal dyspnea*, but it also means *postnasal drip*.
- *RA* means *room air*, but it also means *rheumatoid arthritis* or *right atrium*.

It's Greek to Me! Did you notice that some words have two different combining forms? Combining forms from both Greek and Latin remain a part of medical language today.

Word	Greek	Latin	Medical Word Examples
breathe	spir/o-	hal/o-	respiration, inspiration; inhalation, exhalation
chest	thorac/o- pector/o-	steth/o-	thoracic, expectorant; stethoscope
lung	pneum/o- pneumon/o-	pulmon/o-	pneumothorax, pneumonia; pulmonary
pus	py/o-	purul/o-	empyema, pyothorax; purulent

Career Focus

Meet Susan, a respiratory therapist in a hospital

"I love my job. I've been doing it for 36 years. I probably could retire, but I choose not to. We treat neonates to geriatric patients. We treat asthma, COPD, and pulmonary fibrosis patients and give information to the patients' families. We also manage oxygen therapy, nebulizer therapy, and medication therapy. We do pulmonary function technology and blood gases. I feel that being a respiratory therapist allows me to feel respected and appreciated, not only by the medical staff, but by the patients because you are giving patient care. You are dealing with the patient directly, as well as the physician. You feel good at the end of the day when you leave."

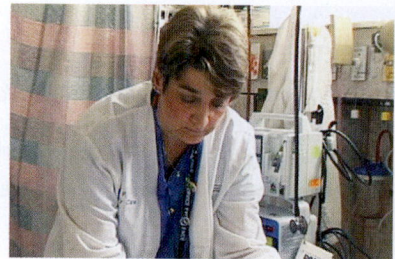

- **Respiratory therapists** are allied health professionals who perform pulmonary function tests and administer respiratory therapy with various types of equipment that provide oxygen or respiratory assistance to a patient.

- **Pulmonologists** are physicians who practice in the medical specialty of pulmonology. They diagnose and treat patients with respiratory problems. Physicians can take additional training and become board certified in the subspecialty of pediatric pulmonology.

- **Thoracic** (or cardiothoracic) **surgeons** perform pulmonary surgery, including surgery for cancer.

- **Oncologists** treat cancer of the lungs with drugs.

therapist (THAIR-ah-pist)
  therap/o- *treatment*
  -ist *person who specializes in*

pulmonologist (PUL-moh-NAW-loh-jist)
  pulmon/o- *lung*
  log/o- *study of; word*
  -ist *person who specializes in*

oncologist (ong-KAW-loh-jist)
  onc/o- *mass; tumor*
  log/o- *study of; word*
  -ist *person who specializes in*

Chapter Review Exercises

Dive In: Medical Language Exercises

Test your knowledge of the chapter by completing these review exercises. Use the Answer Key at the end of the book to check your answers. Note: Each of the numbered exercise headers corresponds to a numbered learning outcome at the beginning of the chapter.

4.1 Anatomy

MATCHING EXERCISE

Match each word or phrase to its description.

1. apex	_____ small passageway that ends in several alveoli
2. turbinates	_____ impulse from this structure causes the diaphragm to contract
3. cilia	_____ projections of bone in the nasal cavity that slow down inhaled air
4. trachea	_____ small hairs in the mucosa that move in waves
5. bronchus	_____ connecting passageway between the trachea and the bronchioles
6. bronchiole	_____ air sacs that are the functional units of the lung
7. alveoli	_____ membranes around the lung and lining the thoracic cavity
8. pleurae	_____ muscular structure that moves on inhalation
9. diaphragm	_____ topmost part of a lung
10. thorax	_____ bony cage surrounding the lungs
11. phrenic nerve	_____ connecting passageway between the larynx and the bronchi

CIRCLE EXERCISE

Circle the correct answer from the choices given.

1. A large division of a lung that is visible on its surface is known as the (**alveolus, apex, lobe**).
2. The (**bronchioles, lungs, pleurae**) have smooth muscle around them that can contract.
3. The bronchus, pulmonary arteries, and pulmonary veins enter and exit the lung at the (**alveolus, hilum, pleural cavity**).
4. The functional part of the lung that is made up of the alveoli is known collectively as the (**bronchioles, mediastinum, parenchyma**).
5. The (**epiglottis, pharynx, turbinates**) prevent(s) swallowed food from entering the trachea and lungs.

TRUE OR FALSE EXERCISE

*Indicate whether each statement is true or false by writing **T** or **F** on the line.*

1. _____ The upper respiratory system includes the nose, throat, and lungs.
2. _____ The pharynx is an air passageway that connects the nasal cavity to the bronchi.
3. _____ The alveoli are divided into lobes.
4. _____ The visceral pleura is a membrane on the surface of the lung.

PLURAL NOUN AND ADJECTIVE EXERCISE

Read the noun and write its plural form and/or adjective form on the line. Only write in the plural noun form if there is a blank line there for it. Be sure to check your spelling. The first one has been done for you.

Singular Noun	Plural Noun	Adjective	Singular Noun	Plural Noun	Adjective
1. **nose**		_nasal_	8. lung	_____	_____
2. alveolus	_____	_____	9. pharynx		_____
3. bronchus	_____	_____	10. pleura	_____	_____
4. diaphragm		_____	11. septum		_____
5. hilum		_____	12. thorax		_____
6. larynx		_____	13. trachea		_____
7. lobe	_____	_____			

DIVIDING WORDS EXERCISE

Separate these words into their component parts (prefix, combining form, suffix). Some words do not contain all three word parts. The first one has been done for you.

Medical Word	Prefix	Combining Form	Suffix	Medical Word	Prefix	Combining Form	Suffix
1. **thoracic**		_thorac/o-_	_-ic_	5. pulmonary		_____	_____
2. diaphragmatic		_____	_____	6. septal		_____	_____
3. epiglottis	_____	_____	_____	7. respiratory	_____	_____	_____
4. nasopharynx		_____	_____	8. turbinate		_____	_____

SPELLING EXERCISE

Read each medical word pronunciation and write the medical word that it represents. Be sure to check your spelling. The first one has been done for you.

1. **(TRAY-kee-al)** _tracheal_
2. (lah-RING-goh-FAIR-ingks) _____
3. (BRONG-kee-OH-lar) _____
4. (al-VEE-oh-lie) _____
5. (pah-RY-eh-tal) _____

4.2 Physiology

CIRCLE EXERCISE

Circle the correct answer from the choices given.

1. (**Carbon dioxide, Oxygen, Surfactant**) keeps the alveoli from collapsing with each breath.
2. The (**diaphragm, phrenic nerve, thorax**) carries an impulse from the respiratory control centers of the brain to initiate inspiration.
3. (**Carbon dioxide, Inhalation, Oxygen**) is a gaseous waste product of cellular metabolism.

TRUE OR FALSE EXERCISE

Indicate whether each statement is true or false by writing **T** or **F** on the line.

1. _____ Inhalation is another word for inspiration.
2. _____ Oxygen is carried in the blood in the form of oxyhemoglobin in a red blood cell.
3. _____ A normal depth and rate of respiration is known as eupnea.
4. _____ Oxygenated blood contains a low level of oxygen.

DIVIDING WORDS EXERCISE

Separate these words into their component parts (prefix, combining form, suffix). Some words do not contain all three word parts. The first one has been done for you.

Medical Word	Prefix	Combining Form	Suffix
1. **respiration**	re-	spir/o-	-ation
2. inhalation	___	_____	_____
3. phrenic		_____	_____
4. intercostal	___	_____	_____
5. metabolism		_____	_____
6. inspiration	___	_____	_____

SPELLING EXERCISE

Read each medical word pronunciation and write the medical word that it represents. Be sure to check your spelling. The first one has been done for you.

1. **(SEL-yoo-lar)**   *cellular*
2. (FREN-ik)   _____
3. (IN-ter-KAW-stal)   _____
4. (AWK-see-HEE-moh-GLOH-bin)   _____
5. (EKS-hah-LAY-shun)   _____

4.3 Diseases

MATCHING EXERCISE

Match each word or phrase to its description.

1. apnea   _____ caused by trauma; treated with a chest tube
2. asthma   _____ blockage of a pulmonary artery by a blood clot or fat globule
3. hemothorax   _____ creates a pleural friction rub
4. pleurisy   _____ premature babies often have this lapse in breathing
5. pneumoconiosis   _____ caused by allergies, exercise, cold air, or stress
6. pulmonary embolus   _____ sternal is a type
7. retraction   _____ caused by taking aspirin during a viral illness
8. Reye syndrome   _____ occupational lung disease

TRUE OR FALSE EXERCISE

*Indicate whether each statement is true or false by writing **T** or **F** on the line.*

1. _____ Bronchospasm occurs during an asthma attack.
2. _____ Patients who have orthopnea use pillows to prop themselves up to sleep.
3. _____ Hemoptysis means *blood in the thoracic cavity*.
4. _____ Asthma is also known as *reactive airway disease*.
5. _____ The two components of COPD are chronic bronchitis and emphysema.
6. _____ Lobar pneumonia is caused by aspirating food while eating.
7. _____ Tuberculosis is spread by airborne droplets from an infected person coughing.
8. _____ Purulent sputum contains pus.
9. _____ Double pneumonia is twice as serious as regular pneumonia.

ADJECTIVE EXERCISE

Read the noun and write its adjective form on the line. Be sure to check your spelling. The first one has been done for you. Item 3 has two adjectives.

Singular Noun	Adjective	Singular Noun	Adjective
1. **apnea**	*apneic*	4. cyanosis	_____
2. asthma	_____	5. dyspnea	_____
3. cancer	_____	6. tachypnea	_____
	_____		

DIVIDING WORDS EXERCISE

Separate these words into their component parts (prefix, combining form, suffix). Some words do not contain all three word parts. The first one has been done for you.

Medical Word	Prefix	Combining Form	Suffix	Medical Word	Prefix	Combining Form	Suffix
1. **anoxia**	*an-*	*ox/o-*	*-ia*	8. hemothorax		_____	_____
2. apneic	_____	_____	_____	9. hypercapnia	_____	_____	_____
3. asthmatic	_____	_____		10. panlobar	_____	_____	_____
4. bronchiectasis		_____	_____	11. pleurisy		_____	_____
5. circumoral	_____	_____	_____	12. pneumonia		_____	_____
6. dyspneic	_____	_____	_____	13. pneumothorax		_____	_____
7. emphysema	_____	_____					

SPELLING EXERCISE

Read each medical word pronunciation and write the medical word that it represents. Be sure to check your spelling. The first one has been done for you.

1. (in-FEK-shun) — *infection*
2. (SPYOO-tum) — _____
3. (az-MAT-ik) — _____
4. (SIS-tik fy-BROH-sihs) — _____
5. (AT-eh-LEK-tah-sihs) — _____
6. (PYOOR-yoo-lent) — _____
7. (IN-floo-EN-zah) — _____
8. (AD-eh-noh-KAR-sih-NOH-mah) — _____
9. (BRONG-koh-noo-MOHN-yah) — _____
10. (hee-MAWP-tih-sihs) — _____
11. (or-THAWP-nee-ah) — _____
12. (as-FIK-see-ah) — _____
13. (SY-ah-NAW-tik) — _____

4.4 Laboratory, Diagnostic, and Radiologic Procedures

MATCHING EXERCISE

Match each word or phrase to its description.

1. ABG
2. carboxyhemoglobin
3. culture and sensitivity
4. MRI
5. pulmonary function test
6. pulse oximeter
7. radiography
8. sleep study
9. tuberculosis tests
10. ventilation/perfusion scan

_____ taking a chest x-ray
_____ carries carbon monoxide in the blood
_____ also known as *polysomnography*
_____ clips on the index finger or earlobe
_____ tine and mantoux
_____ nuclear medicine procedure with inhaled radioactive gas
_____ uses a sputum sample to diagnose a bacterial infection and tell which antibiotic drug to use
_____ measures the FVC and FEV_1
_____ measures the PO_2, PCO_2, and pH
_____ uses magnets to create an image

TRUE OR FALSE EXERCISE

*Indicate whether each statement is true or false by writing **T** or **F** on the line.*

1. _____ A CT scan uses x-rays to create narrow slices of tissue images.

2. _____ The suffix -*metry* means *instrument used to measure.*

3. _____ The patient wears a clip over the nose during a pulmonary function test.

4. _____ A zone of no growth around a drug disk in a C&S means that drug can be prescribed to treat the infection.

DIVIDING WORDS EXERCISE

Separate these words into their component parts (prefix, combining form, suffix). Some words do not contain all three word parts. The first one has been done for you.

Medical Word	Prefix	Combining Form	Suffix
1. **arterial**		*arteri/o-*	*-al*
2. oximeter		_____	_____
3. polysomnography	_____	_____	_____
4. radiography		_____	_____
5. tomography		_____	_____

SPELLING EXERCISE

Read each medical word pronunciation and write the medical word that it represents. Be sure to check your spelling. The first one has been done for you.

1. **(ar-TEER-ee-al)**   *arterial*

2. (kar-BAWK-see-HEE-moh-GLOH-bin)   _____

3. (PAW-lee-sawm-NAW-grah-fee)   _____

4. (awk-SIM-eh-ter)   _____

5. (RAY-dee-AW-grah-fee)   _____

4.5 Medical Procedures, Drugs, and Surgical Procedures

MATCHING EXERCISE

Match each word or phrase to its description.

1. bronchodilator drugs   _____ used to treat a pneumothorax

2. bronchoscopy   _____ incision in the chest

3. chest tube   _____ used to treat asthma, copd, and cystic fibrosis

4. intubation   _____ encourages patients to breathe deeply

5. resuscitation   _____ emergency procedure to ventilate the lungs and circulate the blood

6. spirometer   _____ uses an endotracheal tube

7. thoracotomy   _____ uses a scope to look inside the bronchi

CIRCLE EXERCISE

Circle the correct answer from the choices given.

1. A pneumonectomy involves surgical removal of the (**alveoli, lung, trachea**).

2. Oxygen therapy is administered by using a/an (**ABG, Heimlich maneuver, nasal cannula**).

3. Expectorant drugs are used to treat (**apnea, productive coughs, pneumothorax**).

4. A/An (**endotracheal tube, chest tube, spirometer**) is inserted between the ribs.

TRUE OR FALSE EXERCISE

*Indicate whether each statement is true or false by writing **T** or **F** on the line.*

1. _____ A lobectomy involves removing the entire lung.

2. _____ A ventilator is another name for a respirator.

3. _____ Auscultation uses a stethoscope.

4. _____ A nasal cannula can deliver up to 100 percent oxygen.

5. _____ An MDI is used to deliver a bronchodilator or corticosteroid drug.

6. _____ The suffix *-ectomy* means *process of making an incision*.

DIVIDING WORDS EXERCISE

Separate these words into their component parts (prefix, combining form, suffix). Some words do not contain all three word parts. The first one has been done for you.

Medical Word	Prefix	Combining Form	Suffix
1. **antibiotic**	*anti-*	*bi/o-*	*-tic*
2. antitussive	_____	_____	_____
3. endotracheal	_____	_____	_____
4. expectorant	_____	_____	_____
5. intubation	_____	_____	_____
6. pneumonectomy		_____	_____
7. respirator	_____	_____	_____
8. resuscitation		_____	_____
9. spirometry		_____	_____

SPELLING EXERCISE

Read each medical word pronunciation and write the medical word that it represents. Be sure to check your spelling. The first one has been done for you.

1. **(KAN-yoo-lah)** _____cannula_____

2. (EN-doh-TRAY-kee-al) _____

3. (AWS-kul-TAY-shun) _____

4. (KAR-dee-oh-PUL-moh-NAIR-ee) _____

5. (lah-RING-goh-skohp) _____

6. (spih-RAW-meh-tree) _____

7. (brong-KAW-skoh-pee) _____

8. (THOR-ah-sen-TEE-sihs) _____

9. (TRAY-kee-AW-stoh-mee) _____

10. (eks-PEK-toh-rant) _____

Immerse Yourself: Analyze Medical Reports

Electronic Patient Record #1

This is an Office Visit in the SOAP note format. Read the note and answer the questions.

PEARSON PRIMARY CARE ASSOCIATES

Task   Edit   View   Time Scale   Options   Help

OFFICE VISIT SOAP NOTE

PATIENT NAME: GUPTA, Priya

MEDICAL RECORD NUMBER: 964-43651

DATE OF VISIT: 11/19/xx

SUBJECTIVE: This 45-year-old female has been followed in our office for reactive airway disease. She comes in today with shortness of breath and audible wheezing. This morning it was cold outside; she was in the city and was around someone who was smoking. She did not have her rescue inhaler with her.

OBJECTIVE: Temperature 98.2, heart rate 100, respiratory rate 30, blood pressure 130/80. Oximeter shows a reading of 85 percent. She appears anxious. Auscultation is positive for wheezing.

ASSESSMENT: Asthma attack.

PLAN: A bronchodilator drug was administered via a MDI and the symptoms subsided.

---

1. What type of reactive airway disease did this patient have? _____

2. Why is it important to note the outside temperature, location, and what others were doing around the
   patient? _____

3. What instrument is needed to do auscultation? _____

4. Which result in the Objective section tells you that the patient was tachypneic? _____

5. Divide these words into their word parts and give the meaning of each word part.

   a. Oximeter

Word Part	Meaning
_____	_____
_____	_____

   b. Auscultation

Word Part	Meaning
_____	_____
_____	_____

6. What is a rescue inhaler and what is it used for? _____

7. What does the abbreviation *MDI* stand for? _____

Electronic Patient Record #2

This is a hospital Admission History and Physical Examination report. Read the report and answer the questions.

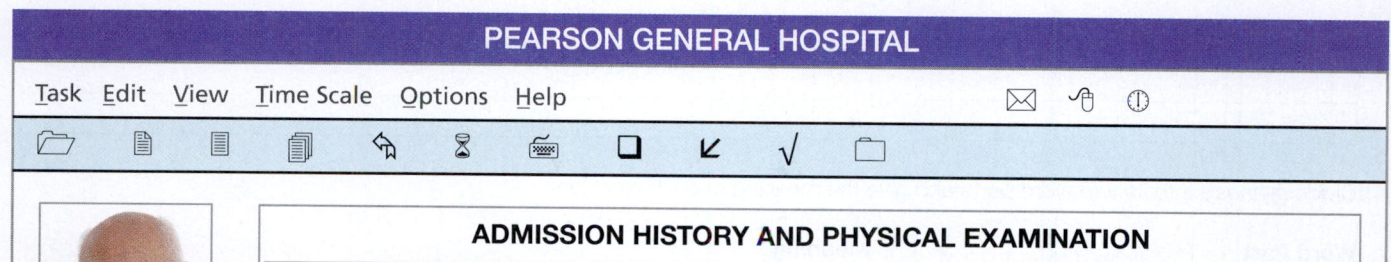

PEARSON GENERAL HOSPITAL

Task   Edit   View   Time Scale   Options   Help

ADMISSION HISTORY AND PHYSICAL EXAMINATION

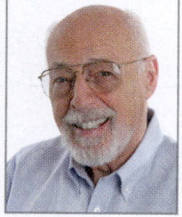

PATIENT NAME: OTT, George

HOSPITAL NUMBER: 208-333-7943

DATE OF ADMISSION: November 19, 20xx

HISTORY OF PRESENT ILLNESS
This 65-year-old male was evaluated by me in the emergency department on the above date, complaining of progressive shortness of breath, coughing, fever, and fatigue.

PAST HISTORY
The patient was a coal miner for 25 years before he retired on disability with black lung disease at age 55. He currently smokes two packs of cigarettes per day and has done so for the past 22 years. Surgical history of an appendectomy in the remote past. Chest x-ray done recently showed a suspicious lesion in the LLL; a bronchoscopy was performed and a biopsy was done, but the biopsy results were negative for malignancy.

PHYSICAL EXAMINATION
VITAL SIGNS: Pulse 110, respiratory rate 42 per minute, temperature 100.6, blood pressure 156/96.
GENERAL: The patient appears older than his stated age and quite tired at this time.
HEENT: Negative, except for slight cyanosis of the lips. The neck is supple and free of any masses.
CHEST: There is an increased anteroposterior diameter to the chest. There are no retractions during inspiration. There are diffuse expiratory wheezes, but no rales or rhonchi.
HEART: Normal heart sounds without murmur, gallop, or rub.
ABDOMEN: Soft and nontender.
EXTREMITIES: Normal with full range of motion noted. There was no clubbing of the fingers noted.

LABORATORY DATA
Complete blood count showed an elevated white blood cell count of 17,600 with 80 segs, 4 bands, and 2 lymphs. Oximeter showed 70 percent saturation. Sputum was sent for C&S. Chest x-ray: Patchy infiltrates from the apex to the midlung on the right with some consolidative changes involving the entire right lower lobe. There is no pleural fluid noted. There is a density seen in the left lower lobe posterolaterally. It is most probably focal scarring or atelectasis from old inflammation.

IMPRESSION
1. Right-sided pneumonia.

2. Chronic obstructive pulmonary disease, secondary to anthracosis and smoking.

Linda C. Warren, M.D.

Linda C. Warren, M.D.

LCW: lcc
D: 11/19/xx
T: 11/19/xx

1. This patient has dyspnea. What phrase in the History of Present Illness says the same thing? _____

2. If you wanted to use the adjective form of *dyspnea*, you would say, "The patient is _____."

3. Divide *bronchoscopy* into its two word parts and give the meaning of each word part.

Word Part	Meaning
_____	_____
_____	_____

4. Divide *cyanosis* into its two word parts and give the meaning of each word part.

Word Part	Meaning
_____	_____
_____	_____

5. What do these abbreviations stand for?

   a. C&S _____

   b. COPD _____

   c. LLL _____

6. What is the medical word for *black lung disease*?

   _____

7. What surgery did the patient have in the remote past?

   _____

8. What two respiratory surgical procedures has the patient had recently?

   _____

9. Circle all of the abnormalities that were seen on the patient's two CXRs.

intercostal muscles	**consolidative changes**	**density in LLL**	**patchy infiltrates**
atelectasis	**cyanosis**	**oximeter**	**pleural fluid**

10. Of the four medical complaints the patient had when he came to the emergency department, which one was directly related to an infection? _____ What infection did the patient have? _____

11. What is the descriptive name that laypersons give for the medical condition of increased anteroposterior diameter of the chest that is seen in patients with chronic obstructive pulmonary disease?

    _____

12. What method of examination would the physician use to hear the patient's expiratory wheezes? (Circle one)

auscultation	**percussion**	**postural drainage**	**oximeter**

13. The patient has an elevated white blood cell count of 17,600, which indicates an infection. This is due to which of the two diagnoses listed in the Impression section? _____

14. Calculate the number of pack-years for this patient's history of smoking.

RELATED COMBINING FORMS EXERCISE

Write the combining form on the line provided. (Hint: See the It's Greek to Me! feature box.)

1. Two combining forms that mean *breathe*. _____ _____

2. Three combining forms that mean *chest*. _____ _____ _____

3. Three combining forms that mean *lung*. _____ _____ _____

You Create the Electronic Health Record

Read the patient's words. Then read the partial sentence in the electronic health record and fill in the blank with the correct medical word.

1. Patient's words: "I have been out of the country, and I think I might have been exposed to tuberculosis."

   You type: "Auscultation using a _____ revealed no abnormal breath sounds. We will perform a M_____ test to check for antibodies from a possible prior exposure to TB."

2. Patient's words: "I just had to come in to see you. I have shortness of breath during the daytime, and I have to sit up on two pillows to sleep."

   You type: "The patient is complaining of _____ during the day and _____ when he tries to sleep. We will order a _____ _____ _____ to measure the capacity of his lungs."

3. Patient's words: "I am here to have a lobe of my lung removed because of lung cancer."

   You type: "The patient was received into the preoperative area and prepared for surgery. A pulse _____ placed on his index finger showed a low level of oxygen saturation. He was given 35 percent oxygen via nasal _____. The patient was taken into surgery and a _____ was performed to remove the lung cancer."

MyLab Medical Terminology™

MyLab Medical Terminology is a premium online homework management system that includes a host of features to help you study. Registered users will find:

- A multitude of quizzes and activities built within the MyLab platform
- Powerful tools that track and analyze your results—allowing you to create a personalized learning experience
- Videos and audio pronunciations to help enrich your progress
- Streaming lesson presentations (guided lectures) and self-paced learning modules
- A space where you and your instructor can check your progress and manage your assignments

5 Cardiology
Cardiovascular System

Cardiology (KAR-dee-AW-loh-jee) is the medical specialty that studies the anatomy and physiology of the cardiovascular system; uses laboratory, diagnostic, and radiologic procedures to diagnose cardiovascular diseases; and uses medical procedures, drugs, and surgical procedures to treat cardiovascular diseases.

∨ Chapter Overview and Learning Outcomes

After you study this chapter, you should be able to demonstrate mastery of the outcomes by successfully completing the exercises.

5.1 Anatomy
Identify the structures of the cardiovascular system.
Demonstrate proficiency in medical language.
5.1 Practice Laps

5.2 Physiology
Describe the functions of the cardiovascular system.
Demonstrate proficiency in medical language.
5.2 Practice Laps
Vocabulary Review

5.3 Diseases
Describe common cardiovascular diseases.
Demonstrate proficiency in medical language.
5.3 Practice Laps

5.4 Laboratory, Diagnostic, and Radiologic Procedures
Describe common cardiovascular laboratory tests, diagnostic procedures, and radiologic procedures.
Demonstrate proficiency in medical language.
5.4 Practice Laps

5.5 Medical Procedures, Drugs, and Surgical Procedures
Describe common cardiovascular medical procedures, drugs, and surgical procedures.
Demonstrate proficiency in medical language.
5.5 Practice Laps
Abbreviations Summary
Career Focus

Chapter Review Exercises
Dive In: Medical Language Exercises (Learning Outcomes 5.1–5.5)

Immerse Yourself: Analyze Medical Reports

Medical Language Key

To unlock the definition of a medical word, first break it into word parts. Then give the meaning of each word part. Put the meanings of the word parts in order, beginning with the meaning of the suffix, then the meaning of the prefix (if there is one), then the meaning of the combining form.

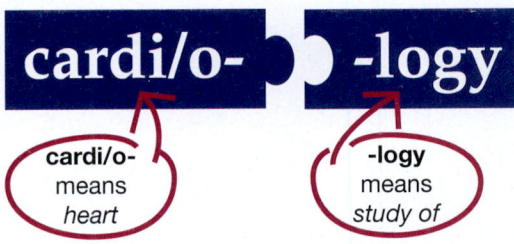

cardi/o- means heart

-logy means study of

Cardiology: ▶ *Study of (the) heart (and related structures).*

The **cardiovascular system** is a continuous, circular pathway that includes the heart and the blood vessels, such as arteries, capillaries, and veins (see Figure 5-1 ■). The study of the cardiovascular system can begin with the heart or with the capillaries, the tiniest blood vessels in the farthest parts of the body. Either starting point takes you through every part of the cardiovascular system and brings you back to where you began.

The function of the cardiovascular system is to transport the blood—and oxygen, carbon dioxide, nutrients, and wastes that are in the blood—to every part of the body. It is also known as the **circulatory system** because it circulates the blood. The blood is described in Chapter 6, Hematology and Immunology.

5.1 Anatomy

Heart

The **heart** is perhaps the best-known organ in the body and certainly one of the most important. The heart is about the size of a person's fist and is located within the thoracic cavity, behind the sternum (breastbone) and between the lungs. The heart has an irregularly shaped external surface with elevated mounds that contrast with grooves that are filled with fat, blood vessels, and nerves. Large blood vessels enter and exit the heart at various points. The inferior tip of the heart is the **apex** (see Figure 5-2 ■).

A double-layered membrane known as the **pericardium** forms a U-shaped **pericardial sac**, and the heart is within that U (see Figure 5-3 ■ and Table 5-1 ■). The membrane next to the surface of the heart is the **epicardium**. The outer membrane is the **parietal pericardium**. In between the two layers is **pericardial fluid**, a slippery, watery fluid that allows the membranes to slide past each other as the heart contracts and relaxes.

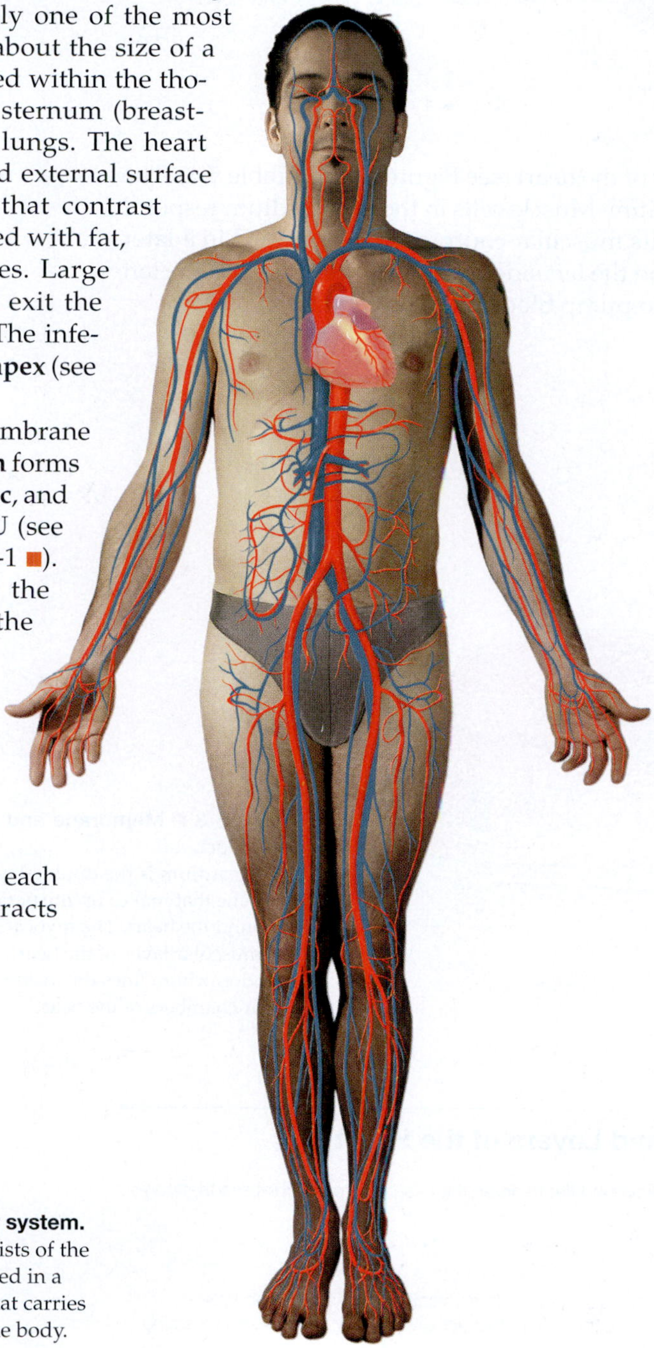

FIGURE 5-1 ■ Cardiovascular system.
The cardiovascular system consists of the heart and blood vessels connected in a continuous, circular pathway that carries blood to and from all parts of the body.

Pronunciation/Word Parts

cardiovascular (KAR-dee-oh-VAS-kyoo-lar)
  cardi/o- *heart*
  vascul/o- *blood vessel*
  -ar *pertaining to*

circulatory (SIR-kyoo-lah-TOR-ee)
  circulat/o- *moving in a circular route*
  -ory *having the function of*

heart (HART)

cardiac (KAR-dee-ak)
  cardi/o- *heart*
  -ac *pertaining to*
Cardiac is the adjective for *heart*. The Latin word *cor*, which means *heart*, is sometimes used in medical reports. The combining form **card/o-** also means *heart*.

apex (AA-peks)

apical (AP-ih-kal)
  apic/o- *apex; tip*
  -al *pertaining to*

pericardium (PAIR-ih-KAR-dee-um)
  peri- *around*
  cardi/o- *heart*
  -um *period of time; structure*

pericardial (PAIR-ih-KAR-dee-al)
  peri- *around*
  cardi/o- *heart*
  -al *pertaining to*

epicardium (EP-ih-KAR-dee-um)
  epi- *above; upon*
  cardi/o- *heart*
  -um *period of time; structure*

parietal (pah-RY-eh-tal)
  pariet/o- *wall of a cavity*
  -al *pertaining to*

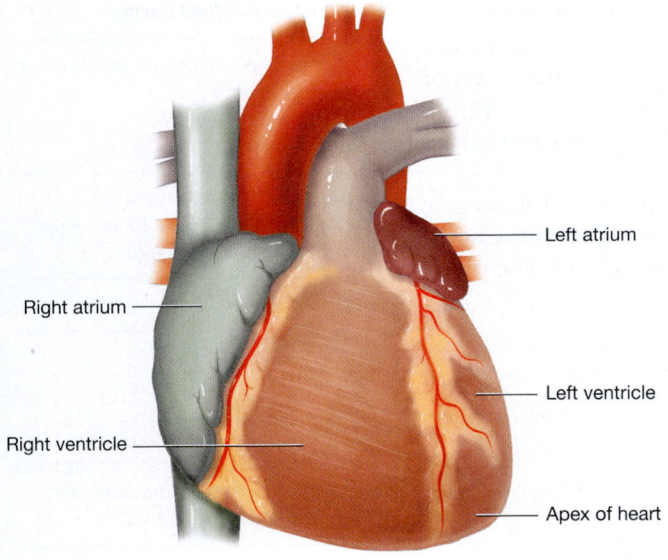

Pronunciation/Word Parts

myocardium (MY-oh-KAR-dee-um)
  my/o- *muscle*
  cardi/o- *heart*
  -um *period of time; structure*

myocardial (MY-oh-KAR-dee-al)
  my/o- *muscle*
  cardi/o- *heart*
  -al *pertaining to*

Right atrium

Right ventricle

Left atrium

Left ventricle

Apex of heart

FIGURE 5-2 ■ Surface of the heart.
The boundaries of the internal chambers of the heart are reflected on the surface of the heart as elevated mounds and grooves that are filled with fat, blood vessels, and nerves.

Heart Muscle

The **myocardium** is the muscular layer of the heart (see Figure 5-3 and Table 5-1). The myocardium lies beneath the pericardium. Muscle cells in the myocardium respond to electrical impulses that coordinate its muscular contractions (described in a later section). The myocardium is thickest on the left side of the heart because it is the left ventricle that must work the hardest to pump blood to the entire body.

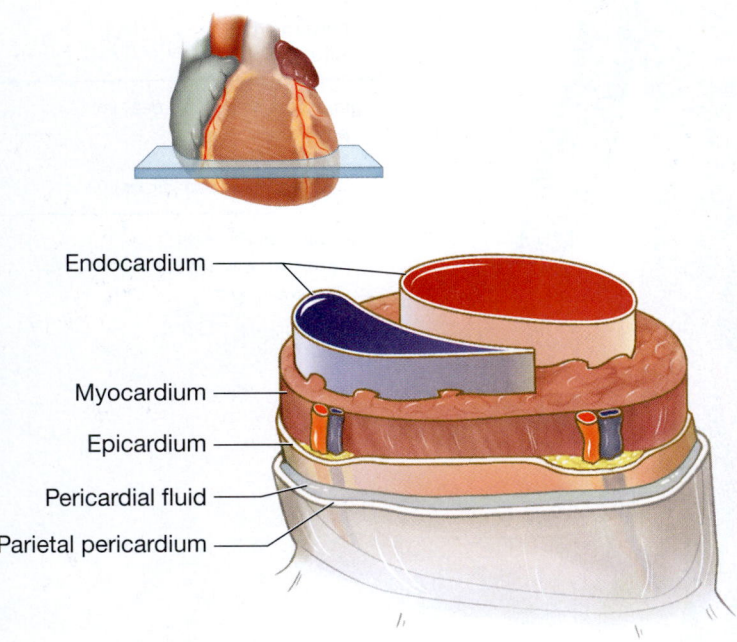

Endocardium

Myocardium

Epicardium

Pericardial fluid

Parietal pericardium

FIGURE 5-3 ■ Membrane and layers of the heart.
The pericardium is the double-layered membrane that makes up the pericardial sac around the heart. The myocardium is the muscular layer of the heart. The endocardium lines the inside of the four chambers of the heart.

Table 5-1 Membrane Around and Layers of the Heart

pericardium	Double-layered membrane around the heart as the U-shaped pericardial sac that contains pericardial fluid
myocardium	Muscular layer of the heart
endocardium	Layer of cells that lines the heart chambers (atria, ventricles) and the heart valves (*Note:* The endocardium also extends into the blood vessels where it is known as the *endothelium* or *intima.*)

Heart Chambers

The heart contains four chambers, two upper chambers and two lower chambers (see Figure 5-4 ■ and also Figure 5-2). Each small upper chamber is an **atrium**—the right atrium (RA) and the left atrium (LA). Each large lower chamber is a **ventricle**—the right ventricle (RV) and the left ventricle (LV). Each chamber is filled with blood and is surrounded by the myocardium that contracts to pump blood through the chamber. Each chamber is lined with **endocardium**. The **septum** is a central wall that divides the heart into right and left sides.

Pronunciation/Word Parts

atrium (AA-tree-um)

atria (AA-tree-ah)
Latin plural noun: Change the singular ending -um to -a.

atrial (AA-tree-al)
  atri/o- atrium; chamber that is open at the top
  -al pertaining to

ventricle (VEN-trih-kul)

ventricular (ven-TRIH-kyoo-lar)
  ventricul/o- chamber that is filled; ventricle
  -ar pertaining to

endocardium (EN-doh-KAR-dee-um)
  end/o- innermost; within
  cardi/o- heart
  -um period of time; structure

septum (SEP-tum)

septal (SEP-tal)
  sept/o- dividing wal; septum
  -al pertaining to

valve (VALV)

valvular (VAL-vyoo-lar)
  valvul/o- valve
  -ar pertaining to
The combining form **valv/o-** also means valve.

tricuspid (try-KUS-pid)
  tri- three
  cusp/o- point; projection
  -id origin; resembling; source

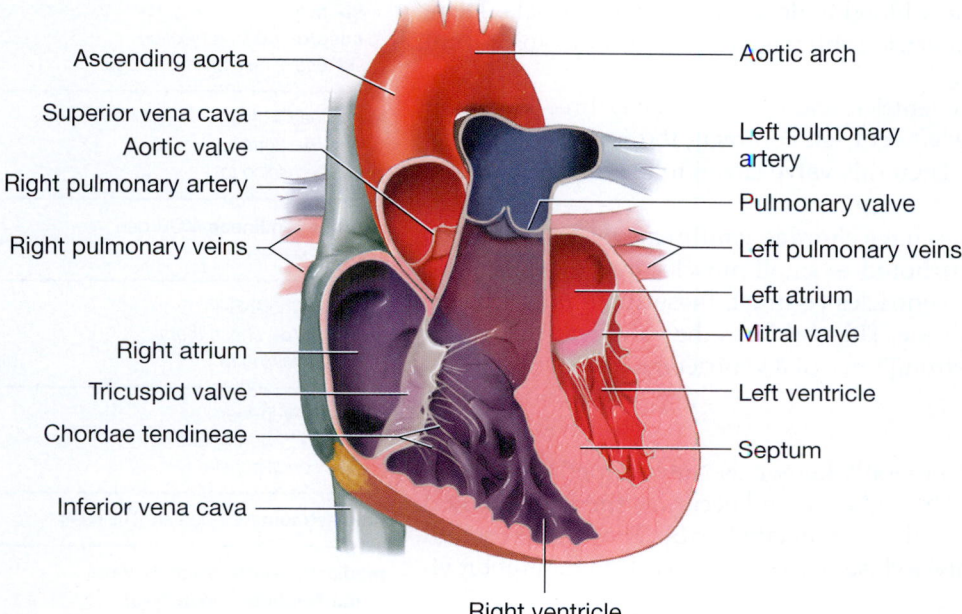

FIGURE 5-4 ■ Chambers and valves of the heart.
The heart has four chambers: right atrium, right ventricle, left atrium, and left ventricle. The heart has four valves: tricuspid valve, pulmonary valve, mitral valve, and aortic valve.

Heart Valves

There are four **valves** that control the flow of blood through the heart: the tricuspid valve, pulmonary valve, mitral valve, and aortic valve (see Figure 5-4).

The **tricuspid valve** is between the right atrium and right ventricle. It has three triangular cusps (leaflets) (see Figure 5-5 ■). As the myocardium around the right

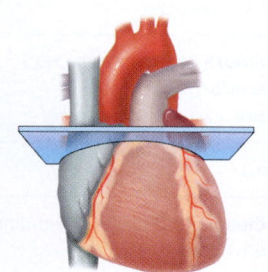

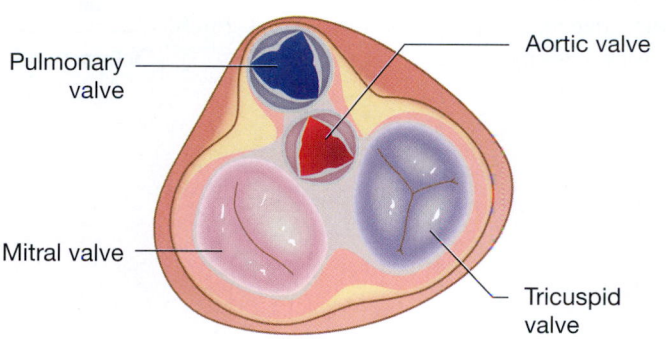

CROSS SECTION THROUGH VALVES (FROM ABOVE)

FIGURE 5-5 ■ Tricuspid valve.
With the three valve leaflets of the tricuspid valve closed (as shown here), their edges seal tightly against one another, preventing the backflow of blood. When the valve leaflets open, blood flows through the tricuspid valve into the right ventricle.

atrium contracts, the tricuspid valve opens to allow blood to flow into the right ventricle. Then, as the myocardium around the right ventricle contracts, this valve closes to prevent blood from returning to the right atrium.

The **pulmonary valve** is between the right ventricle and the pulmonary arteries. As the myocardium around the right ventricle contracts, the pulmonary valve opens to allow blood to flow into the pulmonary arteries. Then this valve closes to prevent blood from returning to the right ventricle.

The **mitral valve** is between the left atrium and left ventricle. It has two cusps and is known as the **bicuspid valve**. As the myocardium around the left atrium contracts, the mitral valve opens to allow blood to flow into the left ventricle. Then, as the myocardium around the left ventricle contracts, this valve closes to prevent blood from returning to the left atrium.

The **aortic valve** is between the left ventricle and the aorta. It has three triangular cusps. As the myocardium around the left ventricle contracts, the aortic valve opens to allow blood to flow into the aorta. Then this valve closes to prevent blood from returning to the left ventricle.

Both the tricuspid and mitral valves have **chordae tendineae**, rope-like strands attached to their valve leaflets and anchored to small muscles in the walls of the ventricles (see Figure 5-4). When the ventricles contract, these small muscles also contract and pull on the chordae tendineae. This stabilizes the valve leaflets to keep them tightly closed, even during the strong force of a ventricular contraction.

Heart Sounds

The sounds of the valves closing are commonly known as "lubb-dupp" (a phonetic approximation of the actual sounds). The "lubb" sound occurs as the tricuspid and mitral valves close. This first heart sound is abbreviated as S_1. The "dupp" sound occurs as the pulmonary and aortic valves close. This second heart sound is abbreviated as S_2.

Thoracic Cavity and Mediastinum

The **thoracic cavity** is a large body cavity within the chest that contains the lungs and the **mediastinum** (see Figure 5-6 ■). The mediastinum contains the heart and parts of the blood vessels that are known as the **great vessels** (aorta, superior vena cava, inferior vena cava, pulmonary arteries and veins), as well as the thymus (described in Chapter 6, Hematology and Immunology), trachea (described in Chapter 4, Pulmonology), and the esophagus (described in Chapter 3, Gastroenterology). The word *cardiothoracic* reflects the anatomic relationship of the heart and the thoracic cavity.

Blood Vessels

The blood vessels are **vascular** channels in which blood circulates throughout the body. **Vasculature** refers to the blood vessels associated with a specific organ. For example, the vasculature of the stomach includes the gastric artery, capillaries, and gastric vein. Blood vessels have a central opening or **lumen** through which the blood flows. They are lined with **endothelium**, a smooth inner lining that promotes the flow of blood. This layer is also known as the **intima**.

There are three kinds of blood vessels: arteries, capillaries, and veins. Each performs a different function in the circulatory system.

Pronunciation/Word Parts

pulmonary (PUL-moh-NAIR-ee)
  pulmon/o- *lung*
  -ary *pertaining to*

mitral (MY-tral)
  mitr/o- *structure with two points*
  -al *pertaining to*

bicuspid (by-KUS-pid)
  bi- *two*
  cusp/o- *point; projection*
  -id *origin; resembling; source*

aortic (aa-OR-tik)
  aort/o- *aorta*
  -ic *pertaining to*

chordae tendineae (KOR-dee TEN-dih-NEE-ee)

thoracic (thor-AS-ik)
  thorac/o- *chest; thorax*
  -ic *pertaining to*

cavity (KAV-ih-tee)
  cav/o- *hollow space*
  -ity *condition; state*

mediastinum (MEE-dee-ah-STY-num)

mediastinal (MEE-dee-ah-STY-nal)
  mediastin/o- *mediastinum*
  -al *pertaining to*

cardiothoracic (KAR-dee-OH-thor-AS-ik)
  cardi/o- *heart*
  thorac/o- *chest; thorax*
  -ic *pertaining to*

vascular (VAS-kyoo-lar)
  vascul/o- *blood vessel*
  -ar *pertaining to*
The combining form **angi/o-** means *blood vessel; lymphatic vessel.*
The combining form **vas/o-** means *blood vessel; vas deferens.*

vasculature (VAS-kyoo-lah-CHUR)
  vascul/o- *blood vessel*
  -ature *system composed of*

lumen (LOO-men)

endothelium (EN-doh-THEE-lee-um)
  end/o- *innermost; within*
  theli/o- *cellular layer*
  -um *period of time; structure*

intima (IN-tih-mah)

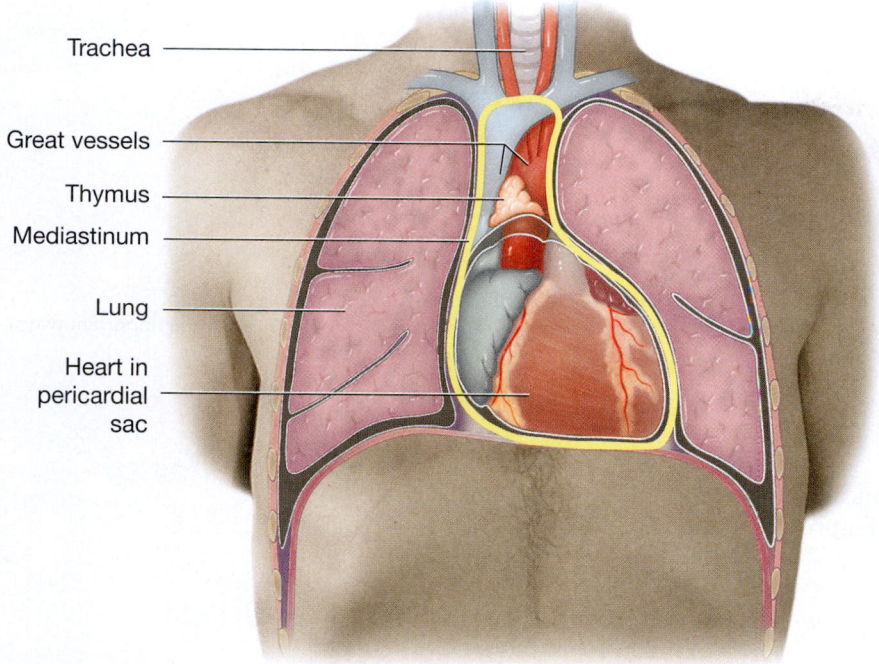

Trachea

Great vessels

Thymus

Mediastinum

Lung

Heart in pericardial sac

FIGURE 5-6 ■ Mediastinum.
The mediastinum holds these structures in place within the thoracic cavity: the heart and pericardial sac and parts of the great vessels, as well as the thymus, trachea, and esophagus.

Arteries

Arteries are large blood vessels that branch into smaller **arterioles**. All arteries and arterioles share some important characteristics and functions.

Characteristics and Functions of Arteries

1. All arteries carry blood away from the heart to the body or to the lungs.

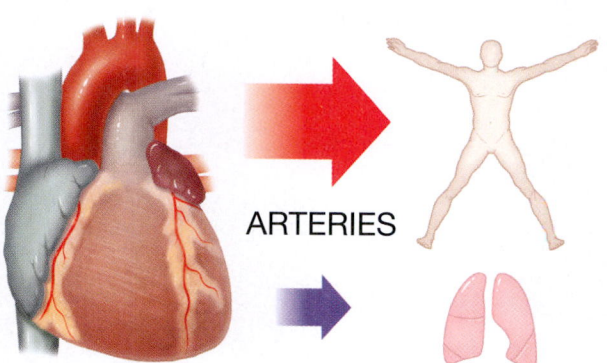

ARTERIES

2. Most arteries carry bright red, **oxygenated** blood that contains a high level of oxygen. The exception is the pulmonary arteries from the heart to the lungs; they carry dark red-purple blood that has a low level of oxygen.

3. Most arteries lie deep beneath the skin. However, a few arteries lie near the skin surface. The walls of these arteries bulge each time the heart contracts, and this can be felt as a **pulse**.

4. All arteries have smooth muscle in their walls. When the smooth muscle contracts, the lumen of the artery decreases in size (**vasoconstriction**), and the pressure of the blood in the artery increases (see Figure 5-7 ■). When the smooth muscle relaxes, the lumen of the artery increases in size (**vasodilation**), and the pressure of the blood in the artery decreases.

Pronunciation/Word Parts

artery (AR-ter-ee)

arterial (ar-TEER-ee-al)
  arteri/o- *artery*
  -al *pertaining to*
The combining form **arter/o-** also means *artery.*

arteriole (ar-TEER-ee-ohl)
  arteri/o- *artery*
  -ole *small thing*

arteriolar (ar-TEER-ee-OH-lar)
  arteriol/o- *arteriole*
  -ar *pertaining to*

oxygenated (AWK-sih-jeh-NAY-ted)
  oxygen/o- *oxygen*
  -ated *composed of; pertaining to a condition*

pulse (PULS)

vasoconstriction
(VAY-soh-con-STRIK-shun)
  vas/o- *blood vessel; vas deferens*
  constrict/o- *drawn together; narrowed*
  -ion *action; condition*

vasodilation (VAY-soh-dy-LAY-shun)
  vas/o- *blood vessel; vas deferens*
  dilat/o- *dilate; widen*
  -ion *action; condition*

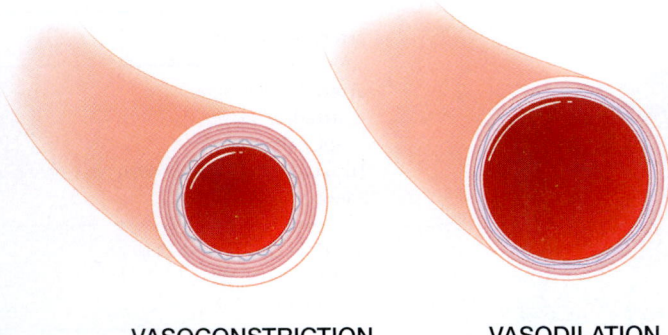

VASOCONSTRICTION   VASODILATION

FIGURE 5-7 ■ Vasoconstriction and vasodilation.
Vasoconstriction and vasodilation of the arteries are important ways in which the body regulates the blood pressure.

Names and Locations of Arteries

Many arteries are named for nearby anatomical structures, such as areas, cavities, bones, muscles, or organs (see Figure 5-8 ■, Figure 5-9 ■, and Table 5-2 ■).

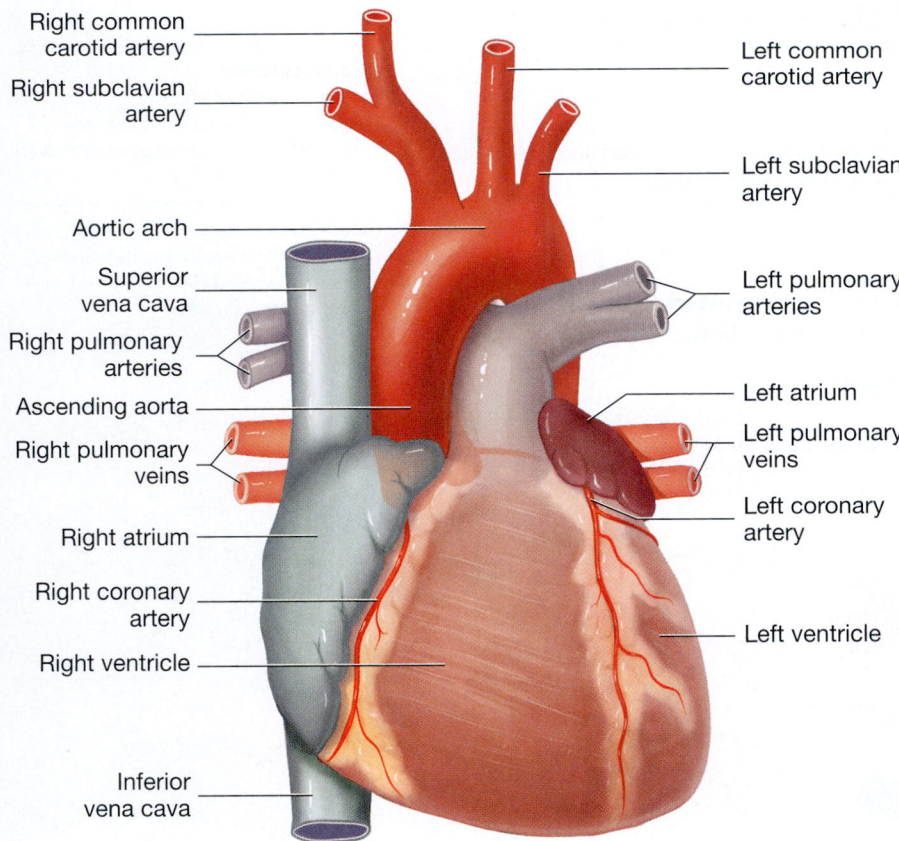

Right common carotid artery
Right subclavian artery
Aortic arch
Superior vena cava
Right pulmonary arteries
Ascending aorta
Right pulmonary veins
Right atrium
Right coronary artery
Right ventricle
Inferior vena cava

Left common carotid artery
Left subclavian artery
Left pulmonary arteries
Left atrium
Left pulmonary veins
Left coronary artery
Left ventricle

FIGURE 5-8 ■ Arteries and veins around the heart.
The aorta is the largest artery in the body. The coronary arteries to the heart are the first to receive oxygenated blood directly from the aorta. The aortic arch contains the first three major branches of arteries. The superior vena cava and inferior vena cava are the largest veins in the body.

Dive Deeper

Even though the chambers of the heart are filled with blood, this blood cannot supply oxygen to the myocardium. The myocardium must obtain its oxygen from blood that flows through the coronary arteries, arteries that branch off directly from the aorta, not from other arteries. This reflects the primary role that the heart muscle plays in maintaining life.

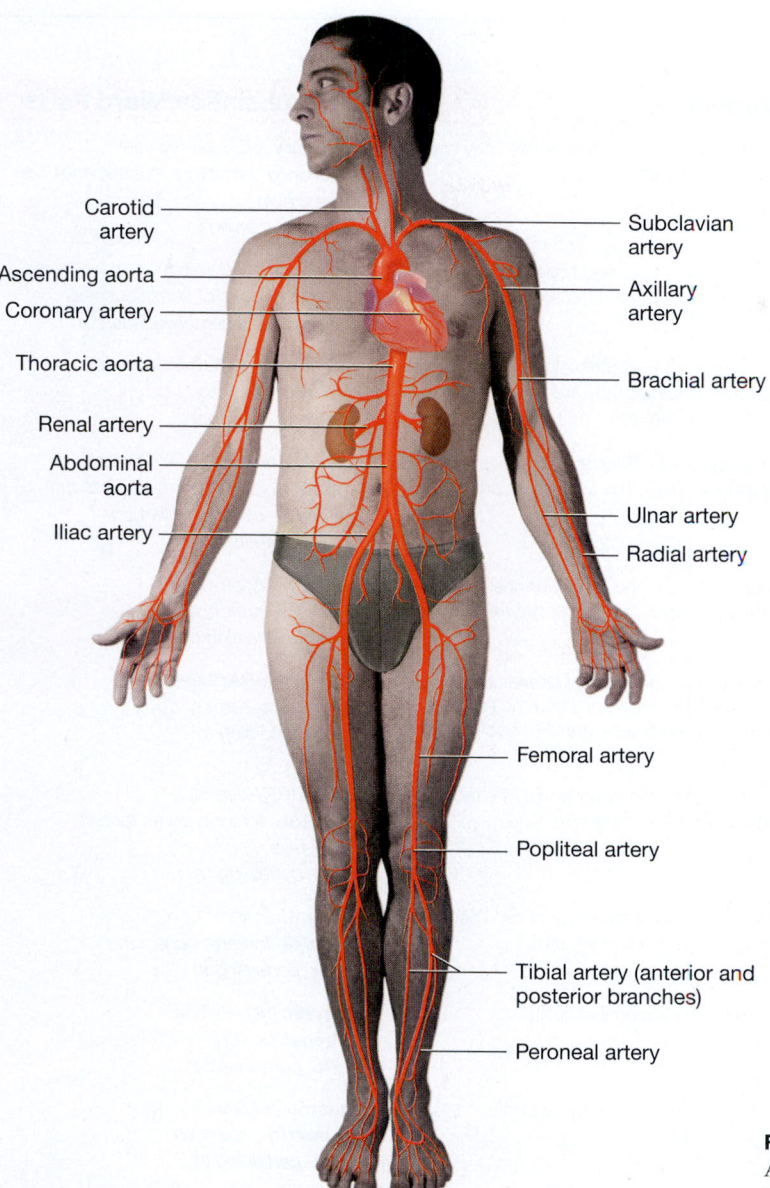

Carotid artery
Ascending aorta
Coronary artery
Thoracic aorta
Renal artery
Abdominal aorta
Iliac artery

Subclavian artery
Axillary artery
Brachial artery
Ulnar artery
Radial artery
Femoral artery
Popliteal artery
Tibial artery (anterior and posterior branches)
Peroneal artery

FIGURE 5-9 ■ Arteries in the body.
Arteries branch off from the aorta and carry oxygenated blood to the head, chest, arms, abdomen, pelvis, and legs.

Table 5-2   Locations and Descriptions of the Arteries

The arteries are listed as they are encountered anatomically, beginning with the aorta.

Arteries	Location and Description	Pronunciation/Word Parts
aorta	The **aorta** is the largest artery in the body. It receives oxygenated blood from the left ventricle of the heart. The **ascending aorta** travels in a superior direction from the heart and then becomes the **aortic arch**, an inverted, U-shaped segment. The ascending aorta brings oxygenated blood to the heart, head, neck, shoulders, and arms. The **thoracic aorta** continues inferiorly through the thoracic cavity of the chest. It branches into arteries that bring oxygenated blood to the esophagus, muscles between the ribs, diaphragm, upper spinal cord, and back. As the thoracic aorta goes through the diaphragm and enters the abdominopelvic cavity, it becomes the **abdominal aorta**. The abdominal aorta brings oxygenated blood to many organs, including the stomach, liver, gallbladder, pancreas, spleen, small intestine, large intestine, adrenal glands, kidneys, ovaries (in a woman), testes (in a man), and the lower spinal cord. Within the pelvic cavity in the area of the hip bones, the abdominal aorta ends as it divides into two branches (a **bifurcation**) to become the right and left iliac arteries that bring oxygenated blood to the legs.	**aorta** (aa-OR-tah) **aortic** (aa-OR-tik) **aort/o-** *aorta* **-ic** *pertaining to* **thoracic** (thor-AS-ik) **thorac/o-** *chest; thorax* **-ic** *pertaining to* **abdominal** (ab-DAW-mih-nal) **abdomin/o-** *abdomen* **-al** *pertaining to* **bifurcation** (BY-fir-KAY-shun) **bifurcat/o-** *divide into two branches* **-ion** *action; condition*

(continued)

Table 5-2   (Continued)

Arteries	Location and Description	Pronunciation/Word Parts
coronary arteries	The **coronary arteries** are the first arteries to branch off from the ascending aorta. They encircle the heart and bring oxygenated blood to all parts of the myocardium.	**coronary** (KOR-oh-NAIR-ee) **coron/o-** *structure that encircles like a crown* **-ary** *pertaining to*
carotid arteries	The **carotid arteries** bring oxygenated blood to the neck, face, head, and brain. The carotid arteries are named for the result of what happens if they are blocked; the person loses consciousness.	**carotid** (kah-RAW-tid) **carot/o-** *loss of consciousness* **-id** *origin; resembling; source*
pulmonary arteries	The **pulmonary arteries** bring deoxygenated blood from the right ventricle of the heart to the lungs. Remember: The pulmonary arteries are the exception because they are the only arteries that carry deoxygenated blood. The adjective for the lung is *pulmonary*.	**pulmonary** (PUL-moh-NAIR-ee) **pulmon/o-** *lung* **-ary** *pertaining to*
subclavian arteries	The **subclavian arteries** bring oxygenated blood to the shoulders. Each subclavian artery goes underneath the clavicle (collarbone) and becomes the axillary artery. The subclavian artery is named for the clavicle (collarbone).	**subclavian** (sub-KLAY-vee-an) **sub-** *below; underneath; less than* **clav/o-** *clavicle; collarbone* **-ian** *pertaining to*
axillary arteries	The **axillary arteries** are a continuation of the subclavian arteries. The axillary arteries bring oxygenated blood to the areas under the arms. The axillary artery is named for the axilla (armpit).	**axillary** (AK-zih-LAIR-ee) **axill/o-** *armpit; axilla* **-ary** *pertaining to*
brachial arteries	The **brachial arteries** are a continuation of the axillary arteries. The brachial arteries bring oxygenated blood to the upper arms. Each brachial artery ends as it divides into the **radial artery** and the **ulnar artery**. The brachial artery is named for the biceps brachii muscle in the upper arm.	**brachial** (BRAY-kee-al) **brachi/o-** *arm* **-al** *pertaining to*
radial arteries	The **radial arteries** bring oxygenated blood to the thumb side of the lower arms. The radial artery is named for the radius bone that is on the thumb side of the lower arm.	**radial** (RAY-dee-al) **radi/o-** *forearm bone; radius; x-rays* **-al** *pertaining to*
ulnar arteries	The **ulnar arteries** bring oxygenated blood to the little finger side of the lower arms. The ulnar artery is named for the ulnar bone that is on the little finger side of the lower arm.	**ulnar** (UL-nar) **uln/o-** *forearm bone; ulna* **-ar** *pertaining to*
hepatic arteries	The **hepatic arteries** bring oxygenated blood to the liver in the abdominal cavity.	**hepatic** (heh-PAT-ik) **hepat/o-** *liver* **-ic** *pertaining to*
gastric arteries	The **gastric arteries** bring oxygenated blood to the stomach in the abdominal cavity.	**gastric** (GAS-trik) **gastr/o-** *stomach* **-ic** *pertaining to*
renal arteries	The **renal arteries** bring oxygenated blood to the kidneys behind the abdominal cavity.	**renal** (REE-nal) **ren/o-** *kidney* **-al** *pertaining to*
iliac arteries	The **iliac arteries** bring oxygenated blood to the hip and groin areas. As it continues into the upper leg, the iliac artery becomes the femoral artery. The iliac artery is named for the ilium (hip bone).	**iliac** (IL-ee-ak) **ili/o-** *ilium* **-ac** *pertaining to*
femoral arteries	The **femoral arteries** are a continuation of the iliac arteries. The femoral arteries bring oxygenated blood to the upper leg. The femoral artery is named for the femur bone in the upper leg. Near the knee joint, the femoral artery continues as the popliteal artery.	**femoral** (FEM-oh-ral) **femor/o-** *femur; thigh bone* **-al** *pertaining to*
popliteal arteries	The **popliteal arteries** are a continuation of the femoral arteries. The popliteal arteries bring oxygenated blood to the knee area. The popliteal artery is named for the popliteus, a small muscle at the back of the knee. The popliteal artery ends as it divides into the **tibial artery** and **peroneal artery**.	**popliteal** (POP-lih-TEE-al) **poplite/o-** *back of the knee* **-al** *pertaining to*
tibial arteries	The **tibial arteries** bring oxygenated blood to the front and back of the lower leg. The tibial artery is named for the tibia bone in the lower leg.	**tibial** (TIB-ee-al) **tibi/o-** *shin bone; tibia* **-al** *pertaining to*
peroneal arteries	The **peroneal arteries** bring oxygenated blood to the little toe side of the lower leg. The peroneal artery is named for the fibula bone in the lower leg. One adjective for the fibula is *peroneal* (the other adjective is *fibular*).	**peroneal** (PAIR-oh-NEE-al) **perone/o-** *fibula* **-al** *pertaining to*

Capillaries

Capillaries are the smallest blood vessels in the body; they lie between the arterioles and the venules. An arteriole branches into a network of capillaries that reaches each cell in the body, and then the capillaries merge into a venule. The lumen of a capillary is so small that blood cells must pass through in single file. Capillaries are not named.

Veins

Small veins, known as **venules**, combine to form a large **vein**. All veins and venules share some important characteristics and functions.

Characteristics and Functions of Veins

1. All veins carry blood from the body and the lungs back to the heart.

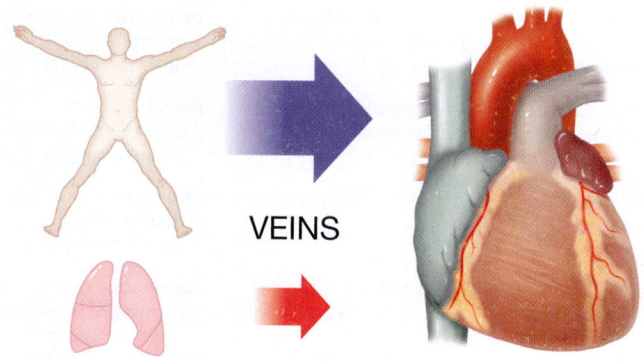

VEINS

2. Most veins carry dark red-purple **deoxygenated** blood that has a low level of oxygen. The exception is the pulmonary veins from the lungs to the heart; they carry bright red blood that has just picked up oxygen in the lungs.

3. The largest veins have valves that keep the blood flowing in one direction—back toward the heart (see Figure 5-10 ■).

4. Many veins are near the surface of the body and can be seen just under the skin as bluish, sometimes bulging lines.

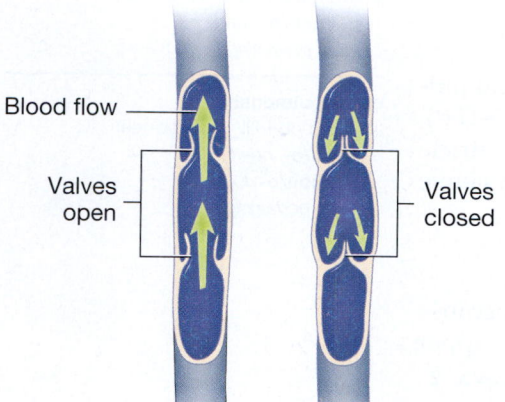

Blood flow

Valves open

Valves closed

FIGURE 5-10 ■ Valves in a vein.
The heart pumps blood through the arteries, but not through the veins. As large muscles in an arm or leg contract, they compress the veins, and this moves blood through the veins back to the heart. Valves in the veins then close to prevent gravity from pulling the blood back to its original location.

Names and Locations of Veins

Just as with arteries, many veins are named for nearby anatomical structures or have names that are the same as those of arteries (see Table 5-3 ■). The two major veins of the body are the superior vena cava and inferior vena cava (see Figure 5-8).

Pronunciation/Word Parts

capillary (KAP-ih-LAIR-ee)
  capill/o- *capillary; hair-like structure*
  -ary *pertaining to*

vein (VAYN)

venous (VEE-nuhs)
  ven/o- *vein*
  -ous *pertaining to*
The combining form **phleb/o-** also means *vein*.

venule (VEN-yool)
  ven/o- *vein*
  -ule *small thing*

deoxygenated (de-AWK-sih-jeh-NAY-ted)
  de- *reversal of; without*
  oxygen/o- *oxygen*
  -ated *composed of; pertaining to a condition*

Table 5-3   Locations and Descriptions of the Veins

The veins are listed as they are encountered anatomically, beginning with the vena cava.

Veins	Location and Description	Pronunciation/Word Parts
superior vena cava	The **superior vena cava** brings deoxygenated blood from the head, neck, chest, and arms to the right atrium. The superior vena cava is named for its location, which is superior to the heart.	**vena cava** (VEE-nah KAY-vah) Latin plural noun: Change the singular ending -a to -ae. Example: The superior and inferior venae cavae
inferior vena cava	The **inferior vena cava** brings deoxygenated blood from the abdomen, pelvis, and legs to the right atrium. The inferior vena cava is named for its location, which is inferior to the heart. In the pelvic cavity in the area of the hip bones, the inferior vena cava ends as it divides to become the right and left iliac veins.	
jugular veins	The **jugular veins** bring deoxygenated blood from the head and neck to the superior vena cava. The jugular vein takes its name from a Latin word that means *neck*.	**jugular** (JUG-yoo-lar) **jugul/o-** *throat* **-ar** *pertaining to*
pulmonary veins	The **pulmonary veins** bring <u>oxygenated</u> blood from the lungs to the left atrium of the heart. Remember: The pulmonary veins are the exception because they are the only veins that carry <u>oxygenated</u> blood. The adjective for the lung is *pulmonary*.	**pulmonary** (PUL-moh-NAIR-ee) **pulmon/o-** *lung* **-ary** *pertaining to*
portal veins	The **portal veins** bring deoxygenated blood from the intestines and liver to the inferior vena cava. The portal vein is named for the porta hepatis, an opening (or portal) in the liver where blood vessels enter and exit.	**portal** (POR-tal) **port/o-** *point of entry* **-al** *pertaining to*
fibular veins	The **fibular veins** bring deoxygenated blood from the little toe side of the lower leg to the femoral veins. The fibular vein is named for the fibula bone in the lower leg.	**fibular** (FIH-byoo-lar) **fibul/o-** *fibula* **-ar** *pertaining to*
saphenous veins	The **saphenous veins** bring deoxygenated blood from the lower legs to the femoral veins. The saphenous vein takes its name from a Latin word that means *clearly visible*, as this vein often can be seen through the skin on the inside lower leg.	**saphenous** (SAF-eh-nuhs) **saphen/o-** *clearly visible* **-ous** *pertaining to*

Circulation

Circulation is a process that moves the blood through a continuous, circular pathway. This pathway has two parts: the systemic circulation and the pulmonary circulation.

1. **Systemic circulation.** This includes arteries, arterioles, capillaries, venules, and veins everywhere in the body, except in the lungs.

2. **Pulmonary circulation.** This includes arteries, arterioles, capillaries, venules, and veins going to, within, and coming from the lungs. The word *cardiopulmonary* reflects the close connection between the heart and the lungs.

This is the route that the blood takes as it travels through the systemic and pulmonary circulations to complete one trip through the entire body (see Figure 5-11 ▪). Each time the heart beats, it simultaneously pumps blood from the right ventricle through the pulmonary circulation and from the left ventricle through the systemic circulation.

Systemic Circulation Beginning in the Capillaries and Veins

Deoxygenated blood coming from the tissues is dark red-purple in color because it has a low level of oxygen. Deoxygenated blood coming from the upper body **1** travels through capillaries, venules, and veins to the superior vena cava **2**. Deoxygenated blood coming from the lower body **3** travels through capillaries, venules, and veins to the inferior vena cava **4**. This deoxygenated blood then enters the right atrium **5**, travels through the tricuspid valve **6**, and into the right ventricle **7**.

Pulmonary Circulation

At that point, the blood enters the pulmonary circulation. The deoxygenated blood travels through the pulmonary valve **8**, through the pulmonary arteries **9**, and into the lungs **10**. In capillaries in the lung, the blood releases carbon dioxide, picks up oxygen, and becomes bright red in color. This oxygenated blood then travels through the pulmonary veins **11** to the left atrium **12** of the heart.

Pronunciation/Word Parts

circulation (SIR-kyoo-LAY-shun)
   circulat/o- *moving in a circular route*
   -ion *action; condition*

systemic (sihs-TEM-ik)
   system/o- *body as a whole*
   -ic *pertaining to*

pulmonary (PUL-moh-NAIR-ee)
   pulmon/o- *lung*
   -ary *pertaining to*

cardiopulmonary
(KAR-dee-oh-PUL-moh-NAIR-ee)
   cardi/o- *heart*
   pulmon/o- *lung*
   -ary *pertaining to*

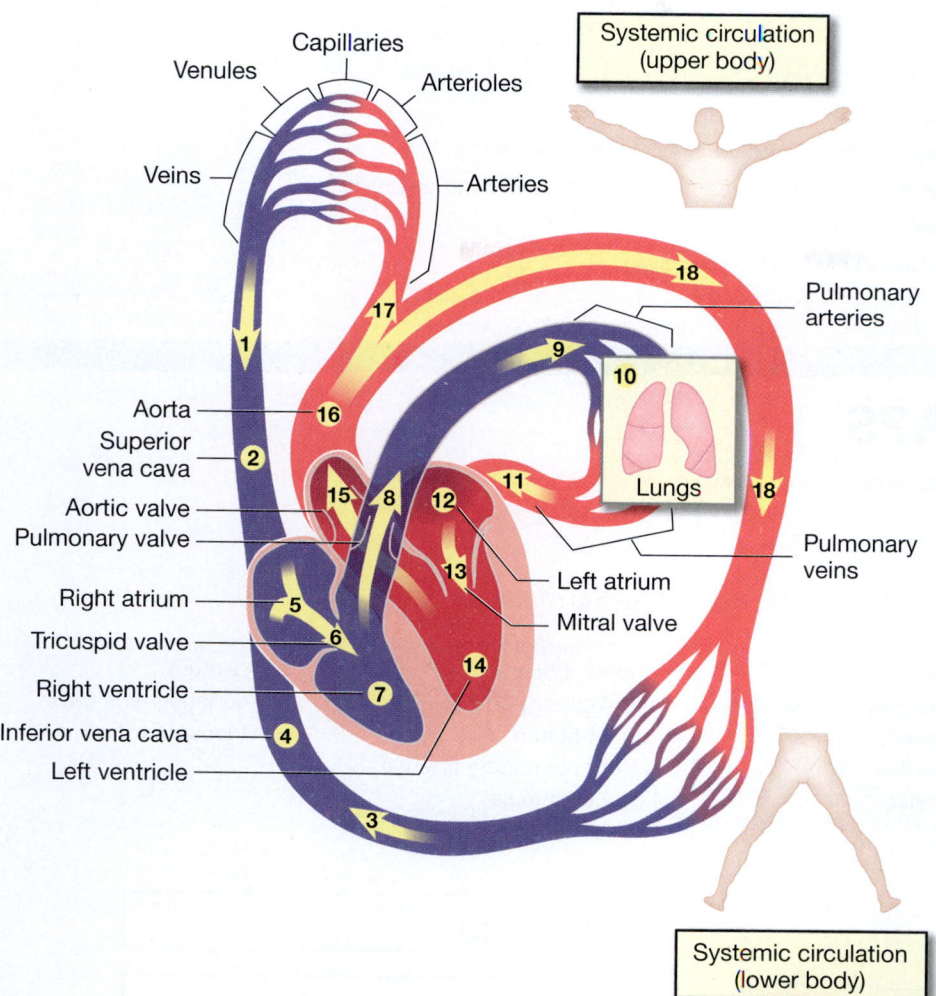

Venules
Capillaries
Veins
Arterioles
Arteries

Systemic circulation (upper body)

18
Pulmonary arteries

17
9
10
Lungs
18
Pulmonary veins

Aorta — 16
Superior vena cava — 2
Aortic valve — 15   8   12   11
Pulmonary valve —
13
Left atrium
Right atrium — 5
Mitral valve
Tricuspid valve — 6
14
Right ventricle — 7
Inferior vena cava — 4
Left ventricle
3
1

Systemic circulation (lower body)

FIGURE 5-11 ■ Circulation of the blood.
Each time the heart beats, it pumps blood from the right ventricle through the pulmonary circulation and from the left ventricle through the systemic circulation.

Systemic Circulation Finishing in the Arteries and Capillaries

Now the blood is back in the systemic circulation. From the left atrium, the blood travels through the mitral valve **13** and into the left ventricle **14**. The blood then travels through the aortic valve **15** and into the aorta **16** to the upper body **17** and the lower body **18**. The arteries, arterioles, and capillaries distribute this oxygenated blood to every part of the body. Then in capillaries within body tissues, the blood releases oxygen and picks up carbon dioxide, and again becomes dark red-purple in color. This completes one trip around the circulatory system.

Clinical Connections

Neonatology. The fetal heart begins to beat just 4 weeks after conception. The circulation of blood in a fetus is different from that of an adult. The fetus receives oxygenated blood and nutrients from the mother through the placenta, via arteries in the umbilical cord that merge with the inferior vena cava of the fetus. The fetal heart has two unique, temporary structures. The **foramen ovale**, a small, oval opening in the septum between the atria, allows some of the oxygenated blood to enter the left side of the heart where it is immediately circulated to the body. The **ductus arteriosus** is a blood vessel that connects the left pulmonary arteries to the descending aorta. This allows oxygenated blood to bypass the not-yet-functioning lungs and go directly to the body. Sometime after birth, these two temporary structures in the fetal heart are no longer needed, and they close automatically because the baby is now breathing.

foramen ovale (foh-RAY-men oh-VAL-ee)

ductus arteriosus (DUK-tuhs ar-TEER-ee-OH-suhs)

Word Alert
Sound-Alike Words

cardia	(noun)	small region of the stomach where the esophagus enters
	Example: *The cardia is the first part of the stomach to receive food from the esophagus.*	
cardiac	(adjective)	pertaining to the heart
	Example: *During a cardiac arrest, the heart stops beating.*	

5.1 PRACTICE LAPS

Use the Answer Key at the end of the book to check your answers.

A. Label Structures

Write each anatomy word or phrase in the correct numbered box. Be sure to check your spelling.

aortic arch	left atrium	myocardium	septum
aortic valve	left pulmonary arteries	pulmonary valve	superior vena cava
ascending aorta	left pulmonary veins	right atrium	tricuspid valve
chordae tendineae	left ventricle	right pulmonary arteries	
inferior vena cava	mitral valve	right ventricle	

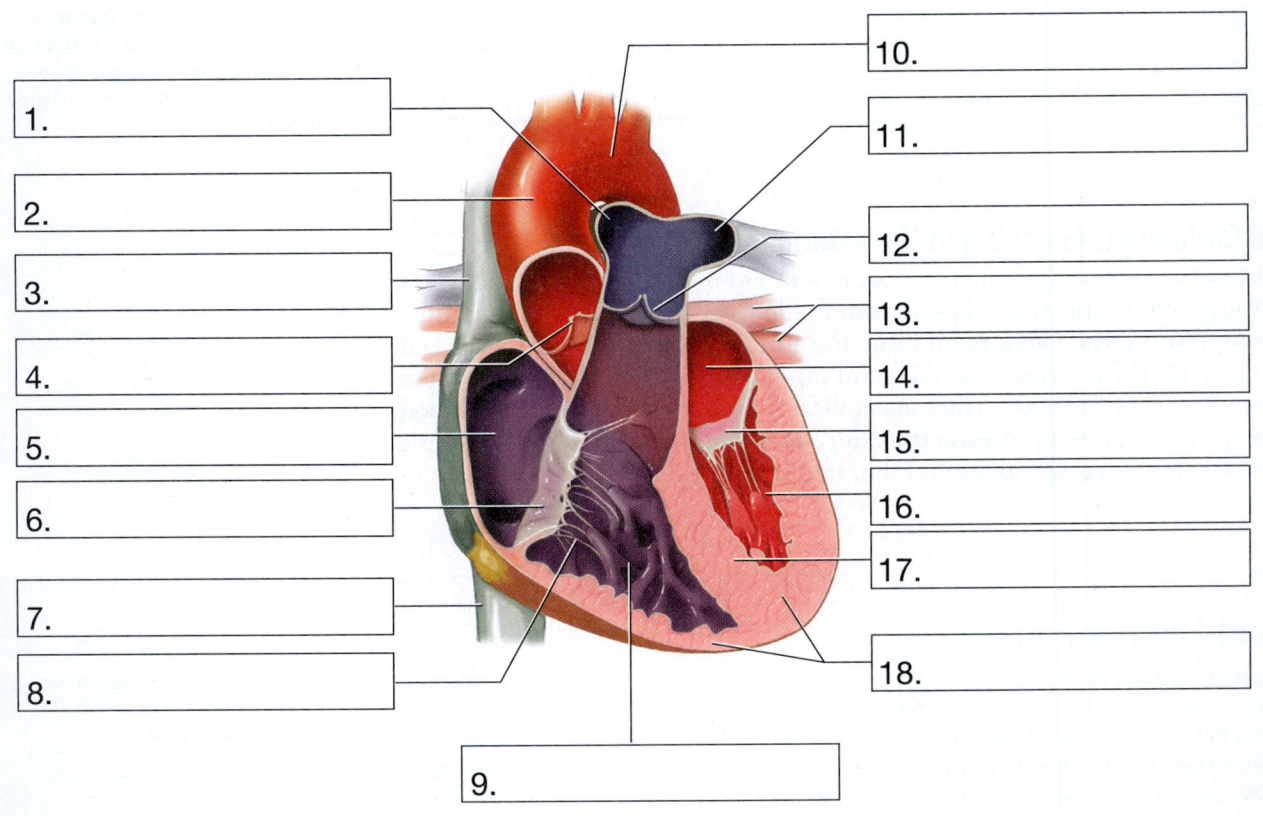

1.

2.

3.

4.

5.

6.

7.

8.

9.

10.

11.

12.

13.

14.

15.

16.

17.

18.

abdominal aorta
ascending aorta
axillary artery
brachial artery

carotid artery
coronary artery
femoral artery
iliac artery

peroneal artery
popliteal artery
radial artery
renal artery

subclavian artery
thoracic aorta
tibial artery
ulnar artery

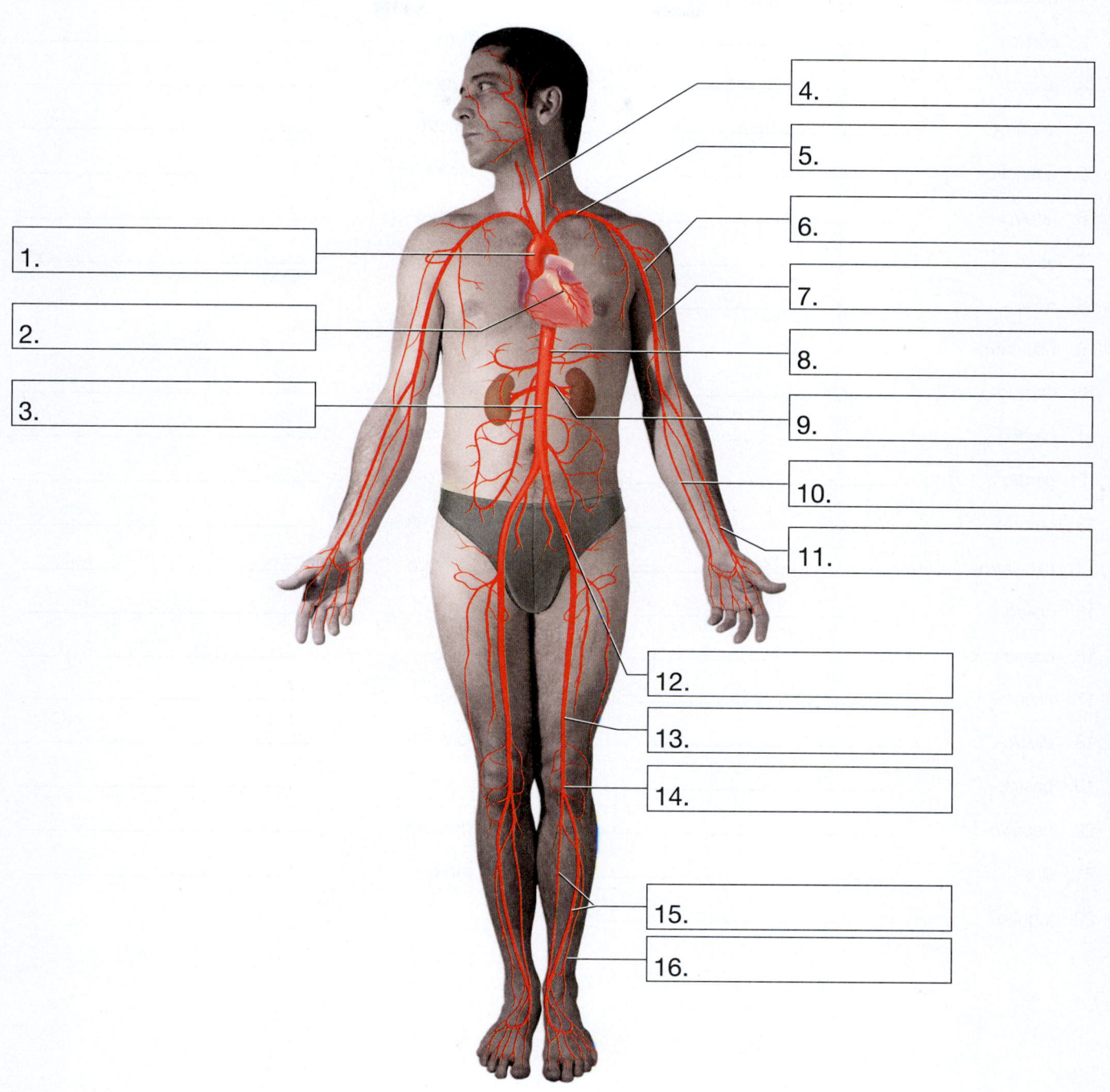

1.

2.

3.

4.

5.

6.

7.

8.

9.

10.

11.

12.

13.

14.

15.

16.

B. Give the Meaning of Combining Forms

Next to each combining form, write its meaning. The first one has been done for you.

Combining Form	Meaning	Combining Form	Meaning
1. **mediastin/o-**	*mediastinum*	23. mitr/o-	
2. aort/o-		24. my/o-	
3. apic/o-		25. oxygen/o-	
4. arteri/o-		26. pariet/o-	
5. arteriol/o-		27. perone/o-	
6. arter/o-		28. phleb/o-	
7. atri/o-		29. poplite/o-	
8. axill/o-		30. port/o-	
9. bifurcat/o-		31. pulmon/o-	
10. capill/o-		32. radi/o-	
11. cardi/o-		33. saphen/o-	
12. card/o-		34. sept/o-	
13. carot/o-		35. system/o-	
14. circulat/o-		36. thorac/o-	
15. clav/o-		37. tibi/o-	
16. constrict/o-		38. uln/o-	
17. cusp/o-		39. valv/o-	
18. dilat/o-		40. valvul/o-	
19. gastr/o-		41. vas/o-	
20. hepat/o-		42. vascul/o-	
21. ili/o-		43. ven/o-	
22. jugul/o-			

C. Build Words

Read the definition of the medical word. Look at the combining form that is given. Select the correct suffix from the Suffix List, and write it on the blank line. Then build the medical word, and write it on the line. (Remember: You may need to remove the combining vowel. Always remove the hyphens and slash.) Be sure to check your spelling.

Suffix List

-ac (pertaining to)
-al (pertaining to)
-ar (pertaining to)
-ary (pertaining to)

-ated (composed of; pertaining to a condition)
-ature (system composed of)
-ic (pertaining to)

-ion (action; condition)
-ole (small thing)
-ory (having the function of)
-ous (pertaining to)

Definition of the Medical Word	Combining Form	Suffix	Build the Medical Word
Example: Pertaining to (the) mediastinum	mediastin/o-	-al	mediastinal

[You think pertaining to (-al) + mediastinum (mediastin/o-). You change the order of the word parts to put the suffix last. You write mediastinal.]

1. Pertaining to (the) heart	cardi/o-		
2. Action (to) divide into two branches	bifurcat/o-		
3. Pertaining to (the) armpit	axill/o-		
4. Small thing (that is an) artery	arteri/o-		
5. Pertaining to (the) throat	jugul/o-		
6. Action (of being) narrowed	constrict/o-		
7. Pertaining to (a) structure with two points	mitr/o-		
8. Having the function of moving in a circular route	circulat/o-		
9. Pertaining to (the) atrium	atri/o-		
10. Pertaining to (a) hair-like structure	capill/o-		
11. Pertaining to (the) aorta	aort/o-		
12. Composed of oxygen	oxygen/o-		
13. System composed (of) blood vessels	vascul/o-		
14. Pertaining to (a) valve	valvul/o-		
15. Pertaining to (a) vein	ven/o-		

5.2 Physiology

The heart contracts and relaxes in a regular rhythm that is coordinated by its **conduction system** (see Figure 5-12 ■). The **sinoatrial (SA) node**, the pacemaker of the heart, is in the posterior wall of the upper right atrium. It initiates the electrical impulse that begins each heartbeat. Muscle cells in the myocardium respond to those electrical impulses by contracting in a coordinated way to pump blood through the heart. First, the myocardium around both atria contracts simultaneously. The electrical impulse then travels through the **atrioventricular (AV) node** (located in the lower right atrium), through the **bundle of His** (in the upper ventricular septum), through the right and left **bundle branches** (in the ventricular septum), finally ending in a network of nerves (the **Purkinje fibers**) (in the walls of the ventricles). This electrical impulse causes both ventricles to contract simultaneously. A **contraction** of the myocardium around the atria and ventricles is known as **systole**, and **diastole** is the resting period between contractions as the heart again fills with blood.

When the SA node is in control of the heart rate, the heart is in **normal sinus rhythm (NSR)**. Besides the SA node, several other areas in the atria and ventricles can produce electrical impulses on their own, although these areas are not part of the normal conduction system. These impulses are usually too weak to override the SA node. However, if the SA node fails to produce its impulses, if its impulses are blocked, or if these other areas become hyperexcited (from excessive amounts of caffeine or smoking), then these **ectopic** sites may produce an abnormal heart rhythm.

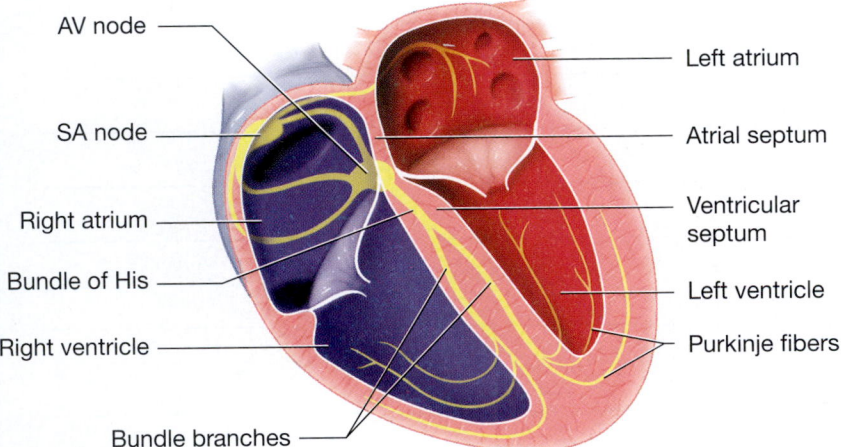

AV node

SA node

Right atrium

Bundle of His

Right ventricle

Bundle branches

Left atrium

Atrial septum

Ventricular septum

Left ventricle

Purkinje fibers

FIGURE 5-12 ■ Conduction system of the heart.
The SA node (pacemaker) initiates an electrical impulse that travels through the AV node, the bundle of His, the right and left bundle branches, and then to the Purkinje fibers, causing the atria and then the ventricles to contract.

Pronunciation/Word Parts

conduction (con-DUK-shun)
  conduct/o- carrying; conveying
  -ion action; condition

sinoatrial (SY-noh-AA-tree-al)
  sin/o- channel; hollow cavity
  atri/o- atrium; chamber that is open at the top
  -al pertaining to

node (NOHD)

atrioventricular
(AA-tree-oh-ven-TRIH-kyoo-lar)
  atri/o- atrium; chamber that is open at the top
  ventricul/o- chamber that is filled; ventricle
  -ar pertaining to

His (HISS)

Purkinje (per-KIN-jee)

contraction (con-TRAK-shun)
  contract/o- pull together
  -ion action; condition

systole (SIS-toh-lee)

systolic (sis-TAW-lik)
  systol/o- contracting
  -ic pertaining to

diastole (dy-AS-toh-lee)

diastolic (DY-ah-STAW-lik)
  diastol/o- dilating
  -ic pertaining to

sinus (SY-nuhs)
The SA node is in a sinus (a recessed area or channel) in the right atrium.

ectopic (ek-TAW-pik)
  ectop/o- outside
  -ic pertaining to

Clinical Connections

Neurology. The heart rate is controlled by the SA node, but the rate is also controlled by the parasympathetic and sympathetic divisions of the nervous system. The SA node generates an impulse of 80–100 beats each minute. The parasympathetic division (through the vagal nerve) releases the neurotransmitter acetylcholine to slow the heart to its normal resting heart rate of 70–80 beats each minute. If needed, the sympathetic division (through spinal cord nerves) releases the neurotransmitter norepinephrine to increase the heart rate. This means that fine adjustments in the heart rate are possible from moment to moment. When the heart needs to beat much faster during times of exercise (see Figure 5-13 ■) or to escape danger (the "fight-or-flight" response), the sympathetic division stimulates the adrenal glands to secrete the hormone **epinephrine**. It travels through the blood to the heart, overrides the normal sinus rhythm, and causes the heart to beat much faster.

epinephrine (EH-pih-NEH-frin)

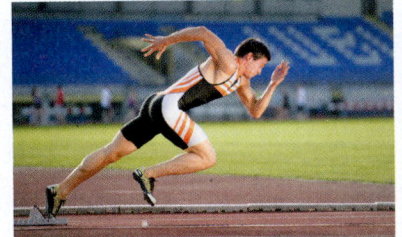

FIGURE 5-13 ■ Exercise increases the heart rate.
During exercise, epinephrine secreted by the adrenal glands (described in Chapter 13, Endocrinology) increases the heart rate and constricts the arteries to increase the blood pressure. Epinephrine also dilates the bronchi to increase airflow into the lungs.

Dive Deeper

On a molecular level, an elegant and intricate system allows the heart to contract tirelessly, approximately 100,000 times each day. An electrical impulse from the SA node changes the permeability of a myocardial cell. Positive sodium ions (Na^+) outside the cell move through the cell membrane, followed by positive calcium ions (Ca^{++}). This gives the inside of the cell a positive electrical charge, which triggers the release of positive calcium ions stored inside the cell. This process is known as **depolarization** because it reverses the normal, slightly negative electrical state of the cell. The calcium ions cause the myocardial cell to contract. As one cell depolarizes and contracts, it triggers the next myocardial cell to do the same.

A contraction ends when positive potassium ions (K^+) move out of the cell, while tiny molecular pumps move sodium ions and some calcium ions out of the cell and move the rest of the calcium ions back into storage within the cell. This process is known as **repolarization**. This restores the normal, slightly negative electrical state of the myocardial cell. The myocardial cell is now ready to respond to another impulse from the SA node.

A myocardial cell cannot respond to another electrical impulse until the full cycle of depolarization and repolarization is complete. This very short period of unresponsiveness is known as the **refractory period**.

depolarization (dee-POH-lar-ih-ZAY-shun)
de- *reversal of; without*
polar/o- *negative state; positive state*
-ization *process of creating; process of inserting; process of making*

repolarization (ree-POH-lar-ih-ZAY-shun)
re- *again and again; backward; unable to*
polar/o- *negative state; positive state*
-ization *process of creating; process of inserting; process of making*

refractory (ree-FRAK-tor-ee)
re- *again and again; backward; unable to*
fract/o- *bend; break up*
-ory *having the function of*
Refractory: *Having the function of (being) unable to break up*

5.2 PRACTICE LAPS

Use the Answer Key at the end of the book to check your answers.

A. Label Structures

Write each anatomy word or phrase in the correct numbered box. Be sure to check your spelling.

atrioventricular node	left atrium	right atrium
bundle branches	left ventricle	right ventricle
bundle of His	Purkinje fibers	sinoatrial node

1. _____

2. _____

3. _____

4. _____

5. _____

6. _____

7. _____

8. _____

9. _____

B. Give the Meaning of Combining Forms

Next to each combining form, write its meaning. The first one has been done for you.

Combining Form	Meaning	Combining Form	Meaning
1. **fract/o-**	*bend; break*	5. ectop/o-	
2. conduct/o-		6. polar/o-	
3. contract/o-		7. sin/o-	
4. diastol/o-		8. systol/o-	

C. Build Words

Read the definition of the medical word. Look at the combining form that is given. Select the correct suffix from the Suffix List, and write it on the blank line. Then build the medical word, and write it on the line. (Remember: You may need to remove the combining vowel. Always remove the hyphens and slash.) Be sure to check your spelling.

Suffix List

-ic (pertaining to)	-ion (action; condition)

Definition of the Medical Word	Combining Form	Suffix	Build the Medical Word
Example: Pertaining to dilating	**diastol/o-**	*-ic*	*diastolic*

[*You think* pertaining to (-ic) + dilating (diastol/o-). You change the order of the word parts to put the suffix last. You write diastolic.]

1. Pertaining to (being on the) outside	ectop/o-		
2. Action (of) conveying	conduct/o-		
3. Pertaining to contracting	systol/o-		
4. Action (of a muscle to) pull together	contract/o-		

Vocabulary Review

Word or Phrase	Description	Combining Forms
Overview		
cardiovascular system	A continuous, circular pathway whose structures include the heart and the blood vessels. The function of the cardiovascular system is to transport blood to every part of the body. Also known as the **circulatory system**.	**cardi/o-** *heart* **vascul/o-** *blood vessel*
circulatory system	Another name for the cardiovascular system that indicates its function of circulation of the blood.	**circulat/o-** *moving in a circular route*

Word or Phrase	Description	Combining Forms
Heart		
apex	The inferior tip of the heart	**apic/o-** *apex; tip*
heart	Organ that pumps blood throughout the body. It is located within the thoracic cavity, behind the sternum, and it contains four chambers, the septum (a center wall), and four valves.	**cardi/o-** *heart* **card/o-** *heart*
myocardium	Muscular layer of the heart	**my/o-** *muscle* **cardi/o-** *heart*
pericardium	Double-layered membrane around the heart. The U-shaped **pericardial sac** is filled with **pericardial fluid**. The layer next to the heart is the **epicardium**. The outer layer is the **parietal pericardium**.	**cardi/o-** *heart* **pariet/o-** *wall of a cavity*
Heart Chambers and Valves		
aortic valve	Heart valve between the left ventricle and the aorta	**aort/o-** *aorta* **valvul/o-** *valve*
atrium	Each of the two upper chambers of the heart	**atri/o-** *atrium; chamber that is open at the top*
chordae tendineae	Rope-like strands attached to the valve leaflets of the tricuspid and mitral valves and anchored to the ventricular walls. These keep the valve leaflets tightly closed when the ventricles contract.	
endocardium	Layer of cells that lines the heart chambers and the heart valves	**cardi/o-** *heart*
mitral valve	Heart valve between the left atrium and the left ventricle. Also known as the **bicuspid valve** because it has two (*bi*-) cusps or leaflets.	**mitr/o-** *structure with two points* **valvul/o-** *valve* **cusp/o-** *point; projection*
pulmonary valve	Heart valve between the right ventricle and the pulmonary arteries	**pulmon/o-** *lung* **valvul/o-** *valve*
septum	Central wall that divides the heart into right and left sides	**sept/o-** *dividing wall; septum*
tricuspid valve	Heart valve between the right atrium and right ventricle. It has three (*tri*-) cusps or leaflets.	**cusp/o-** *point; projection* **valvul/o-** *valve*
valve	Structure that opens and closes to control the flow of blood through the heart or the veins. Heart valves include the tricuspid valve, pulmonary valve, mitral valve, and aortic valve. There are also valves in some of the large veins to prevent backflow of blood.	**valvul/o-** *valve* **valv/o-** *valve*
ventricle	Each of the two large, lower chambers of the heart	**ventricul/o-** *chamber that is filled; ventricle*
Thoracic Cavity and Mediastinum		
cardiothoracic	Pertaining to the heart and thoracic cavity	**cardi/o-** *heart* **thorac/o-** *chest; thorax*
great vessels	Large blood vessels within the mediastinum. They include the aorta, superior vena cava, inferior vena cava, pulmonary arteries, and pulmonary veins.	
mediastinum	Central area in the thoracic cavity that contains the heart and parts of the great vessels, as well as the thymus, trachea, and esophagus	**mediastin/o-** *mediastinum*
thoracic cavity	Body cavity that contains the lungs and the mediastinum	**thorac/o-** *chest; thorax* **cav/o-** *hollow space*

Word or Phrase	Description	Combining Forms
Blood Vessels		
arteriole	Smaller branch of an artery	**arteriol/o-** *arteriole*
artery	Blood vessel that brings bright red, **oxygenated** blood from the heart to the body or to the lungs. (Exception: The pulmonary arteries bring dark red-purple, deoxygenated blood from the heart to the lungs.)	**arteri/o-** *artery* **arter/o-** *artery* **oxygen/o-** *oxygen*
bifurcation	Area where the abdominal aorta ends as it divides into two branches: the right and left iliac arteries	**bifurcat/o-** *divide into two branches*
blood vessels	Large and small **vascular** channels through which the blood flows. These include arteries, arterioles, capillaries, venules, and veins.	**angi/o-** *blood vessel; lymphatic vessel* **vascul/o-** *blood vessel* **vas/o-** *blood vessel; vas deferens*
capillary	Smallest blood vessel in the body. A capillary network connects the arterioles to the venules.	**capill/o-** *capillary; hair-like structure*
endothelium	Smooth layer that lines the inner wall of a blood vessel. Also known as the **intima**.	**theli/o-** *cellular layer*
lumen	Central opening inside a blood vessel through which blood flows	
pulse	The bulging of the wall of an artery located near the surface as blood is pumped by the heart	
vasculature	Blood vessels associated with a specific organ. Example: The vasculature of the stomach includes the gastric artery, capillaries, and gastric vein.	**vascul/o-** *blood vessel*
vasoconstriction	Contraction of smooth muscle in the wall of an artery that causes the lumen to decrease in size and the pressure in the artery to increase	**vas/o-** *blood vessel; vas deferens* **constrict/o-** *drawn together; narrowed*
vasodilation	Relaxation of smooth muscle in the wall of an artery that causes the lumen to increase in size and the pressure in the artery to decrease	**vas/o-** *blood vessel; vas deferens* **dilat/o-** *dilate; widen*
vein	Blood vessel that brings dark red-purple, **deoxygenated** blood from the body back to the heart. (Exception: The pulmonary veins bring bright red, oxygenated blood from the lungs to the heart.) The largest veins have valves that keep the blood flowing in one direction—back to the heart.	**ven/o-** *vein* **phleb/o-** *vein* **oxygen/o-** *oxygen*
venule	Smaller branch of a vein	**ven/o-** *vein*
Arteries		
aorta	Largest artery. It receives oxygenated blood from the left ventricle. It consists of the **ascending aorta**, the **aortic arch**, the **thoracic aorta**, and the **abdominal aorta**.	**aort/o-** *aorta* **thorac/o-** *chest; thorax* **abdomin/o-** *abdomen*
axillary artery	Artery that brings oxygenated blood to the axilla (armpit) area. It continues as the brachial artery.	**axill/o-** *armpit; axilla*
brachial artery	Artery that brings oxygenated blood to the upper arm. It ends as it divides into the radial and ulnar arteries.	**brachi/o-** *arm*
carotid artery	Artery that brings oxygenated blood to the neck, face, head, and brain. If these arteries are blocked, the lack of blood to the brain will cause a person to lose consciousness.	**carot/o-** *loss of consciousness*
coronary artery	Artery that is the first to branch off from the ascending aorta. It brings oxygenated blood to the myocardium.	**coron/o-** *structure that encircles like a crown*

Word or Phrase	Description	Combining Forms
femoral artery	Artery that brings oxygenated blood to the upper leg (along the femur bone). It continues as the popliteal artery.	**femor/o-** *femur; thigh bone*
gastric artery	Artery that brings oxygenated blood to the stomach	**gastr/o-** *stomach*
hepatic artery	Artery that brings oxygenated blood to the liver	**hepat/o-** *liver*
iliac artery	Artery that brings oxygenated blood to the hip and groin areas. It continues as the femoral artery.	**ili/o-** *ilium*
peroneal artery	Artery that brings oxygenated blood to the little toe side of the lower leg (along the fibula bone)	**perone/o-** *fibula*
popliteal artery	Artery that brings oxygenated blood to the back of the knee. It ends as it divides into the tibial and peroneal arteries.	**poplite/o-** *back of the knee*
pulmonary artery	Artery that brings **deoxygenated** blood from the right ventricle to the lungs. The pulmonary artery is the only artery that carries deoxygenated blood.	**pulmon/o-** *lung* **oxygen/o-** *oxygen*
radial artery	Artery that brings oxygenated blood to the thumb side of the lower arm (along the radius bone)	**radi/o-** *forearm bone; radius; x-rays*
renal artery	Artery that brings oxygenated blood to the kidney	**ren/o-** *kidney*
subclavian artery	Artery that brings oxygenated blood to the shoulder. It goes underneath (*sub-*) the clavicle (collarbone) and then becomes the axillary artery.	**clav/o-** *clavicle; collarbone*
tibial artery	Artery that brings oxygenated blood to the front and back of the lower leg (along the tibia bone)	**tibi/o-** *shin bone; tibia*
ulnar artery	Artery that brings oxygenated blood to the little finger side of the lower arm (along the ulna bone)	**uln/o-** *forearm bone; ulna*
Veins		
fibular vein	Vein that brings deoxygenated blood from the little toe side of the lower leg to the femoral vein	**fibul/o-** *fibula*
jugular vein	Vein that brings deoxygenated blood from the head and neck to the superior vena cava	**jugul/o-** *throat*
portal vein	Vein that brings deoxygenated blood from the intestines and liver to the inferior vena cava	**port/o-** *point of entry*
pulmonary vein	Vein that brings **oxygenated** blood from the lungs to the left atrium. The pulmonary vein is the only vein that carries oxygenated blood.	**pulmon/o-** *lung* **oxygen/o-** *oxygen*
saphenous vein	Vein that brings deoxygenated blood from the lower leg to the femoral vein	**saphen/o-** *clearly visible*
vena cava	The **superior vena cava** is a large vein that brings deoxygenated blood from the head, neck, chest, and arms to the right atrium of the heart. The **inferior vena cava** is a large vein that brings deoxygenated blood from the abdomen, pelvis, and legs to the right atrium.	
Circulation		
cardiopulmonary	Pertaining to the heart and lungs	**cardi/o-** *heart* **pulmon/o-** *lung*
ductus arteriosus	Temporary blood vessel in the fetal heart that connects the left pulmonary arteries to the descending aorta. This allows oxygenated blood from the mother to bypass the not-yet-functioning lungs and to the body. The ductus arteriosus closes sometime after birth.	**arteri/o-** *artery*

Word or Phrase	Description	Combining Forms
foramen ovale	Temporary, small, oval opening in the septum between the atria in the fetal heart. It allows some of the oxygenated blood from the mother to enter the left side of the fetal heart and be circulated throughout the body. The foramen ovale closes sometime after birth.	
pulmonary circulation	Arteries, arterioles, capillaries, venules, and veins going to, within, and coming from the lungs	**pulmon/o-** *lung*
systemic circulation	Arteries, arterioles, capillaries, venules, and veins everywhere in the body, except in the lungs	**system/o-** *body as a whole*
Conduction System		
atrioventricular (AV) node	Small area of tissue in the lower right atrium. The AV node is part of the conduction system of the heart and receives electrical impulses from the SA node.	**atri/o-** *atrium; chamber that is open at the top* **ventricul/o-** *chamber that is filled; ventricle*
bundle branches	Part of the conduction system of the heart that branches out from the bundle of His into right and left segments in the ventricular septum	
bundle of His	Part of the conduction system of the heart after the AV node. It splits into the right and left bundle branches.	
conduction system	System that carries the electrical impulses that make the heart beat in a regular and coordinated rhythm. It consists of the SA node, AV node, bundle of His, bundle branches, and Purkinje fibers.	**conduct/o-** *carrying; conveying*
depolarization	Movement of positive sodium ions (Na^+) and positive calcium ions (Ca^{++}) into the myocardial cell followed by the release of positive calcium ions stored in the cell. This causes a contraction of the myocardium.	**polar/o-** *negative state; positive state*
diastole	Resting period between contractions of the heart as the heart again fills with blood	**diastol/o-** *dilating*
ectopic site	Area within the heart that can produce an electrical impulse but is not part of the conduction system. It sometimes overrides the impulse of the SA node and produces an abnormal heart rhythm.	**ectop/o-** *outside*
epinephrine	Hormone from the adrenal glands that causes the heart to beat much faster during times of exercise or emergencies	
normal sinus rhythm	Rhythm of contractions that occurs when the SA node is in control of the heart rate	
Purkinje fibers	A network of nerves in the walls of the ventricles that are a continuation of the right and left bundle branches	
refractory period	Short period of time following repolarization when the myocardial cell cannot respond to an electrical impulse from the SA node	**fract/o-** *bend; break up*
repolarization	Movement of positive potassium ions (K^+), sodium ions (Na^+), and some calcium ions (Ca^{++}) out of the cell; the rest of the calcium ions go back into storage within the cell. The myocardial cell returns to its normal resting state.	**polar/o-** *negative state; positive state*
sinoatrial (SA) node	Small area of tissue in the posterior wall of the upper right atrium. The SA node is the pacemaker of the heart because it initiates the electrical impulse that begins each heartbeat.	**sin/o-** *channel; hollow cavity* **atri/o-** *atrium; chamber that is open at the top*
systole	**Contraction** of the atria and the ventricles	**systol/o-** *contracting* **contract/o-** *pull together*

5.3 Diseases

Word or Phrase	Description	Pronunciation/Word Parts

Heart

Word or Phrase	Description	Pronunciation/Word Parts

acute coronary syndrome	Condition that occurs if the flow of oxygenated blood through a coronary artery to the myocardium is blocked by a blood clot or atherosclerosis. Acute coronary syndrome includes acute **ischemia** of the myocardium, heart attack, or unstable angina.
	Treatment: Nitroglycerin drug; thrombolytic drug if there is a blood clot; oxygen therapy
		ischemia (is-KEE-mee-ah)
		  isch/o- *block; keep back*
		  -emia *condition of the blood; substance in the blood*

angina pectoris	Chest pain. This is a warning sign that the myocardium is not receiving enough oxygenated blood (see Figure 5-14 ■). It occurs when atherosclerosis blocks the flow of oxygenated blood through the coronary arteries to the myocardium. **Anginal** pain is a crushing, squeezing, heaviness, or pressure-like sensation in the chest, with pain that sometimes extends up to the jaw, teeth, neck, back, or down the left arm, often with sweating (diaphoresis) and a sense of doom. Angina pectoris can occur during exercise, stress, after a heavy meal, or even while resting.
	Treatment: Nitroglycerin drug, beta-blocker drug, calcium channel blocker drug; oxygen therapy
		angina (an-JY-nah)
		
		pectoris (PEK-toh-rihs)
		
		anginal (an-JY-nal)
		  angin/o- *angina*
		  -al *pertaining to*
		The combining form **pector/o-** means *chest*.

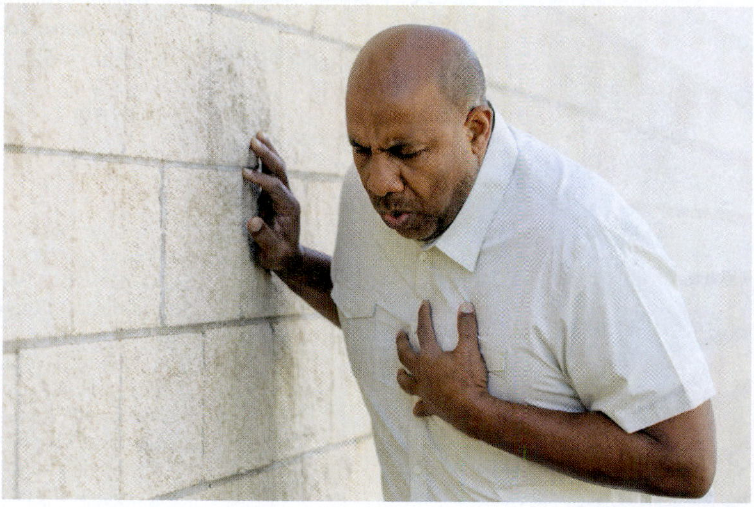

FIGURE 5-14 ■ Angina pectoris. Angina can occur with exercise or stress, after a heavy meal, or even with minimal activity.

Clinical Connections

Public Health. For many years, newspaper and magazine articles described the classic symptoms of angina pectoris in order to raise public awareness and encourage those with angina to promptly seek medical help. Now it is known that those symptoms occur in men, but women can experience angina pectoris as indigestion, nausea, or feeling out of breath.

Word or Phrase	Description	Pronunciation/Word Parts

cardiomegaly	Enlargement of the heart, usually due to congestive heart failure
	Treatment: Correct the underlying cause.
		cardiomegaly (KAR-dee-oh-MEG-ah-lee)
		  cardi/o- *heart*
		  -megaly *enlargement*

cardiomyopathy	Condition of the heart muscle that includes cardiomegaly and heart failure. In some patients, the myocardium around the left ventricle is dilated and stretched so thin that it can no longer contract to pump blood.
	Treatment: Treat the heart failure.
		cardiomyopathy (KAR-dee-oh-my-AW-pah-thee)
		  cardi/o- *heart*
		  my/o- *muscle*
		  -pathy *disease*

Word or Phrase	Description	Pronunciation/Word Parts
congestive heart failure (CHF)	Inability of the heart to pump sufficient amounts of blood. It is caused by coronary artery disease or hypertension. During the early stages of CHF, the myocardium undergoes **hypertrophy** (enlargement). This temporarily improves its ability to pump the blood. In the later stages of CHF, the heart cannot enlarge anymore. Instead, the myocardium becomes flabby and loses its ability to contract. • Right-sided congestive heart failure. The right ventricle cannot adequately pump blood. This causes blood to back up in the superior vena cava, resulting in **jugular venous distention** (dilated jugular veins in the neck). Blood also backs up in the inferior vena cava, resulting in hepatomegaly (enlargement of the liver) and **peripheral edema** in the legs, ankles, and feet as fluid leaves the blood and enters the tissues (see Figure 5-15 ■). • Left-sided congestive heart failure. The left ventricle cannot adequately pump blood. This causes blood to back up in the lungs. Fluid leaves the blood, and this causes pulmonary edema that can be seen on a chest x-ray. There is also shortness of breath, cough, and an inability to sleep while lying flat. Treatment: ACE inhibitor drug, digitalis drug, diuretic drug. Severe left-sided heart failure is life-threatening; it may require surgery for a heart transplantation or a left-ventricular assist device (LVAD).	**congestive** (con-JES-tiv) **congest/o-** *accumulation of fluid* **-ive** *pertaining to* **hypertrophy** (hy-PER-troh-fee) The prefix **hyper-** means *above; more than normal.* The suffix **-trophy** means *process of development.* **jugular** (JUG-yoo-lar) **jugul/o-** *throat* **-ar** *pertaining to* **venous** (VEE-nuhs) **ven/o-** *vein* **-ous** *pertaining to* **distention** (dis-TEN-shun) **distent/o-** *distended; stretched* **-ion** *action; condition* **peripheral** (peh-RIF-eh-ral) **peripher/o-** *outer aspects* **-al** *pertaining to* **edema** (eh-DEE-mah)

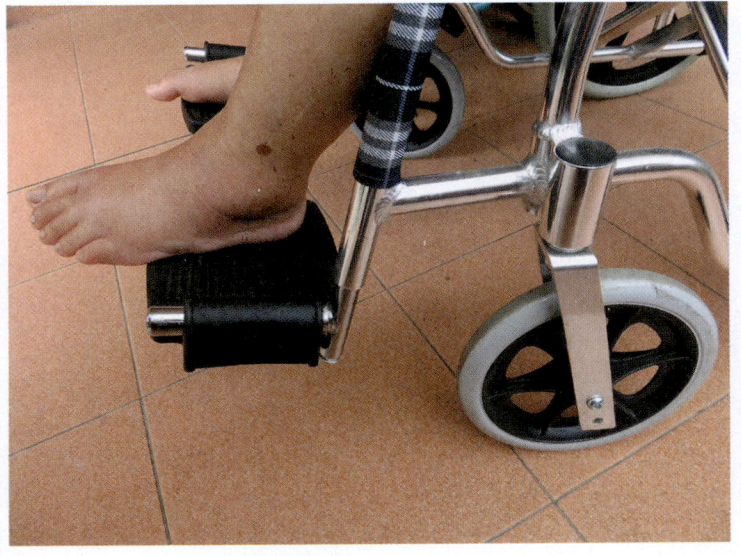

FIGURE 5-15 ■ Peripheral edema. Soft tissue swelling in the feet and lower legs can be a sign of right-sided congestive heart failure. The physician will also examine the patient's neck to look for distention of the jugular veins, another sign of right-sided congestive heart failure. The physician will use a stethoscope to listen to the lungs to detect pulmonary edema, which is a sign of left-sided heart failure.

Word or Phrase	Description	Pronunciation/Word Parts
endocarditis	Bacterial infection and inflammation of the endocardium lining of a heart valve. This occurs in patients who have a structural defect of the valve. Bacteria from an infection elsewhere in the body travel through the blood, are trapped by the structural defect, and cause infection. Acute endocarditis causes a high fever and shock, while **subacute bacterial endocarditis (SBE)** causes fever, fatigue, and aching muscles. Treatment: Antibiotic drug	**endocarditis** (EN-doh-kar-DY-tihs) **end/o-** *innermost; within* **card/o-** *heart* **-itis** *infection of; inflammation of* **subacute** (SUB-ah-KYOOT) The prefix **sub-** means *below; underneath; less than.* Subacute: *Less than acute*
mitral valve prolapse (MVP)	Structural abnormality in which the leaflets of the mitral valve do not close tightly. This can be a congenital condition or can occur if the valve is damaged by infection. There is **regurgitation** as blood flows back into the left atrium with each contraction. Treatment: Valvuloplasty or valve replacement surgery	**prolapse** (PROH-laps) **regurgitation** (ree-GER-jih-TAY-shun) **regurgit/o-** *backward flow* **-ation** *being; having; process*

Word or Phrase	Description	Pronunciation/Word Parts
murmur	Abnormal heart sound created by turbulence as blood leaks through a defective heart valve. Murmurs are described according to their volume (soft or loud), when they occur, and their sound. A murmur can sound like the call of a sea gull, blowing wind, machinery, musical notes, humming, or clicking. Treatment: Mild murmurs do not need treatment; valvuloplasty or valve replacement surgery for a severe murmur	**murmur** (MER-mer)

myocardial infarction (MI)	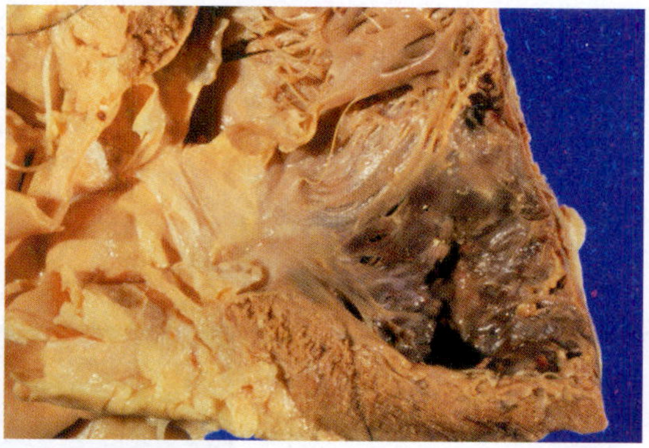 Death of myocardial cells due to a severe lack of oxygenated blood to the myocardium (see Figure 5-16 ■). Also known as a **heart attack**. The flow of oxygenated blood in a coronary artery is blocked by a blood clot or by atherosclerosis. The patient may experience angina pectoris, have mild symptoms similar to indigestion, or have no symptoms at all (a silent MI). The infarcted area of myocardium has dead tissue, the condition of **necrosis**. If the area of necrosis is small, it will eventually be replaced by scar tissue. If the area is large, the heart muscle may be unable to contract, and the patient will die.
	Prevention: Baby aspirin taken daily to prevent an MI or at the first sign of an MI
	Treatment: Thrombolytic drug to dissolve a blood clot during an MI
		myocardial (MY-oh-KAR-dee-al)
		  my/o- _muscle_
		  cardi/o- _heart_
		  -al _pertaining to_
		
		infarction (in-FARK-shun)
		  infarct/o- _small area of dead tissue_
		  -ion _action; condition_
		
		necrosis (neh-KROH-sihs)
		  necr/o- _dead body; dead tissue_
		  -osis _abnormal condition; process_

FIGURE 5-16 ■ Myocardial infarction.
This heart was cut open during an autopsy. It shows dead tissue (necrosis) that died because of a myocardial infarction and a lack of oxygenated blood to that part of the heart muscle.

Word or Phrase	Description	Pronunciation/Word Parts

pericarditis	Infection or inflammation of the pericardial sac that causes a buildup of pericardial fluid. When the fluid compresses the heart to the point that it cannot pump blood to the body, this is known as **cardiac tamponade**.
	Treatment: Antibiotic drug; surgery to remove the fluid (pericardiocentesis)
		pericarditis (PAIR-ee-kar-DY-tihs)
		  peri- _around_
		  card/o- _heart_
		  -itis _infection of; inflammation of_
		
		tamponade (TAM-poh-NAYD)
		  tampon/o- _stop up_
		  -ade _action; process_

rheumatic heart disease	An autoimmune response to a bacterial streptococcal infection, such as strep throat. The body makes antibodies to fight the infection, but the antibodies also attack other areas of the body, particularly the joints and the heart. The joints become inflamed and are swollen with fluid. The mitral and aortic valves of the heart become inflamed and are damaged. Rheumatic heart disease occurs most often in children and is known as _rheumatic fever_.
	Treatment: Antibiotic drug to treat the initial infection; valve replacement surgery. After rheumatic heart disease has occurred, a prophylactic (preventive) antibiotic drug is given prior to any dental or surgical procedure that might release bacteria that could further damage the valves.
		rheumatic (roo-MAT-ik)
		  rheumat/o- _watery discharge_
		  -ic _pertaining to_

Word or Phrase	Description	Pronunciation/Word Parts

Clinical Connections

Neonatology. These congenital abnormalities can occur in the fetal heart as it develops.

- **Atrial septal defect**. An opening in the interatrial septum that allows abnormal circulation of blood.
- **Coarctation of the aorta**. The aorta is abnormally narrow.
- **Tetralogy of Fallot**. There are four different heart defects.
- **Ventricular septal defect**. An opening in the interventricular septum that allows abnormal circulation of blood.

The following abnormalities occur at the time of birth during the change from fetal circulation to normal newborn circulation.

- **Patent ductus arteriosus**. The ductus arteriosus fails to close.
- **Patent foramen ovale**. The foramen ovale fails to close.

coarctation (KOH-ark-TAY-shun)
  coarct/o- *narrowed*
  -ation *being; having; process*

tetralogy (teh-TRAL-oh-jee)
  tetr/a- *four*
  -logy *study of; word*

Fallot (fah-LOH)

patent (PAY-tent)
  pat/o- *open*
  -ent *pertaining to*

Blood Vessels

| aneurysm | Area of dilation and weakness in the wall of an artery (see Figure 5-17 ■). With each heartbeat, the weakened artery wall balloons outward. An aneurysm can rupture without warning. A **dissecting aneurysm** is one that enlarges by tunneling between the layers of the artery wall.
Treatment: Surgery to place a metal clip on the aneurysm to stop blood from flowing through it; coil embolization procedure to insert a metal coil within the aneurysm to create a blood clot there; removal of a large aneurysm (aneurysmectomy) and replacement with a synthetic tubular graft | **aneurysm** (AN-yoor-izm)
The combining form **aneurysm/o-** means *aneurysm; dilation.*

dissecting (dy-SEK-ting)
  dissect/o- *cut apart*
  -ing *doing* |

NORMAL ABDOMINAL AORTA

ABDOMINAL AORTIC ANEURYSM

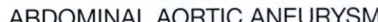
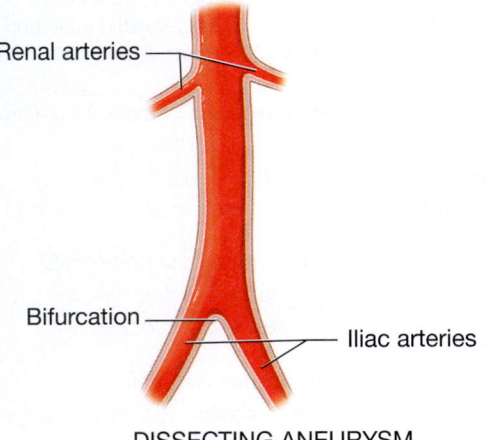

Renal arteries

Bifurcation — Iliac arteries

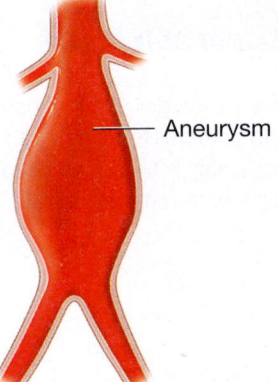

Aneurysm

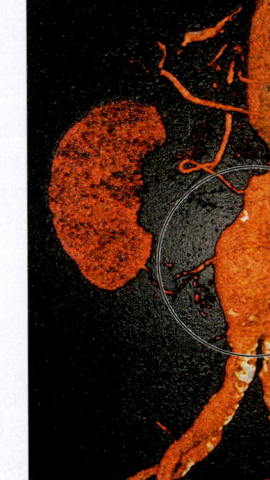

DISSECTING ANEURYSM

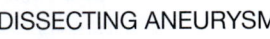
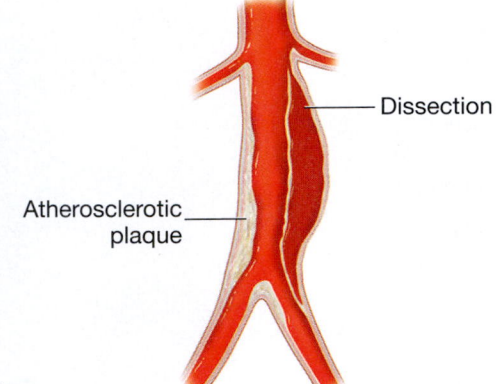

Dissection

Atherosclerotic plaque

B.

A.

FIGURE 5-17 ■ Aneurysm.
A. A normal abdominal aorta, a large abdominal aortic aneurysm, and a dissecting aneurysm that has tunneled between and separated the atherosclerotic plaque from the artery wall. **B.** This colorized CT scan shows a large abdominal aortic aneurysm below the renal arteries to the kidneys but above the bifurcation where the right and left iliac arteries begin.

Word or Phrase	Description	Pronunciation/Word Parts

arteriosclerosis	Degenerative changes over time produce hardened artery walls. Normally, the artery wall is flexible because it contains elastin. As a person ages, the arteries lose elastin and become hard and inflexible. This increases the blood pressure. An artery with arteriosclerosis is said to be **arteriosclerotic**. Also known as **arteriosclerotic cardiovascular disease (ASCVD)**.
	Treatment: Antihypertensive drug
		arteriosclerosis
		(ar-TEER-ee-OH-skleh-ROH-sihs)
		  arteri/o- *artery*
		  scler/o- *hard; sclera*
		  -osis *abnormal condition;*
		    process
		
		arteriosclerotic
		(ar-TEER-ee-OH-skleh-RAW-tik)
		  arteri/o- *artery*
		  scler/o- *hard; sclera*
		  -tic *pertaining to*

atherosclerosis	Fatty deposits in the walls of the arteries that can restrict the flow of blood. Atherosclerosis is a specific type of arteriosclerosis. Atherosclerosis begins with a small tear in the endothelium caused by chronic hypertension, usually related to arteriosclerosis. Then low-density lipoproteins (LDLs) in the blood deposit cholesterol in the tear, and this begins to form an **atheroma** or **atheromatous plaque** inside the artery (see Figure 5-18 ■). As plaque grows on the artery wall, it makes the lumen narrower and narrower. The rough edges of the plaque can also trap red blood cells and form a blood clot.
	
	    Eventually, fatty plaque can completely block the lumen of the artery. In the carotid arteries to the brain, this can cause a stroke. In the coronary arteries to the heart muscle, this can cause angina pectoris and a myocardial infarction. In the renal arteries to the kidney, this can cause kidney failure.
	Treatment: Lipid-lowering drug (also known as a "statin" drug); angioplasty or a stent to press down the plaque or an endarterectomy to remove the plaque
		atherosclerosis
		(ATH-eh-ROH-skleh-ROH-sihs)
		  ather/o- *soft, fatty substance*
		  scler/o- *hard; sclera*
		  -osis *abnormal condition;*
		    process
		
		atheroma (ATH-eh-ROH-mah)
		  ather/o- *soft, fatty substance*
		  -oma *mass; tumor*
		
		atheromatous
		(ATH-eh-ROH-mah-tuhs)
		  atheromat/o- *fatty deposit;*
		    fatty mass
		  -ous *pertaining to*
		
		plaque (PLAK)

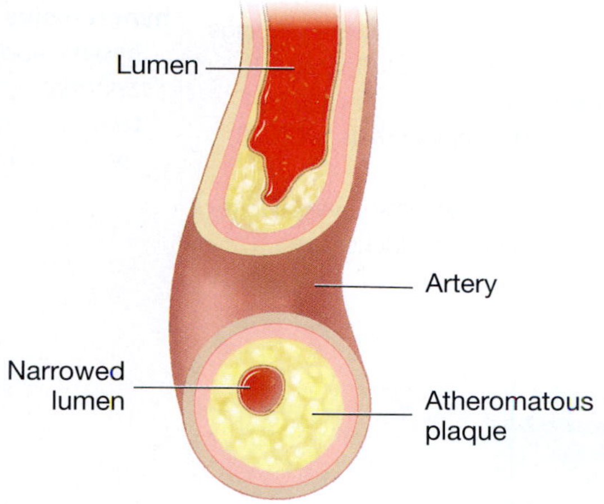

Lumen

Artery

Narrowed lumen

Atheromatous plaque

FIGURE 5-18 ■ Severe atherosclerotic plaque in an artery. The lumen of this artery is so narrowed by atheromatous plaque that little oxygenated blood can flow through it.

Word or Phrase	Description	Pronunciation/Word Parts
bruit	A harsh, rushing sound made by turbulent blood as it passes through an artery that is narrowed by arteriosclerosis or atherosclerosis. The bruit can be heard when a stethoscope is placed over the artery. Treatment: Correct the underlying cause.	**bruit** (BROO-ee)

coronary artery disease (CAD)	Arteriosclerosis of the coronary arteries. They contain atheromatous plaque, and their narrowed lumens cannot carry enough oxygenated blood to the myocardium. This causes angina pectoris. Severe atherosclerosis (or a blood clot that forms on an atherosclerotic plaque) can completely block the lumen of a coronary artery and cause a myocardial infarction.
	Treatment: Lipid-lowering drug (also known as a "statin" drug); percutaneous transluminal coronary angioplasty (PTCA) or a coronary artery bypass graft (CABG)
		coronary
		  coron/o- *structure that*
		    encircles like a crown
		  -ary *pertaining to*

Word or Phrase	Description	Pronunciation/Word Parts

hyperlipidemia	Elevated levels of lipids (fats) in the blood. Lipids include cholesterol and triglycerides. **Hypercholesterolemia** is an elevated level of cholesterol in the blood. **Hypertriglyceridemia** is an elevated level of triglycerides in the blood. Treatment: Lipid-lowering drug (also known as a "statin" drug)	**hyperlipidemia**
		(HY-per-LIP-ih-DEE-mee-ah)
		  hyper- *above; more than*
		    normal
		  lipid/o- *fat; lipid*
		  -emia *condition of the blood;*
		    substance in the blood
		
		hypercholesterolemia
		(HY-per-koh-LES-ter-awl-EE-mee-ah)
		  hyper- *above; more than*
		    normal
		  cholesterol/o- *cholesterol*
		  -emia *condition of the blood;*
		    substance in the blood
		
		hypertriglyceridemia
		(HY-per-try-GLIS-eh-ry-DEE-mee-ah)
		  hyper- *above; more than*
		    normal
		  triglycerid/o- *triglyceride*
		  -emia *condition of the blood;*
		    substance in the blood

hypertension (HTN)	Elevated blood pressure (see Figure 5-19 ■). Essential hypertension, the most common type of hypertension, is one in which the exact cause is not known. Secondary hypertension has a known cause, such as kidney disease. Normal blood pressure in an adult is less than 120/80 mm Hg. Several blood pressure readings, not just one, are needed to make a diagnosis of hypertension.
	• **Hypertension** consists of higher-than-normal blood pressure readings that are categorized in several successive stages (elevated, Stage 1, Stage 2). The patient is said to be **hypertensive**.
	• **Hypertensive crisis**, a blood pressure reading higher than 180/120, requires immediate medical intervention.
	Treatment: Lifestyle changes (decreased salt intake, exercise, weight loss); ACE inhibitor drug, beta-blocker drug, calcium channel blocker drug, diuretic drug
		hypertension (HY-per-TEN-shun)
		  hyper- *above; more than*
		    normal
		  tens/o- *pressure*
		  -ion *action; condition*
		
		hypertensive (HY-per-TEN-siv)
		  hyper- *above; more than*
		    normal
		  tens/o- *pressure*
		  -ive *pertaining to*

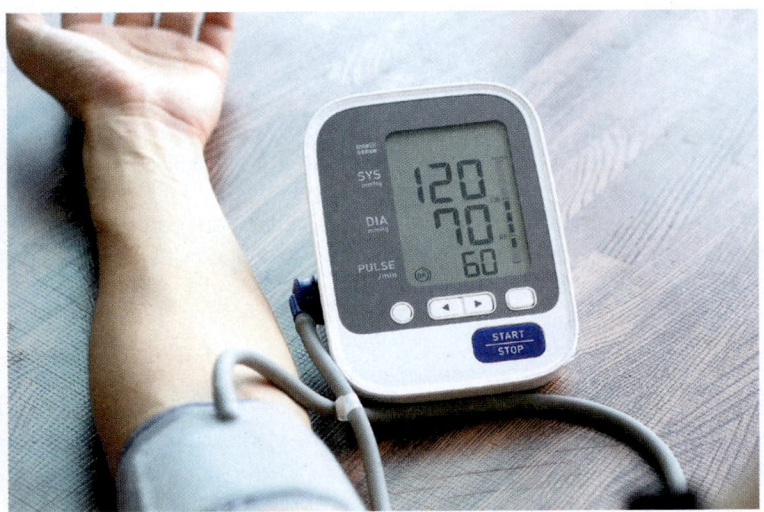

FIGURE 5-19 ■ **Hypertension.**
The American Heart Association recommends home self-monitoring of blood pressure with an automatic device to check the effectiveness of continuing treatment for hypertension in between visits to the doctor.

Word or Phrase	Description	Pronunciation/Word Parts

Dive Deeper

The American College of Cardiology and the American Heart Association issued new guidelines for blood pressure and hypertension in 2017. Normal blood pressure is now anything **less than 120/80.** The new guidelines are illustrated here.

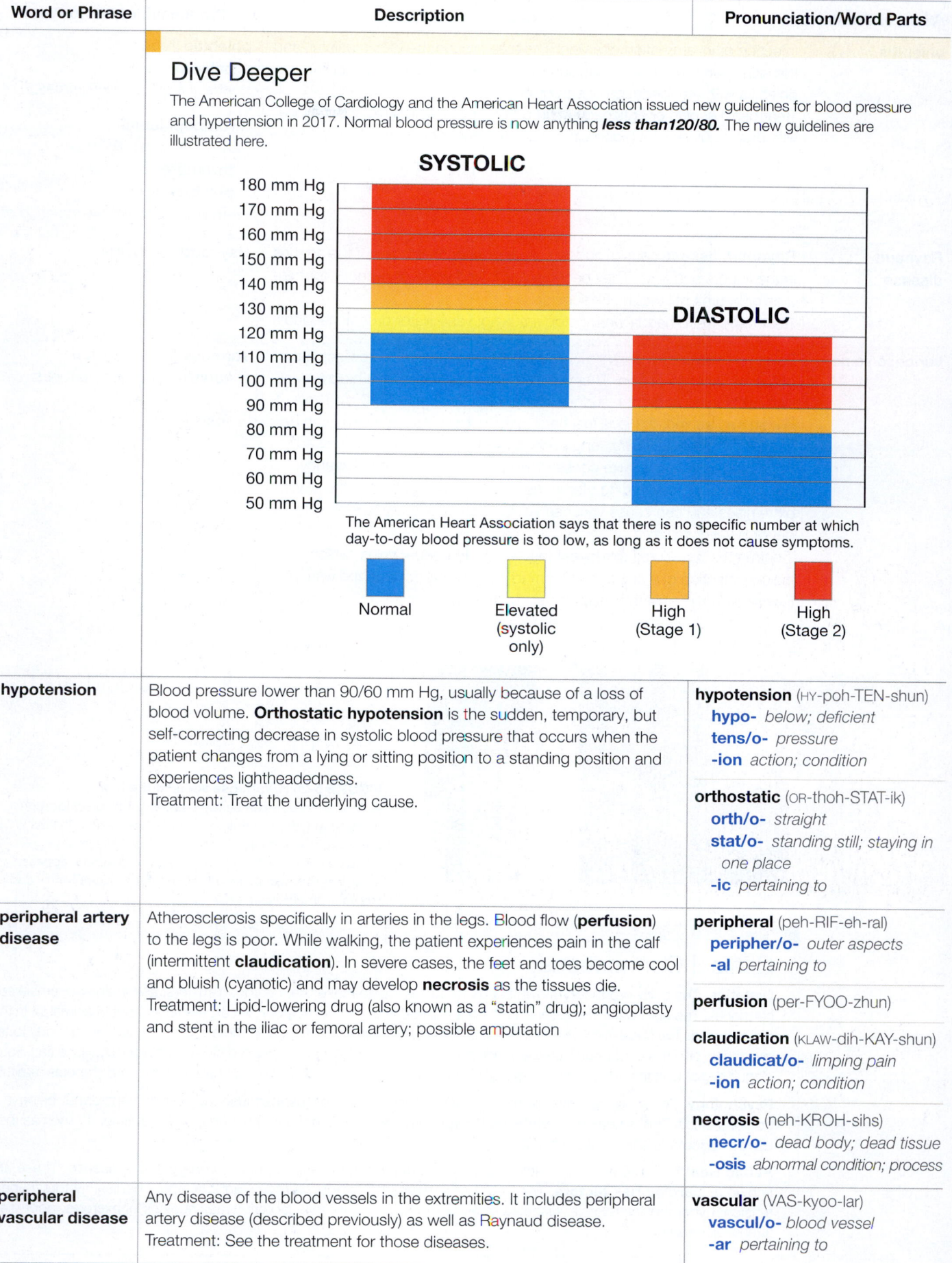

The American Heart Association says that there is no specific number at which day-to-day blood pressure is too low, as long as it does not cause symptoms.

Normal   Elevated (systolic only)   High (Stage 1)   High (Stage 2)

Word or Phrase	Description	Pronunciation/Word Parts

hypotension	Blood pressure lower than 90/60 mm Hg, usually because of a loss of blood volume. **Orthostatic hypotension** is the sudden, temporary, but self-correcting decrease in systolic blood pressure that occurs when the patient changes from a lying or sitting position to a standing position and experiences lightheadedness.
	Treatment: Treat the underlying cause.
		hypotension (HY-poh-TEN-shun)
		  hypo- *below; deficient*
		  tens/o- *pressure*
		  -ion *action; condition*
		
		orthostatic (OR-thoh-STAT-ik)
		  orth/o- *straight*
		  stat/o- *standing still; staying in one place*
		  -ic *pertaining to*

peripheral artery disease	Atherosclerosis specifically in arteries in the legs. Blood flow (**perfusion**) to the legs is poor. While walking, the patient experiences pain in the calf (intermittent **claudication**). In severe cases, the feet and toes become cool and bluish (cyanotic) and may develop **necrosis** as the tissues die.
	Treatment: Lipid-lowering drug (also known as a "statin" drug); angioplasty and stent in the iliac or femoral artery; possible amputation
		peripheral (peh-RIF-eh-ral)
		  peripher/o- *outer aspects*
		  -al *pertaining to*
		
		perfusion (per-FYOO-zhun)
		
		claudication (KLAW-dih-KAY-shun)
		  claudicat/o- *limping pain*
		  -ion *action; condition*
		
		necrosis (neh-KROH-sihs)
		  necr/o- *dead body; dead tissue*
		  -osis *abnormal condition; process*

peripheral vascular disease	Any disease of the blood vessels in the extremities. It includes peripheral artery disease (described previously) as well as Raynaud disease.
	Treatment: See the treatment for those diseases.
		vascular (VAS-kyoo-lar)
		  vascul/o- *blood vessel*
		  -ar *pertaining to*

Word or Phrase	Description	Pronunciation/Word Parts
phlebitis	Infection or inflammation of a vein. The area around the vein is painful, and the skin overlying the vein may show a red streak. **Thrombophlebitis** is phlebitis with the formation of a thrombus (blood clot). Treatment: Aspirin or anticoagulant drug to prevent blood clots; thrombolytic drug to dissolve a blood clot; antibiotic drug for infection	**phlebitis** (fleh-BY-tihs) **phleb/o-** *vein* **-itis** *infection of; inflammation of* **thrombophlebitis** (THRAWM-boh-fleh-BY-tihs) **thromb/o-** *blood clot* **phleb/o-** *vein* **-itis** *infection of; inflammation of*
Raynaud disease	**Raynaud disease** causes sudden, severe vasoconstriction of the arteries in the fingers and toes. They become numb and white or cyanotic for minutes or hours until the attack subsides. Treatment: Keep hands warm; stop smoking; vasodilator drug, if needed	**Raynaud** (ray-NOH)
varicose veins	Damaged valves in a vein allow blood to flow backward and collect in the preceding section of vein. That vein becomes distended with blood, twisting and bulging under the surface of the skin (see Figure 5-20 ■). There is pain and aching; the legs feel heavy and leaden. Varicose veins can be caused by phlebitis, injury, long periods of sitting with the legs crossed, or occupations that require constant standing. Also, during pregnancy, pressure from the enlarging uterus restricts the flow of blood in the lower extremities and can cause varicose veins. There is a family tendency to develop varicose veins. Treatment: Procedures to redirect the blood into deeper veins, which include injection of a solution or foam to harden and occlude the vein (sclerotherapy) or using a laser to destroy the vein	**varicose** (VAIR-ih-kohs) **varic/o-** *enlarged, tortuous vein; varix* **-ose** *full of*

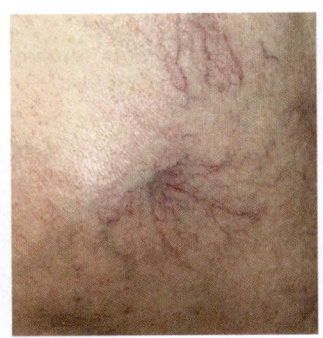 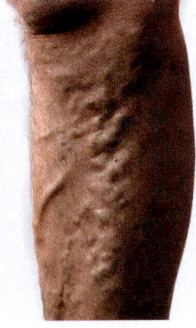

A.   B.

FIGURE 5-20 ■ Varicose veins in the leg.
A. Varicose veins can be tiny, flat, hair-like discolorations of the skin (spider veins). **B.** Protruding varicose veins are unsightly and easily injured. Patients often have varicose veins treated for an improved cosmetic appearance, but this also helps decrease the chance of injury and thrombophlebitis.

Clinical Connections

Dietetics. The body produces its own supply of cholesterol to make bile, neurotransmitters, and male and female sex hormones. The diet contains additional cholesterol in foods from animal sources. An excessive amount of animal fat in the diet increases the cholesterol level in the blood. An excessive amount of sugar in the diet is converted by the body to triglycerides, and this causes an increased triglyceride level in the blood and increased storage as adipose tissue (fat). Fatty plaque deposits in the arteries grow more quickly in patients who eat high-fat diets or have uncontrolled diabetes mellitus.

Psychology. Some people have increased blood pressure readings just because they are nervous about being in a doctor's office. This is known as **white-coat hypertension**. This is not a true hypertension because, as soon as they leave the doctor's office, their blood pressure returns to normal.

Public Health. There are many factors that contribute to the development of coronary artery disease. These are known as **cardiac risk factors**. They include demographic factors (heredity, gender, age), medical factors (hypertension, hypercholesterolemia, diabetes mellitus, obesity), and lifestyle factors (smoking, lack of exercise, poor diet, stress, alcoholism).

Word or Phrase	Description	Pronunciation/Word Parts

Conduction System

arrhythmia	Any type of irregular rate or rhythm of the heart. Arrhythmias include bradycardia, fibrillation, flutter, heart block, premature contraction, sick sinus syndrome, and tachycardia. Electrocardiography is performed to diagnose the type of arrhythmia (see Figure 5-21 ■). Treatment: Antiarrhythmic drug; cardioversion; or implanting a pacemaker in the chest, depending on the type of arrhythmia A. Bradycardia B. Normal sinus rhythm C. Ventricular tachycardia D. Ventricular fibrillation E. Asystole FIGURE 5-21 ■ **Arrhythmias on an ECG tracing.** **A.** Bradycardia with a heart rate of 60 beats per minute. **B.** A normal heart rate at 80 beats per minute. **C.** Ventricular tachycardia at 150 beats per minute. **D.** Ventricular fibrillation. **E.** Asystole is not an arrhythmia because there is no heartbeat.	**arrhythmia** (aa-RITH-mee-ah) **a-** *away from; without* **rrhythm/o-** *rhythm* **-ia** *condition; state; thing* Arrhythmia: *Condition (of being) without (a normal) rhythm*
bradycardia	Arrhythmia in which the heart beats too slowly. A patient with bradycardia is **bradycardic**. Treatment: Antiarrhythmic drug; surgery to insert a pacemaker	**bradycardia** (BRAD-ee-KAR-dee-ah) **brady-** *slow* **card/o-** *heart* **-ia** *condition; state; thing* **bradycardic** (BRAD-ee-KAR-dik) **brady-** *slow* **card/o-** *heart* **-ic** *pertaining to*
fibrillation	Arrhythmia in which there is a very fast, uncoordinated quivering of the myocardium. It can affect the atria or ventricles. Ventricular fibrillation ("V fib"), a life-threatening emergency in which the heart is unable to pump blood, can progress to cardiac arrest. Treatment: Defibrillation	**fibrillation** (FIB-rih-LAY-shun) **fibrill/o-** *muscle fiber; nerve fiber* **-ation** *being; having; process*
flutter	Arrhythmia in which there is a very fast but regular rhythm (250 beats per minute) of the atria or ventricles. The chambers of the heart do not have time to completely fill with blood before the next contraction. Flutter can progress to fibrillation. Treatment: Antiarrhythmic drug; cardioversion	
heart block	Arrhythmia in which electrical impulses from the SA node do not travel normally to the Purkinje fibers. The electrical impulses are delayed, or only some of them reach the ventricles. In complete heart block, no electrical impulses reach the ventricles. Treatment: Antiarrhythmic drug; surgery to insert a pacemaker	

Word or Phrase	Description	Pronunciation/Word Parts
premature contraction	Arrhythmia in which there are one or more extra contractions in between systole and diastole. The extra contraction is known as an **extrasystole**. There are two types of premature contractions: a **premature atrial contraction (PAC)** and a **premature ventricular contraction (PVC)**. A repeating pattern of one premature contraction followed by one normal contraction is **bigeminy**. A repeating pattern of one premature contraction followed by two normal contractions is **trigeminy**. Two premature contractions occurring together is a **couplet**. Treatment: Antiarrhythmic drug; surgery to insert a pacemaker	**contraction** (con-TRAK-shun) **contract/o-** *pull together* **-ion** *action; condition* **extrasystole** (EKS-trah-SIS-toh-lee) **bigeminy** (by-JEM-ih-nee) The prefix **bi-** means *two*. The suffix -**geminy** means *action of pairing*. **trigeminy** (try-JEM-ih-nee) The prefix **tri-** means *three*. **couplet** (KUP-let)
sick sinus syndrome	Arrhythmia in which bradycardia alternates with tachycardia. It occurs when the sinoatrial node and an ectopic site elsewhere in the myocardium compete to be the heart's pacemaker. Treatment: Antiarrhythmic drug; surgery to insert a pacemaker	
tachycardia	Arrhythmia in which there is a fast but regular rhythm (up to 200 beats per minute). A patient with tachycardia is **tachycardic**. Treatment: Antiarrhythmic drug; cardioversion; surgery to insert a pacemaker	**tachycardia** (TAK-ih-KAR-dee-ah) **tachy-** *fast* **card/o-** *heart* **-ia** *condition; state; thing* **tachycardic** (TAK-ih-KAR-dik) **tachy-** *fast* **card/o-** *heart* **-ic** *pertaining to*
asystole	Complete absence of a heartbeat. Also known as **cardiac arrest**. Treatment: Cardiopulmonary resuscitation (CPR)	**asystole** (aa-SIS-toh-lee) The prefix **a-** means *away from; without*. The suffix **-systole** means *process of contracting*.
palpitation	An uncomfortable sensation felt in the chest during a premature contraction of the heart. It is often described as a "thump." Treatment: None, unless it becomes an arrhythmia	**palpitation** (PAL-pih-TAY-shun) **palpit/o-** *quick throbbing* **-ation** *being; having; process*

Word Alert
Sound-Alike Words

palpation	(noun)	a process of touching and feeling
	Example: Palpation allowed the physician to identify a tumor in the abdomen.	
palpitation	(noun)	being or having (the heart to) throb
	Example: Her occasional palpitations concerned the patient until the physician reassured her.	

5.3 PRACTICE LAPS

Use the Answer Key at the end of the book to check your answers.

A. Give the Meaning of Combining Forms

Next to each combining form, write its meaning. The first one has been done for you.

Combining Form	Meaning	Combining Form	Meaning
1. **angin/o-**	*angina*	12. pector/o-	
2. arteri/o-		13. peripher/o-	
3. ather/o-		14. phleb/o-	
4. claudicat/o-		15. regurgit/o-	
5. congest/o-		16. rrhythm/o-	
6. contract/o-		17. scler/o-	
7. coarct/o-		18. tens/o-	
8. infarct/o-		19. thromb/o-	
9. isch/o-		20. varic/o-	
10. lipid/o-		21. vascul/o-	
11. my/o-			

B. Build Words

Read the definition of the medical word. Look at the combining form that is given. Select the correct suffix from the Suffix List, and write it on the blank line. Then build the medical word, and write it on the line. (Remember: You may need to remove the combining vowel. Always remove the hyphens and slash.) Be sure to check your spelling.

Suffix List

-ation (being; having; process)	-ion (action; condition)	-megaly (enlargement)
-emia (condition of the blood;	-itis (infection of; inflammation of)	-oma (mass; tumor)
substance in the blood)	-ive (pertaining to)	-ose (full of)

Definition of the Medical Word	Combining Form	Suffix	Build the Medical Word
Example: Condition of the blood (being) block(ed from the tissues)	**isch/o-**	*-emia*	*ischemia*

[*You think* condition of the blood *(-emia)* + block; keep back *(isch/o-).* You change the order of the word parts to put the suffix last. You write ischemia.]

1. Enlargement (of the) heart	cardi/o-	_____	_____
2. Condition (of a) small area of dead tissue	infarct/o-	_____	_____
3. Having (a) narrowed (aorta)	coarct/o-	_____	_____
4. Pertaining to (an) accumulation of fluid	congest/o-	_____	_____
5. Mass (of a) soft, fatty substance	ather/o-	_____	_____
6. Infection of (or) inflammation of (a) vein	phleb/o-	_____	_____
7. Full of (blood in an) enlarged, tortuous vein	varic/o-	_____	_____
8. Having (a) quick throbbing	palpit/o-	_____	_____
9. Condition (of) limping pain	claudicat/o-	_____	_____

C. Define Abbreviations

1. CAD	_____	5. MVP	_____
2. CHF	_____	6. PAC	_____
3. HTN	_____	7. PVC	_____
4. MI	_____	8. SBE	_____

5.4 Laboratory, Diagnostic, and Radiologic Procedures

Word or Phrase	Description	Pronunciation/Word Parts

Laboratory Tests

Word or Phrase	Description	Pronunciation/Word Parts
cardiac enzymes	Blood test that measures the levels of two enzymes that are released into the blood when myocardial cells die during a myocardial infarction. (These enzymes are not released during angina pectoris.) The higher the levels, the more severe the myocardial infarction and the larger the area of infarction. These cardiac enzymes are measured every few hours for several days. • **Creatine kinase** is an enzyme found in heart, muscle, and brain cells. One specific type, the isoenzyme CK-MB, is found in the heart. The CK-MB level begins to rise 2–6 hours after a myocardial infarction. Also known as *creatine kinase*. • **Lactate dehydrogenase (LDH)** is found in many different cells, including the heart. The LDH level begins to rise 12 hours after a myocardial infarction. An elevated LDH can support the CK-MB results but cannot be the only basis for a diagnosis of myocardial infarction.	**enzyme** (EN-zime) The suffix **-ase** means *enzyme*. **creatine kinase** (KREE-ah-teen KY-nays) **lactate dehydrogenase** (LAK-tayt dee-HY-droh-jeh-NAYS)
C-reactive protein	Blood test that measures the level of inflammation in the body. Inflammation in other areas (such as a urinary tract infection) can produce inflammation of the walls of the blood vessels. This can lead to blood clot formation and a myocardial infarction.	
homocysteine	Blood test that measures the level of this amino acid, which can damage blood vessel walls. An elevated level increases the patient's risk of arteriosclerosis and a blood clot that can cause a heart attack or stroke. This test is included as part of a cardiac risk assessment.	**homocysteine** (HOH-moh-SIS-teen)
lipid profile	Blood test that provides a comprehensive picture of the blood levels of cholesterol and triglycerides and their **lipoprotein** carriers (HDL, LDL, VLDL). Normal blood level for cholesterol is below 200 mg/dL; triglycerides is below 150 mg/dL.	**lipid** (LIP-id) **lip/o-** *fat; lipid* **-id** *origin; resembling; source* **lipoprotein** (LIH-poh-PROH-teen)

Dive Deeper

Lipoproteins are carrier molecules that are produced in the liver. They transport lipids (fats such as cholesterol and triglycerides) in the blood. There are three types of lipoproteins. **High-density lipoprotein (HDL)** carries cholesterol to the liver where it is excreted in the bile. HDL is known by laypersons as "good cholesterol" (even though it is not actually cholesterol). An increased level of HDL is beneficial. **Low-density lipoprotein (LDL)** carries cholesterol but deposits it on the walls of the arteries, and so it is known as "bad cholesterol." **Very-low-density lipoprotein (VLDL)** carries triglycerides and deposits them on the walls of the arteries.

Word or Phrase	Description	Pronunciation/Word Parts
troponin	Blood test that measures the level of two proteins that are released into the blood when myocardial cells die. Troponin I and troponin T are found in myocardial cells and skeletal muscle cells. Cardiac troponin levels begin to rise 4–6 hours after a myocardial infarction. More importantly, they remain elevated for 1–2 weeks, so they can be used to diagnose a myocardial infarction many days after it occurred. Troponin levels are done in conjunction with the cardiac enzymes test (described previously).	**troponin** (TROH-poh-nin)

Word or Phrase	Description	Pronunciation/Word Parts

Diagnostic Procedures

cardiac catheterization	Procedure to study the anatomy and pressures in the heart. A catheter is inserted in the femoral or brachial vein. Also known as a "cardiac cath." • Right heart catheterization. The catheter is threaded to the right atrium and into the pulmonary artery to measure pressures in the right side of the heart and pulmonary artery. Indirect measurement of left heart pressures and cardiac output can also be made. • Left heart catheterization. The catheter is threaded to the left atrium. A contrast dye is injected to show any narrowed areas or blockages in the coronary arteries. If blockage of a coronary artery is present, an angioplasty can be performed at that time.	**catheterization** (KATH-eh-TER-ih-ZAY-shun) **catheter/o-** *catheter* **-ization** *process of creating; process of inserting; process of making*
cardiac exercise stress test	Procedure to evaluate the heart's response to exercise in patients who have chest pain, palpitations, or arrhythmias (see Figure 5-22 ■). The patient walks on a motorized treadmill (**treadmill exercise stress test**) or rides a stationary bicycle while an ECG is performed. The speed of the treadmill and the steepness of its incline (or the resistance of the bicycle) are gradually increased while the patient's heart rate, blood pressure, and ECG are monitored. The procedure is stopped if the patient complains of angina, palpitations, shortness of breath, or tiredness, or if the ECG pattern becomes abnormal. The patient's resting heart rate and maximum heart rate are compared to standards for other people of the same age and sex. Any abnormality in the ECG pattern is analyzed. A **pharmacologic stress test** is performed when the patient is unable to exercise. Instead of exercise, a vasodilator drug is given that will cause normal coronary arteries to dilate. Occluded arteries cannot dilate, and this stresses the heart and causes angina in a way that is similar to an exercise stress test.	**pharmacologic** (FAR-mah-koh-LAW-jik) **pharmac/o-** *drug; medicine* **log/o-** *study of; word* **-ic** *pertaining to*

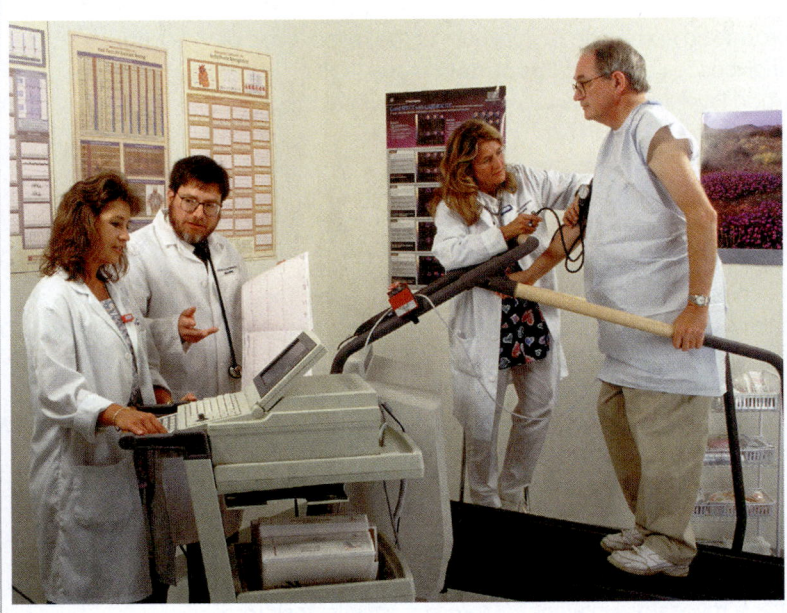

FIGURE 5-22 ■ Treadmill exercise stress test.
This patient is exercising on an inclined treadmill that can be adjusted to become steeper. Electrode patches on his chest pick up the electrical impulses of the heart. The cardiologist watches the computer screen for any arrhythmias. The nurse periodically checks the patient's blood pressure.

Word or Phrase	Description	Pronunciation/Word Parts

electrocardio-graphy (ECG, EKG)	Procedure that records the electrical activity of the heart (see Figure 5-23 ■). Electrodes (metal pieces in adhesive patches) are placed on the limbs (both arms and one leg) to send the electrical impulses of the heart to the ECG machine. These are the three limb leads (leads I–III). Electrodes placed on the chest are known as the **precordial** leads (V_1–V_6).
	• A 12-lead ECG records the electrical activity between different combinations of electrodes to give an electrical picture of the heart from 12 different angles. The record is an **electrocardiogram**.
	• A longer sample of just a single lead tracing (usually lead II) is a **rhythm strip**.
	Note: The *C* in *ECG* comes from the Latin word *cor* (heart). The *K* in *EKG* comes from the Greek word *kardia* (heart).
		electrocardiography
		(ee-LEK-troh-KAR-dee-AW-grah-fee)
		  electr/o- *electricity*
		  cardi/o- *heart*
		  -graphy *process of recording*
		
		precordial (pree-KOR-dee-al)
		The prefix **pre-** means *before; in front of (the heart)*.
		
		electrocardiogram
		(ee-LEK-troh-KAR-dee-oh-GRAM)
		  electr/o- *electricity*
		  cardi/o- *heart*
		  -gram *picture; record*

FIGURE 5-23 ■ Electrocardiography. This portable ECG machine was brought to the patient's bedside. Electrode patches attached to wire leads pick up the electrical impulses of the heart. Interpretation of an ECG includes the heart rate and rhythm and identifying abnormalities in the shape of the electrical pattern.

Word or Phrase	Description	Pronunciation/Word Parts

electrophysiology study	Procedure to map the heart's conduction system to pinpoint the ectopic site that is causing an arrhythmia. While an ECG is performed, catheters are inserted into the femoral vein and subclavian vein. x-rays are used to guide the catheters to the heart. The catheters send out electrical impulses to stimulate the heart and try to pinpoint the ectopic site.	**electrophysiology**
		(ee-LEK-troh-FIZ-ee-AW-loh-jee)
		  electr/o- *electricity*
		  physi/o- *physical function*
		  -logy *study of; word*

Holter monitor	Procedure to document arrhythmias that occur infrequently. The patient's heart rate and rhythm are continuously monitored as an outpatient for 24 hours. The patient wears five electrodes attached to a small portable ECG monitor (carried in a vest or placed in a pocket). The patient also keeps a diary of activities, meals, and symptoms during that time.	**Holter** (HOL-ter)

Word or Phrase	Description	Pronunciation/Word Parts
telemetry	Procedure to monitor a patient's heart rate and rhythm in the hospital. The patient wears electrodes connected to a device that continuously transmits an ECG recording to a central monitoring station in the coronary care unit (CCU) or intensive care unit. A nurse or telemetry technician constantly watches all of the patients' cardiac monitors.	**telemetry** (teh-LEM-eh-tree) **tele/o-** *distance* **-metry** *process of measuring*

Dive Deeper

The electrical image generated by the contraction and relaxation of the heart has a characteristic pattern of waves and a spike (see Figure 5-24 ■). The P wave corresponds to depolarization of the SA node and contractions of both atria. The QRS complex corresponds to depolarization of the septum and contractions of both ventricles. The T wave corresponds to repolarization of the ventricles. (*Note*: The wave that corresponds to repolarization of the atria is hidden by the QRS complex.)

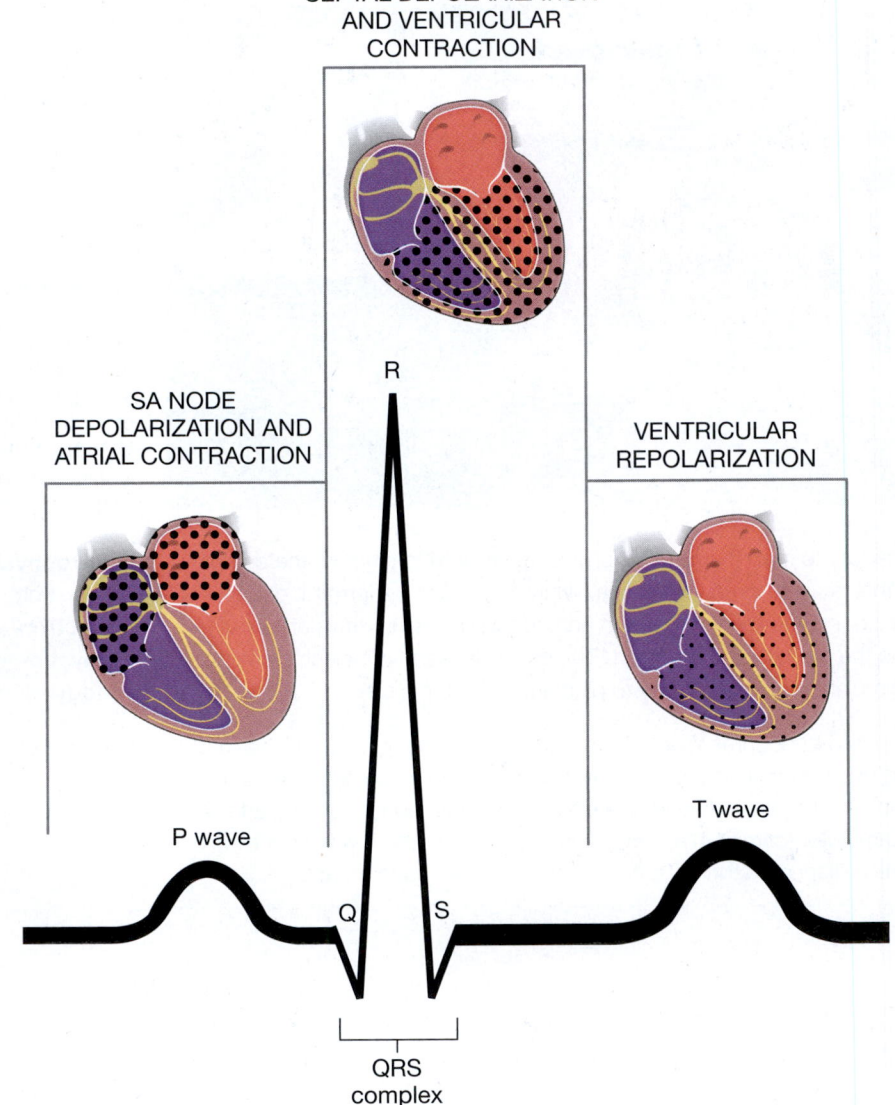

FIGURE 5-24 ■ **ECG tracing.** On an ECG, a normal tracing shows a P wave, QRS complex, and T wave that correspond to depolarization (large dots) and repolarization (small dots) changes going on in the heart. These waves are named to create a simple and universal reference system.

Word or Phrase	Description	Pronunciation/Word Parts

Radiologic and Nuclear Medicine Procedures

| angiography | Radiologic procedure in which radiopaque contrast dye is injected into a blood vessel to outline it. The x-ray image is an **angiogram**.
• **Arteriography**. The dye is injected into an artery to show narrowed areas, blockage, or aneurysms. The image is an **arteriogram**.
• **Venography**. The dye is injected into a vein to show weakened valves and dilated walls. The x-ray image is a **venogram**.
In rotational angiography, multiple x-rays are taken as the x-ray machine goes around the patient. This technique is particularly helpful in documenting tortuous blood vessels in three dimensions.
Digital subtraction angiography combines two x-ray images, one taken without contrast dye and a second image taken with contrast dye. A computer compares the two images and digitally "subtracts" or removes the soft tissues, bones, and muscles, leaving just the image of the arteries. | **angiography**
(AN-jee-AW-grah-fee)
angi/o- *blood vessel; lymphatic vessel*
-graphy *process of recording*

angiogram (AN-jee-oh-GRAM)
angi/o- *blood vessel; lymphatic vessel*
-gram *picture; record*

arteriography
(ar-TEER-ee-AW-grah-fee)
arteri/o- *artery*
-graphy *process of recording*

arteriogram
(ar-TEER-ee-oh-GRAM)
arteri/o- *artery*
-gram *picture; record*

venography (vee-NAW-grah-fee)
ven/o- *vein*
-graphy *process of recording*

venogram (VEE-noh-gram)
ven/o- *vein*
-gram *picture; record* |
| Doppler ultrasonography | Radiologic procedure that uses Doppler technology along with ultra high-frequency sound waves. It is used to image the flow of blood in an artery or vein. Doppler shows how fast the blood is moving by producing an audible sound. The ultrasound image shows blockages or clots.
Color flow duplex ultrasonography combines a color-coded Doppler image with the ultrasound image. Doppler shows variations in blood flow and turbulence, with faster flow in red and slower flow in blue (see Figure 5-25 ■). Color flow duplex ultrasonography is the "gold standard" for evaluating tortuous varicose veins. | **Doppler** (DAW-pler)

ultrasonography
(UL-trah-soh-NAW-grah-fee)
ultra- *beyond; higher*
son/o- *sound*
-graphy *process of recording* |

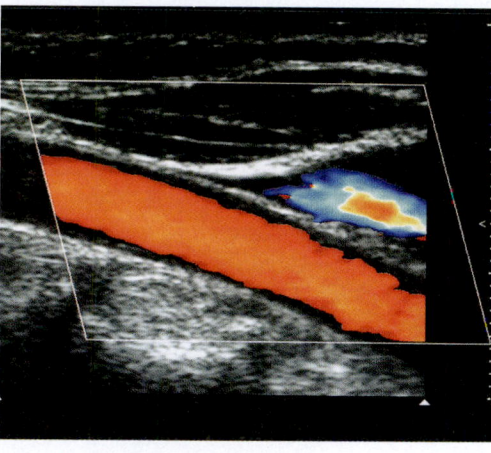

FIGURE 5-25 ■ Color flow duplex ultrasonography.
An ultrasound transducer was positioned over the carotid artery in the patient's neck. Ultrasound was combined with Doppler technology to create this image that shows the anatomy of the artery, but also shows colors that correspond to the velocity and direction of blood flow in that artery.

Word or Phrase	Description	Pronunciation/Word Parts

echocardiography	Radiologic procedure that uses ultra high-frequency sound waves produced by a transducer. The sound waves are bounced off the heart to create an image of the heart and its chambers and valves as it contracts and relaxes. The image is an **echocardiogram** (see Figure 5-26 ■). **Transesophageal echocardiography (TEE)** may be ordered when a standard echocardiogram has a poor-quality image. An ultrasound transducer is passed through the patient's mouth and positioned in the esophagus directly behind, and closer to, the heart for a better image.	**echocardiography**
		(EK-oh-KAR-dee-AW-grah-fee)
		  ech/o- *echo of a sound wave*
		  cardi/o- *heart*
		  -graphy *process of recording*
		
		echocardiogram
		(EK-oh-KAR-dee-oh-GRAM)
		  ech/o- *echo of a sound wave*
		  cardi/o- *heart*
		  -gram *picture; record*
		
		transesophageal
		(TRANS-eh-SAW-fah-JEE-al)
		  trans- *across; through*
		  esophag/o- *esophagus*
		  -eal *pertaining to*

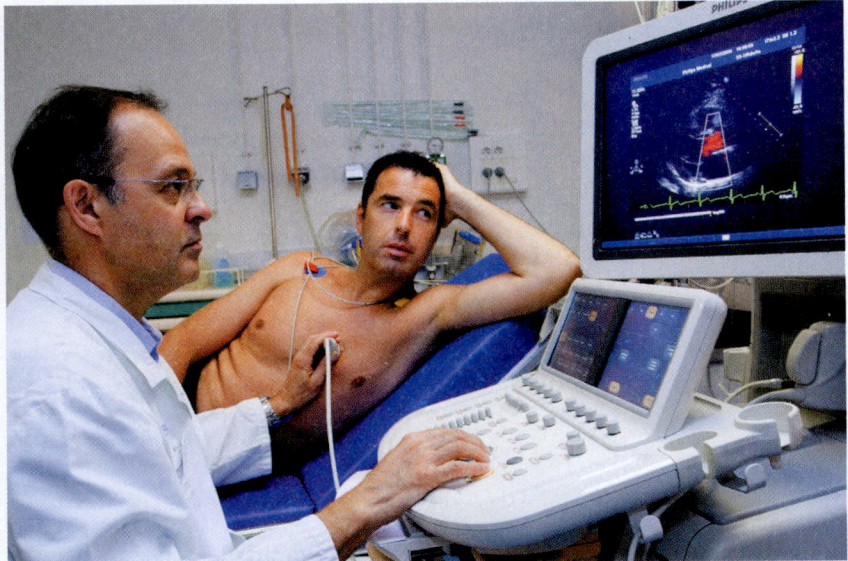

FIGURE 5-26 ■ Echocardiography.
Echocardiography uses sound waves to create images. The ultrasound technician is holding a transducer that produces the sound waves. They bounce off the structures of the heart as echoes that the computer displays on the monitor screen.

Word or Phrase	Description	Pronunciation/Word Parts

multiple-gated acquisition (MUGA) scan	Nuclear medicine procedure that takes images of the heart chambers (with blood and red blood cells in them) at various times. A MUGA scan also calculates the ejection fraction (how much blood the ventricle can eject with one contraction). The ejection fraction is the most accurate indicator of overall heart function. A MUGA scan uses a radioactive tracer that binds to red blood cells. A camera records gamma rays emitted by the radioactive tracer. The camera is coordinated (gated) with the patient's ECG. Also known as a **radionuclide ventriculography.**	**radionuclide**
		(RAY-dee-oh-NOO-klide)
		  radi/o- *forearm bone; radius; x-rays*
		  nucle/o- *nucleus of an atom or a cell*
		  -ide *chemically modified structure*
		
		ventriculography
		(ven-TRIH-kyoo-LAW-grah-fee)
		  ventricul/o- *chamber that is filled; ventricle*
		  -graphy *process of recording*

myocardial perfusion scan	Nuclear medicine procedure that combines a cardiac exercise stress test with an intravenous injection of a radioactive tracer. The radioactive tracer collects in those parts of the myocardium that have the best perfusion (blood flow). A camera records gamma rays emitted by the radioactive tracer and creates a two-dimensional image of the heart. Areas of decreased uptake ("cold spots") indicate poor perfusion from a blocked coronary artery. Areas of no uptake indicate dead tissue from a previous myocardial infarction.	**perfusion** (per-FYOO-zhun)
		  per- *through; throughout*
		  fus/o- *pouring*
		  -ion *action; condition*

5.4 PRACTICE LAPS

Use the Answer Key at the end of the book to check your answers.

A. Give the Meaning of Combining Forms

Next to each combining form, write its meaning. The first one has been done for you.

Combining Form	Meaning	Combining Form	Meaning
1. **cardi/o-**	*heart*	8. pharmac/o-	
2. angi/o-		9. physi/o-	
3. arteri/o-		10. son/o-	
4. catheter/o-		11. tele/o-	
5. ech/o-		12. ven/o-	
6. electr/o-		13. ventricul/o-	
7. lip/o-			

B. Build Words

Read the definition of the medical word. Look at the combining form that is given. Select the correct suffix from the Suffix List, and write it on the blank line. Then build the medical word, and write it on the line. (Remember: You may need to remove the combining vowel. Always remove the hyphens and slash.) Be sure to check your spelling.

Suffix List

-gram (picture; record)	-ization (process of creating; process	-metry (process of measuring)
-graphy (process of recording)	of inserting; process of making)	

Definition of the Medical Word	Combining Form	Suffix	Build the Medical Word
Example: Process of recording (an) artery	**arteri/o-**	*-graphy*	*arteriography*

[You think process of recording (-graphy) + artery (arteri/o-). You change the order of the word parts to put the suffix last. You write arteriography.]

1. Process of recording (a) vein	ven/o-		
2. Process of inserting (a) catheter	catheter/o-		
3. Picture (or) record (of the) ventricle	ventricul/o-		
4. Process of measuring (at a) distance	tele/o-		
5. Picture (or) record (of a) blood vessel	angi/o-		

C. Define Abbreviations

1. ECG, EKG _____   3. TEE _____

2. HDL _____

5.5 Medical Procedures, Drugs, and Surgical Procedures

Word or Phrase	Description	Pronunciation/Word Parts

Medical Procedures

Word or Phrase	Description	Pronunciation/Word Parts
auscultation	Procedure that uses a **stethoscope** to listen to the heart sounds. The stethoscope is placed at the **point of maximum impulse (PMI)**, which is at the apex of the heart. Auscultation can detect arrhythmias and murmurs.	**auscultation** (AWS-kul-TAY-shun) **auscult/o-** *listening* **-ation** *being; having; process* **stethoscope** (STETH-oh-skohp) **steth/o-** *chest* **-scope** *instrument used to examine*
blood pressure (BP)	One of the four vital signs. Blood pressure is measured with a **sphygmomanometer** (see Figure 5-27 ■). Usually this is done by a machine that automatically inflates and deflates the cuff, measures the blood pressure, and displays the digital blood pressure reading. Blood pressure is recorded as two numbers: the **systolic** pressure over the **diastolic** pressure; the pressure is measured in millimeters of mercury (e.g., 120/80 mm Hg). Blood pressure cuffs come in several different sizes to accommodate very thin to very large arms. There are even blood pressure cuffs for newborn and premature infants. The correct-size blood pressure cuff must be used or the blood pressure reading will be either too high or too low.	**sphygmomanometer** (SFIG-moh-mah-NAW-meh-ter) **sphygm/o-** *pulse* **man/o-** *frenzy; thin* **-meter** *instrument used to measure* Sphygmomanometer: *Instrument used to measure (the pressure of the) pulse (by using a) thin (inflatable cuff)* **systolic** (sis-TAW-lik) **systol/o-** *contracting* **-ic** *pertaining to* **diastolic** (DY-ah-STAW-lik) **diastol/o-** *dilating* **-ic** *pertaining to*

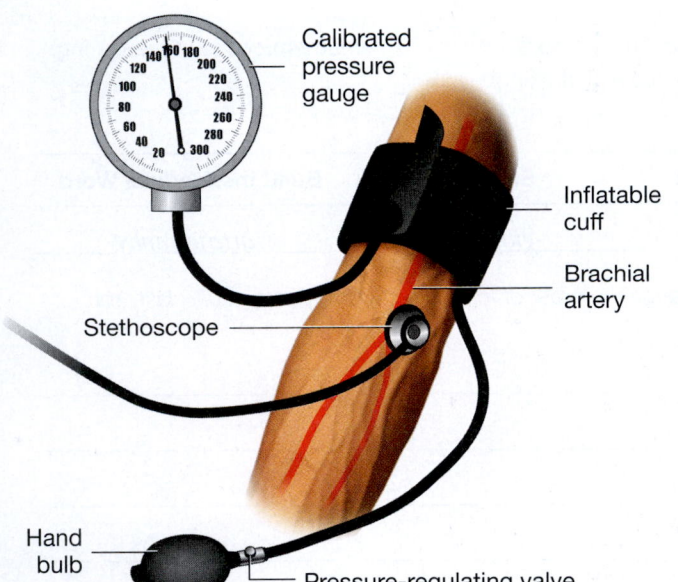

Calibrated pressure gauge

Inflatable cuff

Brachial artery

Stethoscope

Hand bulb

Pressure-regulating valve

FIGURE 5-27 ■ Measuring the blood pressure manually. A manual sphygmomanometer consists of a thin, inflatable cuff that wraps around the arm (or leg), a hand bulb that is pumped to increase the pressure in the cuff, a regulating valve that is opened slowly to release pressure from the cuff, and a calibrated gauge to read the pressure. A stethoscope is placed at the inner elbow over the brachial artery pulse. As the cuff is inflated, the cuff pressure cuts off the flow of blood in the artery. Then the cuff is slowly deflated. When the cuff pressure is lower than the pressure in the artery, the blood spurts through and creates the first sound that is heard through the stethoscope. This is the systolic pressure, the top number in the blood pressure reading, which represents the force of the contraction of the ventricles. When the cuff pressure reaches the resting pressure in the artery, the sound becomes muffled, and this is recorded as the diastolic pressure, the lower number.

Word or Phrase	Description	Pronunciation/Word Parts

cardiopulmonary resuscitation (CPR)	Procedure to circulate the blood after the patient's heart has stopped beating (described in Chapter 4, Pulmonology)	**cardiopulmonary** (KAR-dee-oh-PUL-moh-NAIR-ee)
		  cardi/o- *heart*
		  pulmon/o- *lung*
		  -ary *pertaining to*
		
		resuscitation (ree-SUH-sih-TAY-shun)
		  resuscit/o- *raise up again; revive*
		  -ation *being; having; process*

cardioversion	Procedure to treat an arrhythmia (atrial flutter, atrial fibrillation, or ventricular tachycardia) that cannot be controlled with antiarrhythmic drugs. Two adhesive defibrillator pads are placed on either side of the patient's chest and connected by cables to the machine. The machine generates an electrical shock coordinated with the QRS complex of the patient's heart to restore the heart to a normal rhythm. For a patient with ventricular fibrillation, the same machine is used (it is now called a **defibrillator**) to give a much stronger electrical shock.	**cardioversion** (KAR-dee-oh-VER-zhun)
		  cardi/o- *heart*
		  vers/o- *travel; turn*
		  -ion *action; condition*
		
		defibrillator (dee-FIB-rih-LAY-tor)
		  de- *reversal of; without*
		  fibrill/o- *muscle fiber; nerve fiber*
		  -ator *person who does or produces; thing that does or produces*

Clinical Connections

Health Information Management. An **advance directive** is a legal document that tells healthcare professionals what a person's wishes are in the event that he or she is in a coma, is seriously injured or terminally ill, or is mentally unable to make decisions. A **do not resuscitate (DNR)** order states that a person does not want to have cardiopulmonary resuscitation if the heart or breathing stops.

Public Health. An **automatic external defibrillator (AED)** is a portable computerized device kept on emergency response vehicles and in public places such as airports (see Figure 5-28 ■). It analyzes the patient's heart rhythm and delivers an electrical shock to stimulate the heart in cardiac arrest. An AED is designed to be used by nonmedical persons.

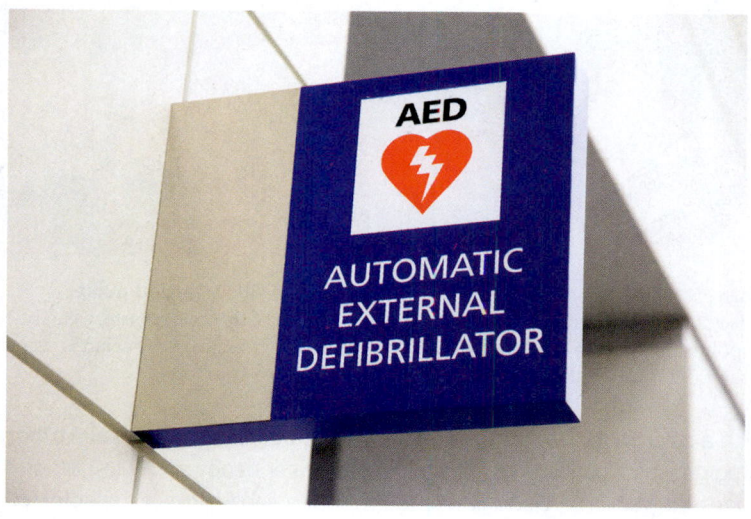

FIGURE 5-28 ■ Automatic external defibrillator (AED).
Signs for an automatic external defibrillator are commonly seen in airports and public places.

Word or Phrase	Description	Pronunciation/Word Parts
pulse rate	One of the four vital signs that include **temperature, pulse, and respirations (TPR)**, as well as blood pressure (BP) (described previously). The pulse rate is measured by counting the **beats per minute (bpm)** by feeling the pulse. The pulse can be felt at pulse points where an artery is close to the skin's surface (see Figure 5-29 ■). The **radial pulse** in the wrist is the most commonly used site. In an emergency, the **carotid pulse** is used (see Figure 5-30 ■) because, if the patient is in shock, there is less blood flow to arteries in the extremities. The **apical pulse** (at the apex of the heart) as heard through a stethoscope is also used to evaluate the heart rhythm and heart sounds. The heart rate for a newborn is 110–150 beats per minute. The heart rate for an adult is 70–80 beats per minute. A well-trained athlete can have a resting heart rate lower than 60 beats per minute.	**radial** (RAY-dee-al) **radi/o-** *forearm bone; radius; x-rays* **-al** *pertaining to* **carotid** (kah-RAW-tid) **carot/o-** *loss of consciousness* **-id** *origin; resembling; source* **apical** (AP-ih-kal) **apic/o-** *apex; tip* **-al** *pertaining to*

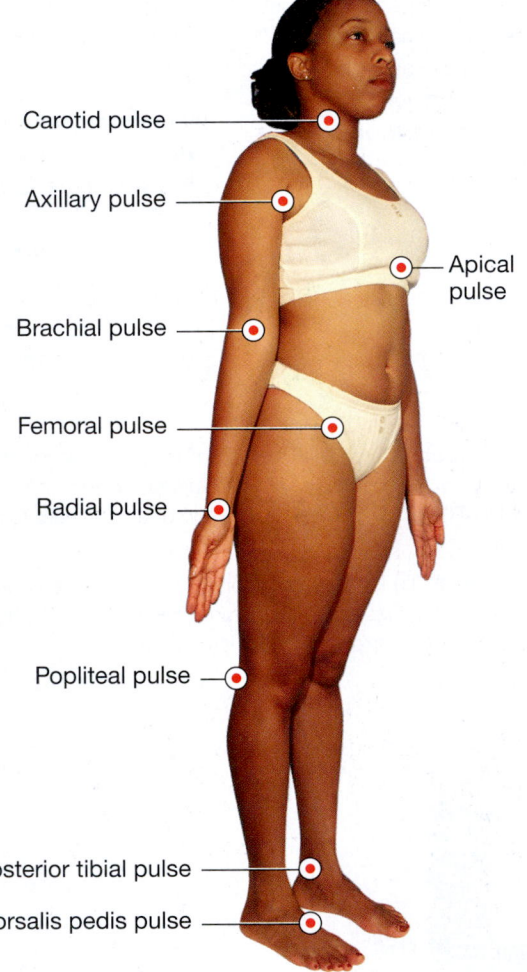

Carotid pulse

Axillary pulse

Apical pulse

Brachial pulse

Femoral pulse

Radial pulse

Popliteal pulse

Posterior tibial pulse

Dorsalis pedis pulse

FIGURE 5-29 ■ Pulse points.
A pulse point is where the pulse of an artery can be felt on the surface of the body. Pulse points are used to determine the heart rate and the amount of flow through the artery.

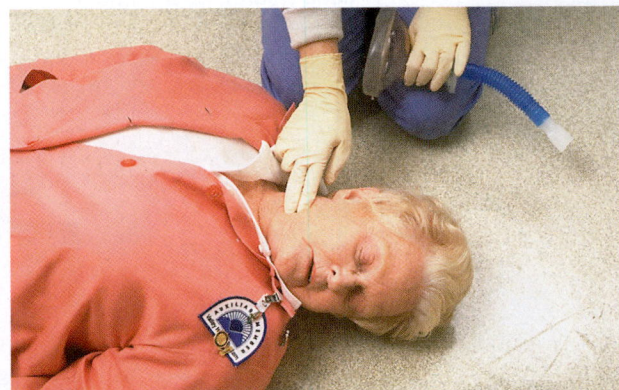

FIGURE 5-30 ■ Carotid pulse.
The pulse of the carotid artery can be felt easily in the neck. This emergency medical technician is using this site to quickly assess the patient's heart rate.

| sclerotherapy | Procedure in which a sclerosing drug (liquid or foam) is injected into a varicose vein. The drug causes irritation and inflammation that later becomes fibrosis that occludes the vein. The blood flow is redirected to another, deeper vein, and the varicose vein is no longer distended. | **sclerotherapy** (SKLAIR-oh-THAIR-ah-pee) **scler/o-** *hard; sclera* **-therapy** *treatment* Sclerotherapy: *Treatment (to make a vein) hard(en)* |

Category	Indication	Pronunciation/Word Parts

Drugs

Category	Indication	Pronunciation/Word Parts
ACE inhibitor drug	Treats congestive heart failure and hypertension. ACE inhibitor drugs produce vasodilation, and this decreases the blood pressure. ACE stands for *angiotensin-converting enzyme*.	**angiotensin** (AN-jee-oh-TEN-sin) **angi/o-** *blood vessel; lymphatic vessel* **tens/o-** *pressure* **-in** *substance*
antiarrhythmic drug	Treats arrhythmias	**antiarrhythmic** (AN-tee-aa-RITH-mik) **anti-** *against* **a-** *away from; without* **rrhythm/o-** *rhythm* **-ic** *pertaining to*
anticoagulant drug	Prevents a blood clot from forming in patients with arteriosclerosis, atrial fibrillation, previous myocardial infarction, or an artificial heart valve	**anticoagulant** (AN-tee-koh-AG-yoo-lant) **anti-** *against* **coagul/o-** *clotting* **-ant** *pertaining to*
antihypertensive drug	Treats hypertension. Includes ACE inhibitor drugs, beta-blocker drugs, calcium channel blocker drugs, and diuretic drugs.	**antihypertensive** (AN-tee-HY-per-TEN-siv) **anti-** *against* **hyper-** *above; more than normal* **tens/o-** *pressure* **-ive** *pertaining to*
aspirin drug	Prevents a heart attack by keeping platelets from sticking together to form a blood clot	
beta-blocker drug	Treats angina pectoris and hypertension. These drugs decrease the heart rate and dilate the arteries by blocking beta receptors.	**beta** (BAY-tah)
calcium channel blocker drug	Treats angina pectoris and hypertension. These drugs block the movement of calcium ions into myocardial cells and smooth muscle cells of artery walls; this causes the heart rate and blood pressure to decrease.	
digitalis drug	Treats congestive heart failure. Digitalis drugs decrease the heart rate and strengthen the heart's contractions (see Figure 5-31 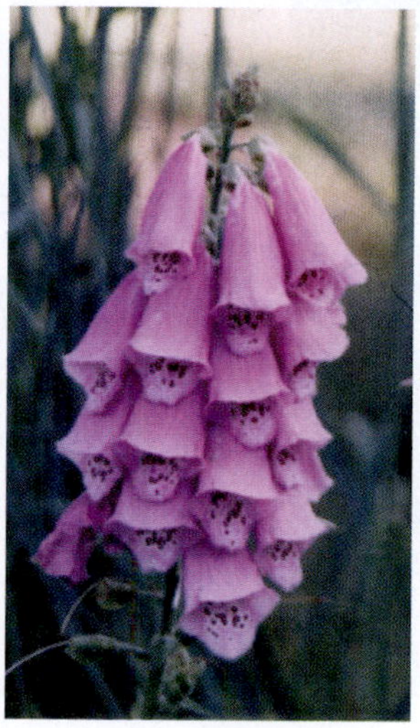 ■).	**digitalis** (DIJ-ih-TAL-is)

FIGURE 5-31 ■ Foxglove plant.
Digitalis drugs originally came from the flowering plant *Digitalis purpurea* (foxglove plant). The plant's scientific name came from the shape of the flowers being like a cap that could fit over a finger (digit) and the color being purple.

Category	Indication	Pronunciation/Word Parts
diuretic drug	Causes sodium to be excreted in the urine. Sodium brings water with it, and this decreases the blood pressure. Diuretic drugs are used to treat hypertension and congestive heart failure. Laypersons call these drugs "water pills."	**diuretic** (DY-yoor-EH-tik) **dia-** *complete; through* **ur/o-** *urinary system; urine* **-etic** *pertaining to* The *a* in *dia-* is deleted when the word is formed.
lipid-lowering drug	Treats hypercholesterolemia. These are often called "statin drugs" because their generic drug names all end in "statin."	
nitroglycerin drug	Treats angina pectoris. These drugs dilate the arteries to decrease the blood pressure.	**nitroglycerin** (NY-troh-GLIH-sair-in)
thrombolytic drug	Breaks apart a blood clot that is blocking blood flow through an artery	**thrombolytic** (THRAWM-boh-LIH-tik) **thromb/o-** *blood clot* **lyt/o-** *break down; destroy* **-ic** *pertaining to*

Word or Phrase	Description	Pronunciation/Word Parts

Surgical Procedures

aneurysmectomy	Procedure to remove an aneurysm and repair the artery. If an aneurysm involves a large segment of artery, a flexible, tubular synthetic graft is used to replace the segment.	**aneurysmectomy** (AN-yoor-iz-MEK-toh-mee) **aneurysm/o-** *aneurysm; dilation* **-ectomy** *surgical removal*
cardiopulmonary bypass	Procedure used during open heart surgery (see Figure 5-32 ■) in which the patient's blood is rerouted through a cannula in the femoral vein to a heart-lung machine. There, the blood is oxygenated, carbon dioxide and waste products are removed, and the blood is pumped back into the patient's body through a cannula in the femoral artery. Cardiopulmonary bypass takes over the functions of the heart and lungs during open heart surgery.	**cardiopulmonary** (KAR-dee-oh-PUL-moh-NAIR-ee) **cardi/o-** *heart* **pulmon/o-** *lung* **-ary** *pertaining to*

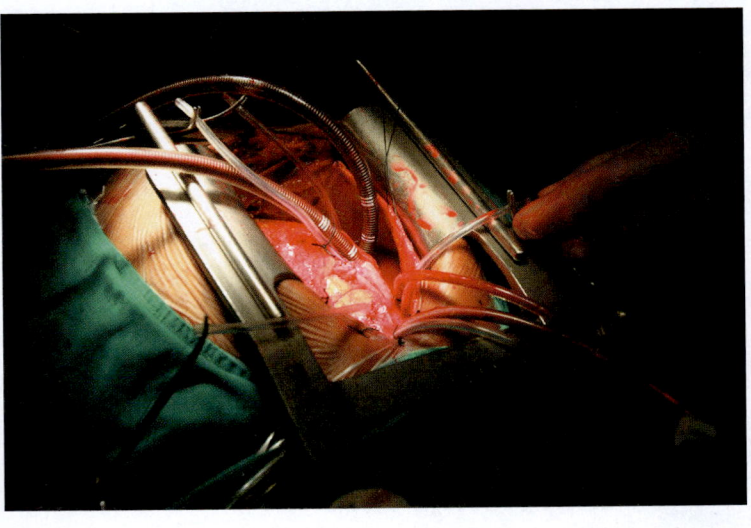

FIGURE 5-32 ■ Open heart surgery.
To perform some types of heart surgery, the sternum (breastbone) is cut in half lengthwise. Metal retractors are used to pull the two halves apart to create an operative field that allows access to the heart. Other surgical procedures on the heart can be done with only small incisions.

Word or Phrase	Description	Pronunciation/Word Parts

carotid endarterectomy	Procedure to remove plaque from an occluded carotid artery. It is used to treat carotid artery **stenosis** due to atherosclerosis.	**endarterectomy** (END-ar-ter-EK-toh-mee)
		  end/o- *innermost; within*
		  arter/o- *artery*
		  -ectomy *surgical removal*
		
		stenosis (steh-NOH-sihs)
		  sten/o- *constriction; narrowness*
		  -osis *abnormal condition; process*

coronary artery bypass graft (CABG)	Procedure to bypass an occluded coronary artery and restore blood flow to the myocardium. A blood vessel (either the saphenous vein from the leg or the internal mammary artery from the chest) is used as the bypass graft. The suturing of one blood vessel to another is an **anastomosis**. Oxygenated blood flows through the blood vessel graft, around the blockage in the coronary artery (bypasses the blockage), and back into the coronary artery.	**anastomosis** (ah-NAS-toh-MOH-sihs)
		  anastom/o- *create an opening between two structures*
		  -osis *abnormal condition; process*

heart transplantation	Procedure to remove a severely damaged heart from a patient with end-stage heart failure and insert a new heart from a **donor** (a person who has recently died). The patient is matched by blood type and tissue type to the donor ("type and crossmatch") (described in Chapter 6, Hematology and Immunology).
	
	While awaiting a donor heart, the patient may have a **left ventricular assist device (LVAD)** temporarily implanted. This battery- or pneumatic-powered pump is placed in the abdomen and connected by tubes to the left ventricle and the aorta. In some patients, it becomes a permanent solution when no donor heart is available. Alternately, some patients receive an artificial heart made of plastic, metal, and other synthetic materials.
		transplantation (TRANS-plan-TAY-shun)
		  transplant/o- *move and put in another place*
		  -ation *being; having; process*
		
		donor (DOH-nor)

pacemaker insertion	Procedure in which an automated device is implanted to control the heart rate and rhythm in a patient with an arrhythmia (see Figure 5-33 ■). A pacemaker uses an electrical impulse and a wire positioned on the heart to coordinate the heartbeat. A. B. **FIGURE 5-33 ■ Pacemaker.** **A.** This pacemaker (programmable pulse generator) is placed under the skin of the anterior chest with its pacemaker wires attached to the heart. **B.** This colorized chest x-ray shows the position of an implanted pacemaker and the pacemaker wires on the heart.	

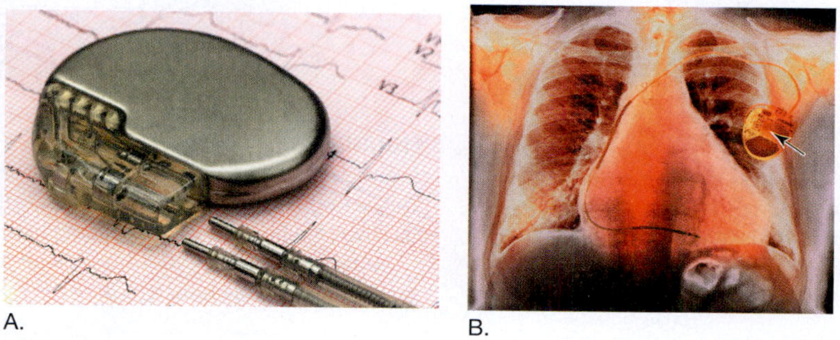

Word or Phrase	Description	Pronunciation/Word Parts

percutaneous transluminal coronary angioplasty (PTCA)	Procedure to reconstruct a coronary artery that is narrowed because of atherosclerosis. A catheter is inserted into the femoral artery and threaded to the site of the stenosis. Then one of two techniques is used.
	• **Balloon angioplasty**. A balloon within the catheter is inflated. It compresses the atheromatous plaque and widens the lumen of the artery. Then the balloon is deflated, and the catheter is removed (see Figure 5-34 ■).
	• **Stent**. Alternately, an intravascular stainless steel mesh stent (unexpanded) is inserted onto the catheter (see Figure 5-35 ■). The stent is expanded, the catheter is removed, and the expanded stent remains in the artery.
		percutaneous
		(PER-kyoo-TAY-nee-uhs)
		  per- *through; throughout*
		  cutane/o- *skin*
		  -ous *pertaining to*
		
		transluminal (trans-LOO-mih-nal)
		  trans- *across; through*
		  lumin/o- *lumen; opening*
		  -al *pertaining to*
		
		angioplasty (AN-jee-oh-PLAS-tee)
		  angi/o- *blood vessel; lymphatic vessel*
		  -plasty *process of reshaping by surgery*

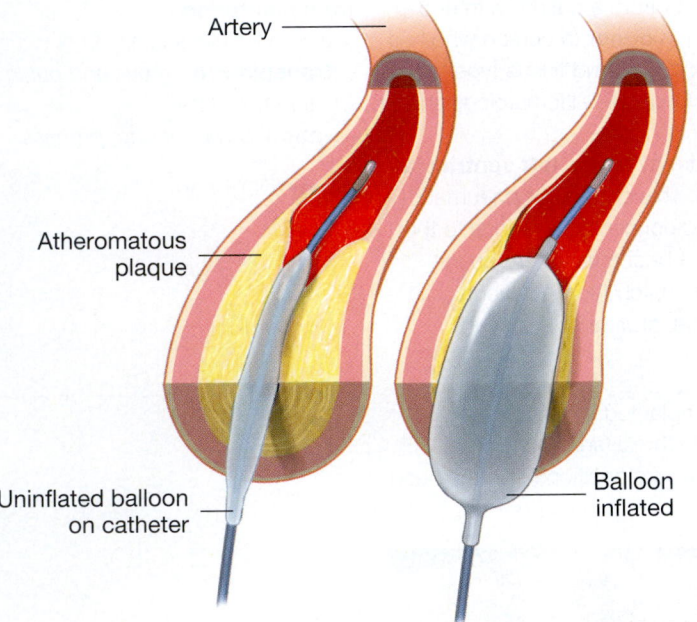

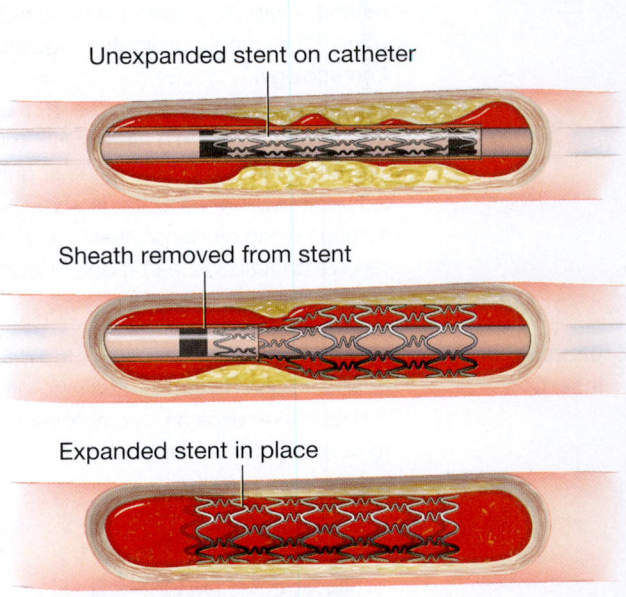

FIGURE 5-34 ■ Balloon angioplasty.
A catheter with an uninflated balloon is able to pass through an artery whose lumen is severely narrowed by atheromatous plaque. When the balloon is inflated, it compresses the atheromatous plaque to open the lumen and increase the flow of oxygenated blood. Then the balloon is deflated, and the catheter is withdrawn.

FIGURE 5-35 ■ Stent.
A catheter with an unexpanded stent is inserted into the artery. The stent is then expanded to compress the atheromatous plaque and increase the flow of oxygenated blood. The stent is left in place as the catheter is withdrawn. The stent provides continuing support to keep the lumen of the artery open over time.

Word or Phrase	Description	Pronunciation/Word Parts

pericardiocentesis	Procedure that uses a needle to puncture the pericardium and withdraw inflammatory fluid accumulated in the pericardial sac. It is used to treat pericarditis and cardiac tamponade.	**pericardiocentesis**
		(PAIR-ih-KAR-dee-oh-sen-TEE-sihs)
		  peri- *around*
		  cardi/o- *heart*
		  -centesis *procedure to puncture*

Word or Phrase	Description	Pronunciation/Word Parts
radiofrequency ablation	Procedure to destroy an ectopic area in the heart that is producing an electrical impulse that causes an arrhythmia. A catheter is inserted into the heart near the ectopic site. Radiofrequency electrical current is used to produce heat to kill the cells causing the arrhythmia.	**ablation** (ah-BLAY-shun) **ablat/o-** *destroy; take away* **-ion** *action; condition*
valve replacement	Procedure to replace a severely damaged or prolapsed heart valve with an artificial valve, also known as a **prosthesis** (see Figure 5-36 ■). There are several types of **prosthetic** heart valves that can be used. 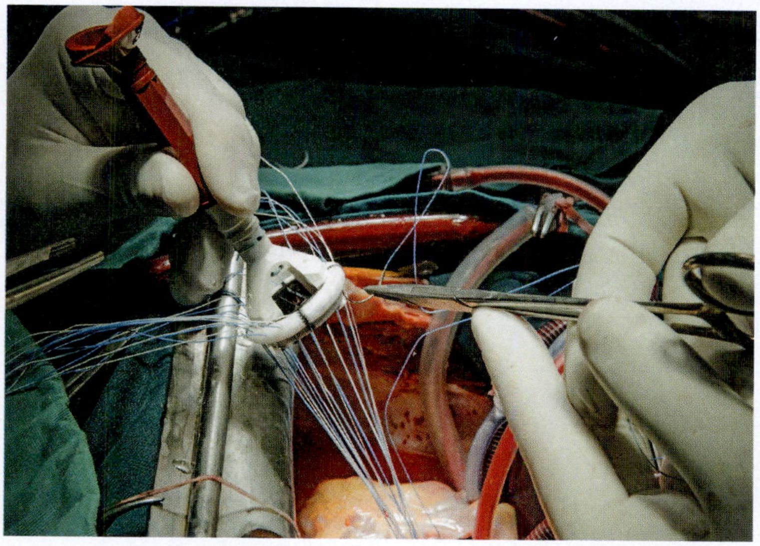 FIGURE 5-36 ■ **Valve replacement.** A white artificial valve is being implanted in the heart. Many sutures are used to attach the valve so that blood will not leak around its edges.	**prosthesis** (praws-THEE-sihs) **prosthetic** (praws-THET-ik) **prosthet/o-** *artificial part* **-ic** *pertaining to*
valvuloplasty	Procedure to reconstruct a heart valve to correct stenosis or prolapse. A **valvulotome** is used to cut the valve.	**valvuloplasty** (VAL-vyoo-loh-PLAS-tee) **valvul/o-** *valve* **-plasty** *process of reshaping by surgery* **valvulotome** (VAL-vyoo-loh-TOHM) **valvul/o-** *valve* **-tome** *area with distinct edges; instrument used to cut*

5.5 PRACTICE LAPS

Use the Answer Key at the end of the book to check your answers.

A. Give the Meaning of Combining Forms

Next to each combining form, write its meaning. The first one has been done for you.

Combining Form	Meaning	Combining Form	Meaning
1. **ablat/o-**	*destroy; take away*	11. prosthet/o-	
2. anastom/o-		12. resuscit/o-	
3. aneurysm/o-		13. scler/o-	
4. angi/o-		14. sphygm/o-	
5. apic/o-		15. systol/o-	
6. auscult/o-		16. tens/o-	
7. coagul/o-		17. thromb/o-	
8. diastol/o-		18. transplant/o-	
9. fibrill/o-		19. valvul/o-	
10. lumin/o-			

B. Build Words

Read the definition of the medical word. Look at the combining form that is given. Select the correct suffix from the Suffix List, and write it on the blank line. Then build the medical word, and write it on the line. (Remember: You may need to remove the combining vowel. Always remove the hyphens and slash.) Be sure to check your spelling.

Suffix List

-al (pertaining to)	-ic (pertaining to)	-plasty (process of reshaping by surgery)	-therapy (treatment)
-ation (being; having; process)	-ion (action; condition)	-scope (instrument used to examine)	-tome (instrument used to cut)
-ectomy (surgical removal)	-osis (abnormal condition; process)		

Definition of the Medical Word	Combining Form	Suffix	Build the Medical Word
Example: Action (to) destroy (or) take away	**ablat/o-**	*-ion*	*ablation*

[*You think* action (-ion) + destroy (or) take away (ablat/o-). You change the order of the word parts to put the suffix last. You write ablation.]

1. Pertaining to (the) apex (or) tip (of the heart)	apic/o-		
2. Process (of) listening	auscult/o-		
3. Process (to) create an opening between two structures	anastom/o-		
4. Surgical removal (of an) aneurysm	aneurysm/o-		

Definition of the Medical Word	Combining Form	Suffix	Build the Medical Word
5. Process (to) raise up again (and) revive	resuscit/o-	_____	_____
6. Instrument used to examine (the) chest	steth/o-	_____	_____
7. Pertaining to contracting	systol/o-	_____	_____
8. Process (to) move and put in another place	transplant/o-	_____	_____
9. Instrument used to cut (a) valve	valvul/o-	_____	_____
10. Treatment (to make a vein) hard(en)	scler/o-	_____	_____
11. Process of reshaping by surgery (on a) valve	valvul/o-	_____	_____
12. Process of reshaping by surgery (on a) blood vessel	angi/o-	_____	_____

C. Define Abbreviations

1. BP _____

2. CABG _____

3. CPR _____

4. DNR _____

5. PMI _____

Abbreviations Summary

ACE	angiotensin-converting enzyme		ECG	electrocardiogram; electrocardiography
AED	automatic external defibrillator		EKG	electrocardiogram; electrocardiography
ASCVD	arteriosclerotic cardiovascular disease		HDL	high-density lipoprotein
AV	atrioventricular		HTN	hypertension
BP	blood pressure		K^+	potassium ion
bpm	beats per minute		LA	left atrium
Ca^{++}	calcium ion		LDH	lactate dehydrogenase
CABG	coronary artery bypass graft (pronounced "cabbage")		LDL	low-density lipoprotein
			LV	left ventricle
CAD	coronary artery disease		LVAD	left ventricular assist device
CCU	coronary care unit		MI	myocardial infarction
CHF	congestive heart failure		mm Hg	millimeters of mercury
CK-MB	creatine kinase		MUGA	multiple-gated acquisition (scan) (pronounced "MUG-ah")
CPR	cardiopulmonary resuscitation			
CV	cardiovascular		MVP	mitral valve prolapse
DNR	do not resuscitate		Na^+	sodium ion

continued on next page

NSR	normal sinus rhythm		S_2	second heart sound
P	pulse (rate)		**SA**	sinoatrial
PAC	premature atrial contraction		**SBE**	subacute bacterial endocarditis
PMI	point of maximum impulse		**TEE**	transesophageal echocardiogram; transesophageal echocardiography
PTCA	percutaneous transluminal coronary angioplasty		**TPR**	temperature, pulse, and respirations
PVC	premature ventricular contraction			
RA	right atrium		**V fib**	ventricular fibrillation (short form)
RV	right ventricle		**V tach**	ventricular tachycardia (short form)
S_1	first heart sound		**VLDL**	very-low-density lipoprotein

Word Alert

Abbreviations. Abbreviations are commonly used in all types of medical documents; however, they can mean different things to different people and their meanings can be misinterpreted. Always verify the meaning of an abbreviation. *RA* means *right atrium*, but it also means *rheumatoid arthritis* or *room air*.

It's Greek to Me! Did you notice that some words have two different combining forms? Combining forms from both Greek and Latin remain a part of medical language today.

Word	Greek	Latin	Medical Word Examples
blood vessel	angi/o-	vas/o-, vascul/o-	angiography; vasoconstriction, vascular
heart	cardi/o-	coron/o-	cardiac; coronary
vein	phleb/o-	ven/o-	thrombophlebitis; venous

Career Focus

Meet Laurie, a cardiac stress test technologist in a hospital

"Cardiology is a very important department. I use medical terminology during all aspects of my job. My daughter was born with a heart defect. Wanting to know more information about what was happening to her, I started to take a class here and a class there, and then I just wound up in a certificate program. The most rewarding part of my job is if I can get a patient through the test and at the end of the test they say, 'You made that so much easier for me.'"

- **Cardiac stress test technologists** are allied health professionals who perform ECGs, Holter monitor tests, and cardiac stress tests in a hospital setting or a cardiologist's office.
- **Cardiologists** are physicians who practice in the medical specialty of cardiology. They diagnose and treat patients with diseases of the heart and circulatory system. When cardiologists perform surgery, they are known as heart surgeons, cardiothoracic surgeons, or cardiovascular surgeons. Physicians can take additional training and become board certified in the subspecialty of pediatric cardiology.

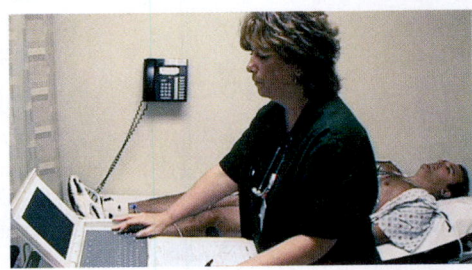

technologist (tek-NAW-loh-jist)
techn/o- *technical skill*
log/o- *study of; word*
-ist *person who specializes in*

cardiologist (KAR-dee-AW-loh-jist)
cardi/o- *heart*
log/o- *study of; word*
-ist *person who specializes in*

Chapter Review Exercises

Dive In: Medical Language Exercises

Test your knowledge of the chapter by completing these review exercises. Use the Answer Key at the end of the book to check your answers. Note: Each of the numbered exercise headers corresponds to a numbered learning outcome at the beginning of the chapter.

5.1 Anatomy

MATCHING EXERCISE

Match each word or phrase to its description.

1. aortic valve
2. bicuspid valve
3. chordae tendineae
4. mediastinum
5. myocardium
6. pericardium
7. septum
8. tricuspid
9. vasculature
10. ventricle

_____ another name for the *mitral valve*

_____ network of blood vessels related to a particular organ

_____ dividing wall between the right and left sides of the heart

_____ double-layered membrane around the heart

_____ bottom chamber of the heart

_____ area behind the breastbone that contains the heart

_____ valve between the right atrium and right ventricle

_____ heart muscle

_____ valve that blood flows through as it leaves the left ventricle

_____ rope-like strands that strengthen the tricuspid and mitral valves

CIRCLE EXERCISE

Circle the correct answer from the choices given.

1. The great vessels include the superior and inferior venae cavae and the (**aorta, artery, mediastinum**).
2. The vascular structures of the body include all of the following *except* (**arteries, capillaries, heart valves, veins**).
3. What unique structure is found only in the fetal heart? (**apex, foramen ovale, vasculature**).
4. This vein brings deoxygenated blood from the head to the superior vena cava: (**jugular, portal, saphenous**).
5. The brachial arteries bring oxygenated blood to the (**armpit, upper arm, upper leg**).
6. The (**axillary, fibular, portal**) veins carry deoxygenated blood from the liver.

TRUE OR FALSE EXERCISE

*Indicate whether each statement is true or false by writing **T** or **F** on the line.*

1. _____ The aorta is the largest vein in the body.
2. _____ Blood flows from the inferior vena cava to the right atrium to the right ventricle and to the pulmonary veins to the lungs.
3. _____ The smallest veins are known as *capillaries*.
4. _____ The interventricular septum is within a ventricle.
5. _____ The epicardium lines the heart chambers.
6. _____ All arteries carry blood away from the heart.
7. _____ The subclavian artery carries blood to the leg.
8. _____ The peroneal artery carries blood to the lateral aspect of the lower leg in the area of the fibula bone.
9. _____ The blood in most veins is a dark red-purple color because it has a low level of oxygen.
10. _____ The systemic circulation carries blood to the whole body, but not to the lungs.
11. _____ Vasodilation is the opposite of vasoconstriction.
12. _____ The myocardium is the muscular layer of the heart.

continued on next page

13. _____ The tricuspid valve is between the right atrium and right ventricle.
14. _____ The coronary arteries bring oxygenated blood to the myocardium.
15. _____ Veins and arteries have valves to keep the blood flowing in one direction.

PLURAL NOUN AND ADJECTIVE EXERCISE

Read the noun and write its plural form and/or adjective form on the line. Only write in the plural noun or adjective if there is a blank line there for it. Be sure to check your spelling. The first one has been done for you.

Singular Noun	Plural Noun	Adjective	Singular Noun	Plural Noun	Adjective
1. **apex**		*apical*	7. pericardium		_____
2. aorta		_____	8. septum		_____
3. artery	_____	_____	9. valve	_____	_____
4. atrium	_____	_____	10. ventricle	_____	_____
5. heart		_____	11. vein	_____	_____
6. myocardium		_____			

DIVIDING WORDS EXERCISE

Separate these words into their component parts (prefix, combining form, suffix). Some words do not contain all three word parts. The first one has been done for you.

Medical Word	Prefix	Combining Form	Suffix	Medical Word	Prefix	Combining Form	Suffix
1. **arteriolar**		*arteriol/o-*	*-ar*	8. pericardium	____	_____	_____
2. aortic		_____	_____	9. pulmonary		_____	_____
3. bifurcation		_____	_____	10. subclavian	____	_____	_____
4. brachial		_____	_____	11. tricuspid	____	_____	_____
5. circulatory		_____	_____	12. valvular		_____	_____
6. coronary		_____	_____	13. ventricular		_____	_____
7. deoxygenated	____	_____	_____				

SPELLING EXERCISE

Read each medical word pronunciation and write the medical word that it represents. Be sure to check your spelling. The first one has been done for you.

1. **(KAR-dee-oh-VAS-kyoo-lar)**   *cardiovascular*
2. (KOR-oh-NAIR-ee) _____
3. (PAIR-ih-KAR-dee-um) _____
4. (POP-lih-TEE-al) _____
5. (thor-AS-ik) _____
6. (VAL-vyoo-lar) _____
7. (VAY-soh-con-STRIK-shun) _____

5.2 Physiology

MATCHING EXERCISE

Match each word or phrase to its description.

1. acetylcholine
2. atria
3. conduction system
4. diastole
5. "fight-or-flight" response
6. pacemaker of the heart
7. Purkinje fibers
8. sodium ion
9. sympathetic

_____ Na⁺ — Na^+

_____ division of the nervous system

_____ contract first during a heartbeat

_____ SA node

_____ system that contracts and relaxes the heart in a coordinated rhythm

_____ neurotransmitter that slows the SA node rate

_____ occurs in times of danger

_____ resting period between heartbeats

_____ network of nerves in the heart

CIRCLE EXERCISE

Circle the correct answer from the choices given.

1. Potassium ions are abbreviated as (**Ca^{++}, K^+, Na^+**).
2. The (**AV node, Purkinje fibers, SA node**) normally initiates the electrical impulse.
3. Depolarization involves the movement of sodium and (**calcium, epinephrine, electrical**) ions.
4. Which of these can take over and produce its own abnormal rhythm? (**ectopic site, epinephrine, SA node**).

TRUE OR FALSE EXERCISE

Indicate whether each statement is true or false by writing **T** *or* **F** *on the line.*

1. _____ The refractory period is the time during which the ventricles contract.
2. _____ The electrical impulse of a heartbeat travels through the AV node and then into the diastole.
3. _____ The SA node is located in the lower right atrium near the septum.
4. _____ A contraction is known as diastole.

DIVIDING WORDS EXERCISE

Separate these words into their component parts (prefix, combining form, suffix). Some words do not contain all three word parts. The first one has been done for you.

Medical Word	Prefix	Combining Form	Suffix	Medical Word	Prefix	Combining Form	Suffix
1. **repolarization**	*re-*	*polar/o-*	*-ization*	5. ectopic	_____	_____	_____
2. conduction	_____	_____		6. refractory	_____	_____	_____
3. depolarization	_____	_____	_____	7. systolic	_____	_____	_____
4. diastolic	_____	_____					

SPELLING EXERCISE

Read each medical word pronunciation and write the medical word that it represents. Be sure to check your spelling. The first one has been done for you.

1. (per-KIN-jee)   *Purkinje*
2. (AA-tree-OH-ven-TRIH-kyoo-lar) _____
3. (dee-POH-lar-ih-ZAY-shun) _____

4. (DY-ah-STAW-lik) _____
5. (ek-TAW-pik) _____
6. (SY-noh-AA-tree-al) _____

5.3 Diseases

MATCHING EXERCISE

Match each word or phrase to its description.

1. arrhythmia
2. asystole
3. atheroma
4. bruit
5. cardiomegaly
6. claudication
7. coarctation
8. hypertension
9. jugular venous distention
10. myocardial infarction
11. necrosis
12. orthostatic hypotension
13. palpitation
14. tetralogy of Fallot
15. thrombus

_____ heart attack

_____ calf pain caused by peripheral artery disease

_____ elevated blood pressure

_____ fatty deposit on the wall of an artery

_____ chest sensation during a premature contraction

_____ dead tissue after a myocardial infarction

_____ a cardiac arrest with no activity seen on an ECG

_____ blood clot

_____ causes lightheadedness when going from lying to sitting position

_____ abnormal narrowing of the aorta in the fetal heart

_____ associated with right-sided congestive heart failure

_____ harsh, rushing sound in artery with arteriosclerosis

_____ sick sinus syndrome is one example of this

_____ enlargement of the heart

_____ four congenital defects in the fetal heart

CIRCLE EXERCISE

Circle the correct answer from the choices given.

1. (**Asystole, Bradycardia, Fibrillation**) is an abnormally slow heart rate.
2. Narrowing of an artery is known as (**aneurysm, endocarditis, stenosis**).
3. A weakness in the wall of an artery is known as a/an (**aneurysm, couplet, varicose vein**).
4. (**Patent foramen ovale, Heart block, Aneurysm**) is a congenital heart defect.
5. Left-sided congestive heart failure is associated with (**arrhythmia, peripheral edema, pulmonary edema**).
6. Mitral valve prolapse is associated with (**aneurysm, arrhythmia, regurgitation**).
7. Coronary artery disease can cause (**angina pectoris, palpitations, varicose veins**).
8. Inflammation of a vein is (**arteriosclerosis, murmur, phlebitis**).
9. Cardiac risk factors include all of the following *except* (**heart attack, heredity, obesity, smoking**).

TRUE OR FALSE EXERCISE

*Indicate whether each statement is true or false by writing **T** or **F** on the line.*

1. _____ Angina pectoris is chest pain that means that myocardial cells have died.
2. _____ Prolapse of a valve is when the leaflets do not close completely.
3. _____ Raynaud disease is severe vasoconstriction of the extremities triggered by cold or emotional stress.
4. _____ Hyperlipidemia includes both hypercholesterolemia and hypertriglyceridemia.
5. _____ Arteriosclerosis is a degenerative change over time that makes an artery hard.
6. _____ Essential hypertension has no known cause.
7. _____ Bradycardia is a very fast, uncoordinated quivering of the myocardium.

ADJECTIVE EXERCISE

Read the noun and write its adjective form on the line. Be sure to check your spelling. The first one has been done for you.

Singular Noun	Adjective		Singular Noun	Adjective
1. **bradycardia**	*bradycardic*		4. atheroma	
2. angina			5. hypertension	
3. arteriosclerosis			6. tachycardia	

DIVIDING WORDS EXERCISE

Separate these words into their component parts (prefix, combining form, suffix). Some words do not contain all three word parts. The first one has been done for you.

Medical Word	Prefix	Combining Form	Suffix	Medical Word	Prefix	Combining Form	Suffix
1. **ischemia**		*isch/o-*	*-emia*	7. hypercholesterolemia			
2. arrhythmia				8. hypotension			
3. atheroma				9. infarction			
4. bradycardia				10. pericarditis			
5. cardiomegaly				11. phlebitis			
6. claudication							

SPELLING EXERCISE

Read each medical word pronunciation and write the medical word that it represents. Be sure to check your spelling. The first one has been done for you.

1. **(MER-mer)**	*murmur*	7. (KAR-dee-OH-my-AW-pah-thee)	
2. (AN-yoor-izm)		8. (KLAW-dih-KAY-shun)	
3. (an-JY-nah)		9. (fleh-BY-tihs)	
4. (aa-SIHS-toh-lee)		10. (try-JEM-ih-nee)	
5. (ATH-eh-ROH-skleh-ROH-sihs)		11. (THRAWM-boh-fleh-BY-tihs)	
6. (BROO-ee)		12. (VAIR-ih-kohs)	

5.4 Laboratory, Diagnostic, and Radiologic Procedures

MATCHING EXERCISE

Match each word or phrase to its description.

1. cardiac catheterization	_____ uses limb leads
2. color flow duplex ultrasonography	_____ can diagnose an MI many days after it occurred
3. CK-MB	_____ used in a cardiac exercise stress test
4. ejection fraction	_____ blood test that is one of the cardiac enzymes
5. EKG	_____ monitors heart rate and rhythm in the CCU
6. Holter monitor	_____ studies anatomy of and pressures in the heart
7. pharmacologic stress test	_____ used when a patient is unable to exercise during a cardiac exercise stress test
8. telemetry	_____ continues for 24 hours
9. treadmill	_____ calculated by a MUGA scan
10. troponin	_____ gold standard for evaluating tortuous varicose veins

CIRCLE EXERCISE

Circle the correct answer from the choices given.

1. A lipid profile test includes all of the following *except* (**HDL, LDL, V₁-V₆**).

2. A longer sample of a lead II tracing is a (**Holter monitor, MUGA scan, rhythm strip**).

3. Angiography includes all of the following *except* (**arteriography, echocardiography, venography**).

4. A MUGA scan uses (**a radioactive tracer, sound waves, x-rays**) to create images of the heart chambers with blood in them.

5. Ultrasonography uses (**radiation, sound waves, x-rays**) to produce an image.

LABORATORY TEST EXERCISE

You need to order the following laboratory tests to be done for a cardiology patient. Find each of these tests on the laboratory form and put a checkmark in the box next to it.

C-reactive protein (CRP)	CK-MB	LDL lipoprotein	troponin
cholesterol, total	digoxin drug level	lipid panel	VLDL lipoprotein
	HDL lipoprotein	triglycerides	

CPT CODE	PANELS AND PROFILES	CPT CODE	PANELS AND PROFILES
80051	Electrolyte panel	85018	Hemoglobin (Hgb)
80053	Metabolic panel, comprehensive	83036	Hemoglobin A1C
80061	Lipid panel	82728	Iron, total
80069	Renal function panel	83615	Lactate dehydrogenase (LDH)
	BLOOD TESTS	83721	LDL lipoprotein
82040	Albumin	83655	Lead, blood
82247	Bilirubin, total	85730	Partial thromboplastin time (PTT)
86900	Blood type	85610	Prothrombin time (PT)
86140	C-reactive protein (CRP)	84443	Thyroid-stimulating hormone (TSH)
82465	Cholesterol, total	84436	Thyroxine (T4), total
85025	Complete blood count (CBC)	84478	Triglycerides
82553	Creatine kinase (CK-MB)	84480	Triiodothyronine (T3), total
82565	Creatinine, blood	84484	Troponin
80162	Digoxin drug level	84550	Uric acid
82947	Glucose, fasting	83719	VLDL lipoprotein
82951	Glucose tolerance test	85025	White blood cell (WBC) count with differential
83718	HDL lipoprotein		
85014	Hematocrit (HCT)		

5.5 Medical Procedures, Drugs, and Surgical Procedures

MATCHING EXERCISE

Match each word or phrase to its description.

1. diastolic	_____ used to treat an arrhythmia
2. diuretic drug	_____ legal form for patient who does not want CPR
3. DNR	_____ where stethoscope is placed at apex of heart
4. heart-lung machine	_____ used during cardiopulmonary bypass surgery
5. nitroglycerin drug	_____ instrument to measure the blood pressure
6. pacemaker	_____ one of the four vital signs
7. point of maximum impulse	_____ surgery to reconstruct a heart valve
8. pulse	_____ bottom number in a blood pressure reading
9. sclerotherapy	_____ used during an angioplasty
10. sphygmomanometer	_____ used to treat angina pectoris
11. stent	_____ treatment for a varicose vein
12. valvuloplasty	_____ also known as a "water pill"

CIRCLE EXERCISE

Circle the correct answer from the choices given.

1. The vital signs include all of the following *except* (**blood pressure, diastolic, pulse, temperature**).
2. (**Aneurysm, Angina, Arrhythmia**) is treated with cardioversion.
3. Suturing one blood vessel to another is a/an (**anastomosis, pacemaker insertion, transplantation**).
4. All of the following are used to compress atheromatous plaque in an artery *except* a (**balloon, prosthesis, stent**).
5. All of these drugs are used to prevent a blood clot from forming *except* a/an (**anticoagulant drug, aspirin, thrombolytic drug**).

TRUE OR FALSE EXERCISE

*Indicate whether each statement is true or false by writing **T** or **F** on the line.*

1. _____ Auscultation is using a stethoscope to listen to the heart sounds.
2. _____ A sphygmomanometer measures the blood pressure in mm Hg.
3. _____ CPR is a procedure to circulate the blood after the patient's heart has stopped.
4. _____ The most commonly used site to take the pulse is the carotid artery.
5. _____ Pericardiocentesis uses a needle to remove fluid from the pericardial sac.
6. _____ Antiarrhythmic drugs are used to treat hypertension.

DIVIDING WORDS EXERCISE

Separate these words into their component parts (prefix, combining form, suffix). Some words do not contain all three word parts. The first one has been done for you.

Medical Word	Prefix	Combining Form	Suffix	Medical Word	Prefix	Combining Form	Suffix
1. **transluminal**	*trans-*	*lumin/o-*	*-al*	7. defibrillator	_____	_____	_____
2. anastomosis		_____	_____	8. pericardiocentesis	_____	_____	_____
3. aneurysmectomy		_____	_____	9. resuscitation		_____	_____
4. angioplasty		_____	_____	10. sclerotherapy		_____	_____
5. anticoagulant	_____	_____	_____	11. stethoscope		_____	_____
6. auscultation		_____	_____	12. valvulotome		_____	_____

PROOFREADING AND SPELLING EXERCISE

Read the following paragraph. Identify each misspelled medical word and write the correct spelling of it on the line provided.

The nurse used a sphigmomanometer to take the patient's blood pressure. He had hypertension in the past. He had a caroted endarterectomy because of atherometous plaque in his artery. He has also had an arhythmia in the past with ventricular takycardia. He just developed congestive heart failure and takes a dijitalis drug for that. We are considering this patient for an angoplasty in the future to keep him from having a myocardal infarcktion. His cardiomegalee is becoming more severe.

1. _____

2. _____

3. _____

4. _____

5. _____

6. _____

7. _____

8. _____

9. _____

10. _____

Immerse Yourself: Analyze Medical Reports

Electronic Patient Record #1

This is an Office Visit SOAP Note. Read the note and answer the questions.

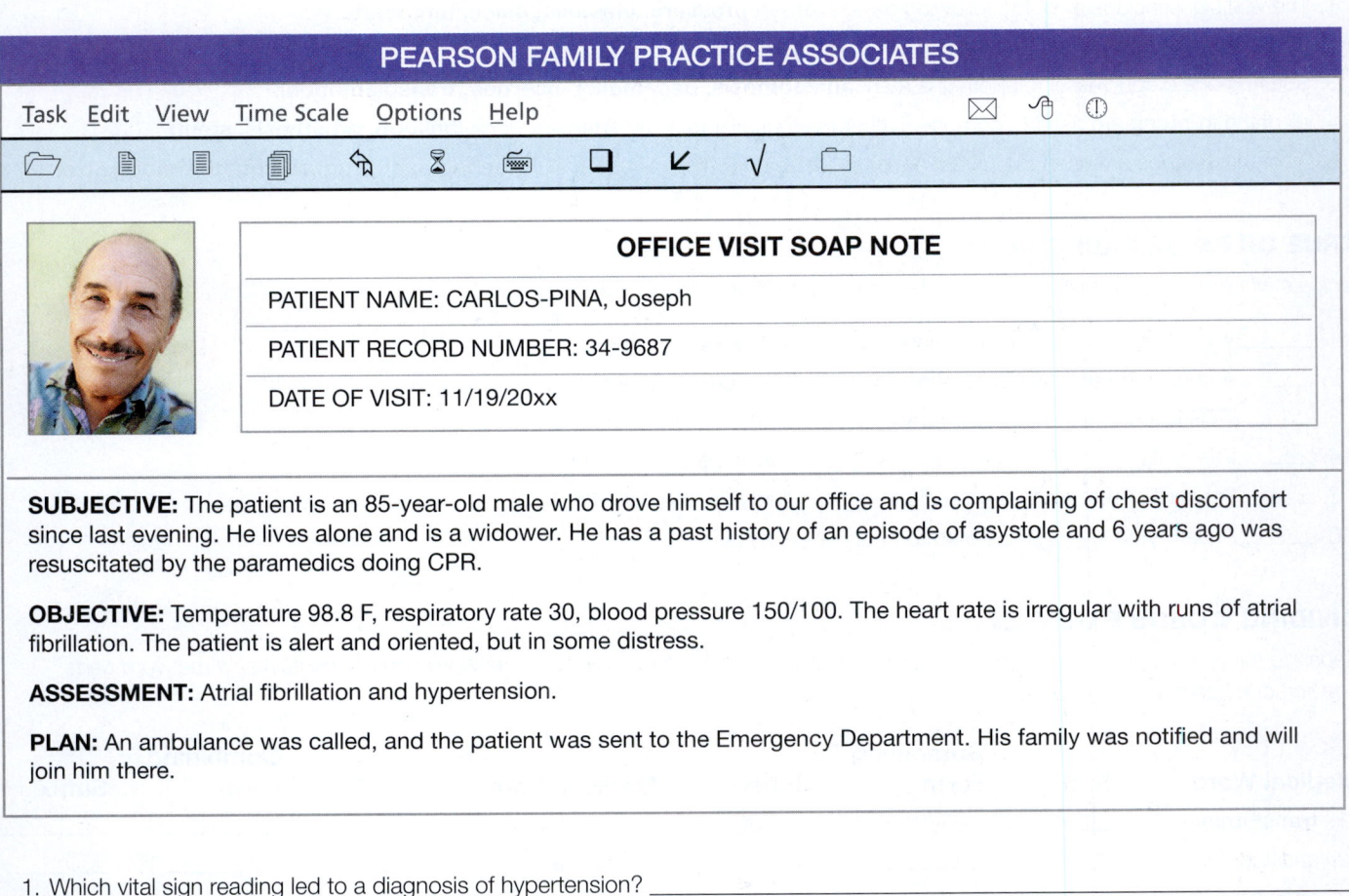

PEARSON FAMILY PRACTICE ASSOCIATES

Task   Edit   View   Time Scale   Options   Help

OFFICE VISIT SOAP NOTE

PATIENT NAME: CARLOS-PINA, Joseph

PATIENT RECORD NUMBER: 34-9687

DATE OF VISIT: 11/19/20xx

SUBJECTIVE: The patient is an 85-year-old male who drove himself to our office and is complaining of chest discomfort since last evening. He lives alone and is a widower. He has a past history of an episode of asystole and 6 years ago was resuscitated by the paramedics doing CPR.

OBJECTIVE: Temperature 98.8 F, respiratory rate 30, blood pressure 150/100. The heart rate is irregular with runs of atrial fibrillation. The patient is alert and oriented, but in some distress.

ASSESSMENT: Atrial fibrillation and hypertension.

PLAN: An ambulance was called, and the patient was sent to the Emergency Department. His family was notified and will join him there.

1. Which vital sign reading led to a diagnosis of hypertension? _____

2. What is the medical definition of asystole? _____

3. How was this patient's asystole treated in the past? _____

4. What does the abbreviation *CPR* mean? _____

Electronic Patient Record #2

This is a hospital Admission History and Physical Examination report. Read the report and answer the questions.

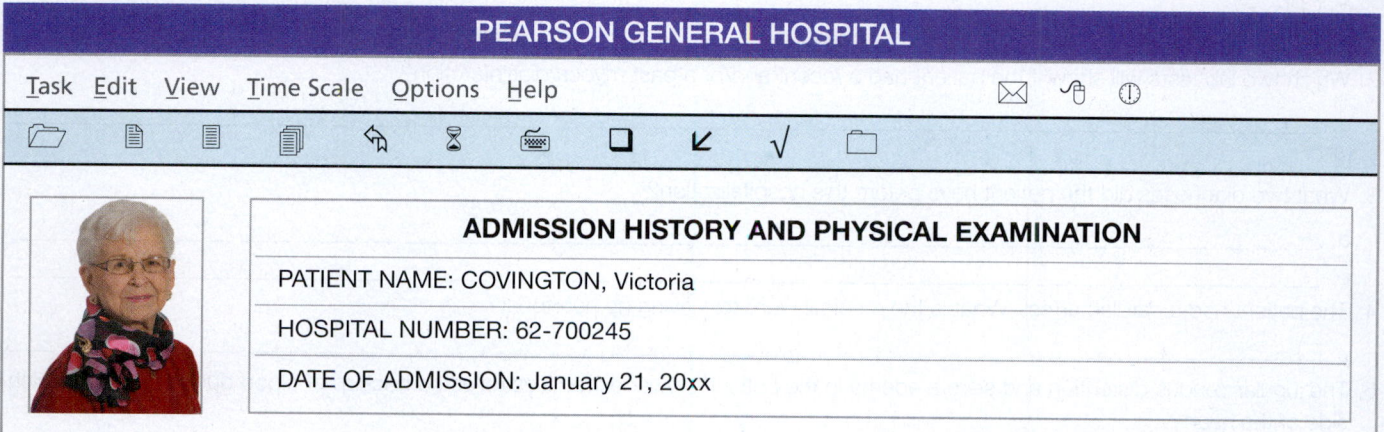

PEARSON GENERAL HOSPITAL

Task Edit View Time Scale Options Help

ADMISSION HISTORY AND PHYSICAL EXAMINATION

PATIENT NAME: COVINGTON, Victoria

HOSPITAL NUMBER: 62-700245

DATE OF ADMISSION: January 21, 20xx

HISTORY OF PRESENT ILLNESS

The patient is a 76-year-old female who was transferred from home via ambulance to this Emergency Department. Apparently, the patient had just finished eating breakfast when her family noticed that she was standing in the middle of the hallway with her walker and seemed dazed. She was assisted to her bed, but rest did not improve her mental status. The family stated that she continued to be confused, incoherent, and unable to answer simple questions. At that point, the family called 911.

PAST MEDICAL HISTORY

The past medical history was obtained from the patient's daughter-in-law. The patient has a history of CHF, which has been slowly worsening over about the past 8 years. She also has a history of HTN. In the past week, the patient has had no appetite, has eaten little, but reportedly gained 2 pounds anyway. The daughter-in-law does not know the names of all of the patient's medications, except that she is taking a diuretic drug. The patient smokes one pack of cigarettes per day and has done so for the past 40+ years. The patient has no known allergies.

PHYSICAL EXAMINATION

The patient is a thin female, lying in bed. She is stuporous, opening her eyes to commands but unable to answer questions. Heart: Regular rate and rhythm. There is jugular venous distention. The breath sounds reveal fluid in the lungs. The abdomen is soft. Physical examination of the lower extremities shows severe edema in both feet and legs.

COURSE IN THE EMERGENCY DEPARTMENT

The patient was placed on a cardiac monitor. Labs were sent for electrolytes, CK-MB, and troponin. A portable chest x-ray in the emergency department showed cardiomegaly with significant pulmonary edema. While we were awaiting the results of the blood chemistries, the patient suddenly went into cardiac arrest. CPR was initiated. She responded to aggressive drug intervention, and we were able to establish a normal sinus rhythm. The patient was then transferred to the CCU in critical condition.

Alfred P. Molina, M.D.

Alfred P. Molina, M.D.

APM:smt

D: 01/21/XX

T: 01/21/XX

1. What do these abbreviations stand for?
   a. CCU _____
   b. CHF _____
   c. CPR _____
   d. HTN _____

2. Which two lab tests will show if the patient had a recent and/or a past myocardial infarction?
   a. _____
   b. _____

3. What two diagnoses did the patient have before this hospitalization?
   a. _____
   b. _____

4. The patient had a cardiac arrest. What is the medical word for having no heartbeat?
   _____

5. The jugular venous distention and severe edema in the patient's lower extremities reflected backup of blood due to failure of which side of the heart?
   _____

6. The pulmonary edema seen on the chest x-ray reflected failure of which side of the heart?
   _____

7. The patient was taking a diuretic drug to treat which condition? (Circle one)

   congestive heart failure   **lack of appetite**   **confusion**

8. If the patient ate little food in the past week, why did she gain 2 pounds?
   _____

You Write the Medical Report

You are a healthcare professional interviewing a patient. Listen to the patient's statements and then enter them in the patient's electronic medical record using medical words and phrases. Be sure to check your spelling. The first one has been done for you.

1. The patient says, "Last night, I had severe pain in my chest that was like a crushing sensation and bad sweating and I felt like something really bad was happening."

   You write: Last night, the patient experienced severe <u>angina pectoris</u> with the pain feeling like a crushing sensation. He also had <u>diaphoresis</u> and a sense of doom.

2. The patient says, "Last year, I went to the emergency room and the doctor told me that my heart was going very fast but was uncoordinated and couldn't pump any blood. They brought this machine in and it had two paddles and they gave me a shock and then my heart rhythm was normal. Today, I could feel my heart do some 'thumps' and then be okay. But the last time this happened, they did hook me up to those electrodes and took a tracing of my heart."

   You write: The patient states that last year she went to the emergency room with ventricular _____. They used a _____ on her, and her heart rhythm returned to normal. The patient says she felt some _____ today, and so, as they did the previous time, we will do an _____ on her in the office today.

3. The patient says, "I know I have a history of my arteries being hard and clogged with fatty stuff, but now I have this new problem and I get on-and-off pain in the calf of my leg when I try to walk very far. My podiatrist said my one toe is black and does not get enough blood to it and the tissue might die."

   You write: The patient has a history of _____ as well as _____ of her arteries. Now she has a new problem of experiencing intermittent _____ when she tries to walk very far. Her podiatrist noted a lack of perfusion to one toe and feels it might develop _____.

4. The nurse's note in the patient's medical record shows that the patient's blood pressure today is 130/88. Previous office visits have shown similar BP results. The patient says, "I am trying to stay on my low-salt diet."

   You write: Based on serial blood pressure measurements today and over the past 3 months, the patient's blood pressure remains in the range of 130/88. Based on these readings, she now has a diagnosis of _____. She has been on a low-salt diet, and we will now add a _____ drug to help her excrete more sodium in her urine and help lower her blood pressure.

MyLab Medical Terminology™

MyLab Medical Terminology is a premium online homework management system that includes a host of features to help you study. Registered users will find:

- A multitude of quizzes and activities built within the MyLab platform

- Powerful tools that track and analyze your results—allowing you to create a personalized learning experience

- Videos and audio pronunciations to help enrich your progress

- Streaming lesson presentations (guided lectures) and self-paced learning modules

- A space where you and your instructor can check your progress and manage your assignments

6 Hematology and Immunology
Blood and Lymphatic System

Hematology (HEE-mah-TAW-loh-jee) is the medical specialty that studies the anatomy and physiology of the blood; uses laboratory, diagnostic, and radiologic procedures to diagnose blood diseases; and uses medical procedures, drugs, and surgical procedures to treat blood diseases.

Immunology (IH-myoo-NAW-loh-jee) is the medical specialty related to the lymphatic system and the immune response.

⌄ Chapter Overview and Learning Outcomes

After you study this chapter, you should be able to demonstrate mastery of the outcomes by successfully completing the exercises.

6.1 Anatomy
Identify the structures of the blood and lymphatic system.
Demonstrate proficiency in medical language.
6.1 Practice Laps

6.2 Physiology
Describe the functions of blood clotting and the immune response.
Demonstrate proficiency in medical language.
6.2 Practice Laps
Vocabulary Review

6.3 Diseases
Describe common blood and lymphatic system diseases.
Demonstrate proficiency in medical language.
6.3 Practice Laps

6.4 Laboratory, Diagnostic, and Radiologic Procedures
Describe common blood and lymphatic laboratory tests, diagnostic procedures, and radiologic procedures.
Demonstrate proficiency in medical language.
6.4 Practice Laps

6.5 Medical Procedures, Drugs, and Surgical Procedures
Describe common blood and lymphatic medical procedures, drugs, and surgical procedures.
6.5 Practice Laps
Abbreviations Summary
Career Focus

Chapter Review Exercises
Dive In: Medical Language Exercises (Learning Outcomes 6.1–6.5)

Immerse Yourself: Analyze Medical Reports

Medical Language Key

To unlock the definition of a medical word, first break it into word parts. Then give the meaning of each word part. Put the meanings of the word parts in order, beginning with the meaning of the suffix, then the meaning of the prefix (if there is one), then the meaning of the combining form.

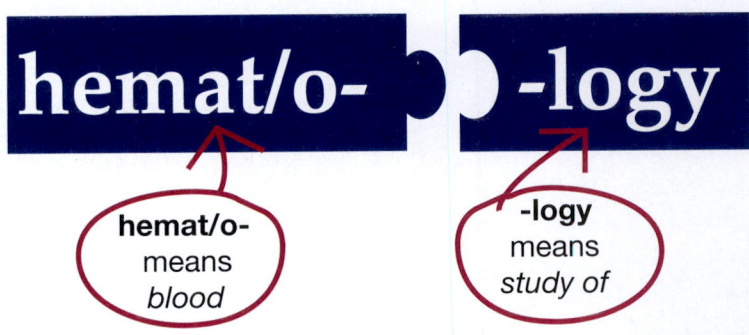

hemat/o- | **-logy**

hemat/o- means *blood*

-logy means *study of*

Hematology: ▶ *Study of (the) blood.*
Immunology: ▶ *Study of (the) immune response.*

The **blood** is essential to the life of the body and to every cell in the body. The blood contains formed elements (red blood cells, white blood cells, thrombocytes), plasma, and other substances. Blood travels within the blood vessels of the cardiovascular system (described in Chapter 5, Cardiology). The blood is categorized as connective tissue because it connects all parts of the body and its blood cells are produced by the bone marrow, a type of connective tissue (see Figure 6-1 ■).

The function of the blood is to continuously transport the formed elements and plasma, as well as nutrients, electrolytes, oxygen, carbon dioxide, clotting factors, and waste products of cellular metabolism.

The **lymphatic system** (see Figure 6-1) consists of the lymphatic vessels, lymph fluid, lymph nodes, lymphoid tissues, and lymphoid organs that form a pathway throughout the body that is separate from the cardiovascular system.

The function of the lymphatic system is to provide an immune response that defends the body against bacteria, viruses, parasites, foreign cells, and cancer cells.

6.1 Anatomy

Anatomy of the Blood

Hematopoiesis

Hematopoiesis is the process by which the formed elements of the blood are produced. Hematopoiesis occurs in the red marrow of certain bones (sternum, ribs, hips, spine, and legs). Each type of blood cell begins in the red bone marrow as a **stem cell**, a very immature cell that gives rise to all the other blood cells, each of which matures in stages until it is finally released into the blood (see Figure 6-2 ■).

Erythrocytes

Erythrocytes or **red blood cells (RBCs)** are the most numerous cells in the blood. Each erythrocyte is a round, somewhat flattened, red disk (see Figure 6-3 ■).

Erythrocytes develop from stem cells that become **erythroblasts**, continue to mature through stages, and are released into the blood in a slightly immature form known as **reticulocytes** (see Figure 6-2). Unlike other body cells, a mature erythrocyte has no nucleus.

Erythrocytes contain **hemoglobin**, a red, iron-containing molecule that binds to and carries oxygen from the lungs to every cell in the body. Hemoglobin bound to oxygen is known as **oxyhemoglobin**. Hemoglobin also binds to and carries carbon dioxide (as carbaminohemoglobin) from the cells back to the lungs.

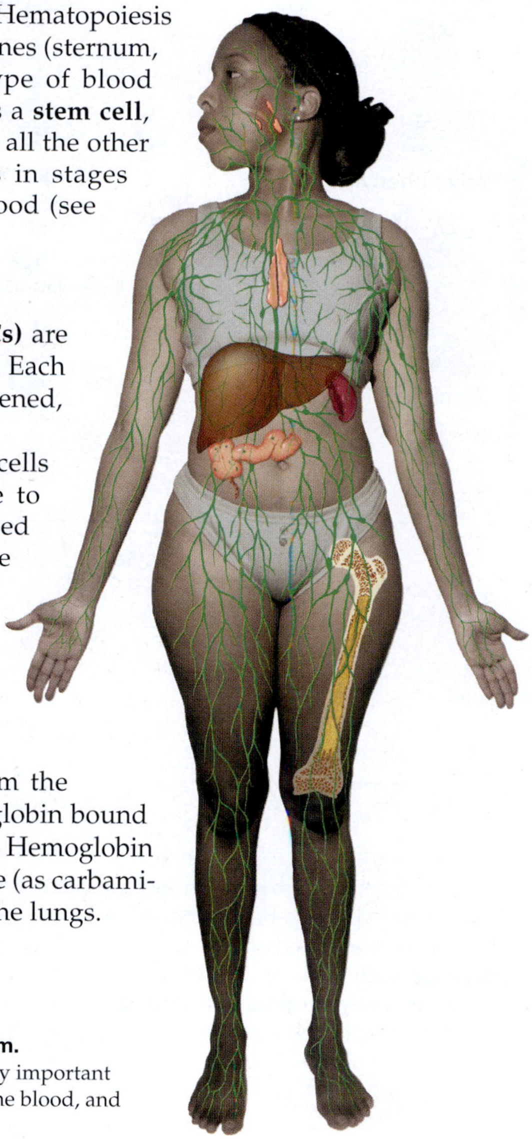

FIGURE 6-1 ■ Blood and the lymphatic system.
These two body systems are responsible for many important body functions: producing blood cells, clotting the blood, and coordinating the body's immune response.

Pronunciation/Word Parts

blood (BLUD)
The combining forms **hemat/o-** and **hem/o-** mean *blood.*

lymphatic (lim-FAH-tik)
   lymph/o- *lymph; lymphatic system*
   -atic *pertaining to*

hematopoiesis (HEE-mah-TOH-poy-EE-sihs)
   hemat/o- *blood*
   -poiesis *process of formation*

stem cell
The stem of something is the source from which all others originate.

erythrocyte (eh-RITH-roh-site)
   erythr/o- *red*
   -cyte *cell*

erythroblast (eh-RITH-roh-blast)
   erythr/o- *red*
   -blast *immature cell*

reticulocyte (reh-TIH-kyoo-loh-SITE)
   reticul/o- *small network*
   -cyte *cell*
A reticulocyte has a network of ribosomes in its cytoplasm.

hemoglobin (HEE-moh-GLOH-bin)
   hem/o- *blood*
   glob/o- *comprehensive; shaped like a globe*
   -in *substance*

oxyhemoglobin
(AWK-see-HEE-moh-GLOH-bin)
   ox/y- *oxygen; quick*
   hem/o- *blood*
   glob/o- *comprehensive; shaped like a globe*
   -in *substance*

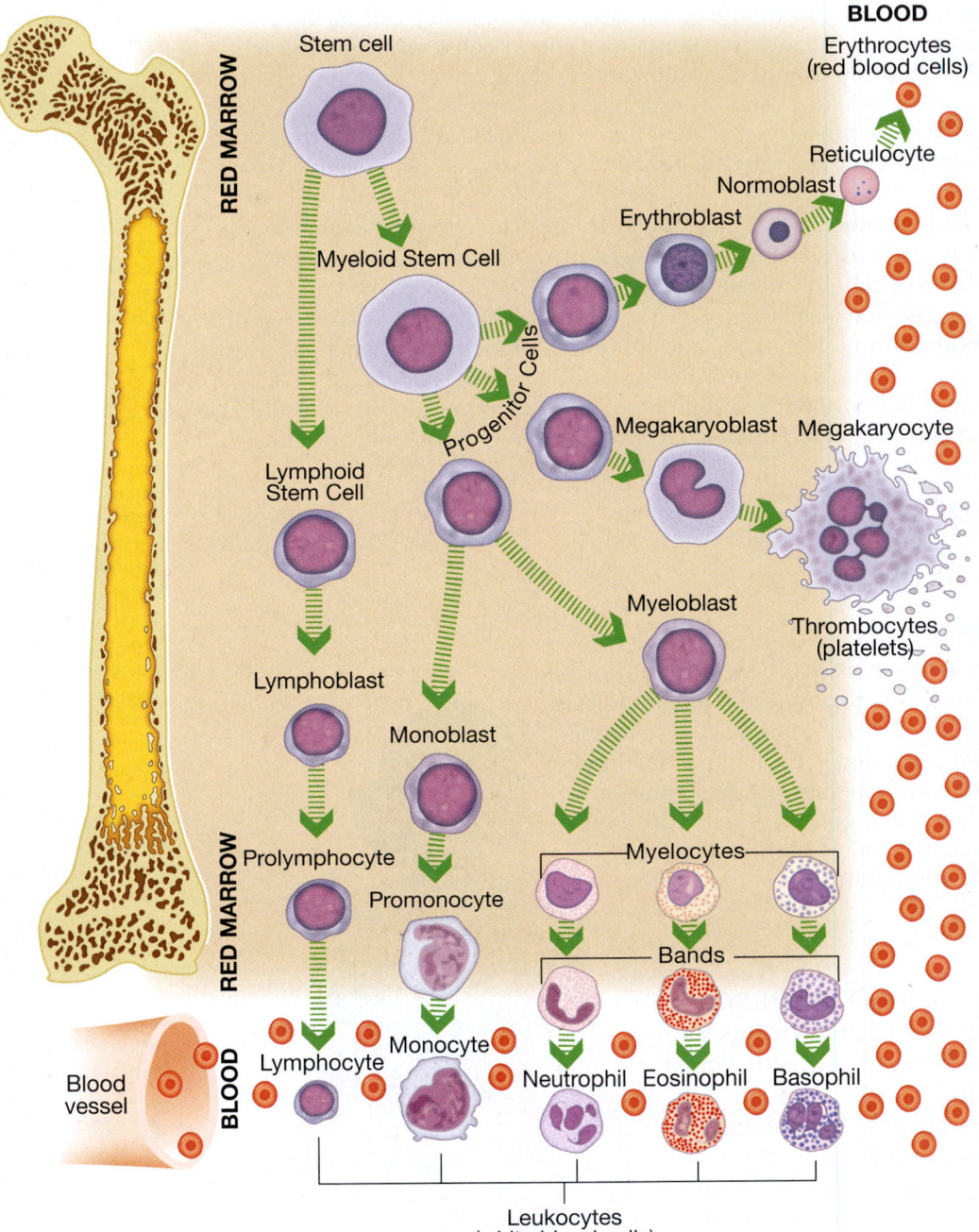

FIGURE 6-2 ■ Hematopoiesis.
All of the formed elements of the blood begin in
the red bone marrow as it produces stem cells that
progress to mature cells, which then enter the blood.

Clinical Connections

Forensic Science. When a person drowns or suffocates, there is a high level of carbon dioxide
(CO_2) in the blood. This causes the skin to have a deep bluish-purple color known as *cyanosis*.
However, when a person dies in a fire or from inhaling the fumes from car exhaust or a faulty space
heater, there is a high level of **carbon monoxide (CO)** in the blood. Unlike oxygen and carbon
dioxide, carbon monoxide binds so tightly and irreversibly to **carboxyhemoglobin** that an erythrocyte is unable to carry any other molecule. Carbon monoxide poisoning causes a characteristic
cherry-red skin color.

carbon monoxide (KAR-bon
mawn-AWK-side)

carboxyhemoglobin
(kar-BAWK-see-HEE-moh-GLOH-bin)
  carbox/y- *carbon monoxide*
  hem/o- *blood*
  glob/o- *comprehensive; shaped like a
    globe*
  -in *substance*

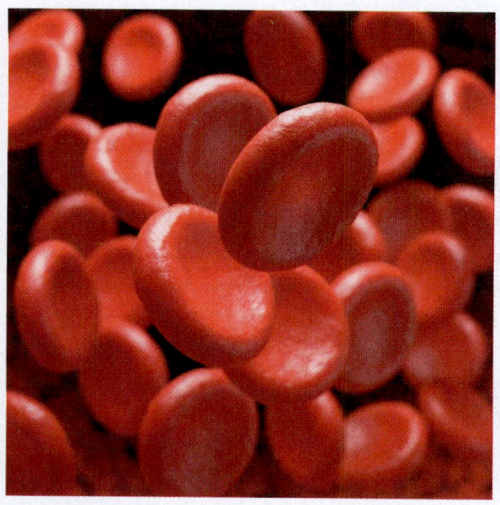

FIGURE 6-3 ■ Erythrocytes.
Notice the characteristic red color of erythrocytes (red blood cells) and their unique "doughnut" shape. Each erythrocyte has a depressed center and no cell nucleus. Because there is no nucleus, an erythrocyte deteriorates and dies after 120 days.

Erythrocytes are unique because, unlike other body cells, an erythrocyte has no cell nucleus when it is mature; this means that it is unable to divide or repair itself, and so it begins to deteriorate and dies after 120 days. Because of this, the supply of erythrocytes must constantly be replenished (the red bone marrow produces several million erythrocytes every second). If a person has anemia with too few erythrocytes or experiences a significant blood loss, the kidneys secrete **erythropoietin**, a hormone that increases the speed at which erythrocytes are produced and become mature. When erythrocytes die, the spleen removes them from the blood and breaks down their hemoglobin into heme and globin molecules. Iron is stripped from the heme molecule and stored in the liver and spleen; it is released to build more erythrocytes if the diet does not contain enough iron. The rest of the heme molecule is used to make bilirubin which is then used by the liver to make bile. The combining form *rub/o-* (red) in *bilirubin* indicates that bilirubin comes from red blood cells. The globin molecule is broken down into amino acids that are used by the body to build proteins.

Pronunciation/Word Parts

erythropoietin (eh-RITH-roh-POY-eh-tin)
   erythr/o- *red*
   -poietin *substance that forms*
Erythropoietin: *Substance that forms red (blood cells)*

Dive Deeper

Erythrocytes contain genetic material that determines a person's **blood type**. Each blood type is named for its **antigen** (protein molecule on the cell membrane of the erythrocyte). The two major blood groups based on these antigens are the ABO blood group and the Rh blood group.

The **ABO blood group** includes four different blood types: A, B, AB, and O. Type A blood contains A antigens on the erythrocytes, type B has B antigens, and type AB has both antigens. Type O blood has neither A nor B antigens on the erythrocytes. Each blood type has antibodies in the plasma against other blood types.

The **Rh blood group** has many different antigens, collectively known as the **Rh factor**. The Rh factor is either present on the erythrocytes or not. When these antigens are present, the blood type is Rh positive. When these antigens are not present, the blood type is Rh negative.

The ABO and the Rh blood groups are always considered together. For example, type AB blood is either AB positive (Rh positive) or AB negative (Rh negative).

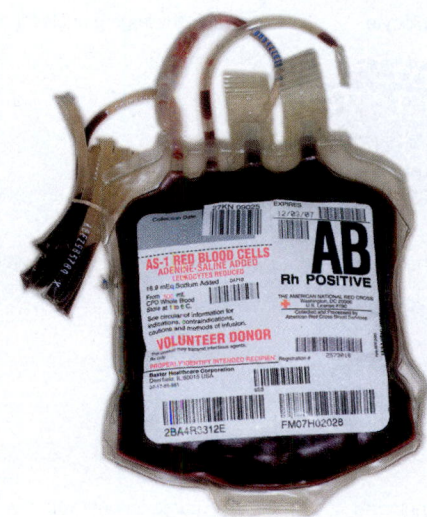

antigen (AN-tih-jen)
Antigen is a combination of part of the word *antibody* and the suffix *-gen* (that which produces).

Rh is an abbreviation for *Rhesus*, a monkey that also has this same blood factor as humans do.

Leukocytes

Leukocytes or **white blood cells (WBCs)** include five distinct types of cells. Leukocytes include neutrophils, eosinophils, basophils, lymphocytes, and monocytes (see Table 6-1 ■).

The type of leukocyte can be identified by the presence or absence of granules in its cytoplasm and by the shape of its nucleus. These differences can be seen when leukocytes are stained and examined under a microscope. Any leukocyte with many large granules in its cytoplasm is categorized as a **granulocyte**. Granulocytes include neutrophils, eosinophils, and basophils. A leukocyte with few or no granules in its cytoplasm is categorized as an **agranulocyte**. Agranulocytes include lymphocytes and monocytes.

Each of the five types of leukocytes has an important, specific role to play in an allergic response or as part of the immune response (described in the Physiology section).

Pronunciation/Word Parts

leukocyte (LOO-koh-site)
  leuk/o- *white*
  -cyte *cell*

granulocyte (GRAN-yoo-loh-SITE)
  granul/o- *granule*
  -cyte *cell*

agranulocyte (aa-GRAN-yoo-loh-SITE)
  a- *away from; without*
  granul/o- *granule*
  -cyte *cell*

Table 6-1   Leukocyte Types and Characteristics

Leukocyte	Category	Cytoplasm	Nucleus
Neutrophil segmented neutrophil, seg, polymorphonuclear leukocyte (PMN), poly	Granulocyte	Many large granules that do not stain either red or blue	Many segments and lobes
Eosinophil eo	Granulocyte	Many large granules that stain bright pink to red	Two lobes
Basophil baso	Granulocyte	Many large granules that stain dark blue to purple	More than one lobe
Lymphocyte lymph	Agranulocyte	Narrow ring with no granules	Large one that is round without lobes
Monocyte mono	Agranulocyte	Large amount with few or no granules	Large one that is kidney bean–shaped

Granulocytes

- **Neutrophils** are the most common leukocyte. They make up 54–62 percent of the leukocytes in the blood. A neutrophil has many large granules in its cytoplasm, but these do not stain when they are exposed to laboratory dye, remaining neutral in color. Its nucleus has many segments and lobes (see Figure 6-4 ■). A neutrophil is also known as a *segmented neutrophil*, *seg*, **polymorphonuclear leukocyte (PMN)**, or *poly*.

Pronunciation/Word Parts

neutrophil (NOO-troh-fil)
  neutr/o- not taking part
  -phil attraction to; fondness for

polymorphonuclear
(PAW-lee-MOR-foh-NOO-klee-ar)
  poly- many; much
  morph/o- shape
  nucle/o- nucleus of an atom or a cell
  -ar pertaining to

eosinophil (EE-oh-SIN-oh-fil)
  eosin/o- eosin; red, acidic dye
  -phil attraction to; fondness for

basophil (BAY-soh-fil)
  bas/o- alkaline; base of a structure
  -phil attraction to; fondness for

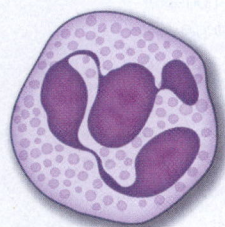

FIGURE 6-4 ■ Neutrophil.
A neutrophil has many large, pale granules in its cytoplasm. These granules do not stain well with either a red, acidic dye (eosin) or with a blue, alkaline dye (hematoxylin). Neutrophils get their name from their neutral reaction to these dyes. The nucleus has many segments and lobes.

Neutrophils develop in the red marrow from stem cells, going through several stages before becoming a **band** (see Figure 6-2). A band is an immature neutrophil that has a nucleus shaped like a curved band. Bands are also known as **stabs** (the German word for *band*). There are always a few bands present in the blood, which then become mature neutrophils.

- **Eosinophils** make up just 1–3 percent of the leukocytes in the blood. An eosinophil has many large granules in its cytoplasm that stain bright pink to red with eosin dye. Its nucleus has two lobes (see Figure 6-5 ■). Eosinophils are also known as *eos*.

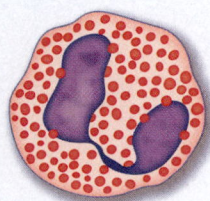

FIGURE 6-5 ■ Eosinophil.
An eosinophil has many large, pink-red granules in its cytoplasm. These granules stain with a red, acidic dye (eosin). Eosinophils get their name from their reaction to this dye. The nucleus has two lobes.

Eosinophils develop in the red marrow from stem cells, going from immature forms to mature eosinophils (see Figure 6-2).

- **Basophils** are the least common leukocyte. They make up just 0.5–1 percent of the leukocytes in the blood. A basophil has many large granules in its cytoplasm that stain dark blue to purple with hematoxylin, an alkaline dye. Its nucleus has more than one lobe (see Figure 6-6 ■). Basophils are also known as *basos*.

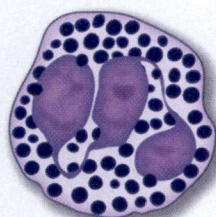

FIGURE 6-6 ■ Basophil.
A basophil has many large granules in its cytoplasm. These granules stain dark blue to purple with a blue, alkaline dye (hematoxylin). Chemically, something that is alkaline is known as a *base*, which is the opposite of an acid.) Basophils get their name from their reaction to this dye, which is a base. The nucleus has more than one lobe.

Basophils develop in the red marrow from stem cells, going from immature forms to mature basophils (see Figure 6-2).

Agranulocytes

- **Lymphocytes** make up 25–33 percent of the leukocytes in the blood. Lymphocytes are the smallest leukocytes. A lymphocyte has a narrow ring of cytoplasm that contains no granules, and its nucleus is round and nearly fills the cell (see Figure 6-7 ■). Some lymphocytes live for just a few days, whereas others live for many years. Lymphocytes are also known as *lymphs*.

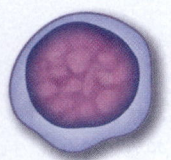

FIGURE 6-7 ■ Lymphocyte.
A lymphocyte has no granules in its cytoplasm, and so it is classified as an agranulocyte. It has little cytoplasm and a nucleus that is round and is without lobes.

Lymphocytes develop in the red marrow from stem cells that become immature **lymphoblasts** (see Figure 6-2). Some lymphoblasts mature and are released into the blood as lymphocytes. Other lymphoblasts mature in the red bone marrow and become B lymphocytes (B cells) (*B* for *bone*) or natural killer (NK) cells. Other lymphoblasts migrate to the thymus and mature there and become T lymphocytes (T cells) (*T* for *thymus*).

- **Monocytes** make up 3–7 percent of the leukocytes in the blood. They are the largest leukocytes. A monocyte has a large amount of cytoplasm that contains few or no granules, and its large nucleus is kidney bean–shaped (see Figure 6-8 ■). Monocytes are also known as *monos*.

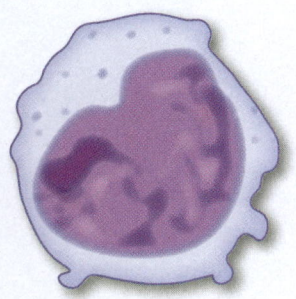

FIGURE 6-8 ■ Monocyte.
A monocyte has few or no granules in its cytoplasm, and so it is classified as an agranulocyte. It has a large amount of cytoplasm and a nucleus that is large and shaped like a kidney bean.

Monocytes develop in the red marrow from stem cells, going through several stages before becoming mature monocytes (see Figure 6-2).

Thrombocytes

Thrombocytes are different from other blood cells because they are only cell fragments. An individual thrombocyte begins in the red marrow as a stem cell, going through several stages before becoming a mature **megakaryocyte**, which is a very large cell with a great deal of cytoplasm (see Figure 6-2). The cytoplasm of the megakaryocyte breaks off into individual fragments that are thrombocytes, and these are released into the blood. Thrombocytes are also known as **platelets**. Platelets play a role in blood clotting (described in the Physiology section).

Plasma

Plasma is a clear, straw-colored liquid that makes up 55 percent of the blood (see Figure 6-9 ■). Erythrocytes, leukocytes, and thrombocytes are carried in the plasma. The plasma transports the nutrients of digested foods from the intestine to all the cells of the body, and it transports the waste products of metabolism (creatinine, urea) from the cells to the kidney to be excreted in the urine. Other important substances in the plasma are albumin and electrolytes (described next).

Pronunciation/Word Parts

lymphocyte (LIM-foh-site)
  lymph/o- *lymph; lymphatic system*
  -cyte *cell*

lymphoblast (LIM-foh-blast)
  lymph/o- *lymph; lymphatic system*
  -blast *immature cell*

monocyte (MAW-noh-site)
  mon/o- *one; single*
  -cyte *cell*
Monocyte: *Cell (that has) one (lobe in its nucleus)*

thrombocyte (THRAWM-boh-site)
  thromb/o- *blood clot*
  -cyte *cell*

megakaryocyte (MEG-ah-KAIR-ee-oh-SITE)
  mega- *large*
  kary/o- *nucleus of a cell*
  -cyte *cell*

platelet (PLAYT-let)

plasma (PLAZ-mah)
The combining form **plasm/o-** means *plasma*.

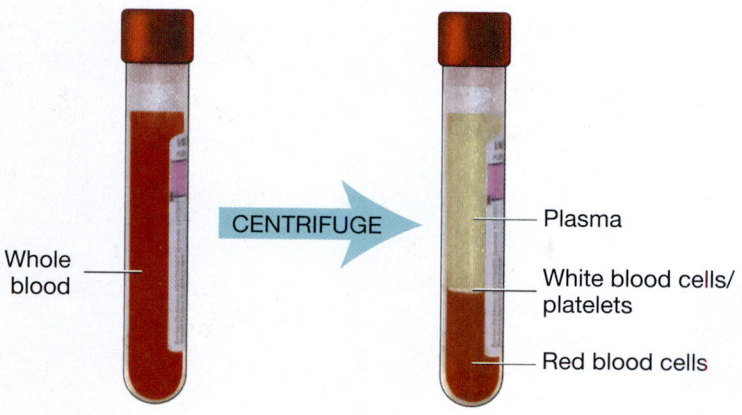

Whole blood

CENTRIFUGE

Plasma

White blood cells/platelets

Red blood cells

FIGURE 6-9 ■ Plasma.
Blood is composed of plasma and formed elements (red blood cells, white blood cells, platelets). When a specimen of whole blood is placed in a centrifuge and spun quickly, the heavier parts (the formed elements) settle to the bottom, and the clear, straw-colored plasma remains on the top.

Dive Deeper

The plasma also contains a number of substances:

- **Albumin** is a protein molecule that is produced by the liver. Albumin exerts osmotic pressure that keeps water from moving out of the blood and into the surrounding tissues. This maintains the volume of the blood and the blood pressure.

- **Electrolytes** are molecules that have a positive or negative electrical charge. Electrolytes in the plasma include **sodium (Na⁺)**, **potassium (K⁺)**, **calcium (Ca⁺⁺)**, **chloride (Cl⁻)**, and **bicarbonate (HCO₃⁻)**. Sodium exerts osmotic pressure that keeps water from moving out of the blood and into the surrounding tissues. This maintains the volume of the blood and the blood pressure. Sodium, potassium, and calcium are important in the contraction of the heart and skeletal muscles. Calcium (factor IV) is part of the process of blood clotting. Calcium is also important in the formation of bone. Bicarbonate acts as a buffer to maintain the normal pH of the blood (acidity vs. alkalinity).

albumin (al-BYOO-min)

electrolyte (ee-LEK-troh-lite)
  electr/o- *electricity*
  -lyte *dissolved substance*

Anatomy of the Lymphatic System

Lymphatic Vessels, Lymph, and Lymph Nodes

Lymphatic vessels are similar in structure to blood vessels, but with an important difference in that lymphatic vessels have a beginning and an end point, whereas blood vessels form a continuous pathway. Lymphatic vessels begin as tiny lymphatic capillaries in the tissues. Tissue fluid enters a lymphatic capillary and becomes **lymph**, the fluid in the lymphatic system. Lymphatic capillaries have large openings in their walls that allow microorganisms and cancer cells to enter. Lymphatic capillaries become larger lymphatic vessels that bring lymph to the lymph nodes. Like veins in the cardiovascular system, lymphatic vessels have valves that keep the lymph flowing in one direction until it reaches its end point at lymphatic ducts that empty into veins in the neck.

Lymph nodes are encapsulated pieces of lymphoid tissue that are round, oval, or bean shaped. They range in size from the head of a pin to 1 inch in length. Lymph nodes are grouped together in chains in areas where there is an increased risk of invasion by microorganisms or cancer cells (see Figure 6-10 ■). Each lymph node filters the lymph, and then special cells in the lymph node destroy any microorganisms or cancer cells that are present. Lymph nodes are also known as **lymph glands**.

Lymphoid Tissues and Lymphoid Organs

Lymphoid tissues include the tonsils and adenoids in the posterior oral cavity (described in Chapter 15, Otolaryngology) and Peyer patches and the appendix in

Pronunciation/Word Parts

lymphatic (lim-FAT-ik)
  lymph/o- *lymph; lymphatic system*
  -atic *pertaining to*

lymph node (LIMF NOHD)
Lymph gland is an alternate name for a *lymph node*, although lymph nodes are not really glands.

lymphoid (LIM-foyd)
  lymph/o- *lymph; lymphatic system*
  -oid *resembling*

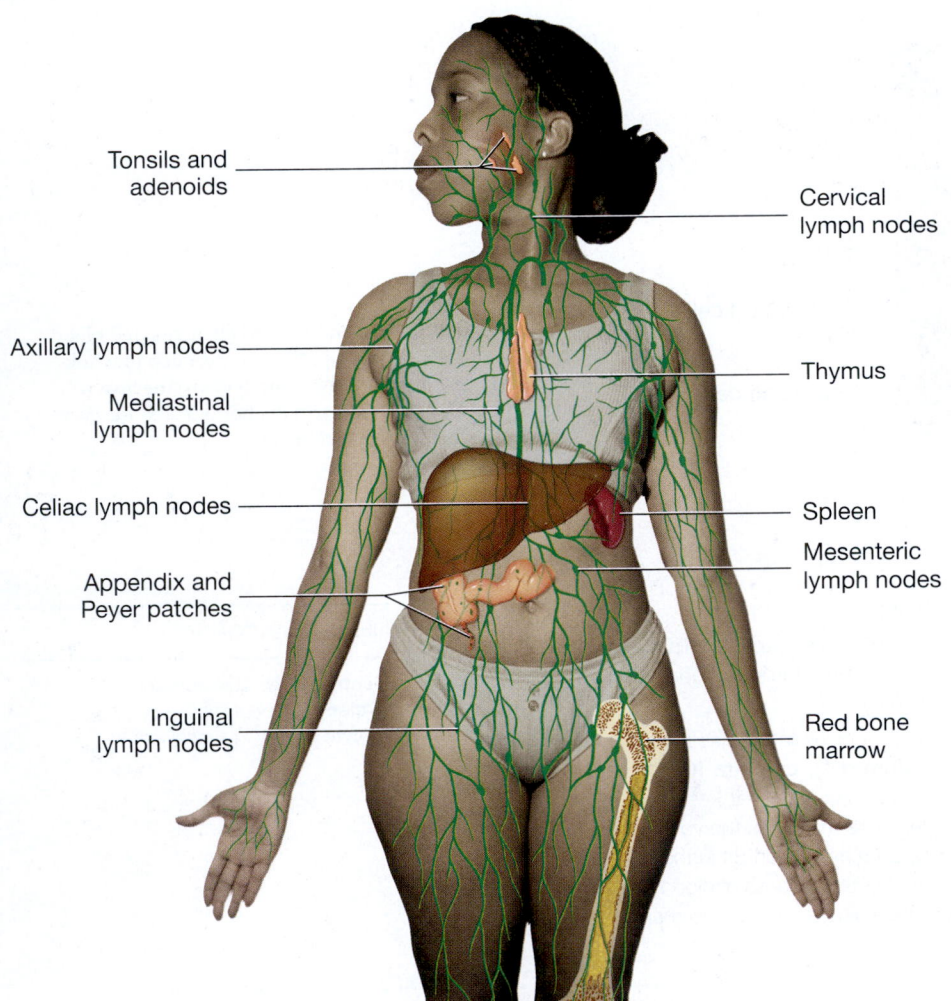

Tonsils and adenoids

Cervical lymph nodes

Axillary lymph nodes

Thymus

Mediastinal lymph nodes

Celiac lymph nodes

Spleen

Mesenteric lymph nodes

Appendix and Peyer patches

Inguinal lymph nodes

Red bone marrow

FIGURE 6-10 ■ Lymphatic system.
The lymphatic system consists of lymphatic vessels, lymph nodes, lymph fluid, lymphoid tissues (tonsils and adenoids in the throat, and Peyer patches and appendix in the intestines), and lymphoid organs (thymus and spleen). White blood cells produced by the red bone marrow are part of the immune response of the lymphatic system.

the intestines (described in Chapter 3, Gastroenterology) (see Figure 6-10). **Lymphoid organs** include the thymus and the spleen. Lymphoid tissues and lymphoid organs contain lymphocytes and macrophages that are active in the immune response (described in the Physiology section).

The **thymus**, a lymphoid organ with a pink color and a grainy consistency, is located within the mediastinum, posterior to the sternum (see Figure 6-10). During childhood and adolescence, the thymus gland is large because it is very active; however, during adulthood, it becomes much smaller. The thymus receives lymphoblasts that migrate from the red bone marrow and helps them mature into several types of T lymphocytes (helper T cells, memory T cells, cytotoxic T cells, and suppressor T cells) that are part of the immune response (the *T* stands for *thymus*). The thymus is also part of the endocrine system because it secretes hormones (**thymosins**) that cause lymphoblasts to become mature T lymphocytes.

The **spleen**, a rounded lymphoid organ, is located posterior to the stomach (see Figure 6-10). The spleen has a firm capsule, but has a soft, pulpy interior. The spleen functions as part of the blood and as part of the immune response of the lymphatic system. The spleen removes and recycles old erythrocytes. The spleen is also a storage area for whole blood. During times of danger or injury, the adrenal glands secrete epinephrine, and this causes the spleen to contract and release its stored blood into the circulatory system. The lymphoid tissue in the spleen contains mature B cell and T cell lymphocytes that are part of the immune response (described in the Physiology section).

Pronunciation/Word Parts

thymus (THY-muhs)

thymic (THY-mik)
  thym/o- *rage; thymus*
  -ic *pertaining to*

thymosins (THY-moh-sins)
  thym/o- *rage; thymus*
  -sin *substance*

spleen (SPLEEN)

splenic (SPLEH-nik)
  splen/o- *spleen*
  -ic *pertaining to*

Clinical Connections

Sports Medicine. Because of its location and pulpy center, the spleen can rupture from sports trauma (or car crashes). A ruptured spleen spills its stored blood into the abdominal cavity. This can cause shock and death unless surgery is done to stop the bleeding, remove the blood from the abdominal cavity, and remove the damaged spleen (splenectomy).

Dermatology. As described in Chapter 2, Dermatology, the skin is the body's first line of defense. Intact skin acts as a protective barrier that stops microorganisms. Openings in the skin (the nose, ears, mouth, urethra, rectum, vagina) are high-risk areas where microorganisms can enter the body, and so lymph nodes are concentrated in those areas.

6.1 PRACTICE LAPS

Use the Answer Key at the end of the book to check your answers.

A. Label Cells and Structures

Write each anatomy word or phrase in the correct numbered box. Be sure to check your spelling.

basophil	lymphocyte	neutrophil
eosinophil	monocyte	

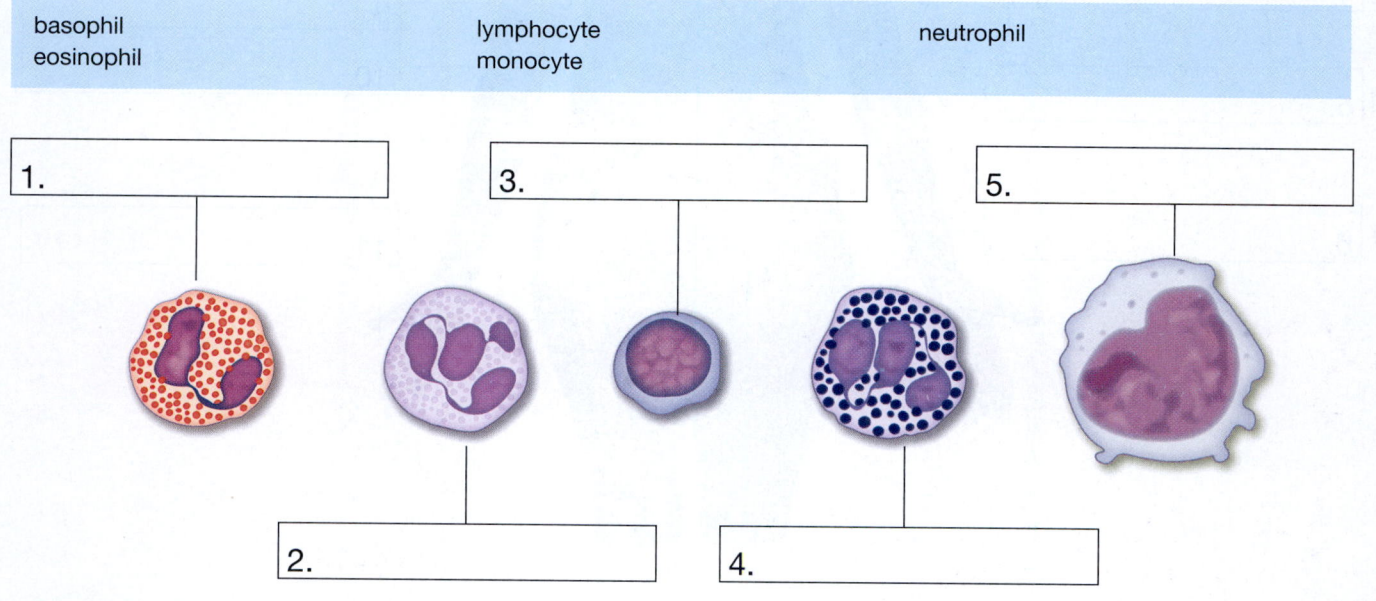

1.

2.

3.

4.

5.

appendix and Peyer patches
axillary lymph nodes
celiac lymph nodes
cervical lymph nodes

inguinal lymph nodes
mesenteric lymph nodes
mediastinal lymph nodes
red bone marrow

spleen
thymus
tonsils and adenoids

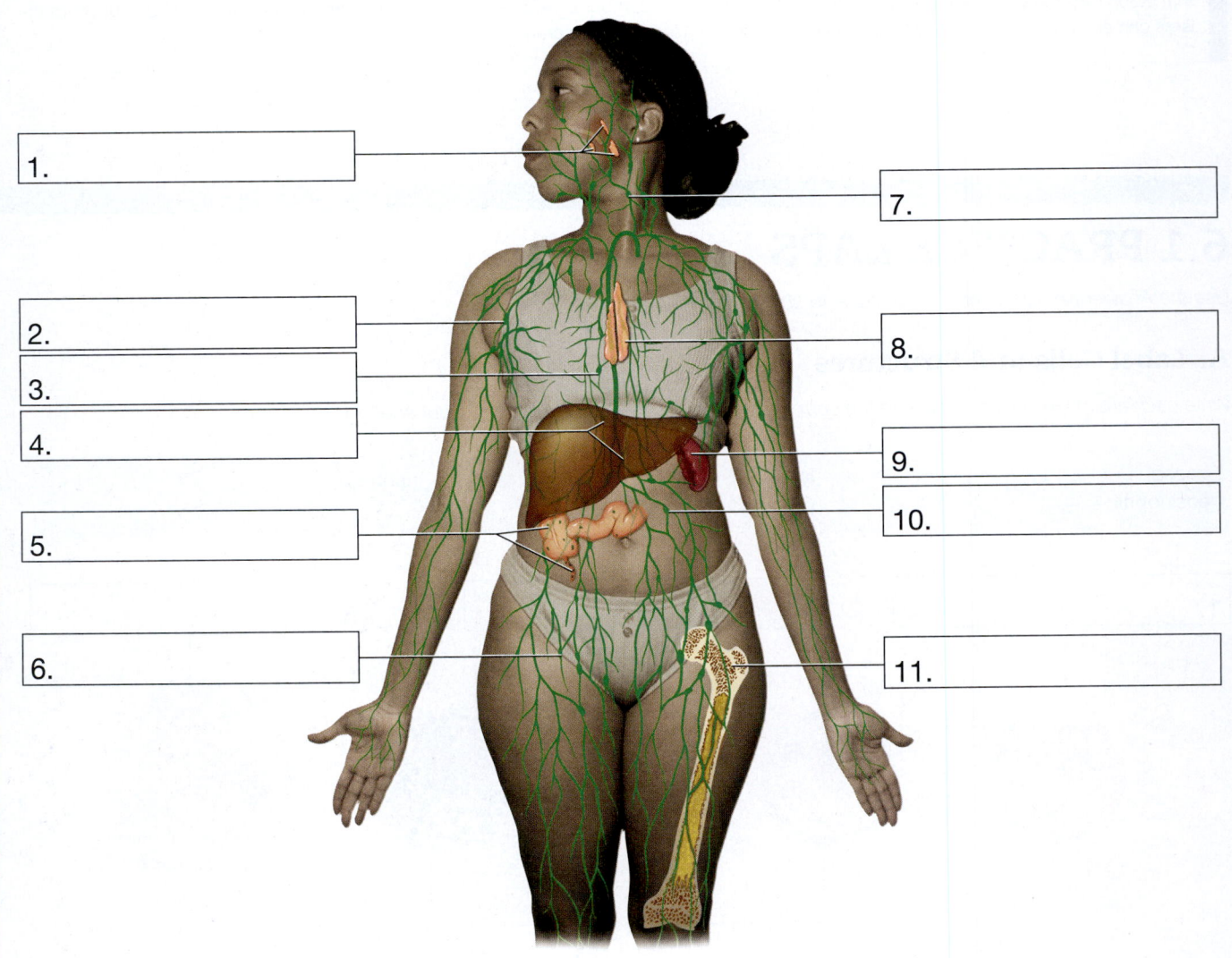

1. _____

2. _____

3. _____

4. _____

5. _____

6. _____

7. _____

8. _____

9. _____

10. _____

11. _____

B. Give the Meaning of Combining Forms

Next to each combining form, write its meaning. The first one has been done for you.

Combining Form	Meaning	Combining Form	Meaning
1. **bas/o-**	*alkaline; base of a structure*	12. lymph/o-	
2. carbox/y-		13. mon/o-	
3. electr/o-		14. morph/o-	
4. erythr/o-		15. neutr/o-	
5. eosin/o-		16. nucle/o-	
6. glob/o-		17. ox/y-	
7. granul/o-		18. plasm/o-	
8. hemat/o-		19. reticul/o-	
9. hem/o-		20. splen/o-	
10. kary/o-		21. thromb/o-	
11. leuk/o-		22. thym/o-	

C. Build Words

Read the definition of the medical word. Look at the combining form that is given. Select the correct suffix from the Suffix List, and write it on the blank line. Then build the medical word, and write it on the line. (Remember: You may need to remove the combining vowel. Always remove the hyphens and slash.) Be sure to check your spelling.

Suffix List

-atic (pertaining to)	-ic (pertaining to)	-poiesis (process of formation)
-blast (immature cell)	-lyte (dissolved substance)	-poetin (substance that forms)
-cyte (cell)	-phil (attraction to; fondness for)	

Definition of the Medical Word	Combining Form	Suffix	Build the Medical Word
Example: Pertaining to (the) thymus	**thym/o-**	*-ic*	*thymic*

[You think pertaining to (-ic) + thymus (thym/o-). You change the order of the word parts to put the suffix last. You write thymic.]

1. Immature cell (that is) red	erythr/o-	_____	_____
2. (Cell that has an) attraction to red, acidic dye	eosin/o-	_____	_____
3. Cell (that is) white	leuk/o-	_____	_____
4. Pertaining to (the) spleen	splen/o-	_____	_____
5. Process of formation (of) blood	hemat/o-	_____	_____
6. Pertaining to (the) lymph	lymph/o-	_____	_____
7. Attraction to (a dye that the cell is) not taking part (in)	neutr/o-	_____	_____
8. Cell (that is of the) lymphatic system	lymph/o-	_____	_____
9. Cell (that forms a) blood clot	thromb/o-	_____	_____
10. Substance that forms red (blood cells)	erythr/o-	_____	_____
11. Cell (that has a) small network (in its cytoplasm)	reticul/o-	_____	_____
12. Cell (that has) granules (in its cytoplasm)	granul/o-	_____	_____
13. (Cell that has an) attraction to alkaline (dye)	bas/o-	_____	_____
14. Cell (that has) one (lobe in its nucleus)	mon/o-	_____	_____
15. Dissolved substance (that has a positive or negative charge of) electricity	electr/o-	_____	_____

6.2 Physiology

Blood Clotting

When the body is injured, the injured blood vessel constricts to decrease the loss of blood. Within seconds of the injury, **thrombocytes** (platelets) form clumps that slow down the flow of blood. This process is known as platelet **aggregation**. The platelets also release several **clotting factors** that are activated by the injured blood vessel. Other clotting factors are released from the liver or from the injured tissue itself.

The clotting factors make strands of **fibrin** that trap erythrocytes and form a **thrombus** (blood clot) (see Figure 6-11 ■). This process is known as **coagulation**, and the cessation of bleeding is known as **hemostasis**. All of the clotting factors must be present and be at normal levels for the blood to clot. There are 12 clotting factors (see Table 6-2 ■), numbered I through XIII (there is no factor VI). Although the clotting factors have a numerical order, they are not activated in that order. The final size of a blood clot is limited by the action of heparin, a natural anticoagulant released from basophils.

When clotting factors in the plasma are activated to form a blood clot, the fluid portion of plasma that remains is known as **serum**.

Pronunciation/Word Parts

thrombocyte (THRAWM-boh-site)

aggregation (AG-reh-GAY-shun)
　aggreg/o- *group crowded together*
　-ation *being; having; process*

fibrin (FY-brin)
　fibr/o- *fiber*
　-in *substance*

thrombus (THRAWM-buhs)

thrombi (THRAWM-by)
Latin plural noun: Change the singular ending -*us* to -*i*.

coagulation (koh-AG-yoo-LAY-shun)
　coagul/o- *clotting*
　-ation *being; having; process*

hemostasis (HEE-moh-STAY-sihs)
　hem/o- *blood*
　-stasis *standing still; staying in one place*

serum (SEER-um)

Clinical Connections

Dietetics. The liver needs vitamin K in order to produce clotting factors. Vitamin K is manufactured by bacteria in the small intestine and is also present in leafy green vegetables, grains, and liver.

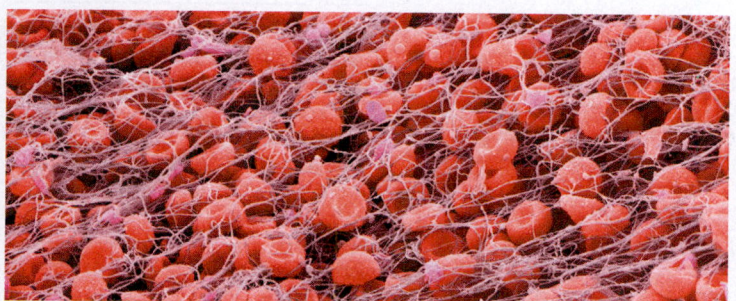

FIGURE 6-11 ■ Blood clot.
The strands of fibrin trap many erythrocytes to form a blood clot.

Table 6-2　Blood Clotting Factors

Note: There are a total of 12 blood clotting factors, numbered as Roman numerals I through XIII. (There is no factor VI). Although the factors have a numerical order, they are not activated in that order. Factors I, II, III, and IV are commonly ordered as diagnostic laboratory tests. Other factors include factors V, VII, IX, X, XI, and XII, which are produced by the liver. Factor VIII is produced by platelets. Factor XIII is produced by both the liver and platelets.

Factor Number and Name	Source	Pronunciation/Word Parts
I fibrinogen	liver	**fibrinogen** (fy-BRIN-oh-jen) 　**fibrin/o-** *fibrin* 　**-gen** *that which produces*
II prothrombin	liver	**prothrombin** (proh-THRAWM-bin) 　**pro-** *before* 　**thromb/o-** *blood clot* 　**-in** *substance* Prothrombin is the clotting factor that is activated just before a thrombus is formed.
III tissue factor (**thromboplastin**)	injured tissue	**thromboplastin** (THRAWM-boh-PLAS-tin) 　**thromb/o-** *blood clot* 　**plast/o-** *formation; growth* 　**-in** *substance*
IV **calcium**	electrolyte in the blood	**calcium** (KAL-see-um)

Allergic Reaction

An **allergy** or an **allergic reaction** is an individual's unique **hypersensitivity** in response to certain **allergens**. Allergens include cells from plants or animals (food, pollen, mold, animal dander), as well as dust, chemicals, and drugs. The basis of the symptoms of an allergic reaction is the release of **histamine** from **basophils** in the blood and from **mast cells** in the connective tissues.

A **local reaction** causes redness, swelling, and itching in one area. Examples include a reaction to the chemicals in deodorant applied to the skin or to pollen in the air that is inhaled into the nose (see Figure 6-12 ■).

A **systemic reaction** occurs when allergens are inhaled, ingested, or injected, causing allergic symptoms in one or more body systems; for example, inhaled pollens trigger asthma attacks or ingested foods cause hives on the skin. **Anaphylaxis** is a severe systemic allergic reaction that is characterized by respiratory distress, hypotension, and shock, and it can be life-threatening; for example, eating peanuts or taking a drug that has caused an allergic reaction in the past.

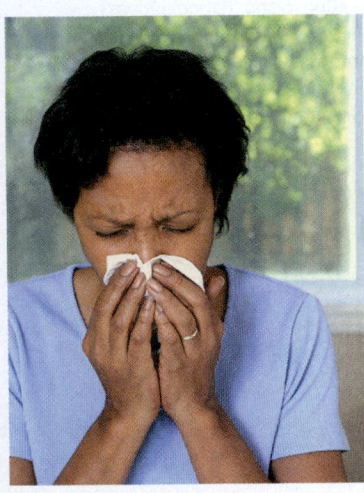

FIGURE 6-12 ■ Allergic reaction.
Sneezing is a sign of a local allergic reaction in mucous membranes of the nose. It can be caused by pollen, mold, animal dander, or dust in the environment.

Immune Response

The **immune response** involves a coordinated effort between leukocytes in the blood and the lymphatic system to identify and destroy microorganisms or foreign cells that invade the body and cancer cells that are produced within the body (see Table 6-3 ■).

Microorganisms (bacteria, viruses, protozoa, fungi, yeasts) that cause disease are known as **pathogens**. Once a pathogen or a cancer cell is detected in the body, the leukocytes attack it in several different ways (described in the next section).

Leukocytes

Neutrophils

Neutrophils function as **phagocytes** that engulf and destroy bacteria. This process is **phagocytosis** (see Figure 6-13 ■). Neutrophils only live for a few days or even just a few hours if they are actively destroying bacteria. One neutrophil can destroy about 10 bacteria before it dies. Neutrophils also engulf wastes and foreign substances in the blood.

Eosinophils

Eosinophils release chemicals that destroy foreign cells (pollen, animal dander, dust) and kill parasites.

Basophils

Basophils release histamine at the site of a tissue injury. **Histamine** dilates blood vessels and increases blood flow, which brings more leukocytes to the area. Histamine causes redness, edema (swelling), and itching.

Pronunciation/Word Parts

allergy (AL-er-jee)

allergic (ah-LER-jik)
  allerg/o- allergy
  -ic pertaining to

hypersensitivity (HY-per-SEN-sih-TIV-ih-tee)
  hyper- above; more than normal
  sensitiv/o- affected by; sensitive to
  -ity condition; state

allergen (AL-er-jen)
  allerg/o- allergy
  -gen that which produces

histamine (HIS-tah-meen)

basophil (BAY-soh-fil)
  bas/o- alkaline; base of a structure
  -phil attraction to; fondness for

local (LOH-kal)
  loc/o- one place
  -al pertaining to

systemic (sis-TEM-ik)
  system/o- body as a whole
  -ic pertaining to

anaphylaxis (AN-ah-fih-LAK-sihs)

anaphylactic (AN-ah-fih-LAK-tik)
  ana- apart; excessive
  phylact/o- guarding; protecting
  -ic pertaining to

immune (ih-MYOON)
The combining form **immun/o-** means immune response.

microorganism (MY-kroh-OR-gan-ism)
  micr/o- one millionth; small
  organ/o- living thing; organ
  -ism disease from a specific cause; process

pathogen (PATH-oh-jen)
  path/o- disease
  -gen that which produces

neutrophil (NOO-troh-fil)

phagocyte (FAG-oh-site)
  phag/o- eating; swallowing
  -cyte cell

phagocytosis (FAG-oh-sy-TOH-sihs)
  phag/o- eating; swallowing
  cyt/o- cell
  -osis abnormal condition; process

eosinophil (EE-oh-SIN-oh-fil)

histamine (HIS-tah-meen)

Table 6-3   Leukocytes and the Immune Response

Leukocyte	Category	Function
Neutrophil segmented neutrophil, seg, polymorphonuclear leukocyte (PMN), poly	Granulocyte	Engulfs and destroys bacteria
Eosinophil eo	Granulocyte	Releases chemicals to destroy foreign cells (pollen, animal dander, dust, etc.) and kill parasites
Basophil baso	Granulocyte	Releases histamine at the site of tissue injury; releases heparin to limit the size of a forming blood clot
Lymphocyte lymph	Agranulocyte	Produces antibodies (immunoglobulins); destroys cancer cells and cells infected with a virus
Monocyte mono	Agranulocyte	Engulfs and destroys microorganisms, cancerous cells, dead leukocytes, and cellular debris

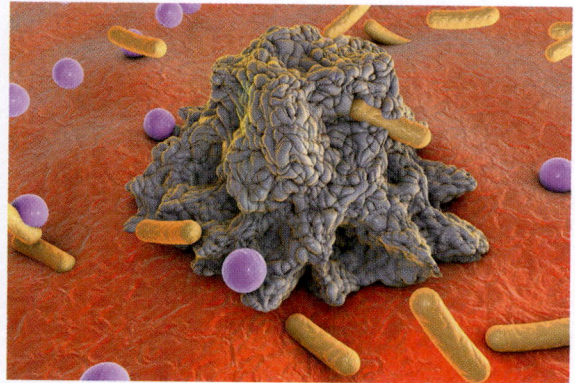

FIGURE 6-13 ■ Phagocytosis.
This white blood cell is eating (phagocytizing) a rod-shaped bacterium that is causing an infection.

Lymphocytes

There are several different lymphocytes that are active in an immune response.

- **NK (natural killer) cells** recognize a cancer cell or a cell infected with a virus and destroy it. NK cells can recognize these cells even before they are coated with antibodies.
- **B cells** are inactive until a monocyte presents them with fragments of a pathogen that the monocyte has engulfed. Then the B cell changes into a plasma cell and produces antibodies.
- **T cells** (lymphocytes that matured in the thymus) have four different types.
  1. **Cytotoxic T cells** kill cells infected with a virus.
  2. **Helper T cells** stimulate the production of cytotoxic T cells. When helper T cells encounter a virus, they produce memory T cells.
  3. **Memory T cells** are inactive until a virus enters the body a second time. Then they remember the virus and become cytotoxic T cells.
  4. **Suppressor T cells** limit the extent and duration of an immune response.

Monocytes

Monocytes engulf and destroy pathogens that have been coated with antibodies in the process of phagocytosis. Monocytes also produce interferon, interleukin, and tumor necrosis factor.

- **Interferon** is produced by monocytes that have engulfed a virus. To keep viral infections from spreading, interferon stimulates other cells to produce substances that prevent a virus from entering other cells and reproducing. Interferon also stimulates NK (natural killer) cells to kill cells already infected with viruses.
- **Interleukin** stimulates B cell and T cell lymphocytes and NK cells. It also produces the fever that is part of the immune response to inflammation and infection. The increased body temperature then stimulates all leukocyte activity.
- **Tumor necrosis factor** destroys **endotoxins** produced by certain bacteria. It also destroys cancer cells.

Antibodies

Antibodies are produced by a B cell when it changes into a plasma cell. Antibodies coat the surface of a bacterium (or virus, or cancer cell, or a cell infected with a virus), and this attracts leukocytes. The antibody coating marks the cell to be destroyed. Antibodies are also known as **immunoglobulins**.

Complement

Complement is a group of proteins (C1–C9) in the plasma. When antibodies coat a bacterium (or virus, or cancer cell, or cell infected with a virus), complement proteins "complement" the effect of antibodies by drilling holes in the foreign cell.

Pronunciation/Word Parts

lymphocyte (LIM-foh-site)

cytotoxic (SY-toh-TAWK-sik)
  cyt/o- cell
  tox/o- poison
  -ic pertaining to

suppressor (soo-PRES-or)
  suppress/o- press down
  -or person who does or produces; thing that does or produces

monocyte (MAW-noh-site)

interferon (IN-ter-FEER-on)

interleukin (IN-ter-LOO-kin)
  inter- between
  leuk/o- white
  -in substance

endotoxin (EN-doh-TAWK-sin)
  end/o- innermost; within
  tox/o- poison
  -in substance

antibody (AN-tee-BAW-dee)
The prefix **anti-** means against.

immunoglobulin
(IH-myoo-noh-GLAW-byoo-lin)
  immun/o- immune response
  globul/o- shaped like a globe
  -in substance

complement (KAWM-pleh-ment)

immunity (ih-MYOO-nih-tee)
  immun/o- immune response
  -ity condition; state

Dive Deeper

There are five classes of **antibodies** or **immunoglobulins**:

- **IgA** is in body secretions (tears, saliva, mucus) and on the skin. IgA is in colostrum, the first milk produced by the mother; this maternal IgA provides **passive immunity** to the breastfeeding baby for all of the diseases that the mother has had, until 18 months of age when the infant begins to make its own antibodies.
- **IgD** is on the surface of a B cell lymphocyte and activates it to become a plasma cell.
- **IgE** is on the surface of a basophil and causes it to release histamine during inflammatory and allergic reactions.
- **IgG** is the most abundant immunoglobulin. It provides active immunity. During pregnancy, IgG crosses the placenta and provides passive immunity to the fetus.
- **IgM** is produced the first time the body encounters a pathogen. It is also produced during a blood transfusion of an incompatible blood type.

6.2 PRACTICE LAPS

Use the Answer Key at the end of the book to check your answers.

A. Give the Meaning of Combining Forms

Next to each combining form, write its meaning. The first one has been done for you.

Combining Form	Meaning	Combining Form	Meaning
1. **tox/o-**	*poison*	11. leuk/o-	
2. aggreg/o-		12. loc/o-	
3. aller/o-		13. micr/o-	
4. allerg/o-		14. organ/o-	
5. coagul/o-		15. path/o-	
6. cyt/o-		16. phag/o-	
7. fibr/o-		17. phylact/o-	
8. globul/o-		18. sensitiv/o-	
9. hem/o-		19. suppress/o-	
10. immun/o-		20. system/o-	

B. Build Words

Read the definition of the medical word. Look at the combining form that is given. Select the correct suffix from the Suffix List, and write it on the blank line. Then build the medical word, and write it on the line. (Remember: You may need to remove the combining vowel. Always remove the hyphens and slash.) Be sure to check your spelling.

Suffix List

-al (pertaining to)	-gen (that which produces)	-ity (condition; state)
-ation (being; having; process)	-ic (pertaining to)	-stasis (standing still; staying in one place)
-cyte (cell)	-in (substance)	

Definition of the Medical Word	Combining Form	Suffix	Build the Medical Word
Example: Pertaining to one place	loc/o-	*-al*	*local*

[You think pertaining to (-al) + one place (loc/o-). You change the order of the word parts to put the suffix last. You write local.]

Definition of the Medical Word	Combining Form	Suffix	Build the Medical Word
1. Staying in one place (as pertains to the) blood	hem/o-		
2. Process (of blood) clotting	coagul/o-		
3. Substance (made of) fiber	fibr/o-		
4. Having (a) group (of platelets) crowded together	aggreg/o-		
5. State (of having an) immune response	immun/o-		
6. That which produces disease	path/o-		
7. Pertaining to (the) body as a whole	system/o-		
8. Pertaining to (an) allergy	allerg/o-		
9. Cell (that is) eating	phag/o-		

Vocabulary Review

Word or Phrase	Description	Combining Forms
Overview		
blood	Structures of the blood include erythrocytes, leukocytes, thrombocytes, plasma, and other substances. Blood is a connective tissue whose function is to continuously transport those substances throughout the body.	**hem/o-** *blood* **hemat/o-** *blood*
lymphatic system	Structures of the lymphatic system include lymphatic vessels, lymph fluid, lymph nodes, lymphoid tissues, and lymphoid organs. The function of the lymphatic system is to provide an immune response that defends the body against bacteria, viruses, parasites, foreign cells, and cancer cells.	**lymph/o-** *lymph; lymphatic system*
Anatomy of the Blood		
agranulocyte	Category of leukocytes with few or no granules in their cytoplasm. It includes lymphocytes and monocytes.	**granul/o-** *granule*
albumin	Protein molecule that is produced by the liver and carried in the plasma. Albumin exerts osmotic pressure that keeps water from moving out of the blood into the surrounding tissues. This maintains the blood volume and blood pressure.	
band	Immature neutrophil in the red bone marrow that has a nucleus shaped like a curved band. Also known as a **stab**.	
basophil	Least common type of leukocyte. It is categorized as a granulocyte because it has many large granules in its cytoplasm. These stain dark blue to purple with an alkaline dye (hematoxylin). The nucleus has more than one lobe. Basophils are also known as *basos*.	**bas/o-** *alkaline; base of a structure*
bicarbonate (HCO$_3^-$)	A negatively charged electrolyte in the plasma. Bicarbonate acts as a buffer to maintain the pH of the blood.	
blood type	Genetic material in erythrocytes that determines a person's blood type. The **ABO blood group** includes four different blood types: A, B, AB, and O. Type A blood contains A **antigens** on the erythrocytes, type B has B antigens, and type AB has both. Type O blood has neither A nor B antigens. Each blood type has antibodies in the plasma against other blood types. The **Rh blood group (Rh factor)** is either present on the erythrocytes (Rh positive) or not present (Rh negative).	
calcium (Ca^{++})	A positively charged electrolyte in the plasma. Calcium is also factor IV in the process of blood clotting.	
carboxyhemo-globin	Hemoglobin that binds to and carries carbon monoxide in the blood	**carbox/y-** *carbon monoxide* **hem/o-** *blood* **glob/o-** *comprehensive; shaped like a globe*
electrolytes	Molecules in the plasma that have a positive or negative electrical charge. Examples: sodium (Na$^+$), potassium (K$^+$), calcium (Ca^{++}), chloride (Cl$^-$), and bicarbonate (HCO$_3^-$).	**electr/o-** *electricity*
eosinophil	A type of leukocyte. It is categorized as a granulocyte because it has many large granules in its cytoplasm. These stain bright pink to red with eosin dye. The nucleus has two lobes. Eosinophils are also known as *eos*.	**eosin/o-** *eosin; red, acidic dye*

Word or Phrase	Description	Combining Forms
erythrocyte	Red blood cell (RBC), a round, somewhat flattened disk with no nucleus. An **erythroblast** is a very immature form that comes from a stem cell. A **reticulocyte** is a slightly immature form that is released into the blood. Because it has no nucleus, a mature erythrocyte only lasts 120 days. Erythrocytes contain hemoglobin that carries oxygen.	**erythr/o-** *red* **reticul/o-** *small network*
erythropoietin	Hormone secreted by the kidneys if the body experiences blood loss. It increases the speed at which erythrocytes are produced and become mature.	**erythr/o-** *red*
granulocyte	Category of leukocytes with many large granules in their cytoplasm. It includes neutrophils, eosinophils, and basophils.	**granul/o-** *granule*
hematopoiesis	Process by which the formed elements of the blood are produced in the red bone marrow, first as very immature cells and then mature cells that are released into the blood.	**hemat/o-** *blood*
hemoglobin	Red, iron-containing molecule in an erythrocyte. Hemoglobin that binds to and carries oxygen from the lungs to the cells is **oxyhemoglobin**. Hemoglobin (as carbaminohemoglobin) carries carbon dioxide from the cells back to the lungs.	**hem/o-** *blood* **glob/o-** *comprehensive; shaped like a globe* **ox/y-** *oxygen; quick*
leukocyte	White blood cell (WBC). There are five distinct types: neutrophils, eosinophils, basophils, lymphocytes, and monocytes. Each has a specific role in an allergic response or in an immune response.	**leuk/o-** *white*
lymphocyte	The smallest leukocyte. It is categorized as an agranulocyte as there are few or no granules in its cytoplasm. A **lymphoblast** is an immature form. Lymphoblasts that mature in the red bone marrow become B lymphocytes (B cells). Lymphoblasts that migrate to the thymus become T lymphocytes (T cells). Lymphocytes are also known as *lymphs*.	**lymph/o-** *lymph; lymphatic system*
monocyte	The largest leukocyte. It is categorized as an agranulocyte as there are few or no granules in its cytoplasm. Its nucleus is shaped like a kidney bean. Monocytes are also known as *monos*.	**mon/o-** *one; single*
neutrophil	Most common type of leukocyte. It is categorized as a granulocyte because it has many large granules in its cytoplasm, but these granules do not stain when they are exposed to laboratory dye, remaining neutral in color. Its nucleus has many segments and lobes. Neutrophils are also known as *segmented neutrophils*, *segs*, **polymorphonuclear leukocytes (PMNs)**, or *polys*.	**neutr/o-** *not taking part* **morph/o-** *shape* **nucle/o-** *nucleus of an atom or a cell*
oxyhemoglobin	Hemoglobin that is carrying oxygen	**ox/y-** *oxygen; quick* **hem/o-** *blood* **glob/o-** *comprehensive; shaped like a globe*
plasma	Clear, straw-colored liquid portion of the blood that transports erythrocytes, leukocytes, and thrombocytes, as well as the nutrients of digested foods and the waste products of metabolism	**plasm/o-** *plasma*
red bone marrow	Type of connective tissue where all blood cells are produced	
Rh blood group	Category of blood type. When the Rh factor is present, the blood is Rh positive. Without the Rh factor, the blood is Rh negative.	
sodium (Na⁺)	A positively charged electrolyte in the plasma. Sodium exerts osmotic pressure that keeps water from moving out of the blood into the surrounding tissues. This maintains the blood volume and blood pressure.	

Word or Phrase	Description	Combining Forms
stem cell	Original, very immature cell in the red bone marrow that gives rise to all other blood cells, each of which matures in stages to finally become a mature erythrocyte, leukocyte, or thrombocyte that is released into the blood	
thrombocyte	Cell fragment that is formed from a **megakaryocyte**, a very large, mature cell with a great deal of cytoplasm. The cytoplasm breaks off into individual thrombocytes. Also known as **platelets**. After an injury, platelets form clumps that slow down the flow of blood (platelet aggregation). The platelets also release several clotting factors.	**thromb/o-** *blood clot* **kary/o-** *nucleus of a cell*
Anatomy of the Lymphatic System		
lymph	Tissue fluid enters a lymphatic capillary and becomes the fluid known as *lymph*. Lymph flows through the lymphatic system.	
lymph nodes	Small, encapsulated pieces of lymphoid tissue. They are grouped together in chains in areas where there is a high rate of invasion by microorganisms or cancer cells. Special cells in the lymph node destroy any microorganisms or cancer cells in the lymph. Also known as **lymph glands**.	**lymph/o-** *lymph; lymphatic system*
lymphatic vessels	Structures that begin as capillaries, carry lymph, continue as larger lymphatic vessels, and bring lymph to the lymph nodes. Lymphatic vessels have valves that keep the lymph flowing in one direction. Lymphatic vessels end at lymphatic ducts that empty into veins in the neck.	**lymph/o-** *lymph; lymphatic system*
lymphoid tissues and organs	Lymphoid tissues include the tonsils and adenoids in the posterior oral cavity, as well as Peyer patches and the appendix in the intestines. Lymphoid organs include the thymus and spleen.	**lymph/o-** *lymph; lymphatic system*
spleen	Lymphoid organ that is posterior to the stomach. The spleen removes old erythrocytes. It is a storage area for whole blood that it releases during times of danger or injury. It contains B cell and T cell lymphocytes.	**splen/o-** *spleen*
thymus	Lymphoid organ in the mediastinum. It receives lymphoblasts that migrate from the red bone marrow, and it helps them mature into several types of T lymphocytes that are part of the immune response. As an endocrine gland, it secretes thymosins, which are hormones that cause lymphoblasts to become mature T lymphocytes.	**thym/o-** *rage; thymus*
Physiology of Blood Clotting		
aggregation	Process of thrombocytes (platelets) forming clumps to slow down the flow of blood	**aggreg/o-** *group crowded together*
clotting factors	There are 12 clotting factors, numbered I through XIII (there is no factor VI). Platelets release several clotting factors that are activated by the injured blood vessel. Other clotting factors are released from the liver and the injured tissue itself. Clotting factors make strands of fibrin that trap erythrocytes and form a thrombus.	
coagulation	Process of the formation of a thrombus (blood clot)	**coagul/o-** *clotting*
fibrin	Strands formed by the clotting factors. Fibrin strands trap erythrocytes to form a thrombus (blood clot).	**fibr/o-** *fiber*
fibrinogen	Blood clotting factor I that is produced by the liver	**fibrin/o-** *fibrin*
hemostasis	The cessation of bleeding	**hem/o-** *blood*
prothrombin	Blood clotting factor II that is produced by the liver. This clotting factor is activated just before a thrombus is formed.	**thromb/o-** *blood clot* **Pro-** means *before*.

Word or Phrase	Description	Combining Forms
serum	Fluid portion of the plasma that remains after the clotting factors are activated to form a blood clot	
thrombocytes	Thrombocytes (platelets) immediately form clumps to slow down the flow of blood after any injury to a blood vessel.	**thromb/o-** *blood clot*
thromboplastin	Blood clotting factor III. Also known as *tissue factor* because it is released from injured tissue.	**thromb/o-** *blood clot* **plast/o-** *formation; growth*
thrombus	A blood clot	**thromb/o-** *blood clot*
Physiology of an Allergic Reaction		
allergen	Cells from plants or animals (food, pollen, mold, animal dander), as well as dust, chemicals, and drugs. Any of these allergens can cause an allergic reaction in a hypersensitive person.	**aller/o-** *other work; strange activity*
allergic reaction	An individual's unique hypersensitivity in response to a certain allergen. Also known as an **allergy**.	**allerg/o-** *allergy*
anaphylaxis	Severe systemic allergic reaction characterized by respiratory distress, hypotension, and shock	**phylact/o-** *guarding; protecting*
basophil	Blood cell that releases histamine during an allergic reaction	**bas/o-** *alkaline; base of a structure*
histamine	The basis of the symptoms of an allergic reaction. Histamine is released from basophils in the blood and from mast cells in the connective tissues.	
hypersensitivity	An individual's unique response to an allergen	**sensitiv/o-** *affected by; sensitive to*
local reaction	An allergic reaction of redness, swelling, and itching in one area. Example: An allergen contacts the skin or is inhaled into the nose (a new deodorant or pollen in the air).	**loc/o-** *one place*
systemic reaction	An allergic reaction throughout the body after an allergen is inhaled, ingested, or injected	**system/o-** *body as a whole*
Physiology of an Immune Response		
active immunity	Immune response that is the body's continuing defense against pathogens it has seen before. It is produced by immunoglobulin G.	**immun/o-** *immune response*
antibody	Antibodies are produced by a B cell when it becomes a plasma cell. Antibodies coat the surface of a bacterium (or virus, or cancer cell, or cell infected with a virus), and this attracts leukocytes to destroy it. Antibodies are also known as *immunoglobulins*.	
B cell	Type of lymphocyte that is inactive until a monocyte presents it with fragments from an eaten pathogen. Then the B cell becomes a **plasma cell** that produces antibodies.	
basophil	Leukocyte that functions in the immune response by releasing histamine	**bas/o-** *alkaline; base of a structure*
complement proteins	Group of proteins in the plasma (C1–C9). When antibodies coat a bacterium (or virus, or cancer cell, or a cell infected with a virus), complement proteins "complement" that effect by drilling holes in them.	
cytotoxic T cell	Type of T cell that kills cells infected with a virus	**cyt/o-** *cell* **tox/o-** *poison*

Word or Phrase	Description	Combining Forms
eosinophil	Leukocyte that functions in the immune response by releasing chemicals that destroy foreign cells (pollen, animal dander, dust) and kill parasites	**eosin/o-** *eosin; red, acidic dye*
helper T cell	Type of T cell that stimulates the production of cytotoxic T cells. When a helper T cell encounters a virus, it produces memory T cells.	
histamine	Released by basophils and mast cells as part of the immune response. It dilates blood vessels and increases blood flow, which brings more leukocytes to the area. Histamine causes redness and edema (swelling).	
IgA	Immunoglobulin A. Antibody in body secretions (tears, saliva, mucus, and breast milk) and on the skin. It gives passive immunity to a breastfeeding infant.	
IgD	Immunoglobulin D. Antibody on the surface of a B cell lymphocyte; it activates the B cell to become a plasma cell.	
IgE	Immunoglobulin E. Antibody on the surface of a basophil. It causes the basophil to release histamine.	
IgG	Immunoglobulin G. Antibody that provides active immunity. During pregnancy, it crosses the placenta and provides passive immunity to the fetus.	
IgM	Immunoglobulin M. Antibody that is produced by plasma cells during the initial exposure to a pathogen. IgM is also produced during a blood transfusion of incompatible blood types.	
immune response	Coordinated effort between leukocytes in the blood and the lymphatic system to identify and destroy invading microorganisms, or foreign cells, or cancer cells produced within the body	**immun/o-** *immune response*
immunoglobulins	Also known as *antibodies*. There are five classes of immunoglobulins: IgA, IgD, IgE, IgG, and IgM.	**immun/o-** *immune response* **globul/o-** *shaped like a globe*
interferon	Substance produced by a monocyte that has engulfed a virus. Interferon stimulates other cells to produce substances that prevent a virus from entering them to reproduce itself.	
interleukin	Substance produced by monocytes. It stimulates NK cells to kill cells already infected with a virus. It stimulates B cell and T cell lymphocytes. It also produces the fever that is part of the immune response to inflammation and infection.	
lymphocyte	Leukocyte that functions in the immune response in many different ways. See *B cells*, *T cells*, and *NK cells*.	**lymph/o-** *lymph; lymphatic system*
memory T cell	Type of T cell that is inactive until a virus enters the body a second time. Then it remembers the virus and becomes a cytotoxic T cell.	
microorganisms	Small living organisms that cause disease. Examples: Bacteria, viruses, protozoa, fungi, and yeasts.	**micr/o-** *one millionth; small* **organ/o-** *living thing; organ*
monocyte	Leukocyte that engulfs and destroys pathogens that have been coated with antibodies in the process of phagocytosis. It also produces interferon, interleukin, and tumor necrosis factor.	**mon/o-** *one; single*
NK (natural killer) cell	Type of lymphocyte that recognizes a cancer cell or a cell infected with a virus and destroys it without the help of an antibody coating	
neutrophil	Leukocyte that functions in the immune response by engulfing and destroying bacteria in the process of phagocytosis. It also engulfs wastes and foreign substances in the blood.	**neutr/o-** *not taking part*

Word or Phrase	Description	Combining Forms
passive immunity	Immune response that occurs when IgG crosses the placenta and gives passive immunity to the fetus. Passive immunity also occurs when IgA in the mother's first breast milk (colostrum) is given to the breastfeeding baby. IgG and IgA provide protection from all the diseases the mother has had.	**immun/o-** *immune response*
pathogen	Microorganism that causes disease	**path/o-** *disease*
phagocyte	A neutrophil that engulfs and destroys bacteria. Also, a monocyte that destroys pathogens that have been coated with antibodies. The process of engulfing and destroying is **phagocytosis**.	**phag/o-** *eating; swallowing* **cyt/o-** *cell*
suppressor T cell	Type of T cell that limits the extent and duration of an immune response	
T cell	Type of lymphocyte that matures in the thymus. There are four different kinds: cytotoxic T cells, helper T cells, memory T cells, and suppressor T cells.	
tumor necrosis factor (TNF)	Substance that destroys **endotoxins** produced by certain bacteria. It also destroys cancer cells.	**tox/o-** *poison*

Abbreviations Review

ABO	A, B, AB, and O blood groups		**IgM**	immunoglobulin M
Ca⁺⁺	calcium		**K⁺**	potassium
Cl⁻	chloride		**Na⁺**	sodium
CO	carbon monoxide		**NK**	natural killer (cell)
HCO₃⁻	bicarbonate		**PMN**	polymorphonuclear leukocyte
IgA	immunoglobulin A		**RBC**	red blood cell
IgD	immunoglobulin D		**Rh**	blood group
IgE	immunoglobulin E		**WBC**	white blood cell
IgG	immunoglobulin G			

6.3 Diseases

Word or Phrase	Description	Pronunciation/Word Parts
Blood		
hemorrhage	Loss of a large amount of blood, either externally or internally, from disease or from an injury. Injury to an artery causes a forceful spurting of a large amount of bright red blood. Treatment: Tourniquet, manual pressure, or suturing to stop the bleeding	**hemorrhage** (HEM-oh-rij) **hem/o-** *blood* **-rrhage** *excessive discharge; excessive flow*
pancytopenia	Decreased numbers of all types of blood cells due to failure of the red bone marrow to produce stem cells. This can be caused by some blood diseases, or it can be a side effect of chemotherapy drugs. Treatment: Correct the underlying cause.	**pancytopenia** (PAN-sy-toh-PEE-nee-ah) **pan-** *all* **cyt/o-** *cell* **-penia** *condition of deficiency*
septicemia	Bacterial infection in the tissues or an organ that spreads to the blood. **Sepsis** is a result of septicemia and occurs when the bacteria and their endotoxins cause severe symptoms, inflammation, and blood clots throughout the entire body. Treatment: Antibiotic drug; drugs to treat other symptoms	**septicemia** (SEP-tih-SEE-mee-ah) **septic/o-** *infection* **-emia** *condition of the blood; substance in the blood* **sepsis** (SEP-sihs)

Word or Phrase	Description	Pronunciation/Word Parts

Erythrocytes

Word or Phrase	Description	Pronunciation/Word Parts
anemia	Anemia is a decrease in the number of erythrocytes. A patient with anemia is **anemic**. Anemia can have several causes. 1. Insufficient amounts of amino acids, folic acid, iron, vitamin B_6, or vitamin B_{12} in the diet 2. Disease, cancer, radiation therapy, or chemotherapy drugs that have damaged or destroyed the red bone marrow 3. Hemolysis with loss of erythrocytes because of increased cell fragility 4. Hemorrhage, excessive menstruation, or chronic blood loss. Anemias can be categorized by the cause of the anemia or by the abnormal size, shape, or color of each erythrocyte. Treatment: Correct the underlying cause.	**anemia** (ah-NEE-mee-ah) The prefix **an-** means *not; without*. The suffix -**emia** means *condition of the blood*. Anemia: *Condition of the blood (of) not (enough red blood cells)* **anemic** (ah-NEE-mik)

aplastic anemia	Anemia caused by failure of the red bone marrow to produce erythrocytes because it has been damaged by disease, cancer, radiation therapy, or chemotherapy drugs. In aplastic anemia, each erythrocyte is **normocytic** (normal in size) and **normochromic** (normal in color), but there are too few erythrocytes.
	Treatment: Blood transfusion; erythropoietin drug to stimulate erythrocyte production; bone marrow transplantation
		aplastic (aa-PLAS-tik)
		  a- *away from; without*
		  plast/o- *formation; growth*
		  -ic *pertaining to*
		
		normocytic (NOR-moh-SIH-tik)
		  norm/o- *normal; usual*
		  cyt/o- *cell*
		  -ic *pertaining to*
		
		normochromic
		(NOR-moh-KROH-mik)
		  norm/o- *normal; usual*
		  chrom/o- *color*
		  -ic *pertaining to*

folic acid deficiency anemia	Anemia caused by a deficiency of folic acid in the diet. This anemia is seen in malnourished persons, older adults with a poor diet, alcoholics, and pregnant women. Each erythrocyte is **macrocytic** (abnormally large).
	Treatment: Balanced diet; folic acid supplement
		macrocytic (MAK-roh-SIH-tik)
		  macr/o- *large*
		  cyt/o- *cell*
		  -ic *pertaining to*

iron deficiency anemia	Anemia caused by a deficiency of iron in the diet or by an increased loss of iron due to menstruation, hemorrhage, or chronic blood loss. The person has pale skin and mucous membranes because iron gives erythrocytes their color. Each erythrocyte is **microcytic** (small in size) and **hypochromic** (pale in color) (see Figure 6-14 ■). Compare to normal red blood cells (see Figure 6-3). Treatment: Infant formula with additional iron; dietary iron supplements; correction of blood loss	**microcytic** (MY-kroh-SIH-tik)
		  micr/o- *one millionth; small*
		  cyt/o- *cell*
		  -ic *pertaining to*
		
		hypochromic
		(HY-poh-KROH-mik)
		  hypo- *below; deficient*
		  chrom/o- *color*
		  -ic *pertaining to*

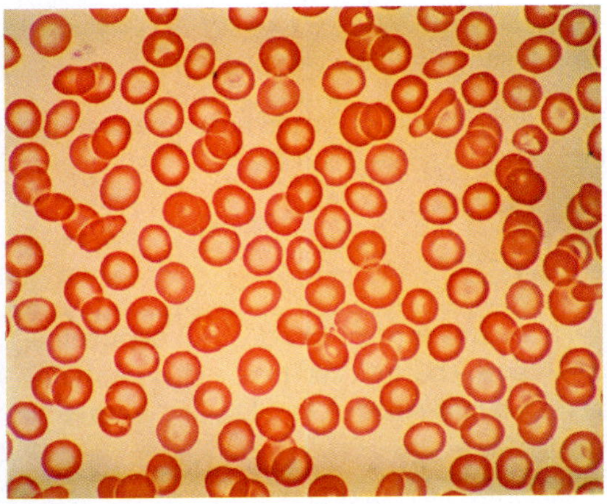

FIGURE 6-14 ■ Microcytic, hypochromic erythrocytes.
Under a microscope, this person's blood shows many centrally pale erythrocytes that are characteristic of iron deficiency anemia.

Word or Phrase	Description	Pronunciation/Word Parts
pernicious anemia	Anemia caused by a lack of vitamin B_{12} in the diet or by a lack of intrinsic factor. Intrinsic factor produced by the stomach helps the body absorb vitamin B_{12}. As a person ages, the stomach produces less intrinsic factor. If untreated, pernicious anemia can cause permanent nerve damage. Each erythrocyte is macrocytic (abnormally large) and is immature. Treatment: Vitamin B_{12} drug as a tablet, nasal spray, or injection	**pernicious** (per-NIH-shuhs)
sickle cell disease	Anemia caused by an inherited genetic abnormality of an amino acid in the hemoglobin. When there is a low level of oxygen in the blood, each erythrocyte distorts to become a crescent or sickle shape (see Figure 6-15 ■). Sickle cells do not flow easily through the blood vessels, and this causes pain (see Figure 6-16 ■). Treatment: Pain medication; avoidance of situations that lower the blood oxygen level; use of a drug that increases the production of erythrocytes that contain fetal hemoglobin and do not sickle	

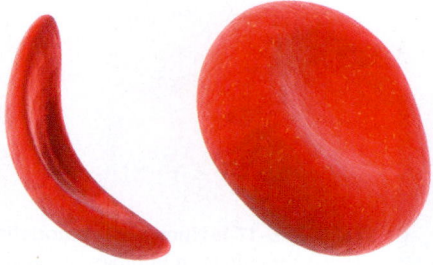

FIGURE 6-15 ■ Sickle cell.
The abnormal crescent shape and sharp edges of this sickled erythrocyte (on the left) are very different from the smooth, rounded contour of a normal erythrocyte (on the right). Repeated sickling causes these fragile erythrocytes to have a shortened life span, resulting in anemia.

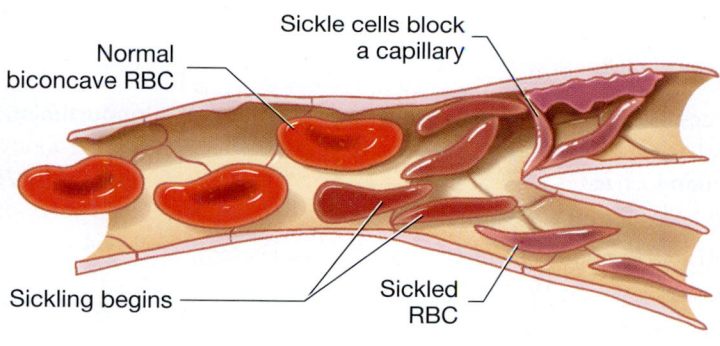

FIGURE 6-16 ■ Sickle cells in a capillary.
Sickle cells do not move easily through the capillaries. They become tangled and block the flow of blood. This causes severe pain and blood clots, particularly in the chest, abdomen, and joints.

Word or Phrase	Description	Pronunciation/Word Parts
transfusion reaction	Reaction that occurs when a person receives a transfusion with the wrong blood type. Antibodies in the person's serum attack antigens on the erythrocytes of the donor blood, causing **hemolysis** of the donor erythrocytes. Fever, chills, and hypotension occur almost immediately. The person has flank pain because the fragments of donor erythrocytes clog the kidneys. A transfusion reaction can be fatal. Treatment: Stop the transfusion immediately and treat the patient's symptoms.	**transfusion** (trans-FYOO-shun) **trans-** *across; through* **fus/o-** *pouring* **-ion** *action; condition* **hemolysis** (hee-MAW-lih-sihs) **hem/o-** *blood* **-lysis** *process to break down or destroy*

Word or Phrase	Description	Pronunciation/Word Parts

Leukocytes

acquired immuno- deficiency syndrome (AIDS)	Severe infection caused by the **human immunodeficiency virus (HIV)**, a retrovirus that infects helper T cell lymphocytes (see Figure 6-17 ■). Initially, there is a fever, night sweats, weight loss, enlarged lymph nodes, and diarrhea. AIDS is usually transmitted by sexual intercourse with an infected person, but it can also be transmitted: • When intravenous drug abusers share needles • When healthcare workers have an accidental needlestick and are exposed to infected blood • From transfusions with infected blood • From an infected mother to the fetus or from the breast milk to a nursing baby. As large numbers of helper T cells are infected and destroyed, the action of suppressor T cell lymphocytes dominates. This suppresses the normal immune response; the person becomes **immunocompromised** and defenseless against infection and cancer. Treatment: Antiretroviral drugs. There is no cure for AIDS.	**immunodeficiency** (IH-myoo-NOH-deh-FIH-shun-see) **immun/o-** *immune response* **defici/o-** *inadequate; lacking* **-ency** *condition of being; condition of having* **immunocompromised** (IH-myoo-noh-KAWM-proh-mizd) **immun/o-** *immune response* **compromis/o-** *exposed to danger* **-ed** *pertaining to*

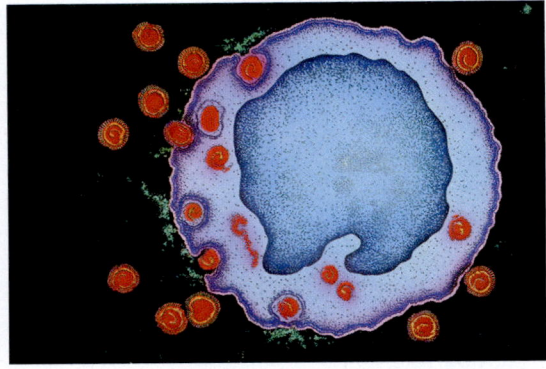

FIGURE 6-17 ■ Human immunodeficiency virus. This color-enhanced photograph taken with an electron microscope shows a helper T cell lymphocyte being invaded by many small human immunodeficiency (HIV) retroviruses. Like all viruses, HIV cannot reproduce itself. It must enter a lymphocyte and use that cell's DNA to reproduce. Then the lymphocyte is destroyed as the new HIV retroviruses are released.

Dive Deeper

A helper T cell lymphocyte is also known as a CD4 cell. A diagnosis of AIDS is made when the CD4 cell count is low and there is an **opportunistic infection** such as:

- *Pneumocystis jiroveci* pneumonia (described in Chapter 4, Pulmonology)
- Oral or esophageal candidiasis (described in Chapter 15, Otolaryngology)
- Cytomegalovirus retinitis (described in Chapter 14, Ophthalmology)
- Kaposi sarcoma (described in Chapter 2, Dermatology).

AIDS wasting syndrome is characterized by weight loss and loss of muscle mass and strength. The universal symbol for AIDS is a red ribbon.

opportunistic
(AW-por-too-NIS-tik)
opportun/o- *taking advantage of an opportunity; well timed*
-ist *person who specializes in; thing that specializes in*
-ic *pertaining to*

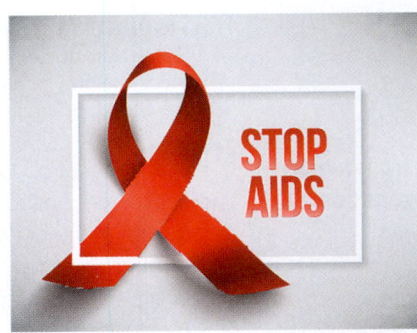

Word or Phrase	Description	Pronunciation/Word Parts
leukemia	Cancer of the leukocytes. Excessive numbers of immature leukocytes crowd out other cells in the red bone marrow, causing anemia (from too few erythrocytes), easy bruising and hemorrhages (from too few thrombocytes), fever, and susceptibility to infection (from too few mature leukocytes). Leukemia is named according to which leukocyte is affected and whether the onset of symptoms is acute or chronic. Leukemia can be caused by exposure to radiation or toxic chemicals and drugs. A diagnosis of leukemia is made by examination of the blood (see Figure 6-18 ■) and by performing a bone marrow aspiration to look at blood cells in the red bone marrow. Treatment: Chemotherapy drug; radiation therapy; bone marrow transplantation or stem cell transplantation	**leukemia** (loo-KEE-mee-ah) **leuk/o-** *white* **-emia** *condition of the blood; substance in the blood* Leukemia: *Condition of the blood (with too many immature) white (blood cells)*

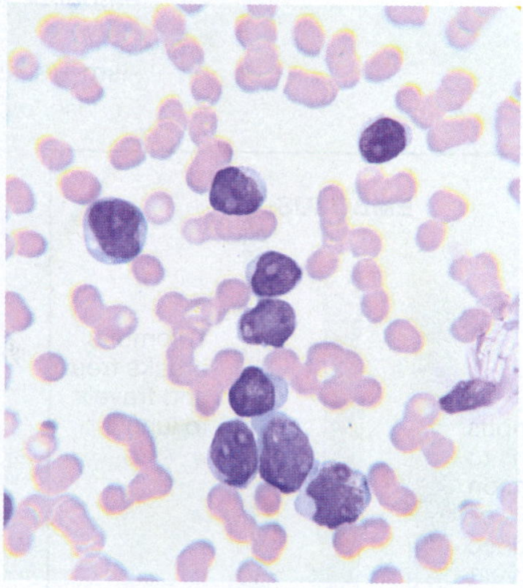

FIGURE 6-18 ■ Acute lymphocytic leukemia.
This blood was taken from a patient with acute lymphocytic leukemia. There is an increase in the number of immature lymphoblasts with some mature lymphocytes being present as well. The pale cells in the background are erythrocytes.

Word or Phrase	Description	Pronunciation/Word Parts
mononucleosis	Infectious disease caused by the **Epstein-Barr virus (EBV)**. There is lymphadenopathy, fever, and fatigue. It is often called the "kissing disease" because it commonly affects young adults and is transmitted through contact with saliva that contains the virus. Also known as *mono*. Treatment: Rest (There is no antiviral drug that is effective against mononucleosis. An antibiotic drug is not effective against a virus.)	**mononucleosis** (MAW-noh-NOO-klee-OH-sihs) **mon/o-** *one; single* **nucle/o-** *nucleus of an atom or a cell* **-osis** *abnormal condition; process* Mononucleosis: *Abnormal condition (of monocytes that have) one (unlobed) nucleus in the cell*
multiple myeloma	Cancer of B cell lymphocytes that would normally become plasma cells and produce antibodies. The decreased number of normal B cells results in weakness, anemia, and increased susceptibility to infections. Multiple tumors in the bone destroy the red bone marrow and cause pain and bone fractures. Bence Jones protein, an abnormal antibody produced by the cancerous B cell lymphocytes, is seen in the urine. Treatment: Radiation therapy; chemotherapy drugs	**myeloma** (MY-eh-LOH-mah) **myel/o-** *bone marrow; myelin; spinal cord* **-oma** *mass; tumor*

Thrombocytes and Blood Clotting

Word or Phrase	Description	Pronunciation/Word Parts
coagulopathy	Any disease that affects the ability of the blood to clot normally. Treatment: Correct the underlying cause.	**coagulopathy** (koh-AG-yoo-LAW-pah-thee) **coagul/o-** *clotting* **-pathy** *disease*

Word or Phrase	Description	Pronunciation/Word Parts
deep venous thrombosis (DVT)	A **thrombus** (blood clot) in one of the deep veins of the lower leg; this often occurs after surgery or in patients who are immobile or on bedrest. Lack of exercise causes the blood to pool in the veins (**venous stasis**) and form a blood clot (see Figure 6-19 ■). If a thrombus in a deep vein detaches from the vein wall and enters the blood, it becomes an **embolus**. Sometimes an embolus travels to the heart but, as it leaves the heart, becomes trapped in the smaller pulmonary artery, where it blocks blood flow to the lung. This condition is a pulmonary **embolism**. Treatment: Anticoagulant drug to prevent another thrombus from forming; thrombolytic enzyme drug to dissolve the embolus	**thrombosis** (thrawm-BOH-sihs) **thromb/o-** *blood clot* **-osis** *abnormal condition; process* **thrombus** (THRAWM-buhs) **thrombi** (THRAWM-by) **stasis** (STAY-sihs) **embolus** (EM-boh-luhs) **embolism** (EM-boh-LIZ-em) **embol/o-** *embolus; occluding plug* **-ism** *disease from a specific cause; process*

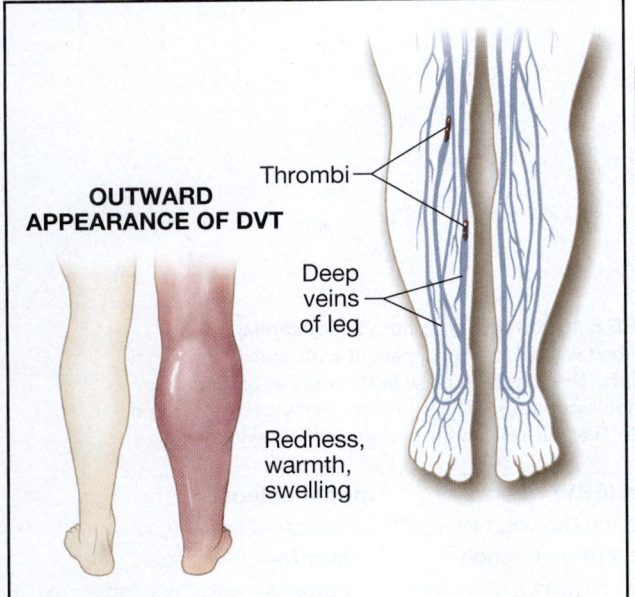

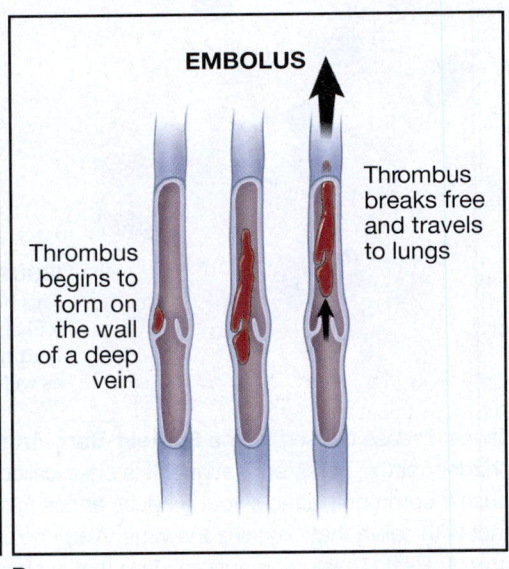

A.

B.

FIGURE 6-19 ■ Deep venous thrombosis.
A. When a blood clot (thrombus) forms in a deep vein in the leg, it causes redness, warmth, and swelling as the blood flow is impaired and the tissues become inflamed. **B.** A thrombus can break free and become an embolus that travels to other parts of the body.

Word or Phrase	Description	Pronunciation/Word Parts
disseminated intravascular coagulation (DIC)	Severe disorder of clotting in which multiple small thrombi are formed throughout the body. These thrombi use up platelets and fibrinogen from the plasma to such an extent that there is spontaneous bleeding from the nose, mouth, IV sites, and incisions. DIC can be triggered by severe injuries, burns, cancer, or systemic infections. Treatment: Intravenous fibrinogen and platelets	**disseminated** (dih-SEM-ih-NAY-ted) **dissemin/o-** *scattered throughout the body* **-ated** *composed of; pertaining to a condition* **intravascular** (IN-trah-VAS-kyoo-lar) **intra-** *within* **vascul/o-** *blood vessel* **-ar** *pertaining to* **coagulation** (koh-AG-yoo-LAY-shun) **coagul/o-** *clotting* **-ation** *being; having; process*

Word or Phrase	Description	Pronunciation/Word Parts
hemophilia	Inherited genetic abnormality that causes a lack or a deficiency of a specific clotting factor. The patient is a **hemophiliac**. When injured, hemophiliac patients continue to bleed for a long period of time. Minor injuries produce large hematomas under the skin and bleeding inside body cavities, joints, and organs. Treatment: Intravenous administration of the specific clotting factor that is lacking	**hemophilia** (HEE-moh-FIL-ee-ah) **hem/o-** *blood* **phil/o-** *attraction to; fondness for* **-ia** *condition; state; thing* Hemophilia: *Condition (of the) blood (in which it has a) fondness for (not clotting)* **hemophiliac** (HEE-moh-FIL-ee-ak) **hem/o-** *blood* **phil/o-** *attraction to; fondness for* **-iac** *pertaining to*
thrombocyto-penia	Deficiency in the number of thrombocytes due to exposure to radiation, chemicals, or drugs that damage stem cells in the red bone marrow. It also occurs when leukemia cells crowd out the stem cells in the red bone marrow that produce thrombocytes. Thrombocytopenia causes **petechiae** (small, pinpoint hemorrhages) or **ecchymoses** (larger hemorrhages) and bruises on the skin. Treatment: Blood or platelet transfusion	**thrombocytopenia** (THRAWM-boh-SY-toh-PEE-nee-ah) **thromb/o-** *blood clot* **cyt/o-** *cell* **-penia** *condition of deficiency* **petechiae** (peh-TEE-kee-ee) **ecchymoses** (EK-ih-MOH-seez)

Lymphatic System

graft-versus-host disease	Immune reaction of donor tissue or a donor organ (graft) against the patient (host). This can occur after a bone marrow transplantation or organ transplantation. Mild symptoms are a rash and fever, but the symptoms can be severe enough to cause death. Treatment: Corticosteroid drug	
lymphadenopathy	Enlarged lymph nodes. Lymph nodes in the neck, axillae, and groin can be felt if they are enlarged. A sore throat causes lymph nodes in the neck to enlarge (see Figure 6-20 ■). A severe infection or cancer will cause the lymph nodes in that area to become enlarged. Cancer cells can travel through the blood and the lymphatic system and cause enlarged lymph nodes in other places in the body. This spread is known as **metastasis**. Treatment: Correct the underlying cause.	**lymphadenopathy** (lim-FAD-eh-NAW-pah-thee) **lymph/o-** *lymph; lymphatic system* **aden/o-** *gland* **-pathy** *disease* **metastasis** (meh-TAS-tah-sihs) The prefix **meta-** means *change*. The suffix **-stasis** means *staying in one place*. Metastasis: *(A cell that is normally) staying in one place (but undergoes) change (to become cancerous and moves to another area)*

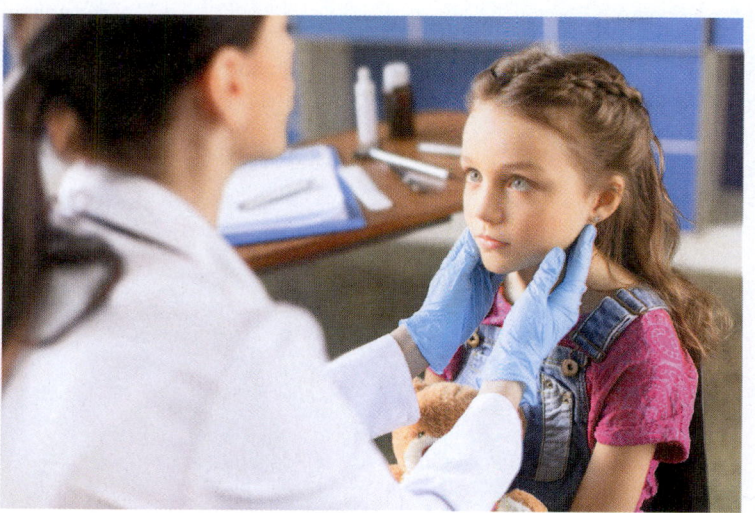

FIGURE 6-20 ■ Lymphadenopathy. The pediatrician is palpating the cervical lymph nodes of this patient. The cervical lymph nodes trap and destroy microorganisms or cancer cells from the nose, mouth, or throat, but large numbers of these eventually can cause enlarged lymph nodes and a complaint of sore throat or difficulty swallowing.

Word or Phrase	Description	Pronunciation/Word Parts
lymphedema	Generalized swelling of an arm or leg that occurs after surgery when a chain of lymph nodes has been removed. Tissue fluid in that area cannot drain into the lymphatic vessels at the normal rate, and this causes edema. Treatment: Elevation of the body part to promote drainage	**lymphedema** (LIMF-eh-DEE-mah) **lymph/o-** *lymph; lymphatic system* **-edema** *swelling*
lymphoma	Cancer of the lymphocytes, lymph nodes, or lymphatic tissue. Hodgkin and non-Hodgkin are two types of lymphomas. *Note*: A lymphoma that originates in a lymph node should not be confused with metastasis to a lymph node from a primary site of cancer located elsewhere. Treatment: Radiation therapy; chemotherapy drug	**lymphoma** (lim-FOH-mah) **lymph/o-** *lymph; lymphatic system* **-oma** *mass; tumor*
Hodgkin lymphoma	Most common type of lymphoma. It often occurs in young adults and is discovered on physical examination as a painless, enlarged cervical lymph node in the neck. There are symptoms of fever, weakness, weight loss, and splenomegaly. A biopsy of the lymph node shows abnormal lymphocytes known as **Reed-Sternberg cells** (see Figure 6-21 ■). Also known as **Hodgkin disease**. 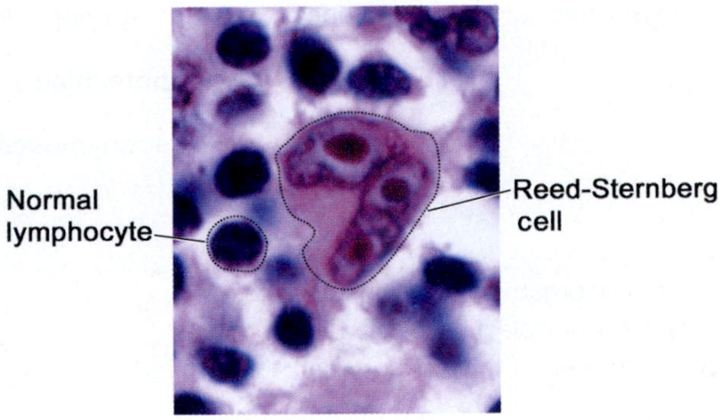 **FIGURE 6-21** ■ **Reed-Sternberg cell.** A normal lymphocyte (on the left) compared to an abnormal Reed-Sternberg cell (on the right) that is seen in Hodgkin lymphoma.	**Hodgkin** (HAWJ-kin)
non-Hodgkin lymphoma	A group of several different types of lymphomas that occur in older adults and do not contain Reed-Sternberg cells	
splenomegaly	Enlargement of the spleen that can be felt on palpation of the abdomen. Causes include mononucleosis, Hodgkin lymphoma, leukemia, and other blood and lymphatic diseases. Treatment: Correct the underlying cause.	**splenomegaly** (SPLEH-noh-MEG-ah-lee) **splen/o-** *spleen* **-megaly** *enlargement*
thymoma	Tumor of the thymus that is usually benign. It may cause a cough and chest pain. It is often seen in patients who already have an autoimmune disorder. Treatment: Thymectomy	**thymoma** (thy-MOH-mah) **thym/o-** *rage; thymus* **-oma** *mass; tumor*

Word or Phrase	Description	Pronunciation/Word Parts

Autoimmune Disorders

Word or Phrase	Description	Pronunciation/Word Parts
autoimmune disorders	Disorders in which the body makes antibodies against its own tissues, causing pain and loss of function. The following are common autoimmune disorders. (*Note*: These autoimmune disorders are described in detail in other chapters, as mentioned.)	**autoimmune** (AW-toh-ih-MYOON) **aut/o-** *self* **-immune** *immune response*

Autoimmune Disorder	Area Affected
diabetes mellitus, type 1	pancreas (Chapter 13, Endocrinology)
Graves disease	thyroid (Chapter 13, Endocrinology)
Hashimoto thyroiditis	
gluten sensitivity enteropathy	intestines (Chapter 3, Gastroenterology)
inflammatory bowel disease	
multiple sclerosis	nerves (Chapter 9, Neurology)
myasthenia gravis	muscles (Chapter 8, Orthopedics—Muscular)
psoriasis	skin (Chapter 2, Dermatology)
vitiligo	
rheumatoid arthritis	joints (Chapter 7, Orthopedics—Skeletal)
scleroderma	skin and blood vessels (Chapter 2, Dermatology)
systemic lupus erythematosus	connective tissue, skin, kidneys, lungs (Chapter 2, Dermatology)

6.3 PRACTICE LAPS

Use the Answer Key at the end of the book to check your answers.

A. Give the Meaning of Combining Forms

Next to each combining form, write its meaning. The first one has been done for you.

Combining Form	Meaning	Combining Form	Meaning
1. **aden/o-**	*gland*	14. micr/o-	
2. aut/o-		15. mon/o-	
3. chrom/o-		16. myel/o-	
4. coagul/o-		17. norm/o-	
5. cyt/o-		18. nucle/o-	
6. defici/o-		19. phil/o-	
7. embol/o-		20. plast/o-	
8. fus/o-		21. septic/o-	
9. hem/o-		22. splen/o-	
10. immun/o-		23. thromb/o-	
11. leuk/o-		24. thym/o-	
12. lymph/o-		25. vascul/o-	
13. macr/o-			

B. Build Words

Read the definition of the medical word. Look at the combining form that is given. Select the correct suffix from the Suffix List, and write it on the blank line. Then build the medical word, and write it on the line. (Remember: You may need to remove the combining vowel. Always remove the hyphens and slash.) Be sure to check your spelling.

Suffix List

-ation (being; having; process)	-ism (disease from a specific	-oma (mass; tumor)
-edema (swelling)	cause; process)	-osis (abnormal condition; process)
-emia (condition of the blood;	-lysis (process to break down or	-pathy (disease)
substance in the	destroy)	-rrhage (excessive discharge;
blood)	-megaly (enlargement)	excessive flow)

Definition of the Medical Word	Combining Form	Suffix	Build the Medical Word
Example: Mass (or) tumor (of the) thymus	**thym/o-**	*-oma*	*thymoma*

[*You think* mass; tumor *(-oma)* + thymus *(thym/o-)*. You change the order of the word parts to put the suffix last. You write thymoma.]

1. Process (of blood) clotting	coagul/o-	_____	_____
2. Disease from a specific cause (of an) embolism	embol/o-	_____	_____
3. Abnormal condition (of having a) blood clot	thromb/o-	_____	_____
4. Enlargement (of the) spleen	splen/o-	_____	_____
5. Condition of the blood (of having) infection	septic/o-	_____	_____
6. Swelling (of the) lymph (nodes)	lymph/o-	_____	_____
7. Disease (of blood) clotting	coagul/o-	_____	_____
8. Excessive flow (of) blood	hem/o-	_____	_____
9. Substance in the blood (of too many) white (cells)	leuk/o-	_____	_____
10. Mass (or) tumor (of the) bone marrow	myel/o-	_____	_____
11. Process to destroy blood (cells)	hem/o-	_____	_____

C. Define Abbreviations

1. AIDS _____

2. DIC _____

3. DVT _____

4. EBV _____

5. HIV _____

6.4 Laboratory, Diagnostic, and Radiologic Procedures

Word or Phrase	Description	Pronunciation/Word Parts

Blood Cell Tests

Word or Phrase	Description	Pronunciation/Word Parts
blood smear	Blood test in which a drop of blood is spread as a thin smear on a glass slide (see Figure 6-22 ■). Then hematoxylin and eosin dyes are used to stain the blood cells. The slide is examined under a microscope to identify characteristics of the erythrocytes and leukocytes. This test is performed to visually investigate an abnormal result from a previous complete blood count (CBC). 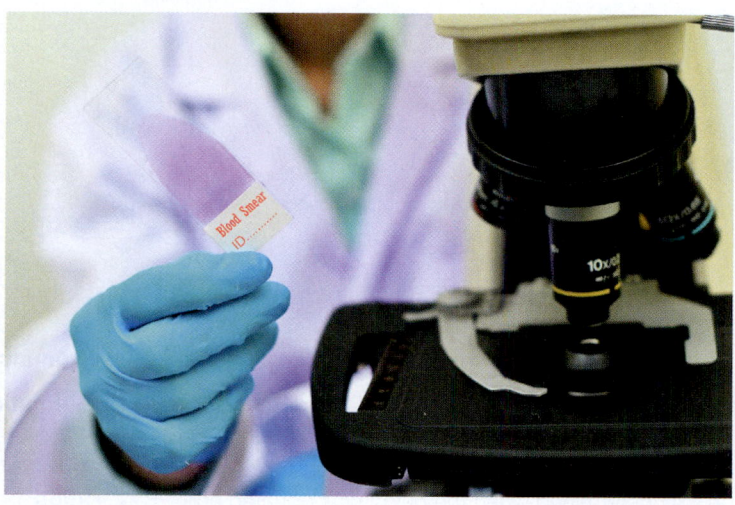 **FIGURE 6-22 ■ Blood smear.** A drop of the patient's blood is put on a glass slide and then smeared to spread out all of the blood cells into a very thin layer that can be viewed under a microscope.	

complete blood count (CBC) with differential	Group of blood tests that are performed by an automated machine. The tests determine the number, type, and characteristics of erythrocytes, the **hematocrit (HCT)** and **hemoglobin (Hgb)**, the number and percentages of the five different (differential) types of leukocytes, and the number of thrombocytes (see Table 6-4 ■).	**differential** (DIF-er-EN-shal)
		  different/o- *different; distinct*
		  -ial *pertaining to*
		
		hematocrit (heh-MAT-oh-krit)
		  hemat/o- *blood*
		  -crit *separation of*
		
		hemoglobin (HEE-moh-GLOH-bin)
		  hem/o- *blood*
		  glob/o- *comprehensive; shaped like a globe*
		  -in *substance*

Table 6-4 Complete Blood Count (CBC) with Differential

Test Name	Description	Pronunciation/Word Parts
Erythrocytes (red blood cells, RBCs)	Number in millions per milliliter (mL) of blood	
Hematocrit (HCT)	Percentage of RBCs in blood sample	**hematocrit** (hee-MAT-oh-krit) **hemat/o-** *blood* **-crit** *separation of*
Hemoglobin (Hgb)	Amount in grams per deciliter (g/dL) of blood	
Red blood cell **indices** **Mean** cell volume (MCV) Mean cell hemoglobin (MCH) Mean cell hemoglobin concentration (MCHC)	Average volume of one RBC Average weight of hemoglobin in one RBC Average concentration of hemoglobin in one RBC	**indices** (IN-dih-seez) *Index* is a Latin singular noun. Form the plural by changing *–ex* to *–ices*. **mean** (MEEN) *Mean* is an arithmetic word that means the *average*.
Leukocytes (white blood cells, WBCs)	Number in thousands per milliliter (k/mL) of blood	The *k* in *k/mL* stands for *kilo-,* a prefix meaning *one thousand.*
WBC differential Neutrophils Eosinophils Basophils Lymphocytes Monocytes	Percentage of each type of WBC per 100 WBCs	
Thrombocytes (platelets)	Number in thousands per milliliter (k/mL) of blood	

Word or Phrase	Description	Pronunciation/Word Parts
type and crossmatch	Blood test to determine the blood type (A, B, AB, or O) and Rh factor (positive or negative) of the patient's blood and to crossmatch the blood to a donor's blood when the patient needs a blood transfusion. The donor's blood type was determined when the blood was donated and stored in the blood bank. The patient's (recipient's) blood type is determined. Then the patient's plasma is crossmatched by mixing it with the donor's red blood cells. If the donor's red blood cells clump together (**agglutination**), the blood types are not compatible.	**agglutination** (ah-GLOO-tih-NAY-shun) **agglutin/o-** *clumping; sticking* **-ation** *being; having; process*

Clinical Connections

Blood Bank. Type O negative blood is known as the **universal donor** because it can be given to patients with any other blood type without causing a reaction. Blood is collected in units and refrigerated until it is needed for a transfusion.

Organ Transplantation. A patient who needs to have an organ transplantation must be matched to the donor not only by blood type but also by tissue type, which is matching for human leukocyte antigen (HLA).

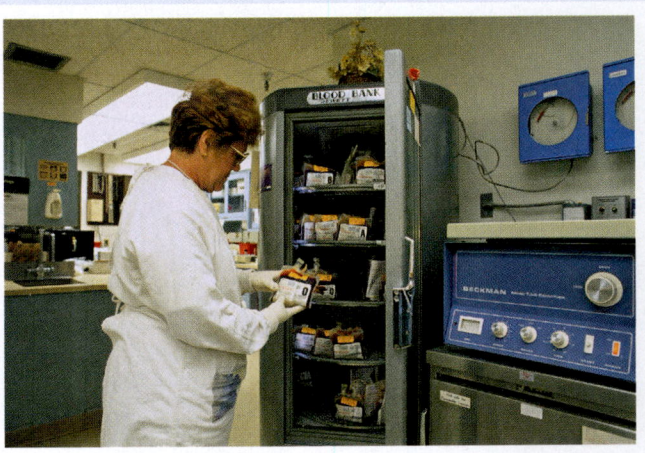

Word or Phrase	Description	Pronunciation/Word Parts

Coagulation Time Tests

Word or Phrase	Description	Pronunciation/Word Parts

coagulation time tests	Coagulation time tests are used to measure the length of time it takes the blood to clot. These tests are used to monitor the effectiveness of various anticoagulant drugs that are given to lengthen the blood clotting time in order to decrease the chance of blood clots forming. These tests include:
	
	• **Activated clotting time (ACT)**
	• **Partial thromboplastin time (PTT)**
	• **Prothrombin time (PT)**.
	
	The **international normalized ratio (INR)** reports the PT value in a standardized way, regardless of which laboratory performed the test.
		coagulation
		(koh-AG-yoo-LAY-shun)
		  coagul/o- *clotting*
		  -ation *being; having; process*

Other Blood Tests

Word or Phrase	Description	Pronunciation/Word Parts
blood chemistries	Blood test used to determine the levels of various substances in the blood (see Figure 6-23 ■). These include electrolytes, albumin, total protein, ALT, AST, BUN, creatinine, bilirubin, glucose, LDH, total cholesterol, uric acid, and alkaline phosphatase. 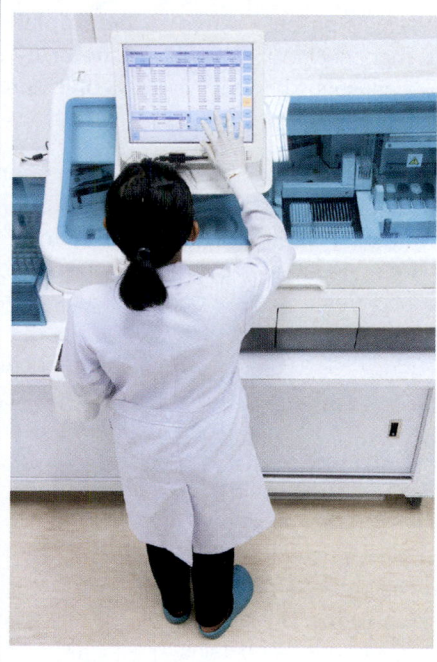 **FIGURE 6-23** ■ **Blood chemistry analyzer.** This clinical laboratory scientist is performing a blood chemistry analysis, the results of which are displayed on the computer screen. Multiple tests can be performed together automatically on this computerized equipment.	

ferritin	Blood test that indirectly measures the amount of iron (ferritin) stored in the body by measuring the small amount that is always present in the blood. This test is used to diagnose iron deficiency anemia.	**ferritin** (FAIR-ih-tin)
		  ferrit/o- *iron*
		  -in *substance*

human immuno-deficiency virus (HIV) tests	Blood tests that detect infection with HIV	
enzyme-linked immunosorbent assay (ELISA)	First screening test done for HIV. It can be done on blood, urine, or saliva samples. The test uses two antibodies. The first binds to HIV, forming a complex; the second reacts to an enzyme in that complex. However, this test can also be positive if the patient has antibodies against some other diseases.	

Word or Phrase	Description	Pronunciation/Word Parts
CD4 count	Blood test that measures the number of helper T cell lymphocytes (CD4 lymphocytes). A diagnosis of AIDS is made when the CD4 cell count is below 200 and the patient also has an opportunistic infection. The CD4 count is used to monitor the progression of AIDS and the patient's response to antiretroviral drugs. The ratio of CD4:CD8 (suppressor T cell lymphocytes) is also monitored.	
OraSure	Quick screening test done in a doctor's office or clinic to detect antibodies to HIV in the saliva.	
p24 antigen test	Blood test that detects p24, an actual protein in HIV. It is used to detect early HIV infection, as the test is positive before there are any antibodies against HIV. It is also a screening test for HIV in units of donated blood.	
viral RNA load test	Blood test that measures the amount of HIV present, as high, medium, or low. This test is used to monitor the progression of the disease and the patient's response to antiretroviral drugs.	
Western blot	Used to confirm a positive ELISA test result, so that a diagnosis of HIV infection can actually be made.	
MonoSpot test	Serum test for mononucleosis. Rapid test that uses the patient's serum mixed with horse erythrocytes. If the patient has mononucleosis, **heterophil antibodies** in the patient's serum will cause the horse's erythrocytes to clump.	**heterophil** (HET-er-oh-FIL) **heter/o-** *other* **-phil** *attraction to; fondness for*
serum protein electrophoresis (SPEP)	Serum test that determines the amount of each of the immunoglobulins (IgA, IgD, IgE, IgG, and IgM) in the blood. A sample of serum is placed in a gel and an electrical current is applied. Each immunoglobulin becomes electrically charged and moves toward the positive or negative electrode. Each travels a different distance through the gel and creates a spike on the graph, depending on its size, electrical charge, and how much of it there is.	**electrophoresis** (ee-LEK-troh-foh-REE-sihs) **electr/o-** *electricity* **phor/o-** *bear; carry; range* **-esis** *abnormal condition; process* Electrophoresis: *Process (of using) electricity (to) carry (immunoglobulins in a gel)*

Urine Tests

Schilling test	Urine test used to diagnose pernicious anemia by measuring the amount of radioactive vitamin B_{12} excreted in the urine. The patient swallows two capsules: one capsule contains intrinsic factor plus vitamin B_{12} labeled with a radioactive tracer and intrinsic factor; the other capsule contains vitamin B_{12} labeled with a different radioactive tracer but with no intrinsic factor. If the patient has pernicious anemia, only the capsule that contained intrinsic factor will have its radioactive vitamin B_{12} absorbed into the blood and then excreted in the urine.	
urine protein electrophoresis (UPEP)	Urine test to determine the amount of Bence Jones protein in order to monitor the course of multiple myeloma. It uses the process of electrophoresis (described previously).	

Word or Phrase	Description	Pronunciation/Word Parts

Radiologic Procedures

lymphangiography	Radiologic procedure in which a radiopaque contrast dye is injected into a lymphatic vessel. X-rays are taken as the dye travels through the lymphatic vessels and lymph nodes. It shows enlarged lymph nodes, lymphomas, and areas of blocked lymphatic drainage. The x-ray image is a **lymphangiogram**.	**lymphangiography** (lim-FAN-jee-AW-grah-fee) **lymph/o-** *lymph; lymphatic system* **angi/o-** *blood vessel; lymphatic vessel* **-graphy** *process of recording* **lymphangiogram** (lim-FAN-jee-oh-GRAM) **lymph/o-** *lymph; lymphatic system* **angi/o-** *blood vessel; lymphatic vessel* **-gram** *picture; record*

6.4 PRACTICE LAPS

Use the Answer Key at the end of the book to check your answers.

A. Give the Meaning of Combining Forms

*Next to each combining form, write its meaning. The first one has been done for you.*continued on next page

Combining Form	Meaning	Combining Form	Meaning
1. **different/o-**	*different; distinct*	7. glob/o-	
2. agglutin/o-		8. hemat/o-	
3. angi/o-		9. hem/o-	
4. coagul/o-		10. heter/o-	
5. electr/o-		11. lymph/o-	
6. ferrit/o-		12. phor/o-	

B. Build Words

Read the definition of the medical word. Look at the combining form that is given. Select the correct suffix from the Suffix List, and write it on the blank line. Then build the medical word, and write it on the line. (Remember: You may need to remove the combining vowel. Always remove the hyphens and slash.) Be sure to check your spelling.

Suffix List

-ation (being; having; process)	-ial (pertaining to)
-crit (separation of)	-in (substance)

Definition of the Medical Word	Combining Form	Suffix	Build the Medical Word
Example: Pertaining to (counting white blood cells that are) different (or) distinct	**different/o-**	_-ial_	_differential_

[*You think* pertaining to *(-ial)* + different; distinct *(different/o-)*. You change the order of the word parts to put the suffix last. You write differential.]

1. Process (of red blood cells) clumping	agglutin/o-	_____	_____
2. Substance (that is) iron	ferrit/o-	_____	_____
3. Separation of (red) blood (cells from other cells)	hemat/o-	_____	_____
4. Process (of blood) clotting	coagul/o-	_____	_____

C. Define Abbreviations

1. ACT _____
2. CBC _____
3. HCT _____

4. Hgb _____
5. PT _____
6. PTT _____

6.5 Medical Procedures, Drugs, and Surgical Procedures

Word or Phrase	Description	Pronunciation/Word Parts

Medical Procedures

Word or Phrase	Description	Pronunciation/Word Parts
blood donation	Procedure in which a unit of whole blood is collected from a donor. The unit is tested and labeled as to blood type and stored in a refrigerated blood bank. A unit of whole blood can be given as a transfusion or the unit can be divided into its component parts (erythrocytes, platelets, plasma), and just that part can be given as a transfusion to meet the needs of a specific patient.	**donation** (doh-NAY-shun) **donat/o-** *gift; giving* **-ion** *action; condition*

Clinical Connections

Public Health. All donated blood must be tested for syphilis, hepatitis, and HIV. The Food and Drug Administration (FDA) is responsible for the safety of blood and blood products used in the United States.

Word or Phrase	Description	Pronunciation/Word Parts
blood transfusion	Procedure in which blood, blood cells, or plasma is given by intravenous transfusion. A transfusion of whole blood (a unit of blood) provides a complete correction of blood loss (see Figure 6-24 ■). **Packed red blood cells (PRBCs)** are a concentrated preparation of RBCs in a small amount of plasma. Platelets are given to patients with thrombocytopenia or to cancer patients whose production of platelets is depressed after radiation therapy or chemotherapy drugs. Plasma is given to hemophiliac patients who need clotting factors.	**transfusion** (trans-FYOO-shun) **trans-** *across; through* **fus/o-** *pouring* **-ion** *action; condition*

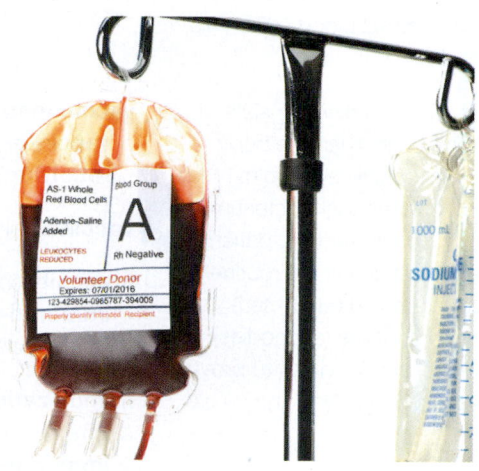

FIGURE 6-24 ■ Blood transfusion.
A unit of blood is collected from a donor and refrigerated until it is needed for a transfusion. One unit of blood contains 500 cc. This is nearly the same as 1 pint. That is why people talk of donating a "pint" of blood. This unit of A negative blood has been hung on an IV pole and is being given through intravenous tubing to a patient.

Dive Deeper

According to the American Red Cross, a physician can write a prescription for a patient to donate a unit of his or her own blood in advance, if blood loss is anticipated during surgery. This is an **autologous blood transfusion**.

At the conclusion of every surgery, the surgeon estimates the amount of blood loss and records this in the patient's operative report.

autologous (aw-TAW-loh-guhs)
aut/o- *self*
log/o- *study of; word*
-ous *pertaining to*

Word or Phrase	Description	Pronunciation/Word Parts
phlebotomy	Procedure that uses a needle and a vacuum tube or syringe to draw a sample of blood from a vein (see Figure 6-25 ■). Also known as **venipuncture**. The vacuum tubes have different-colored rubber stoppers that indicate which additive or anticoagulant is in the tube; this determines what blood test can be performed on the blood in that tube.	**phlebotomy** (fleh-BAW-toh-mee) **phleb/o-** *vein* **-tomy** *process of cutting; process of making an incision* **venipuncture** (VEE-nih-PUNK-chur) **ven/i-** *vein* **punct/o-** *hole; perforation* **-ure** *result of; system*

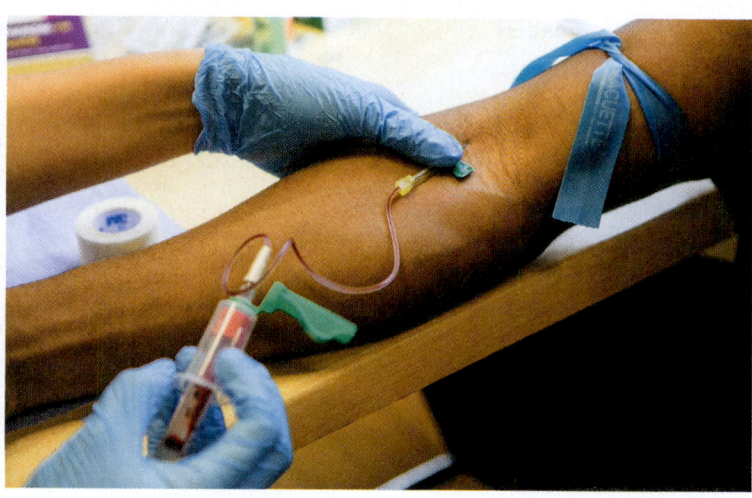

FIGURE 6-25 ■ Phlebotomy.
This patient is having blood drawn. The phlebotomist placed a tourniquet around the patient's upper arm to distend the veins in the lower arm. The patient's arm is supported to keep the elbow straight so that the needle goes into the lumen of the vein, not through it. A vacuum tube is placed into the plastic holder and the vacuum draws blood into the tube. The tubes of blood are sent to a laboratory for testing.

Word or Phrase	Description	Pronunciation/Word Parts
plasmapheresis	Procedure in which plasma is separated from the blood cells. A donor gives a unit of blood, which is rapidly spun in a centrifuge. Centrifugal force pulls the blood cells to the bottom of the unit of blood. The plasma portion at the top is siphoned off. The blood cells are given back to the donor. Then the plasma is processed and pooled with plasma from other donors to make fresh frozen plasma, albumin, or clotting factors.	**plasmapheresis** (PLAZ-mah-feh-REE-sihs) **plasm/o-** *plasma* **apher/o-** *withdrawal* **-esis** *abnormal condition; process*
stem cell transplantation	Procedure to give stem cells from a matched donor's red bone marrow to a patient. The stem cells are given intravenously; they then migrate to the patient's red bone marrow and begin producing normal blood cells. This procedure is used to treat leukemia or lymphoma.	
vaccination	Procedure that injects a **vaccine** into the body. The vaccine consists of dead or weakened bacteria, viruses, or cell fragments. Then the body produces antibodies and memory B lymphocytes specifically against that bacterium or virus. If the vaccinated patient encounters that bacterium or virus again, the body has a targeted immune response, and the patient will have mild or no symptoms of the disease. Vaccinations are routinely used to provide **active immunity** to diseases that could cause serious disability (polio, diphtheria, tetanus). Immunoglobulins (antibodies) against some diseases (such as rabies or tetanus) can be given to provide **passive immunity** if the person has just been exposed. Also known as **immunization**.	**vaccination** (VAK-sih-NAY-shun) **vaccin/o-** *vaccine* **-ation** *being; having; process* **vaccine** (vak-SEEN) **immunity** (ih-MYOO-nih-tee) **immun/o-** *immune response* **-ity** *condition; state* **immunization** (IH-myoo-nih-ZAY-shun) **immun/o-** *immune response* **-ization** *process of creating; process of inserting; process of making*

Across the Life Span

Pediatrics. Childhood immunizations against measles, mumps, rubella, polio, diphtheria, pertussis, and tetanus use a vaccine made of dead or weakened pathogens or inactivated endotoxins. The vaccination causes B lymphocytes to become plasma cells and produce antibodies, and this gives active immunity without exposure to the actual disease. The human papillomavirus vaccine is recommended for adolescents. The meningococcal meningitis vaccine is recommended for college students living in dormitories.

Middle Age. Adult immunizations include annual vaccinations for influenza (the flu) and periodic boosters for tetanus.

Geriatrics. Influenza, pneumococcal pneumonia, and shingles vaccinations are recommended for older adults.

Drugs

Category	Indication	Pronunciation/Word Parts
anticoagulant drug	Prevents blood clots from forming by inhibiting the clotting factors or by inhibiting vitamin K that is needed to make the clotting factors	**anticoagulant** (AN-tee-koh-AG-yoo-lant) **anti-** *against* **coagul/o-** *clotting* **-ant** *pertaining to*
corticosteroid drug	Anti-inflammatory drug that suppresses the immune response and decreases inflammation. Also given to organ transplant patients to prevent rejection of the donor organ.	**corticosteroid** (KOR-tih-koh-STAIR-oyd) **cortic/o-** *cortex; outer region* **-steroid** *steroid*
erythropoietin drug	Stimulates the red bone marrow to make erythrocytes	**erythropoietin** (eh-RITH-roh-POY-eh-tin) **erythr/o-** *red* **-poietin** *substance that forms*

Category	Indication	Pronunciation/Word Parts
immunosuppressant drug	Suppresses the immune response to prevent rejection of a transplanted organ	**immunosuppressant** (IH-myoo-NOH-soo-PRES-ant) **immun/o-** *immune response* **suppress/o-** *press down* **-ant** *pertaining to*
nucleoside reverse transcriptase inhibitor drug	Antiretroviral drug that inhibits reverse transcriptase, an enzyme that HIV needs to reproduce itself	**nucleoside** (NOO-klee-oh-SIDE) **transcriptase** (trans-KRIP-tays)
platelet aggregation inhibitor drug	Prevents platelets from aggregating (clumping together), the first step in forming a blood clot	**inhibitor** (in-HIB-ih-tor) **inhibit/o-** *block; hold back* **-or** *person who does or produces; thing that does or produces*
protease inhibitor drug	Antiretroviral drug that inhibits protease, an enzyme that HIV needs to reproduce itself	**protease** (PROH-tee-ays) **prote/o-** *protein* **-ase** *enzyme*
thrombolytic enzyme drug	Breaks fibrin strands to dissolve a blood clot that has already formed	**thrombolytic** (THRAWM-boh-LIT-ik) **thromb/o-** *blood clot* **lyt/o-** *break down; destroy* **-ic** *pertaining to*
tissue plasminogen activator (TPA) drug	Activates plasminogen to become an enzyme that breaks fibrin strands and dissolves a blood clot that has already formed	**plasminogen** (plaz-MIN-oh-jen)
vitamin B₁₂ drug	Treats pernicious anemia. It is given by intramuscular injection, by nasal spray, or sublingually (under the tongue).	

Word or Phrase	Description	Pronunciation/Word Parts

Surgical Procedures

bone marrow aspiration	Procedure using a needle and syringe to aspirate and remove a sample of red bone marrow from the posterior iliac crest of the hip bone. This is done for one of two reasons: 1. To diagnose leukemia or lymphoma and to monitor its progression by examining the different stages of cell development (stem cell to mature cell) 2. To harvest red bone marrow from a healthy, compatible donor to give to a patient who needs a bone marrow transplantation (see Figure 6-26 ■).	**aspiration** (AS-pih-RAY-shun) **aspir/o-** *breath in; suck in* **-ation** *being; having; process*

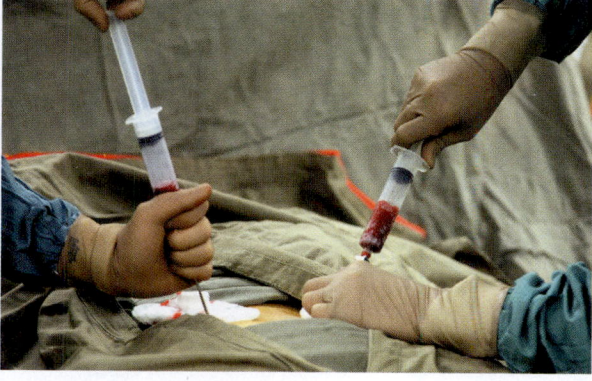

FIGURE 6-26 ■ Bone marrow aspiration.
A large needle is inserted into the red bone marrow, and the red marrow is drawn out by suction into a syringe.

Word or Phrase	Description	Pronunciation/Word Parts
bone marrow transplantation	Procedure used to treat patients with leukemia or lymphoma. The bone marrow donor and the recipient patient are matched for blood type and also for tissue type: **human leukocyte-associated (HLA) antigens**. Red bone marrow is harvested by aspirating it from the hip bone of a matched donor (see Figure 6-26). The patient is treated with chemotherapy drugs or radiation to destroy all cancer cells (this also destroys the patient's red bone marrow cells). The donor's bone marrow cells are given intravenously to the patient; the cells travel through the patient's blood to the bones where they implant. After 2–4 weeks, the patient's red bone marrow again begins to produce normal blood cells.	**transplantation** (TRANS-plan-TAY-shun) **transplant/o-** *move and put in another place* **-ation** *being; having; process*
lymph node biopsy	Procedure that uses a fine needle to aspirate tissue from a lymph node. The tissue is examined under a microscope to look for cancer cells. The lymph node may also be completely removed by doing an **excisional biopsy**.	**biopsy** (BY-awp-see) **bi/o-** *living organism; living tissue* **-opsy** *process of viewing* **excisional** (ek-SIH-zhun-al) **ex-** *away from; out* **cis/o-** *cut* **-ion** *action; condition* **-al** *pertaining to*
lymph node dissection	Surgical procedure to separate (dissect) lymph nodes from tissue and remove several or all of the lymph nodes in a lymph node chain to look for metastasis of a cancer from its original site elsewhere in the body	**dissection** (dy-SEK-shun) **dissect/o-** *cut apart* **-ion** *action; condition*
splenectomy	Procedure to remove the spleen when it has ruptured due to trauma	**splenectomy** (spleh-NEK-toh-mee) **splen/o-** *spleen* **-ectomy** *surgical removal*
thymectomy	Procedure to remove the thymus because of a benign thymoma tumor	**thymectomy** (thy-MEK-toh-mee) **thym/o-** *rage; thymus* **-ectomy** *surgical removal*

6.5 PRACTICE LAPS

Use the Answer Key at the end of the book to check your answers.

A. Give the Meaning of Combining Forms

Next to each combining form, write its meaning. The first one has been done for you.

Combining Form	Meaning	Combining Form	Meaning
1. **aspir/o-**	*breathe in; suck in*	14. lyt/o-	
2. apher/o-		15. phleb/o-	
3. aut/o-		16. plasm/o-	
4. bi/o-		17. prote/o-	
5. cis/o-		18. punct/o-	
6. coagul/o-		19. splen/o-	
7. cortic/o-		20. suppress/o-	
8. dissect/o-		21. thromb/o-	
9. donat/o-		22. thym/o-	
10. erythr/o-		23. transplant/o-	
11. fus/o-		24. vaccin/o-	
12. immun/o-		25. ven/i-	
13. inhibit/o-			

B. Build Words

Read the definition of the medical word. Look at the combining form that is given. Select the correct suffix from the Suffix List, and write it on the blank line. Then build the medical word, and write it on the line. (Remember: You may need to remove the combining vowel. Always remove the hyphens and slash.) Be sure to check your spelling.

Suffix List

-ation (being; having; process) -ectomy (surgical removal) -ion (action; condition)	-ity (condition; state) -ization (process of making) -opsy (process of viewing)	-or (thing that does or produces) -poietin (substance that forms)	-tomy (process of cutting; process of making an incision)

Definition of the Medical Word	Combining Form	Suffix	Build the Medical Word
Example: Surgical removal (of the) thymus	**thym/o-**	*-ectomy*	*thymectomy*

[*You think* surgical removal (-ectomy) + thymus (thym/o-). You change the order of the word parts to put the suffix last. You write thymectomy.]

1. Action (of) giving (blood)	donat/o-	_____	_____
2. Substance that forms red (blood cells)	erythr/o-	_____	_____
3. State (of having an) immune response	immun/o-	_____	_____
4. Process of cutting (into a) vein	phleb/o-	_____	_____
5. Surgical removal (of the) spleen	splen/o-	_____	_____
6. Process (of receiving a) vaccine	vaccin/o-	_____	_____
7. Process of viewing living tissue	bi/o-	_____	_____
8. Process of making (an) immune response	immun/o-	_____	_____
9. Process (to) move and put in another place	transplant/o-	_____	_____
10. Thing (drug) that does block	inhibit/o-	_____	_____
11. Process (to) suck in	aspir/o-	_____	_____
12. Action (to) cut apart	dissect/o-	_____	_____

Abbreviations Summary

A	blood type A in the ABO blood group	**IgE**	immunoglobulin E
AB	blood type AB in the ABO blood group	**IgG**	immunoglobulin G
ACT	activated clotting time	**IgM**	immunoglobulin M
AIDS	acquired immunodeficiency syndrome	**INR**	international normalized ratio
B	blood type B in the ABO blood group	**K$^+$**	potassium (an electrolyte)
basos	basophils (short form)	**lymphs**	lymphocytes (short form)
Ca^{++}	calcium (an electrolyte)	**mono**	mononucleosis (short form)
CBC	complete blood count	**monos**	monocytes (short form)
CD4	helper T cell	**Na$^+$**	sodium (an electrolyte)
CD8	suppressor T cell	**O**	blood type O in the ABO blood group
Cl$^-$	chloride (an electrolyte)	**PMN**	polymorphonuclear (leukocyte)
DIC	disseminated intravascular coagulation	**polys**	polymorphonuclear leukocytes (short form)
DVT	deep venous thrombosis	**PRBCs**	packed red blood cells
EBV	Epstein-Barr virus	**pro time**	prothrombin time (short form)
ELISA	enzyme-linked immunosorbent assay	**PT**	prothrombin time
eos	eosinophils (short form)	**PTT**	partial thromboplastin time
H&H	hemoglobin and hematocrit	**RBC**	red blood cell
HCO$_3^-$	bicarbonate (an electrolyte)	**segs**	segmented neutrophils (short form)
HCT	hematocrit	**SPEP**	serum protein electrophoresis (pronounced "S-pep")
Hgb	hemoglobin		
HIV	human immunodeficiency virus	**UPEP**	urine protein electrophoresis (pronounced "U-pep")
HLA	human leukocyte antigen		
IgA	immunoglobulin A	**WBC**	white blood cell
IgD	immunoglobulin D		

Word Alert

Abbreviations. Abbreviations are commonly used in all types of medical documents; however, they can mean different things to different people and their meanings can be misinterpreted. Always verify the meaning of an abbreviation.
Monos is a short form that means *monocytes*, but the short form *mono* means *mononucleosis*.
PT means *prothrombin time*, but it also means *physical therapist* or *physical therapy*.

It's Greek to Me! Did you notice that some words have two different combining forms? Combining forms from both Greek and Latin remain a part of medical language today.

Word	Greek	Latin	Medical Word Examples
cell	cyt/o-	cellul/o-	cytoplasm; cellular
nucleus	kary/o-	nucle/o-	megakaryocyte; polymorphonuclear
red	erythr/o-	rub/o-	erythrocyte; bilirubin
vein	phleb/o-	ven/o-	phlebotomy; venipuncture

Career Focus

Meet Adriana, a phlebotomist in a hospital

"A phlebotomist's job description is to draw blood, the collection of blood. On a daily basis, I draw blood from about 30 to 50 patients. Every time it's someone different, so every time it's a different challenge. That's why I love it."

- **Phlebotomists** are allied health professionals who use venipuncture techniques to draw blood. They follow procedures for storing and transporting blood specimens for diagnostic testing in the laboratory.
- **Hematologists** are physicians who practice in the medical specialty of hematology. They diagnose and treat patients with diseases of the blood. Malignancies of the blood and lymphatic system are treated medically by an oncologist or surgically by a general surgeon.
- **Immunologists** are physicians, or they are scientists who have a Ph.D. in cellular biology or pharmacology. They practice in the medical specialty of immunology. Clinical immunologists diagnose and treat patients who have autoimmune diseases, immunodeficiency diseases, cancer, or who are undergoing transplantation (organ, bone marrow, or stem cell).
- **Oncologists** are physicians who treat patients with cancer of the blood or immune system.

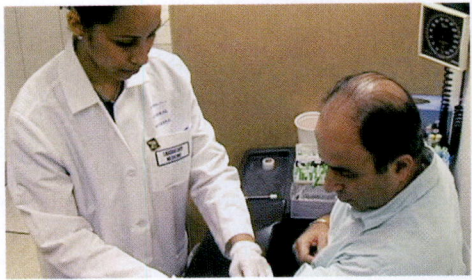

phlebotomist (fleh-BAW-toh-mist)
  phleb/o- *vein*
  tom/o- *cut; layer; slice*
  -ist *person who specializes in; thing that specializes in*

hematologist (HEE-mah-TAW-loh-jist)
  hemat/o- *blood*
  log/o- *study of; word*
  -ist *person who specializes in; thing that specializes in*

immunologist (IH-myoo-NAW-loh-jist)
  immun/o- *immune response*
  log/o- *study of; word*
  -ist *person who specializes in; thing that specializes in*

Chapter Review Exercises

Dive In: Medical Language Exercises

Test your knowledge of the chapter by completing these review exercises. Use the Answer Key at the end of the book to check your answers. Note: Each of the numbered exercise headers corresponds to a numbered learning outcome at the beginning of the chapter.

6.1 Anatomy

MATCHING EXERCISE

Match each word or phrase to its description.

1. band
2. basophil
3. blood type
4. erythrocytes
5. hematopoiesis
6. lymph node
7. lymphocyte
8. megakaryocyte
9. neutrophil
10. oxyhemoglobin
11. plasma
12. sodium
13. spleen
14. stem cell
15. thrombocyte

_____ encapsulated lymphoid tissue
_____ how blood cells and cell fragments are produced
_____ cell fragment
_____ matures either in the red bone marrow or the thymus
_____ clear, straw-colored part of the blood
_____ hemoglobin bound to oxygen
_____ also known as a stab
_____ named for antigens on the erythrocyte
_____ the electrolyte Na^+
_____ least common leukocyte
_____ removes and recycles old erythrocytes
_____ red blood cells
_____ immature cell in the red bone marrow
_____ does not readily take on laboratory stain
_____ its cytoplasm breaks away to create platelets

CIRCLE EXERCISE

Circle the correct answer from the choices given.

1. An immature RBC is a/an (**erythroblast, erythrocyte, hemoglobin**).
2. (**Carboxyhemoglobin, Erythropoietin, Granulocyte**) is a hormone that stimulates red blood cell production.
3. Agranulocytes include all of the following *except* (**eosinophils, lymphocytes, monocytes**).
4. This leukocyte has large, red-pink granules in its cytoplasm (**basophil, eosinophil, monocyte**).
5. A (**lymphocyte, monocyte, neutrophil**) is the most common type of leukocyte.
6. All of the following are electrolytes in the blood *except* (**albumin, calcium, sodium**).

TRUE OR FALSE EXERCISE

*Indicate whether each statement is true or false by writing **T** or **F** on the line.*

1. _____ Blood is categorized as a connective tissue.
2. _____ The lymph circulates in the same blood vessels as the blood does.
3. _____ Hemoglobin contains an iron molecule.
4. _____ A leukocyte is another name for a platelet.
5. _____ A neutrophil is also known as a PMN or a poly.
6. _____ Monocytes are the largest leukocytes.
7. _____ Unlike blood vessels, lymphatic vessels have a beginning and an end point.
8. _____ Lymphoid organs include the appendix and the spleen.
9. _____ A mature erythrocyte has no nucleus.

DIVIDING WORDS EXERCISE

Separate these words into their component parts (prefix, combining form, suffix). Some words do not contain all three word parts. The first one has been done for you.

Medical Word	Prefix	Combining Form	Suffix	Medical Word	Prefix	Combining Form	Suffix
1. **erythropoietin**		*erythr/o-*	*-poietin*	6. lymphatic		_____	_____
2. agranulocyte	_____	_____	_____	7. lymphocyte		_____	_____
3. electrolyte		_____	_____	8. megakaryocyte	_____	_____	_____
4. erythrocyte		_____	_____	9. neutrophil		_____	_____
5. hemoglobin		_____	_____				

SPELLING EXERCISE

Read each medical word pronunciation and write the medical word that it represents. Be sure to check your spelling. The first one has been done for you.

1. **(ee-LEK-troh-lite)** _____ *electrolyte* _____
2. (eh-RITH-roh-site) _____
3. (HEE-moh-GLOH-bin) _____
4. (EE-oh-SIN-oh-fil) _____
5. (aa-GRAN-yoo-loh-SITE) _____
6. (THRAWM-boh-site) _____
7. (LIM-foyd) _____

6.2 Physiology

MATCHING EXERCISE

Match each word or phrase to its description.

1. anaphylaxis
2. antibody
3. basophil
4. fibrin
5. cytotoxic T cell
6. endotoxins
7. hemostasis
8. IgA
9. local allergic reaction
10. neutrophil
11. NK cell
12. thrombocyte
13. virus
14. vitamin K

_____ phagocyte that engulfs and destroys bacteria
_____ releases histamine during an allergic reaction
_____ a platelet
_____ strands that are made by clotting factors
_____ produced by certain bacteria
_____ needed by the liver in order to make clotting factors
_____ in the colostrum in mother's milk (mother's first breast milk)
_____ cessation of bleeding
_____ example of a microorganism
_____ swelling and itching in one area
_____ severe systemic allergic reaction
_____ can recognize a cancer cell even if it is not coated with antibodies
_____ kills cells infected with a virus
_____ also known as an immunoglobulin

CIRCLE EXERCISE

Circle the correct answer from the choices given.

1. The immune response is directed against all of the following *except* (**bacteria, cancer cells, fibrin**).
2. The process of platelets forming into clumps is known as (**aggregation, coagulation, hemostasis**).
3. A blood clot is known as a (**basophil, pathogen, thrombus**).
4. Allergens include all of the following *except* (**antibodies, food, pollen**).
5. A pathogen causes (**coagulation, disease, phagocytosis**).
6. Interferon is produced by monocytes that have engulfed a (**bacterium, thrombus, virus**).

TRUE OR FALSE EXERCISE

*Indicate whether each statement is true or false by writing **T** or **F** on the line.*

1. _____ Platelets release several clotting factors.
2. _____ Coagulation is the process of fibrin strands trapping leukocytes to form a blood clot.
3. _____ Hypersensitivity is an individual's unique response to allergens.
4. _____ Anaphylaxis can occur when a person who is allergic to peanuts eats them.
5. _____ Helper T cells limit the extent and duration of an immune response.
6. _____ IgG is the most abundant immunoglobulin.

DIVIDING WORDS EXERCISE

Separate these words into their component parts (prefix, combining form, suffix). Some words do not contain all three word parts. The first one has been done for you.

Medical Word	Prefix	Combining Form	Suffix	Medical Word	Prefix	Combining Form	Suffix
1. **local**		*loc/o-*	*-al*	7. immunity			
2. aggregation				8. interleukin			
3. allergen				9. pathogen			
4. anaphylactic				10. phagocyte			
5. hemostasis				11. systemic			
6. hypersensitivity							

SPELLING EXERCISE

Read each medical word pronunciation and write the medical word that it represents. Be sure to check your spelling. The first one has been done for you.

1. (AL-er-jee)   _____*allergy*_____
2. (ih-MYOO-nih-tee)   _____
3. (THRAWM-boh-site)   _____
4. (koh-AG-yoo-LAY-shun)   _____
5. (PATH-oh-jen)   _____
6. (IH-myoo-noh-GLAW-byoo-lin)   _____

6.3 Diseases

MATCHING EXERCISE

Match each word or phrase to its description.

1. AIDS
2. aplastic anemia
3. Bence Jones protein
4. embolus
5. hemophilia
6. hemorrhage
7. lymphoma
8. pancytopenia
9. Reed-Sternberg cells
10. septicemia
11. sickle cells
12. splenomegaly
13. transfusion reaction
14. thrombus

_____ abnormal protein in the urine seen in multiple myeloma
_____ caused by exposure to radiation therapy or chemotherapy drugs
_____ cancer of a lymph node
_____ a thrombus in the deep veins that detaches and travels to the heart
_____ cells seen in Hodgkin lymphoma
_____ enlargement of the spleen
_____ causes hemolysis of erythrocytes
_____ genetic abnormality with lack of a specific clotting factor
_____ loss of a large amount of blood
_____ crescent-shaped red blood cells
_____ severe bacterial infection in the blood
_____ sexually transmitted disease caused by a retrovirus
_____ a blood clot
_____ decreased numbers of all types of blood cells because the bone marrow does not produce stem cells

CIRCLE EXERCISE

Circle the correct answer from the choices given.

1. A severe bacterial infection that spreads to the blood and then the entire body is (**anemia, folic acid deficiency, sepsis**).
2. Anemia can be caused by all of the following *except* (**chronic blood loss, hemorrhage, lymphadenopathy**).
3. A transfusion reaction causes hemolysis of the (**platelets, red blood cells, white blood cells**).
4. Mononucleosis is caused by (**an opportunistic infection, Epstein-Barr virus, sickle cell disease**).
5. Patients with pernicious anemia lack (**folic acid, intrinsic factor, iron**).
6. All of the following are autoimmune disorders *except* (**hemorrhage, multiple sclerosis, psoriasis**).

TRUE OR FALSE EXERCISE

Indicate whether each statement is true or false by writing **T** *or* **F** *on the line.*

1. _____ Folic acid anemia is seen in malnourished persons.
2. _____ An erythrocyte that is macrocytic is abnormally small.
3. _____ Genetically abnormal erythrocytes can sickle when there is a low level of oxygen.
4. _____ HIV is caused by a retrovirus.
5. _____ Coagulopathy is any disease that affects the ability of the blood to clot normally.
6. _____ In iron deficiency anemia, the erythrocytes are microcytic and hypochromic.
7. _____ Opportunistic infections cause disease in patients who already have hemophilia.
8. _____ Lymphadenopathy is the medical word for enlarged lymph nodes.
9. _____ A low oxygen level in a person with sickle cell disease can cause the red blood cells to become sickled.
10. _____ All patients with HIV also have AIDS.
11. _____ AIDS is a sexually transmitted disease that is also known as the "kissing disease."
12. _____ A thymoma is a tumor of the thymus that is usually benign.

DIVIDING WORDS EXERCISE

Separate these words into their component parts (prefix, combining form, suffix). Some words do not contain all three word parts. The first one has been done for you.

Medical Word	Prefix	Combining Form	Suffix	Medical Word	Prefix	Combining Form	Suffix
1. **hypochromic**	*hypo-*	*chrom/o-*	*-ic*	7. leukemia		_____	_____
2. coagulopathy		_____	_____	8. lymphoma		_____	_____
3. embolism		_____	_____	9. pancytopenia	_____	_____	_____
4. hemolysis		_____	_____	10. septicemia	_____	_____	_____
5. hemorrhage		_____	_____	11. splenomegaly	_____	_____	_____
6. intravascular	_____	_____	_____	12. transfusion	_____	_____	_____

SPELLING EXERCISE

Read each medical word pronunciation and write the medical word that it represents. Be sure to check your spelling. The first one has been done for you.

1. (ah-NEE-mee-ah) _____ *anemia* _____
2. (HEM-oh-rij) _____
3. (loo-KEE-mee-ah) _____
4. (MAW-noh-NOO-klee-OH-sihs) _____
5. (koh-AG-yoo-LAW-pah-thee) _____
6. (thrawm-BOH-sihs) _____
7. (HEE-moh-FIL-ee-ah) _____

6.4 Laboratory, Diagnostic, and Radiologic Procedures

MATCHING EXERCISE

Match each word or phrase to its description.

1. blood chemistries
2. blood smear
3. blood type
4. ferritin
5. differential
6. hematocrit
7. lymphangiography
8. MonoSpot test
9. Schilling test

_____ part of a CBC test

_____ drop of blood spread thin and examined under a microscope

_____ used to diagnose mononucleosis

_____ includes electrolytes, albumin, cholesterol, glucose, and other tests

_____ uses radiopaque contrast dye to outline the lymphatic system

_____ used to diagnose pernicious anemia

_____ percentage of erythrocytes in a sample of blood

_____ includes both the ABO and Rh factor

_____ blood test for amount of iron stored in the body

CIRCLE EXERCISE

Circle the correct answer from the choices given.

1. The physician would order a (**ferritin level, lymphangiography, type and crossmatch**) to see if a patient had iron deficiency anemia.
2. All of the following are coagulation tests *except* (**ACT, HCT, INR**).
3. What test uses gel and an electrical current to separate proteins? (**electrophoresis, prothrombin time, Schilling test**)
4. Which blood type is the universal donor? (**B negative, AB positive, O negative**).
5. All of the following are tests for HIV *except* (**CD4 count, ELISA, Hgb**).

TRUE OR FALSE EXERCISE

*Indicate whether each statement is true or false by writing **T** or **F** on the line.*

1. _____ A blood smear is done to investigate the results of an abnormal CBC.
2. _____ A CBC includes tests for the HCT and Hgb.
3. _____ Agglutination refers to clumping together of the clotting factors.
4. _____ The INR reports the PT value in a standardized way.
5. _____ OraSure is a quick screening test that detects antibodies to HIV in the patient's urine.
6. _____ SPEP determines the levels of each of the five immunoglobulins.

LABORATORY TEST EXERCISE

Review the form below for ordering laboratory tests for a hematology patient. Find each of the following tests and put a checkmark next to it.

albumin	carboxyhemoglobin	HCT	sodium
blood group	CBC	PT	total iron
	electrolyte panel		WBC count

CPT CODE	LABORATORY TESTS	CPT CODE	LABORATORY TESTS
82040	Albumin	82330	Calcium
82307	Blood alcohol	82375	Carboxyhemoglobin
84520	Blood urea nitrogen (BUN)	82378	Carcinoembryonic antigen (CEA)
82247	Bilirubin, total	82465	Cholesterol
87040	Blood culture	85025	Complete blood count (CBC) with
86900	Blood group		differential

continued on next page

CPT CODE	LABORATORY TESTS	CPT CODE	LABORATORY TESTS
82553	Creatine kinase (CK-MB)	84144	Progesterone
82565	Creatinine, blood	85610	Prothrombin time (PT)
82575	Creatinine clearance	84295	Sodium
80051	Electrolyte panel	84403	Testosterone, total
82670	Estradiol	84443	Thyroid-stimulating hormone (TSH)
82947	Glucose	84436	Thyroxine (T4), total
82951	Glucose tolerance test	84478	Triglycerides
85014	Hematocrit (HCT)	84481	Triiodothyronine (T3), free
83036	Hemoglobin A1c	84550	Uric acid
84702	Human chorionic gonadotropin (hCG)	81001	Urinalysis
82728	Iron, total	87086	Urine culture
84132	Potassium	85048	White blood cell (WBC) count

6.5 Medical Procedures, Drugs, and Surgical Procedures

MATCHING EXERCISE

Match each word or phrase to its description.

1. anticoagulant drug
2. autologous
3. excisional biopsy
4. phlebotomy
5. PRBCs
6. splenectomy
7. vaccination
8. vitamin B$_{12}$ drug

_____ surgical removal of a lymph node
_____ concentrated red blood cells in a small amount of plasma
_____ also known as *immunization*
_____ patient donates a unit of his or her own blood
_____ drug that prevents blood clots from forming
_____ used to treat pernicious anemia
_____ venipuncture
_____ surgery to remove a ruptured spleen

CIRCLE EXERCISE

Circle the correct answer from the choices given.

1. A bone marrow aspiration is done by taking red bone marrow from the (**blood, iliac crest of the hip bone, spleen**).
2. (**Anticoagulant, Antiretroviral, Thrombolytic**) drugs are used to break apart an already formed blood clot.
3. Donated blood must be tested for all of the following *except* (**hepatitis, HIV, immunity, syphilis**).
4. (**Anticoagulant, Corticosteroid, Protease inhibitor**) drugs are anti-inflammatory drugs used to suppress the immune response.
5. All of the following vaccinations are recommended for older adults *except* (**influenza, pneumococcal pneumonia, polio**).

TRUE OR FALSE EXERCISE

Indicate whether each statement is true or false by writing **T** *or* **F** *on the line.*

1. _____ A unit of blood divided into erythrocytes, platelets, and plasma can each be given separately as a transfusion, as needed.
2. _____ Different-colored rubber stoppers on vacuum tubes indicate the type of blood test.
3. _____ Plasmapheresis uses a centrifuge to separate the red blood cells from the white blood cells.
4. _____ A vaccine contains dead or weakened bacteria, viruses, or cell fragments.
5. _____ A thrombolytic enzyme drug prevents blood clots from forming.
6. _____ Matching for tissue type involves testing for HLA antigens.

DIVIDING WORDS EXERCISE

Separate these words into their component parts (prefix, combining form, suffix). Some words do not contain all three word parts. The first one has been done for you.

Medical Word	Prefix	Combining Form	Suffix		Medical Word	Prefix	Combining Form	Suffix
1. **aspiration**		*aspir/o-*	*-ation*		6. immunity			
2. anticoagulant					7. phlebotomy			
3. biopsy					8. splenectomy			
4. dissection					9. transplantation			
5. erythropoietin					10. vaccination			

SPELLING EXERCISE

Read each medical word pronunciation and write the medical word that it represents. Be sure to check your spelling. The first one has been done for you.

1. **(doh-NAY-shun)** *donation*
2. (trans-FYOO-shun)
3. (fleh-BAW-toh-mee)
4. (VEE-nih-PUNK-chur)

5. (VAK-sih-NAY-shun)
6. (KOR-tih-koh-STAIR-oyd)
7. (THRAWM-boh-LIT-ik)
8. (TRANS-plan-TAY-shun)

Immerse Yourself: Analyze Medical Reports

Electronic Patient Record #1

This is a laboratory report. Read the report and answer the questions.

PEARSON OUTPATIENT LABORATORY REPORT

Task   Edit   View   Time Scale   Options   Help

Test	Result	Normal Range	Technician
Complete Blood Count (CBC)			
RBC	4.7 m/mL	4.2–5.7 m/mL	JRT
Hemoglobin	14.7 g/dL	12.6–16.6 g/dL	JRT
Hematocrit	42.9%	38.0–50.0%	JRT
MCV	91.2 fL	80–100 fL	JRT
MCH	31.3 pg	28.0–33.0 pg	JRT
MCHC	34.3 g/dL	32–36 g/dL	JRT
WBC	7.7 k/mL	4.3–10.5 k/mL	JRT
Platelets	130 k/mL	150–450 k/mL	JRT

1. What is the name of the group of tests that was done on this patient? _____

2. What unit of measurement is used to report erythrocytes? _____

3. What individual test result was not within the normal range of values? _____

Electronic Patient Record #2

Read this Emergency Department Report and answer the questions.

PEARSON GENERAL HOSPITAL

Task	Edit	View	Time Scale	Options	Help

ADMISSION HISTORY AND PHYSICAL EXAMINATION

PATIENT NAME: RICE, Xavier

HOSPITAL NUMBER: 93-66805

DATE OF ADMISSION: November 19, 20xx

HISTORY OF PRESENT ILLNESS
This 40-year-old male presented to the emergency room today with complaints of dysphagia, extreme weakness, fevers, diarrhea, and weight loss.

PAST MEDICAL HISTORY
He has a prior history of intravenous heroin use for many years and was diagnosed with HIV about 6 years ago. At that time, he tested HIV positive, but was asymptomatic. His CD4 count then was 500. He was subsequently lost to follow-up until recently. In the last few months, his health has deteriorated rapidly, but he refused to seek medical attention. Last month, however, he was admitted to this hospital through the Emergency Department in respiratory distress with a CD4 count of 100 and had *Pneumocystis jiroveci* pneumonia and was diagnosed with AIDS. He was discharged on a three-drug antiretroviral drug regimen. Today he states that he has been noncompliant with his drug therapy, stating that he does not take it on a regular basis.

PHYSICAL EXAMINATION
General: Physical examination today showed a male, very thin, appearing much older than his stated age. Temperature 101.2, pulse 100, respirations 26, blood pressure 110/76. Height: 5 feet 11 inches. Weight: 108 pounds. HEENT exam: Normocephalic, atraumatic. Eyes: Sclerae and conjunctivae pale and nonicteric. Mouth: White plaque coating on the tongue and underneath is beefy red and bleeds slightly. Neck: The neck is supple. There are enlarged lymph nodes in his neck on both sides (cervical lymphadenopathy).
HEART: Regular rate and rhythm.
CHEST: Clear.
ABDOMEN: Soft, nontender, with normal bowel sounds.
EXTREMITIES: Wasting of the extremities. Extreme weakness with muscle strength decreased on both sides. The skin shows no evidence of Kaposi sarcoma.

DIAGNOSES

1. Oral candidiasis

2. Wasting syndrome, secondary to acquired immunodeficiency syndrome (AIDS)

3. Acquired immunodeficiency syndrome (AIDS)

4. Past history of *Pneumocystis jiroveci* pneumonia

PLAN
Bloodwork was sent for CBC and differential and CD4 total count. The patient was restarted on his antiretroviral three-drug regimen. He was given nystatin oral suspension 5 cc q.i.d., swish and swallow, to treat his oral candidiasis. He will be started on a drug to stimulate his appetite and help him gain weight.

Joseph K. McAdams, M.D.

Joseph K. McAdams, M.D.

JKM:ltt
D: 11/19/xx
T: 11/19/xx

1. Six years ago, the patient was "asymptomatic," which means that

   a. he did not have an HIV infection.

   b. he did not have any symptoms of an HIV infection.

   c. he was healthy.

2. What was the patient's CD4 count 6 years ago? _____

   What was the patient's CD4 count when he was diagnosed with AIDS? _____

3. What does the physical examination show about the patient's lymph nodes in his neck? _____

4. What is the probable source of the patient's HIV infection? _____

5. When the patient was admitted to the hospital last month with *Pneumocystis jiroveci* pneumonia, why was his diagnosis changed from HIV positive to AIDS? _____

6. What two different opportunistic infections has the patient had in the past and has now? _____

7. The patient's skin shows no evidence of what opportunistic infection? _____

MyLab Medical Terminology™

MyLab Medical Terminology is a premium online homework management system that includes a host of features to help you study. Registered users will find:

- A multitude of quizzes and activities built within the MyLab platform

- Powerful tools that track and analyze your results—allowing you to create a personalized learning experience

- Videos and audio pronunciations to help enrich your progress

- Streaming lesson presentations (guided lectures) and self-paced learning modules

- A space where you and your instructor can check your progress and manage your assignments

7 Orthopedics
Skeletal System

Orthopedics (OR-thoh-PEE-diks) is the medical specialty that studies the anatomy and physiology of the skeletal and muscular systems; uses laboratory, diagnostic, and radiologic procedures to diagnose skeletal and muscular diseases; and uses medical procedures, drugs, and surgical procedures to treat skeletal and muscular diseases. In this chapter, you will study orthopedics from the perspective of the skeletal system. In Chapter 8, you will study the muscular system.

Chapter Overview and Learning Outcomes

After you study this chapter, you should be able to demonstrate mastery of the outcomes by successfully completing the exercises.

7.1 Anatomy
Identify the structures of the skeletal system.
Demonstrate proficiency in medical language.
7.1 Practice Laps

7.2 Physiology
Describe the functions of the skeletal system.
Demonstrate proficiency in medical language.
7.2 Practice Laps
Vocabulary Review

7.3 Diseases
Describe common skeletal diseases.
Demonstrate proficiency in medical language.
7.3 Practice Laps

7.4 Laboratory, Diagnostic, and Radiologic Procedures
Describe common skeletal laboratory tests, diagnostic procedures, and radiologic procedures.
Demonstrate proficiency in medical language.
7.4 Practice Laps

7.5 Medical Procedures, Drugs, and Surgical Procedures
Describe common skeletal medical procedures, drugs, and surgical procedures.
Demonstrate proficiency in medical language.
7.5 Practice Laps
Abbreviations Summary
Career Focus

Chapter Review Exercises
Dive In: Medical Language Exercises (Learning Outcomes 7.1–7.5)

Immerse Yourself: Analyze Medical Reports

Medical Language Key

To unlock the definition of a medical word, first break it into word parts. Then give the meaning of each word part. Put the meanings of the word parts in order, beginning with the meaning of the suffix, then the meaning of the prefix (if there is one), then the meaning of the combining form.

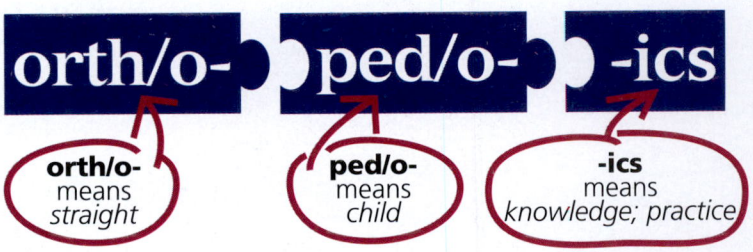

orth/o-) ped/o-) -ics

orth/o- means *straight*

ped/o- means *child*

-ics means *knowledge; practice*

Orthopedics: ▶ *Knowledge and practice (of producing) straight(ness) of the bones and muscles in a) child (or adult).*

The **skeletal system** is the body system that supports the body, and its structures include connective tissues of bones, cartilage, ligaments, and joints. The **skeleton**, the **bony** framework on which the body is built, consists of 206 bones (see Figure 7-1 ■), which can be divided into two areas: the axial skeleton and the appendicular skeleton.

The **axial skeleton** forms the central bony structure of the body around which other parts move. It consists of the bones of the head (cranium, facial bones), associated bones of the head and neck (ossicles in the middle ear, hyoid bone in the neck), the chest (sternum, ribs), and the spine (vertebrae, sacrum, coccyx). The **appendicular skeleton** consists of the limbs, including the bones of the shoulders (clavicle, scapula), upper extremities (humerus, radius, ulna, carpal bones, metacarpal bones, phalanges), the hip (ilium, ischium, pubic bone), and the lower extremities (femur, patella, tibia, fibula, tarsal bones, metatarsal bones, phalanges).

The functions of the skeletal system are to provide structural support for the body and protection for the body's soft tissues and internal organs. The bones are also a storage site for calcium and phosphorus. The skeletal system works in conjunction with the muscular system (described in Chapter 8, Orthopedics: Muscular System) to maintain body posture and produce movement, and so it is known as the **musculoskeletal system** because of the close working relationship between the bones and muscles. The skeletal system is also the site of blood cell production. All types of blood cells are produced in the red marrow within the bones of the skull, scapula, sternum, rib, vertebra, ilium, humerus, and femur (described in Chapter 6, Hematology and Immunology).

7.1 Anatomy

Bones of the Axial Skeleton

The axial skeleton consists of the bones of the head, associated bones of the head and neck, bones of the chest, and bones of the spine.

Bones of the Head
The **skull** is the bony structure of the head. It includes both the cranial bones and facial bones.

CRANIUM   The **cranium** is the dome-like bone around the top of the head. Within the cranium is the **cranial cavity**, which contains the brain and other structures (described in Chapter 9, Neurology). The cranium consists of eight bones (see Figure 7-2 ■ and Figure 7-3 ■). A **suture** is the joint where two cranial bones meet.

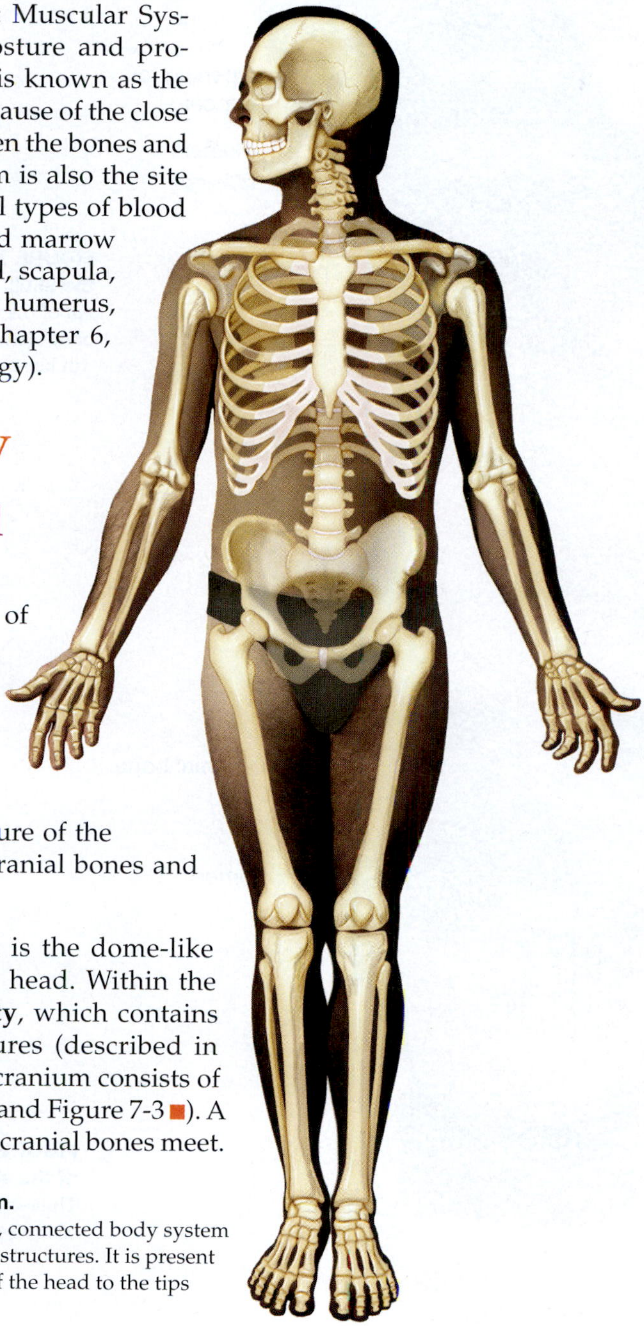

FIGURE 7-1 ■ The skeletal system.
The skeletal system is a widespread, connected body system that consists of 206 bones and other structures. It is present throughout the body from the top of the head to the tips of the fingers and toes.

Pronunciation/Word Parts

skeleton (SKEL-eh-ton)

skeletal (SKEL-eh-tal)
   skelet/o- *skeleton*
   -al *pertaining to*

bony (BOH-nee)
Osseous and *osteal* are also adjectives for *bone*. The combining forms **osse/o-**, **oss/i-**, and **oste/o-** mean *bone*.

axial (AK-see-al)
   axi/o- *axis*
   -al *pertaining to*

appendicular (AP-en-DIH-kyoo-lar)
   appendicul/o- *limb; small attached part*
   -ar *pertaining to*

musculoskeletal
(MUS-kyoo-loh-SKEL-eh-tal)
   muscul/o- *muscle*
   skelet/o- *skeleton*
   -al *pertaining to*

skull (SKUHL)

cranium (KRAY-nee-um)
   crani/o- *cranium; top part of the skull*
   -um *period of time; structure*

cranial (KRAY-nee-al)
   crani/o- *cranium; top part of the skull*
   -al *pertaining to*

cavity (KAV-ih-tee)
   cav/o- *hollow space*
   -ity *condition; state*

suture (SOO-chur)

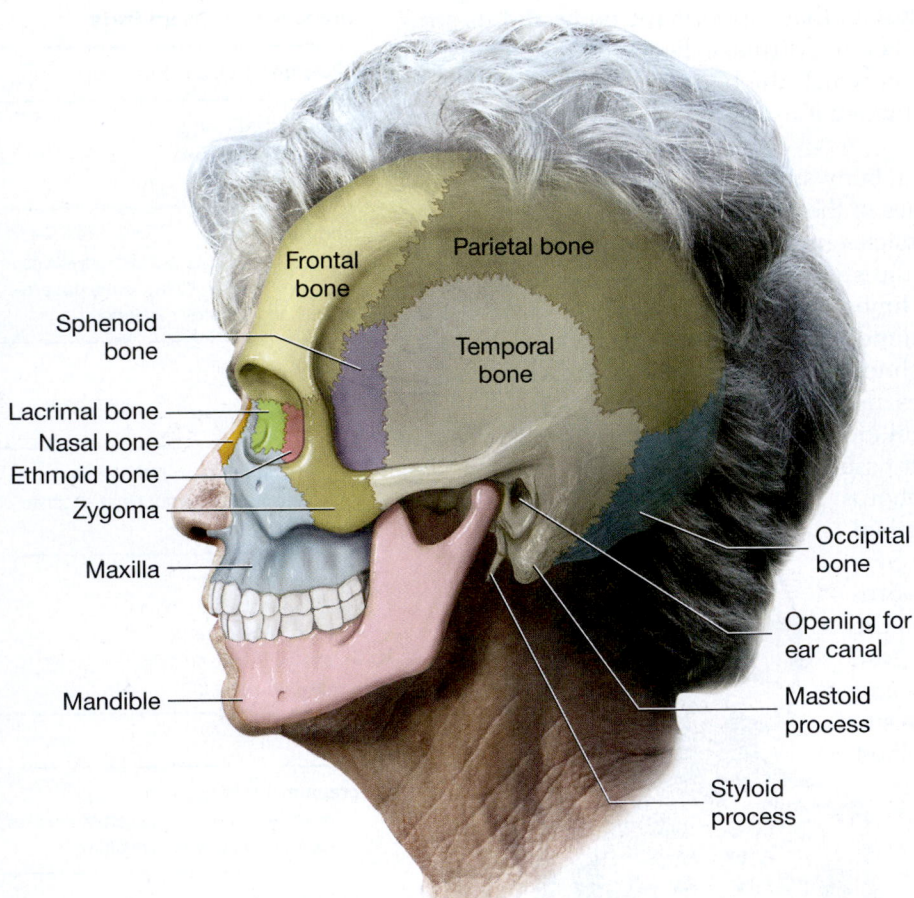

FIGURE 7-2 ■ Lateral view of the bones of the skull.
All of the cranial bones and most of the facial bones (except the vomer and palatine bones) can be seen in this lateral view.

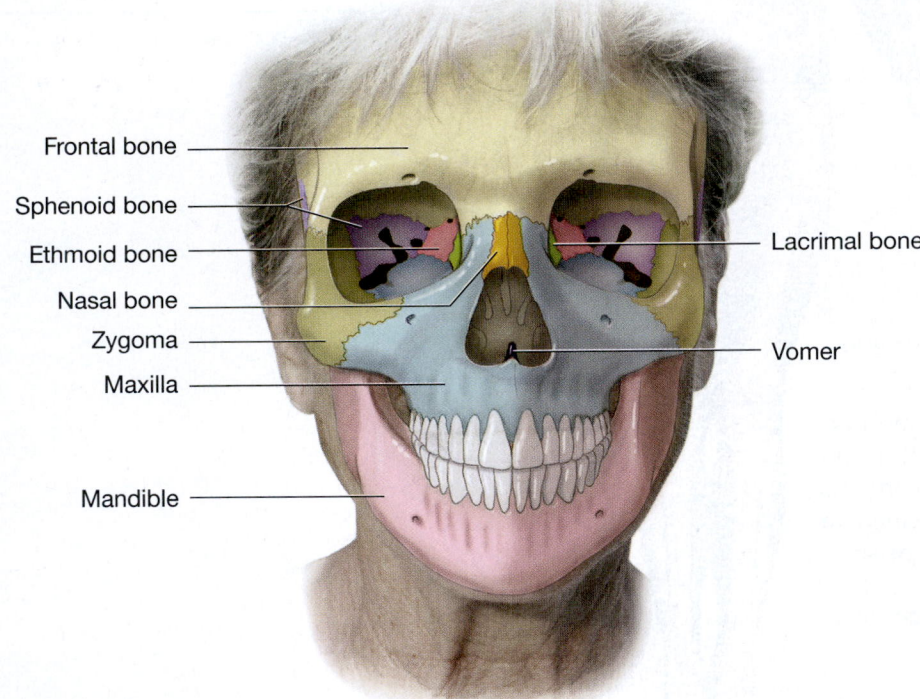

FIGURE 7-3 ■ Frontal view of the bones of the skull.
The facial bones connect to each other and to the bones of the cranium.

The **frontal bone** forms the forehead and top of the cranium, and it ends at the **coronal suture** (see Figure 7-15). The two **parietal bones** form the superior sides and posterior part of the cranium. These bones join at the **sagittal suture**, which runs from the top center to the back of the cranium. The **occipital bone** forms the posterior base of the cranium. It contains the **foramen magnum**, a large, round opening through which the spinal cord passes to join the brain. The two **temporal bones** form the inferior sides of the cranium. Bony landmarks on the temporal bone include the **mastoid process**, a bony projection just behind the ear, and the pointed **styloid process**, the site of attachment for ligaments to the hyoid bone (described later). The **sphenoid bone**, a large, irregularly shaped bone, forms part of the central base and sides of the cranium and the posterior walls of the eye sockets. A bony cup in the sphenoid bone holds the pituitary gland (described in Chapter 13, Endocrinology). The **ethmoid bone** forms the posterior nasal septum and the medial walls of the eye sockets.

FACIAL BONES The facial bones support the nose, cheeks, and lips and protect the eyes and internal structures of the nose, mouth, and upper throat. There are 14 bones in the face (see Figure 7-2 and Figure 7-3). The two **nasal bones** form the bridge of the nose and the roof of the nasal cavity. Within the nasal cavity is the nasal septum. The tip of the nose and most of the nasal septum are made of cartilage. The **vomer** is a narrow bone that forms the most inferior part of the nasal septum, and then it widens as it continues posteriorly to join the ethmoid bone. Also within the nasal cavity are the two bones of the **inferior nasal conchae** that project inwardly from the wall of the nasal cavity. (The superior and middle nasal conchae are part of the ethmoid bone, but the inferior nasal conchae are facial bones.) The two **lacrimal bones** are small, flat bones within the eye sockets, near the lacrimal (tear) glands of the eye. Each **zygoma** or **zygomatic bone** is a cheekbone on either side of the face.

Clinical Connections

Otolaryngology. In each temporal bone is a bony opening for the external auditory canal of the ear and the hollow cavity of the middle ear. The frontal bone and sphenoid bones contain hollow cavities that are sinuses. The ethmoid bones contain many small, hollow air spaces as sinuses. The maxillary bones contain hollow cavities that are sinuses. All of the nasal conchae in the nasal cavity are also known as *turbinates*.

Neonatology. In a newborn baby, the bones of the cranium have large areas of fibrous connective tissue between them. These are **fontanels** (commonly known as "soft spots" because of the difference in firmness that is felt when touching the baby's head) (see Figure 7-4 ■). Fontanels allow the cranial bones to move together as the head goes through the birth canal and move apart as the brain grows during childhood. The bony edges finally fuse together at a suture line, and the cranial bones become immobile in early adulthood.

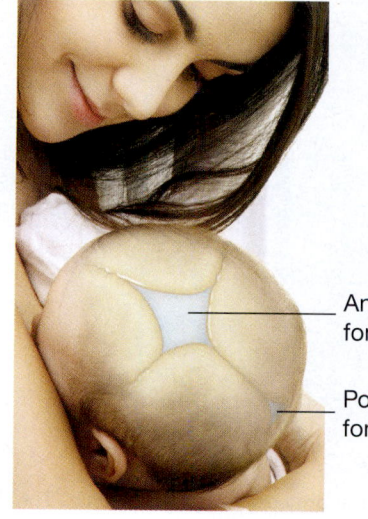

Anterior fontanel

Posterior fontanel

FIGURE 7-4 ■ Fontanel.
This fetal cranium shows a large open space (the anterior fontanel) between the two frontal bones and the two parietal bones. The translucent membrane in the fontanel is fibrous connective tissue.

Pronunciation/Word Parts

frontal (FRUN-tal)
 front/o- *front*
 -al *pertaining to*

coronal (koh-ROH-nal)
 coron/o- *structure that encircles like a crown*
 -al *pertaining to*

parietal (pah-RY-eh-tal)
 pariet/o- *wall of a cavity*
 -al *pertaining to*

sagittal (SAJ-ih-tal)
 sagitt/o- *front to back*
 -al *pertaining to*

occipital (awk-SIH-pih-tal)
 occipit/o- *back of the head; occiput*
 -al *pertaining to*

foramen magnum (foh-RAY-min MAG-num)

temporal (TEM-poh-ral)
 tempor/o- *side of the head; temple*
 -al *pertaining to*

mastoid (MAS-toyd)
 mast/o- *breast; mastoid process*
 -oid *resembling*
This rounded, downward-pointing bone was thought to resemble a female breast.

process (PRAW-sehs)

styloid (STY-loyd)
 styl/o- *stake*
 -oid *resembling*

sphenoid (SFEE-noyd)
 sphen/o- *wedge shaped*
 -oid *resembling*

ethmoid (ETH-moyd)
 ethm/o- *sieve*
 -oid *resembling*
The ethmoid bone has many small, hollow spaces like a sieve.

nasal (NAY-zal)
 nas/o- *nose*
 -al *pertaining to*

vomer (VOH-mer)

conchae (CON-kee)

lacrimal (LAK-rih-mal)
 lacrim/o- *tears*
 -al *pertaining to*

zygoma (zy-GOH-mah)

zygomatic (zy-goh-MAT-ik)
 zygomat/o- *cheekbone; zygoma*
 -ic *pertaining to*

fontanel (FAWN-tah-NEL)

The **maxilla** is the upper jaw bone that consists of two **maxillary bones** fused in the midline. It contains the roots of the upper teeth. The two **palatine bones** are small, flat bones that form the hard palate in the oral cavity. The **mandible** is the lower jaw bone. It contains the roots of the lower teeth. The mandible is the only movable bone in the skull. Each side of the mandible ends in two bony tips; one tip is under the zygoma, while the other tip forms a movable joint (the temporomandibular joint) with the temporal bone just anterior to the ear.

Associated Bones of the Head and Neck

These bones are part of the axial skeleton, but are not cranial or facial bones, as previously described.

The **ossicles** are three tiny bones in the middle ear cavity of each ear: the **malleus, incus**, and **stapes**. Collectively, these are the ossicular chain because they are arranged in a row (described in Chapter 15, Otolaryngology). These bones function in the process of hearing.

The **hyoid bone** is a flat, U-shaped bone in the anterior neck. It does not connect directly to any other bones, but its ends are attached by ligaments to the styloid process of each temporal bone. It is also the point of attachment for the tendons of several muscles in the mouth and neck.

Bones of the Chest

The chest or **thorax** is the area between the neck and the diaphragm (see Figure 7-5 ■). The rib cage makes up the bony wall of the thorax. The **sternum** or **breastbone** is a vertical bone in the center of the anterior rib cage. It consists of the triangular-shaped **manubrium**, the body of the sternum, and the inferior tip or **xiphoid process**. The clavicle (described later) and some of the ribs are attached to the sternum.

Pronunciation/Word Parts

maxilla (mak-SIL-ah)

maxillary (MAK-sih-LAIR-ee)
  maxill/o- *maxilla; upper jaw*
  -ary *pertaining to*

palatine (PAL-ah-tyne)
  palat/o- *palate*
  -ine *pertaining to*

mandible (MAN-dih-bul)

mandibular (man-DIH-byoo-lar)
  mandibul/o- *lower jaw; mandible*
  -ar *pertaining to*

ossicle (AW-sih-kul)
  oss/i- *bone*
  -cle *small thing*

malleus (MAL-ee-uhs)

incus (ING-kuhs)

stapes (STAY-peez)

hyoid (HY-oyd)
  hy/o- *U-shaped structure*
  -oid *resembling*

thorax (THOR-aks)

thoracic (thor-AS-ik)
  thorac/o- *chest; thorax*
  -ic *pertaining to*

sternum (STER-num)

sternal (STER-nal)
  stern/o- *breastbone; sternum*
  -al *pertaining to*

manubrium (mah-NOO-bree-um)

xiphoid (ZY-foyd)
  xiph/o- *sword*
  -oid *resembling*

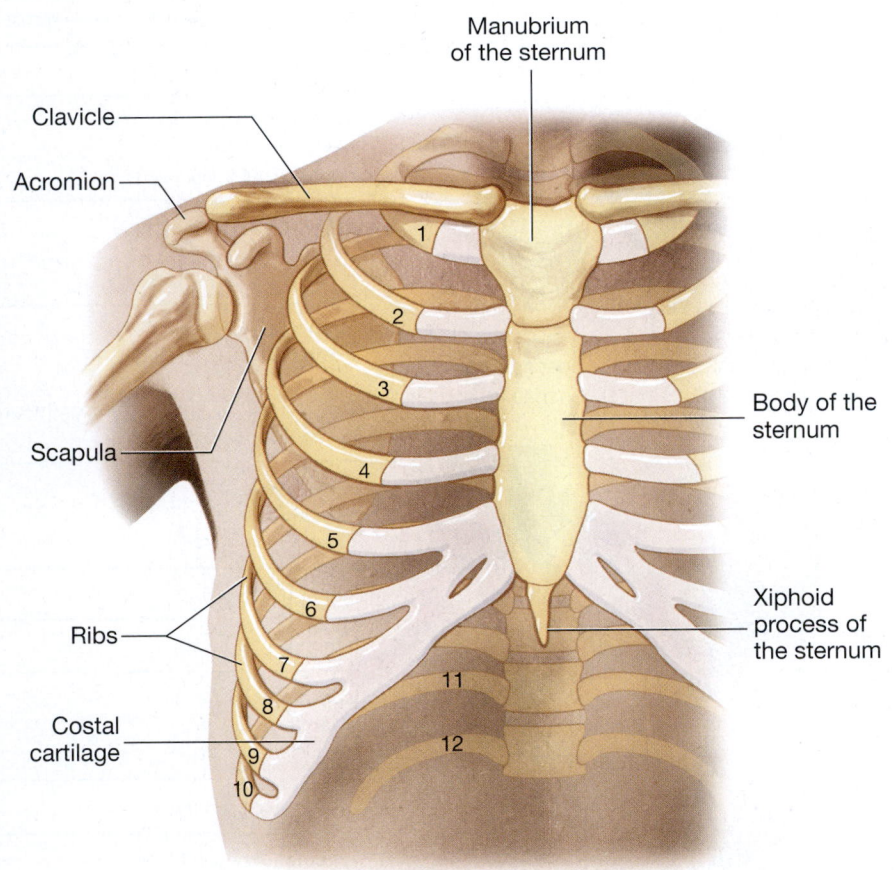

FIGURE 7-5 ■ Bones of the chest and shoulder.
The sternum and ribs form the thorax, a bony cage that protects the heart and lungs. The clavicle and scapula are part of the bones of each shoulder.

There are 12 pairs of **ribs**. Rib pairs 1–7 (true ribs) are attached posteriorly to the vertebrae of the spine and anteriorly to the sternum by **costal cartilage**. This cartilage is a firm but flexible connective tissue. The **costochondral joint** is where the cartilage meets the rib. Rib pairs 8–10 (false ribs) are attached posteriorly to the vertebrae, but are only indirectly attached to the sternum by long lengths of costal cartilage. Rib pairs 11 and 12 (floating ribs) are attached posteriorly to the vertebrae but are not attached to the sternum. The area between two ribs is the **intercostal space**.

Within the thorax is the **thoracic cavity**, which contains the heart, lungs, and other structures.

Bones of the Spine

The **spine** or **backbone**, a vertical column that consists of the bones of the **vertebrae**, is also known as the **spinal column** or **vertebral column** (see Figure 7-6 ■). The vertebral column supports the weight of the head, neck, and trunk of the body and protects the spinal cord.

The spine contains 26 bones that are divided into five regions: the cervical vertebrae, the thoracic vertebrae, the lumbar vertebrae, the sacrum, and the coccyx. The **cervical vertebrae (C1–C7)** are in the neck. The first cervical vertebra (C1, the **atlas**) is directly below the occipital bone of the cranium. Its appearance is different from the other cervical vertebrae because it must form a joint that allows the head to move up and down. The second cervical vertebra (C2, the **axis**) fits into the atlas to form a joint that allows the head to move from side to side. The **thoracic vertebrae (T1–T12)** are in the chest. Each thoracic vertebra joins with one pair of the 12 pairs of ribs. The **lumbar vertebrae (L1–L5)** are in the lower back. The lumbar vertebrae are larger than the cervical or thoracic vertebrae because they bear the weight of the head, neck, and trunk of the body. The **sacrum** is a group of five fused vertebrae that

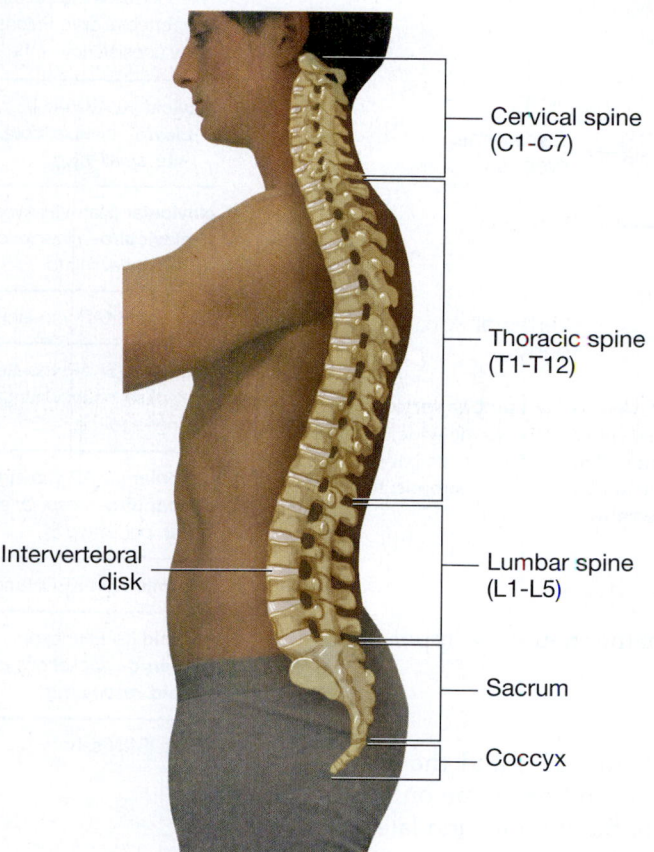

Intervertebral disk

Cervical spine (C1-C7)

Thoracic spine (T1-T12)

Lumbar spine (L1-L5)

Sacrum

Coccyx

FIGURE 7-6 ■ Bones of the spine.
The vertebral column consists of five regions: cervical vertebrae, thoracic vertebrae, lumbar vertebrae, and the sacrum and coccyx. Notice how the vertebrae become progressively larger from top to bottom as they bear more and more of the weight of the body.

Clinical Connections

Medical History. *Atlas* was the name given to the mythological Greek god who was forced to hold the world on his shoulders. In anatomy, a person's head was imagined as a round globe and so the first vertebra was named the *atlas*.

Cardiology. The sternum is used as a landmark to ensure the correct placement of the hands to perform cardiopulmonary resuscitation. The sternum and the ribs are used as landmarks to ensure the correct placement of electrode pads before an electrocardiogram (EKG) is performed.

Pulmonology. The ribs and the fifth intercostal space are used as landmarks when inserting a chest tube to treat a collapsed lung.

are not individually numbered, except for the first sacral vertebra (**S1**). The sacrum joins with the hip bones in the posterior pelvis. The **coccyx** or **tailbone** is a group of several small, fused vertebrae that are not individually numbered.

Many of the vertebrae share common features (see Figure 7-7 ■). These include a vertebral body (circular, flat area), a **spinous process** (a long, bony projection that juts out in the midline along the back), two **transverse processes** (bony projections to each side), and a vertebral **foramen** (the hole through which the spinal cord passes). Between most vertebrae are **intervertebral disks** that act as cushions to absorb impact during body movements. The outer wall of each disk is fibrocartilage, and the inside is filled with **nucleus pulposus**, a gelatinous substance.

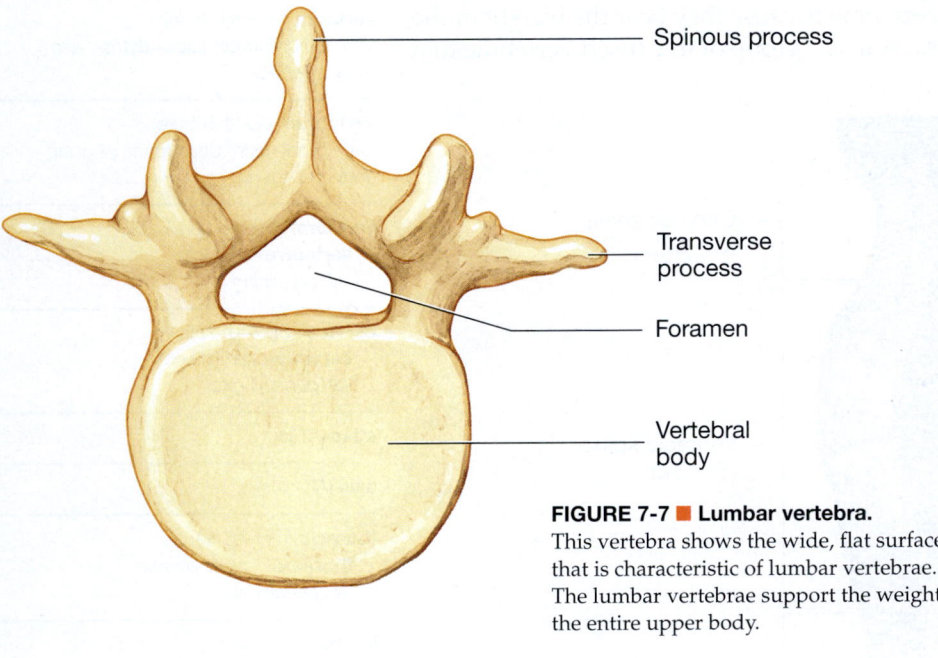

Spinous process

Transverse process

Foramen

Vertebral body

FIGURE 7-7 ■ Lumbar vertebra.
This vertebra shows the wide, flat surface that is characteristic of lumbar vertebrae. The lumbar vertebrae support the weight of the entire upper body.

Bones of the Appendicular Skeleton

The appendicular skeleton consists of the bones of the shoulders, upper extremities, hip, and lower extremities.

Bones of the Shoulders

The shoulder bones include the clavicle (see Figure 7-5) and the scapula (see Figure 7-8 ■). The **clavicle** or **collarbone** is a thin, rod-like bone on each side of the anterior neck. It connects to the manubrium of the sternum and laterally to the scapula. The **scapula** or **shoulder blade** is a triangular-shaped bone on each side of the spine in the upper back. It has a long, bony blade across its upper half that ends in a flat projection (the **acromion**) that connects to the clavicle. The **glenoid fossa**, a shallow depression, is where the head of the humerus (upper arm bone) joins the scapula to form the shoulder joint.

Pronunciation/Word Parts

sacral (SAY-kral)
  sacr/o- *sacrum*
  -al *pertaining to*

coccyx (KAWK-siks)

coccygeal (kawk-SIH-jee-al)
  coccyg/o- *coccyx; tailbone*
  -eal *pertaining to*

spinous (SPY-nuhs)
  spin/o- *backbone; spine*
  -ous *pertaining to*

process (PRAW-sehs)

transverse (trans-VERS)
  The prefix **trans-** means *across; through*, and the suffix **-verse** means *travel; turn*.

foramen (foh-RAY-min)

intervertebral (IN-ter-VER-teh-bral)
  inter- *between*
  vertebr/o- *vertebra*
  -al *pertaining to*

disk (DISK)

nucleus pulposus (NOO-klee-uhs pul-POH-sihs)
  The nucleus is the central part of an intervertebral disk. *Pulposus* refers to the pulpy consistency of the contents.

clavicle (KLAV-ih-kul)
  clav/o- *clavicle; collarbone*
  -cle *small thing*

clavicular (klah-VIH-kyoo-lar)
  clavicul/o- *clavicle; collarbone*
  -ar *pertaining to*

scapula (SKAP-yoo-lah)

scapulae (SKAP-yoo-lee)
  Latin plural noun: Change the singular ending -a to -ae.

scapular (SKAP-yoo-lar)
  scapul/o- *scapula; shoulder blade*
  -ar *pertaining to*

acromion (ah-KROH-mee-on)

glenoid (GLEH-noyd)
  glen/o- *socket of a joint*
  -oid *resembling*

fossa (FAW-sah)

Bones of the Upper Extremities

UPPER AND LOWER ARM   The arm consists of the upper arm and lower arm (forearm) (see Figure 7-9 ■). The upper arm contains the long bone of the **humerus**. The head of the humerus fits into the glenoid fossa of the scapula to form the shoulder joint. At its distal end, the humerus joins with both the radius and the ulna to form the elbow joint.

Pronunciation/Word Parts

humerus (HYOO-mer-uhs)

humeri (HYOO-mer-eye)
Latin plural noun: Change the singular ending -us to -i.

humeral (HYOO-mer-al)
   humer/o- humerus; upper arm bone
   -al pertaining to

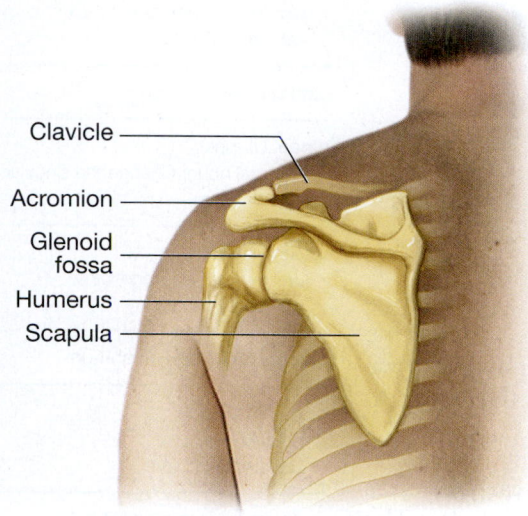

Clavicle
Acromion
Glenoid fossa
Humerus
Scapula

FIGURE 7-8 ■ Bones of the shoulder.
This posterior view shows the scapula joining the humerus (upper arm bone) at the glenoid fossa. The acromion of the scapula is connected to the clavicle. The scapula itself is not connected to the ribs or vertebral column. This allows it to move freely in several directions as the shoulder moves.

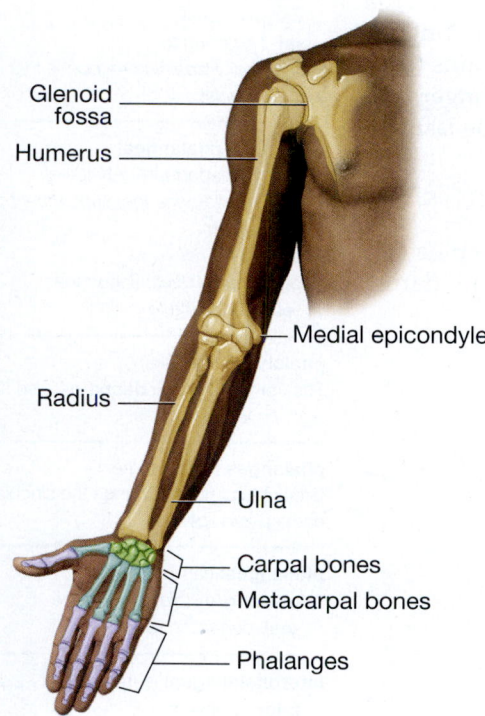

Glenoid fossa
Humerus
Medial epicondyle
Radius
Ulna
Carpal bones
Metacarpal bones
Phalanges

FIGURE 7-9 ■ Bones of the upper extremity.
The humerus of the upper arm joins with both the radius and the ulna, the bones of the forearm. The radius and ulna rotate around each other to allow the hand to turn the palm up or down. The carpal bones in the wrist are connected to the metacarpal bones in the hand. Each finger contains three phalanges; the thumb contains only two.

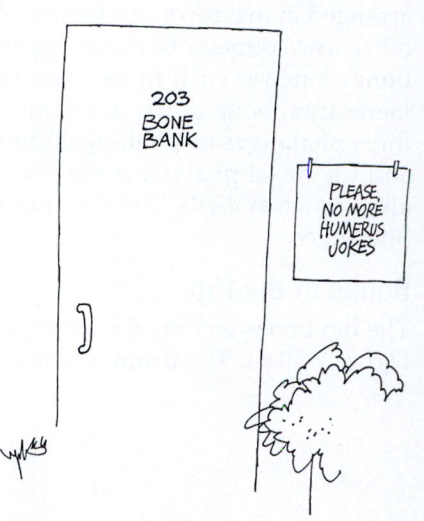

203 BONE BANK

PLEASE, NO MORE HUMERUS JOKES

Dive Deeper

The "funny bone" is not a bone at all. The ulnar nerve travels across a rounded, bony projection (medial epicondyle) on the distal humerus. When you accidentally bump this area, you hit the ulnar nerve, and this sends a shock wave (that is in no way "funny") through your entire upper extremity.

Word Alert
Sound-Alike Words

humerus	(noun)	bone of the upper arm
		Example: The patient sustained a fracture of the humerus.
humorous	(adjective)	English word meaning *funny*
		Example: It is not very humorous when you fracture a bone.
humeral	(adjective)	pertaining to the humerus of the upper arm
		Example: The x-ray showed a humeral fracture.
humoral	(adjective)	pertaining to immunity to infection that comes from antibodies in the blood
		Example: Humoral immunity occurs when B cell lymphocytes attack pathogens.

The lower arm or forearm contains the bones of the radius and ulna. The **radius** is on the thumb side of the forearm. At its distal end, it connects to the bones of the wrist. The **ulna** is on the little finger side of the forearm. At the proximal end of the ulna is the **olecranon**, a large, square projection that forms the point of the elbow. At its distal end, the ulna connects to the bones of the wrist.

WRIST, HAND, AND FINGERS   The wrist contains eight small **carpal bones** arranged in two rows (see Figure 7-9). One row connects to the radius and ulna. The other row connects to the bones of the hand. Each hand contains five **metacarpal bones**, one for each finger. The **metacarpophalangeal (MCP)** joint is between a metacarpal bone of the hand and a **phalanx** or finger bone. Each finger contains three **phalanges** or **phalangeal bones** (except for the thumb, which contains two), and the distal phalanx is the final bone at the end of each finger. The fingers are also known as *digits*. The **distal interphalangeal (DIP)** joint is between the last two phalanges.

Bones of the Hip

The hip bones include the ilium, ischium, and pubis on each side of the spine (see Figure 7-10 ■). The **ilium**, the most superior of the hip bones, has a broad, flaring

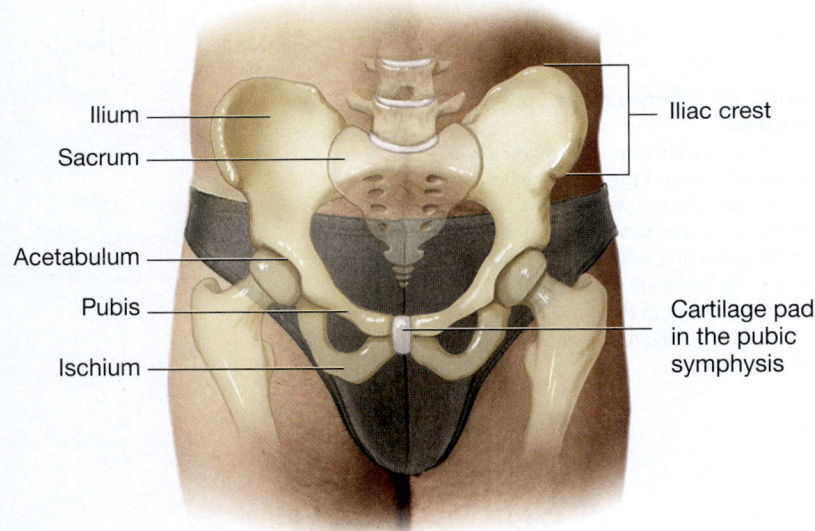

Ilium
Sacrum
Acetabulum
Pubis
Ischium

Iliac crest

Cartilage pad in the pubic symphysis

FIGURE 7-10 ■ **Bones of the hip.**
The ilium, ischium, and pubis on each side of the hip flow into each other without visible sutures or joints. However, the main part of each bone can be identified by its bony landmarks.

---

radius (RAY-dee-uhs)

radii (RAY-dee-eye)
Latin plural noun: Change the singular ending -*us* to -*i*.

radial (RAY-dee-al)
 radi/o- *forearm bone; radius; x-rays*
 -al *pertaining to*

ulna (UL-nah)

ulnae (UL-nee)
Latin plural noun: Change the singular ending -*a* to -*ae*.

ulnar (UL-nar)
 uln/o- *forearm bone; ulna*
 -ar *pertaining to*

olecranon (oh-LEH-krah-non)

carpal (KAR-pal)
 carp/o- *wrist*
 -al *pertaining to*

metacarpal (MET-ah-KAR-pal)
 meta- *after; change; subsequent to; transition*
 carp/o- *wrist*
 -al *pertaining to*
Metacarpal: *Pertaining to (bones that are) after (the) wrist*

metacarpophalangeal
(MEH-tah-KAR-poh-fah-LAN-jee-al)
 meta- *after; change; subsequent to; transition*
 carp/o- *wrist*
 phalang/o- *digit; finger; toe*
 -eal *pertaining to*

phalanx (FAY-langks)
The combining form **dactyl/o-** also means *digit; finger; toe.*

phalanges (fah-LAN-jeez)
Greek plural noun: Change the singular ending -*x* to -*ges*.

phalangeal (fah-LAN-jee-al)
 phalang/o- *digit; finger; toe*
 -eal *pertaining to*

interphalanageal (IN-ter-fah-LAN-jee-al)
 inter- *between*
 phalang/o- *digit; finger; toe*
 -eal *pertaining to*

ilium (IL-ee-um)
There are two ilia, but the plural form is seldom used.

rim known as the **iliac crest**. Posteriorly, each ilium joins the sacrum of the spine. The **ischium** is the most inferior of the hip bones. Each ischium is one of the "seat bones" that you sit on. The **pubis** or **pubic bone**, a small bridge-like bone, is the most anterior hip bone. Its two halves meet in the midline, where they form the **pubic symphysis**, a nearly immobile joint that has a cartilage pad between the bone ends. Parts of the ilium, ischium, and pubis join together to form the **acetabulum**, the cup-shaped, deep socket of the hip joint. The **pelvis** collectively includes the hip bones as well as the sacrum and coccyx of the spine.

Word Alert
Sound-Alike Words

ilium   (noun)   superior flaring part of the hip bone

Example: During the car accident, she sustained a hip fracture that involved the ilium.

ileum   (noun)   third part of the small intestine

Example: Inflammation in the ileum can also extend to other parts of the small bowel.

ileus   (noun)   abnormal absence of contractions in the small intestine

Example: A postoperative ileus can occur after abdominal surgery.

Bones of the Lower Extremities

UPPER AND LOWER LEG   The leg consists of the upper leg (thigh) and lower leg (see Figure 7-11 ■). The upper leg contains the long, weight-bearing bone of the **femur** or **thigh bone**. The head of the femur fits into the acetabulum to form the hip joint.

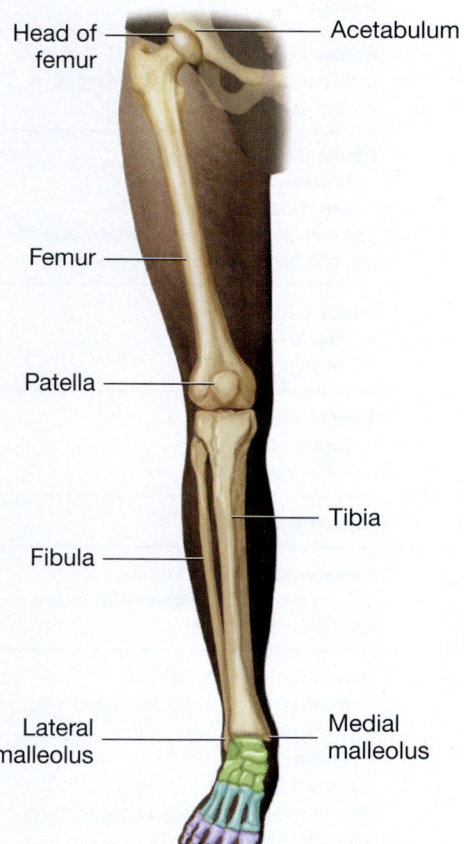

Head of femur
Acetabulum
Femur
Patella
Tibia
Fibula
Lateral malleolus
Medial malleolus

FIGURE 7-11 ■ Bones of the lower extremity. The femur of the upper leg joins the tibia of the lower leg to support the weight of the body. The fibula, the smaller of the two bones in the lower leg, is on the little toe side. The patella is a small, round bone that protects the anterior knee joint.

Pronunciation/Word Parts

iliac (IL-ee-ak)
   ili/o- *ilium*
   -ac *pertaining to*

ischium (IS-kee-um)
There are two ischia, but the plural form is seldom used.

ischial (IS-kee-al)
   ischi/o- *ischium*
   -al *pertaining to*

pubis (PYOO-bihs)

pubic (PYOO-bik)
   pub/o- *hip bone; pubis*
   -ic *pertaining to*

symphysis (SIM-fih-sihs)
The prefix **sym-** means *together; with*, and the suffix **-physis** means *state of growing*.

acetabulum (AS-eh-TAB-yoo-lum)

acetabular (AS-eh-TAB-yoo-lar)
   acetabul/o- *socket of the hip joint*
   -ar *pertaining to*

pelvis (PEL-vihs)

pelvic (PEL-vik)
   pelv/o- *hip bone; pelvis; renal pelvis*
   -ic *pertaining to*

femur (FEE-mur)

femora (FEM-oh-rah)
Femur is a Latin singular noun. The plural form is *femora*.

femoral (FEM-oh-ral)
   femor/o- *femur; thigh bone*
   -al *pertaining to*

The **patella** or **kneecap** is a thick, round bone anterior to the knee joint. It is most prominent in thin people and when the knee is partially bent.

The lower leg contains the bones of the tibia and fibula. The **tibia** or **shin bone** is the long, weight-bearing bone on the medial (great toe) side of the lower leg. At its distal end, it has a bony prominence known as the **medial malleolus**. The **fibula** is the thin bone on the lateral (little toe) side of the lower leg. Its proximal end connects to the tibia, not to the femur, and so it is not a weight-bearing bone. Its distal end has a bony prominence known as the **lateral malleolus**. The medial and lateral malleoli are often mistakenly called the *ankle bones*.

ANKLE, FOOT, AND TOES Each ankle contains seven **tarsal bones** (see Figure 7-12 ■). The first tarsal bone is the **talus**, and the largest tarsal bone is the **calcaneus** or **heel bone**. The midfoot contains five **metatarsal bones**, one for each toe. The instep or arch of the foot contains both tarsal bones and metatarsal bones. Each toe or digit contains three phalangeal bones or phalanges (except for the great toe, which contains two). The distal phalanx is at the very tip of the toe. The toes are also known as *digits*. The great toe is the **hallux**.

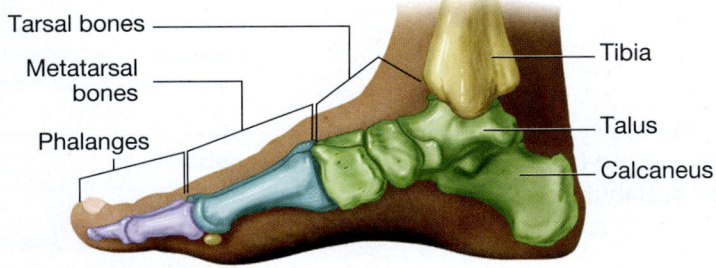

Tarsal bones
Metatarsal bones
Phalanges
Tibia
Talus
Calcaneus

FIGURE 7-12 ■ Bones of the ankle and foot.
The tarsal bones in the ankle are connected to the metatarsal bones in the midfoot. Each toe contains three phalanges; the great toe or hallux contains only two. In all, each foot contains 26 bones and 150 ligaments.

Clinical Connections

Medical Illustration. Andreas Vesalius (1514–1564) was born in Belgium and was educated in medical universities in France and Italy. At that time, medical textbooks contained almost no illustrations. He studied and illustrated a human skeleton by removing a dead body after a public hanging and dissecting it. His masterpiece, *De Humani Corporis Fabrica (The Structure of the Human Body)*, was published in 1543. Its illustrations showed dissected bodies in natural poses with scenery in the background. These beautiful, highly detailed, anatomically correct, and occasionally whimsical illustrations educated many generations of physicians (see Figure 7-13 ■). Today, a medical illustrator is a professional artist who has extensive training in anatomy, physiology, and the sciences in order to communicate complex technical and scientific information in visual images.

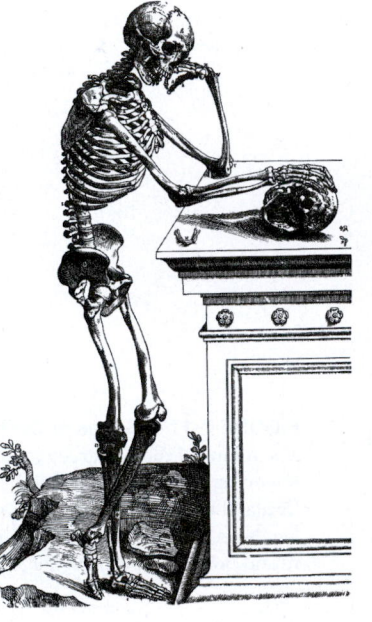

FIGURE 7-13 ■ The skeleton.

Pronunciation/Word Parts

patella (pah-TEL-ah)

patellae (pah-TEL-ee)
Latin plural noun: Change the singular ending -a to -ae.

patellar (pah-TEL-ar)
  patell/o- kneecap; patella
  -ar pertaining to

tibia (TIB-ee-ah)

tibiae (TIB-ee-ee)
Latin plural noun: Change the singular ending -a to -ae.

tibial (TIB-ee-al)
  tibi/o- shin bone; tibia
  -al pertaining to

medial (MEE-dee-al)
  medi/o- middle
  -al pertaining to

malleolus (mah-LEE-oh-luhs)

malleoli (mah-LEE-oh-lie)
Latin plural noun: Change the singular ending -us to -i.

malleolar (mah-LEE-oh-lar)
  malleol/o- malleolus
  -ar pertaining to

fibula (FIH-byoo-lah)

fibulae (FIH-byoo-lee)
Latin plural noun: Change the singular ending -a to -ae.

fibular (FIH-byoo-lar)
  fibul/o- fibula
  -ar pertaining to
The combining form **perone/o-** means *fibula*, and *peroneal* is an adjective for *fibula*.

lateral (LAT-er-al)
  later/o- side
  -al pertaining to

tarsal (TAR-sal)
  tars/o- ankle
  -al pertaining to

talus (TAY-luhs)

calcaneus (kal-KAY-nee-uhs)
The combining form **calcane/o-** means *calcaneus; heel bone*.

metatarsal (MET-ah-TAR-sal)
  meta- after; change; subsequent to; transition
  tars/o- ankle
  -al pertaining to
Metatarsal: *Pertaining to (bones that are) after (the) ankle*

hallux (HAL-uks)

The Structure of Bone

Bone or **osseous tissue** is a type of connective tissue. The surface of a bone is covered with **periosteum**, a thick, fibrous membrane (see Figure 7-14 ■). A long bone such as the humerus or femur has a straight shaft or **diaphysis**. Inside the shaft is a layer of dense compact **cortical bone** for weight bearing and an inner **medullary cavity** filled with yellow bone marrow that contains fatty tissue. A long bone has two widened ends—the proximal **epiphysis** and the distal epiphysis. It is at the **epiphyseal plates** that bone growth takes place. Each epiphysis contains **cancellous bone** or *spongy bone*, which is less dense than compact bone, and the spaces in it are filled with red bone marrow. There are small foramina (openings) in the bones where the blood vessels go through to the bone marrow.

Clinical Connections

Hematology and Immunology. Red bone marrow produces stem cells that eventually become mature blood cells and enter the blood. Red bone marrow is found in the ends of the long bones and in the skull, clavicles, sternum, ribs, vertebrae, and hip bones.

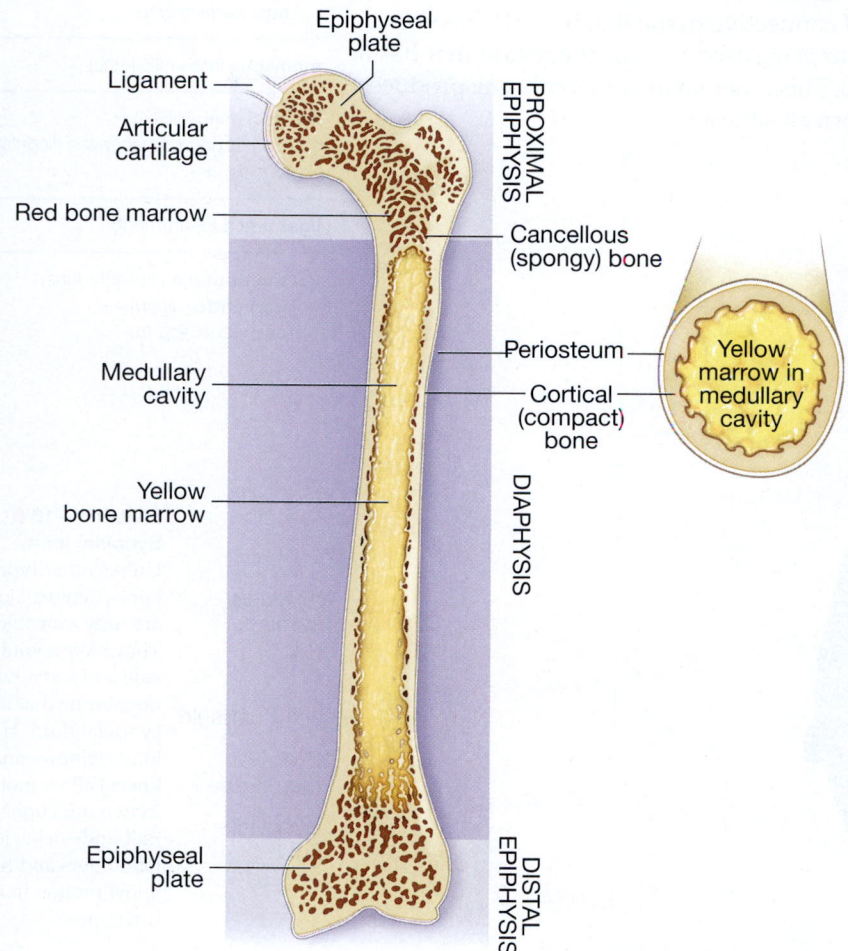

FIGURE 7-14 ■ Structure of a bone.
A long bone has a diaphysis (shaft) and epiphyses (ends). The internal structure has dense cortical bone for weight bearing, a medullary cavity that contains yellow marrow, and bone ends of cancellous bone filled with red bone marrow that produces blood cells.

Pronunciation/Word Parts

osseous (AW-see-uhs)
  osse/o- *bone*
  -ous *pertaining to*

periosteum (PAIR-ee-AW-stee-um)

periosteal (PAIR-ee-AW-stee-al)
  peri- *around*
  oste/o- *bone*
  -al *pertaining to*

diaphysis (dy-AF-ih-sihs)

diaphyseal (DY-ah-FIZ-ee-al)
  diaphys/o- *shaft of a bone*
  -eal *pertaining to*

cortical (KOR-tih-kal)
  cortic/o- *cortex; outer region*
  -al *pertaining to*

medullary (MEH-dyoo-LAIR-ee)
  medull/o- *inner region; medulla*
  -ary *pertaining to*

cavity (KAV-ih-tee)
  cav/o- *hollow space*
  -ity *condition; state*

epiphysis (eh-PIF-ih-sihs)

epiphyses (eh-PIF-ih-seez)
Greek plural noun: Change the singular ending *-is* to *-es*.

epiphyseal (EP-ih-FIZ-ee-al)
  epiphys/o- *enlarged end of long bone*
  -eal *pertaining to*

cancellous (kan-SEL-uhs)
  cancell/o- *lattice structure*
  -ous *pertaining to*

Joints, Cartilage, and Ligaments

A **joint** or **articulation** is where two bones come together, whether those bones move or not. There are three types of joints: suture, symphysis, and synovial.

1. A **suture joint** between two bones is immovable and contains no cartilage (see Figure 7-15 ■). The cranial bones and most of the facial bones have suture joints.

2. A **symphysis joint** is a slightly movable joint with a cartilage pad or disk between the bones (see Figure 7-6 and Figure 7-11). The pubis symphysis and the joints between the vertebrae are symphysis joints.

3. A **synovial joint** is a fully movable joint that joins two bones whose ends are covered with **articular** cartilage (see Figure 7-16 ■). There are two kinds of synovial joints.

   • hinge joints (elbow and knee) allow motion in two directions

   • ball-and-socket joints (shoulder and hip) allow motion in many directions

   The temporomandibular joint of the jaw is a combination of a hinge joint and a ball-and-socket joint.

Cartilage in the joints is composed of collagen fibers that are densely packed together. Articular cartilage covers the bone ends in a synovial joint. A **meniscus** is a crescent-shaped cartilage pad found in some synovial joints, such as the knee. It cushions the joint and protects the bone ends from wear and tear. There are no blood vessels in cartilage, and so damaged cartilage in a joint does not heal easily.

Ligaments are strong fibrous bands of connective tissue that hold the two bones together in a synovial joint. The entire joint is encased in a **joint capsule** that has a fibrous outer layer and an inner membrane. This inner **synovial membrane** produces **synovial fluid**, a clear, thick fluid that lubricates the joint.

Pronunciation/Word Parts

joint (JOYNT)

articulation (ar-TIH-kyoo-LAY-shun)
  articul/o- *joint*
  -ation *being; having; process*
The combining form **arthr/o-** also means *joint*.

suture (SOO-chur)

symphysis (SIM-fih-sihs)

synovial (sih-NOH-vee-al)
  synovi/o- *joint membrane; synovium*
  -al *pertaining to*
The combining form **synov/o-** also means *joint membrane; synovium.*

articular (ar-TIH-kyoo-lar)
  articul/o- *joint*
  -ar *pertaining to*

cartilage (KAR-tih-lij)

cartilaginous (KAR-tih-LAJ-ih-nuhs)
  cartilagin/o- *cartilage*
  -ous *pertaining to*

meniscus (meh-NIS-kuhs)

menisci (meh-NIS-ki)
Latin plural noun: Change the singular ending *-us* to *-i.*

ligament (LIG-ah-ment)

ligamentous (LIG-ah-MEN-tuhs)
  ligament/o- *ligament*
  -ous *pertaining to*

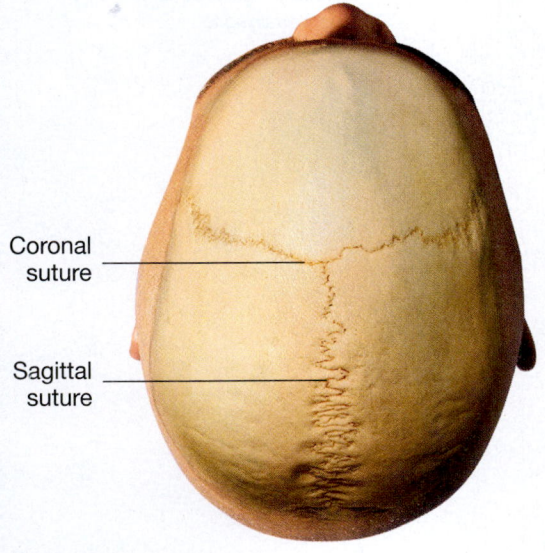

FIGURE 7-15 ■ Suture joint.
In an adult, the coronal suture is an immovable joint that joins the frontal and parietal bones. The sagittal suture joins the two parietal bones on either side of the posterior cranium. A suture is not a straight line because the two bones grow together more quickly in some areas than others.

Coronal suture

Sagittal suture

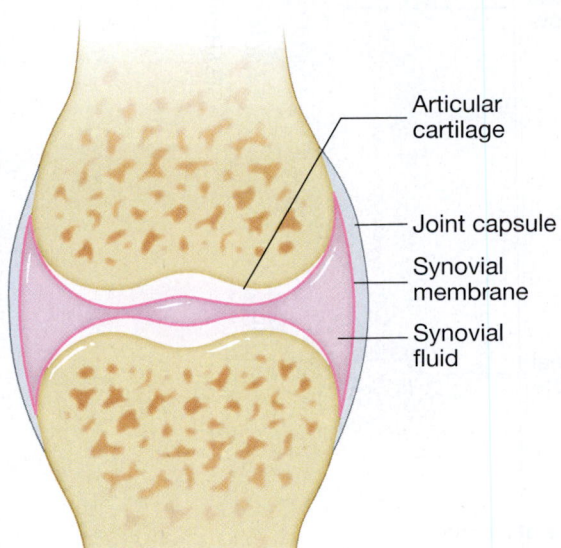

Articular cartilage

Joint capsule

Synovial membrane

Synovial fluid

FIGURE 7-16 ■
Synovial joint.
Unlike other types of joints, synovial joints are fully movable. They have a joint capsule and a synovial membrane that makes synovial fluid. Hinge joints (elbows and knees) allow motion in two directions. Ball-and-socket joints (shoulders and hips) allow motion in many directions.

7.1 PRACTICE LAPS

Use the Answer Key at the end of the book to check your answers.

A. Label Structures

Write each anatomy word or phrase in the correct numbered box. Be sure to check your spelling.

coronal suture	lacrimal bone	nasal bone	sphenoid bone
ethmoid bone	mandible	occipital bone	temporal bone
frontal bone	maxilla	parietal bone	zygoma

1.

2.

3.

4.

5.

6.

7.

8.

9.

10.

11.

12.

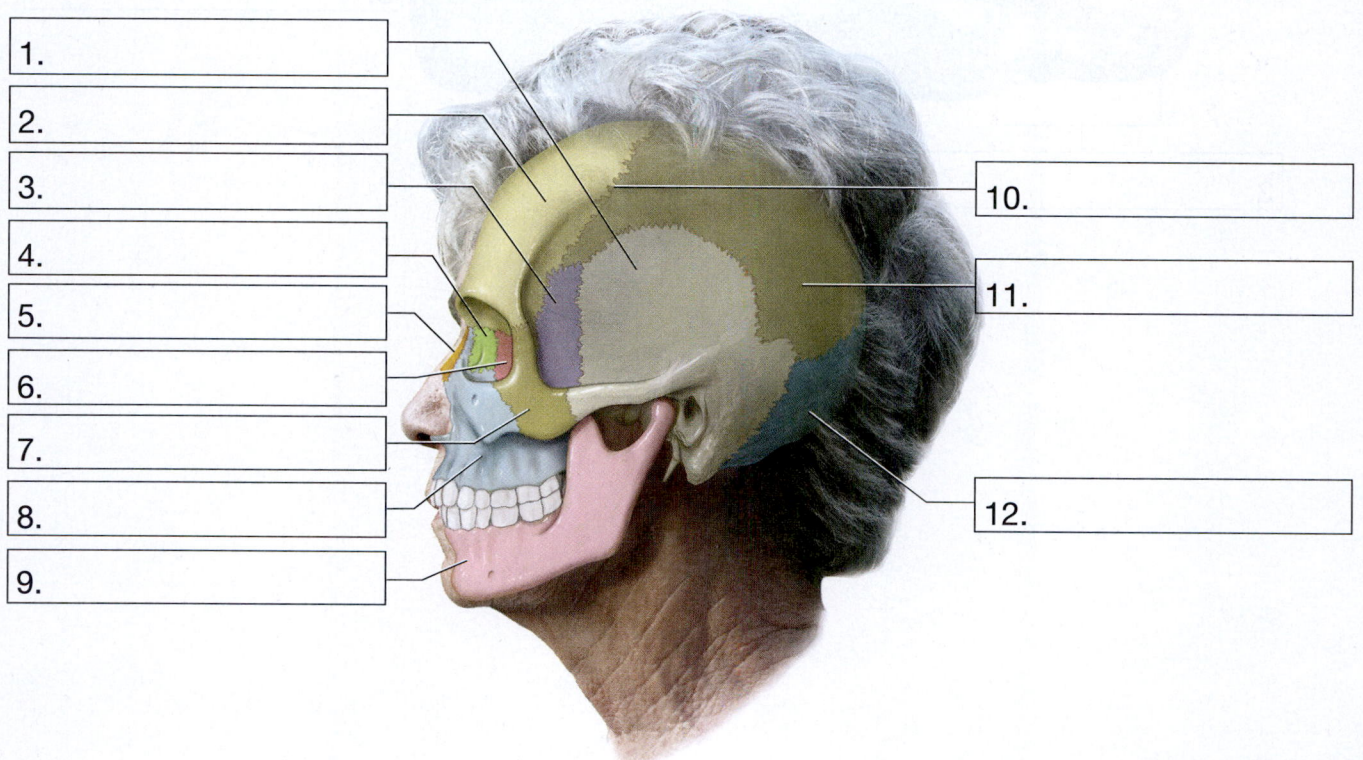

continued on next page

calcaneus   metatarsal bones   phalanges   talus   tarsal bones   tibia

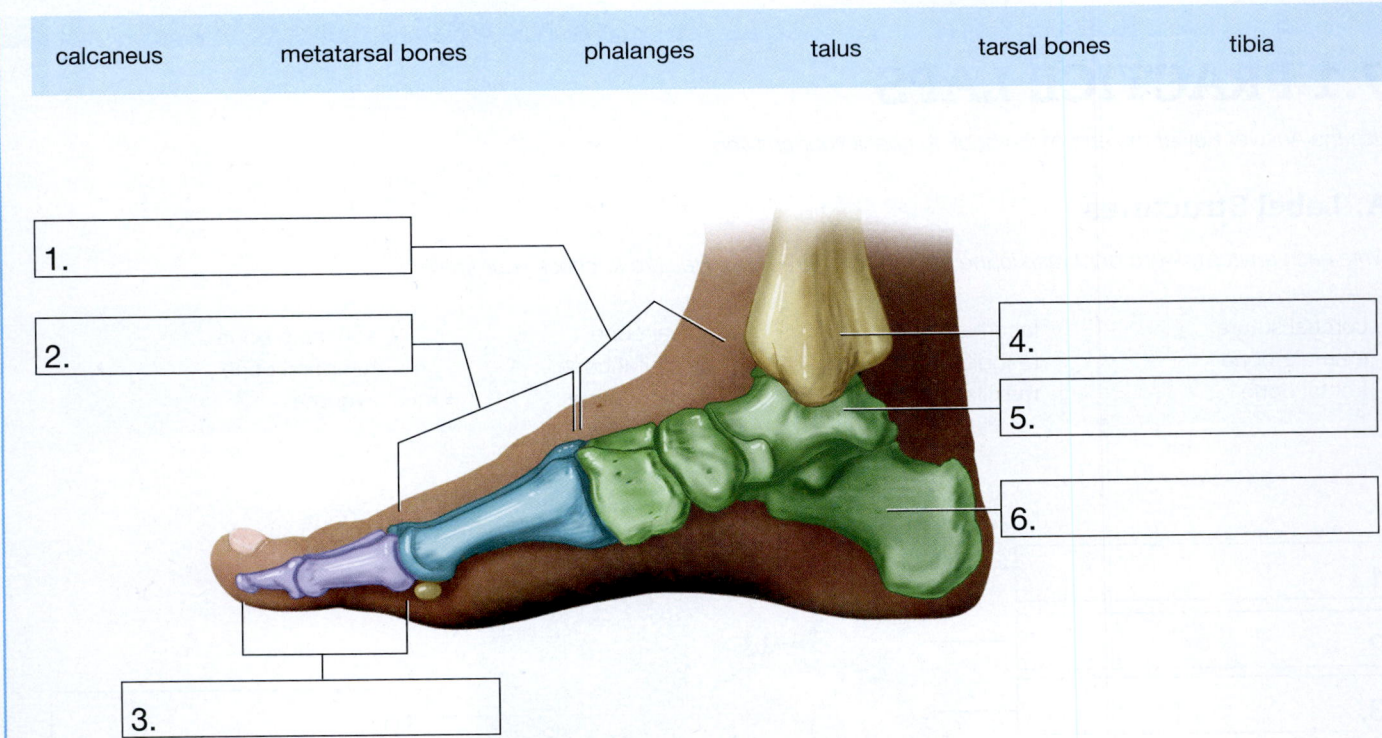

1.

2.

3.

4.

5.

6.

carpal bones	glenoid fossa	patella	sternum
clavicle	humerus	phalanges	tibia
coccyx	ilium	pubic bone	ulna
costal cartilage	ischium	radius	vertebra
femur	manubrium	rib	xiphoid process
fibula	metacarpal bones	sacrum	

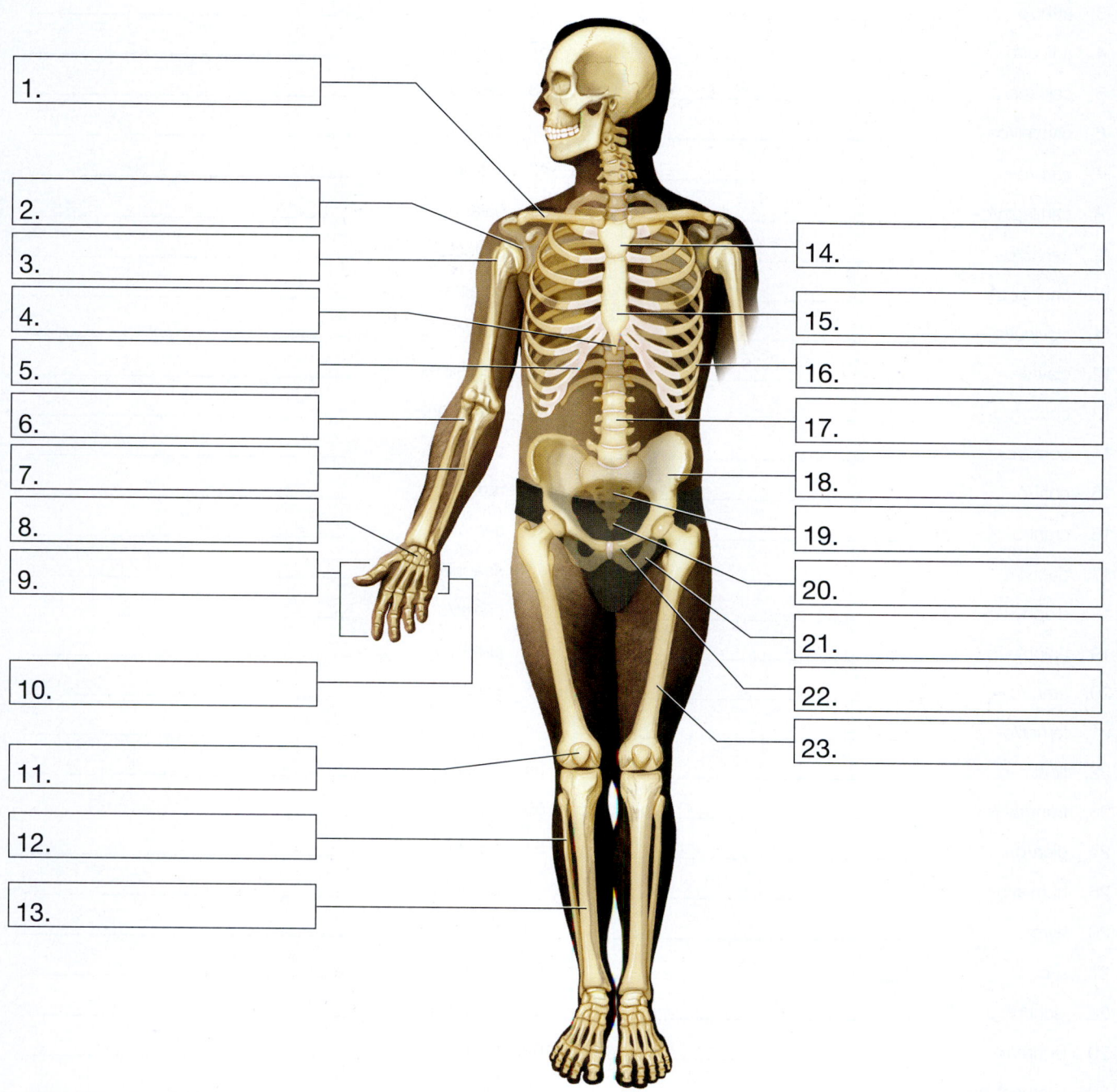

1.

2.

3.

4.

5.

6.

7.

8.

9.

10.

11.

12.

13.

14.

15.

16.

17.

18.

19.

20.

21.

22.

23.

continued on next page

B. Give the Meaning of Combining Forms

Next to each combining form, write its meaning. The first one has been done for you.

Combining Form	Meaning	Combining Form	Meaning
1. **acetabul/o-**	*socket of the hip joint*	34. maxill/o-	
2. appendicul/o-		35. medull/o-	
3. arthr/o-		36. nas/o-	
4. articul/o-		37. occipit/o-	
5. calcane/o-		38. osse/o-	
6. cancell/o-		39. oss/i-	
7. carp/o-		40. oste/o-	
8. cartilagin/o-		41. palat/o-	
9. cervic/o-		42. pariet/o-	
10. chondr/o-		43. patell/o-	
11. clavicul/o-		44. pelv/o-	
12. clav/o-		45. perone/o-	
13. coccyg/o-		46. phalang/o-	
14. coron/o-		47. pub/o-	
15. cost/o-		48. radi/o-	
16. crani/o-		49. sacr/o-	
17. dactyl/o-		50. scapul/o-	
18. diaphys/o-		51. skelet/o-	
19. epiphys/o-		52. sphen/o-	
20. ethm/o-		53. spin/o-	
21. femor/o-		54. spondyl/o-	
22. fibul/o-		55. stern/o-	
23. front/o-		56. styl/o-	
24. glen/o-		57. synovi/o-	
25. humer/o-		58. synov/o-	
26. hy/o-		59. tars/o-	
27. ili/o-		60. tempor/o-	
28. ischi/o-		61. thorac/o-	
29. lacrim/o-		62. tibi/o-	
30. ligament/o-		63. uln/o-	
31. lumb/o-		64. vertebr/o-	
32. mandibul/o-		65. xiph/o-	
33. mast/o-		66. zygomat/o-	

C. Build Words

Read the definition of the medical word. Look at the combining form that is given. Select the correct suffix from the Suffix List, and write it on the blank line. Then build the medical word, and write it on the line. (Remember: You may need to remove the combining vowel. Always remove the hyphens and slash.) Be sure to check your spelling.

Suffix List

-al (pertaining to)	-ation (being; having; process)	-ine (pertaining to)
-ar (pertaining to)	-eal (pertaining to)	-oid (resembling)
-ary (pertaining to)	-ic (pertaining to)	-ous (pertaining to)

Definition of the Medical Word	Combining Form	Suffix	Build the Medical Word
Example: Pertaining to (the) cranium	**crani/o-**	*-al*	*cranial*

[*You think* pertaining to (-al) + cranium (crani/o-). *You change the order of the word parts to put the suffix last. You write* cranial.]

Definition of the Medical Word	Combining Form	Suffix	Build the Medical Word
1. Pertaining to (the) thorax	thorac/o-		
2. Pertaining to (the) rib	cost/o-		
3. Pertaining to (the) mandible	mandibul/o-		
4. Pertaining to (a) ligament	ligament/o-		
5. Pertaining to (the) pelvis	pelv/o-		
6. Pertaining to (a) finger (or) toe	phalang/o-		
7. Pertaining to bone	osse/o-		
8. Being (or) having (a) joint	articul/o-		
9. Pertaining to (the) vertebra	vertebr/o-		
10. Pertaining to (the) lower back	lumb/o-		
11. Pertaining to (the) ulna	uln/o-		
12. Pertaining to (the) fibula	fibul/o-		
13. (A bone) resembling (a) sieve	ethm/o-		
14. Pertaining to (the) sternum	stern/o-		
15. Pertaining to (the) neck	cervic/o-		
16. Pertaining to (the) clavicle	clavicul/o-		
17. Pertaining to (the) humerus	humer/o-		
18. Pertaining to (the) pubis	pub/o-		
19. Pertaining to (the) wrist	carp/o-		
20. Pertaining to (the) kneecap	patell/o-		
21. Pertaining to (the) coccyx	coccyg/o-		
22. Pertaining to (the) upper jaw	maxill/o-		
23. Pertaining to (the) palate	palat/o-		
24. (A bone) resembling (a) stake	styl/o-		
25. Pertaining to (the) shaft of a bone	diaphys/o-		

continued on next page

Definition of the Medical Word	Combining Form	Suffix	Build the Medical Word
26. Pertaining to (the) tibia	tibi/o-	_____	_____
27. (A bone) resembling (a) sword	xiph/o-	_____	_____
28. Pertaining to (the) inner region (of a bone)	medull/o-	_____	_____
29. Resembling (a) U-shaped structure	hy/o-	_____	_____

C. Define Abbreviations

1. C1–C7 _____

2. DIP _____

3. L1–L5 _____

4. MCP _____

5. S1 _____

6. T1–T12 _____

7.2 Physiology

Osteocytes are bone cells that are located in small spaces within the bone. These cells do not divide or move, and so nearby blood vessels bring nutrients to these cells and remove the waste products of cellular metabolism. The function of osteocytes is to maintain and monitor the mineral content (calcium, phosphorus) of the bone. Bone is composed of several types of calcium salts, which are hard and form a bony matrix, as well as collagen fibers, which are flexible. Almost all of the body's calcium is stored in the bones, but it can be released to help maintain a normal blood level of calcium that is needed for contractions of the heart and skeletal muscles. Calcium in the blood also comes from foods. In addition, calcium is released into the blood when areas of damaged bone are broken down (described in the next section).

Although mature bone is a hard substance, it is also a living tissue that undergoes change. About 10 percent of the entire skeleton is broken down and rebuilt each year. This process occurs in areas of the bone that are damaged or have been subjected to mechanical stress and need to be rebuilt. **Osteoclasts**, large cells that have 50 or more nuclei, secrete acid and enzymes that break down and dissolve areas of damaged bone. In order to rebuild those areas, immature stem cells located in the periosteum and in medullary cavities within the bone become osteoblasts. **Osteoblasts** build a protein matrix (framework) and cause calcium salts to be deposited there, forming new bone tissue. This process is called **osteogenesis**. As the new bone forms around an osteoblast, it changes to become an osteocyte within the new, permanent bone.

Pronunciation/Word Parts

osteocyte (AW-stee-oh-SITE)
 oste/o- *bone*
 -cyte *cell*

osteoclast (AW-stee-oh-KLAST)
 oste/o- *bone*
 -clast *cell that breaks down*

osteoblast (AW-stee-oh-BLAST)
 oste/o- *bone*
 -blast *cell that builds; immature cell*

osteogenesis (AW-stee-oh-JEN-eh-sihs)
 oste/o- *bone*
 gen/o- *arising from; produced by*
 -esis *abnormal condition; process*

Clinical Connections

Endocrinology. The calcium level in the blood is controlled by parathyroid hormone secreted by the parathyroid glands and by calcitonin hormone secreted by the thyroid gland. Parathyroid hormone raises the calcium level by stimulating osteoclasts to break down bone. Calcitonin has the opposite effect. Estradiol (a female hormone) and other hormones stimulate bone formation. Growth hormone from the pituitary gland influences the rate of bone growth.

Space Medicine. Astronauts who live in a weightless environment for prolonged periods of time lose bone mass. The lack of weight-bearing stress on the bones decreases new bone formation while the rate of bone breakdown remains the same. The astronauts have a regular exercise program that includes resistance exercises to exert weight-bearing force on the bones.

Across the Life Span

Pediatrics. During birth, it is not unusual for the clavicle to break as the baby goes through the birth canal. This fracture does not need to be treated, as it heals by itself within a matter of days because of the high rate of bone growth. Babies are born without kneecaps! These bones develop between 2 and 6 years of age. **Ossification** is the gradual replacing of cartilage with bone that takes place during childhood and adolescence. In addition, new bone is formed along the epiphyseal growth plates at the ends of long bones as the body grows taller. From childhood through adolescence, new bone formation exceeds bone breakdown, as cartilage is continuously replaced by mature bone. The height and weight of a child are important indicators of health and are measured at regular intervals by the pediatrician and recorded on a standardized pediatric growth chart in the child's electronic health record (see Figure 7-17 ■).

During adolescence, the rate of bone growth accelerates (a "growth spurt") because of growth hormone secreted by the anterior pituitary gland.

Middle Age. During adulthood, the rate of new bone formation equals the rate of bone breakdown. In all stages of life, formation of new bone is dependent on having enough calcium and phosphorus in the diet.

Geriatrics. In older adults, the rate of bone breakdown is faster than new bone formation, and the bones can become fragile and prone to fracture. Patients confined to bed who are unable to do any weight-bearing exercises to stimulate new bone formation have an increased rate of bone loss. Osteoporosis or "thinning of the bones" occurs in both men and women.

Pronunciation/Word Parts

ossification (AW-sih-fih-KAY-shun)
  ossific/o- *changing into bone*
  -ation *being; having; process*

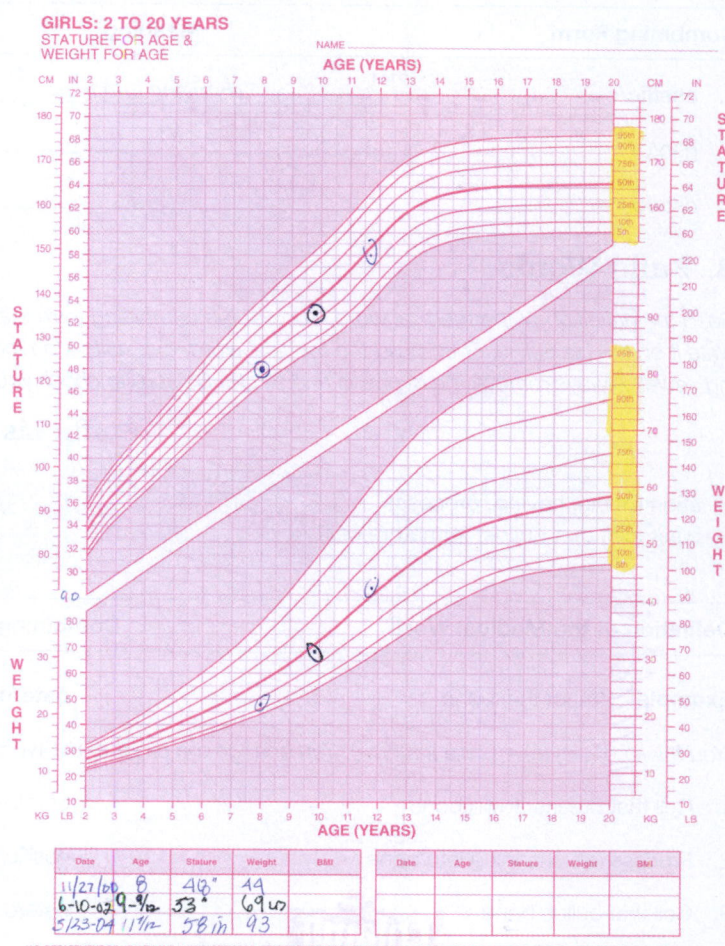

FIGURE 7-17 ■ Pediatric growth chart.
This chart tracks height and weight for girls ages 2–20 years and assigns percentiles. On the initial office visit with the pediatrician, this 8-year-old child had a diagnosis of malnutrition and was in about the 15th percentile for both height (stature) and weight. After 3 years of good nutrition, her office visit at age 11 years, 7 months, showed that she was in the 40th percentile for height and the 55th percentile for weight.

7.2 PRACTICE LAPS

Use the Answer Key at the end of the book to check your answers.

A. Give the Meaning of Combining Forms

Next to each combining form, write its meaning. The first one has been done for you.

Combining Form	Meaning
1. **ossific/o-**	*changing into bone*
2. gen/o-	
3. oste/o-	

B. Build Words

Read the definition of the medical word. Look at the combining form that is given. Select the correct suffix from the Suffix List, and write it on the blank line. Then build the medical word, and write it on the line. (Remember: You may need to remove the combining vowel. Always remove the hyphens and slash.) Be sure to check your spelling. The first one has been done for you.

Suffix List

-ation (being; having; process)   -clast (cell that breaks down)
-blast (cell that builds; immature cell)   -cyte (cell)

Definition of the Medical Word	Combining Form	Suffix	Build the Medical Word
Example: Cell (of the) bone	**oste/o-**	*-cyte*	*osteocyte*

[You think cell (-cyte) + bone (oste/o-). You change the order of the word parts to put the suffix last. You write osteocyte.]

1. Cell that breaks down bone	oste/o-		
2. Process (of) changing into bone	ossific/o-		
3. Cell that builds bone	oste/o-		

Vocabulary Review

Word or Phrase	Description	Combining Forms
Overview		
appendicular skeleton	The limbs, including the bones of the shoulders, upper extremities, hip, and lower extremities	**appendicul/o-** *limb; small attached part*
axial skeleton	Central bony structure of the body. It consists of the bones of the head, associated bones of the head and neck, the chest, and the spine	**axi/o-** *axis*
bones	The framework on which the body is built. The 206 individual pieces of the skeleton. Bone is known as **osseous tissue**. *Bony* and *osteal* are also adjectives for *bone*.	**osse/o-** *bone* **oste/o-** *bone*

Word or Phrase	Description	Combining Forms
musculoskeletal system	The combined systems of the muscles and bones. The bones provide structural support for the body and work in conjunction with the muscles to maintain body posture and produce movement.	**muscul/o-** *muscle* **skelet/o-** *skeleton*
skeletal system	Body system that consists of all of the bones, cartilage, ligaments, and joints in the body. It provides structural support and protection for soft tissues and internal organs. It is a storage site for calcium and phosphorus. The red bone marrow is the site of blood cell production.	**skelet/o-** *skeleton*
skeleton	Bony framework of the body that consists of 206 bones	**skelet/o-** *skeleton*
Anatomy of the Skeletal System		
Bones of the Cranium		
coronal suture	Immovable joint on top of the cranium, extending from one side to the other, where the frontal bone and the parietal bones meet	**coron/o-** *structure that encircles like a crown*
cranium	Dome-like bone at the top of the skull that contains the **cranial cavity** with the brain and other structures	**crani/o-** *cranium; top part of the skull*
ethmoid bone	Bone that forms the posterior nasal septum and the medial walls of the eye sockets. The superior and medial conchae of the ethmoid bone are bony projections within the nasal cavity. The ethmoid bone contains many small, hollow air spaces of the ethmoid sinus.	**ethm/o-** *sieve*
fontanel	"Soft spot" on a baby's head where the cranial sutures are still open and there is only fibrous connective tissue	
foramen magnum	Large hole in the occipital bone. The spinal cord goes through it to join with the brain.	
frontal bone	Bone that forms the forehead and top of the cranium and ends at the coronal suture. It contains the hollow cavities of the frontal sinuses.	**front/o-** *front*
occipital bone	Bone that forms the posterior base of the cranium. It contains the large opening of the foramen magnum.	**occipit/o-** *back of the head; occiput*
parietal bones	Bones that form the superior sides and posterior part of the cranium. They join at the sagittal suture.	**pariet/o-** *wall of a cavity*
sagittal suture	Immovable joint from the top center to the back of the cranium between the two parietal bones	**sagitt/o-** *front to back*
skull	Bony structure of the head that includes the cranium and facial bones	
sphenoid bone	Large, irregularly shaped bone that forms the central base and sides of the cranium and the posterior walls of the eye sockets. It contains the hollow cavities of the sphenoid sinuses. A bony cup in the sphenoid bone holds the pituitary gland (of the endocrine system).	**sphen/o-** *wedge shaped*
suture	Type of joint where one cranial bone meets another. It is an immovable joint that contains no cartilage. Examples: Coronal suture, sagittal suture	
temporal bones	Bones that form the inferior sides of the cranium. Each temporal bone has a bony opening for the external ear canal and contains the hollow cavity of the middle ear. Bony landmarks include the **mastoid process** behind the ear and the pointed **styloid process**, a site of attachment for ligaments to the hyoid bone.	**tempor/o-** *side of the head; temple* **mast/o-** *breast; mastoid process* **styl/o-** *stake*

Word or Phrase	Description	Combining Forms
Facial Bones		
inferior nasal conchae	Facial bones that project inwardly from the side of the nasal cavity	**nas/o-** *nose*
lacrimal bones	Facial bones within the eye socket. They are small, flat bones near the lacrimal glands (of the eyes that produce tears).	**lacrim/o-** *tears*
mandible	Facial bone that is the lower jaw bone and contains the roots of the lower teeth. It is the only movable bone in the skull. Together with the temporal bone, the movable mandible forms the temporomandibular joint located just anterior to the ear.	**mandibul/o-** *lower jaw; mandible*
maxilla	Facial bone that is the upper jaw bone. It contains the roots of the upper teeth and the hollow cavities of the maxillary sinuses. The maxilla consists of two fused **maxillary bones**.	**maxill/o-** *maxilla; upper jaw*
nasal bones	Facial bones that form the bridge of the nose and the roof of the nasal cavity	**nas/o-** *nose*
palatine bones	Facial bones that are small and flat and join in the midline to form the hard palate in the oral cavity	**palat/o-** *palate*
vomer	Facial bone that is the most inferior part of the nasal septum and continues posteriorly to join the sphenoid bone	
zygoma	Facial bone that is a cheekbone and goes to the edge of the eye socket. Also known as the **zygomatic bone**.	**zygomat/o-** *cheekbone; zygoma*
Associated Bones of the Head and Neck		
hyoid bone	Flat, U-shaped bone in the anterior neck. It is attached by ligaments to the styloid process of each temporal bone. The tendons of several muscles in the mouth and neck are attached to the hyoid bone.	**hy/o-** *U-shaped structure*
ossicles	Three tiny bones in the middle ear cavity (**malleus**, **incus**, **stapes**) that function in the process of hearing. Collectively, they are the ossicular chain.	**oss/i-** *bone*
Bones of the Chest		
costal cartilage	Firm, but flexible connective tissue that joins the ribs to the sternum at the **costochondral joint**	**cost/o-** *rib* **chondr/o-** *cartilage* **cartilagin/o-** *cartilage*
ribs	Twelve pairs of bones that form the sides of the rib cage. There are true ribs, false ribs, and floating ribs. The area between two ribs is the **intercostal space**.	**cost/o-** *rib*
sternum	Vertical bone in the center of the anterior rib cage. Also known as the **breastbone**. The **manubrium** is the triangular-shaped, superior part of the sternum, while the **xiphoid process** is the inferior tip. The clavicle and some of the ribs are attached to the sternum.	**stern/o-** *breastbone; sternum* **xiph/o-** *sword*
thoracic cavity	Area within the rib cage that contains the heart, lungs, and other structures	**thorac/o-** *chest; thorax*
thorax	Area between the neck and the diaphragm. The wall of the thorax is the **rib cage**.	**thorac/o-** *chest; thorax*
Bones of the Spine		
cervical vertebrae	Vertebrae C1–C7 of the vertebral column in the neck. C1 is the **atlas**; C2 is the **axis**.	**cervic/o-** *cervix; neck* **vertebr/o-** *vertebra*

Word or Phrase	Description	Combining Forms
coccyx	Group of several small, fused vertebrae inferior to the sacrum. Also known as the **tailbone**.	**coccyg/o-** *coccyx; tailbone*
foramen	Hole in each vertebrae where the spinal cord goes through	
intervertebral disk	Disk between two vertebrae. It consists of an outer wall of fibrocartilage and an inner gelatinous substance, the **nucleus pulposus**, that acts as a cushion.	**vertebr/o-** *vertebra*
lumbar vertebrae	Vertebrae L1–L5 of the vertebral column in the lower back	**lumb/o-** *lower back*
sacrum	Group of five fused vertebrae inferior to the lumbar vertebrae. The first one is S1, but the others are not numbered.	**sacr/o-** *sacrum*
spine	Bony column of vertebrae that supports the weight of the head, neck, and trunk of the body and protects the spinal cord. Also known as the **vertebral column**, **spinal column**, or **backbone**. It is divided into five regions: cervical vertebrae, thoracic vertebrae, lumbar vertebrae, sacrum, and coccyx.	**spin/o-** *backbone; spine* **vertebr/o-** *vertebra*
thoracic vertebrae	Vertebrae T1–T12 of the vertebral column in the area of the chest. Each vertebra joins with one pair of ribs.	**thorac/o-** *chest; thorax* **vertebr/o-** *vertebra*
vertebrae	Bony structure in the spine. Most vertebrae have a vertebral body (flat, circular area), **spinous process** (bony projection along the midback), two **transverse processes** (bony projections to each side), and a **foramen** (hole where the spinal cord passes through).	**vertebr/o-** *vertebra* **spondyl/o-** *vertebra* **spin/o-** *backbone; spine*
Bones of the Shoulders		
clavicle	Thin, rod-like bone on each side of the anterior neck. It connects to the manubrium of the sternum and the acromion of the scapula. Also known as the **collarbone**.	**clavicul/o-** *clavicle; collarbone*
glenoid fossa	Shallow depression in the scapula where the head of the humerus joins the scapula to make the shoulder joint	**glen/o-** *socket of a joint*
scapula	Triangular-shaped bone in the upper back on each side of the spine. Also known as the **shoulder blade**. It contains the **acromion**, a flat, bony projection that connects to the clavicle.	**scapul/o-** *scapula; shoulder blade*
Bones of the Upper Extremities		
carpal bones	The eight small bones of the wrist joint. They connect the radius and ulna to the metacarpal bones.	**carp/o-** *wrist*
humerus	Long bone of the upper arm. The head of the humerus fits into the glenoid fossa of the scapula to form the shoulder joint. The distal end connects to the radius and ulna of the forearm.	**humer/o-** *humerus; upper arm bone*
metacarpal bones	The five bones of the hand, one corresponding to each finger. They connect the carpal bones to the phalanges at the **metacarpophalangeal joint (MCP)**.	**carp/o-** *wrist* **phalang/o-** *digit; finger; toe*
phalanx	Each of the individual bones of a finger. The **distal interphalangeal joint (DIP)** is between the last two phalanges. A finger or toe is a digit.	**phalang/o-** *digit; finger; toe* **dactyl/o-** *digit; finger; toe*
radius	Forearm bone located along the thumb side of the lower arm. Its proximal end connects to the humerus. At its distal end, it connects to the carpal bones.	**radi/o-** *forearm bone; radius; x-rays*

Word or Phrase	Description	Combining Forms
ulna	Forearm bone located along the little finger side of the lower arm. Its proximal end connects to the humerus. The **olecranon** (point of the elbow) is a large, square, bony projection on the proximal ulna. At its distal end, it connects to the carpal bones.	**uln/o-** *forearm bone; ulna*
Bones of the Hip		
acetabulum	Cup-shaped, deep socket of the hip joint that is made up of the bones of the ilium, ischium, and pubis. The head of the femur fits into the acetabulum to form the hip joint.	**acetabul/o-** *socket of the hip joint*
ilium	Most superior hip bone. It has a broad, flaring **iliac crest**. Posteriorly, each ilium joins the sacrum.	**ili/o-** *ilium*
ischium	Most inferior hip bone. Each ischium is one of the "seat bones."	**ischi/o-** *ischium*
pelvis	The hip bones as well as the sacrum and coccyx of the vertebral column	**pelv/o-** *hip bone; pelvis; renal pelvis*
pubis	Small bridge-like bone that is the most anterior hip bone. The **pubic symphysis** is a nearly immobile joint that has a cartilage pad between the two **pubic bones**.	**pub/o-** *hip bone; pubis*
Bones of the Lower Extremities		
calcaneus	Largest of the ankle bones. Also known as the **heel bone**.	**calcane/o-** *calcaneus; heel bone*
femur	Long, weight-bearing bone of the upper leg. Also known as the **thigh bone**. The head of the femur fits into the acetabulum to form the hip joint. Its distal end connects to the tibia.	**femor/o-** *femur; thigh bone*
fibula	Thin bone on the lateral (little toe side) of the lower leg. Its proximal end connects to the tibia. At its distal end is the bony prominence of the lateral malleolus.	**fibul/o-** *fibula* **perone/o-** *fibula*
hallux	The great toe	
malleolus	Bony projection of the distal tibia (**medial malleolus**) or the distal fibula (**lateral malleolus**). Often mistakenly called the *ankle bones*.	**malleol/o-** *malleolus* **medi/o-** *middle* **later/o-** *side*
metatarsal bones	The five bones of the midfoot, one corresponding to each toe. They connect the ankle bones to the phalanges.	**tars/o-** *ankle*
patella	Thick, round bone anterior to the knee joint. Also known as the **kneecap**.	**patell/o-** *kneecap; patella*
phalanx	Each of the individual bones of a toe. A toe is a digit.	**phalang/o-** *digit; finger; toe* **dactyl/o-** *digit; finger; toe*
tarsal bones	The seven bones of the ankle joint. The first is the **talus**; the largest is the calcaneus.	**tars/o-** *ankle*
tibia	Long, weight-bearing bone on the medial (great toe) side of the lower leg. Its proximal end connects to the femur. At its distal end is the bony prominence of the medial malleolus. Its distal end connects to the metatarsal bones. Also known as the **shin bone**.	**tibi/o-** *shin bone; tibia*
Structure of the Bones		
cancellous bone	Spongy bone in the epiphyses of long bones. Its spaces are filled with red bone marrow that produces stem cells that mature to become all types of blood cells. Cancellous bone is also found in the skull, clavicles, sternum, ribs, vertebrae, and each ilium.	**cancell/o-** *lattice structure*

Word or Phrase	Description	Combining Forms
cortical bone	Dense, compact, weight-bearing bone inside the shaft of a long bone	**cortic/o-** *cortex; outer region*
diaphysis	The straight shaft of a long bone, such as the humerus or femur	**diaphys/o-** *shaft of a bone*
epiphysis	Widened ends of a long bone that contain cancellous bone filled with red bone marrow. The **epiphyseal plate** is where bone growth takes place.	**epiphys/o-** *enlarged end of long bone*
foramen	Small opening in the bone where a blood vessel goes through to the bone marrow	
medullary cavity	Cavity within the shaft of a long bone. It contains yellow bone marrow (fatty tissue).	**medull/o-** *inner region; medulla*
osseous tissue	Bone, a type of connective tissue	**osse/o-** *bone*
periosteum	Thick, fibrous membrane that covers the surface of a bone	**oste/o-** *bone*
Joints, Cartilage, and Ligaments		
cartilage	Densely packed collagen fibers that do not contain blood vessels. Articular cartilage covers the bone ends in a synovial joint. A meniscus is a cartilage pad in some synovial joints.	**cartilagin/o-** *cartilage*
joint	Area where two bones come together. Also known as an **articulation**. There are three types of joints: suture, symphysis, and synovial.	**articul/o-** *joint* **arthr/o-** *joint*
ligament	Fibrous band that holds two bone ends together in a synovial joint	**ligament/o-** *ligament*
meniscus	Crescent-shaped cartilage pad found in some synovial joints, such as the knee joint	
suture joint	Immovable joint that contains no cartilage, such as the joint between the cranial bones and most of the facial bones	
symphysis joint	Slightly movable joint that contains a cartilage pad or disk between the bones, such as the joint between the two pubic bones (the pubic symphysis) and between the vertebrae	
synovial joint	Fully movable joint that contains two bones whose ends are covered with **articular cartilage**. There are two types: hinge joints (elbow and knee) and ball-and-socket joints (shoulder and hip). Ligaments hold the bone ends together. The joint is encased in a **joint capsule** that is lined with a **synovial membrane** that produces **synovial fluid** to lubricate the joint.	**synovi/o-** *joint membrane; synovium* **synov/o-** *joint membrane; synovium* **articul/o-** *joint* **cartilagin/o-** *cartilage*
Physiology of the Skeletal System		
ossification	Process by which cartilage is gradually replaced with bone from childhood through adolescence	**ossific/o-** *changing into bone*
osteoblast	Bone cell that builds a protein matrix and stimulates calcium salts to deposit there to build new bone	**oste/o-** *bone*
osteoclast	Bone cell that secretes acid and enzymes to break down and dissolve areas of old or damaged bone	**oste/o-** *bone*
osteocyte	Bone cell that maintains and monitors the mineral content (calcium, phosphorus) of bone	**oste/o-** *bone*
osteogenesis	Process of new bone being built on a protein matrix with deposits of calcium salts. This forms around an osteoblast that then becomes an osteocyte within the new, permanent bone.	**oste/o-** *bone* **gen/o-** *arising from; produced by*

7.3 Diseases

Word or Phrase	Description	Pronunciation/Word Parts

Bones and Cartilage

Word or Phrase	Description	Pronunciation/Word Parts
avascular necrosis	Death of cells in the epiphysis of a long bone, often in the femur. This is caused by an injury, fracture, or dislocation that damages nearby blood vessels or by a blood clot that interrupts the blood supply to the bone. Treatment: Surgery to remove the dead bone, followed by a bone graft; for large areas of avascular necrosis, joint replacement surgery is done.	**avascular** (aa-VAS-kyoo-lar) **a-** *away from; without* **vascul/o-** *blood vessel* **-ar** *pertaining to* **necrosis** (neh-KROH-sihs) **necr/o-** *dead body; dead tissue* **-osis** *abnormal condition; process*
bone tumor	A bone tumor can be benign (not cancerous) or cancerous. • **Osteoma** is a benign tumor of the bone. • **Osteosarcoma** is a cancerous bone tumor in which osteoblasts, the cells that form new bone, multiply uncontrollably. Also known as **osteogenic sarcoma**. • **Ewing sarcoma** is a cancerous bone tumor that occurs mainly in young men. Treatment: Surgical removal of a benign bone tumor; amputation of the limb followed by radiation therapy or chemotherapy drugs for a cancerous tumor	**osteoma** (AW-stee-OH-mah) **oste/o-** *bone* **-oma** *mass; tumor* **osteosarcoma** (AW-stee-OH-sar-KOH-mah) **oste/o-** *bone* **sarc/o-** *connective tissue* **-oma** *mass; tumor* **osteogenic** (AW-stee-oh-JEN-ik) **oste/o-** *bone* **gen/o-** *arising from; produced by* **-ic** *pertaining to* **Ewing** (YOO-ing)
chondroma	Benign tumor of the cartilage Treatment: Surgical removal, if it is large	**chondroma** (con-DROH-mah) **chondr/o-** *cartilage* **-oma** *mass; tumor*
chondromalacia patellae	Abnormal softening of the patella because of thinning and uneven wear. The thigh muscle pulls the patella in a twisted path that wears away the underside of the bone. Treatment: Strengthening of the thigh muscle to correct the direction of its contraction	**chondromalacia** (CON-droh-mah-LAY-shah) **chondr/o-** *cartilage* **malac/o-** *softening* **-ia** *condition; state; thing* **patellae** (pah-TEL-ee)

Word or Phrase	Description	Pronunciation/Word Parts
fracture (FX, Fx)	Broken bone due to an accident, an injury, or a disease. Some fractures are categorized according to how the bone breaks (see Figure 7-18 ■ and Table 7-1 ■). Other types of fractures include a **stress fracture** (caused by force or torsion during an accident or sports activity) and a **pathologic fracture** (caused by a disease process such as osteoporosis, bone cancer, or metastases to the bone). Fractures that are allowed to heal without treatment often show malunion or **malalignment** of the fracture fragments. Treatment: Closed reduction and manipulation to align the fracture pieces with application of a cast Surgery: Open reduction and internal fixation using wires, pins, screws, or plates **FIGURE 7-18 ■ Bone fracture.** These x-rays show lateral and anteroposterior (AP) views of a fracture of the forearm that involves both the radius and the ulna.	**fracture** (FRAK-chur) **fract/o-** *bend; break up* **-ure** *result of; system* **pathologic** (PATH-oh-LAW-jik) **path/o-** *disease* **log/o-** *study of; word* **-ic** *pertaining to* **malalignment** (MAL-ah-LINE-ment) **mal-** *bad; inadequate* **align/o-** *arranged in a straight line* **-ment** *action; state*

Table 7-1   Fracture Names and Descriptions

Fracture Name	Description	Illustration	Pronunciation/Word Parts
closed fracture	Broken bone does not break through the overlying skin		
open fracture	Broken bone breaks through the overlying skin. It is also known as a **compound fracture**.		
nondisplaced fracture	Broken bone remains in its normal anatomical alignment	Non-displaced fracture / Displaced fracture	**nondisplaced** (non-dihs-PLAYSD) The prefix **non-** means *not*. The prefix **dis-** means *away from*; *lack of*.
displaced fracture	Broken bone is pulled out of its normal anatomical alignment		**displaced** (dis-PLAYSD)

(continued)

Table 7-1 (Continued)

Fracture Name	Description	Illustration	Pronunciation/Word Parts
Colles fracture	Distal radius is broken by falling onto an outstretched hand	Colles fracture	**Colles fracture** (KOH-leez)
comminuted fracture	Bone is crushed into several small pieces	Comminuted fracture	**comminuted** (KAWM-ih-NYOO-ted) **comminut/o-** *break into small pieces* **-ed** *pertaining to*
compression fracture	Vertebrae are compressed together when a person falls onto the buttocks or when a vertebra collapses in on itself because of disease	Compression fracture	**compression** (com-PREH-shun) **compress/o-** *press together* **-ion** *action; condition*
depressed fracture	Cranium is fractured inward toward the brain	Depressed fracture	**depressed** (dee-PRESD) **depress/o-** *press down* **-ed** *pertaining to*
greenstick fracture	Bone is broken on only one side. This occurs in children because part of the bone is still flexible cartilage.	Greenstick fracture	

Fracture Name	Description	Illustration	Pronunciation/Word Parts
hairline fracture	Very thin fracture line with the bone pieces still together. It is difficult to detect except on an x-ray.	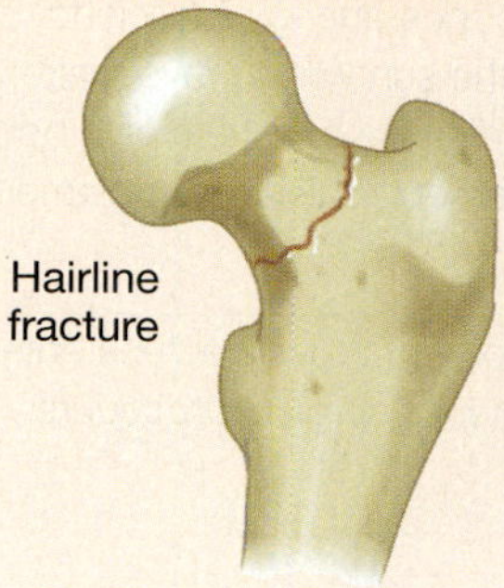 Hairline fracture	
oblique fracture	Bone is broken on an oblique angle (see also Figure 7-18)	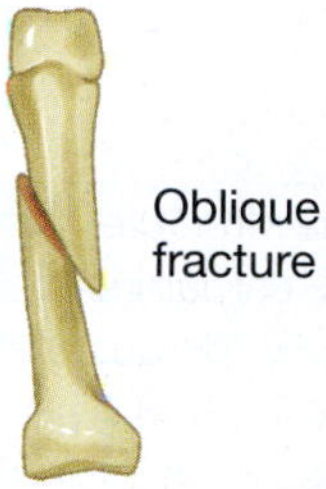 Oblique fracture	**oblique** (oh-BLEEK)
spiral fracture	Bone is broken in a spiral because of a twisting force	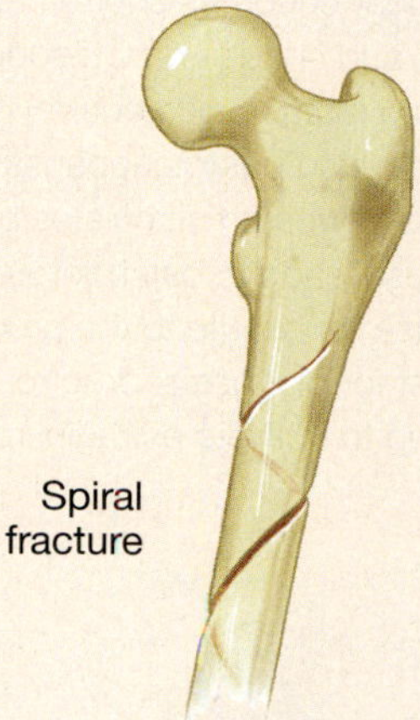 Spiral fracture	**spiral** (SPY-ral) **spir/o-** *breathe; coil* **-al** *pertaining to*
transverse fracture	Bone is broken in a transverse plane perpendicular to its long axis	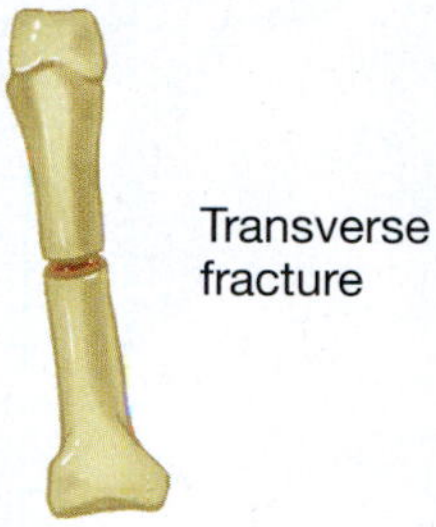 Transverse fracture	**transverse** (trans-VERS) The prefix **trans-** means *across; through.* The suffix **-verse** means *travel; turn.*

Word or Phrase	Description	Pronunciation/Word Parts
osteomalacia	Abnormal softening of the bones due to a deficiency of vitamin D in the diet or inadequate exposure to the sun whose rays make vitamin D in the skin. In children, this causes the disease of rickets with bone pain and fractures. Treatment: Vitamin D supplement; calcium supplement; sun exposure	**osteomalacia** (AW-stee-OH-mah-LAY-shah) **oste/o-** *bone* **malac/o-** *softening* **-ia** *condition; state; thing*
osteomyelitis	Infection of the bone and bone marrow. Bacteria enter the bone following an open fracture, crush injury, or surgical procedure. Treatment: Antibiotic drug	**osteomyelitis** (AW-stee-oh-MY-eh-LY-tihs) **oste/o-** *bone* **myel/o-** *bone marrow; myelin; spinal cord* **-itis** *infection of; inflammation of* Osteomyelitis: *Infection of (the) bone (and) bone marrow*
osteoporosis	Abnormal thinning of the bone structure. When bone breakdown exceeds new bone formation, calcium and phosphorus are lost, and the bone becomes osteoporotic (porous) with many small areas of **demineralization** (see Figure 7-19 ■). This can cause a compression fracture as a vertebra collapses in on itself. The vertebral column decreases in height, the patient becomes shorter, and there is an abnormal curvature of the upper back and shoulders. Osteoporosis can also cause a spontaneous fracture (pathologic fracture) of the hip or femur. Osteoporosis occurs most often in postmenopausal women but can also occur in older men. Estradiol in women stimulates bone formation, and loss of estradiol at menopause leads to osteoporosis. A lack of dietary calcium and a lack of exercise contribute to the process. Treatment: Bone density test for diagnosis; drug to decrease the rate of bone breakdown or a drug to activate estradiol receptors; calcium supplement 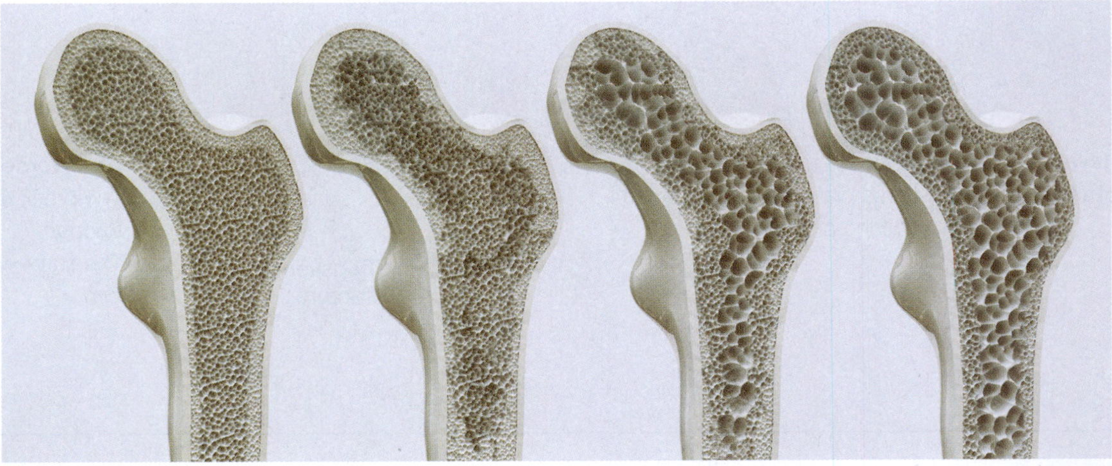	**osteoporosis** (AW-stee-OH-poh-ROH-sihs) **oste/o-** *bone* **por/o-** *pores; small openings* **-osis** *abnormal condition; process* **demineralization** (dee-MIN-er-AL-ih-ZAY-shun) **de-** *reversal of; without* **mineral/o-** *electrolyte; mineral* **-ization** *process of creating; process of inserting; process of making*

FIGURE 7-19 ■ Normal bone versus bone with osteoporosis.
The image on the left, a cross-section of the head and body of the femur, shows normal bone mineralization and density. The other images show progressively more osteoporosis with mild-to-severe demineralization and loss of bone density. Osteoporotic bone is extremely prone to fracture.

Word or Phrase	Description	Pronunciation/Word Parts

Bones of the Chest

pectus excavatum	Congenital deformity in which the sternum, particularly the xiphoid process, is bent inward, creating a hollow depression in the anterior chest Treatment: Surgical correction, if severe	**pectus excavatum** (PEK-tuhs EKS-kah-VAH-tum)

Bones of the Spine

ankylosing spondylitis	Chronic inflammation of the vertebrae that leads to fibrosis, fusion, and restriction of movement of the spine Treatment: Nonsteroidal anti-inflammatory drug	**ankylosing** (ANG-kih-LOH-sing) **ankyl/o-** *fused together; stiff* **-osing** *abnormal condition of making* **spondylitis** (SPAWN-dih-LY-tihs) **spondyl/o-** *vertebra* **-itis** *infection of; inflammation of*
kyphosis	Abnormal, excessive, posterior curvature of the thoracic spine. It is commonly known as **humpback** or **hunchback**. The back is said to have a **kyphotic** curvature. **Kyphoscoliosis** is a complex curvature with components of both kyphosis and scoliosis. Treatment: Back brace; surgery to fuse and straighten a severely curved spine	**kyphosis** (ky-FOH-sihs) **kyph/o-** *bent; humpbacked* **-osis** *abnormal condition; process* **kyphotic** (ky-FAW-tik) **kyph/o-** *bent; humpbacked* **-tic** *pertaining to* **kyphoscoliosis** (KY-foh-SKOH-lee-OH-sihs) **kyph/o-** *bent; humpbacked* **scoli/o-** *crooked; curved* **-osis** *abnormal condition; process*
lordosis	Abnormal, excessive, anterior curvature of the lumbar spine. It is commonly known as **swayback**. The back is said to have a **lordotic** curvature. Treatment: Back brace or surgery to fuse and straighten a severely curved spine	**lordosis** (lor-DOH-sihs) **lord/o-** *swayback* **-osis** *abnormal condition; process* **lordotic** (lor-DAW-tik) **lord/o-** *swayback* **-tic** *pertaining to*

Word or Phrase	Description	Pronunciation/Word Parts
scoliosis	Abnormal, excessive, C-shaped or S-shaped lateral curvature of the spine (see Figure 7-20 ■). The back is said to have a **scoliotic** curvature. A **dextroscoliosis** curves to the patient's right, while a **levoscoliosis** curves to the patient's left. Scoliosis can be congenital but most often the cause is unknown. The incidence of scoliosis is the same in males and females, but females are 10 times more likely to develop severe scoliosis. Scoliosis develops during childhood and may continue to progress during adolescence. It impairs movement, posture, and breathing. An x-ray shows the degree of curvature. Treatment: Back brace; surgery to fuse and straighten a severely curved spine	**scoliosis** (SKOH-lee-OH-sihs) **scoli/o-** *crooked; curved* **-osis** *abnormal condition; process* **scoliotic** (SKOH-lee-AW-tik) **scoli/o-** *crooked; curved* **-tic** *pertaining to* **dextroscoliosis** (DEKS-troh-SKOH-lee-OH-sihs) **dextr/o-** *right; sugar* **scoli/o-** *crooked; curved* **-osis** *abnormal condition; process* **levoscoliosis** (LEE-voh-SKOH-lee-OH-sihs) **lev/o-** *left* **scoli/o-** *crooked; curved* **-osis** *abnormal condition; process*

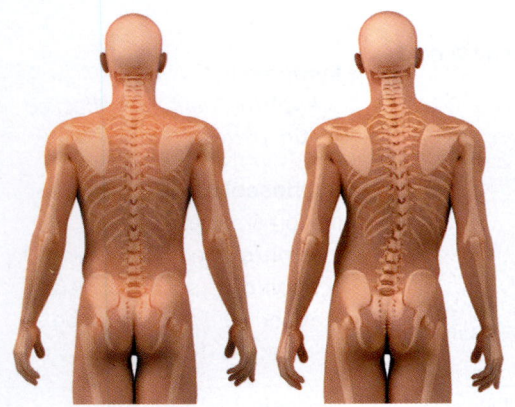
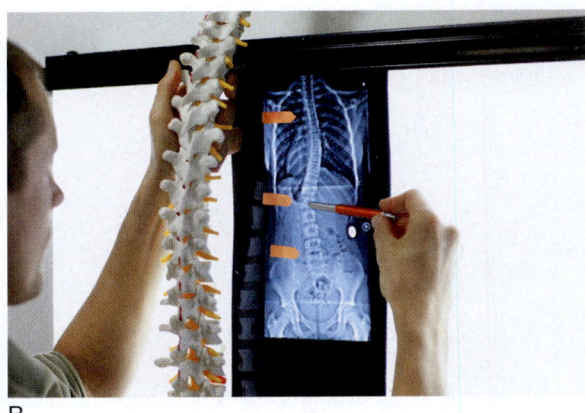

A.   B.

FIGURE 7-20 ■ Scoliosis.
A. The patient on the left has a straight spine with no evidence of scoliosis. The patient on the right has moderate dextroscoliosis of the thoracic and lumbar spine with the characteristic tilt of the shoulders and hips, uneven scapulae, and a difference in arm lengths. **B.** X-rays of the spine in three dimensions, a model of the spine, and the computer are used to measure the degree of scoliosis and prepare an individualized treatment plan.

Clinical Connections

Public Health. Scoliosis screening of schoolchildren was mandatory in many states, but has been gradually discontinued. However, the American Academy of Pediatrics and the American Academy of Orthopedic Surgeons still recommend early routine screening (see Figure 7-21 ■) as the best way to prevent later cases of undetected serious scoliosis.

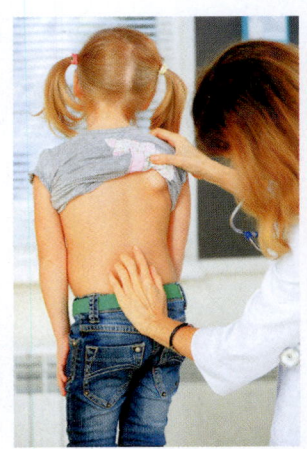

FIGURE 7-21 ■ Scoliosis screening.
A pediatrician is evaluating this elementary schoolchild for signs of scoliosis. The child's back is observed while standing and then while doing a forward-bend test. Some cases of scoliosis become more apparent with bending over as one side of the back becomes noticeably higher and one scapula is prominent.

Word or Phrase	Description	Pronunciation/Word Parts
spondylolisthesis	Degenerative condition of the spine in which one vertebra moves anteriorly and slips out of proper alignment due to degeneration of the intervertebral disk. It can also occur because of a sports injury or a compression fracture of the vertebra from osteoporosis. Treatment: Back brace or surgery to relieve a pinched spinal nerve; analgesic drug; nonsteroidal anti-inflammatory drug; intra-articular injection of a corticosteroid drug	**spondylolisthesis** (SPAWN-dih-LOH-lihs-THEE-sihs) **spondyl/o-** *vertebra* **-listhesis** *abnormal condition of slipping*

Bones of the Lower Extremity

genu valgum	Congenital deformity in which the knees are rotated toward the midline and are abnormally close together with the lower legs bent laterally. Also known as **knock-knee**. Treatment: Surgical correction, if severe	**genu valgum** (JEE-noo VAL-gum)
genu varum	Congenital deformity in which the knees are rotated laterally away from each other and the lower legs are bent toward the midline. Also known as **bowleg**. Treatment: Surgical correction, if severe	**genu varum** (JEE-noo VAR-um)
hallux valgus	Deformity in which the great toe is angled laterally toward the other toes (see Figure 7-22 ■). There is swelling and inflammation at the base of the great toe. It can be caused by an inherited defect in the foot, an injury, rheumatoid arthritis, or wearing pointy-toed shoes. Also known as a **bunion**. Treatment: Wide-toed shoes; bunionectomy	**hallux valgus** (HAL-uks VAL-guhs) **bunion** (BUN-yun)

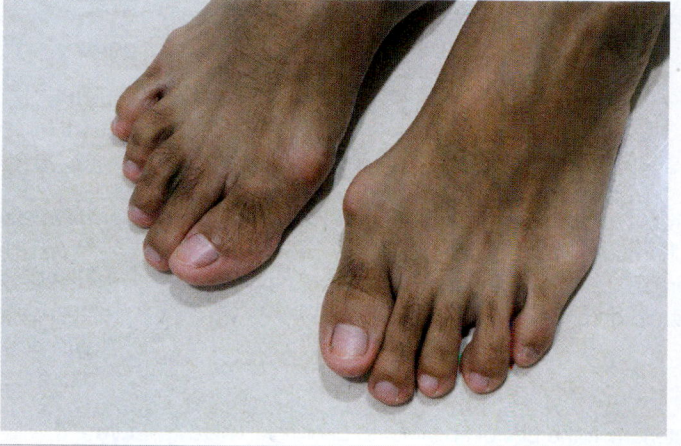

FIGURE 7-22 ■ Hallux valgus and bunion.
This patient's great toes are both angled away from the midline, and there are reddened, enlarged, and painful bunions on the medial sides of both feet.

talipes equinovarus	Congenital deformity in which the foot is pulled downward and toward the midline. Also known as **clubfoot**. One or both feet can be affected (see Figure 7-23 ■). Treatment: Casts applied to progressively straighten the foot; surgical correction, if severe	**talipes equinovarus** (TAY-lih-peez ee-KWY-noh-VAR-uhs)

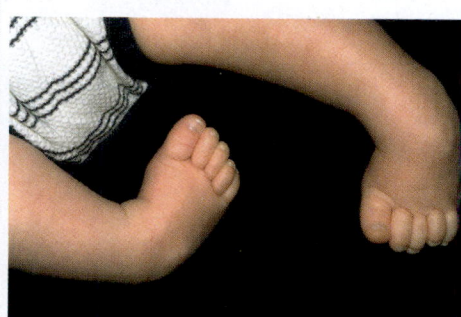

FIGURE 7-23 ■ Bilateral clubfeet.
This child was born with bilateral clubfeet. Although all newborns' feet are rotated medially due to the confining environment of the uterus, their feet can easily be moved into an anatomically correct position. In this child, the position of the feet cannot be straightened and would remain this way throughout childhood and adulthood unless surgery was performed.

Word or Phrase	Description	Pronunciation/Word Parts

Joints, Cartilage, and Ligaments

Word or Phrase	Description	Pronunciation/Word Parts

arthralgia	Pain in a joint due to injury, inflammation, or infection from various causes
	Treatment: Correct the underlying cause.
		arthralgia (ar-THRAL-jah)
		  arthr/o- *joint*
		  alg/o- *pain*
		  -ia *condition; state; thing*

arthropathy	Disease of a joint from any cause
	Treatment: Correct the underlying cause.
		arthropathy
		(ar-THRAW-pah-thee)
		  arthr/o- *joint*
		  -pathy *disease*

dislocation	Displacement of the end of a bone from its normal position within a joint. This is usually caused by injury or trauma. **Congenital dislocation of the hip (CDH)** is present at birth because the acetabulum is poorly formed or the ligaments are loose.
	Treatment: Manipulate and return the bone to its normal position; congenital dislocation of the hip is treated with a splint or with surgery to correct the shape of the acetabulum or to tighten the ligaments.
		dislocation (DIS-loh-KAY-shun)
		  dis- *away from; lack of*
		  locat/o- *place*
		  -ion *action; condition*
		
		congenital (con-JEN-ih-tal)
		  congenit/o- *present at birth*
		  -al *pertaining to*

gout	Metabolic disorder that occurs most often in men. There is a high level of uric acid in the blood. An acute attack causes sudden, severe pain after uric acid moves from the blood into the soft tissues and forms crystals known as **tophi**. Historically, patients with gout have been pictured with throbbing big toes, although tophi can form in the joints of the ankle, knee, wrist, or fingers. Tophi in the joints causes **gouty arthritis**.
	Treatment: Avoid foods that increase the uric acid level; drug to decrease the uric acid level
		gout (GOWT)
		
		tophus (TOH-fuhs)
		
		tophi (TOH-fi)
		Latin plural noun: Change the singular ending *-us* to *-i*.
		
		gouty (GOW-tee)
		
		arthritis (ar-THRY-tihs)
		  arthr/o- *joint*
		  -itis *infection of; inflammation of*

hemarthrosis	Blood in the joint cavity from blunt trauma or a penetrating wound. It also occurs spontaneously in hemophiliac patients.
	Treatment: Temporary immobilization of the joint, aspiration of blood from the joint cavity; corticosteroid drug; surgery of an arthroscopy
		hemarthrosis
		(HEE-mar-THROH-sihs)
		  hem/o- *blood*
		  arthr/o- *joint*
		  -osis *abnormal condition; process*

Lyme disease	Arthritis caused by a bacterium in the bite of an infected deer tick. There is an erythematous rash that expands outward from the bite for several weeks (bull's-eye rash) but is not itchy; there is joint pain, fever, chills, and fatigue. If untreated, Lyme disease can cause severe fatigue and affect the nervous system (numbness, severe headache) and the heart. Treatment: Antibiotic drug	**Lyme** (LIME)

Word or Phrase	Description	Pronunciation/Word Parts

osteoarthritis (OA)	Chronic inflammatory disease of the joints, particularly the large weight-bearing joints (knees, hips) and joints that move repeatedly (shoulders, neck, hands). Osteoarthritis usually begins in middle age but can develop sooner in a joint that has been overused or injured. There is joint pain and stiffness with inflammation from constant wear and tear, and this is worsened if the patient is overweight. The normally smooth cartilage becomes roughened and then wears away in spots (see Figure 7-24 ■). The bone ends rub against each other, causing additional inflammation and **crepitus**, a grinding sound. New bone sometimes forms abnormally as an **osteophyte**, a sharp bone spur that causes pain. Osteoarthritis is also known as **degenerative joint disease (DJD)**.
	Treatment: Analgesic drug; nonsteroidal anti-inflammatory drug; intra-articular injection of a corticosteroid drug; joint replacement surgery
		osteoarthritis
		(AW-stee-OH-ar-THRY-tihs)
		  oste/o- bone
		  arthr/o- joint
		  -itis infection of; inflammation of
		
		crepitus (KREP-ih-tuhs)
		
		osteophyte (AW-stee-oh-FITE)
		  oste/o- bone
		  -phyte growth
		
		degenerative (dee-JEN-er-ah-TIV)
		  de- reversal of; without
		  gener/o- creation; production
		  -ative pertaining to

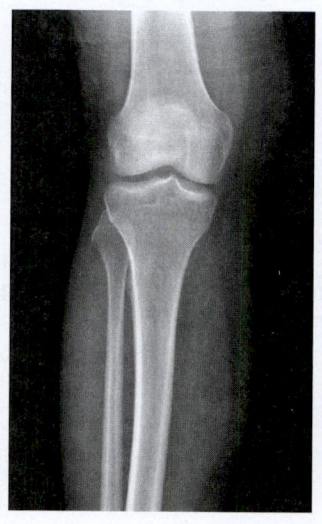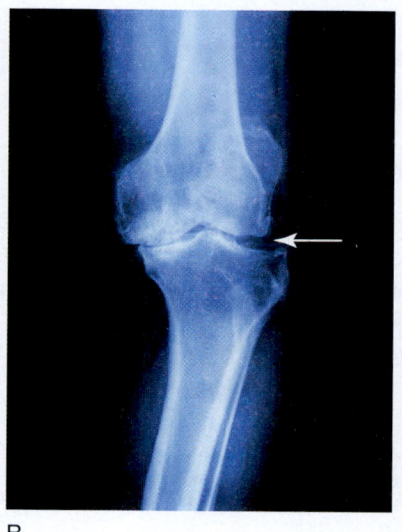

A. **B.**

FIGURE 7-24 ■ Osteoarthritis.
A. This patient's knee x-ray shows a normal knee joint. **B.** This patient's knee x-ray shows loss of the articular cartilage and narrowing of the joint space between the bone ends on one side more than the other. This narrowing is characteristic of degenerative joint disease.

rheumatoid arthritis (RA)	Acute and chronic inflammatory disease of connective tissue, particularly of the joints. This is an autoimmune disorder in which the patient's own antibodies attack cartilage and connective tissue. Patients are usually young to middle-aged females. There is redness and swelling of the joints, most often of the hands and feet. The joint cartilage is slowly destroyed by inflammation. The symptoms flare and subside over time, and there is progressive deformity of the joints (see Figure 7-25 ■).
	Treatment: Corticosteroid drug; gold compound drug; joint replacement surgery
		rheumatoid (ROO-mah-toyd)
		  rheumat/o- watery discharge
		  -oid resembling
		
		arthritis (ar-THRY-tihs)
		  arthr/o- joint
		  -itis infection of; inflammation of

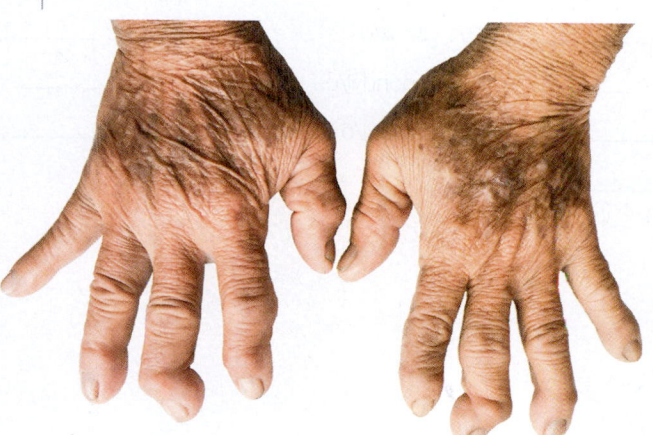

FIGURE 7-25 ■ Rheumatoid arthritis.
This patient has severe joint deformities of the hand that are characteristic of rheumatoid arthritis.

Word or Phrase	Description	Pronunciation/Word Parts
sprain	Overstretching or tearing of a ligament around a joint Treatment: Rest or surgery to repair the ligament	**sprain** (SPRAYN)
subluxation	A partial dislocation with slight displacement of the end of a bone from its normal position within a joint. It is not always visible on an x-ray. Treatment: Closed reduction to manipulate the bone into a normal position; immobilization; analgesic drug	**subluxation** (SUB-luk-SAY-shun) **sub-** *below; underneath; less than* **luxat/o-** *displacement* **-ion** *action; condition*
torn meniscus	Tear of the cartilage pad of the knee because of an injury Treatment: Arthroscopy and repair	**meniscus** (meh-NIHS-kuhs)

7.3 PRACTICE LAPS

Use the Answer Key at the end of the book to check your answers.

A. Give the Meaning of Combining Forms

Next to each combining form, write its meaning. The first one has been done for you.

Combining Form	Meaning	Combining Form	Meaning
1. **gen/o-**	*arising from; produced by*	16. lord/o-	
2. alg/o-		17. luxat/o-	
3. align/o-		18. malac/o-	
4. ankyl/o-		19. mineral/o-	
5. arthr/o-		20. myel/o-	
6. chondr/o-		21. necr/o-	
7. congenit/o-		22. oste/o-	
8. dextr/o-		23. path/o-	
9. fract/o-		24. por/o-	
10. gener/o-		25. rheumat/o-	
11. hem/o-		26. sarc/o-	
12. kyph/o-		27. scoli/o-	
13. lev/o-		28. spondyl/o-	
14. locat/o-		29. vascul/o-	
15. log/o-			

B. Build Words

Read the definition of the medical word. Look at the combining form that is given. Select the correct suffix from the Suffix List, and write it on the blank line. Then build the medical word, and write it on the line. (Remember: You may need to remove the combining vowel. Always remove the hyphens and slash.) Be sure to check your spelling.

Suffix List

-al (pertaining to)	-osing (abnormal condition of making)	-phyte (growth)
-itis (infection of; inflammation of)	-osis (abnormal condition; process)	-ure (result of; system)
-oma (mass; tumor)	-pathy (disease)	

Definition of the Medical Word	Combining Form	Suffix	Build the Medical Word
Example: Abnormal condition (of being) humpbacked	**kyph/o-**	*-osis*	*kyphosis*

[*You think* abnormal condition *(-osis)* + humpbacked *(kyph/o-)*. *You change the order of the word parts to put the suffix last. You write* kyphosis.]

	Definition	Combining Form	Suffix	Build the Medical Word
1.	Tumor (made of) cartilage	chondr/o-		
2.	Pertaining to (being) present at birth	congenit/o-		
3.	Result of (bone) break(ing) up	fract/o-		
4.	Abnormal condition of making (the spine) fused together	ankyl/o-		
5.	Infection of (or) inflammation of (a) joint	arthr/o-		
6.	Abnormal condition (of having) swayback	lord/o-		
7.	Disease (of a) joint	arthr/o-		
8.	Infection of (or) inflammation of (a) vertebra	spondyl/o-		
9.	Tumor (of a) bone	oste/o-		
10.	Abnormal condition (of) dead tissue	necr/o-		
11.	Growth (on a) bone	oste/o-		
12.	Abnormal condition (of being) curved	scoli/o-		

C. Define Abbreviations

1. DJD _____

2. OA _____

3. RA _____

7.4 Laboratory, Diagnostic, and Radiologic Procedures

Word or Phrase	Description	Pronunciation/Word Parts

Laboratory Tests and Diagnostic Procedures

Word or Phrase	Description	Pronunciation/Word Parts
anti-CCP test	Blood test that measures the level of antibodies. It is always increased in patients with rheumatoid arthritis.	
rheumatoid factor (RF)	Blood test that is usually positive in patients with rheumatoid arthritis.	
uric acid	Blood test that has an elevated level in patients with gout and gouty arthritis	**uric acid** (YOOR-ik AS-id)

Radiologic and Nuclear Medicine Procedures

Word or Phrase	Description	Pronunciation/Word Parts
arthrography	Procedure that uses a radiopaque contrast dye that is injected into a joint. It coats and outlines the bone ends and joint capsule. An x-ray, **CT (computerized tomography) scan**, or MRI scan is done. The x-ray, CT, or MRI image is an **arthrogram**.	**arthrography** (ar-THRAW-grah-fee) **arthr/o-** *joint* **-graphy** *process of recording* **arthrogram** (AR-throh-gram) **arthr/o-** *joint* **-gram** *picture; record*
bone density tests	Procedure that measures the **bone mineral density (BMD)** to determine if demineralization from osteoporosis has occurred (see Figure 7-26 ■). The heel or wrist bone can be tested, but the hip and spine bones give a more accurate result. Also known as **bone densitometry**. There are two types of bone density tests: DEXA scan and quantitative computerized tomography. • A **DEXA scan** (dual-energy x-ray absorptiometry) uses two (dual) x-ray beams with different energy levels to create a two-dimensional image. This scan can detect as little as a 1 percent loss of bone. • **Quantitative computerized tomography (QCT)** uses an x-ray beam and a CT scan to create a three-dimensional image. QCT can measure the density of both cancellous and cortical bone. Cancellous bone is the first to be affected by osteoporosis and the first to respond to therapy.	**densitometry** (DEN-sih-TAW-meh-tree) **densit/o-** *density* **-metry** *process of measuring* **DEXA** (DEK-sah) *DEXA* stands for *dual-energy x-ray absorptiometry.* **tomography** (toh-MAW-grah-fee) **tom/o-** *cut; layer; slice* **-graphy** *process of recording*

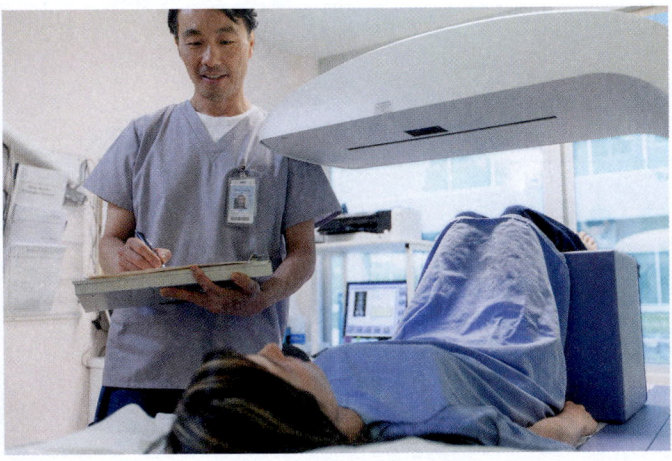

FIGURE 7-26 ■ Bone densitometry.
A. This patient is having a bone mineral density test performed. The radiologic technician has positioned the patient with a foam block under the knees so that the hip is at a 90-degree angle to the spine. He is verifying the patient's identity and medical information, and then he will explain the test procedure and answer any questions that she has.

A.

Word or Phrase	Description	Pronunciation/Word Parts
	  B. **FIGURE 7-26 ■ (continued)** **B.** The x-ray on the left shows the hip with a rectangular box around the neck of the femur, an area that has been found to be the optimum site for predicting the risk of hip fracture from osteoporosis. The same image on the right is color-coded, with green related to areas of bone that are the least dense and white related to those that are the most dense.	
bone scintigraphy	Nuclear medicine procedure in which a phosphate compound is tagged with the radioactive tracer technetium-99m and injected intravenously. This is taken up into the bone, and a gamma scintillation camera detects gamma rays from the radioactive tracer. Areas of increased uptake ("hot spots") indicate arthritis, fracture, osteomyelitis, cancerous tumors of the bone, or areas of bony metastasis. The nuclear medicine image is a **scintigram**.	**scintigraphy** (sin-TIH-grah-fee) 　**scint/i-** *point of light* 　**-graphy** *process of recording* **scintigram** (SIN-tih-gram) 　**scint/i-** *point of light* 　**-gram** *picture; record*
x-ray	Procedure that uses x-rays to diagnose bony abnormalities in any part of the body. X-rays are the primary means for diagnosing fractures, dislocations, and bone tumors.	**x-ray** (EKS-ray)

Clinical Connections

Radiology. Magnetic resonance imaging (MRI) uses a strong magnetic field to align protons in the atoms of the patient's body. The protons emit signals to form a series of thin, successive images or "slices" of a body structure. An MRI scan can be done with or without contrast dye.

A standard x-ray is not used to measure bone mineral density because patients must lose at least 30 percent of their bone mass before the loss can be detected on an x-ray image. After menopause, a woman can lose 1–2 percent of her bone mass each year.

7.4 PRACTICE LAPS

Use the Answer Key at the end of the book to check your answers.

A. Give the Meaning of Combining Forms

Next to each combining form, write its meaning. The first one has been done for you.

Combining Form	Meaning
1. **scint/i-**	*point of light*
2. arthr/o-	
3. densit/o-	
4. tom/o-	

continued on next page

B. Build Words

Read the definition of the medical word. Look at the combining form that is given. Select the correct suffix from the Suffix List, and write it on the blank line. Then build the medical word, and write it on the line. (Remember: You may need to remove the combining vowel. Always remove the hyphens and slash.) Be sure to check your spelling.

Suffix List

-gram (picture; record)	-graphy (process of recording)	-metry (process of measuring)

Definition of the Medical Word	Combining Form	Suffix	Build the Medical Word
Example: Picture (generated by many) point(s) of light	**scint/i-**	*-gram*	*scintigram*

[*You think* picture (-gram) + point of light *(scint/i-). You change the order of the word parts to put the suffix last. You write* scintigram.]

1. Process of recording (a) joint	arthr/o-		
2. Process of measuring (the bone) density	densit/o-		
3. Process of recording (a) slice (of an image)	tom/o-		
4. Picture (of a) joint	arth/o-		

C. Define Abbreviations

1. BMD _____	3. RF _____
2. CT _____	4. MRI _____

7.5 Medical Procedures, Drugs, and Surgical Procedures

Word or Phrase	Description	Pronunciation/Word Parts

Medical Procedures

cast	Procedure in which a layer of plaster or fiberglass is applied around a fractured bone and adjacent areas to immobilize the fracture in a fixed position and facilitate healing (see Figure 7-27 ■ and Figure 7-28 ■). For fractures of the leg, the physician may order the patient to be non–weight bearing (putting no weight on the affected leg), toe touch (partial weight bearing), or full weight bearing (with a walking cast). Patients with leg casts are instructed in the use of crutches.	**cast** (KAST)

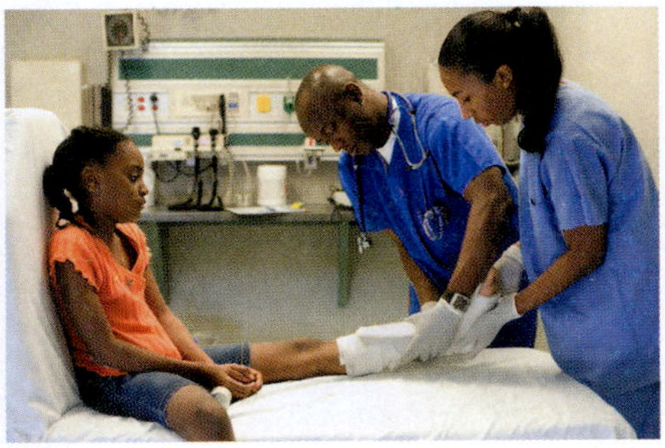

FIGURE 7-27 ■ **Application of a cast.**
This patient sustained a fractured fibula from a bike accident. The emergency department physician is applying padding, which will be followed by a plaster cast.

Word or Phrase	Description	Pronunciation/Word Parts
	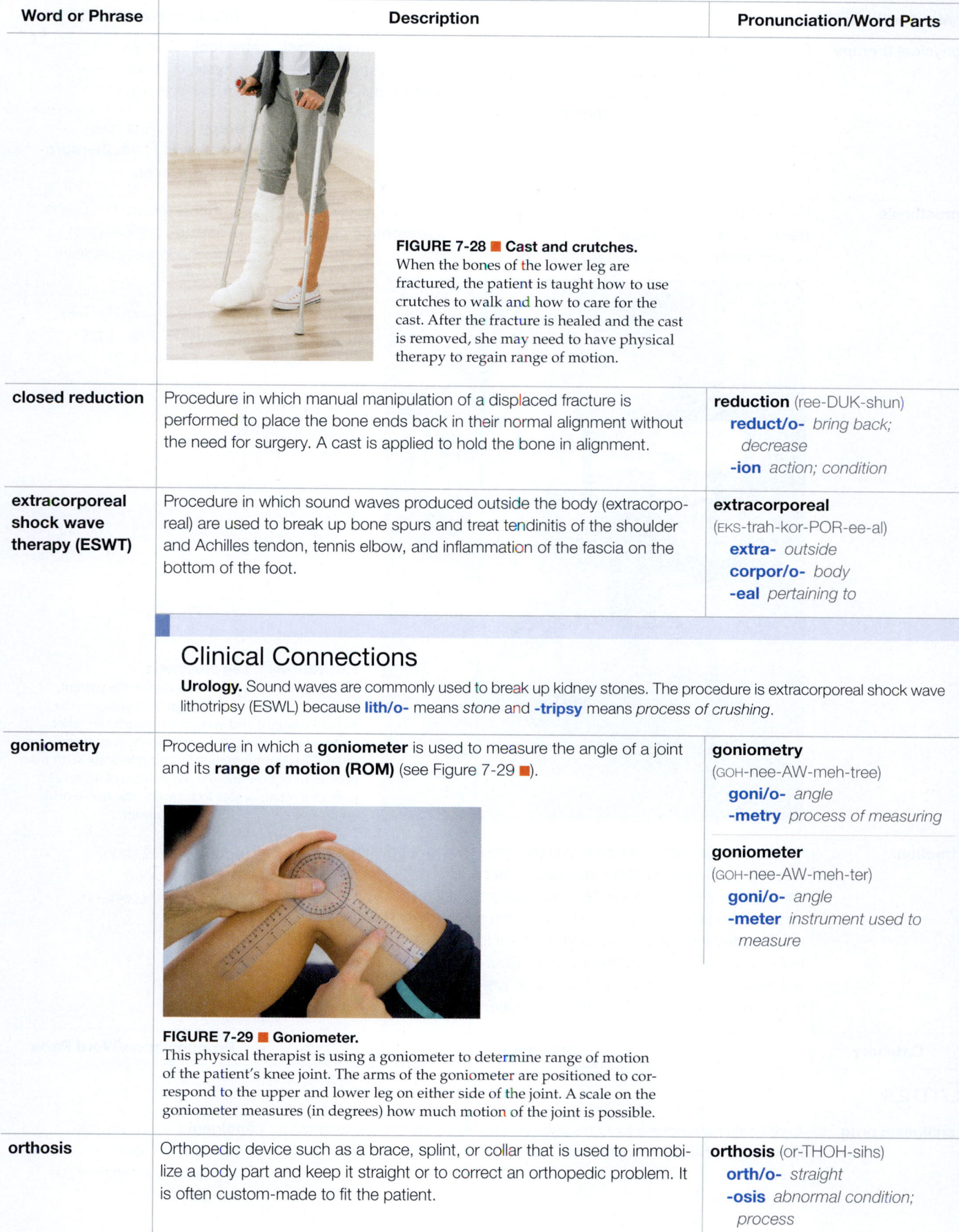 **FIGURE 7-28 ■ Cast and crutches.** When the bones of the lower leg are fractured, the patient is taught how to use crutches to walk and how to care for the cast. After the fracture is healed and the cast is removed, she may need to have physical therapy to regain range of motion.	
closed reduction	Procedure in which manual manipulation of a displaced fracture is performed to place the bone ends back in their normal alignment without the need for surgery. A cast is applied to hold the bone in alignment.	**reduction** (ree-DUK-shun) **reduct/o-** *bring back; decrease* **-ion** *action; condition*
extracorporeal shock wave therapy (ESWT)	Procedure in which sound waves produced outside the body (extracorporeal) are used to break up bone spurs and treat tendinitis of the shoulder and Achilles tendon, tennis elbow, and inflammation of the fascia on the bottom of the foot.	**extracorporeal** (EKS-trah-kor-POR-ee-al) **extra-** *outside* **corpor/o-** *body* **-eal** *pertaining to*

Clinical Connections

Urology. Sound waves are commonly used to break up kidney stones. The procedure is extracorporeal shock wave lithotripsy (ESWL) because **lith/o-** means *stone* and **-tripsy** means *process of crushing*.

goniometry	Procedure in which a **goniometer** is used to measure the angle of a joint and its **range of motion (ROM)** (see Figure 7-29 ■). 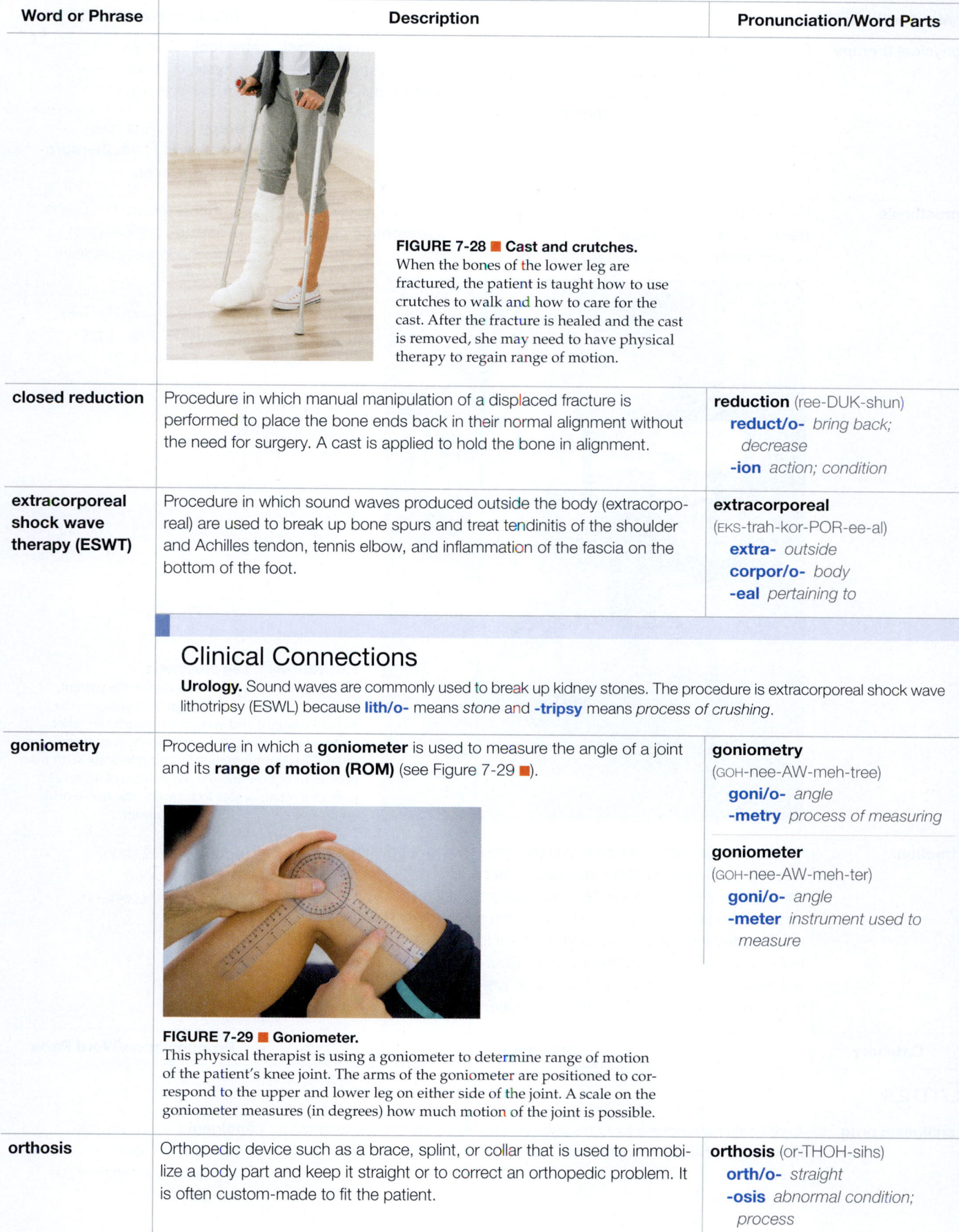 **FIGURE 7-29 ■ Goniometer.** This physical therapist is using a goniometer to determine range of motion of the patient's knee joint. The arms of the goniometer are positioned to correspond to the upper and lower leg on either side of the joint. A scale on the goniometer measures (in degrees) how much motion of the joint is possible.	**goniometry** (GOH-nee-AW-meh-tree) **goni/o-** *angle* **-metry** *process of measuring* **goniometer** (GOH-nee-AW-meh-ter) **goni/o-** *angle* **-meter** *instrument used to measure*
orthosis	Orthopedic device such as a brace, splint, or collar that is used to immobilize a body part and keep it straight or to correct an orthopedic problem. It is often custom-made to fit the patient.	**orthosis** (or-THOH-sihs) **orth/o-** *straight* **-osis** *abnormal condition; process*

Word or Phrase	Description	Pronunciation/Word Parts
physical therapy	Procedure that uses exercises to improve a patient's range of motion, joint mobility, strength, and balance. Active exercises are done by the patient. Passive exercises are done by the therapist who moves the patient's body.	**physical** (FIZ-ih-kal) **physic/o-** *body* **-al** *pertaining to* **therapy** (THAIR-ah-pee) The combining form **therap/o-** means *treatment*.
prosthesis	Orthopedic device such as an artificial leg for a patient who has had amputation of a limb (see Figure 7-30 ■). Also known as a **prosthetic device**. An implanted artificial joint is also a prosthetic device. **FIGURE 7-30** ■ **Leg prosthesis.** Each prosthesis is custom-built for the patient, using computer-aided design, according to the patient's height and weight (to match the other leg) and according to where the leg was amputated. This young man is learning to walk with his prosthetic leg on the uneven surface of a gravel path in a rehab center to simulate the real-world environment he will soon encounter.	**prosthesis** (praws-THEE-sihs) **prosth/o-** *artificial part* **-esis** *abnormal condition; process* **prosthetic** (praws-THET-ik) **prosth/o-** *artificial part* **-etic** *pertaining to*
traction	Procedure that uses a weight to pull the bone ends of a fracture into correct alignment. Skin traction uses elastic wraps, straps, halters, or skin adhesives connected to a pulley and a weight. Skeletal traction uses pins, wires, or tongs inserted into the bone during surgery. Halo traction uses pins inserted into the cranium and attached to a circular metal frame that forms a halo around the patient's head. Bars connect the halo to a rigid vest that immobilizes the chest and back while exerting upward traction on the head to straighten a fracture of the spine.	**traction** (TRAK-shun) **tract/o-** *pulling* **-ion** *action; condition*

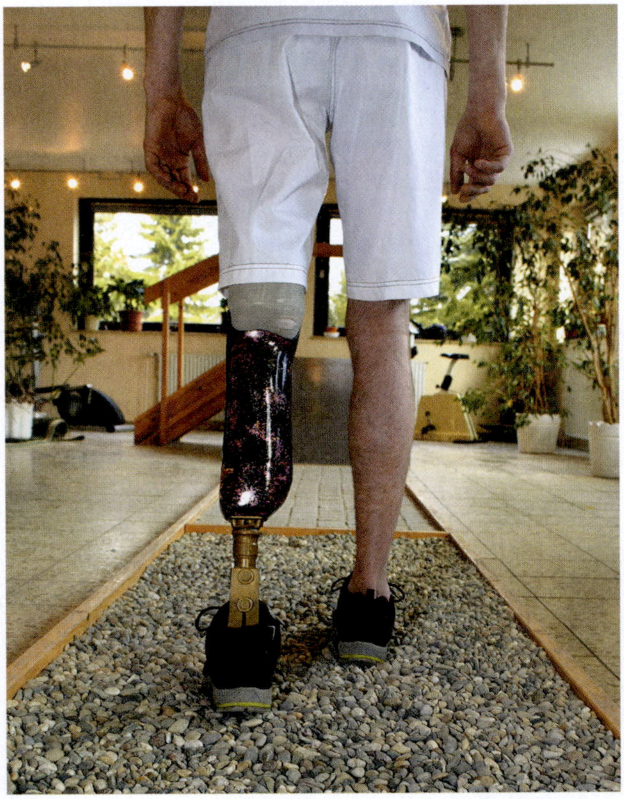

Category	Indication	Pronunciation/Word Parts

Drugs

analgesic drug	Treats pain from bone injury or surgery. Over-the-counter drugs treat mild-to-moderate pain. Prescription narcotic drugs are used to treat severe pain.	**analgesic** (AN-al-JEE-zik) **an-** *not; without* **alges/o-** *sensation of pain* **-ic** *pertaining to*

Category	Indication	Pronunciation/Word Parts
bone resorption inhibitor drug	Inhibits osteoclasts from breaking down bone; used to prevent and treat osteoporosis	**resorption** (ree-SORP-shun) **re-** *again and again; backward; unable to* **sorpt/o-** *absorb* **-ion** *action; condition*
corticosteroid drug	Decreases severe inflammation. Given orally or by **intra-articular injection** into a joint to treat osteoarthritis and rheumatoid arthritis.	**corticosteroid** (KOR-tih-koh-STAIR-oyd) **cortic/o-** *cortex; outer region* **-steroid** *steroid* **intra-articular** (IN-trah-ar-TIH-kyoo-lar) **intra-** *within* **articul/o-** *joint* **-ar** *pertaining to*
gold compound drug	Inhibits the autoimmune response that attacks the joints and connective tissue in patients with rheumatoid arthritis. These drugs actually contain gold.	
nonsteroidal anti-inflammatory drug (NSAID)	Treats mild-to-moderate inflammation and pain due to osteoarthritis and orthopedic injuries	**nonsteroidal** (NON-steh-ROY-dal) **non-** *not* **steroid/o-** *steroid* **-al** *pertaining to* **anti-inflammatory** (AN-tee-in-FLAM-ah-TOR-ee) **anti-** *against* **inflammat/o-** *redness and warmth* **-ory** *having the function of*

Word or Phrase	Description	Pronunciation/Word Parts

Surgical Procedures

amputation	Procedure to remove all or part of an extremity because of trauma, cardiovascular disease, or diabetes mellitus. A **below-the-knee amputation (BKA)** is at the level of the tibia and fibula. An **above-the-knee amputation (AKA)** is at the level of the femur. A muscle flap is wrapped over the end of the amputated limb to provide a cushion and some bulk so the patient can be fitted with an artificial limb (prosthesis). A patient who has had an amputation is an **amputee**.	**amputation** (AM-pyoo-TAY-shun) **amput/o-** *cut off* **-ation** *being; having; process* **amputee** (AM-pyoo-tee) **amput/o-** *cut off* **-ee** *person who is the object of an action; thing that is the object of an action*
arthrocentesis	Procedure to remove an accumulation of fluid from an injured joint by using a needle inserted into the joint space. It is also done to inject a drug to control inflammation and pain.	**arthrocentesis** (AR-throh-sen-TEE-sihs) **arthr/o-** *joint* **-centesis** *procedure to puncture*
arthrodesis	Procedure to fuse the bones in a deteriorated, unstable joint	**arthrodesis** (AR-throh-DEE-sihs) **arthr/o-** *joint* **-desis** *procedure to fuse together*

Word or Phrase	Description	Pronunciation/Word Parts
arthroscopy	Procedure that uses an **arthroscope** to visualize structures inside the joint (see Figure 7-31 ■). Other instruments can be inserted through the arthroscope to scrape or cut damaged cartilage or smooth sharp bone edges. 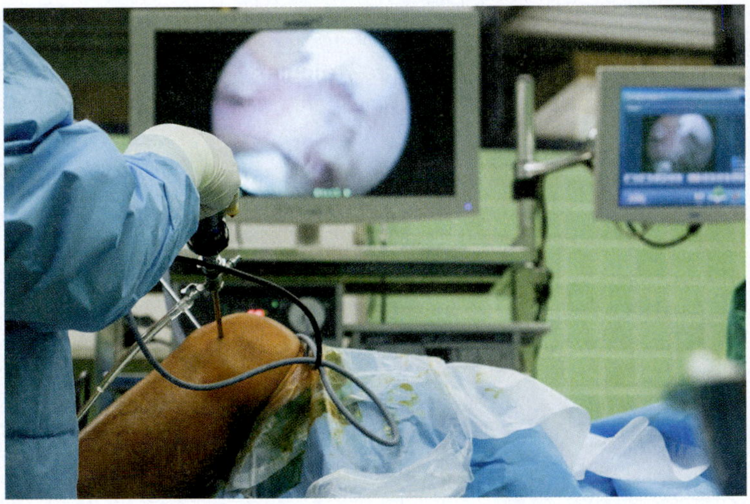 **FIGURE 7-31 ■ Arthroscopic surgery.** The arthroscope was inserted into the knee joint through a surgically created portal (opening in the skin). Other portals were created to insert other instruments. A fiberoptic light and magnifying lens on the arthroscope allow the surgeon to see inside the joint, and the image is also displayed on a computer screen in the operating room.	**arthroscopy** (ar-THRAW-skoh-pee) **arthr/o-** *joint* **-scopy** *process of using an instrument to examine* **arthroscope** (AR-throh-skohp) **arthr/o-** *joint* **-scope** *instrument used to examine* **arthroscopic** (AR-throh-SKAW-pik) **arthr/o-** *joint* **scop/o-** *examine with an instrument* **-ic** *pertaining to*
bone graft	Procedure that uses whole bone or bone chips to repair fractures with extensive bone loss or defects due to bone cancer. Bone taken from the patient's own body is an **autograft**. Frozen or freeze-dried bone taken from a cadaver is an **allograft**.	**graft** (GRAFT) **autograft** (AW-toh-graft) **aut/o-** *self* **-graft** *tissue for implant or transplant* **allograft** (AL-oh-graft) **all/o-** *other; strange* **-graft** *tissue for implant or transplant*
bunionectomy	Procedure to remove the prominent part of the metatarsal bone that is causing a bunion in patients with hallux valgus	**bunionectomy** (BUN-yun-EK-toh-mee) **bunion/o-** *bunion* **-ectomy** *surgical removal*
cartilage transplantation	Procedure that replaces damaged cartilage as an alternative to a total knee replacement. It is used to treat middle-aged adults (as opposed to older adults) with degenerative joint disease of the knee who have an active lifestyle.	**transplantation** (TRANS-plan-TAY-shun) **transplant/o-** *move and put in another place* **-ation** *being; having; process*
external fixation	Procedure used to treat a complicated fracture. An external fixator orthopedic device has metal pins that are inserted into the bone on either side of the fracture and connected to a metal frame. This immobilizes the fracture. A similar device is used to perform a **leg lengthening** to treat a congenitally short leg. It has screws that are turned daily, pulling the cut ends of bone apart so that new bone grows in the gap and lengthens the leg.	**external** (eks-TER-nal) **extern/o-** *outside* **-al** *pertaining to* **fixation** (fik-SAY-shun) **fixat/o-** *make stable* **-ion** *action; condition*

Word or Phrase	Description	Pronunciation/Word Parts
joint replacement surgery	Procedure to replace a joint that has been destroyed by trauma or osteoarthritis. A metal or plastic joint prosthesis is inserted (see Figure 7-32 ■). This surgery is done on the hips as a **total hip replacement (THR)**, or the knees, shoulders, or small joints of the fingers. For a total hip replacement, the head of the patient's femur is removed. The stem (long metal projection) of the prosthesis is hammered into the cut end of the femur. The head (ball) of the prosthesis is matched to the size of the patient's acetabulum. The cup of the prosthesis is used to replace the patient's acetabulum, and the ball is inserted into the cup. Also known as an **arthroplasty**.	**arthroplasty** (AR-throh-PLAS-tee) **arthr/o-** *joint* **-plasty** *process of reshaping by surgery*

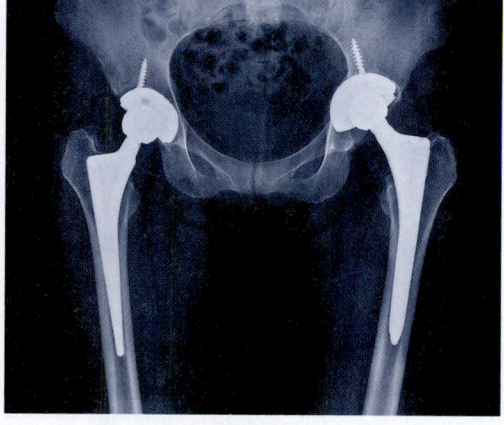

FIGURE 7-32 ■ Hip prostheses.
This patient had two total hip replacement surgeries at different times and now has bilateral hip prostheses. The metal components of each prosthesis stand out clearly on an x-ray.

Word or Phrase	Description	Pronunciation/Word Parts
open reduction and internal fixation (ORIF)	Procedure to treat a complicated fracture. An incision is made to open the skin and visualize the fracture, the fracture is reduced (realigned), and an internal fixation procedure is done using screws, nails, or plates to hold the fracture fragments in correct anatomical alignment (see Figure 7-33 ■).	**reduction** (ree-DUK-shun) **reduct/o-** *bring back; decrease* **-ion** *action; condition*

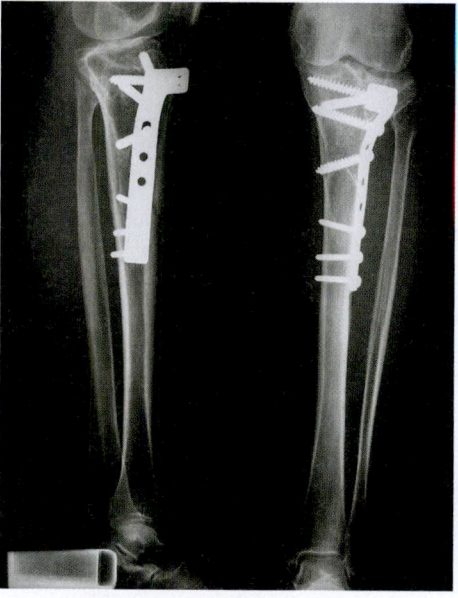

FIGURE 7-33 ■ Orthopedic plate and screws.
These x-rays show two different patients who had fractures of the tibia that were repaired in different ways using metal plates or multiple screws to stabilize the bone fragments.

Dive Deeper

Orthopedic surgery is not unlike carpentry, but instead of wood, the surgeon works on bone. Surgical orthopedic instruments include hammers, nails, screws, metal plates, chisels, mallets, gouges, and saws. An **osteotome** is used to cut bone. A **rongeur** is a forceps that is used to remove small bone fragments.

osteotome (AW-stee-oh-TOHM)
oste/o- *bone*
-tome *area with distinct edges; instrument used to cut*
rongeur (rawn-ZHUR)

7.5 PRACTICE LAPS

Use the Answer Key at the end of the book to check your answers.

A. Give the Meaning of Combining Forms

Next to each combining form, write its meaning. The first one has been done for you.

Combining Form	Meaning	Combining Form	Meaning
1. **steroid/o-**	*steroid*	12. goni/o-	
2. alges/o-		13. inflammat/o-	
3. all/o-		14. orth/o-	
4. amput/o-		15. physic/o-	
5. arthr/o-		16. prosth/o-	
6. articul/o-		17. reduct/o-	
7. aut/o-		18. scop/o-	
8. bunion/o-		19. sorpt/o-	
9. corpor/o-		20. therap/o-	
10. cortic/o-		21. tract/o-	
11. fixat/o-		22. transplant/o-	

B. Build Words

Read the definition of the medical word. Look at the combining form that is given. Select the correct suffix from the Suffix List, and write it on the blank line. Then build the medical word, and write it on the line. (Remember: You may need to remove the combining vowel. Always remove the hyphens and slash.) Be sure to check your spelling.

Suffix List

-al (pertaining to)
-ation (being; having; process)
-centesis (procedure to puncture)
-desis (procedure to fuse together)
-ectomy (surgical removal)
-ee (person who is the object of an action)

-esis (abnormal condition; process)
-etic (pertaining to)
-graft (tissue for implant or transplant)
-ion (action; condition)
-meter (instrument used to measure)
-metry (process of measuring)

-osis (abnormal condition; process)
-plasty (process of reshaping by surgery)
-scope (instrument used to examine)
-scopy (process of using an instrument to examine)

Definition of the Medical Word	Combining Form	Suffix	Build the Medical Word
Example: Pertaining to (the) body	**physic/o-**	*-al*	*physical*

[*You think* pertaining to (-al) + body (physic/o-). You change the order of the word parts to put the suffix last. You write physical.]

1. Pertaining to (an) artificial part	prosth/o-		
2. Instrument used to examine (a) joint	arthr/o-		

Definition of the Medical Word	Combining Form	Suffix	Build the Medical Word
3. Surgical removal (of a) bunion	bunion/o-	_____	_____
4. Person who is the object of an action (to) cut off	amput/o-	_____	_____
5. Process of measuring (the joint) angle	goni/o-	_____	_____
6. Process (of using a device to make a bone) straight	orth/o-	_____	_____
7. Procedure to fuse (a) joint	arthr/o-	_____	_____
8. Process of reshaping by surgery (on a) joint	arthr/o-	_____	_____
9. Process (of a body part being) cut off	amput/o-	_____	_____
10. Tissue for implant (from one's) self	aut/o-	_____	_____
11. Action (to) bring back (bone alignment)	reduct/o-	_____	_____
12. Process (to) move and put in another place	transplant/o-	_____	_____
13. Process of using an instrument to examine (a) joint	arthr/o-	_____	_____
14. Instrument used to measure (a joint) angle	goni/o-	_____	_____
15. Process (of having an) artificial part (of the body)	prosth/o-	_____	_____
16. Action (to) make stable	fixat/o-	_____	_____
17. Procedure to puncture (a) joint	arthr/o-	_____	_____
18. Tissue for implant (from some) other (person)	all/o-	_____	_____

C. Define Abbreviations

1. ESWT _____

2. NSAID _____

3. ROM _____

4. THR _____

Abbreviations Summary

AKA	above-the-knee amputation		**LUE**	left upper extremity
anti-CCP	anti-cyclic citrullinated peptide		**MCP**	metacarpophalangeal (joint)
BKA	below-the-knee amputation		**MRI**	magnetic resonance imaging
BMD	bone mineral density		**NSAID**	nonsteroidal anti-inflammatory drug
C1	first cervical vertebra (atlas)		**OA**	osteoarthritis
C2	second cervical vertebra (axis)		**ORIF**	open reduction and internal fixation
C1–C7	cervical vertebrae		**ortho**	orthopedics (short form)
CT	computerized tomography		**PT**	physical therapist; physical therapy
D.C.	Doctor of Chiropracty		**QCT**	quantitative computerized tomography
DEXA	dual-energy x-ray absorptiometry		**RA**	rheumatoid arthritis
DIP	distal interphalangeal (joint)		**RF**	rheumatoid factor
DJD	degenerative joint disease		**RLE**	right lower extremity
D.O.	Doctor of Osteopathy		**ROM**	range of motion
D.P.M.	Doctor of Podiatric Medicine		**RUE**	right upper extremity
ESWT	extracorporeal shock wave therapy		**S1**	first sacral vertebra
FX, Fx	fracture		**T1–T12**	thoracic vertebrae
L1–L5	lumbar vertebrae		**THR**	total hip replacement
LLE	left lower extremity		**tib-fib**	tibia-fibula (short form)

Word Alert

Abbreviations. Abbreviations are commonly used in all types of medical documents; however, they can mean different things to different people and their meanings can be misinterpreted. Always verify the meaning of an abbreviation.

- *AKA* means *above-the-knee amputation*, but it also means the English phrase *also known as*.
- *OA* means *osteoarthritis*, but it also means *Overeaters Anonymous*.
- *PT* means *physical therapist* and *physical therapy*, but it also means *prothrombin time*.
- *RA* means *rheumatoid arthritis*, but it also means *right atrium* (of the heart) or *room air*.
- *ROM* means *range of motion*, but it also means *rupture of membranes* (before the birth of a baby).

It's Greek To Me! Did you notice that some words have two different combining forms? Combining forms from both Greek and Latin remain a part of medical language today.

Word	Greek	Latin	Medical Word Examples
bone	oste/o-	osse/o-, oss/i-	osteoarthritis; osseous, ossicle
cartilage	chondr/o-	cartilagin/o-	costochondral; cartilaginous
fibula	perone/o-	fibul/o-	peroneal; fibular
joint	arthr/o-	articul/o-	arthroscopy; articulation
vertebra	spondyl/o-	vertebr/o-	spondylolisthesis; vertebral

Career Focus

Meet Jennifer, a radiologic technologist

"I became an x-ray technologist because I wanted to be in a profession where I worked with all different patients. You get to work in the emergency room; you get to work doing procedures alongside a physician, dealing with acutely ill patients. You also get to go to the operating room. We also deal with outpatients. We not only do routine x-rays, but we're also involved in minor procedures, along with assisting the radiologists during upper GIs, barium enemas, etc. You're not in any single area all the time, and it's just very nice to see every aspect of the hospital. We use medical terminology every day in our profession. When reading the requisitions that are sent in from the doctors' offices or notifying nurses if we have questions about a patient's exam, we need to use appropriate medical terminology."

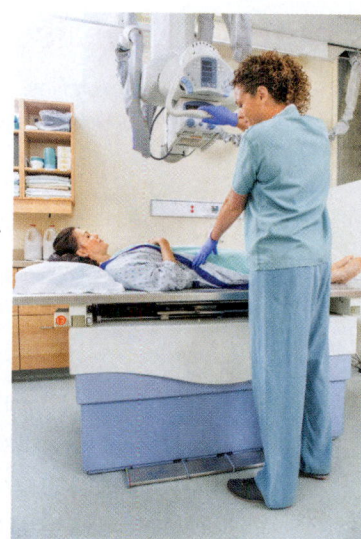

- **Radiologic technologists** are allied health professionals who perform and document a variety of radiologic procedures and assist the radiologist in the radiology and nuclear medicine department in a hospital or in a diagnostic imaging outpatient facility.

- **Radiologists** are physicians who practice in the medical specialty of radiology. They view and interpret the results of radiologic procedures to diagnose conditions of all body systems. Nuclear medicine physicians practice in the medical specialty of nuclear medicine. They view and interpret the results of nuclear medicine procedures.

- **Orthopedists** are physicians who practice in the medical specialty of orthopedics. They diagnose and treat patients with skeletal and muscular problems. Orthopedists are physicians who have an M.D. (Doctor of Medicine) degree. When they perform surgery, they are known as orthopedic surgeons. Physicians can take additional training and become board certified in the subspecialty of pediatric orthopedics.

- **Rheumatologists** are physicians who specialize in treating inflammatory and degenerative diseases of the joints.

- **Osteopaths** have a D.O. (Doctor of **Osteopathy** or Osteopathic Medicine). They diagnose and treat patients based on prevention, the use of nutrition, and keeping the body structures in a normal anatomical relationship.

- **Chiropractors** have a D.C. (Doctor of Chiropracty or Chiropractic Medicine). They diagnose and treat patients with injuries of the bones, muscles, and nerves by manipulating the alignment of the vertebral column.

- **Podiatrists** have a D.P.M. (Doctor of **Podiatry** or Podiatric Medicine). They diagnose and treat medical and surgical conditions of the foot.

- Malignancies of the musculoskeletal system are treated medically by an oncologist or surgically by an orthopedic surgeon.

---

radiologic (RAY-dee-oh-LAW-jik)
  radi/o- forearm bone; radius; x-rays
  log/o- study of; word
  -ic pertaining to

technologist (tek-NAW-loh-jist)
  techn/o- technical skill
  log/o- study of; word
  -ist person who specializes in; thing that specializes in

radiologist (RAY-dee-AW-loh-jist)
  radi/o- forearm bone; radius; x-rays
  log/o- study of; word
  -ist person who specializes in; thing that specializes in

orthopedist (OR-thoh-PEE-dist)
  orth/o- straight
  ped/o- child
  -ist person who specializes in; thing that specializes in

rheumatologist (ROO-mah-TAW-loh-jist)
  rheumat/o- watery discharge
  log/o- study of; word
  -ist person who specializes in; thing that specializes in

osteopath (AW-stee-oh-PATH)
  oste/o- bone
  -path person treating disease

osteopathy (AW-stee-AW-pah-thee)
  oste/o- bone
  -pathy disease

chiropractor (KY-roh-PRAK-tor)
  chir/o- hand
  pract/o- medical practice
  -or person who does or produces; thing that does or produces
Chiropractor: *Person who does or produces (manipulation and alignment of the body with the) hands (to perform) medical practice*

podiatrist (poh-DY-ah-trist)
  pod/o- foot
  iatr/o- medical treatment; physician
  -ist person who specializes in; thing that specializes in

podiatry (poh-DY-ah-tree)
  pod/o- foot
  -iatry medical treatment

Chapter Review Exercises

Dive In: Medical Language Exercises

Test your knowledge of the chapter by completing these review exercises. Use the Answer Key at the end of the book to check your answers. Note: Each of the numbered exercise headers corresponds to a numbered learning outcome at the beginning of the chapter.

7.1 Anatomy

MATCHING EXERCISE

Match each word or phrase to its description.

1. acetabulum
2. calcaneus
3. carpal bones
4. coronal
5. diaphysis
6. foramen magnum
7. humerus
8. ilium
9. ligaments
10. mandible
11. medial malleolus
12. occipital bone
13. patella
14. radius
15. scapula
16. symphysis
17. thorax
18. xiphoid process

_____ kneecap
_____ suture between the frontal bone and parietal bones
_____ cranial bone that forms the posterior base of the skull
_____ facial bone that moves up and down when you chew
_____ pointed tip at the inferior end of the sternum
_____ opening in the base of the skull where the spinal cord enters
_____ contains the glenoid fossa area of the shoulder joint
_____ fibrous bands that connect bone to bone
_____ bone of the upper arm
_____ lower arm bone that is on the same side as the thumb
_____ bones of the wrist
_____ area between the neck and the diaphragm
_____ part of the hip bone where the head of the femur sits
_____ bony projection on the distal tibial bone
_____ heel bone
_____ slightly movable joint that joins the two pubic bones
_____ shaft of a long bone
_____ one of the hip bones

CIRCLE EXERCISE

Circle the correct answer from the choices given.

1. The bone of the upper arm is the (**acetabulum, fibula, humerus**).
2. The hip bone that has a large crest on it is the (**ilium, intervertebral disk, ischium**).
3. The tarsal bones are in the (**ankle, elbow, hand**).
4. If you hit your "funny bone," you would have hit the nerve that runs across the (**glenoid fossa, lateral malleolus, medial epicondyle**).
5. The olecranon is located in the (**ankle, elbow, hip**).
6. (**Parietal, Periosteum, Peroneal**) is an adjective for *fibula*.
7. The (**clavicle, coccyx, cranium**) is another name for the *collarbone*.

TRUE OR FALSE EXERCISE

*Indicate whether each statement is true or false by writing **T** or **F** on the line.*

1. _____ The parietal and temporal bones are in the cranium.
2. _____ The olecranon is a large, square bony projection on the ulna.
3. _____ The *humorous* is the name of the upper arm bone.

4. _____ The adjective form for *rib* is *costal*.

5. _____ The fibula is in the lower leg on the side of the little toe.

6. _____ The patella is a small bone that protects the knee joint.

PLURAL NOUN AND ADJECTIVE EXERCISE

Read the noun and write its plural form and/or adjective form on the line. Only write in the plural noun form if there is a blank line there for it. Be sure to check your spelling. The first one has been done for you.

Singular Noun	Plural Noun	Adjective	Singular Noun	Plural Noun	Adjective
1. **ligament**	*ligaments*	*ligamentous*	16. maxilla		
2. axis			17. nose		
3. bone			18. patella		
			19. pelvis		
			20. phalanx		
4. cartilage			21. pubis		
5. clavicle			22. radius		
6. cranium			23. rib		
7. coccyx			24. sacrum		
8. diaphysis			25. scapula		
9. femur			26. skeleton		
10. fibula			27. spine		
			28. sternum		
11. humerus			29. thorax		
12. ilium			30. tibia		
13. ischium			31. ulna		
14. malleolus			32. vertebra		
15. mandible			33. zygoma		

DIVIDING WORDS EXERCISE

Separate these words into their component parts (prefix, combining form, suffix). Some words do not contain all three word parts. The first one has been done for you.

Medical Word	Prefix	Combining Form	Suffix	Medical Word	Prefix	Combining Form	Suffix
1. **skeletal**		*skelet/o-*	*-al*	12. lumbar			
2. appendicular				13. mastoid			
3. articulation				14. maxillary			
4. cartilaginous				15. metacarpal			
5. cavity				16. osseous			
6. cervical				17. periosteal			
7. clavicular				18. sagittal			
8. coccygeal				19. sphenoid			
9. intercostal				20. synovial			
10. interphalangeal				21. thoracic			
11. lacrimal							

SPELLING EXERCISE

Read each medical word pronunciation and write the medical word that it represents. Be sure to check your spelling. The first one has been done for you.

1. **(pah-RY-eh-tal)** _____ *parietal* _____
2. (KAWK-siks) _____
3. (MUS-kyoo-loh-SKEL-eh-tal) _____
4. (zy-GOH-mah) _____
5. (klah-VIH-kyoo-lar) _____
6. (man-DIH-byoo-lar) _____
7. (ZY-foyd) _____

7.2 Physiology

CIRCLE EXERCISE

Circle the correct answer from the choices given.

1. Calcium in the blood comes from all of the following sources *except* (**foods, damaged bone that is broken down, calcitonin hormone**).
2. Gradually replacing cartilage with hard bone is the process of (**articulation, costochondral, ossification**).
3. Cells that maintain and monitor the minerals in the bones are (**osteoblasts, osteoclasts, osteocytes**).
4. In (**adolescence, adulthood, old age**), new bone formation exceeds bone breakdown.
5. (**Bone matrix, calcitonin, parathyroid hormone**) stimulates osteoclasts to break down bone.

TRUE OR FALSE EXERCISE

*Indicate whether each statement is true or false by writing **T** or **F** on the line.*

1. _____ Osteoblasts do not divide or move from within permanent bone.
2. _____ Bone is composed of several calcium salts and collagen fibers.
3. _____ Ossification takes place during childhood and adolescence.
4. _____ New bone forms along the epiphyseal growth plates.
5. _____ An astronaut's weightless environment increases new bone formation.

DIVIDING WORDS EXERCISE

Separate these words into their component parts (combining form, suffix). The first one has been done for you.

Medical Word	Combining Form	Suffix
1. **osteoblast**	*oste/o-*	*-blast*
2. osteocyte	_____	_____
3. ossification	_____	_____
4. osteoclast	_____	_____

SPELLING EXERCISE

Read each medical word pronunciation and write the medical word that it represents. Be sure to check your spelling. The first one has been done for you.

1. **(AW-stee-oh-KLAST)** _____ *osteoclast* _____
2. (AW-stee-oh-JEN-eh-sihs) _____
3. (AW-stee-oh-SITE) _____
4. (AW-sih-fih-KAY-shun) _____

7.3 Diseases

MATCHING EXERCISE

Match each word or phrase to its description.

1. arthralgia	_____ demineralization of the bone
2. arthropathy	_____ wear-and-tear disease of the joints
3. bunion	_____ bowleg
4. chondroma	_____ blood in the joint
5. comminuted	_____ dextro and levo are forms of this
6. compound	_____ pain in the joints
7. genu varum	_____ infection in the bone and bone marrow
8. gout	_____ malignant tumor of the bone
9. hemarthrosis	_____ caused by disease in the bone
10. osteoarthritis	_____ high level of uric acid
11. osteomyelitis	_____ fracture with bone crushed into pieces
12. osteoporosis	_____ common name for hallux valgus
13. osteosarcoma	_____ fracture where bone breaks the overlying skin
14. pathologic fracture	_____ benign tumor of cartilage
15. scoliosis	_____ one vertebra slips anteriorly over another
16. spondylolisthesis	_____ disease of a joint

CIRCLE EXERCISE

Circle the correct answer from the choices given.

1. Infection in the bone and bone marrow is known as (**osteoarthritis, osteomyelitis, osteoporosis**).
2. An injury that disrupts the blood flow to a bone can cause (**ankylosing spondylitis, avascular necrosis, bone tumor**).
3. (**Demineralization, Levoscoliosis, Malalignment**) is seen in patients with osteoporosis.
4. Trauma or hemophilia can cause (**chondromalacia, hemarthrosis, scoliosis**).
5. A congenital bony abnormality that affects the chest is (**gout, lordosis, pectus excavatum**).
6. Spondylolisthesis involves slipping of the (**joints, sutures, vertebrae**).
7. A (**comminuted, hairline, transverse**) fracture is one that is difficult to detect except on an x-ray.
8. Lyme disease is associated with all of the following *except* (**bull's-eye rash, clubfoot, infected deer tick**).
9. The grinding sound of bone rubbing against bone is (**arthralgia, crepitus, necrosis**).

TRUE OR FALSE EXERCISE

Indicate whether each statement is true or false by writing **T** *or* **F** *on the line.*

1. _____ Hallux valgus can be caused by wearing pointy-toed shoes.
2. _____ Gout is characterized by tophi.
3. _____ An osteophyte is a sharp bone spur that causes pain.
4. _____ Rheumatoid arthritis is a congenital disease that is present at birth.
5. _____ A torn meniscus is a tear of the cartilage pad between the vertebrae.
6. _____ Overstretching of a ligament around a joint causes a bone tumor.
7. _____ Ewing sarcoma is a cancerous bone tumor that occurs in young men.
8. _____ An osteoma is a malignant tumor of the bone.
9. _____ A Colles fracture is usually caused by a car accident.
10. _____ Osteoporosis can occur in both men and women.
11. _____ Scoliosis is an abnormal posterior curvature of the thoracic spine.

12. _____ Blood in a joint is hemarthrosis.

13. _____ Osteoarthritis is an autoimmune disease in which the body attacks its own cartilage.

14. _____ Pectus excavatum is another name for clubfoot.

DIVIDING WORDS EXERCISE

Separate these words into their component parts (prefix, combining form, suffix). Some words do not contain all three word parts. The first one has been done for you.

Medical Word	Prefix	Combining Form	Suffix	Medical Word	Prefix	Combining Form	Suffix
1. **congenital**		_congenit/o-_	_-al_	7. dislocation	_____	_____	_____
2. arthropathy		_____	_____	8. fracture		_____	_____
3. avascular	_____	_____	_____	9. kyphosis		_____	_____
4. chondroma		_____	_____	10. malalignment	_____	_____	_____
5. degenerative	_____	_____	_____	11. osteophyte		_____	_____
6. demineralization	_____	_____	_____				

SPELLING EXERCISE

Read each medical word pronunciation and write the medical word that it represents. Be sure to check your spelling. The first one has been done for you.

1. **(ar-THRY-tihs)** _____arthritis_____
2. (con-DROH-mah) _____
3. (FRAK-chur) _____

4. (ky-FOH-sihs) _____
5. (ar-THRAL-jah) _____
6. (AW-stee-oh-MY-eh-LY-tihs) _____

7.4 Laboratory, Diagnostic, and Radiologic Procedures

CIRCLE EXERCISE

Circle the correct word from the choices given.

1. A DEXA scan is also known as a/an (**arthrogram, bone densitometry, uric acid**).
2. A radiologic procedure that uses contrast dye injected into a joint is (**arthrography, bone density test, x-ray**).
3. To diagnose rheumatoid arthritis, the physician would check the (**bone density, rheumatoid factor, uric acid**).
4. All of the following are bone density tests *except* (**arthrogram, DEXA scan, quantitative computerized tomography**).

TRUE OR FALSE EXERCISE

Indicate whether each statement is true or false by writing **T** or **F** on the line.

1. _____ Bone density test results are most accurate when done on the heel or wrist bone.
2. _____ RF is a blood test that measures the level of antibodies in patients with rheumatoid arthritis.
3. _____ A picture of a joint using radiopaque contrast dye is an arthrogram.
4. _____ A standard x-ray can be used to measure bone mineral density.
5. _____ Bone scintigraphy can detect areas of increased uptake from arthritis, fractures, and cancer.
6. _____ An MRI uses a strong magnetic field to align protons in the atoms in the body.

SPELLING EXERCISE

Read each medical word pronunciation and write the medical word that it represents. Be sure to check your spelling. The first one has been done for you.

1. **(toh-MAW-grah-fee)** _____tomography_____
2. (EKS-ray) _____
3. (sin-TIH-grah-fee) _____

4. (ar-THRAW-grah-fee) _____
5. (DEN-sih-TAW-meh-tree) _____

7.5 Medical Procedures, Drugs, and Surgical Procedures

MATCHING EXERCISE

Match each word or phrase to its description.

1. analgesic drug
2. amputee
3. arthrocentesis
4. arthroplasty
5. cast
6. physical therapy
7. prosthesis

_____ immobilizes a fracture

_____ needle inserted into a joint to remove fluid

_____ treats mild-to-moderate pain

_____ has had an amputation

_____ procedure to replace a joint

_____ uses exercises to improve range of motion

_____ artificial leg

CIRCLE EXERCISE

Circle the correct answer from the choices given.

1. The degree of joint movement is measured with a/an (**arthroscope, goniometer, osteotome**).
2. A patient with an amputated limb would be fitted with a (**brace, cast, prosthesis**).
3. A surgical procedure to fuse a degenerated, unstable joint is known as an (**allograft, arthrocentesis, arthrodesis**).
4. Gold compound drugs are used to treat (**fractures, osteoarthritis, rheumatoid arthritis**).
5. An orthopedic device such as a brace or splint is known as a/an (**cast, external fixation, orthosis**).
6. A transplant of bone from a cadaver is known as an (**allograft, arthroscopy, autograft**).
7. A bone resorption drug (**decreases severe inflammation, inhibits osteoclasts, treats pain**).

TRUE OR FALSE EXERCISE

*Indicate whether each statement is true or false by writing **T** or **F** on the line.*

1. _____ An arthroscope and a rongeur are surgical instruments.
2. _____ A goniometer is used to measure bone density.
3. _____ Traction uses weights to pull the bone ends of a fracture into alignment.
4. _____ Gold compound drugs are used to treat osteoporosis.
5. _____ A bunionectomy is used to treat a patient who has hallux valgus.
6. _____ ESWT uses sound waves to break up bone spurs.

DIVIDING WORDS EXERCISE

Separate these words into their component parts (prefix, combining form, suffix). Some words do not contain all three word parts. The first one has been done for you.

Medical Word	Prefix	Combining Form	Suffix	Medical Word	Prefix	Combining Form	Suffix
1. **nonsteroidal**	*non-*	*steroid/o-*	*-al*	6. bunionectomy		_____	_____
2. amputation		_____	_____	7. goniometer		_____	_____
3. analgesic		_____	_____	8. intra-articular	_____	_____	_____
4. arthrocentesis		_____	_____	9. orthosis		_____	_____
5. arthroscope		_____	_____	10. traction		_____	_____

SPELLING EXERCISE

Read each medical word pronunciation and write the medical word that it represents. Be sure to check your spelling. The first one has been done for you.

1. (ree-DUK-shun) _____*reduction*_____
2. (GOH-nee-AW-meh-tree) _____
3. (praws-THEE-sihs) _____
4. (AM-pyoo-TAY-shun) _____
5. (BUN-yun-EK-toh-mee) _____

RELATED COMBINING FORMS EXERCISE

Write the combining forms on the line provided. (Hint: See the It's Greek to Me! feature box.)

1. Three combining forms that mean *bone*. _____ _____ _____

2. Two combining forms that mean *cartilage*. _____ _____

3. Two combining forms that mean *joint*. _____ _____

4. Two combining forms that mean *vertebra*. _____ _____

5. Two combining forms that mean *fibula*. _____ _____

Immerse Yourself: Analyze Medical Reports

Electronic Patient Record #1

This is an Office Visit Note. Read the note and answer the questions.

PEARSON PRIMARY CARE ASSOCIATES

Task Edit View Time Scale Options Help

OFFICE VISIT NOTE

PATIENT NAME:	LOWE, James
PATIENT NUMBER:	63-1004
DATE OF VISIT:	November 19, xx

HISTORY

This is a 35-year-old male who has been having problems with intermittent low back pain for several years now. He leads an active lifestyle and his job requires him to do a lot of lifting and walking. The pain is getting worse, and he would like to get some definitive treatment at this time. He has been told in the past by a physician that his pelvis is tilted up on the left. However, he does not believe this was ever diagnosed as a leg-length discrepancy. He denies any radiation of the pain to his buttocks or legs, and he says he has not noticed any tingling in his lower extremities.

PHYSICAL EXAMINATION

Left leg: The leg length from the iliac crest to the medial malleolus is 106 cm. Right leg: The leg length from the iliac crest to the medial malleolus is 103 cm. Examination of his back reveals diffuse tenderness over the spinous processes in the lumbar region. I also noticed a dextroscoliosis in the lower thoracic region, which seemed to be significant. Neurologically, the patient had normal reflexes and normal strength in the lower extremities.

ASSESSMENT

Chronic back pain due to a significant leg-length discrepancy. He also has a dextroscoliosis, although the exact number of degrees of curvature was not measured.

PLAN

1. Refer to an orthopedist for a definitive diagnosis and measurement of the scoliosis.

2. Over-the-counter nonsteroidal anti-inflammatory drug.

Lien T. Nguyen, M.D.

Lien T. Nguyen, M.D.

LTN: lcc
D: 11/19/xx
T: 11/19/xx

1. Divide *dextroscoliosis* into its three word parts and give the meaning of each word part.

   Word Part   **Meaning**

   _____   _____

   _____   _____

   _____   _____

2. The adjective *spinal* refers to the spine or backbone while the adjective *spinous* refers to a bony process. True False

3. Divide *orthopedist* into its three word parts and give the meaning of each word part.

   Word Part   **Meaning**

   _____   _____

   _____   _____

   _____   _____

4. The patient's leg length was measured using what two anatomical structures? _____ _____

5. The medial malleolus is located on the distal end of what bone? _____

6. Which leg was shorter, the patient's right leg or left leg? _____

7. The spinous processes are located on what bones? _____

8. What is the single-letter designation for the vertebrae in the lumbar region? _____

9. Which way did the patient's spine curve? To the right or to the left? _____

10. What will the orthopedist measure that this physician did not measure during the office visit? _____

Electronic Patient Record #2

This is a Radiology Report. Read the report and answer the questions.

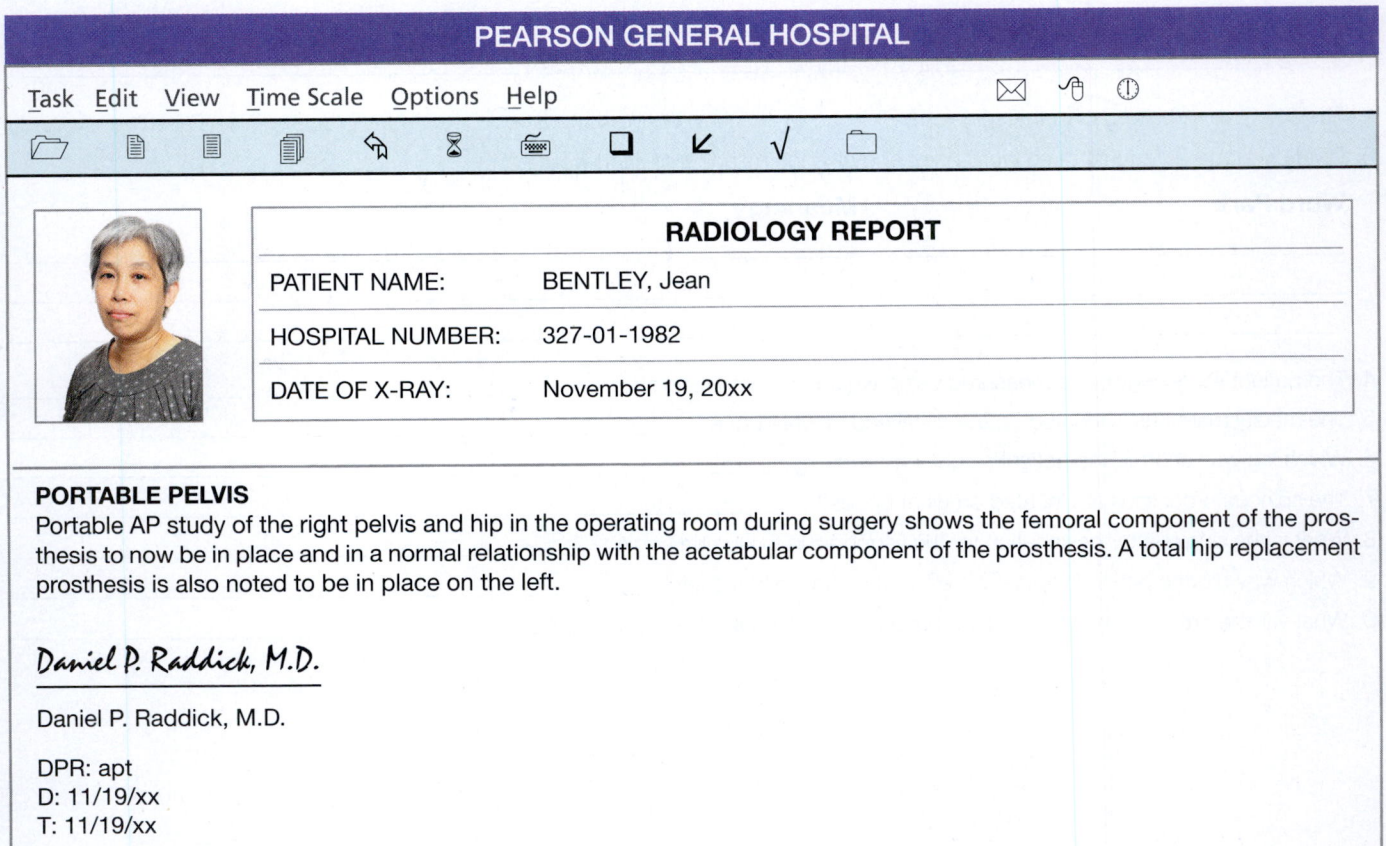

PEARSON GENERAL HOSPITAL

Task   Edit   View   Time Scale   Options   Help

RADIOLOGY REPORT

PATIENT NAME:	BENTLEY, Jean
HOSPITAL NUMBER:	327-01-1982
DATE OF X-RAY:	November 19, 20xx

PORTABLE PELVIS
Portable AP study of the right pelvis and hip in the operating room during surgery shows the femoral component of the prosthesis to now be in place and in a normal relationship with the acetabular component of the prosthesis. A total hip replacement prosthesis is also noted to be in place on the left.

Daniel P. Raddick, M.D.

Daniel P. Raddick, M.D.

DPR: apt
D: 11/19/xx
T: 11/19/xx

1. Where did the radiologic technologist have to go to take this x-ray? _____

2. When this x-ray was taken, the patient was undergoing a total hip replacement in which hip?   **Right   Left**

3. Define *prosthesis*. _____

4. The prosthesis had two parts: a _____ component and an _____ component.

MyLab Medical Terminology™

MyLab Medical Terminology is a premium online homework management system that includes a host of features to help you study. Registered users will find:

- A multitude of quizzes and activities built within the MyLab platform

- Powerful tools that track and analyze your results—allowing you to create a personalized learning experience

- Videos and audio pronunciations to help enrich your progress

- Streaming lesson presentations (guided lectures) and self-paced learning modules

- A space where you and your instructor can check your progress and manage your assignments

8 Orthopedics
Muscular System

Orthopedics (OR-thoh-PEE-diks) is the medical specialty that studies the anatomy and physiology of the skeletal and muscular systems; uses laboratory, diagnostic, and radiologic procedures to diagnose skeletal and muscular diseases; and uses medical procedures, drugs, and surgical procedures to treat skeletal and muscular diseases. In this chapter, you will study orthopedics from the perspective of the muscular system.

∨ Chapter Overview and Learning Outcomes

After you study this chapter, you should be able to demonstrate mastery of the outcomes by successfully completing the exercises.

8.1 Anatomy
Identify the structures of the muscular system.
Demonstrate proficiency in medical language.
8.1 Practice Laps

8.2 Physiology
Describe the functions of the muscular system.
Demonstrate proficiency in medical language.
8.2 Practice Laps
Vocabulary Review

8.3 Diseases
Describe common muscular diseases.
Demonstrate proficiency in medical language.
8.3 Practice Laps

8.4 Laboratory, Diagnostic, and Radiologic Procedures
Describe common muscular laboratory tests, diagnostic procedures, and radiologic procedures.
Demonstrate proficiency in medical language.
8.4 Practice Laps

8.5 Medical Procedures, Drugs, and Surgical Procedures
Describe common muscular medical procedures, drugs, and surgical procedures.
Demonstrate proficiency in medical language.
8.5 Practice Laps
Abbreviations Summary
Career Focus

Chapter Review Exercises
Dive In: Medical Language Exercises
(Learning Outcomes 8.1–8.5)

Immerse Yourself: Analyze Medical Reports

Medical Language Key

To unlock the definition of a medical word, first break it into word parts. Then give the meaning of each word part. Put the meanings of the word parts in order, beginning with the meaning of the suffix, then the meaning of the prefix (if there is one), then the meaning of the combining form.

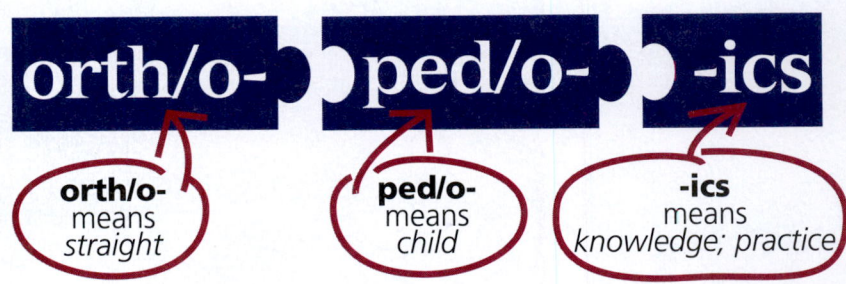

orth/o- ⬭ ped/o- ⬭ -ics

orth/o- means *straight*

ped/o- means *child*

-ics means *knowledge; practice*

Orthopedics: ▶ *Knowledge and practice (of producing) straight(ness of the bones and muscles in a) child (or adult).*

The **muscular system** is the body system that moves the bony framework of the body (see Figure 8-1 ■). There are approximately 700 skeletal **muscles** in the body, as well as tendons and other structures. The contours of some skeletal muscles are visible under the skin, particularly when they contract. Others are located more deeply, but their movements can be felt. All of the skeletal muscles in the body (or the muscles in a particular part of the body) are the **musculature**.

The functions of the muscular system are to help maintain body position and produce movements of the bony framework. The muscular system is also known as the **musculoskeletal system** because it works in conjunction with the skeletal system (described in Chapter 7, Orthopedics: Skeletal System). Without the muscles, the bones would not be able to move, and, without the bones, the muscles would lack support. The muscles also work in conjunction with the nervous system. The muscles contract in response to conscious thought as the brain sends electrical impulses through the nerves to cause the muscles to contract.

8.1 Anatomy

Types of Muscles

There are three types of muscles: skeletal muscles, the cardiac muscle, and smooth muscles (see Figure 8-2 ■). Each type of muscle has its own unique characteristics. Of the three types of muscles, only skeletal muscle belongs to the muscular system. In the rest of this chapter, the word *muscle* should be understood to mean *skeletal muscle*.

- **Skeletal muscles:** Skeletal muscles provide the means by which the body moves. Skeletal muscles are **voluntary muscles** that contract and relax in response to conscious thought. Each muscle cell has multiple nuclei and **striations** (bands of color) when seen under a microscope.
- **Cardiac muscle:** The cardiac muscle of the heart pumps blood through the circulatory system (described in Chapter 5, Cardiology). It is an involuntary muscle that is not under conscious control. Each cardiac muscle cell has a single nucleus and fewer and less prominent striations than a skeletal muscle cell.
- **Smooth muscles:** Smooth muscles form a continuous, thin layer around many body organs and structures (blood vessels, bronchi, intestines, etc.). These are involuntary muscles that are not under conscious control. Smooth muscle cells have a single nucleus and no striations.

Tendons and Related Structures

A muscle is attached to a bone by a **tendon**, a cord-like, nonelastic, white fibrous band of connective tissue (see Figure 8-3 ■). Each muscle is wrapped in **fascia**, a thin connective tissue that merges into the tendon. An **aponeurosis** is a wide, white fibrous sheet of connective tissue, sometimes

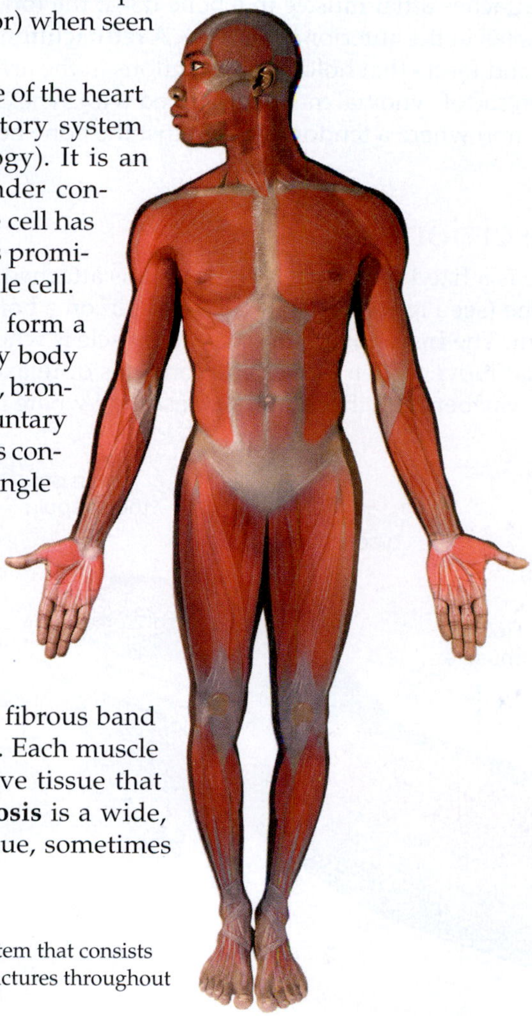

FIGURE 8-1 ■ Muscular system.
The muscular system is a widespread body system that consists of the voluntary skeletal muscles and other structures throughout the body.

Pronunciation/Word Parts

muscular (MUS-kyoo-lar)
  muscul/o- *muscle*
  -ar *pertaining to*
The combining forms **my/o-** and **myos/o-** also mean *muscle.*

muscle (MUS-el)

musculature (MUS-kyoo-lah-CHUR)
  muscul/o- *muscle*
  -ature *system composed of*

musculoskeletal
(MUHS-kyoo-loh-SKEL-eh-tal)
  muscul/o- *muscle*
  skelet/o- *skeleton*
  -al *pertaining to*

skeletal (SKEL-eh-tal)
  skelet/o- *skeleton*
  -al *pertaining to*

voluntary (VAW-lun-TAIR-ee)
  volunt/o- *one's own will*
  -ary *pertaining to*

striation (stry-AA-shun)
  stri/o- *parallel stripes*
  -ation *being; having; process*

cardiac (KAR-dee-ak)
  cardi/o- *heart*
  -ac *pertaining to*

tendon (TEN-dun)

tendinous (TEN-dih-nuhs)
  tendin/o- *tendon*
  -ous *pertaining to*
The combining form **ten/o-** also means *tendon.*

fascia (FASH-ee-ah)

fascial (FASH-ee-al)
  fasci/o- *fascia*
  -al *pertaining to*

aponeurosis (AP-oh-nyoor-OH-sihs)

FIGURE 8-2 ■ Types of muscle.
There are three types of muscles—skeletal muscles, the cardiac muscle, and smooth muscles. Each has a different appearance under a microscope. Note the very prominent color bands (striations) and multiple nuclei in each skeletal muscle cell. Cardiac muscle cells have fewer and less prominent bands, and smooth muscle cells have no bands.

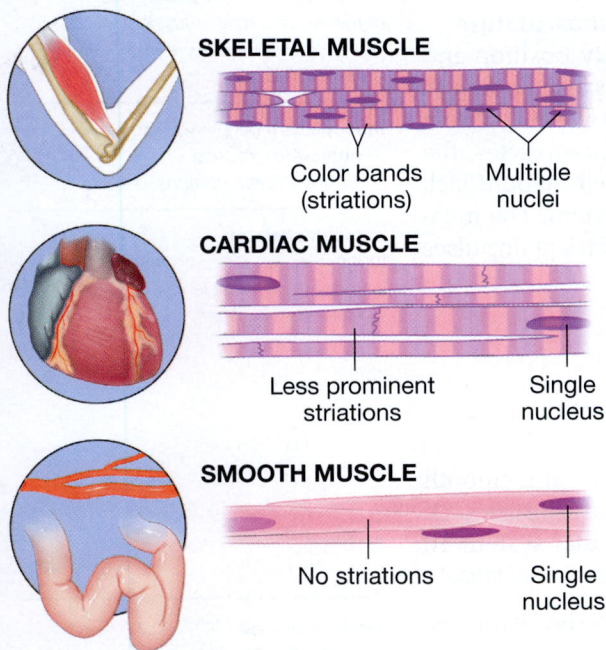

SKELETAL MUSCLE
Color bands (striations)   Multiple nuclei

CARDIAC MUSCLE
Less prominent striations   Single nucleus

SMOOTH MUSCLE
No striations   Single nucleus

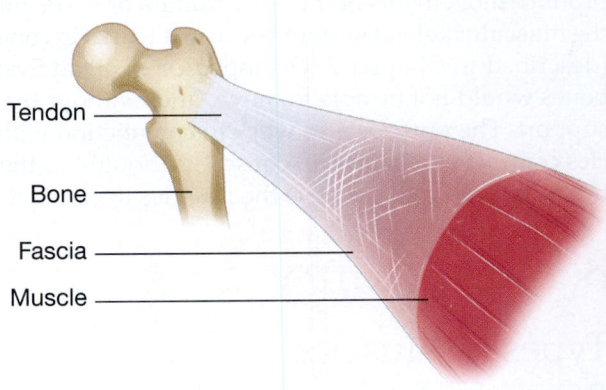

Tendon
Bone
Fascia
Muscle

FIGURE 8-3 ■ Tendon
At their origins and insertions, most muscles are attached to the bone by a tendon. As the muscle transitions to the tendon, the red color of the muscle is replaced by the white fibrous tissue of the tendon. The fascia that surrounds the muscle also merges with the tendon.

composed of several tendons, that attaches a flat muscle to a bone (as at the top of the skull) or to other, deeper muscles (as in the anterior abdomen). A **retinaculum** is a translucent band of fibrous tissue and fascia that holds down tendons in the areas of the wrist and ankle. A **bursa**, a thin sac of synovial membrane filled with synovial fluid, acts as a cushion to reduce friction where a tendon rubs against the bone near a synovial joint.

Muscle Origins and Insertions

The **origin** or beginning of a muscle is a fixed point where its tendon is attached to a stationary or nearly stationary bone (see Figure 8-4 ■). From its origin on a bone, the muscle often travels across a joint. The **insertion** or ending of a muscle is where its tendon is attached to the bone that moves when the muscle contracts or relaxes. The **belly** of a muscle is usually midway between the origin and insertion where the muscle mass is the greatest.

Pronunciation/Word Parts

retinaculum (RET-ih-NAK-yoo-lum)

bursa (BER-sah)

bursae (BER-see)
Latin plural noun: Change the singular ending *-a* to *-ae*.

bursal (BER-sal)
　burs/o- *bursa*
　-al *pertaining to*

origin (OR-ih-jin)

insertion (in-SER-shun)
　insert/o- *introduce; put in*
　-ion *action; condition*

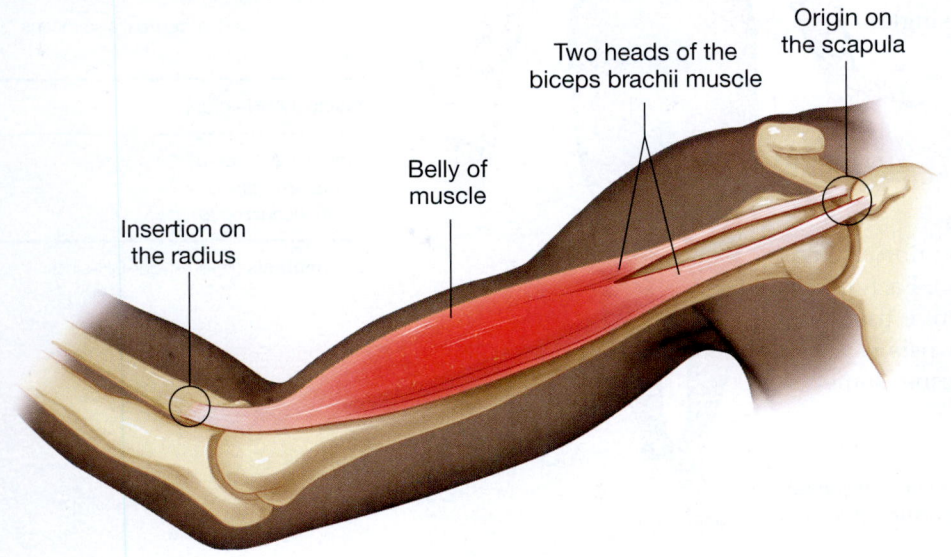

Two heads of the biceps brachii muscle
Origin on the scapula
Belly of muscle
Insertion on the radius

FIGURE 8-4 ■ Origin and insertion of a muscle.
Every muscle has at least one point of origin on a stationary (or nearly stationary) bone and an insertion on a bone that moves when the muscle contracts. The biceps brachii muscle has two origins whose tendons are right next to each other but are on different parts of the scapula bone. The other tendon of this muscle crosses the elbow joint and ends at its insertion on the radius. When the biceps brachii muscle contracts, the radius is pulled toward the upper arm and the arm flexes.

Types of Muscle Movement

Muscles function in pairs whose movements are antagonistic or synergistic to each another. **Antagonism** occurs when one muscle contracts and another muscle relaxes to allow movement or partially contracts to control the movement. Contraction of the biceps muscle and simultaneous relaxation of the triceps muscle in the arm (described in a later section) is an example of antagonism. **Synergism** occurs when one muscle contracts and other nearby muscles also contract to produce the same but greater combined movement. Contraction of the biceps muscle and simultaneous contraction of the brachioradialis muscle in the arm is an example of synergism. **Flexion** and **extension**, **abduction** and **adduction**, **rotation** to the right and to the left, **supination** and **pronation**, and **eversion** and **inversion** are opposite movements that are controlled by muscle pairs (see Figures 8-5 ■ through 8-7 ■ and Table 8-1).

Pronunciation/Word Parts

antagonism (an-TAG-oh-nizm)
　antagon/o- *opposing effect*
　-ism *disease from a specific cause; process*

synergism (SIN-er-jizm)
　synerg/o- *joined, enhanced effect*
　-ism *disease from a specific cause; process*

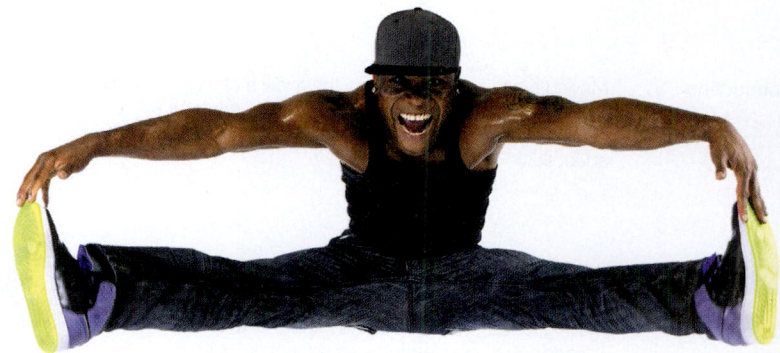

FIGURE 8-5 ■ Extension, abduction, pronation, and dorsiflexion.
This dancer has his arms and legs in extension and abduction. His hands are in pronation, and his feet are in dorsiflexion.

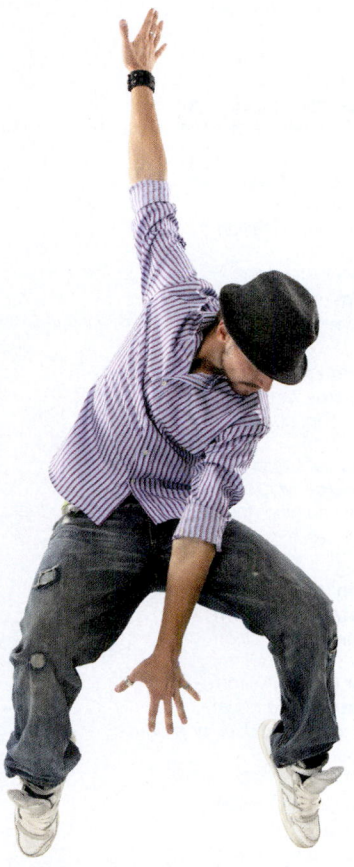

FIGURE 8-6 ■ Extension, adduction, abduction, flexion, plantar flexion, and rotation.
This dancer has his arms in extension with his left arm in adduction. His thighs are in abduction with his knees in flexion and his feet in plantar flexion. His head is rotated to the left.

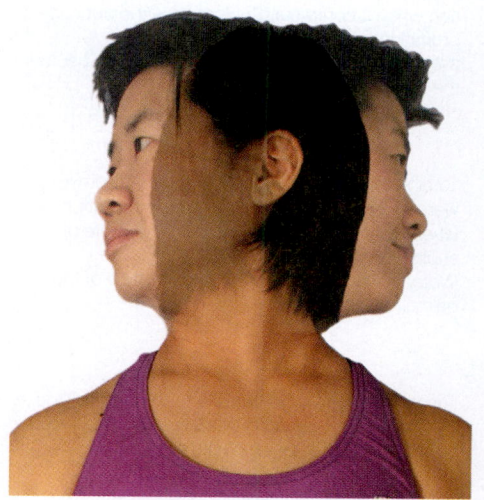

FIGURE 8-7 ■ Rotation.
The head rotates to the right and left around its axis, which is the vertebral column.

Table 8-1 Types of Muscle Movement

Movement	Description	Muscle Type	Pronunciation/Word Parts
flexion	Bending a joint to decrease the angle between two bones or two body parts. A **flexor** muscle produces flexion when it contracts. Flexion is the opposite of extension. (*Note*: Plantar flexion of the foot causes the toes to point downward. Dorsiflexion of the foot causes the toes to point upward.)	flexor	**flexion** (FLEK-shun) **flex/o-** *bending* **-ion** *action; condition* **flexor** (FLEK-sor) **flex/o-** *bending* **-or** *person who does or produces; thing that does or produces*
extension	Straightening and extending a joint to increase the angle between two bones or two body parts. An **extensor** muscle produces extension when it contracts. Extension is the opposite of flexion.	extensor	**extension** (eks-TEN-shun) **extens/o-** *straightening* **-ion** *action; condition* **extensor** (eks-TEN-sor) **extens/o-** *straightening* **-or** *person who does or produces; thing that does or produces*
abduction	Moving a body part away from the midline of the body. An **abductor** muscle produces abduction when it contracts. Abduction is the opposite of adduction.	abductor	**abduction** (ab-DUK-shun) **ab-** *away from* **duct/o-** *bring; duct; move* **-ion** *action; condition* **abductor** (ab-DUK-tor) **ab-** *away from* **duct/o-** *bring; duct; move* **-or** *person who does or produces; thing that does or produces*
adduction	Moving a body part toward the midline of the body. An **adductor** muscle produces adduction when it contracts. Adduction is the opposite of abduction.	adductor	**adduction** (ad-DUK-shun) **ad-** *toward* **duct/o-** *bring; duct; move* **-ion** *action; condition* **adductor** (ad-DUK-tor) **ad-** *toward* **duct/o-** *bring; duct; move* **-or** *person who does or produces; thing that does or produces*
rotation	Moving a body part around its axis. A **rotator** muscle produces rotation when it contracts.	rotator	**rotation** (roh-TAY-shun) **rotat/o-** *rotate* **-ion** *action; condition* **rotator** (ROH-tay-tor) **rotat/o-** *rotate* **-or** *person who does or produces; thing that does or produces*
supination	Turning the palm of the hand superiorly or upward. A **supinator** muscle produces supination when it contracts. Supination is the opposite of pronation. (*Note:* Here, *lying on the back* refers to the back of the hand.)	supinator	**supination** (soo-pih-NAY-shun) **supinat/o-** *lying on the back* **-ion** *action; condition* **supinator** (SOO-pih-NAY-tor) **supinat/o-** *lying on the back* **-or** *person who does or produces; thing that does or produces*
pronation	Turning the palm of the hand inferiorly or downward. A **pronator** muscle produces pronation when it contracts. Pronation is the opposite of supination. (*Note:* Here, *face down* refers to the face of the palm.)	pronator	**pronation** (proh-NAY-shun) **pronat/o-** *face down* **-ion** *action; condition* **pronator** (proh-NAY-tor) **pronat/o-** *face down* **-or** *person who does or produces; thing that does or produces*
eversion	Turning a body part outward and toward the side. An **evertor** muscle produces eversion when it contracts. Eversion is the opposite of inversion.	evertor	**eversion** (ee-VER-zhun) **e-** *out; without* **vers/o-** *travel; turn* **-ion** *action; condition* **evertor** (ee-VER-tor) **e-** *out; without* **vert/o-** *travel; turn* **-or** *person who does or produces; thing that does or produces*

Movement	Description	Muscle Type	Pronunciation/Word Parts
inversion	Turning a body part inward. An **invertor** muscle produces inversion when it contracts. Inversion is the opposite of eversion.	invertor	**inversion** (in-VER-zhun) **in-** *in; not; within* **vers/o-** *travel; turn* **-ion** *action; condition* **invertor** (in-VER-tor) **in-** *in; not; within* **vert/o-** *travel; turn* **-or** *person who does or produces; thing that does or produces*

Muscle Names

Muscle names can seem complex because they are in Latin, but they relate to some of the Latin words for the bones, or they describe where the muscle is located, its shape, its size, or what action it performs (see Table 8-2).

Table 8-2   Examples of Muscle Names and Their Meanings

Muscle Name	What the Muscle Name Tells You	Pronunciation/Word Parts
biceps brachii	Shape: Origin of the muscle has two parts or heads (*biceps*) Location: Arm (*brachii*)	**biceps** (BY-seps) The prefix **bi-** means *two*. The suffix **-ceps** is from the Latin word *caput* (head). **brachii** (BRAY-kee-eye)
brachioradialis	Location: Radial bone (*radialis*) in the arm (*brachii*)	**brachioradialis** (BRAY-kee-oh-RAY-dee-AL-ihs) **brachi/o-** *arm* **radi/o-** *forearm bone; radius; x-rays* **-alis** *pertaining to*
extensor digitorum	Action: Extends Location: Digits (*digitorum*)	**extensor** (eks-TEN-sor) **extens/o-** *straightening* **-or** *person who does or produces; thing that does or produces* **digitorum** (DIJ-ih-TOR-um)
flexor hallucis brevis	Action: Flexes Location: Big toe (*hallux*) Size: Short (*brevis*)	**flexor** (FLEK-sor) **flex/o-** *bending* **-or** *person who does or produces; thing that does or produces* **hallucis** (HAL-yoo-sihs) **brevis** (BREV-ihs)
gluteus maximus	Location: Buttocks (*gluteus*) Size: Large (*maximus*)	**gluteus** (GLOO-tee-uhs) **maximus** (MAK-sih-muhs)
rectus abdominis	Orientation: Straight up and down (*rectus*) Location: Abdomen (*abdominis*)	**rectus** (REK-tuhs) **abdominis** (ab-DAW-mih-nihs)
temporalis	Location: Temporal bone (*temporalis*) of the cranium	**temporalis** (TEM-poh-RAY-lihs) **tempor/o-** *side of the head; temple* **-alis** *pertaining to*
triceps brachii	Shape: Origin of the muscle has three parts or heads (*triceps*) Location: Arm (*brachii*)	**triceps** (TRY-seps) The prefix **tri-** means *three*.

Muscles of the Head and Neck

These are the most important muscles of the head and neck (see Figure 8-8 ■).

- **Frontalis**: Moves the eyebrows and wrinkles the forehead skin.
- **Orbicularis oculi**: Closes the eyelids and presses them together.
- **Orbicularis oris**: Closes the lips and presses them together.
- **Buccinator**: Moves the cheeks.
- **Temporalis**: Moves the mandible (lower jaw) upward and backward.
- **Masseter**: Moves the mandible (lower jaw) upward.
- **Platysma**: Moves the mandible (lower jaw) down.
- **Sternocleidomastoid**: Bends the head toward the sternum (flexion) and turns the head to either side (rotation).

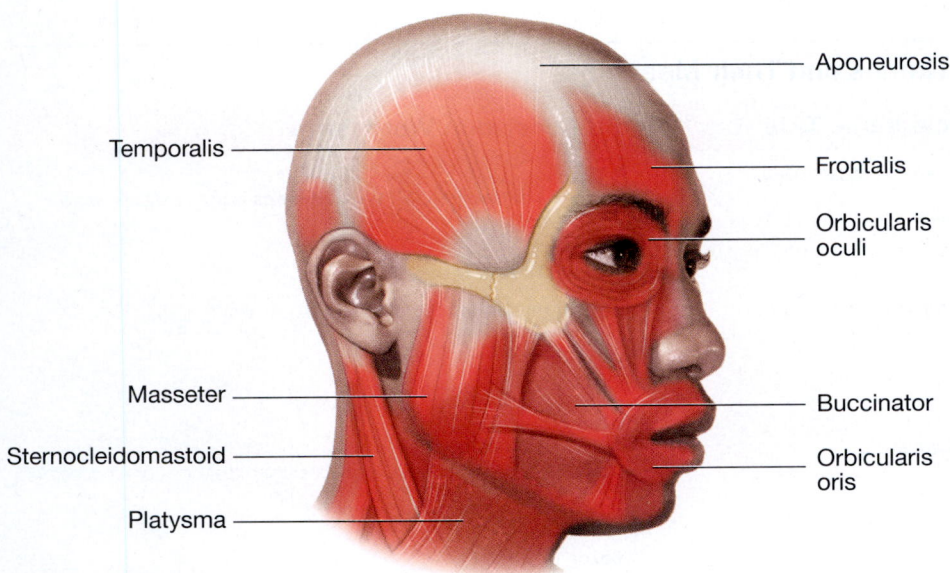

Temporalis

Masseter

Sternocleidomastoid

Platysma

Aponeurosis

Frontalis

Orbicularis oculi

Buccinator

Orbicularis oris

FIGURE 8-8 ■ Muscles of the head and neck.
These muscles contract and relax when you close your eyes, make facial expressions, chew food, or move your head.

Pronunciation/Word Parts

frontalis (frun-TAY-lihs)
  front/o- *front*
  -alis *pertaining to*

orbicularis (or-BIH-kyoo-LAIR-ihs)
  orbicul/o- *small circle*
  -aris *pertaining to*

oculi (AW-kyoo-lie)

oris (OR-ihs)

buccinator (BUK-sih-NAY-tor)
  buccin/o- *cheek*
  -ator *person who does or produces; thing that does or produces*

temporalis (TEM-poh-RAY-lihs)
  tempor/o- *side of the head; temple*
  -alis *pertaining to*

masseter (MAS-eh-ter)
  masset/o- *chewing*
  -er *person who does or produces; thing that does or produces*

platysma (plah-TIZ-mah)

sternocleidomastoid
(STER-noh-KLY-doh-MAS-toyd)
  stern/o- *breastbone; sternum*
  cleid/o- *clavicle; collarbone*
  mast/o- *breast; mastoid process*
  -oid *resembling*
Note: The origin of this muscle has two heads, one on the sternum and one on the clavicle. Its insertion is on the mastoid process of the temporal bone behind the ear.

Muscles of the Shoulders, Chest, and Back

These are the most important muscles of the shoulders, chest, and back (see Figure 8-9 ■ and Figure 8-10 ■).

- **Trapezius**: Raises the shoulder, pulls the shoulder blades together, and elevates the clavicle. Turns the head from side to side (rotation). Moves the head posteriorly (extension).
- **Deltoid**: Raises the arm and moves the arm away from the body (abduction).
- **Pectoralis major**: Moves the arm anteriorly and medially across the chest (adduction).
- **Latissimus dorsi**: Moves the arm posteriorly and medially toward the vertebral column (adduction).
- **Intercostal muscles**: Muscle pairs between the ribs; one contracts during inspiration to spread the ribs apart; the other contracts during forced expiration, coughing, or sneezing to pull the ribs together.

Pronunciation/Word Parts

trapezius (trah-PEE-zee-uhs)
This muscle is shaped like a trapezoid, a geometric figure that has two parallel sides and two nonparallel sides.

deltoid (DEL-toyd)
delt/o- triangle
-oid resembling
This muscle is shaped like a triangle. In the Greek alphabet, the capital letter *delta* is in the shape of a triangle.

pectoralis (PEK-toh-RAY-lihs)
pector/o- chest
-alis pertaining to

latissimus (lah-TIH-sih-muhs)

dorsi (DOR-sigh)

intercostal (IN-ter-KAW-stal)
inter- between
cost/o- rib
-al pertaining to

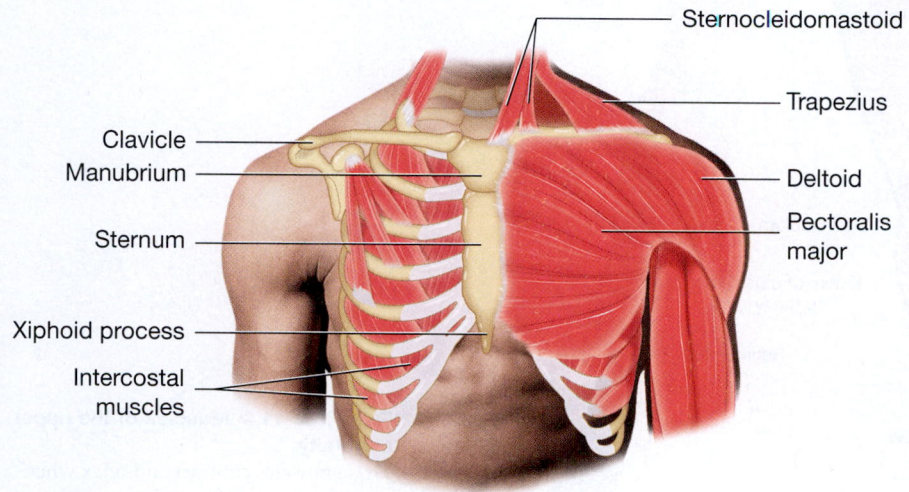

Sternocleidomastoid
Trapezius
Clavicle
Manubrium
Deltoid
Sternum
Pectoralis major
Xiphoid process
Intercostal muscles

FIGURE 8-9 ■ Muscles of the shoulders and chest.
These muscles contract and relax when you raise your arms, move your arms and shoulders toward the midline to hug someone, or rotate your arms inwardly.

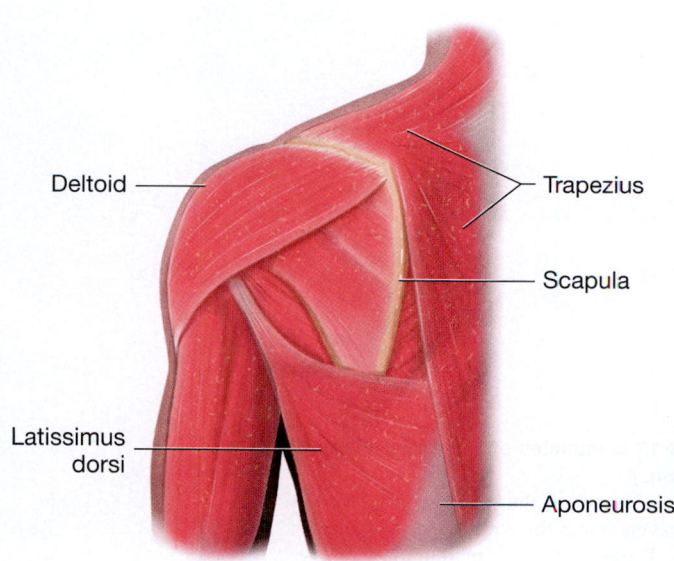

Deltoid
Trapezius
Scapula
Latissimus dorsi
Aponeurosis

FIGURE 8-10 ■ Muscles of the shoulders and back.
These muscles contract and relax when you shrug your shoulders or pull your shoulder blades together to sit up straight. They also move your head backward and to the side and turn your trunk to the right or left.

Muscles of the Upper Extremity

These are the most important muscles of the arm and hand (see Figure 8-11 ■ and Figure 8-12 ■).

- **Biceps brachii**: Bends the upper arm toward the shoulder (flexion) and bends the lower arm toward the upper arm (flexion).
- **Brachioradialis**: Bends the lower arm toward the upper arm (flexion).
- **Triceps brachii**: Straightens the lower arm (extension).
- **Thenar muscles**: Bend the thumb (flexion) and move it toward the palm (adduction).

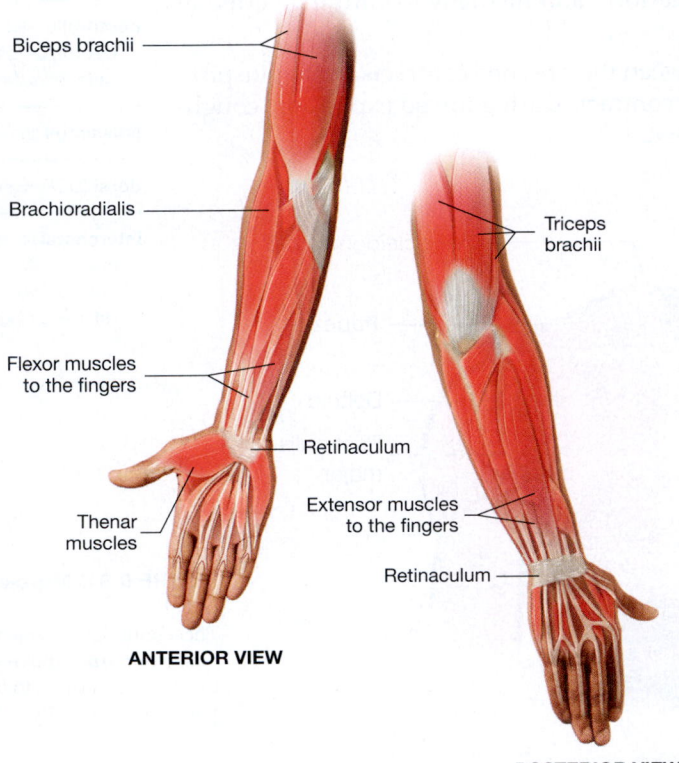

Biceps brachii

Brachioradialis

Flexor muscles to the fingers

Thenar muscles

Retinaculum

ANTERIOR VIEW

Triceps brachii

Extensor muscles to the fingers

Retinaculum

POSTERIOR VIEW

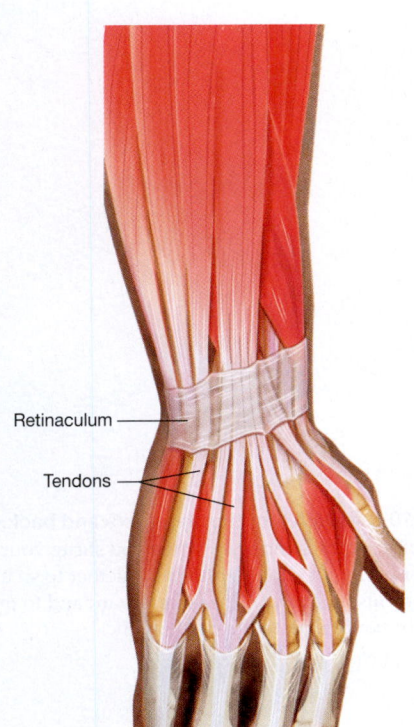

Retinaculum

Tendons

Pronunciation/Word Parts

biceps (BY-seps)
The origin of the biceps muscle has two parts (**bi-**) or heads (**-ceps**).

brachii (BRAY-kee-eye)

brachioradialis
(BRAY-kee-oh-RAY-dee-AL-ihs)
    brachi/o- *arm*
    radi/o- *forearm bone; radius; x-rays*
    -alis *pertaining to*

triceps (TRY-seps)
The origin of the triceps muscle has three parts (**tri-**) or heads (**-ceps**).

thenar (THEE-nar)
    then/o- *thumb*
    -ar *pertaining to*

FIGURE 8-11 ■ **Muscles of the upper extremity.**
These muscles contract and relax when you lift a heavy box, straighten your arms to do a handstand, shake hands, make a fist, or play the piano.

FIGURE 8-12 ■ **Muscles of the forearm and the retinaculum.**
Each extensor muscle of the forearm has a long tendon that travels across the wrist to one or more of the fingers. These tendons are held in place by the retinaculum, a translucent band of tissue. When the extensor muscles in the forearm contract, they pull the tendons, which then pull on the finger bones to straighten and extend the fingers.

Muscles of the Abdomen

These are the most important muscles of the abdomen (see Figure 8-13 ■).

- **External abdominal oblique**: Bends the upper body forward (flexion), rotates the side of the body medially, and compresses the side of the abdominal wall.

- **Internal abdominal oblique**: Bends the upper body forward (flexion), rotates the side of the body medially, and compresses the side of the abdominal wall.

- **Rectus abdominis**: Bends the upper body forward (flexion) and compresses the anterior abdominal wall.

Pronunciation/Word Parts

external (eks-TER-nal)
  extern/o- *outside*
  -al *pertaining to*

abdominal (ab-DAW-mih-nal)
  abdomin/o- *abdomen*
  -al *pertaining to*

oblique (oh-BLEEK)

internal (in-TER-nal)
  intern/o- *inside*
  -al *pertaining to*

rectus (REK-tuhs)

abdominis (ab-DAW-mih-nihs)

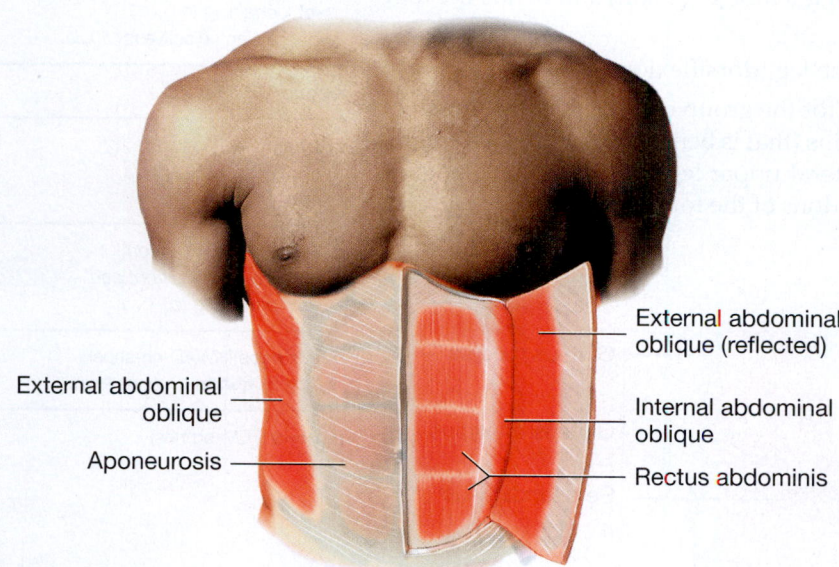

External abdominal oblique

Aponeurosis

External abdominal oblique (reflected)

Internal abdominal oblique

Rectus abdominis

FIGURE 8-13 ■ **Muscles of the abdomen.**
These muscles contract and relax when you rotate the trunk of your body from side to side, flatten your abdomen, bend forward, do a sit-up, or take a bow for learning medical language!

Word Alert
Sound-Alike Words

rectus   (noun)   Latin word meaning *straight*. The segments of the rectus abdominis muscle are in a straight vertical column, top to bottom, on the abdomen.

Example: When the rectus abdominis muscle contracts, it pulls the chest toward the legs.

rectum   (noun)   straight part of the large intestine that comes after the curving S-shaped sigmoid colon

Example: Digested food travels through the colon, through the rectum, through the anus, and is then expelled from the body.

Muscles of the Lower Extremity

These are the most important muscles of the lower extremity (see Figure 8-14 ■).

Anterior Leg

These muscles are in the anterior upper and lower leg.

- **Rectus femoris**: Bends the upper leg toward the abdomen (flexion); straightens the lower leg (extension).
- **Sartorius**: Bends the upper leg toward the abdomen (flexion) and rotates it laterally.
- **Vastus lateralis** and **vastus medialis**: Bend the upper leg toward the abdomen (flexion); straighten the lower leg (extension).
- **Peroneus longus**: Raises the lateral edge of the foot (eversion) and bends the foot downward (plantar flexion).
- **Tibialis anterior**: Bends the foot toward the leg (dorsiflexion).

Quadriceps femoris is a collective name for the group of four muscles—the rectus femoris, vastus lateralis, vastus intermedius (that is beneath the vastus lateralis), and vastus medialis—in the anterior and lateral upper leg. The origins of some of these muscles are on the femur bone. The tendons of the four heads of these muscles join together and insert on the tibia.

Pronunciation/Word Parts

rectus (REK-tuhs)

femoris (FEM-oh-rihs)

sartorius (sar-TOR-ee-uhs)

vastus lateralis (VAS-tuhs LAT-er-AL-ihs)

vastus medialis (VAS-tuhs MEE-dee-AL-ihs)

peroneus (PAIR-oh-NEE-uhs)

peroneal (PAIR-oh-NEE-al)
  perone/o- *fibula*
  -al *pertaining to*
Peroneal is an adjective for *fibula*.

longus (LONG-guhs)

tibialis (TIB-ee-AL-ihs)
  tibi/o- *shin bone; tibia*
  -alis *pertaining to*

anterior (an-TEER-ee-or)
  anter/o- *before; front part*
  -ior *pertaining to*

quadriceps (KWAD-rih-seps)
The prefix **quadri-** means *four*.

femoris (FEM-oh-rihs)

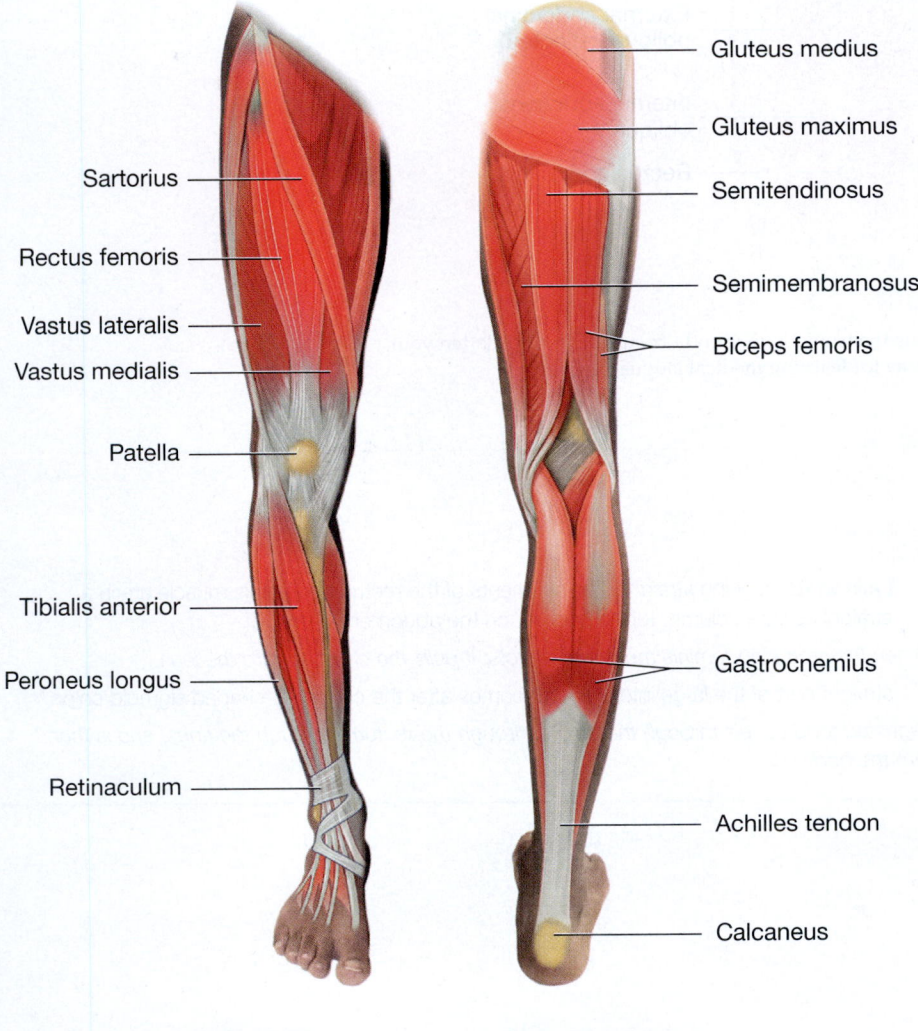

Sartorius

Rectus femoris

Vastus lateralis

Vastus medialis

Patella

Tibialis anterior

Peroneus longus

Retinaculum

Gluteus medius

Gluteus maximus

Semitendinosus

Semimembranosus

Biceps femoris

Gastrocnemius

Achilles tendon

Calcaneus

ANTERIOR VIEW   **POSTERIOR VIEW**

FIGURE 8-14 ■ Muscles of the lower extremity.
The muscles of the legs and buttocks contract and relax when you move your legs in any direction, bend your knees, walk on tiptoe, climb the stairs, or get up from a sitting position.

Posterior Leg

These muscles are in the posterior upper and lower leg.

- **Gluteus maximus**: Moves the upper leg posteriorly (extension) and rotates it laterally.
- **Biceps femoris**: Moves the upper leg posteriorly (extension) and bends the lower leg toward the buttocks (flexion).
- **Semitendinosus** and **semimembranosus**: Move the upper leg posteriorly (extension), bend the lower leg toward the buttocks (flexion), and rotate the leg medially.
- **Gastrocnemius**: Bends the foot downward (plantar flexion).

Hamstrings is a collective name for the group of three muscles—the biceps femoris, semitendinosus, and semimembranosus—in the posterior upper leg.

Pronunciation/Word Parts

gluteus (GLOO-tee-uhs)

maximus (MAK-sih-muhs)

biceps (BY-seps)

femoris (FEM-oh-rihs)

semitendinosus
(SEM-eye-TEN-dih-NOH-suhs)

semimembranosus
(SEM-eye-MEM-brah-NOH-suhs)

gastrocnemius (GAS-trawk-NEE-mee-uhs)
  gastr/o- *stomach*
  -cnemius *leg*
The gastrocnemius muscle is shaped somewhat like a stomach filled with food, which may be how it got its name.

Dive Deeper

The gastrocnemius muscle has its insertion on the calcaneus (heel bone). This tendon is known as the *Achilles tendon* in reference to Achilles, the mythical Greek hero who was wounded in the heel, his only vulnerable spot. The hamstrings take their name from an Old English word, *ham*, which means *hollow at the back of the knee*; *strings* refers to the cord-like tendons of these muscles.

Across the Life Span

Pediatrics. Babies are evaluated by a pediatrician for their ability to attain developmental milestones. A 1-month-old baby can lift its head only briefly. By 3 months of age, a baby has developed the muscular coordination to turn over in bed. One of the next developmental milestones is being able to lift up the head and chest (see Figure 8-15 ■).

Geriatrics. Throughout life, regular exercise is an important part of wellness and physical fitness. Aging and chronic disease can limit mobility and decrease muscle strength. The size and strength of the muscles decrease over time. There is less flexibility because elastic muscle tissue is replaced by fibrous connective tissue, but active exercise helps maintain muscle strength and flexibility.

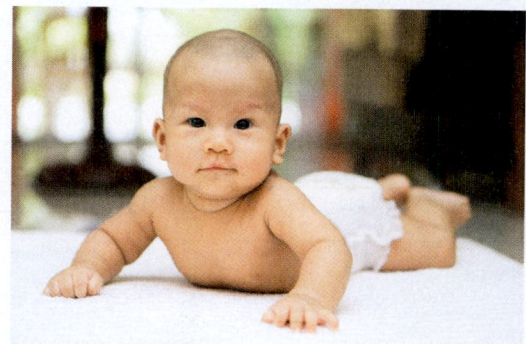

FIGURE 8-15 ■ Growth and development milestones.
This baby can lift his head and support his entire upper body with his arms, an activity that requires strength and coordination of the muscles of the neck, shoulders, and arms.

8.1 PRACTICE LAPS

Use the Answer Key at the end of the book to check your answers.

A. Label Structures

Write each anatomy phrase in the correct numbered box. Be sure to check your spelling.

biceps brachii muscle	gastrocnemius muscle	rectus abdominis muscle	temporalis muscle
brachioradialis muscle	gluteus maximus muscle	rectus femoris muscle	tibialis anterior muscle
deltoid muscle	masseter muscle	sternocleidomastoid	trapezius muscle
external oblique muscle	pectoralis major muscle	muscle	triceps brachii muscle
frontalis muscle	peroneus longus muscle		

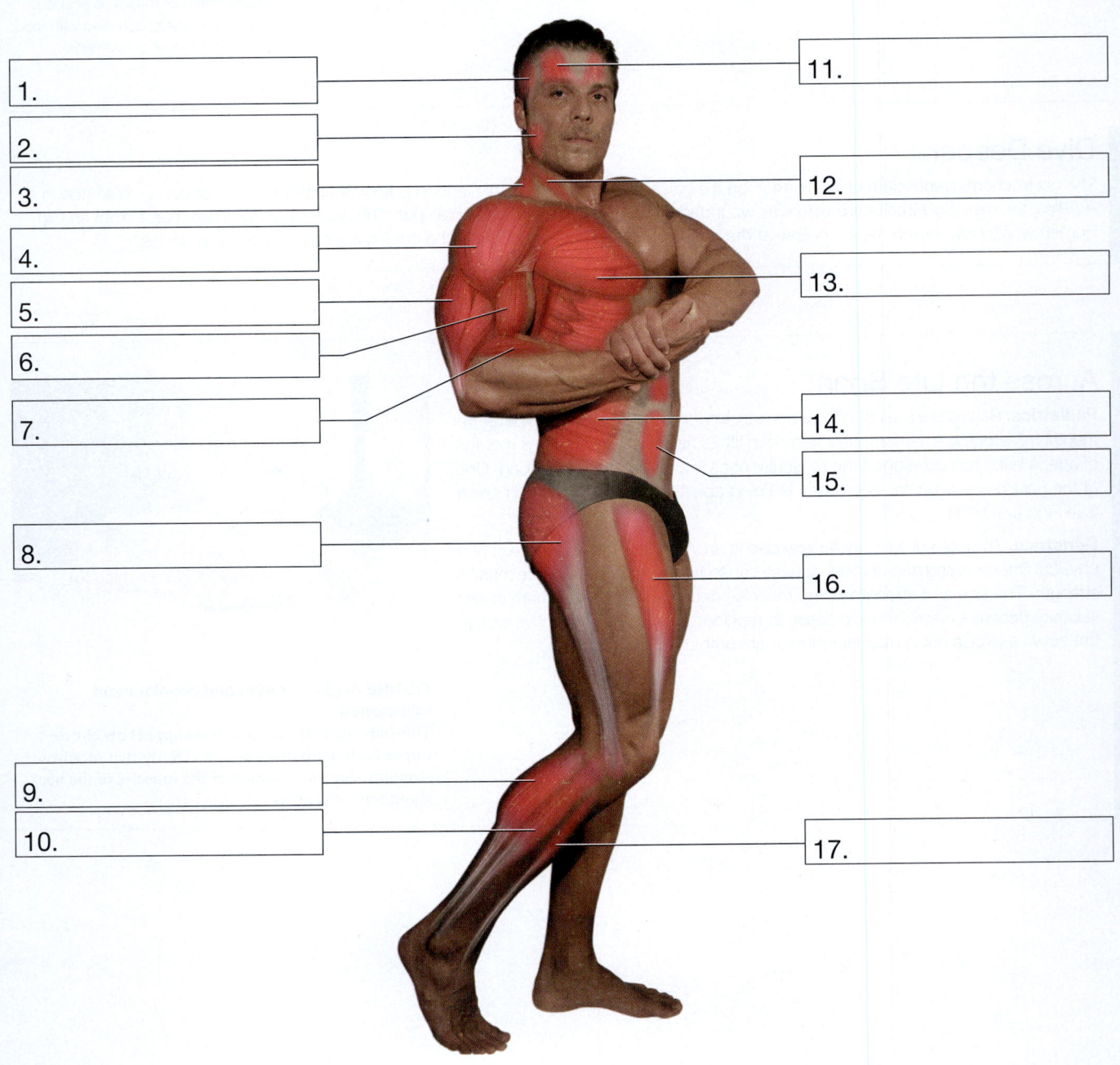

1.

2.

3.

4.

5.

6.

7.

8.

9.

10.

11.

12.

13.

14.

15.

16.

17.

A. Label Movements

extension	plantar flexion	rotation
extension and abduction	pronation	slight flexion
flexion and adduction		

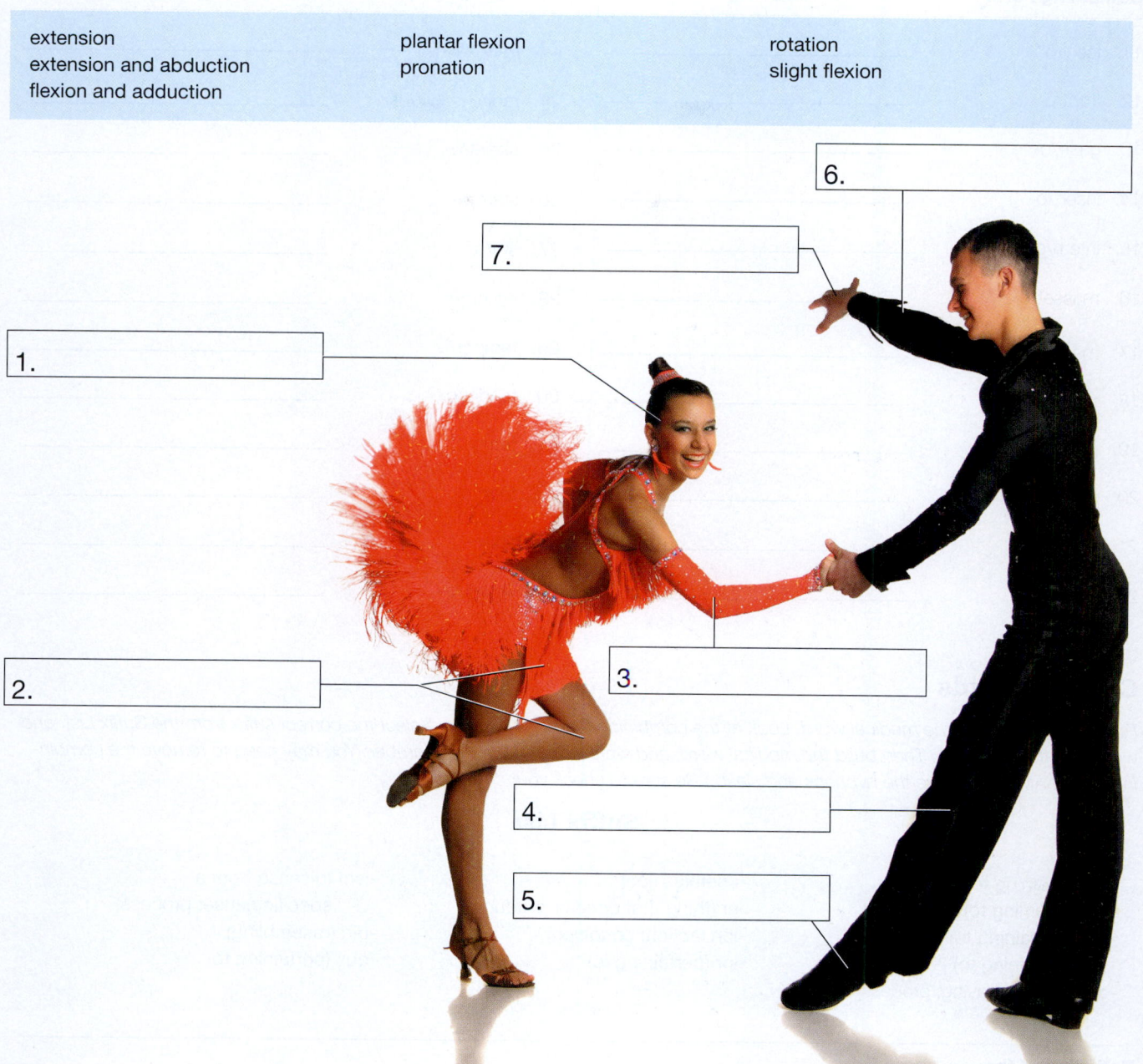

6. _____

7. _____

1. _____

2. _____

3. _____

4. _____

5. _____

B. Give the Meaning of Combining Forms

Next to each combining form, write its meaning. The first one has been done for you.

Combining Form	Meaning	Combining Form	Meaning
1. **abdomin/o-**	*abdomen*	6. burs/o-	_____
2. antagon/o-	_____	7. cleid/o-	_____
3. anter/o-	_____	8. cost/o-	_____
4. brachi/o-	_____	9. delt/o-	_____
5. buccin/o-	_____	10. extern/o-	_____

continued on next page

Combining Form	Meaning	Combining Form	Meaning
11. fasci/o-	_____	23. perone/o-	_____
12. front/o-	_____	24. radi/o-	_____
13. gastr/o-	_____	25. skelet/o-	_____
14. insert/o-	_____	26. stern/o-	_____
15. intern/o-	_____	27. stri/o-	_____
16. masset/o-	_____	28. synerg/o-	_____
17. mast/o-	_____	29. tempor/o-	_____
18. muscul/o-	_____	30. tendin/o-	_____
19. my/o-	_____	31. ten/o-	_____
20. myos/o-	_____	32. then/o-	_____
21. orbicul/o-	_____	33. tibi/o-	_____
22. pector/o-	_____	34. volunt/o-	_____

C. Build Words

Read the definition of the medical word. Look at the combining form that is given. Select the correct suffix from the Suffix List, and write it on the blank line. Then build the medical word, and write it on the line. (Remember: You may need to remove the combining vowel. Always remove the hyphens and slash.) Be sure to check your spelling.

Suffix List

-al (pertaining to)	-cnemius (leg)	-ism (disease from a
-ar (pertaining to)	-er (thing that does or produces)	specific cause; process)
-aris (pertaining to)	-ion (action; condition)	-oid (resembling)
-ary (pertaining to)	-ior (pertaining to)	-ous (pertaining to)
-ation (being; having; process)		

Definition of the Medical Word	Combining Form	Suffix	Build the Medical Word
Example: Pertaining to (the) outside	**extern/o-**	*-al*	*external*

[*You think* pertaining to (-al) + outside (extern/o-). You change the order of the word parts to put the suffix last. You write external.]

1. Pertaining to (the) fascia	fasci/o-	_____	_____
2. (Muscle in the) leg (that looks like food in the) stomach	gastr/o-	_____	_____
3. Action (of a tendon to) put in	insert/o-	_____	_____
4. Pertaining to inside	intern/o-	_____	_____

Definition of the Medical Word	Combining Form	Suffix	Build the Medical Word
5. Pertaining to (a) muscle	muscul/o-	_____	_____
6. Pertaining to (a) tendon	tendin/o-	_____	_____
7. Pertaining to (the) thumb	then/o-	_____	_____
8. Pertaining to one's free will	volunt/o-	_____	_____
9. Thing that does or produces chewing	masset/o-	_____	_____
10. Pertaining to (a muscle that is a) small circle	orbicul/o-	_____	_____
11. (Muscle) resembling (a) triangle	delt/o-	_____	_____
12. Pertaining to (the) front part	anter/o-	_____	_____
13. Pertaining to (a) bursa	burs/o-	_____	_____
14. Pertaining to (the) fibula	perone/o-	_____	_____
15. Having parallel stripes	stri/o-	_____	_____
16. Action (to) rotate	rotat/o-	_____	_____
17. Process (of muscles in a) joined, enhanced effect	synerg/o-	_____	_____

Clinical Connections

Sports Medicine. Professional athletes depend on their muscles to help them compete and win. The muscle fibers of a marathon runner are different from those of a sprinter. Marathon runners have mostly slow-twitch muscle fibers that can contract many times without becoming fatigued. Sprinters have fast-twitch muscle fibers that can contract very quickly and repeatedly, but soon become tired. Because of the effect of the male hormone testoster-one, men have larger muscles than women and a bulkier muscu-lature, but vigorous weight train-ing can increase the size of a muscle (**muscle hypertro-phy**) in either sex. Bodybuild-ers work to enlarge, define, and sculpt their muscles (see Figure 8-16 ■). Some athletes try to enhance their performance with the use of illicit drugs, particularly ana-bolic steroid drugs that add bulk to the muscles.

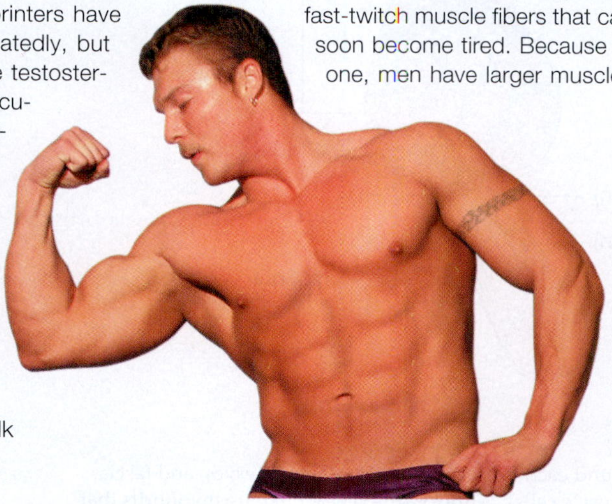

hypertrophy (hy-PER-troh-fee)
The prefix **hyper-** means *above; more than normal*. The suffix **-trophy** means *process of development*.

FIGURE 8-16 ■ Muscle strength and size.
This bodybuilder has highly developed muscles: the biceps brachii of the flexed right arm, the deltoid muscle of the shoulder, and the well-defined pectoral muscle of the chest. The individual segments of the rectus abdominis muscles can be seen on either side of the umbilicus.

8.2 Physiology

A **muscle** is composed of several muscle **fascicles**, each of which is individually wrapped in fascia (see Figure 8-17 ■). Each muscle fascicle is composed of bundles of individual muscle fibers. These run parallel to each other so that, when they contract, they all pull in the same direction. A **muscle fiber** (which is actually one long muscle cell) has hundreds of nuclei along its length to speed up the chemical processes that occur as it contracts. Each muscle fiber is composed of **myofibrils** that contain thin strands of the protein actin and thick strands of the protein myosin that give skeletal muscle its characteristic striated (striped) appearance under a microscope.

A muscle contracts in response to an electrical impulse from a nerve. On a microscopic level, each muscle fiber (muscle cell) is connected to a single nerve cell at a **neuromuscular junction**. The nerve cell releases the **neurotransmitter acetylcholine**, a chemical messenger that changes the permeability of the muscle fiber and allows sodium ions to flow into it. This releases calcium ions from a storage site within the muscle fiber. Calcium causes the thin strands (actin) to slide between the thick strands (myosin), which shortens the muscle and produces a muscle **contraction**. The muscle eventually relaxes when acetylcholine is inactivated by an enzyme and the calcium ions are pumped back into the storage site.

Even when not actively moving, the muscles are in a state of mild, partial contraction because of nerve impulses from the brain and spinal cord. This produces muscle tone that keeps the muscles firm and ready to act. This is the only aspect of skeletal muscle activity that is not under conscious control.

Pronunciation/Word Parts

muscle (MUS-el)
The combining forms **muscul/o-**, **my/o-**, and **myos/o-** mean *muscle*.

fascicle (FAS-ih-kul)
  fasci/o- *fascia*
  -cle *small thing*

myofibril (MY-oh-FY-bril)
  my/o- *muscle*
  fibr/o- *fiber*
  -il *small thing*

neuromuscular (NYOOR-oh-MUS-kyoo-lar)
  neur/o- *nerve*
  muscul/o- *muscle*
  -ar *pertaining to*

neurotransmitter
(NYOOR-oh-TRANS-mih-ter)
  neur/o- *nerve*
  transmitt/o- *send across; send through*
  -er *person who does or produces; thing that does or produces*

acetylcholine (AS-eh-til-KOH-leen)

contraction (con-TRAK-shun)
  contract/o- *pull together*
  -ion *action; condition*

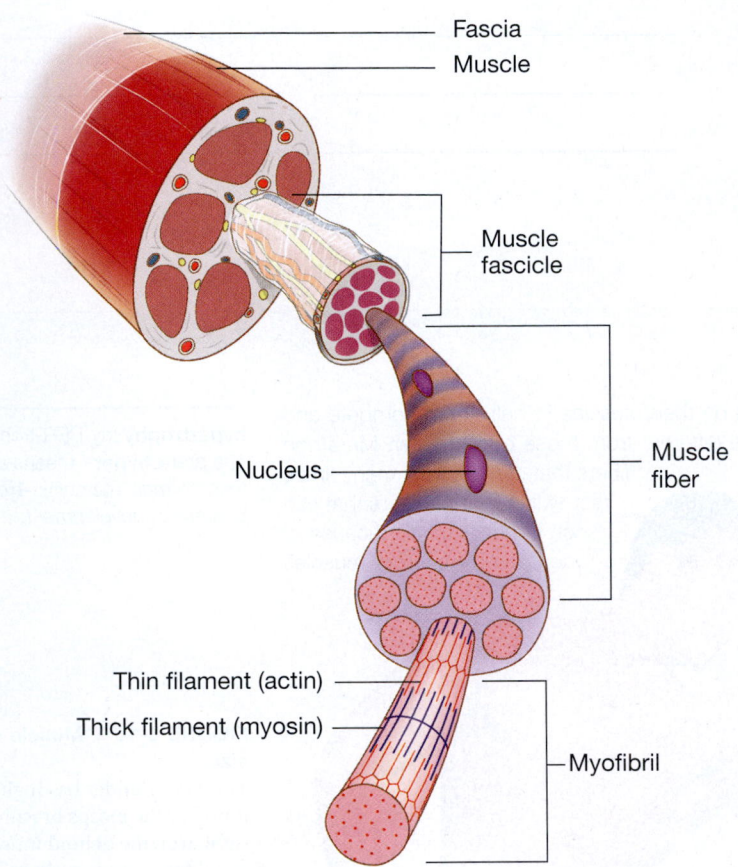

Fascia
Muscle
Muscle fascicle
Nucleus
Muscle fiber
Thin filament (actin)
Thick filament (myosin)
Myofibril

FIGURE 8-17 ■ **Parts of a muscle.**
A muscle is composed of muscle fascicles. Around each fascicle are arteries, veins, nerves, and fascia. Each fascicle contains several muscle fibers (muscle cells). Within each muscle fiber are myofibrils that contain thin strands of actin and thick strands of myosin.

8.2 PRACTICE LAPS

Use the Answer Key at the end of the book to check your answers

A. Give the Meaning of Combining Forms

Next to each combining form, write its meaning. The first one has been done for you.

Combining Form	Meaning	Combining Form	Meaning
1. **fibr/o-**	*fiber*	5. my/o-	
2. contract/o-		6. neur/o-	
3. fasci/o-		7. transmitt/o-	
4. muscul/o-			

B. Build Words

Read the definition of the medical word. Look at the combining form that is given. Select the correct suffix from the Suffix List, and write it on the blank line. Then build the medical word, and write it on the line. (Remember: You may need to remove the combining vowel. Always remove the hyphens and slash.) Be sure to check your spelling. The first one has been done for you.

Suffix List

-ar (pertaining to)	-cle (small thing)	-ion (action; condition)

Definition of the Medical Word	Combining Form	Suffix	Build the Medical Word
Example: Pertaining to (a) muscle	**muscul/o-**	*-ar*	*muscular*

[*You think* pertaining to (-ar) + muscle (muscul/o-). You change the order of the word parts to put the suffix last. You write muscular.]

Definition of the Medical Word	Combining Form	Suffix	Build the Medical Word
1. Small thing (wrapped in) fascia	fasci/o-		
2. Action (of a muscle to) pull together	contract/o-		

Vocabulary Review

Word or Phrase	Description	Combining Forms
Overview		
muscles	Structures that produce movement of body parts. There are approximately 700 muscles.	**muscul/o-** *muscle* **my/o-** *muscle* **myos/o-** *muscle*
muscular system	Body system that consists of skeletal muscles, tendons, and other structures. The functions of the muscular system are to help maintain body position and produce movement of the bony framework of the body. Also known as the **musculoskeletal system**.	**muscul/o-** *muscle* **skelet/o-** *skeleton*

Word or Phrase	Description	Combining Forms
musculature	All of the skeletal muscles or all of the skeletal muscles in one part of the body	**muscul/o-** *muscle*

Anatomy of the Muscular System		
Types of Muscles		
cardiac muscle	Heart muscle that pumps blood through the circulatory system; it is an involuntary muscle. Each cardiac muscle cell has a single nucleus and fewer and less prominent striations than a skeletal muscle cell.	**cardi/o-** *heart*
skeletal muscle	Muscles that move parts of the body. These are **voluntary** muscles that contract or relax in response to conscious thought. Each skeletal muscle cell has multiple nuclei and **striations** (bands of color) seen under a microscope.	**skelet/o-** *skeleton* **volunt/o-** *one's free will* **stri/o-** *parallel stripes*
smooth muscles	Muscles that form a continuous, thin layer around many body organs and structures. These are involuntary muscles that are not under conscious control. Each smooth muscle cell has a single nucleus and no striations.	
Tendons and Related Structures		
aponeurosis	Wide, white fibrous sheet of connective tissue (sometimes composed of several tendons) that attaches a flat muscle to a bone or to deeper muscles	
bursa	Thin sac of synovial membrane filled with synovial fluid. It decreases friction where a tendon rubs against a bone near a synovial joint.	**burs/o-** *bursa*
fascia	Thin connective tissue around each muscle. It merges into the tendon.	**fasci/o-** *fascia*
retinaculum	Thin, translucent band of fibrous tissue and fascia that holds down tendons in the areas of the wrist and ankle	
tendon	Cord-like, nonelastic, white fibrous band of connective tissue that attaches a muscle to a bone	**tendin/o-** *tendon* **ten/o-** *tendon*
Muscle Origins and Insertions		
belly of a muscle	Area of greatest mass, usually midway between the origin and insertion	
insertion	Ending of a muscle where its tendon is attached to the bone that moves when the muscle contracts or relaxes	**insert/o-** *introduce; put in*
origin	Beginning of a muscle, a fixed point where its tendon is attached to a stationary (or nearly stationary) bone	
Types of Muscle Movements		
abduction	Moving a body part away from the midline. It is the opposite of adduction. An **abductor** muscle produces abduction when it contracts.	**duct/o-** *bring; duct; move*

Word or Phrase	Description	Combining Forms
adduction	Moving a body part toward the midline. It is the opposite of abduction. An **adductor** muscle produces adduction when it contracts.	**duct/o-** *bring; duct; move*
antagonism	Process in which one muscle contracts and another muscle relaxes to allow movement	**antagon/o-** *opposing effect*
eversion	Turning a body part outward and toward the side. It is the opposite of inversion. An **evertor** muscle produces eversion when it contracts.	**vers/o-** *travel; turn* **vert/o-** *travel; turn*
extension	Straightening and extending a joint to increase the angle between two bones or two body parts. It is the opposite of flexion. An **extensor** muscle produces extension when it contracts.	**extens/o-** *straightening*
flexion	Bending a joint to decrease the angle between two bones or two body parts. It is the opposite of extension. A **flexor** muscle produces flexion when it contracts.	**flex/o-** *bending*
inversion	Turning a body part inward. It is the opposite of eversion. An **invertor** muscle produces inversion when it contracts.	**vers/o-** *travel; turn* **vert/o-** *travel; turn*
pronation	Turning the palm of the hand inferiorly or downward. It is the opposite of supination. A **pronator** muscle produces pronation when it contracts.	**pronat/o-** *face down*
rotation	Moving a body part around its axis. A **rotator** muscle produces rotation when it contracts.	**rotat/o-** *rotate*
supination	Turning the palm of the hand superiorly or upward. It is the opposite of pronation. A **supinator** muscle produces supination when it contracts.	**supinat/o-** *lying on the back*
synergism	Process in which one muscle contracts and other nearby muscles contract to produce a greater combined movement	**synerg/o-** *joined, enhanced effect*
Muscles of the Head and Neck		
buccinator muscle	Muscle of the side of the face that moves the cheek	**buccin/o-** *cheek*
frontalis muscle	Muscle of the forehead that moves the eyebrows and forehead skin	**front/o-** *front*
masseter muscle	Muscle of the side of the jaw that moves the mandible upward	**masset/o-** *chewing*
orbicularis oculi muscle	Muscle around the eye that closes the eyelids	**orbicul/o-** *small circle*
orbicularis oris muscle	Muscle around the mouth that closes the lips	**orbicul/o-** *small circle*
platysma muscle	Muscle of the neck that moves the mandible down	
sternocleidomastoid muscle	Muscle of the neck that bends the head toward the sternum (flexion) and turns the head to either side (rotation). Its origin is at two muscle heads on the sternum and clavicle. Its insertion is at the mastoid process of the temporal bone behind the ear.	**stern/o-** *breastbone; sternum* **cleid/o-** *clavicle; collarbone* **mast/o-** *breast; mastoid process*

Word or Phrase	Description	Combining Forms
temporalis muscle	Muscle of the side of the head that moves the mandible upward and backward	**tempor/o-** *side of the head; temple*
Muscles of the Shoulders, Chest, and Back		
deltoid muscle	Muscle of the shoulder that raises the arm and moves the arm away from the body (abduction)	**delt/o-** *triangle*
intercostal muscles	Muscles between the ribs that work in pairs to spread the ribs apart during inspiration and pull the ribs together during forced expiration, coughing, or sneezing	**cost/o-** *rib*
latissimus dorsi muscle	Muscle of the back that moves the arm posteriorly and medially toward the vertebral column (adduction)	
pectoralis major muscle	Muscle of the chest that moves the arm anteriorly and medially across the chest (adduction)	**pector/o-** *chest*
trapezius muscle	Muscle of the shoulder that raises the shoulder, pulls the shoulder blades together, and elevates the clavicle. It turns the head from side to side (rotation) and moves the head posteriorly (extension).	
Muscles of the Upper Extremity		
biceps brachii muscle	Muscle of the anterior upper arm that bends the upper arm toward the shoulder (flexion) and bends the lower arm toward the upper arm (flexion). The origin of this muscle has two (**bi-**) heads (**-ceps**).	
brachioradialis muscle	Muscle of the anterior lower arm that bends the lower arm toward the upper arm (flexion)	**brachi/o-** *arm* **radi/o-** *forearm bone; radius; x-rays*
thenar muscles	Group of muscles in the palm side of the hand that bends the thumb (flexion) and moves it toward the palm (adduction)	**then/o-** *thumb*
triceps brachii muscle	Muscle of the posterior upper arm that straightens the lower arm (extension). The origin of this muscle has three (**tri-**) heads (**-ceps**).	
Muscles of the Abdomen		
external abdominal oblique muscle	Muscle of the side of the abdomen that bends the upper body forward (flexion), rotates the side of the body medially, and compresses the side of the abdominal wall. The **internal abdominal oblique muscle** lies directly beneath it and performs the same movements, but its muscle fibers are oriented in the opposite direction.	**extern/o-** *outside* **abdomin/o-** *abdomen* **intern/o-** *inside*
rectus abdominis muscle	Muscle of the anterior abdomen that bends the upper body forward (flexion) and compresses the anterior abdominal wall	

Word or Phrase	Description	Combining Forms
Muscles of the Lower Extremity		
biceps femoris muscle	Muscle of the posterior upper leg that moves the upper leg posteriorly (extension) and bends the lower leg toward the buttocks (flexion). The origin of this muscle has two (**bi-**) heads (**-ceps**).	
gastrocnemius muscle	Muscle of the posterior lower leg that bends the foot downward (plantar flexion)	**gastr/o-** *stomach* *Note:* The shape of this muscle is somewhat like a stomach filled with food.
gluteus maximus muscle	Muscle of the buttocks that moves the upper leg posteriorly (extension) and rotates it laterally	
hamstrings	Collective name for three muscles in the posterior upper leg: biceps femoris, semitendinosus, and semimembranosus muscles	
peroneus longus muscle	Muscle of the lateral lower leg that raises the lateral edge of the foot (eversion) and bends the foot downward (plantar flexion)	**perone/o-** *fibula*
quadriceps femoris	Collective name for four muscles in the anterior and lateral upper leg: rectus femoris, vastus lateralis, vastus intermedius, and vastus medialis muscles. The origins of some of these muscles are on the femur bone (femoris). The tendons of the four (**quadri-**) heads (**-ceps**) of these muscles join together and insert on the tibia.	
rectus femoris muscle	Muscle of the anterior upper leg that bends the upper leg toward the abdomen (flexion) and straightens the lower leg (extension)	
sartorius muscle	Muscle of the anterior upper leg that bends the upper leg toward the abdomen (flexion) and rotates it laterally	
semitendinosus muscle	Muscle of the posterior upper leg that moves the upper leg posteriorly (extension), bends the lower leg toward the buttocks (flexion), and rotates the leg medially. The **semimembranosus muscle** has the same action.	
tibialis anterior muscle	Muscle of the anterior lower leg that bends the foot toward the leg (dorsiflexion)	**tibi/o-** *shin bone; tibia* **anter/o-** *before; front part*
vastus lateralis muscle	Muscle of the lateral upper leg that bends the upper leg toward the abdomen (flexion) and straightens the lower leg (extension). The **vastus medialis muscle** on the medial upper leg has the same action.	

Word or Phrase	Description	Combining Forms
Physiology of the Muscular System		
acetylcholine	Neurotransmitter that initiates a muscle contraction by changing the permeability of the muscle fibers	
contraction	Shortening of the length of all the muscle fibers within a muscle and of the muscle itself as thin strands of actin slide between thick strands of myosin.	**contract/o-** *pull together*
fascicle	Structures within a muscle that are individually wrapped in fascia. Each fascicle contains bundles of individual muscle fibers.	**fasci/o-** *fascia*
muscle	Structure that contains several muscle fascicles	**muscul/o-** *muscle* **my/o-** *muscle* **myos/o-** *muscle*
muscle fiber	One long muscle cell. Each muscle fiber is composed of myofibrils.	
muscle hypertrophy	An increase in the size of a muscle	
myofibril	Structure within a muscle fiber that contains thin strands of the protein actin and thick strands of the protein myosin that give a characteristic **striated** appearance under a microscope	**my/o-** *muscle* **fibr/o-** *fiber* **stri/o-** *parallel stripes*
neuromuscular junction	Area on a muscle fiber where a single nerve cell is connected to it	**neur/o-** *nerve* **muscul/o-** *muscle*
neurotransmitter	Chemical messenger between nerves and muscle cells	**neur/o-** *nerve* **transmitt/o-** *send across; send through*

8.3 Diseases

Word or Phrase	Description	Pronunciation/Word Parts
Diseases of the Muscles		
atrophy	Loss of muscle bulk in one or more muscles (see Figure 8-18 ■). It is caused by a lack of use, by paralysis in which the muscles receive no electrical impulses from the nerves, by a lack of a muscle protein in muscular dystrophy, or by severe malnutrition. The muscle is **atrophic**. Also known as **muscle wasting**. Treatment: Correct the underlying cause.	**atrophy** (AT-roh-fee) **atrophic** (aa-TROH-fik) **a-** *away from; without* **troph/o-** *development* **-ic** *pertaining to*

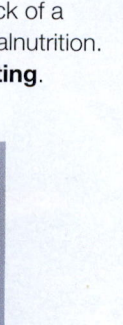

FIGURE 8-18 ■ Muscle atrophy.
Malnutrition can cause severe weight loss with muscle wasting and weakness.

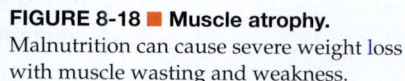

Clinical Connections

Psychiatry. Anorexia nervosa is a psychiatric illness characterized by an extreme, chronic fear of being fat and an obsession with becoming thinner. The patient voluntarily decreases food intake to the point of starvation, and yet denies being too thin. Most of the subcutaneous fat on the body is gone and there is muscle wasting and prominence of the bones (see Figure 8-19 ■).

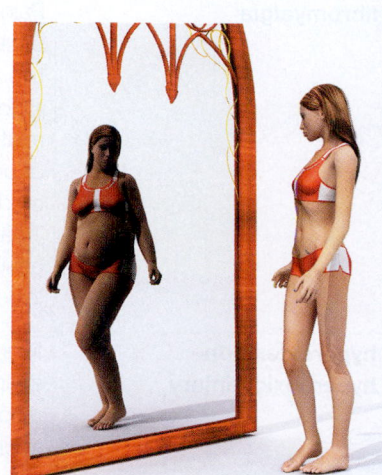

FIGURE 8-19 ■ Anorexia nervosa.
A patient with anorexia nervosa denies being too thin and would, in fact, appear to herself as being fat if she looked in a mirror.

Word or Phrase	Description	Pronunciation/Word Parts
avulsion	Condition in which the muscle tears away from the tendon or the tendon tears away from the bone Treatment: Surgical repair (myorrhaphy or tenorrhaphy)	**avulsion** (ah-VUL-shun) **a-** *away from; without* **vuls/o-** *tear* **-ion** *action; condition*
compartment syndrome	Severe blunt or crushing injury causes bleeding in the muscles of the arm or leg. The fascia acts as a compartment, holding in the accumulating blood. The increased pressure causes muscle and nerve damage and tissue death. Treatment: Fasciotomy to allow the blood and fluid to drain out	

Word or Phrase	Description	Pronunciation/Word Parts
contracture	Condition in which a muscle becomes progressively more flexed. As it continues to receive nerve impulses, it finally becomes flexed in an immovable position. Contractures are seen in nursing home patients in wheelchairs or in bed and in patients with some muscular and neurological diseases (see Figure 8-20 ■). Treatment: Range of motion (ROM) exercises **FIGURE 8-20 ■ Muscle contracture.** This man has a neurological condition that causes the muscles to contract into the fixed position of a contracture.	**contracture** (con-TRAK-chur) **contract/o-** *pull together* **-ure** *result of; system*

Word Alert
Sound-Alike Words

contraction	(noun)	the normal shortening of a muscle in response to a nerve impulse *Example: It requires a strong contraction of the arm muscles to lift a heavy box.*
contracture	(noun)	abnormal, fixed position in which the muscle is permanently flexed *Example: Range-of-motion exercises help prevent a contracture from occurring.*

Word or Phrase	Description	Pronunciation/Word Parts
fibromyalgia	Pain located at specific trigger points in the muscles of the neck, back, or hips. The trigger points are hyperirritable, hypersensitive areas that are tender and cause musculoskeletal pain when touched. The cause of fibromyalgia is not known, but may be related to an overreaction to painful stimuli with a possible history of prior injury or a genetic predisposition. Fibromyalgia is associated with disturbed sleep patterns and sometimes depression. Treatment: Analgesic drug; muscle relaxant drug; drug that affects calcium channels in the skeletal muscles; trigger point injections with a local anesthetic drug; massage therapy	**fibromyalgia** (FY-broh-my-AL-jah) **fibr/o-** *fiber* **my/o-** *muscle* **alg/o-** *pain* **-ia** *condition; state; thing*
hyperextension–hyperflexion injury	Injury that occurs during a car accident as a person's head snaps backward (extension) and then forward (flexion) in response to the car's changing speed. This causes a muscle strain or muscle tear, as well as damage to the nerves. Also known as **acceleration–deceleration injury** or more commonly as **whiplash**. Treatment: Soft cervical collar to support the neck; analgesic drug; nonsteroidal anti-inflammatory drug	**hyperextension** (HY-per-eks-TEN-shun) **hyper-** *above; more than normal* **extens/o-** *straightening* **-ion** *action; condition* **hyperflexion** (HY-per-FLEK-shun) **hyper-** *above; more than normal* **flex/o-** *bending* **-ion** *action; condition*
muscle contusion	Condition in which blunt trauma causes bleeding in the muscle. Also known as a **bruise**. Treatment: Analgesic drug	**contusion** (con-TOO-shun) **contus/o-** *bruising* **-ion** *action; condition*

Word or Phrase	Description	Pronunciation/Word Parts

muscle spasm	Painful but temporary condition with a sudden, severe, involuntary contraction of a muscle, often in the legs. It can be brought on by overexercise. Also known as a **muscle cramp**. **Torticollis** is a painful spasm of the muscles on one side of the neck. Also known as **wryneck**.
	Treatment: Massage; muscle relaxant drug; analgesic drug
		spasm (SPAZM)
		torticollis (TOR-tih-KOH-lihs)
		  tort/i- *twisted position*
		  -collis *condition of the neck*

muscle strain	Overstretching or tearing of a muscle or its tendon, often due to physical overexertion. This causes **inflammation**, pain, swelling, and bruising as capillaries in the muscle are torn. Also known as a **pulled muscle**.
	Treatment: Rest; analgesic drug; nonsteroidal anti-inflammatory drug
		strain (STRAYN)
		
		inflammation (IN-flah-MAY-shun)
		  inflammat/o- *redness and warmth*
		  -ion *action; condition*

muscular dystrophy (MD)	A group of muscle diseases caused by a genetic mutation of the gene that normally makes the muscle protein dystrophin. Without dystrophin, the muscles weaken and then atrophy. It begins in early childhood with weakness in the lower extremities and then the upper extremities (see Figure 8-21 ■). The most common and most severe form is **Duchenne muscular dystrophy**. Weakness of the diaphragm with an inability to breathe is the most frequent cause of death. Treatment: Supportive care	**dystrophy** (DIS-troh-fee) The prefix **dys-** means *abnormal; difficult; painful*. The suffix **-trophy** means *process of development*. **Duchenne** (doo-SHEN)

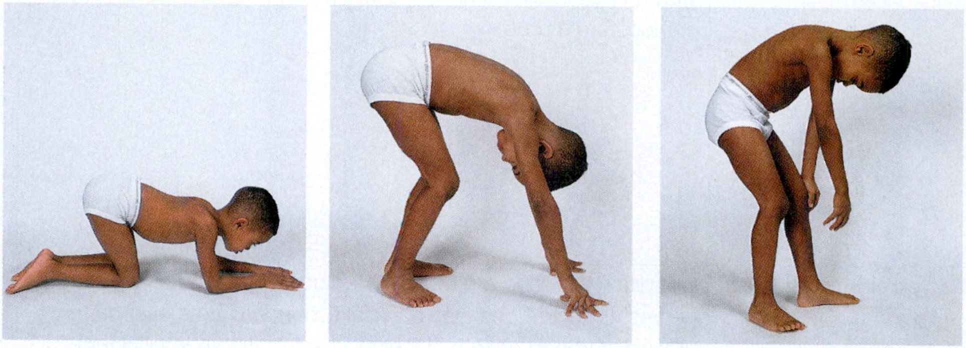

FIGURE 8-21 ■ Muscular dystrophy.
Weakness of the muscles in the legs causes this patient with muscular dystrophy to stand up in a way that is characteristic of this disease. The legs and arms must work together to raise the body. Because muscular dystrophy is a progressive disease, soon this patient may not be able to walk at all.

Word or Phrase	Description	Pronunciation/Word Parts

myalgia	Pain in a muscle due to injury or muscle disease. **Polymyalgia** is pain in several muscle groups.
	Treatment: Analgesic drug; massage
		myalgia (my-AL-jah)
		  my/o- *muscle*
		  alg/o- *pain*
		  -ia *condition; state; thing*
		
		polymyalgia (PAW-lee-my-AL-jah)
		  poly- *many; much*
		  my/o- *muscle*
		  alg/o- *pain*
		  -ia *condition; state; thing*

Word or Phrase	Description	Pronunciation/Word Parts
myasthenia gravis	Autoimmune disorder in which the body produces antibodies against its own acetylcholine receptors on the muscle fibers, and the antibodies destroy many of the receptors. There is a normal level of acetylcholine, but too few receptors to produce a muscle contraction. This causes abnormal and rapid fatigue of the muscles, particularly the muscles of the face, where there is **ptosis** (drooping) of the eyelids. The weakness worsens during the day, but is relieved by rest. Treatment: Thymectomy to remove the thymus because it contributes to the abnormal immune response; drug that prolongs the action of acetylcholine; plasmapheresis to remove antibodies from the blood	**myasthenia gravis** (MY-as-THEE-nee-ah GRAV-ihs) **my/o-** *muscle* **asthen/o-** *lack of strength* **-ia** *condition; state; thing* **ptosis** (TOH-sihs)
myopathy	Category that includes many different diseases of the muscles Treatment: Correct the underlying cause.	**myopathy** (my-AW-pah-thee) **my/o-** *muscle* **-pathy** *disease*
myositis	Inflammation of a muscle with localized swelling and tenderness. It can be caused by injury or strain. **Polymyositis** is a chronic, progressive disease that causes widespread inflammation of muscles with weakness and fatigue. The cause is unknown, although it may be an autoimmune disorder. **Dermatomyositis** causes a skin rash as well as muscle weakness and inflammation. Treatment: Analgesic drug; nonsteroidal anti-inflammatory drug; corticosteroid drug	**myositis** (MY-oh-SY-tihs) **myos/o-** *muscle* **-itis** *infection of; inflammation of* **polymyositis** (PAW-lee-MY-oh-SY-tihs) **poly-** *many; much* **myos/o-** *muscle* **-itis** *infection of; inflammation of* **dermatomyositis** (DER-mah-toh-MY-oh-SY-tihs) **dermat/o-** *skin* **myos/o-** *muscle* **-itis** *infection of; inflammation of*
repetitive strain injury (RSI)	Condition affecting the muscles, tendons, and sometimes the nerves. It occurs because of repetitive movements over an extended period of time. It includes tennis elbow, carpal tunnel syndrome, and other disorders. Also known as **cumulative trauma disorder (CTD)**. Treatment: Rest; analgesic drug; nonsteroidal anti-inflammatory drug	

Clinical Connections

Occupational Health. The **Occupational Safety and Health Administration (OSHA)** educates healthcare professionals about workplace-related injuries. Lifting, carrying, pulling, or pushing something heavy and not using proper body mechanics can cause injury, as can repetitive motions done constantly, such as typing on a computer.

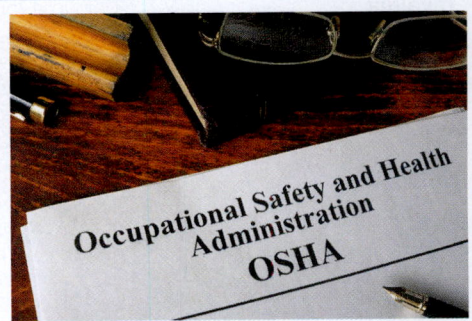

Word or Phrase	Description	Pronunciation/Word Parts

rhabdomyoma	**Benign** (not cancerous) tumor in a muscle
	Treatment: Surgical removal, if needed
		rhabdomyoma
		(RAB-doh-my-OH-mah)
		  rhabd/o- *rod shaped*
		  my/o- *muscle*
		  -oma *mass; tumor*
		Note: This tumor contains immature rod-shaped cells in the muscle.
		
		benign (bee-NINE)

rhabdomyosarcoma	Cancerous tumor in a muscle. This **cancer** usually occurs in children and young adults. A sarcoma is always a cancerous tumor.
	Treatment: Surgical removal; chemotherapy drug; radiation therapy
		rhabdomyosarcoma
		(RAB-doh-MY-oh-sar-KOH-mah)
		  rhabd/o- *rod shaped*
		  my/o- *muscle*
		  sarc/o- *connective tissue*
		  -oma *mass; tumor*
		
		cancer (KAN-ser)
		
		cancerous (KAN-ser-uhs)
		  cancer/o- *cancer*
		  -ous *pertaining to*

rotator cuff tear	Tear in the rotator muscles of the shoulder that surround the head of the humerus. These muscles help to abduct the arm. The tear can be caused by acute trauma or repetitive overuse, particularly motions in which the arm is above the head. Treatment: Surgical repair	

Clinical Connections

Forensic Science. Rigor mortis is not a muscle disease of the living, but rather a normal condition of the muscles that occurs several hours after death. As each muscle fiber dies, its stored calcium is released, and this causes the muscle fibers—and then each muscle of the body—to contract. The muscle fiber is no longer able to pump calcium ions back into the storage site (as a living muscle would do), and so the muscles remain contracted for about 72 hours until the muscle fibers begin to decompose. Also known as **postmortem rigidity**. Forensic scientists use the presence or absence of rigor mortis to help determine the time of death.

rigor mortis (RIG-or MOR-tihs)

postmortem (post-MOR-tem)

Movement Disorders

| ataxia | Incoordination of the muscles during movement, particularly incoordination of the gait. It is caused by a disease of the brain or spinal cord, cerebral palsy, or an adverse reaction to a drug. The patient is **ataxic**.
Treatment: Correct the underlying cause; leg braces or crutches, if needed | **ataxia** (ah-TAK-see-ah)
  a- *away from; without*
  tax/o- *coordination*
  -ia *condition; state; thing*

ataxic (ah-TAK-sik)
  a- *away from; without*
  tax/o- *coordination*
  -ic *pertaining to* |

Word or Phrase	Description	Pronunciation/Word Parts
bradykinesia	Abnormally slow muscle movements or a decrease in the number of spontaneous muscle movements. It is usually associated with Parkinson disease, a neurologic disease of the brain. Treatment: Drug for Parkinson disease	**bradykinesia** (BRAD-ee-kih-NEE-zha) **brady-** *slow* **kines/o-** *movement* **-ia** *condition; state; thing*
dyskinesia	Abnormal motions that occur because of difficulty controlling the voluntary muscles. Attempts at movement become tics, muscle spasms, muscle jerking (**myoclonus**), or slow, wandering, purposeless writhing of the hand (**athetoid movements**) in which some muscles of the fingers are flexed and others are extended. It is associated with neurologic disorders (Parkinson disease, Huntington chorea, cerebral palsy, etc.). Treatment: Correct the underlying cause.	**dyskinesia** (DIHS-kih-NEE-zha) **dys-** *abnormal; difficult; painful* **kines/o-** *movement* **-ia** *condition; state; thing* Dyskinesia: *Condition of abnormal movement* **myoclonus** (MY-oh-KLOH-nuhs) **my/o-** *muscle* **-clonus** *rapid contracting and relaxing* **athetoid** (ATH-eh-toyd) **athet/o-** *without position or purpose* **-oid** *resembling* Athetoid: *Resembling (movement that is wandering and) without position or purpose*

Clinical Connections

Neurology. Cerebral palsy is caused by a lack of oxygen to parts of a fetus's brain before or during birth. The extent of the symptoms varies but can include spastic muscles; dyskinesia; lack of coordination in walking, eating, and talking; or even muscle paralysis.

Word or Phrase	Description	Pronunciation/Word Parts
hyperkinesis	An abnormally increased amount of muscle movements. Restlessness. It can be a side effect of a drug. Treatment: Correct the underlying cause.	**hyperkinesis** (HY-per-kih-NEE-sihs) The prefix **hyper-** means *above; more than normal*. The suffix **-kinesis** means *abnormal condition of movement*.
restless legs syndrome (RLS)	An uncomfortable restlessness and twitching of the muscles of the legs, particularly the calf muscles, along with an indescribable tingling, aching, or crawling-insect sensation. This usually occurs at night and can interfere with sleep. The exact cause is unknown but may be related to the presence of chronic diseases and inflammation. Treatment: Analgesic drug; iron supplement; sedative drug for sleep	
tremor	Small, involuntary, sometimes jerky, back-and-forth movements of the hands, head, jaw, or extremities. These are continuous and cannot be controlled by the patient and are usually due to essential familial tremor, an inherited condition. Treatment: Beta-blocker drug	**tremor** (TREM-or)

Word or Phrase	Description	Pronunciation/Word Parts

Diseases of the Bursa, Fascia, or Tendon

bursitis	Inflammation of the bursal sac because of repetitive muscle contractions or pressure on the bone underneath the bursa. It can occur with any joint that has a bursa, but most often occurs in the shoulders and knees. Prolonged periods of kneeling cause bursitis known as **housemaid's knee**.
	Treatment: Rest; analgesic drug; nonsteroidal anti-inflammatory drug
		bursitis (ber-SY-tihs)
		  burs/o- bursa
		  -itis infection of; inflammation of

Dupuytren contracture	Disease in which collagen fibers in the fascia in the palm of the hand become progressively thickened and shortened. This causes a contracture and flexion deformity of the finger (see Figure 8-22 ■). The cause is not known, but many patients have other family members who are affected by it.
	Treatment: Injection of a drug to dissolve the collagen fibers; surgery to remove the fascia (fasciectomy)
		Dupuytren (DOO-pyoo-tren)
		
		contracture (con-TRAK-chur)
		  contract/o- pull together
		  -ure result of; system

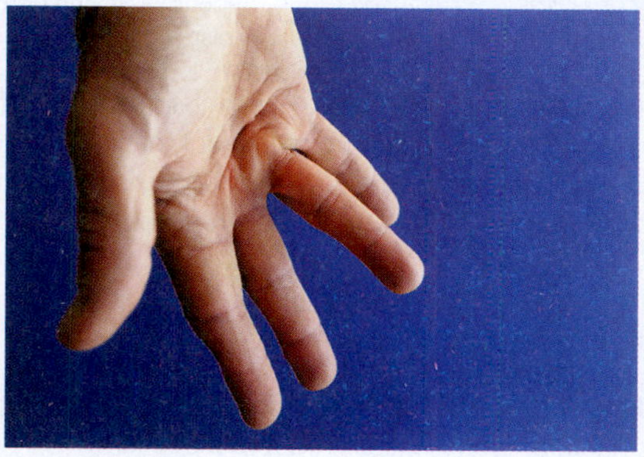

FIGURE 8-22 ■ Dupuytren contracture.
This progressive disease most commonly affects the ring finger and/or the little finger.

epicondylitis	Inflammation and pain of muscles and their tendons that originate on an epicondyle, a rounded protrusion of bone on each side (lateral and medial) of the distal humerus.
	
	• **Lateral epicondylitis** involves the muscles of the forearm where their tendons originate on the lateral epicondyle of the humerus (by the elbow joint). It is an overuse injury caused by repeated extension and pronation of the wrist. Also known as **tennis elbow** (see Figure 8-23 ■).
		epicondylitis
		(EH-pih-CON-dih-LY-tihs)
		  epi- above; upon
		  condyl/o- rounded prominence
		  -itis infection of; inflammation of
		
		lateral (LAT-er-al)
		  later/o- side
		  -al pertaining to
		
		medial (MEE-dee-al)
		  medi/o- middle
		  -al pertaining to

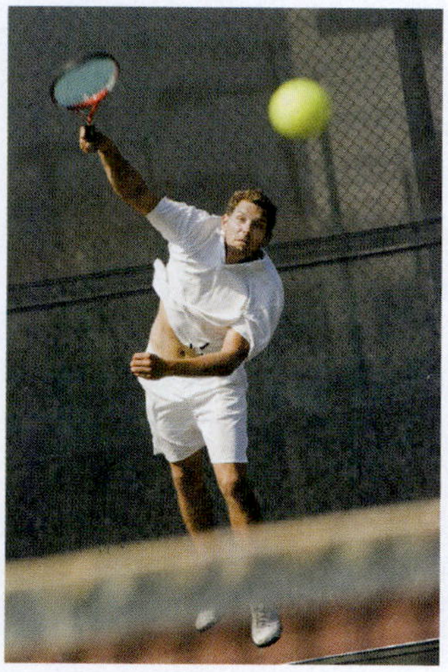

FIGURE 8-23 ■ Lateral epicondylitis.
Tennis elbow is an overuse injury caused by repetitive extension and pronation of the wrist, a movement that is characteristic of a tennis service.

Word or Phrase	Description	Pronunciation/Word Parts
	• **Medial epicondylitis** involves the muscles of the forearm where their tendons originate on the medial epicondyle of the humerus. This is an overuse injury caused by repeated flexing of the wrist while the fingers tightly grasp an object. Also known as **golfer's elbow** or **pitcher's elbow** (see Figure 8-24 ■). Treatment: Rest; analgesic drug; nonsteroidal anti-inflammatory drug	
	FIGURE 8-24 ■ **Medial epicondylitis.** Pitcher's elbow is an overuse injury caused by repetitive flexing of the wrist while the fingers tightly grasp a baseball.	
fasciitis	Inflammation of the fascia around a muscle. Plantar fasciitis is inflammation of the fascia on the bottom of the foot that is caused by excessive running or exercise. There is aching or stabbing pain around the heel. It is the most common cause of heel pain. Treatment: Analgesic drug; nonsteroidal anti-inflammatory drug; injection of a corticosteroid drug into the fascia	**fasciitis** (FASH-ee-EYE-tihs) **fasci/o-** *fascia* **-itis** *infection of; inflammation of*
ganglion	Semisolid or fluid-containing cyst that develops on a tendon, often in the wrist, hand, or foot. A ganglion is a rounded lump under the skin that may or may not be painful. Treatment: Needle aspiration of fluid from the ganglion or surgical removal (ganglionectomy)	**ganglion** (GANG-glee-awn)
shin splints	Pain and inflammation of the tendons of the flexor muscles of the anterior lower leg over the tibia (shin bone). It is an overuse injury common to athletes who run. Treatment: Rest; analgesic drug; nonsteroidal anti-inflammatory drug	
tendinitis	Inflammation of any tendon from injury or overuse. Treatment: Rest; analgesic drug; nonsteroidal anti-inflammatory drug	**tendinitis** (TEN-dih-NY-tihs) **tendin/o-** *tendon* **-itis** *infection of; inflammation of*
tenosynovitis	Inflammation and pain due to overuse of a tendon and inability of the synovium to produce enough lubricating fluid. Treatment: Rest; analgesic drug; nonsteroidal anti-inflammatory drug	**tenosynovitis** (TEN-oh-SIN-oh-VY-tihs) **ten/o-** *tendon* **synov/o-** *joint membrane; synovium* **-itis** *infection of; inflammation of*

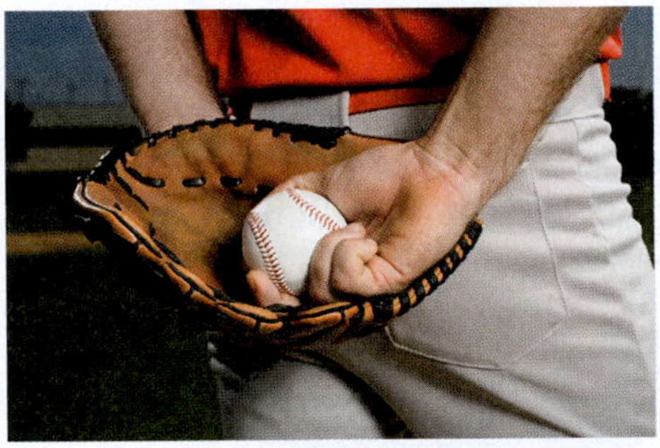

8.3 PRACTICE LAPS

Use the Answer Key at the end of the book to check your answers.

A. Give the Meaning of Combining Forms

Next to each combining form, write its meaning. The first one has been done for you.

Combining Form	Meaning	Combining Form	Meaning
1. **athet/o-**	*without position or purpose*	15. later/o-	
2. alg/o-		16. medi/o-	
3. asthen/o-		17. my/o-	
4. burs/o-		18. myos/o-	
5. cancer/o-		19. rhabd/o-	
6. condyl/o-		20. sarc/o-	
7. contract/o-		21. synov/o-	
8. contus/o-		22. tax/o-	
9. dermat/o-		23. tendin/o-	
10. extens/o-		24. ten/o-	
11. fibr/o-		25. tort/i-	
12. flex/o-		26. troph/o-	
13. inflammat/o-		27. vuls/o-	
14. kines/o-			

B. Build Words

Read the definition of the medical word. Look at the combining form that is given. Select the correct suffix from the Suffix List, and write it on the blank line. Then build the medical word, and write it on the line. (Remember: You may need to remove the combining vowel. Always remove the hyphens and slash.) Be sure to check your spelling.

Suffix List

-al (pertaining to)	-collis (condition of the neck)	-itis (infection of; inflammation of)	-pathy (disease)
-clonus (rapid contracting and relaxing)	-ion (action; condition)	-oid (resembling)	-ure (result of; system)

Definition of the Medical Word	Combining Form	Suffix	Build the Medical Word
Example: Resembling (movement that is) without position or purpose	**athet/o-**	*-oid*	*athetoid*

[*You think* resembling (-oid) + without position or purpose (athet/o-). You change the order of the word parts to put the suffix last. *You write* athetoid.]

Definition of the Medical Word	Combining Form	Suffix	Build the Medical Word
1. Infection of (or) inflammation of (the) fascia	fasci/o-		
2. Result of (a muscle being) pull(ed) together	contract/o-		
3. Pertaining to (the) side	later/o-		
4. Condition (of) redness and warmth	inflammat/o-		
5. Disease (of the) muscle	my/o-		
6. Infection of (or) inflammation of (a) bursa	burs/o-		
7. Condition of the neck (in a) twisted position	tort/i-		
8. Infection of (or) inflammation of (a) tendon	tendin/o-		
9. Pertaining to (the) middle	medi/o-		
10. Condition (of) bruising	contus/o-		
11. Rapid contracting and relaxing (of a) muscle	my/o-		
12. Infection of (or) inflammation of (the) muscle	myos/o-		

C. Define Abbreviations

1. CTD _____

2. MD _____

3. OSHA _____

4. RLS _____

5. RSI _____

8.4 Laboratory, Diagnostic, and Radiologic Procedures

Word or Phrase	Description	Pronunciation/Word Parts
Blood Tests		
acetylcholine receptor antibody test	Test that detects antibodies that the body produces against its own acetylcholine receptors. It is used to diagnose myasthenia gravis.	**antibody** (AN-tih-BAW-dee) The prefix **anti-** means *against*.
creatine phosphokinase (CPK-MM)	Test that measures the level of serum CPK-MM, an isoenzyme found in the muscles. A high blood level of CPK-MM is present in various diseases, particularly muscular dystrophy, in which muscle tissue is being destroyed.	**creatine phosphokinase** (KREE-ah-teen FAWS-foh-KY-nays)
Muscle Tests		
edrophonium test	Procedure in which the drug edrophonium is given to confirm a diagnosis of myasthenia gravis. The drug temporarily increases the amount of acetylcholine that is available to stimulate the fewer number of acetylcholine receptors that are characteristic of myasthenia gravis. Patients with myasthenia gravis show temporarily increased muscle strength during the test.	**edrophonium** (EH-droh-FOH-nee-um)
electromyography (EMG)	Procedure to diagnose muscle disease or nerve damage. A needle electrode inserted into a muscle records electrical activity as the muscle contracts and relaxes. The electrical activity is displayed as waveforms on a computer screen and recorded as an **electromyogram**.	**electromyography** (ee-LEK-troh-my-AW-grah-fee) **electr/o-** *electricity* **my/o-** *muscle* **-graphy** *process of recording* **electromyogram** (ee-LEK-troh-MY-oh-gram) **electr/o-** *electricity* **my/o-** *muscle* **-gram** *picture; record*

8.4 PRACTICE LAPS

Use the Answer Key at the end of the book to check your answers.

A. Give the Meaning of Combining Forms

Next to each combining form, write its meaning.

Combining Form	Meaning
1. electr/o-	
2. my/o-	

B. Define Abbreviations

1. CPK _____

2. EMG _____

8.5 Medical Procedures, Drugs, and Surgical Procedures

Word or Phrase	Description	Pronunciation/Word Parts

Medical Procedures

Word or Phrase	Description	Pronunciation/Word Parts
braces and adaptive devices	A brace is an orthopedic device that supports and straightens a body part and keeps it in anatomical alignment while still permitting movement (see Figure 8-25 ■). Also known as an **orthosis**. An adaptive or assistive device increases **mobility** and independence by helping a physically challenged patient perform **activities of daily living (ADLs)**. Examples of adaptive or assistive devices: A grasper to extend the reach, spoons that can be attached to the wrist, and extra-large pens that can be easily grasped.	**orthosis** (or-THOH-sihs) **orth/o-** *straight* **-osis** *abnormal condition; process* **mobility** (moh-BIL-ih-tee) **mobil/o-** *movement* **-ity** *condition; state*

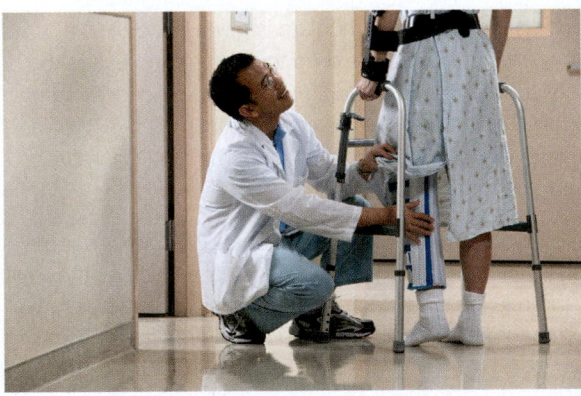

FIGURE 8-25 ■ Braces.
Braces provide support and stability. The physical therapist is instructing and assisting this patient in how to safely walk with a walker and a knee brace.

Dive Deeper

The **Americans with Disabilities Act (ADA)** of 1990 is a federal law that prohibits discrimination against disabled persons. It provides guidelines and requirements for accommodating persons with disabilities at work and in public buildings and transportation vehicles. Instead of *handicapped*, the correct phrase is *physically challenged*.

Word or Phrase	Description	Pronunciation/Word Parts
deep tendon reflexes (DTRs)	Procedure that tests whether the muscular–nervous pathway is functioning normally. Tapping briskly on a tendon should cause an involuntary, automatic contraction of the muscle connected to that tendon. This test can be done in several places, but the most common site is at the knee (see Figure 8-26 ■). Also known as the **knee jerk** or **patellar reflex** because it is near the patella bone (kneecap).	**reflex** (REE-fleks)

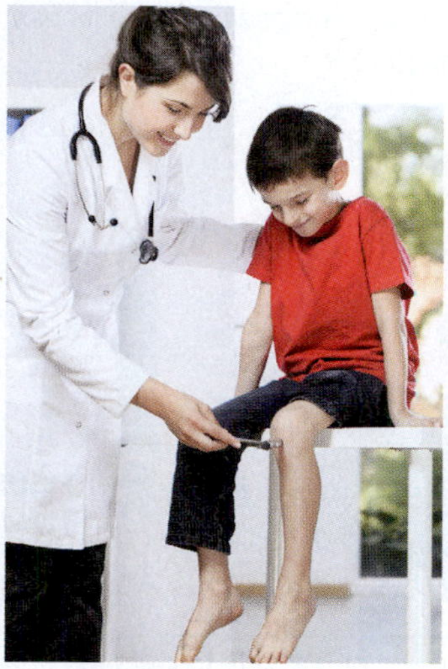

FIGURE 8-26 ■ Deep tendon reflex.
A percussion hammer with a rounded rubber end is used to tap just below the patella on the combined tendons of the quadriceps femoris muscle group. A normal response is a sudden involuntary contraction of the muscles that briskly extends the lower leg. The response in both legs is tested and compared.

Word Alert
Sound-Alike Words

reflex   (noun)   involuntary, automatic response of the muscular–nervous pathway
Example: The patient's knee jerk reflexes were equal bilaterally.

reflux   (noun)   backward flowing of fluid
Example: Acid reflux from the stomach can cause inflammation and ulcers in the esophagus.

Word or Phrase	Description	Pronunciation/Word Parts
muscle strength test	Procedure used to test the **motor strength** of certain muscle groups. For muscles in the legs and feet, the physician presses against the lower leg or foot and asks the patient to extend the leg or dorsiflex the foot upward. For muscles in the shoulder, the physician presses down, and the patient tries to shrug the shoulders. For muscles in the hand, the patient grasps two of the physician's fingers and squeezes them as tightly as possible. Muscle strength is measured on a scale of 0 to 5, with 0 being an inability to move the muscles being tested and 5 being normal strength.	**motor** (MOH-tor) **mot/o-** *movement* **-or** *person who does or produces; thing that does or produces*

Word or Phrase	Description	Pronunciation/Word Parts
rehabilitation exercises	Physical therapy that includes exercises to increase muscle strength and improve coordination and balance. It is prescribed as part of a rehabilitation plan. In active exercise, the patient exercises with supervision but without assistance (see Figure 8-27 ■). In passive exercise, a physical therapist or nurse performs **range-of-motion (ROM)** exercises for a patient who is unable to do the movements. Passive exercise does not increase muscle strength, but it does decrease muscle stiffness and spasticity and prevent contractures. FIGURE 8-27 ■ **Active exercise.** These patients are part of a physical therapy group. Even patients confined to wheelchairs benefit from regular exercise.	**rehabilitation** (REE-hah-BIL-ih-TAY-shun) **re-** *again and again; backward; unable to* **habilit/o-** *give ability* **-ation** *being; having; process* Rehabilitation: *Process (of) again and again (doing exercises to) give ability.* During rehabilitation, exercises are repeated again and again.
RICE treatment for minor injuries	Standard advice given by physicians and sports trainers for treating muscle sprains and soft tissue injuries to prevent further injury and swelling: **R**est the injured part **I**ce applied to the injured part **C**ompression bandage on the injured part **E**levate the injured part.	
trigger point injections	Procedure to treat fibromyalgia. A local anesthetic drug and a corticosteroid drug are injected into each fibromyalgia trigger point to relieve pain and decrease inflammation.	

Category	Indication	Pronunciation/Word Parts

Drugs

Category	Indication	Pronunciation/Word Parts
analgesic drug	Treats mild-to-moderate inflammation and pain (over-the-counter drugs). Used to treat minor injuries, muscle strains, tendinitis, bursitis, and muscle overuse. Prescription narcotic analgesic drugs are used to treat chronic, severe pain.	**analgesic** (AN-al-JEE-zik) **an-** *not; without* **alges/o-** *sensation of pain* **-ic** *pertaining to*
beta-blocker drug	Blocks the action of epinephrine to suppress essential familial tremor	
corticosteroid drug	Decreases severe inflammation. Given orally or injected into the muscle or fascia.	**corticosteroid** (KOR-tih-koh-STAIR-oyd) **cortic/o-** *cortex; outer region* **-steroid** *steroid*
dopamine stimulant drug	Stimulates dopamine receptors to treat restless legs syndrome	
drugs for fibromyalgia	Relieve pain (oral analgesic drug); relax muscles (oral muscle relaxant drug); affect calcium channels in skeletal muscle; relieve trigger point pain (injection of a local anesthetic drug)	

Category	Indication	Pronunciation/Word Parts
drug for myasthenia gravis	Inhibits the enzyme that normally breaks down acetylcholine	
muscle relaxant drug	Relieves muscle spasm and stiffness. Used to treat muscle injuries and muscle spasms in patients with fibromyalgia and neurologic diseases such as multiple sclerosis and cerebral palsy.	**relaxant** (ree-LAKS-ant) **relax/o-** *relax* **-ant** *pertaining to*
nonsteroidal anti-inflammatory drug (NSAID)	Decreases mild-to-moderate inflammation and pain. Used to treat minor injuries, muscle strains, tendinitis, bursitis, and muscle overuse.	**nonsteroidal** (NON-steh-ROYD-al) **non-** *not* **steroid/o-** *steroid* **-al** *pertaining to* **anti-inflammatory** (AN-tee-in-FLAM-ah-TOR-ee) **anti-** *against* **inflammat/o-** *redness and warmth* **-ory** *having the function of*

Clinical Connections

Pharmacology. Some drugs are administered by **intramuscular (IM) injection**. IM injections are given in a large muscle that is not near a large artery, vein, or nerve. In adults, these sites include the deltoid muscle (lateral upper arm), the vastus lateralis (anterolateral thigh), the gluteus medius muscle (lateral hip), and the gluteus maximus (upper outer quadrant of the buttocks). In infants, the only suitable site for an intramuscular injection is in the anterolateral thigh (see Figure 8-28 ■).

intramuscular
 (IN-trah-MUS-kyoo-lar)
 intra- *within*
 muscul/o- *muscle*
 -ar *pertaining to*

injection (in-JEK-shun)
 inject/o- *insert; put in*
 -ion *action; condition*

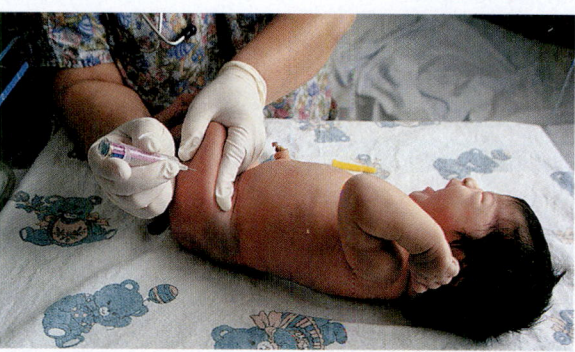

FIGURE 8-28 ■ Intramuscular injection.
The thigh muscles are the largest muscles in a baby's body, and immunizations are injected there.

Word or Phrase	Description	Pronunciation/Word Parts

Surgical Procedures

Word or Phrase	Description	Pronunciation/Word Parts
fasciectomy	Procedure to partially or totally remove the fascia that is causing Dupuytren contracture	**fasciectomy** (FASH-ee-EK-toh-mee) **fasci/o-** *fascia* **-ectomy** *surgical removal*
fasciotomy	Procedure to cut the fascia and release pressure from built-up blood and tissue fluid in a patient with compartment syndrome	**fasciotomy** (FASH-ee-AW-toh-mee) **fasci/o-** *fascia* **-tomy** *process of cutting; process of making an incision*

Word or Phrase	Description	Pronunciation/Word Parts
ganglionectomy	Procedure to remove a ganglion from a tendon	**ganglionectomy** (GANG-glee-oh-NEK-toh-mee) **ganglion/o-** *ganglion* **-ectomy** *surgical removal*
muscle biopsy	Procedure to diagnose muscle weakness that could be caused by many different muscular diseases. An incision is made in the muscle and a piece of tissue is removed and sent to the pathology department for examination under a microscope. This is an **incisional biopsy** or open biopsy. Alternatively, a needle is inserted, and some muscle tissue is aspirated through the needle; this is a closed biopsy.	**biopsy** (BY-awp-see) **bi/o-** *living organism; living tissue* **-opsy** *process of viewing* **incisional** (in-SIH-zhun-al) **in-** *in; not; within* **cis/o-** *cut* **-ion** *action; condition* **-al** *pertaining to*
myorrhaphy	Procedure to suture together a torn muscle after an injury	**myorrhaphy** (my-OR-ah-fee) **my/o-** *muscle* **-rrhaphy** *procedure of suturing*
tenorrhaphy	Procedure to suture together a torn tendon after an injury	**tenorrhaphy** (teh-NOR-ah-fee) **ten/o-** *tendon* **-rrhaphy** *procedure of suturing*
thymectomy	Procedure to remove the thymus gland. It is used to treat patients with myasthenia gravis because, after a thymectomy, the patient produces fewer antibodies against the remaining acetylcholine receptors.	**thymectomy** (thy-MEK-toh-mee) **thym/o-** *rage; thymus* **-ectomy** *surgical removal* Thymectomy: *Surgical removal (of the) thymus*

8.5 PRACTICE LAPS

Use the Answer Key at the end of the book to check your answers.

A. Give the Meaning of Combining Forms

Next to each combining form, write its meaning. The first one has been done for you.

Combining Form	Meaning	Combining Form	Meaning
1. **steroid/o-**	*steroid*	9. mobil/o-	
2. alges/o-		10. mot/o-	
3. bi/o-		11. my/o-	
4. cis/o-		12. orth/o-	
5. fasci/o-		13. relax/o-	
6. ganglion/o-		14. ten/o-	
7. habilit/o-		15. thym/o-	
8. inflammat/o-			

B. Build Words

Read the definition of the medical word. Look at the combining form that is given. Select the correct suffix from the Suffix List, and write it on the blank line. Then build the medical word, and write it on the line. (Remember: You may need to remove the combining vowel. Always remove the hyphens and slash.) Be sure to check your spelling.

Suffix List

-ant (pertaining to) -ectomy (surgical removal) -ity (condition; state) -opsy (process of viewing)	-or (person who does or produces; thing that does or produces)	-osis (abnormal condition; process) -rrhaphy (procedure of suturing)	-tomy (process of cutting; process of making an incision)

Definition of the Medical Word	Combining Form	Suffix	Build the Medical Word
Example: Thing that does or produces movement	**mot/o-**	*-or*	*motor*

[*You think* thing that does or produces (-or) + movement (mot/o-). You change the order of the word parts to put the suffix last. You write motor.]

1.	Process (to help the body be) straight	orth/o-	_____	_____
2.	Pertaining to (a drug to make muscles) relax	relax/o-	_____	_____
3.	Procedure of suturing (of a) tendon	ten/o-	_____	_____
4.	Surgical removal (of the) thymus	thym/o-	_____	_____
5.	State (of) movement	mobil/o-	_____	_____
6.	Surgical removal (of) fascia	fasci/o-	_____	_____
7.	Process of viewing living tissue	bi/o-	_____	_____
8.	Surgical removal (of a) ganglion	ganglion/o-	_____	_____
9.	Process of making an incision (in the) fascia	fasci/o-	_____	_____
10.	Procedure of suturing (a) muscle	my/o-	_____	_____

C. Define Abbreviations

1. ADA _____

2. ADLs _____

3. DTRs _____

4. NSAID _____

5. ROM _____

Abbreviations Summary

ADA	Americans with Disabilities Act		**OSHA**	Occupational Safety and Health Administration
ADLs	activities of daily living		**OT**	occupational therapist; occupational therapy
CPK-MM	creatine phosphokinase-MM		**PM&R**	physical medicine and rehabilitation
DTRs	deep tendon reflexes		**PT**	physical therapist; physical therapy
EMG	electromyogram; electromyography		**rehab**	rehabilitation (short form)
IM	intramuscular		**RICE**	rest, ice, compression, and elevation
LLE	left lower extremity		**RLE**	right lower extremity
LUE	left upper extremity		**ROM**	range of motion
MD	muscular dystrophy		**RSI**	repetitive strain injury
NSAID	nonsteroidal anti-inflammatory drug		**RUE**	right upper extremity
ortho	orthopedics (short form)			

Word Alert

Abbreviations. Abbreviations are commonly used in all types of medical documents; however, they can mean different things to different people and their meanings can be misinterpreted. Always verify the meaning of an abbreviation.

- *ADA* means *Americans with Disabilities Act*, but it also means *American Diabetes Association*, *American Dental Association*, or *American Dietetic Association*.

- *MD* means *muscular dystrophy*, but it also means *macular degeneration (of the eye)* or *Doctor of Medicine (M.D.)*.

- *ROM* means *range of motion*, but it also means *rupture of membranes* (prior to delivery of a baby).

It's Greek to Me! Did you notice that some words have two different combining forms? Combining forms from both Greek and Latin remain a part of medical language today.

Word	Greek	Latin	Medical Word Examples
movement	kines/o-	mobil/o-, mot/o-	dyskinesia; mobility, motor strength
muscle	my/o-	muscul/o-, myos/o-	fibromyalgia; muscular, myositis
tendon	ten/o-	tendin/o-	tenorrhaphy; tendinitis

Career Focus

Meet Sara, a physical therapist in an outpatient physical therapy department

"I always knew I wanted to work in health care. My mom was a nurse. I became aware of other careers in health care, and physical therapy was one of them. It sounded interesting to me, and I enjoyed anatomy. We use a lot of medical terminology on the job, in our daily practice, and particularly in our documentation. That's the way we communicate with physicians, other healthcare providers, and our patients or clients."

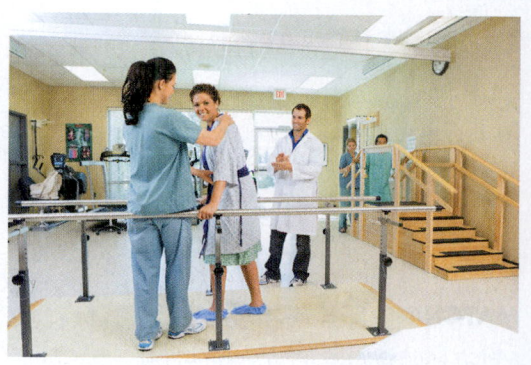

- **Physical therapists (PTs)** are allied health professionals who develop treatment and rehabilitation plans based on a physician's diagnosis of the patient. In most states, physical therapists have the option to practice with or without a physician referral. Physical therapists use strengthening exercises and assistive devices (crutches, canes, wheelchairs, and so forth) to help patients improve and maintain balance and mobility. They work in hospitals, outpatient clinics, rehabilitation centers, long-term care facilities, home health agencies, and sports and fitness facilities; many physical therapists have their own private practices. Most physical therapy programs award a doctoral degree.

- **Occupational therapists (OTs)** are allied health professionals who develop treatment and rehabilitation plans based on a physician's diagnosis of the patient. Occupational therapists help patients with disabilities, injuries, or cognitive decline improve their ability to perform the normal activities of daily living and regain their independence. The word *occupation* refers to all aspects of self-care, work, and play and leisure. Occupational therapists work in hospitals, outpatient clinics, rehabilitation centers, long-term care facilities, and home health agencies.

- **Massage therapists** are allied health professionals who use pressure and manipulation of the muscles and soft tissues to relieve stress and prevent or treat muscular injuries. Massage therapy is known for its relaxation qualities, but more and more people are understanding that it increases circulation, increases range of motion, and reduces pain. The education for massage therapists begins with intense anatomy and physiology, as well as ethics training. Massage therapists work in athletic clubs, resorts, chiropractic or orthopedic offices, or in their own private offices.

- **Physiatry** is the medical specialty that diagnoses and treats musculoskeletal diseases and acute and chronic pain by using the physical properties of cold, heat, light, and water in conjunction with exercise and some drugs. It is also known as the field of **physical medicine and rehabilitation (PM&R)**.

- **Sports medicine** encompasses the prevention, treatment, and rehabilitation of musculoskeletal injuries from sports, as well as athletic training and endurance, biomechanics, nutrition, and psychology. A physician (M.D.) or Doctor of Osteopathy can take additional training and become board certified in physical medicine and rehabilitation or in sports medicine.

physical (FIZ-ih-kal)
  physic/o- *body*
  -al *pertaining to*

therapist (THAIR-ah-pist)
  therap/o- *treatment*
  -ist *person who specializes in; thing that specializes in*

occupational (AW-kyoo-PAY-shun-al)
  occupat/o- *work*
  -ion *action; condition*
  -al *pertaining to*

physiatry (fih-ZY-ah-tree)
  physi/o- *physical function*
  -iatry *medical treatment*

physiatrist (fih-ZY-ah-trist)
  physi/o- *physical function*
  iatr/o- *medical treatment; physician*
  -ist *person who specializes in*

Chapter Review Exercises

Dive In: Medical Language Exercises

Test your knowledge of the chapter by completing these review exercises. Use the Answer Key at the end of the book to check your answers. Note: Each of the numbered exercise headers corresponds to a numbered learning outcome at the beginning of the chapter.

8.1 Anatomy

MATCHING EXERCISE

Match each phrase to its description.

1. biceps brachii muscle
2. biceps femoris muscle
3. deltoid muscle
4. gastrocnemius muscle
5. gluteus maximus muscle
6. latissimus dorsi muscle
7. masseter muscle
8. pectoralis major muscle
9. rectus abdominis muscle
10. rectus femoris muscle
11. sternocleidomastoid muscle
12. tibialis anterior muscle
13. trapezius muscle

_____ posterior aspect of the lower leg

_____ on the chest by the sternum

_____ triangular muscle of the shoulder

_____ from the shoulder to along one side of the back

_____ anterior aspect of the upper leg

_____ side of the neck behind the ear to the clavicle

_____ anterior aspect of the upper arm

_____ anterior aspect of the lower leg

_____ on either side of the midline of the abdomen

_____ shoulder and down one side of the back

_____ on the side of the face and the lower jaw

_____ large muscle in the buttocks

_____ posterior aspect of the upper leg

CIRCLE EXERCISE

Circle the correct answer from the choices given.

1. The (**belly, insertion, origin**) is where the muscle is attached to a stationary bone.
2. The (**aponeurosis, bursa, fascia**) is a wide, white sheet of fibrous connective tissue that attaches a muscle to a bone.
3. The (**muscle, musculature, musculus**) is a group of muscles in one body part.
4. Skeletal muscle is (**involuntary, nonstriated, striated**).
5. The (**deltoid, pectoralis, rectus**) muscle is shaped like a triangle.
6. The prefix (**bi-, quadri-, tri-**) means *three*.

TRUE OR FALSE EXERCISE

*Indicate whether each statement is true or false by writing **T** or **F** on the line.*

1. _____ A tendon is a thin connective tissue that merges into a muscle.
2. _____ Smooth muscles contract and relax to produce body movement.
3. _____ The belly of the muscle is midway between the origin and insertion.
4. _____ The muscle name gluteus maximus tells you that it is a large muscle of the buttocks.
5. _____ Extension decreases the angle between two bones or two body parts.
6. _____ The muscle name triceps brachii tells you that it has three heads and is located in the arm.
7. _____ The latissimus dorsi muscle is in the shoulder.
8. _____ Supination is turning the palm of the hand downward.
9. _____ The intercostal muscles are located between the ribs.
10. _____ The thenar muscles are located in the cheek area.

PLURAL NOUN AND ADJECTIVE EXERCISE

Read the noun and write its plural form and/or adjective form on the line. Only write in the plural noun form if there is a blank line there for it. Be sure to check your spelling. The first one has been done for you.

Singular Noun	Plural Noun	Adjective
1. **muscle**	*muscles*	*muscular*
2. tendon	_____	_____
3. bursa	_____	_____
4. fascia		_____

DIVIDING WORDS EXERCISE

Separate these words into their component parts (prefix, combining form, suffix). Some words do not contain all three word parts. The first one has been done for you.

Medical Word	Prefix	Combining Form	Suffix	Medical Word	Prefix	Combining Form	Suffix
1. **bursal**		*burs/o-*	*-al*	6. gastrocnemius		_____	_____
2. muscular		_____	_____	7. deltoid		_____	_____
3. intercostal	_____	_____	_____	8. insertion		_____	_____
4. peroneal		_____	_____	9. masseter		_____	_____
5. anterior		_____	_____	10. tendinous		_____	_____

SPELLING EXERCISE

Read each medical word pronunciation and write the medical word that it represents. Be sure to check your spelling. The first one has been done for you.

1. **(FASH-ee-ah)**   *fascia*
2. (RET-ih-NAK-yoo-lum)   _____
3. (STER-noh-KLY-doh-MAS-toyd) _____
4. (trah-PEE-zee-uhs)   _____
5. (oh-BLEEK)   _____
6. (GAS-trawk-NEE-mee-uhs)   _____

8.2 Physiology

MATCHING EXERCISE

Match each word or phrase to its description.

1. acetylcholine
2. actin and myosin
3. calcium
4. contraction
5. fascia
6. fascicle
7. muscle fiber
8. neuromuscular junction
9. striations
10. myofibrils

_____ characteristic of skeletal muscle

_____ muscle becomes shorter

_____ a neurotransmitter

_____ area where a muscle fiber is connected to a nerve cell

_____ ion that plays a role in muscle contraction

_____ a single cell of a muscle

_____ thin connective tissue wrapped around a muscle

_____ contain actin and myosin

_____ composed of bundles of muscle fibers

_____ thin and thick strands of protein that slide together as the muscle contracts

TRUE OR FALSE EXERCISE

*Indicate whether each statement is true or false by writing **T** or **F** on the line.*

1. _____ A muscle fiber has hundreds of nuclei along its length.

2. _____ A nerve impulse contracts in response to an electrical impulse from a muscle.

3. _____ Acetylcholine changes the permeability of the muscle fiber to let sodium ions flow in.

4. _____ The muscle fibers of a marathon runner are different from those of a sprinter.

5. _____ Weight training can produce muscle hypertrophy in either sex.

6. _____ In the word *fascicle*, the suffix *-cle* means *small thing*.

SPELLING EXERCISE

Read each medical word pronunciation and write the medical word that it represents. Be sure to check your spelling. The first one has been done for you.

1. **(con-TRAK-shun)** _____*contraction*_____

2. (hy-PER-troh-fee) _____

3. (NYOOR-oh-TRANS-mih-ter) _____

4. (MY-oh-FY-bril) _____

8.3 Diseases

MATCHING EXERCISE

Match each word or phrase to its description.

1. acceleration–deceleration injury

2. ataxia

3. atrophy

4. contusion

5. cumulative trauma disorder

6. muscular dystrophy

7. myopathy

8. myositis

9. polymyalgia

10. torticollis

11. tremor

12. restless legs syndrome

_____ wryneck

_____ incoordination of muscle movement

_____ bruise

_____ category including many muscle diseases

_____ pain in many muscle groups

_____ small, involuntary muscle movements

_____ inflammation of a muscle with swelling

_____ Duchenne is one type

_____ repetitive strain injury

_____ whiplash

_____ muscle wasting

_____ tingling, crawling-insect sensation at night

CIRCLE EXERCISE

Circle the correct answer from the choices given.

1. (**Ataxia, Atrophy, Contracture**) is a type of movement disorder.

2. A ganglion develops on a (**muscle, nerve, tendon**).

3. A slow, writhing movement of the hand is described as (**athetoid, myalgia, tendinitis**).

4. An injury in which the muscle is torn away from the tendon is a/an (**avulsion, compartment syndrome, contusion**).

5. Which is a type of muscular dystrophy? (**Duchenne, Dupuytren, torticollis**).

6. A (**ganglion, rhabdomyosarcoma, tenosynovitis**) is a malignant tumor of the muscle.

7. Housemaid's knee is known by the medical word/phrase (**bursitis, compartment syndrome, shin splints**).

TRUE OR FALSE EXERCISE

*Indicate whether each statement is true or false by writing **T** or **F** on the line.*

1. _____ Myalgia means inflammation in a muscle.
2. _____ Muscular dystrophy is a genetic disorder.
3. _____ Involuntary muscle jerking is known as *bradykinesia*.
4. _____ Muscle wasting is also known as *muscle atrophy*.
5. _____ The two types of muscular dystrophy are Duchenne and Dupuytren.
6. _____ Patients with fibromyalgia may also develop rigor mortis.
7. _____ Myasthenia gravis is caused by antibodies that destroy acetylcholine receptors.
8. _____ Golfer's elbow is a type of overuse injury that is similar to pitcher's elbow.
9. _____ A contracture is a fixed state of flexion of a muscle.
10. _____ Muscular dystrophy causes pain at certain trigger points.

DIVIDING WORDS EXERCISE

Separate these words into their component parts (prefix, combining form, suffix). Some words do not contain all three word parts. The first one has been done for you.

Medical Word	Prefix	Combining Form	Suffix
1. **contusion**		*contus/o-*	*-ion*
2. ataxia	_____	_____	_____
3. avulsion	_____	_____	_____
4. bradykinesia	_____	_____	_____
5. bursitis		_____	_____
6. contracture		_____	_____
7. dyskinesia	_____	_____	_____
8. hyperextension	_____	_____	_____
9. torticollis		_____	_____
10. myopathy		_____	_____
11. polymyositis	_____	_____	_____
12. tendinitis		_____	_____

SPELLING EXERCISE

Read each medical word pronunciation and write the medical word that it represents. Be sure to check your spelling. The first one has been done for you.

1. **(ah-TROH-fik)**   *atrophic*
2. (FY-broh-my-AL-jah)   _____
3. (con-TOO-shun)   _____
4. (my-AL-jah)   _____
5. (PAW-lee-MY-oh-SY-tihs)   _____
6. (FASH-ee-EYE-tihs)   _____

ENGLISH AND MEDICAL WORD EQUIVALENTS EXERCISE

For each English word, write its equivalent medical word. Be sure to check your spelling. The first one has been done for you.

English Word	Medical Word
1. **housemaid's knee**	*bursitis*
2. muscle wasting	_____
3. wryneck	_____
4. pulled muscle	_____
5. whiplash	_____
6. bruise	_____
7. pitcher's elbow	_____
8. tennis elbow	_____

8.4 Laboratory, Diagnostic, and Radiologic Procedures

TRUE OR FALSE EXERCISE

*Indicate whether each statement is true or false by writing **T** or **F** on the line.*

1. _____ The body produces antibodies against its own acetylcholine receptors in myasthenia gravis.

2. _____ An edrophonium test is used to confirm a diagnosis of muscular dystrophy.

3. _____ Electromyography is used to diagnose muscle disease or nerve damage.

4. _____ CPK-MM is an isoenzyme found in the muscles.

8.5 Medical Procedures, Drugs, and Surgical Procedures

MATCHING EXERCISE

Match each word or phrase to its description.

1. ADA	_____ treatment for Dupuytren contracture
2. ADLs	_____ a brace
3. beta-blocker drug	_____ active or passive
4. corticosteroid drug	_____ federal law about discrimination
5. deep tendon reflex	_____ knee jerk test
6. fasciectomy	_____ used to treat essential familial tremor
7. motor strength	_____ helped with adaptive and assistive devices
8. orthosis	_____ tested by squeezing the physician's fingers
9. rehabilitation exercise	_____ used to treat severe inflammation

CIRCLE EXERCISE

Circle the correct answer from the choices given.

1. Trigger point injections are used to treat (**bursitis, fibromyalgia, tendinitis**).

2. Exercises where the therapist moves the extremity for the patient are (**active, passive, reflex**) exercises.

3. A (**muscle biopsy, tenorrhaphy, thymectomy**) is used to treat myasthenia gravis.

4. A surgical procedure to remove a piece of muscle for examination is a/an (**fasciotomy, incisional biopsy, tenorrhaphy**).

5. RICE stands for all of the following *except* (**compression, elevate, exercise, ice, rest**).

6. In infants, the intramuscular injection of a drug is given (**in the anterolateral thigh, in the deltoid muscle, orally**).

TRUE OR FALSE EXERCISE

*Indicate whether each statement is true or false by writing **T** or **F** on the line.*

1. _____ A muscle biopsy is used to diagnose the cause of muscle weakness.

2. _____ An adaptive device increases mobility and independence for a physically challenged patient.

3. _____ Physically challenged is the newer way of referring to someone who is handicapped.

4. _____ DTR tests whether the muscular–nervous pathway is functioning correctly.

5. _____ An analgesic drug is used to treat mild-to-moderate inflammation and pain from minor injuries such as muscle strains and muscle overuse.

6. _____ A fasciotomy is used to release blood and fluid in a patient with compartment syndrome.

DIVIDING WORDS EXERCISE

Separate these words into their component parts (prefix, combining form, suffix). Some words do not contain all three word parts. The first one has been done for you.

Medical Word	Prefix	Combining Form	Suffix
1. **nonsteroidal**	*non-*	*steroid/o-*	*-al*
2. orthosis		_____	_____
3. mobility		_____	_____
4. rehabilitation	_____	_____	_____
5. analgesic	_____	_____	_____
6. fasciotomy		_____	_____
7. biopsy		_____	_____
8. myorrhaphy		_____	_____

RELATED COMBINING FORMS EXERCISE

Write the combining forms on the lines provided. (Hint: See the It's Greek to Me! feature box.)

1. Three combining forms that mean *movement.* _____ _____ _____

2. Three combining forms that mean *muscle.* _____ _____ _____

3. Two combining forms that mean *tendon.* _____ _____

PROOFREADING AND SPELLING EXERCISE

Read the following paragraph. Identify each misspelled medical word and write the correct spelling of it on the line provided.

Orothopedics is the study of the bones and muscles. A tendin connects the bone to the muscle and the facsia around it. The rectis femoris is in the leg. Fibromialgia has pain at trigger points, while bersitis is inflamation of a fluid-filled sac. A ganglian forms on a tendon. A muscle biopsee is used to diagnose muscular dystrophee. A tenorhaphy sews together a tendon after an injury.

1. _____

2. _____

3. _____

4. _____

5. _____

6. _____

7. _____

8. _____

9. _____

10. _____

11. _____

Immerse Yourself: Analyze Medical Reports

This contains two related reports: an Operative Report and a Pathology Report. Read both reports and answer the questions.

Electronic Patient Record #1

PEARSON GENERAL HOSPITAL OPERATIVE REPORT

Task   Edit   View   Time Scale   Options   Help

PATIENT NAME: PHELPS, George R.

HOSPITAL NUMBER: 42-51-55

DATE OF OPERATION: November 19, 20xx

PREOPERATIVE DIAGNOSIS
Myopathy of undetermined etiology

POSTOPERATIVE DIAGNOSIS
Myopathy of undetermined etiology

PROCEDURE
Right quadriceps muscle biopsy

ANESTHESIA
Xylocaine 1% local anesthetic with IV sedation

SPECIMEN
Muscle biopsy x3

COMPLICATIONS
None

CLINICAL HISTORY
The patient is a 68-year-old male who has had progressive lower back and right leg weakness for approximately 6 months. He notes difficulty climbing stairs or getting up from a chair or bed. He moves slowly. There is mild eyelid ptosis noted.

OPERATIVE TECHNIQUE
After the induction of IV sedation, the right thigh skin was prepped with a topical antibiotic solution and draped with surgical drapes in a sterile fashion. After infiltration of the skin with local anesthesia, a longitudinal incision was made over the anterolateral aspect of the thigh. The incision was deepened through subcutaneous tissue to the quadriceps fascia, which was incised. Three muscle specimens were obtained for biopsy as per Armed Forces Institute of Pathology (AFIP) protocol. A thin core of muscle, approximately the thickness of a pencil, going deep into the muscle was submitted for the first biopsy. Then two muscle segments were grasped with biopsy clamps and excised. Pressure was held over the muscle for hemostasis. The wound was irrigated with warm saline solution, and the fascia was reapproximated with two interrupted sutures of #2-0 Vicryl. The subcutaneous tissue was approximated with interrupted sutures of #3-0 Vicryl. The skin was approximated with skin staples. A sterile dressing was applied. The patient was transferred to the recovery room in stable condition. Blood loss during the procedure was minimal.

Jamison R. Smith, M.D.

Jamison R. Smith, M.D.

JRS: srd
D: 11/19/xx
T: 11/19/xx

Electronic Patient Record #2

PEARSON GENERAL HOSPITAL PATHOLOGY REPORT

Task   Edit   View   Time Scale   Options   Help

PATIENT NAME: PHELPS, George R.

HOSPITAL NUMBER: 42-51-55

DATE OF REPORT: November 19, 20xx

OPERATION PERFORMED
Right quadriceps muscle biopsy

CLINICAL HISTORY
Myopathy

GROSS SPECIMEN
Received on ice are three specimen jars. One is a porcelain jar labeled "without a clamp, for freezing" and it contains a thin core of red-tan muscle wrapped in gauze, 0.7 × 0.7 × 2.0 cm. There are also two glass jars. One is labeled "formalin" and within the jar is a large clamp with a fragment of red-tan muscle, 1.8 × 1.3 × 1.3 cm. The other jar is labeled "glutaraldehyde" and contains a small clamp to which is attached a fragment of red-tan muscle measuring about 1.8 × 1.2 × 1.3 cm. All three containers are sent on ice to the Armed Forces Institute of Pathology for processing and diagnosis.

MICROSCOPIC SPECIMEN
Biopsy of right quadriceps muscle. Await forthcoming report from the Armed Forces Institute of Pathology.

Ralph A. Stanley, M.D.

Ralph A. Stanley, M.D.

RAS: drc
D: 11/19/xx
T: 11/19/xx

1. Divide *myopathy* into its two word parts and give the meaning of each word part.

Word Part	**Meaning**

2. Divide *biopsy* into its two word parts and give the meaning of each word part.

Word Part	**Meaning**

3. What operative procedure was performed?

4. Where is that muscle group located?

5. How many specimens were taken?

_____

6. What two ADLs does the report specifically mention that the patient had difficulty doing before surgery?

_____

_____

7. What color is the muscle biopsy specimen?

_____

8. What was this patient's postoperative diagnosis?

_____

9. In what order were these structures encountered when the incision was performed? Circle the correct answer.

   a. Quadriceps muscle, skin, fascia, subcutaneous tissue

   b. Skin, subcutaneous tissue, fascia, quadriceps muscle

   c. Fascia, skin, subcutaneous tissue, quadriceps muscle

10. Formalin and glutaraldehyde are _____.

   a. used to prep and drape the skin

   b. used as preservatives for biopsy specimens

   c. local anesthetic drugs

11. When will the etiology be determined?

_____

MyLab Medical Terminology™

MyLab Medical Terminology is a premium online homework management system that includes a host of features to help you study. Registered users will find:

- A multitude of quizzes and activities built within the mylab platform

- Powerful tools that track and analyze your results—allowing you to create a personalized learning experience

- Videos and audio pronunciations to help enrich your progress

- Streaming lesson presentations (guided lectures) and self-paced learning modules

- A space where you and your instructor can check your progress and manage your assignments

9 Neurology

Nervous System

Neurology (nyoor-AW-loh-jee) is the medical specialty that studies the anatomy and physiology of the nervous system; uses laboratory, diagnostic, and radiologic procedures to diagnose nervous system diseases; and uses medical procedures, drugs, and surgical procedures to treat nervous system diseases.

⋁ Chapter Overview and Learning Outcomes

After you study this chapter, you should be able to demonstrate mastery of the outcomes by successfully completing the exercises.

9.1 Anatomy
Identify the structures of the nervous system.
Demonstrate proficiency in medical language.
9.1 Practice Laps

9.2 Physiology
Describe the functions of the nervous system.
Demonstrate proficiency in medical language.
9.2 Practice Laps
Vocabulary Review

9.3 Diseases
Describe common nervous system diseases.
Demonstrate proficiency in medical language.
9.3 Practice Laps

9.4 Laboratory, Diagnostic, and Radiologic Procedures
Describe common nervous system laboratory tests, diagnostic procedures, and radiologic procedures.
Demonstrate proficiency in medical language.
9.4 Practice Laps

9.5 Medical Procedures, Drugs, and Surgical Procedures
Describe common nervous system medical procedures, drugs, and surgical procedures.
Demonstrate proficiency in medical language.
9.5 Practice Laps
Abbreviations Summary
Career Focus

Chapter Review Exercises
Dive In: Medical Language Exercises
(Learning Outcomes 9.1–9.5)
Immerse Yourself: Analyze Medical Reports

Medical Language Key

To unlock the definition of a medical word, break it into word parts. Give the meaning of each word part. Put the meanings of the word parts in order, beginning with the meaning of the suffix, then the meaning of the prefix (if there is one), then the meaning of the combining form.

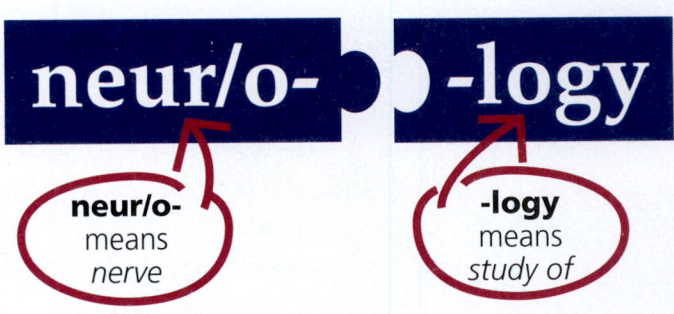

neur/o- means *nerve*

-logy means *study of*

Neurology: ▶ *Study of (the) nerves (and related structures).*

The **nervous system** is a body system that is present in and communicates with every part of the body from the head to the tips of the fingers and toes (see Figure 9-1 ■). The nervous system contains **neural tissue**, a specialized tissue that can conduct electrical impulses.

The structures of the nervous system can be divided into two main areas: the central nervous system and the peripheral nervous system (see Figure 9-2 ■) with its divisions. The **central nervous system (CNS)** consists of the brain and the spinal cord. These structures are protected by the bones of the cranium and vertebrae. The **peripheral nervous system** consists of the cranial nerves and the spinal nerves. The peripheral nervous system is divided into the autonomic nervous system and the somatic nervous system. The autonomic nervous system is further divided into the parasympathetic and sympathetic divisions.

The functions of the nervous system are to receive, process, and interpret sensory information from the internal body and the environment around the body. Based on this information, the nervous system then sends motor commands to muscles and other structures in the body. This information can be acted on immediately, if needed, or it can be stored for future reference in the memory. The brain is also the site of conscious awareness, thinking, memory, creativity, emotions, planning, and the ability to learn.

The nervous system works in conjunction with the muscular and skeletal systems to initiate and coordinate the body's voluntary movements. With the input of sensory information from the inner ear, visual information from the eyes, and sensory information from the muscles about body position, the nervous system helps to maintain the body's sense of balance. The nervous system works in conjunction with the skin by relaying sensory information from nerves in the skin to the spinal cord and brain. The nervous system works in conjunction with several body systems to regulate automatic functions such as the heart rate, blood pressure, breathing, and digestion. The nervous system works in conjunction with the endocrine system (described in Chapter 13, Endocrinology) as the pituitary gland (an endocrine gland that secretes hormones) is located in the brain.

9.1 Anatomy

Central Nervous System

The central nervous system consists of the brain, with its many structures, and the spinal cord.

Brain

The **brain** is the largest part of the central nervous system. It is located within the bony **cranium**, and it fills the **cranial cavity**. The brain consists of the cerebrum (and its lobes) and additional structures of the ventricles, thalamus, hypothalamus, hippocampus, amygdaloid bodies, brainstem, and cerebellum—all of which are surrounded by the meninges (layers of membranes) (described in a later section).

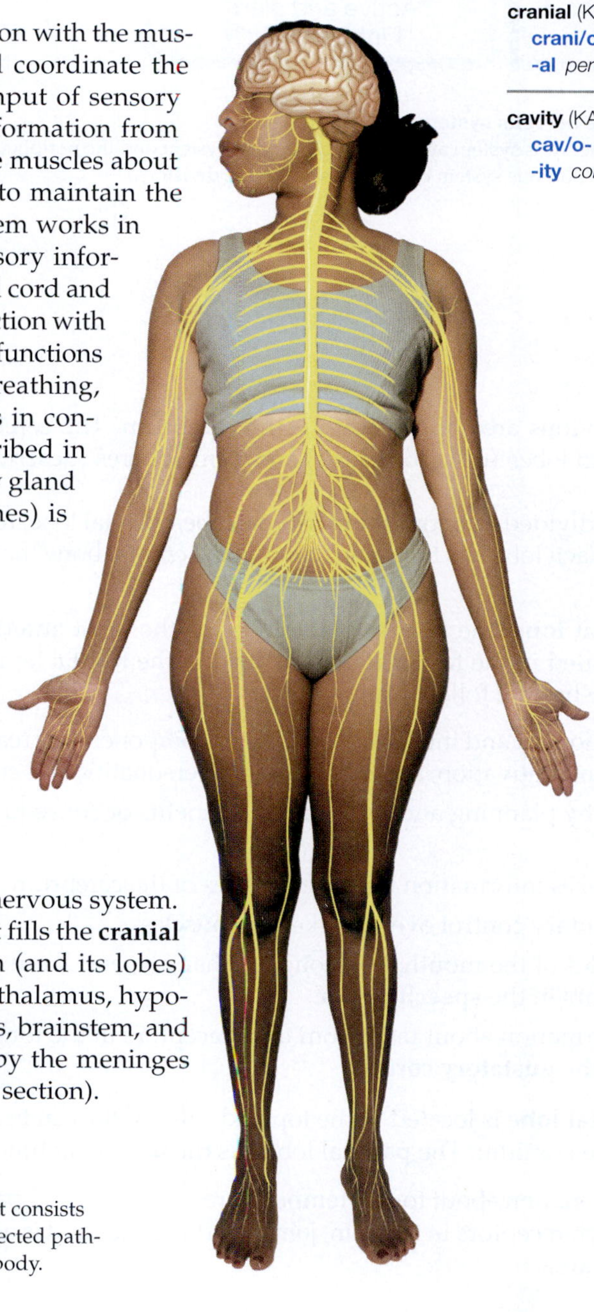

FIGURE 9-1 ■ Nervous system.
The nervous system is a widespread body system that consists of the brain, spinal cord, and nerves that form a connected pathway on which nerve impulses travel throughout the body.

Pronunciation/Word Parts

nervous (NER-vuhs)
  nerv/o- *nerve*
  -ous *pertaining to*

neural (NYOOR-al)
  neur/o- *nerve*
  -al *pertaining to*

central (SEN-tral)

peripheral (peh-RIF-eh-ral)
  peripher/o- *outer aspects*
  -al *pertaining to*

brain (BRAYN)
The combining form **encephal/o-** means *brain*.

cranium (KRAY-nee-um)

cranial (KRAY-nee-al)
  crani/o- *cranium; top part of the skull*
  -al *pertaining to*

cavity (KAV-ih-tee)
  cav/o- *hollow space*
  -ity *condition; state*

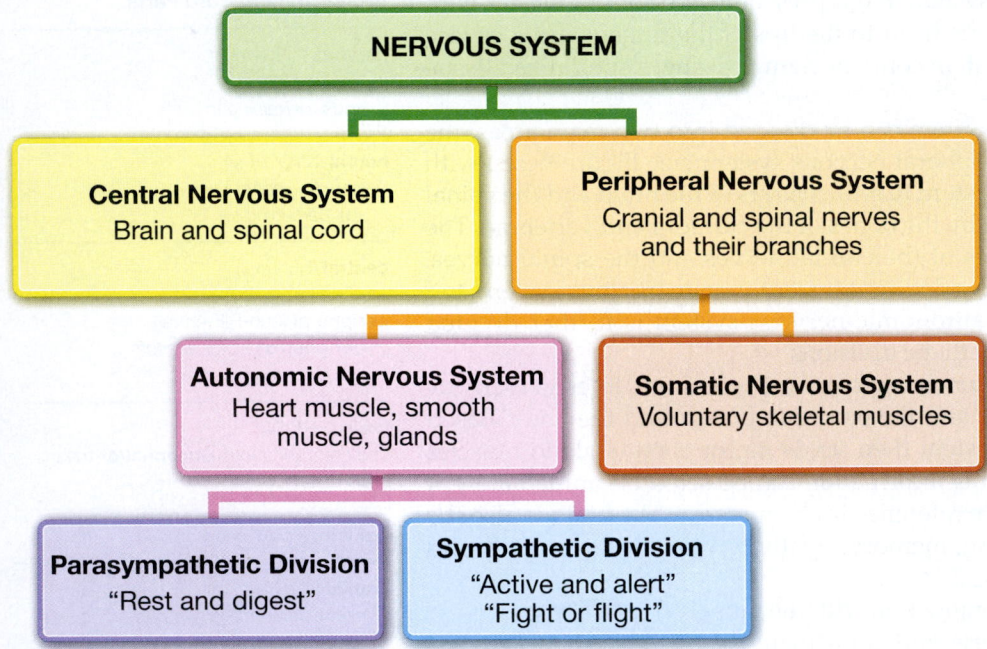

FIGURE 9-2 ■ **Divisions of the nervous system.**
The two main divisions of the nervous system are the central nervous system and the peripheral nervous system. The peripheral nervous system contains several other divisions.

Cerebrum

The largest and most obvious area of the brain is the **cerebrum**. The cerebrum is divided in two ways: into lobes (described here) and hemispheres (described in a later section).

The cerebrum can be divided into four **lobes**: frontal lobe, parietal lobe, temporal lobe, and occipital lobe. Each lobe has the same name as the cranial bone that is next to it (see Figure 9-3 ■).

Frontal Lobe. The **frontal lobe**, the largest of the lobes, is the most anterior lobe of the cerebrum. It is located in the forehead region, next to the frontal bone of the cranium. The frontal lobe has the following functions:

- Originates conscious thought and intelligence and their components of reasoning, judgment, organization, motivation, abstract thinking, personality, and creativity
- Predicts future events by planning and weighing the benefits or consequences of actions
- Coordinates and analyzes information from other lobes of the cerebrum
- Exerts conscious, voluntary control over the skeletal muscles
- Coordinates the muscles of the mouth, lips, tongue, pharynx, and larynx to produce speech. This occurs in the **speech center.**
- Analyzes sensory information about taste from taste receptors in the tongue and throat. This occurs in the **gustatory cortex.**

Parietal Lobe. The **parietal lobe** is located in the top and sides of the cerebrum next to the parietal bone of the cranium. The parietal lobe has the following functions:

- Analyzes sensory information about touch, temperature, vibration, and pain. This information comes from receptors in the skin, joints, and muscles and is analyzed in the **somatosensory area.**

Pronunciation/Word Parts

cerebrum (seh-REE-brum)

cerebral (seh-REE-bral)
  cerebr/o- *cerebrum*
  -al *pertaining to*

lobe (LOHB)

frontal (FRUN-tal)
  front/o- *front*
  -al *pertaining to*

gustatory (GUS-tah-TOR-ee)
  gustat/o- *sense of taste*
  -ory *having the function of*

cortex (KOR-teks)

parietal (pah-RY-eh-tal)
  pariet/o- *wall of a cavity*
  -al *pertaining to*

somatosensory
(soh-MAH-toh-SEN-soh-ree)
  somat/o- *body*
  sens/o- *feeling*
  -ory *having the function of*
The combining forms **esthes/o-** and **esthet/o-** mean *feeling; sensation.*

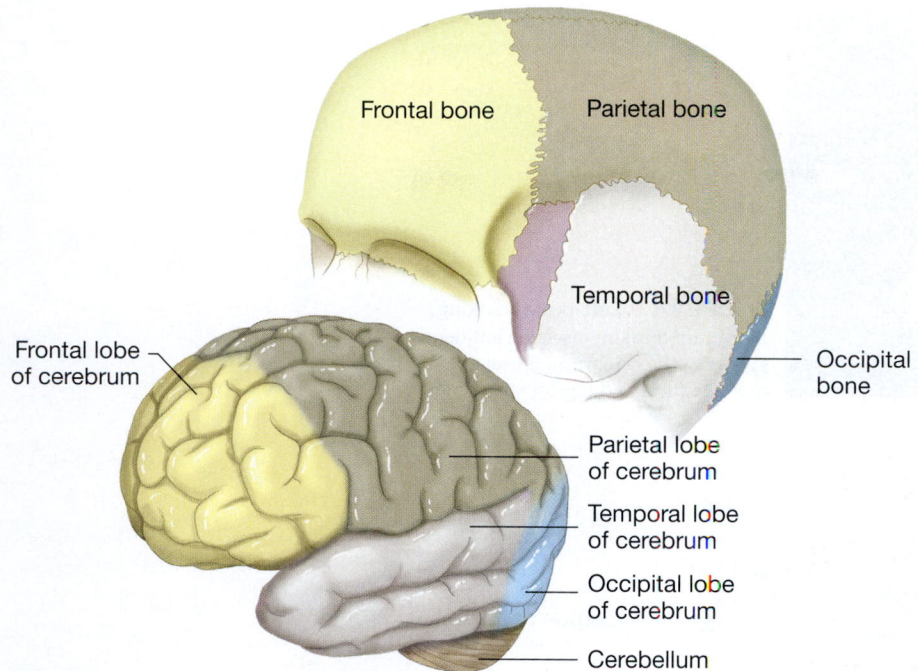

FIGURE 9-3 ■ Lobes of the cerebrum.
Each lobe of the cerebrum takes its name from the bone of the cranium that is next to it.

Temporal Lobe. The **temporal lobe** is located on the sides of the cerebrum beneath the temporal bone of the cranium. The temporal lobe has the following functions:

- Analyzes sensory information about hearing from receptors in the cochlea of the inner ear. This occurs in the **auditory cortex.** (The auditory cortex of the right temporal lobe analyzes sensory information from the left ear and vice versa.)
- Analyzes sensory information about smells from olfactory receptors in the nose. This occurs in the **olfactory cortex.**

Occipital Lobe. The **occipital lobe** is located at the lower back of the brain next to the occipital bone of the cranium. The occipital lobe has the following functions:

- Analyzes sensory information about vision from receptors in the retina of the eye. This occurs in the **visual cortex.** (The visual cortex of the right occipital lobe analyzes sensory information from some parts of both eyes, and vice versa, to produce three-dimensional vision.)

The cerebrum can also be divided into **hemispheres**. There is a very deep, anterior-to-posterior **fissure** in the top surface of the cerebrum that divides it into right and left sides or hemispheres. The **corpus callosum**, a band of nerve fibers, connects the two hemispheres and allows them to communicate with each other and coordinate their activities. Each hemisphere receives sensory information from the other side and sends motor commands to coordinate movements on that side. In general, the left hemisphere of the cerebrum is active in recalling memories and in speech, writing, language, reasoning, problem solving, science, and mathematics (see Figure 9-4 ■). The right hemisphere is active in analyzing the environment in three dimensions, recognizing faces and patterns, interpreting the emotional content of words (but not the actual words), and understanding music and art.

The surface of the cerebrum has elevated folds (**gyri**) and narrow grooves (**sulci**) (see Figure 9-5 ■). The **cerebral cortex** or gray matter is the outermost layer of tissue that follows the curves of the gyri and sulci. The gray matter is composed of the cell bodies of neurons (described in a later section). Beneath the gray matter, the white matter of the cerebrum is composed of the axons of neurons. Most of these axons are covered by a fatty, white insulating layer of myelin, which gives the white matter of the cerebrum its color. Besides the cerebrum and its hemispheres and lobes, the brain

Pronunciation/Word Parts

temporal (TEM-poh-ral)
  tempor/o- *side of the head; temple*
  -al *pertaining to*

auditory (AW-dih-TOR-ee)
  audit/o- *sense of hearing*
  -ory *having the function of*

olfactory (ohl-FAK-toh-ree)
  olfact/o- *sense of smell*
  -ory *having the function of*

occipital (awk-SIH-pih-tal)
  occipit/o- *back of the head; occiput*
  -al *pertaining to*

visual (VIH-shoo-al)
  vis/o- *sight; vision*
  -ual *pertaining to*

hemisphere (HEM-ih-sfeer)
The prefix **hemi-** means *one half*. The suffix **-sphere** means *ball; sphere.*

fissure (FIH-shur)
  fiss/o- *splitting*
  -ure *result of; system*

corpus callosum (KOR-puhs kah-LOH-sum)

gyrus (JY-ruhs)

gyri (JY-rye)
Latin plural noun: Change the singular ending *-us* to *-i.*

sulcus (SUL-kuhs)

sulci (SUL-sigh)
Latin plural noun: Change the singular ending *-us* to *-i.*

cerebral (seh-REE-bral)
  cerebr/o- *cerebrum*
  -al *pertaining to*

cortex (KOR-teks)

cortical (KOR-tih-kal)
  cortic/o- *cortex; outer region*
  -al *pertaining to*

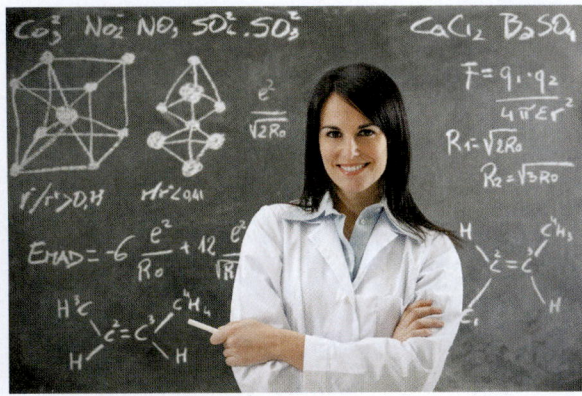

FIGURE 9-4 ■ **Left-brain thinking.**
Left-brain thinking uses the left hemisphere of the cerebrum, the site of mathematical and logical reasoning.

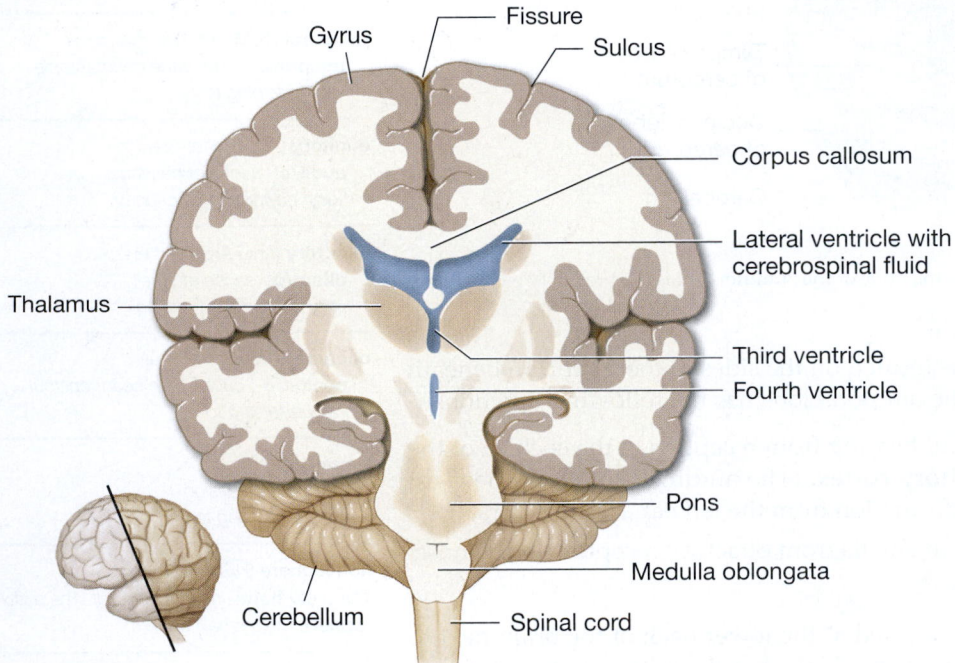

FIGURE 9-5 ■ **Gyri, sulci, and ventricles.**
(The anterior part of the cerebrum has been removed.) The gyri and sulci are visible on the surface of the cerebrum. The fissure that divides the right and left hemispheres of the cerebrum can be seen at the top. The corpus callosum is the white connecting bridge between the hemispheres. The right and left lateral ventricles, as well as the small third and fourth ventricles, are filled with cerebrospinal fluid. The medulla oblongata, the most posterior part of the brainstem, merges with the spinal cord.

also contains these structures: ventricles, thalamus, hypothalamus, hippocampus, amygdaloid bodies, brainstem, cerebellum, and meninges.

Ventricles

The **ventricles** are four interconnected cavities in the brain. The largest of these are the lateral ventricles, one in each hemisphere, that meet in the midline just below the corpus callosum (see Figure 9-5). The third ventricle, a small central cavity that is an inferior extension of the lateral ventricles, lies between the two lobes of the thalamus. The fourth ventricle is a long, narrow cavity that connects to the spinal canal. The ventricles are lined with **ependymal cells** that produce **cerebrospinal fluid (CSF)**, a clear fluid that cushions and protects the brain and contains glucose and other nutrients. CSF circulates through the ventricles and spinal canal and returns to the brain and the subarachnoid space in the meninges where it is absorbed into the blood of large veins nearby.

Thalamus

The **thalamus** is located near the center of the cerebrum, and its two lobes form the walls of the third ventricle (see Figure 9-5 and Figure 9-6 ■). The thalamus acts as a relay

Pronunciation/Word Parts

ventricle (VEN-trih-kul)

ventricular (ven-TRIH-kyoo-lar)
  ventricul/o- *chamber that is filled; ventricle*
  -ar *pertaining to*

ependymal (eh-PEN-dih-mal)
  ependym/o- *cellular lining*
  -al *pertaining to*

cerebrospinal (seh-REE-broh-SPY-nal)
  cerebr/o- *cerebrum*
  spin/o- *backbone; spine*
  -al *pertaining to*

thalamus (THAL-ah-muhs)

thalamic (thah-LAM-ik)
  thalam/o- *thalamus*
  -ic *pertaining to*

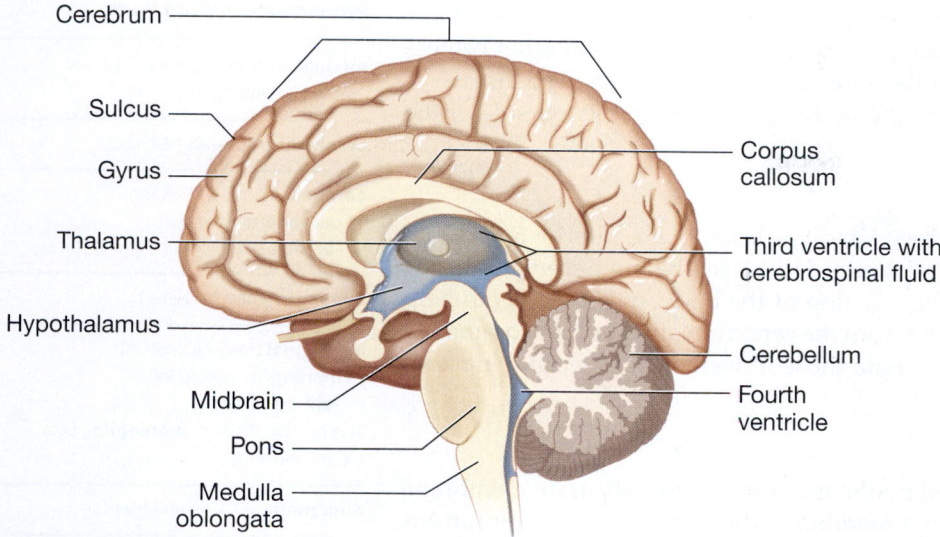

FIGURE 9-6 ■ Midline cut section of the brain.
This cut section shows the right half of the brain. The large size of the cerebrum is seen in comparison to the cerebellum and other structures. Many gyri and sulci are visible on the surface of the cerebrum. The thalamus, hypothalamus, midbrain, pons, medulla oblongata, and cerebellum can be seen in this view.

station, receiving sensory information from the five senses (sight, hearing, taste, smell, and touch) via the cranial nerves and the spinal nerves. The thalamus simultaneously relays this information (1) to the midbrain (which generates motor commands if the sensory information suggests immediate danger) and (2) to the cerebrum (which analyzes the sensory information, compares it with memories, and uses it to plan future actions).

Hypothalamus

The **hypothalamus**, as its name indicates, is located below the thalamus (see Figure 9-6) and forms the floor and part of the walls of the third ventricle. The hypothalamus coordinates the activities of the pons and medulla oblongata, structures that control the heart rate, blood pressure, and respiratory rate. It also regulates body temperature and sensations of thirst and hunger as it contains the **feeding center** and the **satiety center.** The hypothalamus controls emotions of pleasure, excitement, fear, anger, sexual arousal, and bodily responses to these emotions.

Hippocampus

The **hippocampus** is an elongated structure located in both temporal lobes. It is active in the learning process because it causes short-term memories to become permanent long-term memories.

Amygdaloid Body

The **amygdaloid body** is an almond-shaped area in each temporal lobe. It correlates visual images with long-term memories as it interprets facial expressions and new social situations to detect danger. The amygdaloid body is most active during the intense emotions of fear, anger, and rage.

Brainstem

The **brainstem** is a column of tissue that begins in the center of the brain and continues inferiorly until it meets the spinal cord. The brainstem consists of three parts: the midbrain, the pons, and the medulla oblongata (see Figure 9-5 and Figure 9-6).

The **midbrain** is the most superior part of the brainstem. It keeps the mind conscious. It coordinates immediate reflex responses to sudden events. It maintains muscle tone and the position of the extremities. It contains the **substantia nigra**, a gray-to-black pigmented area that produces the neurotransmitter dopamine that regulates muscle tone.

The **pons** is the next part of the brainstem. It relays nerve impulses from the spinal cord to the midbrain and other parts of the brain.

Pronunciation/Word Parts

hypothalamus (HY-poh-THAL-ah-muhs)

hypothalamic (HY-poh-thah-LAM-ik)
  hypo- *below; deficient*
  thalam/o- *thalamus*
  -ic *pertaining to*

satiety (sah-TY-ih-tee)

hippocampus (HIP-oh-KAM-puhs)

amygdaloid (ah-MIG-dah-loyd)
  amygdal/o- *almond shape*
  -oid *resembling*

brainstem (BRAYN-stem)

substantia nigra (sub-STAN-shee-ah NY-grah)

pons (PAWNZ)

The **medulla oblongata** is the most inferior part of the brainstem. It contains the **respiratory centers** that automatically set the respiratory rate and other centers that control the heart rate. (In the medulla oblongata, nerve tracts cross so that nerve impulses coming from the right side of the body are relayed to the left side of the cerebrum, and vice versa.)

Cerebellum

The **cerebellum** is a separate, rounded section of the brain that is inferior and posterior to the cerebrum (see Figures 9-3, 9-5, and 9-6). The cerebellum receives sensory information about muscle tone and the position of the body and uses this to help maintain balance. It receives information from the cerebrum about motor commands and makes minor adjustments to coordinate those movements, especially intricate movements such as typing or skiing.

Meninges

The brain is surrounded and protected by the **meninges**, three separate membrane layers (see Figure 9-7 ■). The outermost membrane (beneath the bony cranium) is the **dura mater**, a tough, fibrous layer that protects the brain. The second membrane layer is the **arachnoid**. Beneath the arachnoid is the **subarachnoid space**, which is filled with cerebrospinal fluid and contains branching fibers (like a spiderweb) that connect the arachnoid to the pia mater membrane beneath it. The innermost layer is the **pia mater**, a thin, delicate membrane that covers the surface of the brain; it contains a network of small blood vessels.

Spinal Cord

The **spinal cord** is the other part of the central nervous system. It begins at the medulla oblongata of the brain (see Figure 9-5). The spinal cord is a long, narrow column of neural tissue that travels inferiorly through the **spinal canal** (also known as the *spinal cavity*), a bony cavity created by the opening (foramen) in each vertebra of the neck and back (see Figure 9-8 ■). The spinal cord is protected and nourished by the three layers of the meninges. Between the dura mater layer of the meninges and the bone of the vertebra is the **epidural space**, which is filled with fatty tissue and blood vessels. Within the spinal cord itself is the **central canal** (a narrow passageway) lined with **ependymal cells** that produce cerebrospinal fluid. At its inferior end, which is at the level of the second lumbar vertebra, the spinal cord separates into a group of nerve roots known as the **cauda equina**.

Pronunciation/Word Parts

medulla oblongata (meh-DUL-ah AWB-long-GAW-tah)

cerebellum (SAIR-eh-BEL-um)

cerebellar (SAIR-eh-BEL-ar)
  cerebell/o- *cerebellum*
  -ar *pertaining to*

meninges (meh-NIN-jeez)

meningeal (meh-NIN-jee-al)
  mening/o- *meninges*
  -eal *pertaining to*
The combining form **meningi/o-** also means *meninges.*

dura mater (DOOR-ah MAH-ter)

dural (DOOR-al)
  dur/o- *dura mater*
  -al *pertaining to*

arachnoid (ah-RAK-noyd)
  arachn/o- *spider; spiderweb*
  -oid *resembling*

subarachnoid (SUB-ah-RAK-noyd)
  sub- *below; underneath; less than*
  arachn/o- *spider; spiderweb*
  -oid *resembling*

pia mater (PEE-ah MAH-ter)

spinal (SPY-nal)
  spin/o- *backbone; spine*
  -al *pertaining to*
The combining form **myel/o-** means *bone marrow; myelin; spinal cord.*

canal (kah-NAL)

epidural (EP-ih-DOOR-al)
  epi- *above; upon*
  dur/o- *dura mater*
  -al *pertaining to*

ependymal (eh-PEN-dih-mal)
  ependym/o- *cellular lining*
  -al *pertaining to*

cauda equina (KAW-dah ee-KWY-nah)

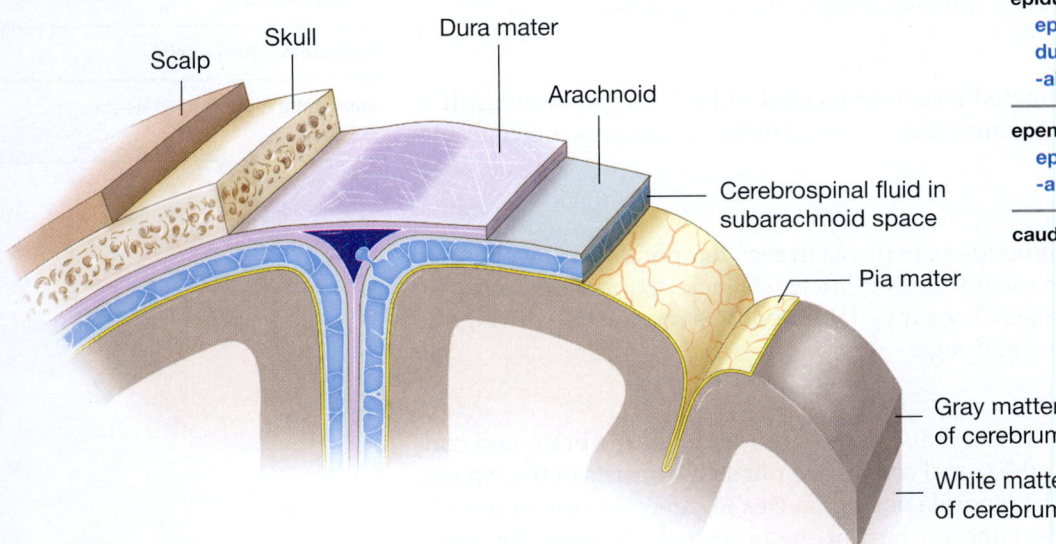

FIGURE 9-7 ■ Meninges.
The meninges have three membrane layers: the dura mater, arachnoid, and pia mater. Between the arachnoid and the pia mater is the subarachnoid space, which is filled with cerebrospinal fluid.

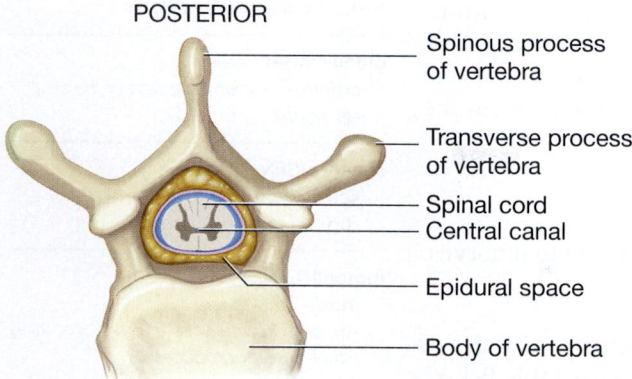

POSTERIOR

- Spinous process of vertebra
- Transverse process of vertebra
- Spinal cord
- Central canal
- Epidural space
- Body of vertebra

FIGURE 9-8 ■ Spinal cord.
The spinal cord passes through the foramen (opening) within each vertebra. It is protected by the bony vertebra, a layer of fat in the epidural space, and then the dura mater and rest of the meninges.

Clinical Connections

Psychiatry. An emotion is an intense state of feelings connected to a particular situation that imprints deeply in long-term memory. Later, when that situation is remembered, it brings with it those same intense emotions. The **limbic system** controls emotion, mood, memory, motivation, and behavior and links the conscious mind to the unconscious mind. Structurally, the limbic system consists of the thalamus, hypothalamus, hippocampus, amygdaloid bodies, fornix, and limbic lobe (a curved area that includes parts of the right and left hemispheres and parts of each lobe of the cerebrum). (See Figure 9-9 ■.)

Endocrinology. The hypothalamus has a stalk of blood vessels and nerves that connects it to the pituitary gland, an endocrine gland (see Figure 9-9). As part of the endocrine system, the hypothalamus secretes hormones that control the hormones from the anterior pituitary gland; the hypothalamus also produces two hormones that are stored in the posterior pituitary gland (described in Chapter 13, Endocrinology). During times of fear or anger, the hypothalamus sends nerve impulses to the sympathetic division of the nervous system to trigger the adrenal gland to secrete the hormone epinephrine for the "fight-or-flight" response to danger.

Pronunciation/Word Parts

limbic (LIM-bik)
  limb/o- *border; edge*
  -ic *pertaining to*

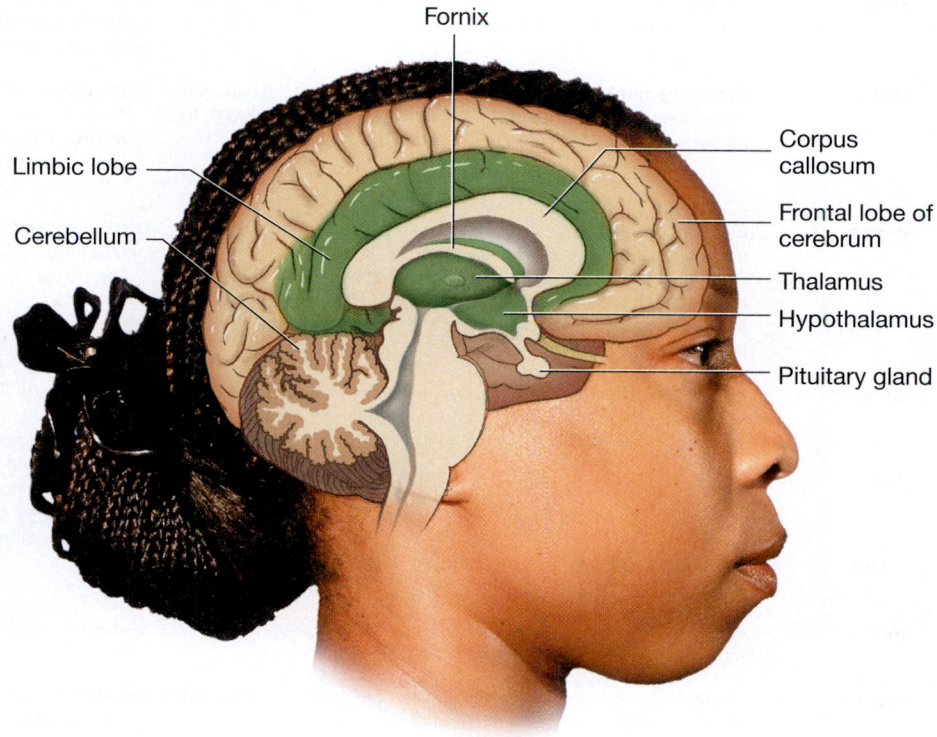

Fornix

- Limbic lobe
- Cerebellum
- Corpus callosum
- Frontal lobe of cerebrum
- Thalamus
- Hypothalamus
- Pituitary gland

FIGURE 9-9 ■ Limbic system.
This midsagittal section of the brain shows the limbic lobe and some of the structures of the limbic system. The structures of the hippocampus and amygdaloid body are part of the limbic system, but they are not visible on this view.

The gray matter of the spinal cord is composed of the cell bodies of neurons. The white matter of the spinal cord is composed of the axons of neurons bundled together as an ascending tract that carries sensory information from a sensory spinal nerve to the brain or as a descending tract that carries motor commands from the brain to a motor spinal nerve connected to a muscle.

Peripheral Nervous System

The peripheral nervous system consists of the cranial nerves and the spinal nerves.

Cranial Nerves

The **cranial nerves** are part of the peripheral nervous system. There are 12 pairs of cranial nerves that begin in the brain or at receptors in the body (see Table 9-1 ■). Sometimes their names reflect the part of the body where they are located. Each pair consists of a cranial nerve to the right side of the body and one to the left. Some cranial nerves receive nerve impulses as **sensory information** from the body (visual images, sounds, smells, tastes, touch, pressure, vibration, temperature, pain, or position). Other cranial nerves send nerve impulses as **motor commands** from the brain to voluntary muscles (to move the face, head, and neck) or to involuntary muscles (to slow the heart rate, to cause peristalsis in the digestive tract, to cause the bronchioles to constrict, or to cause the lacrimal or salivary glands to secrete tears or saliva). Some cranial nerves carry both sensory and motor nerve impulses.

Pronunciation/Word Parts

cranial (KRAY-nee-al)
  crani/o- cranium; top part of the skull
  -al pertaining to

sensory (SEN-soh-ree)
  sens/o- feeling
  -ory having the function of

motor (MOH-tor)
  mot/o- movement
  -or person who does or produces; thing that does or produces

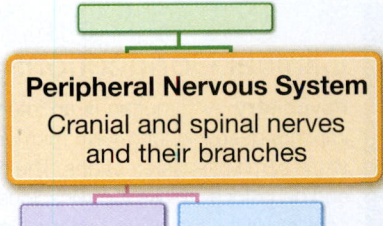

Peripheral Nervous System
Cranial and spinal nerves and their branches

Table 9-1   Cranial Nerves

Cranial Nerve	Type of Nerve	Function	Pronunciation/Word Parts
I olfactory nerve	sensory	**Smell.** Receives sensory information about smells from olfactory receptors in the nose	**olfactory** (ohl-FAK-toh-ree) **olfact/o-** sense of smell **-ory** having the function of
II optic nerve	sensory	**Vision.** Receives sensory information about light, dark, and color from rods and cones in the retina of the eye	**optic** (AWP-tik) **opt/o-** eye; vision **-ic** pertaining to
III oculomotor nerve	motor	**Eye movement.** Carries motor commands to four of the extraocular muscles that move the eye; to muscles that move the eyelid; to muscles of the iris that change the size of the pupil	**oculomotor** (aw-kyoo-loh-MOH-tor) **ocul/o-** eye **mot/o-** movement **-or** person who does or produces; thing that does or produces
IV trochlear nerve	motor	**Eye movement.** Carries motor commands to one extraocular muscle (superior oblique muscle) to move the eye A ligament loop is attached to the bone of the eye socket. When an impulse from the trochlear nerve stimulates the superior oblique muscle, it contracts, pulling its tendon through that ligament loop like the rope of a pulley, and this moves the eye.	**trochlear** (TROH-klee-ar) **trochle/o-** pulley-shaped structure **-ar** pertaining to
V trigeminal nerve	sensory	**Facial sensation.** Receives sensory information about touch, temperature, vibration, and pain from the skin of the face, eyes, nasal cavity, oral cavity, gums, teeth, tongue, and palate	**trigeminal** (try-JEM-ih-nal) **tri-** three **gemin/o-** group; set **-al** pertaining to The trigeminal nerve is a group of three nerve branches: the ophthalmic, maxillary, and mandibular nerves.
	motor	**Chewing.** Carries motor commands to move the muscles for chewing	
VI abducens nerve	motor	**Eye movement.** Carries motor commands to one extraocular muscle (lateral rectus muscle) to move the eye	**abducens** (ab-DOO-senz)
VII facial nerve	sensory	**Taste.** Receives sensory information about taste (sweet, sour, bitter, etc.) from taste receptors in the front of the tongue	**facial** (FAY-shal) **faci/o-** face **-al** pertaining to
	motor	**Facial movement.** **Tears and saliva production.** Carries motor commands to move the facial muscles; to muscles around the lacrimal glands to contract and release tears; to contract muscles around the salivary glands to contract and release saliva	

Cranial Nerve	Type of Nerve	Function	Pronunciation/Word Parts
VIII vestibulocochlear nerve	sensory	**Hearing and balance.** Receives sensory information about sounds from the cochlea (in the inner ear); from the semicircular canals to maintain body balance	**vestibulocochlear** (ves-TIH-byoo-loh-KOH-klee-ar) **vestibul/o-** entrance; vestibule **cochle/o-** cochlea; spiral-shaped structure **-ar** pertaining to
IX glossopharyngeal nerve	sensory	**Taste.** Receives sensory information about taste (sweet, sour, bitter, etc.) from taste receptors at the back of the tongue, palate, and pharynx; receives sensory information about the blood pressure and oxygen/carbon dioxide levels in arterial blood from pressure receptors in the carotid artery	**glossopharyngeal** (GLAW-soh-fah-RIN-jee-al) **gloss/o-** tongue **pharyng/o-** pharynx; throat **-eal** pertaining to
	motor	**Swallowing.** Carries motor commands to move the muscles involved in swallowing **Saliva.** Carries motor commands to move the muscles around the parotid gland to contract and release saliva	
X vagus nerve	sensory	**Taste.** Receives sensory information about taste (sweet, sour, bitter, etc.) from taste receptors in the soft palate and pharynx **Ear, chest, and abdomen sensation.** Receives sensory information about touch, temperature, vibration, and pain from receptors in the ear, diaphragm, and organs in the thoracic cavity and abdominopelvic cavity	**vagus** (VAY-guhs) **vagal** (VAY-gal) **vag/o-** vagus nerve; wandering **-al** pertaining to
	motor	**Heart rate.** Carries motor commands to slow the heart rate **Bronchi.** Carries motor commands to contract smooth muscle around the bronchi **Peristalsis.** Carries motor commands to contract smooth muscle in the gastrointestinal tract to produce peristalsis	
XI accessory nerve	motor	**Swallowing.** Carries motor commands to move the muscles involved in swallowing **Vocal cord and neck movement.** Carries motor commands to move the vocal cords and move the muscles of the neck and upper back The accessory nerve supplements the functions of the vagus nerve.	**accessory** (ak-SEH-soh-ree) **access/o-** contributing part; supplemental part **-ory** having the function of
XII hypoglossal nerve	motor	**Tongue movement.** Carries motor commands to move the tongue	**hypoglossal** (HY-poh-GLAW-sal) **hypo-** below; deficient **gloss/o-** tongue **-al** pertaining to

Spinal Nerves

The **spinal nerves** are part of the peripheral nervous system because they are found in the periphery of the body (those parts away from the center). There are 31 pairs of spinal nerves that originate at regular intervals along the spinal cord. Each pair consists of a spinal nerve to the right side of the body and a spinal nerve to the left side of the body. Each pair of spinal nerves is named according to the vertebra next to it.

Each spinal nerve has two different groups of nerve roots that connect it to the spinal cord: dorsal nerve roots and ventral nerve roots (see Figure 9-10 ■).

Pronunciation/Word Parts

spinal (SPY-nal)
  spin/o- backbone; spine
  -al pertaining to

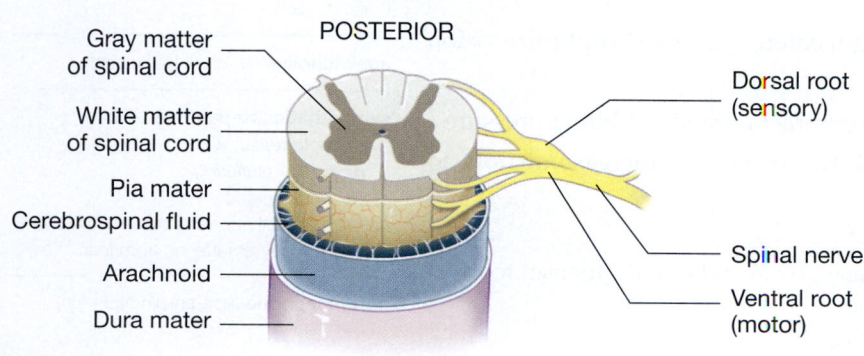

Gray matter of spinal cord
White matter of spinal cord
Pia mater
Cerebrospinal fluid
Arachnoid
Dura mater
POSTERIOR
Dorsal root (sensory)
Spinal nerve
Ventral root (motor)

FIGURE 9-10 ■ Spinal nerves.
The spinal nerves originate at regular intervals along the spinal cord. Each spinal nerve consists of dorsal nerve roots that receive sensory information from the body and ventral nerve roots that carry motor commands to the body.

The **dorsal nerve roots** enter the posterior (dorsal) part of the spinal cord. They receive sensory information (touch, pressure, vibration, temperature, pain, and body position) from a specific area of the skin known as a *dermatome* (described in Chapter 2, Dermatology). Dermatomes are important in the diagnosis of nerve injuries because they correlate a specific spinal nerve and its dermatome to an area of the skin where there is pain or loss of sensation or movement. The dorsal nerve roots also receive sensory information from the muscles and joints. Dorsal nerve roots and their spinal nerve are an **afferent nerve** because they carry nerve impulses from the body to the spinal cord.

The **ventral nerve roots** exit from the anterior (ventral) part of the spinal cord. They carry motor commands from the spinal cord to skeletal muscles and involuntary smooth muscles within organs, glands, and other structures. Ventral nerve roots and their spinal nerve are an **efferent nerve** because they carry nerve impulses away from the spinal cord to the body.

A **reflex** is a rapid, involuntary muscle reaction that is controlled by the spinal cord. The spinal cord reacts immediately to certain types of sensory information (sudden pain or when a physician uses a percussion hammer to tap on a tendon that stretches a muscle) (see Figure 8-26). For example, if you touch something hot, the sensory and motor nerves immediately cause you to move your hand, even before your brain understands what is wrong. This circuit is known as a **reflex arc**. Later, the sensory information is analyzed by the cerebrum, and you say, "Ouch."

Autonomic Nervous System

The **autonomic nervous system** automatically controls the contractions of involuntary cardiac muscle in the heart, as well as smooth muscles around organs, glands, and other structures. The autonomic nervous system can be further broken down into two divisions: the parasympathetic division and the sympathetic division.

The **parasympathetic division** is active when the body is sleeping, resting, eating, or doing light activity (so-called "rest-and-digest" activities). The neurotransmitter of the parasympathetic division is **acetylcholine**. The actions of the parasympathetic division and acetylcholine are to:

- Decrease the heart rate, blood pressure, and metabolic rate
- Increase or decrease the diameter of the pupils in response to changing levels of light
- Increase peristalsis in the gastrointestinal tract
- Cause the secretion of saliva, digestive enzymes, and insulin
- Prepare the body for sexual activity
- Contract the bladder for urination.

The **sympathetic division** is active when the body is active or exercising. The neurotransmitter of the sympathetic division is **norepinephrine**. The actions of the sympathetic division and norepinephrine are to:

- Increase mental alertness
- Dilate the pupils to increase the amount of light entering the eye to optimize vision
- Increase the heart rate and metabolic rate
- Cause the smooth muscles in the arteries to contract to raise the blood pressure
- Cause the smooth muscles in the bronchioles to relax to increase airflow to the lungs
- Increase the respiratory rate
- Cause the skeletal muscles and liver to release glycogen (stored glucose) to meet increased energy needs.

Pronunciation/Word Parts

dorsal (DOR-sal)
  dors/o- *back; dorsum*
  -al *pertaining to*

nerve root (NERV ROOT)
The combining forms **radicul/o-** and **rhiz/o-** mean *spinal nerve root.*

afferent (AF-eh-rent)
  affer/o- *toward the center*
  -ent *pertaining to*

ventral (VEN-tral)
  ventr/o- *abdomen; front*
  -al *pertaining to*

efferent (EF-eh-rent)
  effer/o- *away from the center*
  -ent *pertaining to*

reflex (REE-fleks)

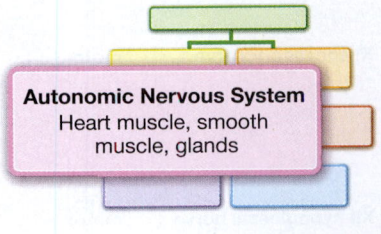

Autonomic Nervous System
Heart muscle, smooth muscle, glands

autonomic (AW-toh-NAW-mik)
  autonom/o- *independent; self-governing*
  -ic *pertaining to*

parasympathetic
(PAIR-ah-SIM-pah-THEH-tik)
  para- *abnormal; apart from; beside; two parts of a pair*
  sym- *together; with*
  pathet/o- *suffering*
  -ic *pertaining to*
The parasympathetic division is one of two parts of a pair in the autonomic nervous system. It works together with the sympathetic division.

acetylcholine (AS-eh-til-KOH-leen)

sympathetic (SIM-pah-THEH-tik)
  sym- *together; with*
  pathet/o- *suffering*
  -ic *pertaining to*
The sympathetic nervous system is active when the body is suffering from fear.

norepinephrine (NOR-eh-pih-NEH-frin)

During stress, anxiety, fear, or anger, the hypothalamus sends nerve impulses to the sympathetic division, which then stimulates the medulla of the adrenal gland (a gland in the endocrine body system) to secrete the hormone **epinephrine** into the blood to prepare the body for more intense activity as in "fight or flight."

Somatic Nervous System

The **somatic nervous system** controls the voluntary movements of skeletal muscles. Cranial nerves and spinal nerves send nerve impulses as motor commands to skeletal muscles and cause them to contract. These motor commands are the result of conscious thoughts in the brain, and the movements produced are voluntary movements. For example, if you decide to open this book and begin studying, your brain sends nerve impulses as motor commands through specific spinal nerves to the skeletal muscles in your arms and hands, and you open the book and find the correct page. Then your brain sends nerve impulses as motor commands through specific cranial nerves to the extraocular muscles of the eyes, and your eyes move across the page as you read.

Neurons and Neuroglia

All of the structures of the nervous system are composed of neural tissue. **Neural tissue** is made up of two categories of cells: neurons and neuroglia.

A **neuron** is an individual nerve cell that conducts electrical impulses; it is the functional unit of the nervous system. **Nerves** are bundles of neurons.

Neuroglia are a group of cells that do not conduct electrical impulses like neurons do. Instead, they perform specialized tasks that assist neurons in doing their work (see Table 9-2 ■). Cancers of the nervous system arise from the neuroglia, not from the neurons.

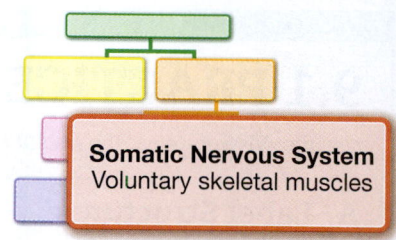

Somatic Nervous System
Voluntary skeletal muscles

Pronunciation/Word Parts

epinephrine (EH-pih-NEH-frin)

somatic (soh-MAT-ik)
  somat/o- *body*
  -ic *pertaining to*

neural (NYOOR-al)
  neur/o- *nerve*
  -al *pertaining to*

neuron (NYOOR-on)
  neur/o- *nerve*
  -on *structure; substance*

nerve (NERV)
The combining forms **nerv/o-** and **neur/o-** mean *nerve*.

neuroglia (nyoor-OH-glee-ah)
  neur/o- *nerve*
  -glia *group of cells that support*

Table 9-2   Neuroglia

Cell Name	Description and Function	Pronunciation/Word Parts
astrocytes	Cells with branches that radiate outward like a star. They support the dendrites of neurons and connect them to capillaries. Astrocytes form the blood–brain barrier that keeps certain harmful substances in the blood from entering the brain.	**astrocyte** (AS-troh-site) **astr/o-** *star-like structure* **-cyte** *cell*
ependymal cells	Cells that line the ventricles of the brain and the narrow, central canal within the spinal cord; they produce cerebrospinal fluid	**ependymal** (eh-PEN-dih-mal) **ependym/o-** *cellular lining* **-al** *pertaining to*
microglia	Cells that move throughout the tissues of the brain and spinal cord. They engulf and destroy dead cells and pathogens (bacteria, viruses, etc.). Microglia are the smallest of all the neuroglia.	**microglia** (my-KROH-glee-ah) **micr/o-** *one millionth; small* **-glia** *group of cells that support*
oligodendroglia	Cells that provide structural support. They also produce myelin that is around the larger axons of neurons in the brain and spinal cord.	**oligodendroglia** (OH-lih-GOH-den-DROH-glee-ah) **olig/o-** *few; scanty* **dendr/o-** *branching structure* **-glia** *group of cells that support* Oligodendroglia: *Group of cells that support (a neuron but have) few branching structures.*
Schwann cells	Cells that produce myelin that is around the larger axons of neurons in the cranial nerves and spinal nerves	**Schwann** (SHVAWN)

9.1 PRACTICE LAPS

Use the Answer Key at the end of the book to check your answers.

A. Label Structures

Write each anatomy word or phrase in the correct numbered box. Be sure to check your spelling.

cerebellum	frontal lobe	occipital lobe	parietal lobe	temporal lobe

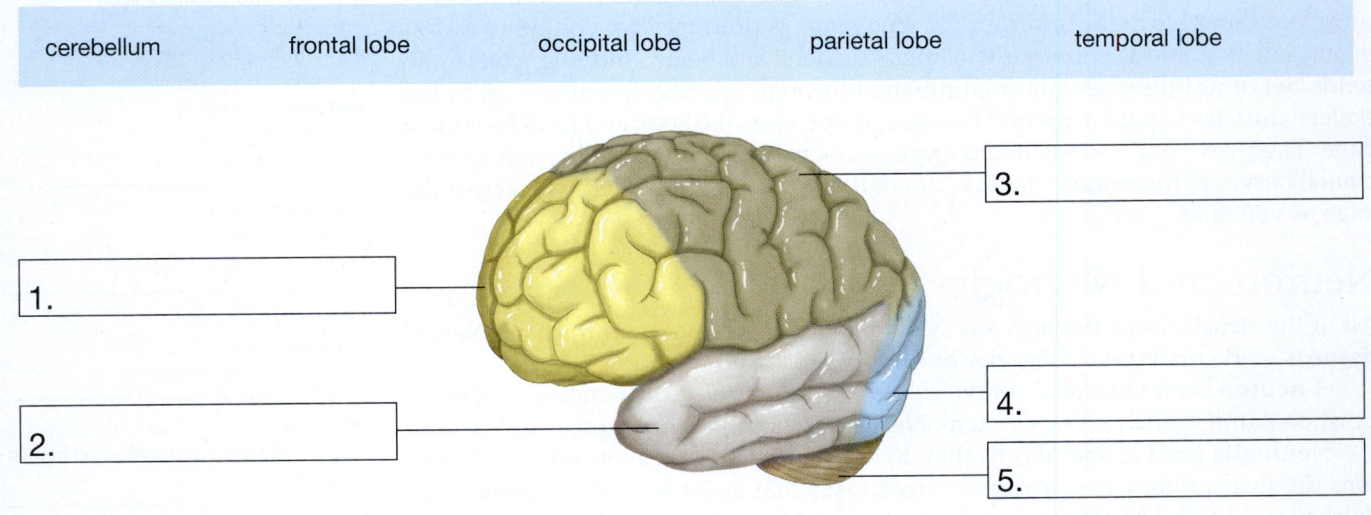

1.

2.

3.

4.

5.

arachnoid
cranium
dura mater
gray matter of the cerebral cortex

pia mater
subarachnoid space
white matter of the cerebrum

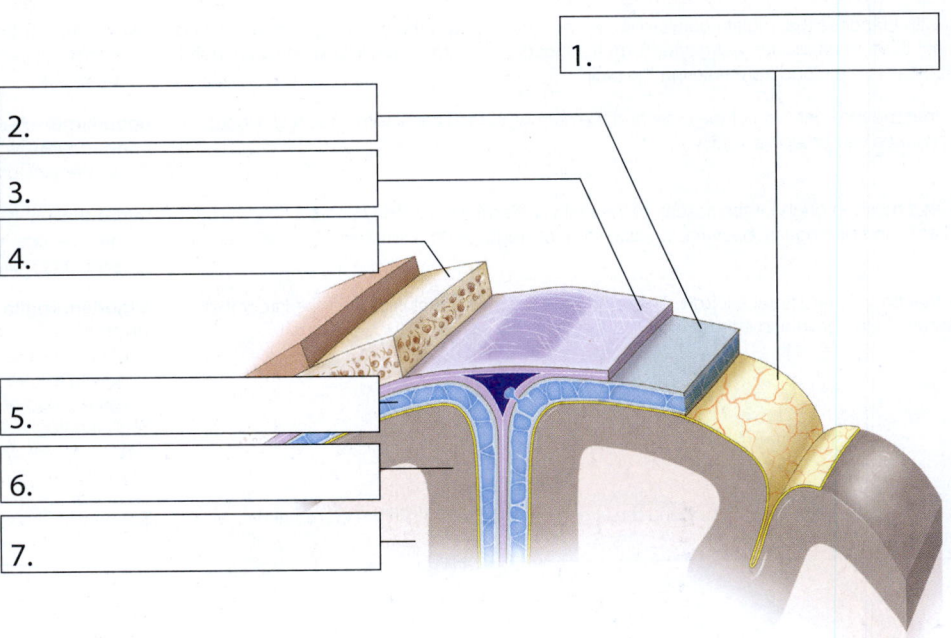

1.

2.

3.

4.

5.

6.

7.

cerebellum   fourth ventricle   medulla oblongata   sulcus
cerebrum   gyrus   midbrain   thalamus
corpus callosum   hypothalamus   pons   third ventricle with cerebrospinal fluid

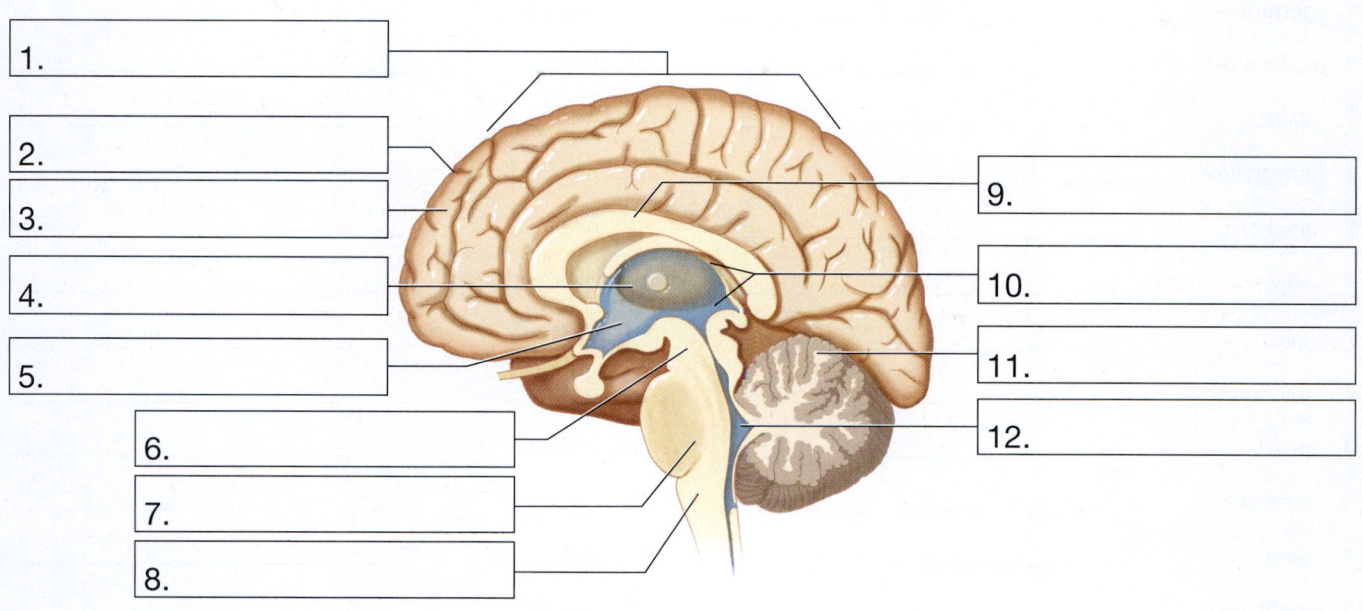

1.

2.

3.

4.

5.

6.

7.

8.

9.

10.

11.

12.

B. Give the Meaning of Combining Forms

Next to each combining form, write its meaning. The first one has been done for you.

Combining Form	Meaning	Combining Form	Meaning
1. **gemin/o-**	*group; set*	30. mening/o-	
2. access/o-		31. micr/o-	
3. affer/o-		32. mot/o-	
4. amygdal/o-		33. myel/o-	
5. arachn/o-		34. nerv/o-	
6. astr/o-		35. neur/o-	
7. audit/o-		36. occipit/o-	
8. autonom/o-		37. ocul/o-	
9. cav/o-		38. olfact/o-	
10. cerebell/o-		39. olig/o-	
11. cerebr/o-		40. opt/o-	
12. cochle/o-		41. pariet/o-	
13. cortic/o-		42. pathet/o-	
14. crani/o-		43. peripher/o-	
15. dendr/o-		44. pharyng/o-	
16. dors/o-		45. radicul/o-	
17. dur/o-		46. rhiz/o-	
18. effer/o-		47. sens/o-	
19. encephal/o-		48. somat/o-	
20. ependym/o-		49. spin/o-	
21. esthes/o-		50. tempor/o-	
22. esthet/o-		51. thalam/o-	
23. faci/o-		52. trochle/o-	
24. fiss/o-		53. vag/o-	
25. front/o-		54. ventricul/o-	
26. gloss/o-		55. ventr/o-	
27. gustat/o-		56. vestibul/o-	
28. limb/o-		57. vis/o-	
29. meningi/o-			

C. Build Words

Read the definition of the medical word. Look at the combining form that is given. Select the correct suffix from the Suffix List, and write it on the blank line. Then build the medical word, and write it on the line. (Remember: You may need to remove the combining vowel. Always remove the hyphens and slash.) Be sure to check your spelling.

Suffix List

-al (pertaining to)	-glia (group of cells that support)	-on (structure; substance)	-ory (having the function of)
-ar (pertaining to)	-ic (pertaining to)	-or (person who does or produces; thing that does or produces)	-ual (pertaining to)
-cyte (cell)	-ity (condition; state)		-ure (result of; system)
-eal (pertaining to)	-oid (resembling)		
-ent (pertaining to)			

Definition of the Medical Word	Combining Form	Suffix	Build the Medical Word
Example: (Division of the nervous system) pertaining to (the) body	**somat/o-**	*-ic*	*somatic*

[*You think* pertaining to (*-ic*) + body (*somat/o-*). *You change the order of the word parts to put the suffix last. You write* somatic.]

1. Pertaining to (the) cerebrum	cerebr/o-		
2. Pertaining to (the) top part of the skull	crani/o-		
3. Pertaining to nerve (tissue)	neur/o-		
4. Having the function of (the) sense of hearing	audit/o-		
5. Pertaining to (the) ventricle (in the brain)	ventricul/o-		
6. Resembling (a) spiderweb	arachn/o-		
7. Pertaining to (the) meninges	mening/o-		
8. Pertaining to (the) spine	spin/o-		
9. Pertaining to away from the center	effer/o-		
10. (Structure that is the) result of splitting	fiss/o-		
11. Pertaining to (the) outer aspects (of the body)	peripher/o-		
12. Pertaining to (the) thalamus	thalam/o-		
13. Having the function of feeling	sens/o-		
14. Pertaining to independent or self-governing	autonom/o-		
15. Structure (of a single) nerve (cell)	neur/o-		
16. Pertaining to (the) side of the head	tempor/o-		
17. Having the function of (the) sense of smell	olfact/o-		
18. Pertaining to (the) cerebellum	cerebell/o-		
19. Group of cells that support (the neuron of a) nerve	neur/o-		
20. Pertaining to (a) cellular lining	ependym/o-		

continued on next page

Definition of the Medical Word	Combining Form	Suffix	Build the Medical Word
21. Pertaining to (the) back of the head	occipit/o-	_____	_____
22. Condition (of being a) hollow space	cav/o-	_____	_____
23. Thing that produces movement	mot/o-	_____	_____
24. Having the function of (the) sense of taste	gustat/o-	_____	_____
25. (Structure) resembling (an) almond shape	amygdal/o-	_____	_____
26. Pertaining to sight (and) vision	vis/o-	_____	_____
27. Cell (with a) star-like structure	astr/o-	_____	_____

D. Define Abbreviations

1. CNS   _____

2. CSF   _____

9.2 Physiology

Neurons and Neurotransmitters

A **neuron** is the functional unit of the nervous system. It consists of three parts: dendrites, the cell body, and an axon (see Figure 9-11 ■). The **dendrites** are multiple branching structures at the beginning of the neuron. Astrocytes are specialized cells that support the dendrites and connect them to nearby capillaries. The cell body contains the **nucleus** of the neuron, which directs cellular activities. The cell body also contains **cytoplasm**, a gel-like substance; structures in the cytoplasm produce neurotransmitters. The **axon** is an elongated extension of cytoplasm at the end of the neuron. Large axons are covered by a fatty, white insulating layer of **myelin**; small axons are not covered with myelin. Myelin increases the speed of an electrical impulse along the neuron. Oligodendroglia are specialized cells that produce the myelin that is around the axons of neurons in the brain and spinal cord. Schwann cells produce the myelin that is around the axons of neurons of cranial and spinal nerves.

The axon of one neuron does not connect directly to the dendrites of the next neuron. Instead, there is a space or **synapse** between the two neurons. (There is also a synapse between a neuron and other structures, such as the cell of a muscle, organ, or gland.) An electrical impulse travels long the axon. At the tip of the axon are vesicles (fluid-filled sacs) that store a **neurotransmitter**. The electrical impulse stimulates the vesicles to release a neurotransmitter, which acts as a chemical messenger that travels across the synapse and binds to a **receptor**, a structure on the cell membrane of the next dendrite. There, the neurotransmitter's chemical message is converted into an electrical impulse that travels to the end of that neuron. All of these events happen in a fraction of a second.

There are many different neurotransmitters in the nervous system. The most common ones are described in Table 9-3 ■.

Pronunciation/Word Parts

dendrite (DEN-dryt)
  dendr/o- *branching structure*
  -ite *thing that pertains to*

nucleus (NOO-klee-us)

cytoplasm (SY-toh-plazm)
  cyt/o- *cell*
  -plasm *formed substance; growth*

axon (AK-sawn)

myelin (MY-eh-lin)

myelinated (MY-eh-lih-NAY-ted)
  myelin/o- *myelin*
  -ated *composed of; pertaining to a condition*

synapse (SIN-aps)

neurotransmitter
(NYOOR-oh-TRANS-mih-ter)
  neur/o- *nerve*
  transmitt/o- *send across; send through*
  -er *person who does or produces; thing that does or produces*

receptor (ree-SEP-tor)
  recept/o- *receive*
  -or *person who does or produces; thing that does or produces*

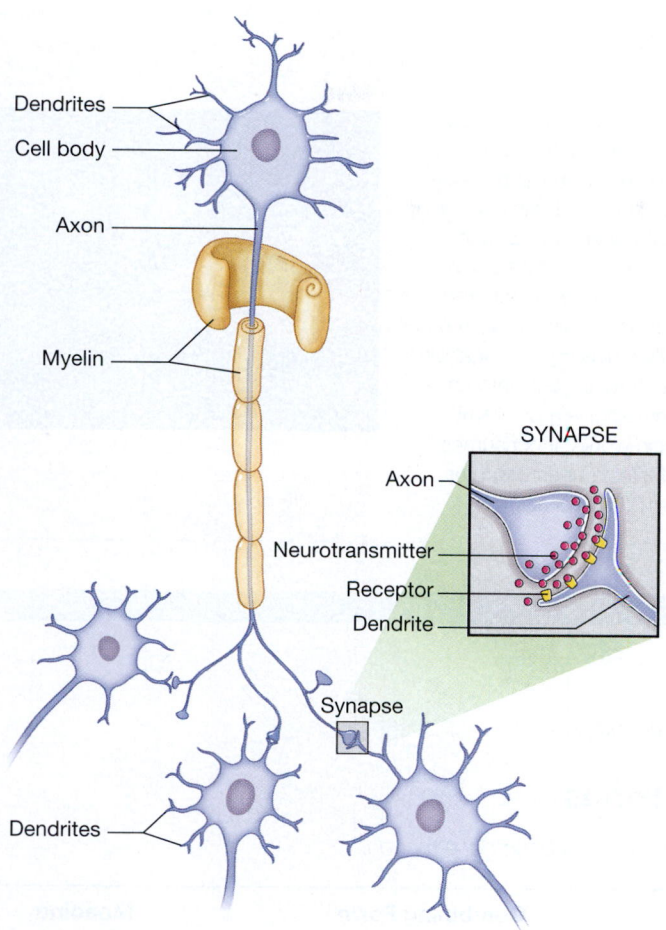

FIGURE 9-11 ■ Neuron.
A neuron consists of several dendrites, a cell body, and an axon. The dendrites receive electrical impulses from other neurons. The cell body contains the nucleus of the neuron. The axon transmits electrical impulses to other neurons (or to a muscle fiber, to a cell in an organ, or to a cell in a gland). Larger axons are covered with myelin to increase the speed of electrical impulses.

Table 9-3   Neurotransmitters, Neuromodulators, and Hormones

Substance	Location	Pronunciation/Word Parts
acetylcholine	Neurotransmitter between neurons of the parasympathetic division. It is also in the somatic nervous system in synapses between a motor neuron and a voluntary skeletal muscle.	**acetylcholine** (AS-eh-til-KOH-leen)
dopamine	Neurotransmitter in the brain between neurons in the cerebral cortex, hypothalamus, midbrain, and limbic system. Produced by the substantia nigra of the midbrain.	**dopamine** (DOH-pah-meen)
endorphins	Neuromodulators in the brain between neurons in the hypothalamus, thalamus, and brainstem. They are one of several natural pain relievers produced by the brain.	**endorphins** (en-DOR-finz)
epinephrine	Hormone secreted by the adrenal gland and released into the blood. It stimulates neurons in the sympathetic division during times of anxiety, fear, or anger to prepare the body for "fight or flight."	**epinephrine** (EH-pih-NEH-frin)
norepinephrine	Neurotransmitter of the sympathetic division. It is also found between neurons in the cerebral cortex, hypothalamus, cerebellum, brainstem, and spinal cord. It is also a hormone secreted by the adrenal gland.	**norepinephrine** (NOR-eh-pih-NEH-frin)
serotonin	Neurotransmitter between neurons of the limbic system, hypothalamus, and cerebellum in the brain and in the spinal cord	**serotonin** (SAIR-oh-TOH-nin)

Dive Deeper

The latest computers are amazing in their ability to process large amounts of data, as computer chips can now process in parallel (as the brain does) rather than sequentially. According to *Scientific American* magazine, the world's most powerful supercomputer does computations four times faster than the human brain and can hold 10 times as much data. Even an everyday computer can hear your spoken questions and answer them verbally, drive a car by itself, monitor your home and notify you remotely of intruders, and so on. The human brain has been compared to a computer, but that comparison falls short in important ways. The brain excels in other areas: self-awareness, emotions, pattern recognition, creative thinking, and analyzing complex tasks. In fact, it is human thinking that translates a complex task into an algorithm of step-by-step instructions that allow a computer to solve a problem! And here is another important difference. As the human brain works, it consumes only 20 watts of power (less than one lightbulb), while the fastest supercomputer consumes about a million watts (amount needed to power 10,000 homes).

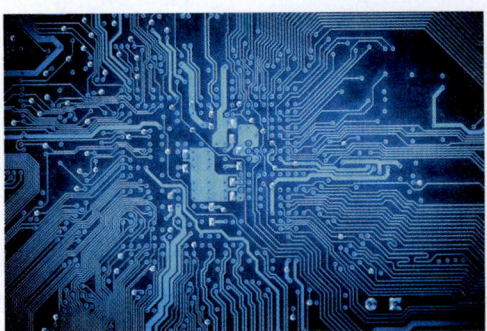

9.2 PRACTICE LAPS

Use the Answer Key at the end of the book to check your answers.

A. Give the Meaning of Combining Forms

Next to each combining form, write its meaning. The first one has been done for you.

Combining Form	Meaning	Combining Form	Meaning
1. **cyt/o-**	*cell*	4. neur/o-	
2. dendr/o-		5. recept/o-	
3. myelin/o-		6. transmitt/o-	

B. Build Words

Read the definition of the medical word. Look at the combining form that is given. Select the correct suffix from the Suffix List, and write it on the blank line. Then build the medical word, and write it on the line. (Remember: You may need to remove the combining vowel. Always remove the hyphens and slash.) Be sure to check your spelling.

Suffix List

-ated (composed of; pertaining to a condition)   -or (person who does or produces; thing that does or produces)
-ite (thing that pertains to)   -plasm (formed substance; growth)

Definition of the Medical Word	Combining Form	Suffix	Build the Medical Word
Example: Formed substance (in a) cell	**cyt/o-**	*-plasm*	*cytoplasm*

[*You think* formed substance (*-plasm*) + cell (*cyt/o-*). You put the suffix last. You combine the word parts and write cytoplasm.]

1. Thing that pertains to (a) branching structure	dendr/o-		
2. Thing that does receive	recept/o-		
3. Composed of myelin	myelin/o-		

Vocabulary Review

Word or Phrase	Description	Combining Forms
Overview		
autonomic nervous system	Division of the peripheral nervous system that controls the contractions of involuntary muscles. It includes the divisions of the parasympathetic and sympathetic nervous systems.	**autonom/o-** *independent; self-governing*
central nervous system (CNS)	Division of the nervous system that consists of the brain and the spinal cord	**nerv/o-** *nerve*
nerve	Bundle of individual neurons	**neur/o-** *nerve* **neur/o-** *nerve*
nervous system	Body system that consists of the brain, spinal cord, cranial nerves, and spinal nerves. It includes the central nervous system as well as the peripheral nervous system and its further divisions. The nervous system's structures are made of neural tissue. The functions of the nervous system are to receive and process sensory information and send motor commands.	**nerv/o-** *nerve* **neur/o-** *nerve*
neural tissue	Specialized tissue of the nervous system that can conduct electrical impulses. The two types are neurons and neuroglia.	**neur/o-** *nerve*
neuroglia	Type of neural tissue whose cells perform specialized tasks that assist neurons in doing their work. Types of neuroglia include astrocytes, ependymal cells, microglia, oligodendroglia, and Schwann cells.	**neur/o-** *nerve*
neuron	An individual nerve cell, which is the functional unit of the nervous system	**neur/o-** *nerve*
parasympathetic nervous system	Division of the autonomic nervous system. It is active when the body is sleeping, resting, eating, or doing light activities. Its neurotransmitter is **acetylcholine.**	**pathet/o-** *suffering*
peripheral nervous system	Division of the nervous system that consists of the cranial nerves and the spinal nerves. It is divided into the autonomic nervous system and the somatic nervous system.	**peripher/o-** *outer aspects*
somatic nervous system	Division of the peripheral nervous system that controls the voluntary movements of skeletal muscles	**somat/o-** *body*
sympathetic nervous system	Division of the autonomic nervous system. It works when the body is active or exercising. Its neurotransmitter is **norepinephrine**. During danger or stress ("fight or flight"), it stimulates the adrenal gland to release the hormone **epinephrine** into the blood.	**pathet/o-** *suffering*
Anatomy of the Central Nervous System		
Brain		
arachnoid	Thin, middle layer of the meninges. It is a spiderweb-like network of fibers that goes into the subarachnoid space and connects the arachnoid to the pia mater layer.	**arachn/o-** *spider; spiderweb*
auditory cortex	Area in the temporal lobe that analyzes sensory information from receptors in the cochlea for the sense of hearing	**audit/o-** *sense of hearing*
brain	Largest part of the central nervous system. It is located in the cranial cavity.	**encephal/o-** *brain*

Word or Phrase	Description	Combining Forms
brainstem	Column of tissue from the center of the brain to the spinal cord. It consists of three parts: the midbrain, pons, and medulla oblongata.	
cerebellum	Smaller, separate, rounded structure of the brain that is inferior and posterior to the cerebrum. It helps maintain balance and adjusts intricate muscle movements.	**cerebell/o-** *cerebellum*
cerebral cortex	The outermost layer of the cerebrum. It consists of gray matter that contains the cell bodies of neurons.	**cortic/o-** *cortex; outer region*
cerebrospinal fluid (CSF)	Clear fluid that is produced by the ependymal cells that line the ventricles in the brain and the central canal within the spinal cord. CSF circulates through the ventricles, flows through the spinal canal, and returns to the brain and the subarachnoid space in the meninges where it is absorbed into the blood of large veins nearby. CSF cushions and protects the brain and contains glucose and other nutrients.	**cerebr/o-** *cerebrum* **spin/o-** *backbone; spine*
cerebrum	The largest and most visible part of the brain. Its surface contains gyri and sulci, and it is divided into four lobes and two hemispheres.	**cerebr/o-** *cerebrum*
corpus callosum	Connecting band of nerve fibers between the two hemispheres of the cerebrum that allows them to communicate and coordinate their activities	
cranial cavity	Hollow cavity inside the bony cranium that contains the brain	**crani/o-** *cranium; top part of the skull* **cav/o-** *hollow space*
dura mater	Tough, outermost layer of the meninges. The dura mater lies just beneath the bones of the cranium and within the foramen of each vertebra.	**dur/o-** *dura mater*
ependymal cells	Cells that line the ventricles of the cerebrum and the narrow central canal in the spinal cord and produce cerebrospinal fluid	**ependym/o-** *cellular lining*
fissure	Deep division that runs in an anterior-to-posterior direction through the superior surface of the cerebrum and divides it into right and left hemispheres	**fiss/o-** *splitting*
frontal lobe	Lobe of the cerebrum next to the frontal bone of the cranium. It originates conscious thought and intelligence and predicts future events and consequences. It exerts conscious control over the skeletal muscles. It contains the speech center that coordinates muscles for speaking and the gustatory cortex for the sense of taste.	**front/o-** *front*
gray matter	Tissue of the cerebral cortex that contains the cell bodies of neurons	
gustatory cortex	Area in the frontal lobe that receives and analyzes sensory information from taste receptors in the tongue for the sense of taste	**gustat/o-** *sense of taste*
gyrus	One of the many elevated folds on the surface of the cerebrum	
hemisphere	One-half of the cerebrum. The right hemisphere recognizes faces, patterns, three-dimensional structures, and the emotional content of words. The left hemisphere deals with recalling memories and is active in speaking, writing, language, reasoning, problem solving, science, and mathematics.	

Word or Phrase	Description	Combining Forms
hypothalamus	Structure in the cerebrum just below the thalamus. It coordinates the activities of the pons and medulla oblongata. It controls body temperature and sensations of hunger and thirst. The hypothalamus controls emotions and bodily responses to emotions. The hypothalamus contains the **feeding center** and the **satiety center**. The hypothalamus is also part of the limbic system and the endocrine system.	**thalam/o-** *thalamus*
lobe	Large area of the cerebrum. Each lobe is named for the bone of the cranium that is next to it: frontal lobe, parietal lobe, temporal lobe, and occipital lobe.	
medulla oblongata	Most inferior part of the brainstem that connects to the spinal cord. It contains the respiratory centers that control the respiratory rate and other centers that control the heart rate.	
meninges	Three separate membranes that surround and protect the entire brain and spinal cord. The meninges include the dura mater, arachnoid, and pia mater.	**meningi/o-** *meninges* **mening/o-** *meninges*
midbrain	Most superior part of the brainstem. It keeps the mind conscious and coordinates reflex responses. It contains the substantia nigra.	
occipital lobe	Lobe of the cerebrum next to the occipital bone of the cranium. It receives and analyzes sensory information from the eyes. It contains the visual cortex for the sense of sight.	**occipit/o-** *back of the head; occiput*
olfactory cortex	Area in the temporal lobe of the cerebrum that analyzes sensory information from receptors in the nose for the sense of smell	**olfact/o-** *sense of smell*
parietal lobe	Lobe of the cerebrum next to the parietal bone of the cranium. It receives and analyzes sensory information about touch, temperature, vibration, and pain from the skin, joints, and muscles. It contains the somatosensory area.	**pariet/o-** *wall of a cavity*
pia mater	Thin, delicate, innermost layer of the meninges. It covers the surface of the brain and contains many small blood vessels.	
pons	Middle part of the brainstem. It relays nerve impulses from the spinal cord to the brain.	
somatosensory area	Area of the parietal lobe that receives and analyzes sensory information (touch, temperature, vibration, and pain) from receptors in the skin, joints, and muscles	**somat/o-** *body* **esthes/o-** *feeling; sensation* **esthet/o-** *feeling; sensation* **sens/o-** *feeling*
speech center	Area in the frontal lobe that coordinates muscles of the mouth, lips, tongue, pharynx, and larynx to produce speech	
subarachnoid space	Space beneath the arachnoid layer of the meninges. It is filled with cerebrospinal fluid.	**arachn/o-** *spider; spiderweb*
substantia nigra	Gray-to-black pigmented area in the midbrain of the brainstem that produces the neurotransmitter **dopamine**	
sulcus	One of many grooves on the surface of the cerebrum	

Word or Phrase	Description	Combining Forms
temporal lobe	Lobe of the cerebrum next to the temporal bone of the cranium. It receives and analyzes sensory information about hearing and smells. It contains the auditory cortex for the sense of hearing and the olfactory cortex for the sense of smell.	**tempor/o-** *side of the head; temple*
thalamus	Area in the center of the cerebrum that forms the walls of the third ventricle. It acts as a relay station, receiving sensory information from the cranial nerves and the spinal nerves and sending it to the midbrain and the cerebrum.	**thalam/o-** *thalamus*
ventricle	One of four interconnected cavities in the brain that contains cerebrospinal fluid. The two lateral ventricles are in the right and left hemispheres of the cerebrum. The small third ventricle is between the two lobes of the thalamus. The long, narrow fourth ventricle connects to the spinal canal.	**ventricul/o-** *chamber that is filled; ventricle*
visual cortex	Area in the occipital lobe that receives and analyzes sensory information from the retina of each eye for the sense of sight	**vis/o-** *sight; vision*
white matter	Tissue layer beneath the gray matter of the cerebral cortex. It contains the axons of neurons, and the myelin around the axons gives the tissue its white color.	
Spinal Cord		
cauda equina	Group of nerve roots that begin where the spinal cord ends and continue inferiorly within the spinal canal. They look like the tail (Latin word *cauda*) of a horse (Latin word *equina*).	
central canal	Narrow passageway within the spinal cord. It is lined with ependymal cells.	
ependymal cells	Cells that line the ventricles of the cerebrum and the narrow central canal in the spinal cord and produce cerebrospinal fluid	**ependym/o-** *cellular lining*
epidural space	Area between the bone of the vertebra and the dura mater. It is filled with fatty tissue and blood vessels.	**dur/o-** *dura mater*
spinal canal	Bony cavity created by the opening (foramen) in each vertebra of the neck and back. It contains the spinal cord.	**spin/o-** *backbone; spine* **cav/o-** *hollow space*
spinal cord	Part of the central nervous system. It begins at the medulla oblongata of the brain and extends inferiorly within the bony spinal canal. It ends at the second lumbar vertebra, where it separates into nerve roots (cauda equina). It contains gray and white matter.	**spin/o-** *backbone; spine* **myel/o-** *bone marrow; myelin; spinal cord*
Anatomy of the Peripheral Nervous System		
Cranial Nerves		
abducens nerve	Cranial nerve VI. Motor nerve for movement of one of the extraocular muscles (lateral rectus muscle) of the eye.	
accessory nerve	Cranial nerve XI. Motor nerve for swallowing, movement of the vocal cords, and movement of the muscles of the neck and upper back.	**access/o-** *contributing part; supplemental part*
cranial nerves	Part of the peripheral nervous system. Twelve pairs of nerves (I–XII) that begin in the brain or at receptors in the body. They carry nerve impulses as **sensory information** from the body to the brain and/or nerve impulses as **motor commands** from the brain to voluntary and involuntary muscles in the body.	**crani/o-** *cranium; top part of the skull* **sens/o-** *feeling* **mot/o-** *movement*

Word or Phrase	Description	Combining Forms
facial nerve	Cranial nerve VII. Sensory nerve for the sense of taste. Motor nerve for movement of the facial muscles, production of tears by the lacrimal gland, and production of saliva by the sublingual and submandibular salivary glands.	**faci/o-** *face*
glossopharyngeal nerve	Cranial nerve IX. Sensory nerve for the sense of taste. Motor nerve for swallowing and the production of saliva by the parotid salivary glands.	**gloss/o-** *tongue* **pharyng/o-** *pharynx; throat*
hypoglossal nerve	Cranial nerve XII. Motor nerve for movement of the tongue.	**gloss/o-** *tongue*
oculomotor nerve	Cranial nerve III. Motor nerve for movement for four of the extraocular muscles of the eye, the eyelids, and the iris (to change the size of the pupil).	**ocul/o-** *eye* **mot/o-** *movement*
olfactory nerve	Cranial nerve I. Sensory nerve for the sense of smell.	**olfact/o-** *sense of smell*
optic nerve	Cranial nerve II. Sensory nerve for the sense of vision.	**opt/o-** *eye; vision*
trigeminal nerve	Cranial nerve V. Sensory nerve for sensation of the face and mouth. Motor nerve for movement of the muscles for chewing. It consists of three branches: ophthalmic nerve, maxillary nerve, mandibular nerves.	**gemin/o-** *group; set*
trochlear nerve	Cranial nerve IV. Motor nerve for movement of one extraocular muscle (superior oblique muscle) of the eye.	**trochle/o-** *pulley-shaped structure*
vagus nerve	Cranial nerve X. Sensory nerve for the sense of taste from the soft palate and pharynx. Sensory nerve for the feelings in the ears, diaphragm, and the internal organs. Motor nerve that controls the heart rate and the smooth muscles around the bronchi and gastrointestinal tract.	**vag/o-** *vagus nerve; wandering*
vestibulocochlear nerve	Cranial nerve VIII. Sensory nerve for the sense of hearing and balance.	**vestibul/o-** *entrance; vestibule* **cochle/o-** *cochlea; spiral-shaped structure* **audit/o-** *sense of hearing*
Spinal Nerves		
afferent nerves	Dorsal nerve roots and their spinal nerve that carry sensory information as nerve impulses from the body to the spinal cord	**affer/o-** *toward the center*
dorsal nerve roots	Spinal nerve roots that enter the posterior (dorsal) part of the spinal cord. They receive sensory information from a specific area of the skin (a dermatome).	**dors/o-** *back; dorsum*
efferent nerves	Ventral nerve roots and their spinal nerve that carry motor commands as nerve impulses away from the spinal cord or brain to the body	**effer/o-** *away from the center*
reflex	Rapid, involuntary muscle reaction that is controlled by the spinal cord (without conscious thought). In response to sudden pain or muscle stretching, the spinal cord immediately sends a motor command to move. The entire circuit that the nerve impulse travels is known as a **reflex arc**.	
spinal nerves	Part of the peripheral nervous system. There are 31 pairs of spinal nerves. Each pair joins the spinal cord in the area between two vertebrae. An individual spinal nerve consists of dorsal nerve roots and ventral nerve roots.	**spin/o-** *backbone; spine* **radicul/o-** *spinal nerve root* **rhiz/o-** *spinal nerve root*
ventral nerve roots	Spinal nerve roots that exit from the anterior (ventral) part of the spinal cord. They carry motor commands as nerve impulses to the body.	**ventr/o-** *abdomen; front*

Word or Phrase	Description	Combining Forms
Neuroglia		
astrocyte	Star-like structure that provides structural support for neurons, connects them to capillaries, and forms the blood–brain barrier	**astr/o-** *star-like structure*
ependymal cells	Cells that line the walls of the ventricles and the central canal within the spinal cord and produce cerebrospinal fluid	**ependym/o-** *cellular lining*
microglia	Cells that move, engulf, and destroy pathogens anywhere in the central nervous system	**micr/o-** *one millionth; small*
neuroglia	Cells that hold neurons in place and perform specialized tasks. Neuroglia include astrocytes, ependymal cells, microglia, oligodendroglia, and Schwann cells.	**neur/o-** *nerve*
oligodendroglia	Cells that form the myelin around larger axons in the brain and spinal cord. These cells have few branching structures.	**olig/o-** *few; scanty* **dendr/o-** *branching structure*
Schwann cells	Cells that form the myelin around larger axons of the cranial and spinal nerves	
Physiology of the Nervous System		
Neurons		
axon	Part of the neuron that is a single, elongated extension of cytoplasm at the opposite end from the dendrites. It conducts the electrical impulse and releases neurotransmitters into the synapse. Larger axons are covered by an insulating layer of myelin.	
cytoplasm	Gel-like substance in the cell body of a neuron; it contains structures that produce a neurotransmitter and energy for the neuron	**cyt/o-** *cell*
dendrites	Multiple branches at the beginning of a neuron whose receptors bind with a neurotransmitter and convert it to an electrical impulse	**dendr/o-** *branching structure*
myelin	Fatty, white insulating layer around larger axons. It increases the speed that an electrical impulse can travel along the axon. An axon with myelin is myelinated. Myelin around larger axons in the brain and spinal cord is produced by oligodendroglia. Myelin around larger axons in the cranial and spinal nerves is produced by the Schwann cells.	**myelin/o-** *myelin*
neuron	An individual nerve cell. The functional unit of the nervous system.	**neur/o-** *nerve*
neurotransmitter	Chemical messenger that is released from vesicles on the axon and travels across the synapse and binds with a receptor	**neur/o-** *nerve* **transmitt/o-** *send across; send through*
nucleus	Structure in the cell body of a neuron that directs cellular activities	
receptor	Structure on the cell membrane of a dendrite (or on a muscle, organ, or gland) where a neurotransmitter binds	**recept/o-** *receive*
synapse	Space between the axon of one neuron and the dendrites of the next neuron (or between the axon and the cell of a muscle, organ, or gland)	
Neurotransmitters, Neuromodulators, and Hormones		
acetylcholine	Neurotransmitter of the parasympathetic division. It is also in the somatic nervous system between motor neurons and voluntary skeletal muscles.	

Word or Phrase	Description	Combining Forms
dopamine	Neurotransmitter between neurons in the brain. It is produced by the substantia nigra of the midbrain.	
endorphins	Neuromodulators that are one of several natural pain relievers produced by the brain	
epinephrine	Hormone secreted by the adrenal gland when stimulated by the sympathetic division. It prepares the body for "fight or flight."	
neurotransmitter	Chemical messenger that travels across the synapse between neurons	**neur/o-** *nerve* **transmitt/o-** *send across; send through*
norepinephrine	Neurotransmitter of the sympathetic division. It is also secreted by the adrenal gland.	
serotonin	Neurotransmitter between neurons in the limbic system, brain, and spinal cord	

9.3 Diseases

Word or Phrase	Description	Pronunciation/Word Parts

Brain

| amnesia | Partial or total loss of memory of recent or remote (past) experiences. It is often a consequence of brain injury or a stroke that damages the hippocampus where short-term memories are converted to long-term memories. In **retrograde amnesia**, the patient cannot remember events that occurred in the past (before the onset of the amnesia). In **anterograde amnesia**, the patient cannot remember events that occurred after the onset of the amnesia. In **global amnesia**, all memories (past and present) are lost.
 Treatment: Correct the underlying cause. Some memories may return over time. | **amnesia** (am-NEE-zha)
 amnes/o- *memory loss*
 -ia *condition; state; thing*

 retrograde (REH-troh-grayd)
 The prefix **retro-** means *backward; behind.*

 anterograde (AN-ter-oh-GRAYD)
 The combining form **anter/o-** means *before; front part.*

 global (GLOH-bal)
 glob/o- *comprehensive; shaped like a globe*
 -al *pertaining to* |
| anencephaly | Rare congenital condition in which some or all of the cranium and cerebrum are missing. The newborn breathes, because the respiratory centers in the medulla oblongata are present, but only survives a few hours or days.
 Treatment: None | **anencephaly** (AN-en-SEF-ah-lee)
 The prefix **an-** means *not; without.* The suffix **-encephaly** means *condition of the brain.* |

Word or Phrase	Description	Pronunciation/Word Parts
aphasia	Loss of the ability to communicate verbally or in writing. Aphasia can occur with head trauma, a stroke, or a neurocognitive disorder when there is injury to or deterioration of the areas of the brain that deal with language and the interpretation of sounds and symbols. Patients with aphasia are said to be **aphasic**. **Expressive aphasia** is the inability to verbally express thoughts. **Receptive aphasia** is the inability to understand the spoken or written word. Patients with both types are said to have **global aphasia**. Limited impairment that involves some difficulty speaking or understanding words is known as **dysphasia**. Treatment: Correct the underlying cause; speech therapy	**aphasia** (ah-FAY-zha) **a-** *away from; without* **phas/o-** *speech* **-ia** *condition; state; thing* **aphasic** (ah-FAY-sik) **a-** *away from; without* **phas/o-** *speech* **-ic** *pertaining to* **expressive** (eks-PREH-siv) **express/o-** *communicate* **-ive** *pertaining to* **receptive** (ree-SEP-tiv) **recept/o-** *receive* **-ive** *pertaining to* **global** (GLOH-bal) **glob/o-** *comprehensive; shaped like a globe* **-al** *pertaining to* **dysphasia** (dis-FAY-zha) **dys-** *abnormal; difficult; painful* **phas/o-** *speech* **-ia** *condition; state; thing*
arteriovenous malformation (AVM)	Abnormality in which arteries in the brain connect directly to veins (rather than to capillaries), forming a twisted nest of abnormal blood vessels with weak walls. An AVM can rupture and cause a stroke. Treatment: Targeted radiation to destroy the AVM or occlusion of the blood vessel (embolization) to block blood flow to the AVM; surgical removal, if needed	**arteriovenous** (ar-TEER-ee-oh-VEE-nuhs) **arteri/o-** *artery* **ven/o-** *vein* **-ous** *pertaining to* **malformation** (MAL-for-MAY-shun) **mal-** *bad; inadequate* **format/o-** *arrangement; structure* **-ion** *action; condition*
brain death	Condition in which there is irreversible loss of all brain function as confirmed by an electroencephalogram (EEG) that is flat, showing no brain wave activity of any kind for 30 minutes. The patient is said to be "brain dead." Treatment: None	
brain tumor	**Benign** or **malignant** tumor in any area of the brain. Brain tumors arise from the neuroglia or meninges (not from the neurons), and they are named according to the type of cell from which they originated (see Table 9-4 ■). Malignant brain tumors can also be secondary tumors that metastasized from a primary malignant tumor elsewhere in the body. Because the cranium is rigid, the enlarging benign or malignant tumor causes increased **intracranial pressure (ICP)**, cerebral edema, and sometimes seizures. The pressure compresses and destroys brain tissue. Treatment: Surgery to remove or debulk the tumor; chemotherapy drugs or radiation therapy for malignant tumors	**benign** (bee-NINE) *Note:* A benign tumor is one that is not malignant (cancerous). **malignant** (mah-LIG-nant) **malign/o-** *cancer* **-ant** *pertaining to* **intracranial** (IN-trah-KRAY-nee-al) **intra-** *within* **crani/o-** *cranium; top part of the skull* **-al** *pertaining to*

Table 9-4 Types of Brain Tumors

Brain Tumor	Characteristic	Originating Cell or Structure	Pronunciation/Word Parts
astrocytoma (see Figure 9-12 ■)	malignant	astrocyte in the cerebrum	**astrocytoma** (AS-troh-sy-TOH-mah) **astr/o-** *star-like structure* **cyt/o-** *cell* **-oma** *mass; tumor*
ependymoma	benign	ependymal cells that line the ventricles and the narrow central canal in the spinal cord	**ependymoma** (eh-PEN-dih-MOH-mah) **ependym/o-** *cellular lining* **-oma** *mass; tumor*
glioblastoma multiforme	malignant	immature astrocyte in the cerebrum	**glioblastoma multiforme** (GLY-oh-blas-TOH-mah MUL-tih-FOR-may) **gli/o-** *supporting cells* **blast/o-** *embryonic; immature* **-oma** *mass; tumor*
glioma (see Figure 9-13 ■)	benign or malignant	any neuroglial cell	**glioma** (glee-OH-mah) **gli/o-** *supporting cells* **-oma** *mass; tumor*
lymphoma	malignant	microglia in the cerebrum	**lymphoma** (lim-FOH-mah) **lymph/o-** *lymph; lymphatic system* **-oma** *mass; tumor*
meningioma	benign	meninges around the brain or spinal cord	**meningioma** (meh-NIN-jee-OH-mah) **meningi/o-** *meninges* **-oma** *mass; tumor*
neurofibrosarcoma	malignant	Schwann cells that produce myelin around neurons of the cranial and spinal nerves	**neurofibrosarcoma** (NYOOR-oh-FY-broh-sar-KOH-mah) **neur/o-** *nerve* **fibr/o-** *fiber* **-oma** *mass; tumor*
oligodendroglioma	malignant	oligodendroglia in the cerebrum	**oligodendroglioma** (OH-lih-GOH-den-DROH-glee-OH-mah) **olig/o-** *few; scanty* **dendr/o-** *branching structure* **gli/o-** *supporting cells* **-oma** *mass; tumor*
schwannoma	benign	Schwann cells that produce myelin around the neurons of the cranial and spinal nerves	**schwannoma** (shwah-NOH-mah)

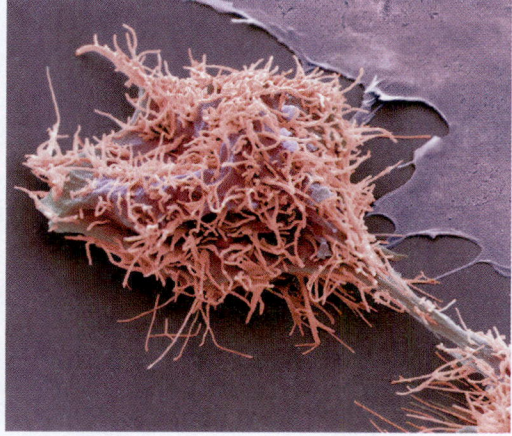

FIGURE 9-12 ■ Astrocytoma.
This is a cancerous astrocyte that has just divided.
It is one of many rapidly dividing cells in a malignant
astrocytoma tumor.

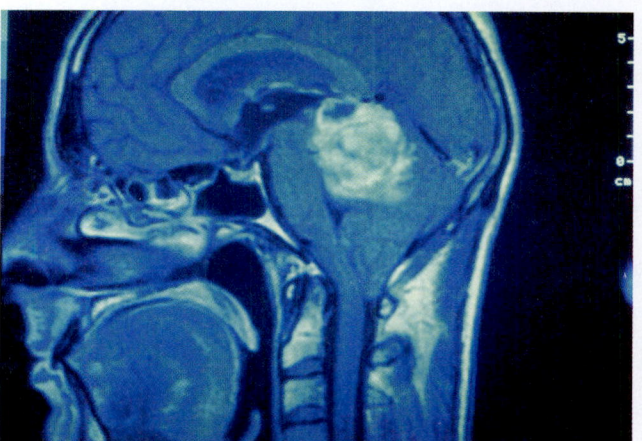

FIGURE 9-13 ■ Glioma.
This patient's MRI scan of the brain shows a large glioma that is
pressing on the cerebellum and midbrain. This tumor would affect
the patient's ability to keep his balance and coordinate movements.

Word or Phrase	Description	Pronunciation/Word Parts
cephalalgia	Pain in the head. Commonly known as a **headache**. It can be caused by eyestrain, muscle tension in the face or neck, generalized infections such as the flu, migraine headaches, sinus infections, hypertension, or by more serious conditions such as head trauma, meningitis, or brain tumors. Treatment: Correct the underlying cause.	**cephalalgia** (SEF-al-AL-jah) **cephal/o-** *head* **alg/o-** *pain* **-ia** *condition; state; thing*
cerebral palsy (CP)	Cerebral palsy is caused by abnormal development of the fetus's brain or sometimes from a lack of oxygen during birth. This can cause spastic muscles; lack of coordination in walking, eating, and talking; muscle paralysis; seizures; or intellectual disability. Treatment: Braces; muscle relaxant drug; physical therapy; occupational therapy; speech therapy	**cerebral** (seh-REE-bral) **cerebr/o-** *cerebrum* **-al** *pertaining to* **palsy** (PAWL-zee)
cerebrovascular accident (CVA)	Disruption or blockage of blood flow to the brain, which causes tissue death and an area of necrosis known as an **infarct**. A CVA can be caused by blocking or disrupting the blood flow. An embolus (a blood clot that travels through the blood) can become lodged in a small artery to the brain, blocking the blood flow. High blood pressure can cause an artery, aneurysm, or arteriovenous malformation to rupture and hemorrhage and disrupt the blood flow. A CVA is also known as a **stroke** or **brain attack**. A **transient ischemic attack (TIA)**, a temporary lack of oxygenated blood to an area of the brain, is like a CVA, but its effects last only 24 hours. A **reversible ischemic neurologic deficit (RIND)** is a TIA whose effects last for several days. TIAs and RINDs are precursors to an impending CVA. The severity and symptoms of the CVA depend on how much brain tissue dies. A CVA can result in **hemiparesis**, which is muscle weakness on one side of the body. **Hemiplegia** is paralysis on one side of the body, and the patient is said to be **hemiplegic** (see Figure 9-14 ■). A cerebrovascular accident on the left side of the brain affects the right side of the body and vice versa (see Figure 9-15 ■). A CVA can also cause amnesia, aphasia, dysphasia, or dysphagia (difficulty swallowing). Prevention: Antihypertensive drug to control the blood pressure; carotid endarterectomy or aneurysmectomy Treatment: Thrombolytic drug to break up an embolus that is occluding the artery; physical therapy; occupational therapy; speech therapy	**cerebrovascular** (seh-REE-broh-VAS-kyoo-lar) **cerebr/o-** *cerebrum* **vascul/o-** *blood vessel* **-ar** *pertaining to* **infarct** (IN-farkt) **infarction** (in-FARK-shun) **infarct/o-** *small area of dead tissue* **-ion** *action; condition* **ischemia** (is-KEE-mee-ah) **isch/o-** *block; keep back* **-emia** *condition of the blood; substance in the blood* **ischemic** (is-KEE-mik) **isch/o-** *block; keep back* **-emic** *pertaining to a condition of the blood; pertaining to a substance in the blood* **neurologic** (NYOOR-oh-LAW-jik) **neur/o-** *nerve* **log/o-** *study of; word* **-ic** *pertaining to* **hemiparesis** (HEM-ee-pah-REE-sihs) The prefix **hemi-** means *one-half*. *Paresis* is a Greek word that means *condition of weakness*. **hemiplegia** (HEM-ee-PLEE-jah) **hemi-** *one-half* **pleg/o-** *paralysis* **-ia** *condition; state; thing* **hemiplegic** (HEM-ee-PLEE-jik) **hemi-** *one half* **pleg/o-** *paralysis* **-ic** *pertaining to*

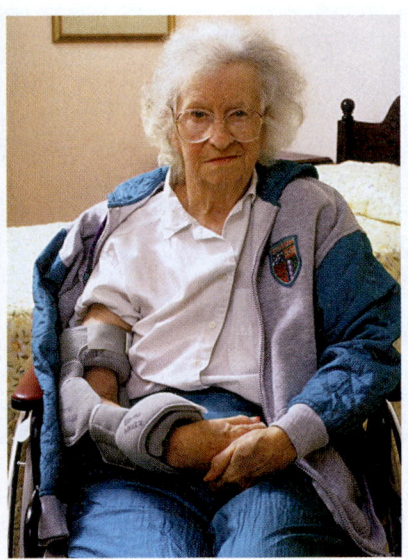

FIGURE 9-14 ■ Patient with a cerebrovascular accident. This patient had a cerebrovascular accident on the left side of her brain that has paralyzed the right side of her body. Notice the drooping of the right side of her mouth and her right shoulder. The elbow and wrist of her right arm are covered with protective padding. She is using her functioning left hand to hold her paralyzed right hand in her lap and move her right arm from time to time.

Word or Phrase	Description	Pronunciation/Word Parts

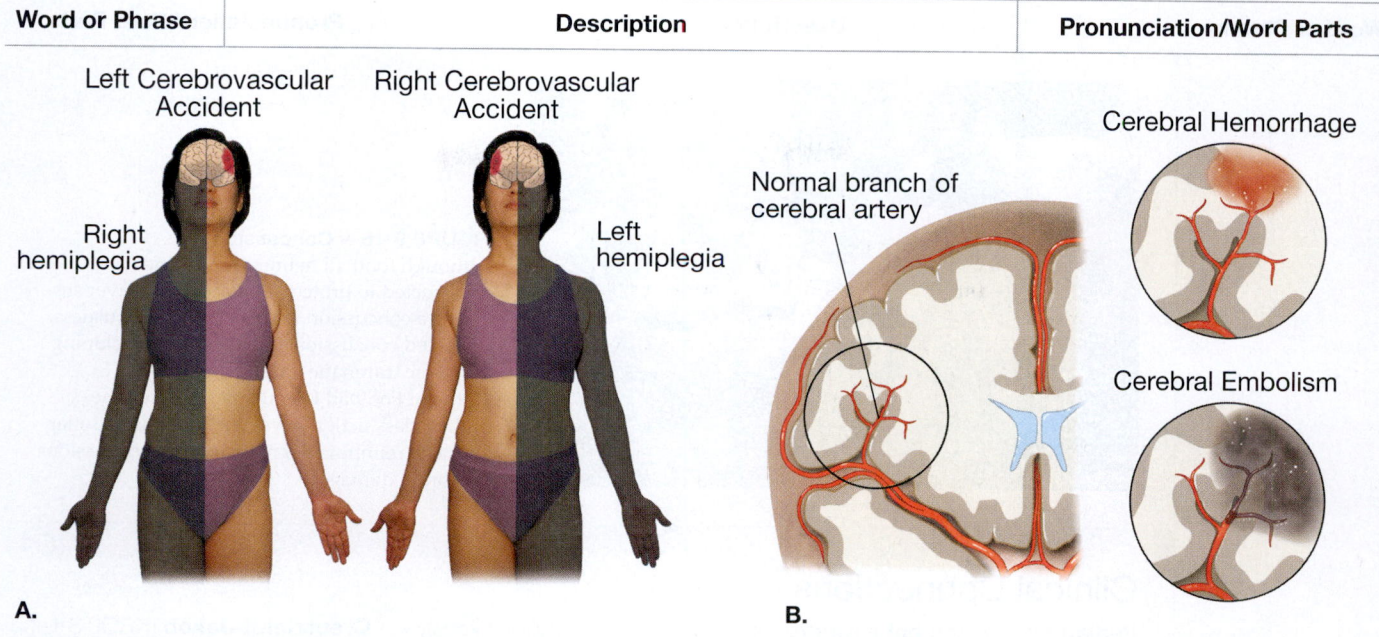

FIGURE 9-15 ■ Cerebrovascular accident.
A. A cerebrovascular accident on the left side of the brain affects the right side of the body and vice versa. **B.** A cerebrovascular accident can occur when hemorrhage of an aneurysm disrupts blood flow to the brain or when an embolus blocks blood flow to the brain.

Word or Phrase	Description	Pronunciation/Word Parts

coma	Deep state of unconsciousness and unresponsiveness caused by trauma or disease in the brain, by metabolic imbalance with accumulation of waste products in the blood (hepatic coma), or by too little glucose in the blood (hypoglycemia). A coma may be temporary or permanent. The patient is said to be **comatose**.
	Treatment: Correct the underlying cause.
		coma (KOH-mah)
		
		comatose (KOH-mah-tohs)
		  comat/o- *unconsciousness*
		  -ose *full of*

concussion	Traumatic injury to the brain in which the brain suddenly impacts the inside of the cranium. This results in an immediate **loss of consciousness (LOC)** for a brief or prolonged period of time (see Figure 9-16 ■). Even after consciousness returns, the patient must be watched closely for signs of a slowly enlarging hemorrhage in the brain. These signs include sleepiness or irritability, a vacant stare, slowness in answering questions, inability to follow commands, disorientation to time and place, slurred speech, or a lack of coordination. A **contusion** is a traumatic injury to the brain or spinal cord. There is no loss of consciousness, but there is bruising with some bleeding in the tissues.	**concussion** (con-KUH-shun)
		  concuss/o- *violent impact*
		  -ion *action; condition*
		
		contusion (con-TOO-shun)
		  contus/o- *bruising*
		  -ion *action; condition*

Word or Phrase	Description	Pronunciation/Word Parts

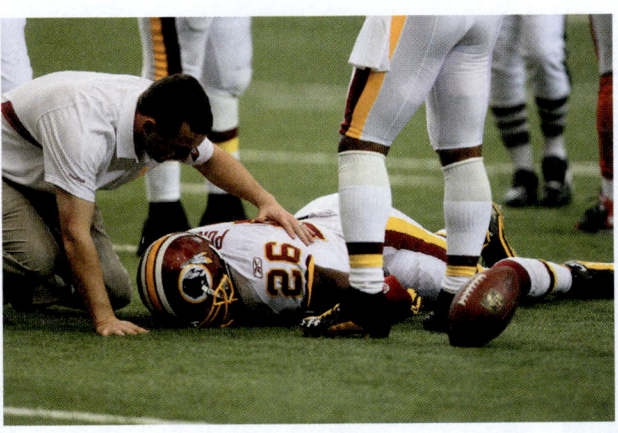

FIGURE 9-16 ■ **Concussion.**
Although football helmets are padded and constructed to protect the head, this player sustained a concussion with loss of consciousness. Repeated concussions can result in developing a chronic traumatic encephalopathy (CTE). National Football League players sued the NFL in class-action lawsuits for a billion-dollar financial reimbursement because of concussions and brain damage.

Clinical Connections

Pediatrics. Shaken baby syndrome is caused by an adult vigorously shaking an infant in anger or to discipline. Because the infant's head is large and the neck muscles are weak, severe shaking causes the head to whip back and forth. This can cause a brain contusion, concussion, hemorrhage, intellectual disability, coma, or even death.

Public Health. New variant **Creutzfeldt-Jakob disease**, a fatal neurologic disorder, is caused by a prion (a small infectious protein particle). This disease is contracted from cows infected with mad cow disease (bovine spongiform encephalopathy), which was first discovered in Great Britain. It is transmitted to cows when they eat animal feed contaminated with the processed brains and spinal cords of infected cows. All such animal feed has been banned in the United States. The disease can be transmitted to humans who eat meat from the infected cows, and so the Food and Drug Administration prohibits people who have lived or traveled extensively in England from donating blood to prevent transmission of this disease.

Creutzfeldt-Jakob (KROITS-felt YAH-kohp)

| delirium | Acute confusion, disorientation, and agitation due to toxic levels of chemicals, drugs, or alcohol in the blood that affect the brain. These acute symptoms slowly subside as the substances in the blood are metabolized and excreted from the body. | **delirium** (deh-LEER-ee-um) |

Clinical Connections

Psychiatry. Delirium tremens (DT) is caused by withdrawal symptoms from alcoholic intoxication. Symptoms include restlessness, tremors of the hands, hallucinations, sweating, and an increased heart rate.
Treatment: Antianxiety drug

Word or Phrase	Description	Pronunciation/Word Parts
Down syndrome	A random error in cell division creates a genetic defect in which there are three of chromosome 21 instead of the normal two. This defect affects every cell in the body, but is most obvious as mild-to-severe **intellectual disability** and the characteristic physical features of a large, protruding tongue, short fingers, and a single transverse crease on the palm of the hand (see Figure 9-17 ■). Previously known as *mental retardation*. Prenatal test: Amniocentesis of fluid around the developing fetus 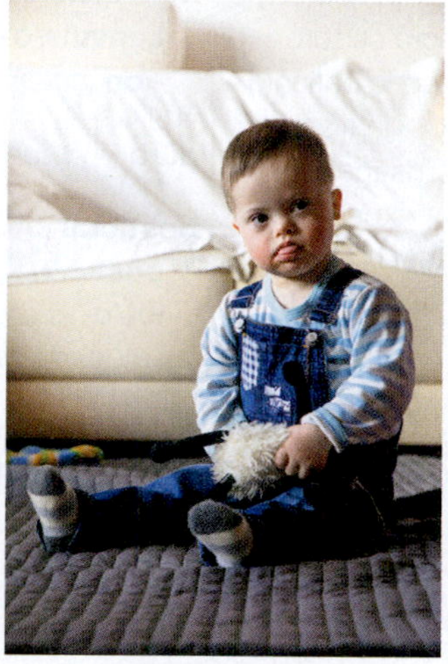 **FIGURE 9-17 ■ Down syndrome.** This young patient shows the characteristic features of the face and hands that are typical of Down syndrome.	**disability** (dihs-ah-BIL-ih-tee) The prefix **dis-** means *away from; lack of.*
dyslexia	Difficulty reading and writing words even though visual acuity and intelligence are normal (see Figure 9-18 ■). Dyslexia tends to run in families and is more prevalent in left-handed persons and in males. It is caused by an abnormality in the occipital lobe of the cerebrum as it interprets moving visual images (as the eye moves quickly across the page). A person with dyslexia is said to be **dyslexic**. Treatment: Educational techniques that help a child learn to compensate or overcome this difficulty; occupational therapy 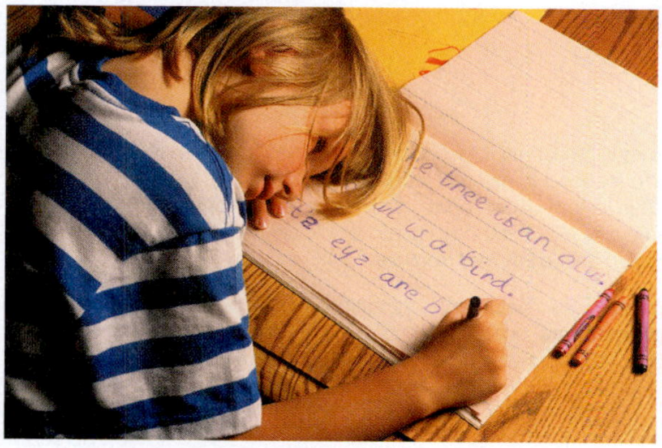 **FIGURE 9-18 ■ Dyslexia.** A child with dyslexia may write certain alphabet letters backward or may change the order of the letters in a word.	**dyslexia** (dis-LEK-see-ah) **dys-** *abnormal; difficult; painful* **lex/o-** *word* **-ia** *condition; state; thing* **dyslexic** (dis-LEK-sik) **dys-** *abnormal; difficult; painful* **lex/o-** *word* **-ic** *pertaining to*
encephalitis	Inflammation and infection of the brain caused by a virus. Herpes simplex virus is the most common cause of encephalitis, but others include herpes zoster virus, West Nile virus, and cytomegalovirus. There is fever, headache, stiff neck, lethargy, vomiting, irritability, and **photophobia**. Treatment: Corticosteroid drug to decrease inflammation of the brain. Only encephalitis caused by the herpes virus responds to an antiviral drug. Antibiotic drugs are not effective against viruses.	**encephalitis** (en-SEF-ah-LY-tihs) **encephal/o-** *brain* **-itis** *infection of; inflammation of* **photophobia** (FOH-toh-FOH-bee-ah) **phot/o-** *light* **phob/o-** *avoidance; fear* **-ia** *condition; state; thing*

Word or Phrase	Description	Pronunciation/Word Parts

epilepsy	Recurring condition in which a group of neurons in the brain spontaneously sends out electrical impulses in an abnormal, uncontrolled way. These impulses spread from neuron to neuron. A seizure can be triggered by a flashing light, stress, lack of sleep, alcohol or drugs, or the cause can be unknown. The type and extent of the seizures depend on the number and location of the affected neurons. A patient with epilepsy is said to be **epileptic**. Also known as **seizures** or **convulsions**.
	
	There are four common types of epilepsy (see Table 9-5 ■). With each type of epilepsy, the patient displays a specific EEG pattern during a seizure (see Figure 9-19 ■). Before the onset of a seizure, some epileptic patients experience an **aura**—a visual, olfactory, sensory, or auditory sign (flashing lights, strange odor, tingling, or buzzing sound)—that warns them of an impending seizure. After a tonic-clonic seizure, the patient experiences sleepiness and confusion. This is known as the **postictal state**. Over time, seizures can cause memory loss and personality changes. **Status epilepticus** is a prolonged, continuous seizure or repeated seizures that occur without the patient regaining consciousness.
	
	Treatment: Antiepileptic drug; sometimes surgery, if a tumor or a specific area of the brain is causing the seizures
		epilepsy (EP-ih-LEP-see)
		
		epileptic (EP-ih-LEP-tik)
		  epilept/o- *seizure*
		  -ic *pertaining to*
		
		seizure (SEE-zher)
		
		convulsion (con-VUL-shun)
		  convuls/o- *seizure*
		  -ion *action; condition*
		
		aura (AW-rah)
		
		postictal (post-IK-tal)
		  post- *after; behind*
		  ict/o- *seizure*
		  -al *pertaining to*
		
		status epilepticus (STAT-us EP-ih-LEP-tih-kuhs)

Table 9-5   Seizures

Type of Seizure	Description	Pronunciation/Word Parts

tonic-clonic	Unconsciousness with excessive motor activity. The body alternates between excessive muscle tone with rigidity (tonic) and jerking muscle contractions (clonic) in the extremities, with tongue biting and sometimes incontinence. This lasts 1–2 minutes. Also known as a **grand mal seizure**.	**tonic** (TAW-nik)
		  ton/o- *pressure; tone*
		  -ic *pertaining to*
		
		clonic (KLAW-nik)
		  clon/o- *identical group derived from one; rapid contracting and relaxing*
		  -ic *pertaining to*
		
		grand mal (GRAN MAWL)
		This is a French phrase that means *large sickness*.

absence	Impaired consciousness with slight or no muscle activity. Muscle tone is retained, and the patient does not fall down, but is unable to respond to external stimuli. There is vacant staring, repetitive blinking, or facial tics. This lasts 5–15 seconds, after which the patient resumes activities and is unaware of the seizure. A patient can have many absence seizures during the course of a day. Also known as a **petit mal seizure**.	**absence** (AB-sens) **petit mal** (peh-TEE MAWL) This is a French phrase that means *small sickness*.

complex partial	Some degree of impairment of consciousness with involuntary contractions of one or several muscle groups. There can be **automatisms**, such as lip smacking or repetitive muscle movements. This lasts 1–2 minutes. Also known as a **psychomotor seizure**.	**automatism** (aw-TAW-mah-tizm)
		
		psychomotor (SY-koh-MOH-tor)
		  psych/o- *mind*
		  mot/o- *movement*
		  -or *person who does or produces; thing that does or produces*

simple partial	No impairment of consciousness. The patient is aware of the seizure but is unable to stop the involuntary motor activity, such as jerking of one hand or turning of the head. There can also be sensory hallucinations. This lasts 1–2 minutes. Also known as a **focal motor seizure**.	**focal** (FOH-kal)
		  foc/o- *point of activity*
		  -al *pertaining to*

Word or Phrase	Description	Pronunciation/Word Parts

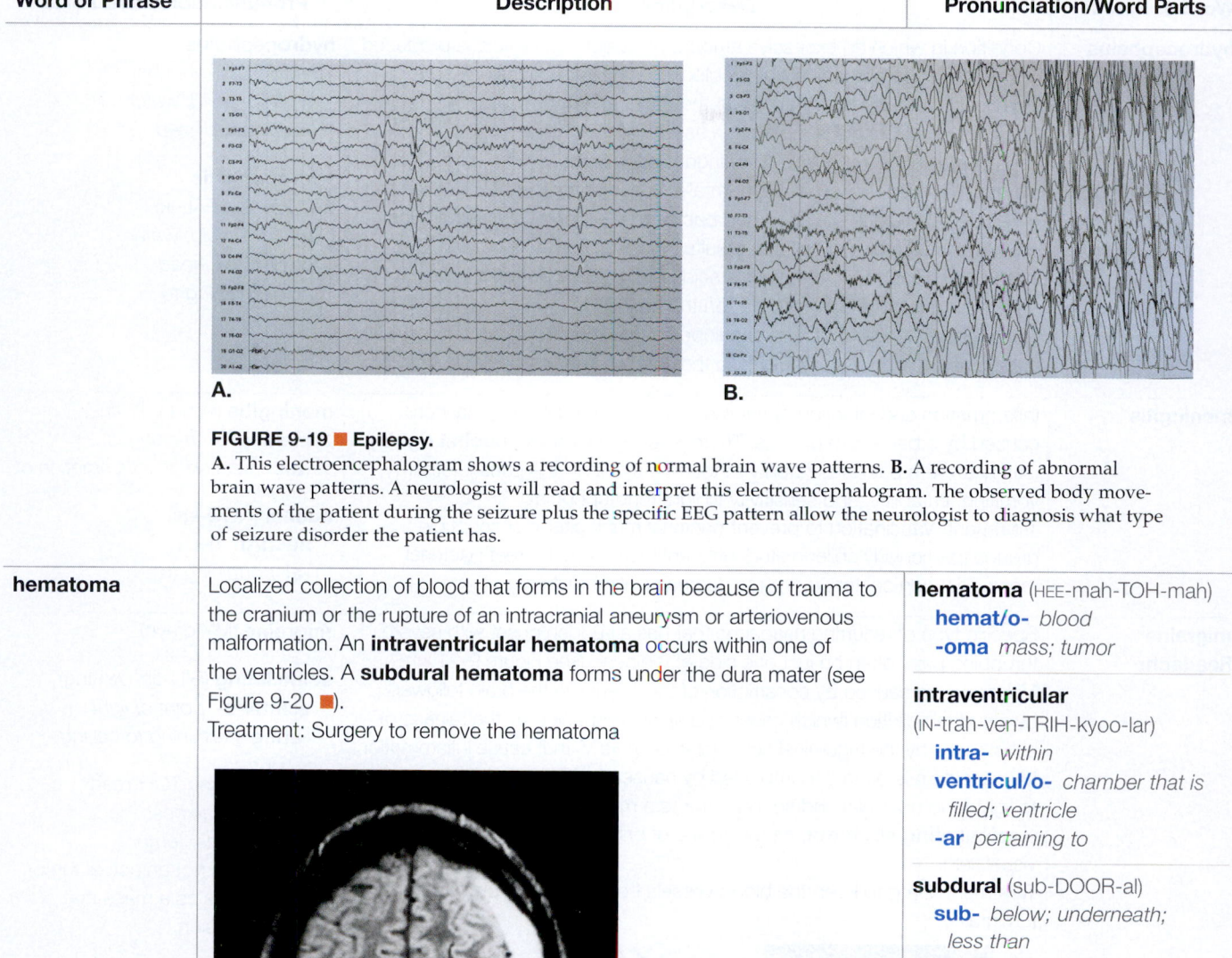

FIGURE 9-19 ■ Epilepsy.
A. This electroencephalogram shows a recording of normal brain wave patterns. **B.** A recording of abnormal brain wave patterns. A neurologist will read and interpret this electroencephalogram. The observed body movements of the patient during the seizure plus the specific EEG pattern allow the neurologist to diagnosis what type of seizure disorder the patient has.

| **hematoma** | Localized collection of blood that forms in the brain because of trauma to the cranium or the rupture of an intracranial aneurysm or arteriovenous malformation. An **intraventricular hematoma** occurs within one of the ventricles. A **subdural hematoma** forms under the dura mater (see Figure 9-20 ■).
Treatment: Surgery to remove the hematoma

FIGURE 9-20 ■ Subdural hematoma.
This patient developed a subdural hematoma after trauma to the side of the head. His MRI scan shows how the hematoma has compressed the brain on that side. | **hematoma** (HEE-mah-TOH-mah)
  hemat/o- *blood*
  -oma *mass; tumor*

intraventricular
(IN-trah-ven-TRIH-kyoo-lar)
  intra- *within*
  ventricul/o- *chamber that is filled; ventricle*
  -ar *pertaining to*

subdural (sub-DOOR-al)
  sub- *below; underneath; less than*
  dur/o- *dura mater*
  -al *pertaining to* |
| **Huntington chorea** | Progressive inherited degenerative disease of the brain that begins in middle age. It is characterized by dementia with spasms of the extremities and face (chorea), alternating with slow writhing movements of the hands and feet (**athetoid movements**).
Treatment: None | **Huntington** (HUN-ting-ton)

chorea (kor-EE-ah)

athetoid (ATH-eh-toyd)
  athet/o- *without position or purpose*
  -oid *resembling*
Athetoid: *Resembling (movement that is wandering and) without position or purpose* |

Word or Phrase	Description	Pronunciation/Word Parts
hydrocephalus	Condition in which an excessive amount of cerebrospinal fluid is produced or the flow of cerebrospinal fluid is blocked. The intracranial pressure increases, distends the ventricles in the brain, and compresses the brain tissue. Hydrocephalus is most often associated with the congenital conditions of meningocele or myelomeningocele (described in the next section), although it can occur in adults (normal-pressure hydrocephalus) when the cerebrospinal fluid is not absorbed back into the blood. Untreated hydrocephalus in infants and children results in a grossly enlarged head and intellectual disability. The patient is said to be **hydrocephalic**. A layman's phrase for this condition is "water on the brain." Treatment: Placement of a ventriculoperitoneal shunt to move excess cerebrospinal fluid from the ventricles in the cerebrum to the peritoneal cavity	**hydrocephalus** (HY-droh-SEF-ah-luhs) **hydr/o-** *fluid; water* **-cephalus** *head* **hydrocephalic** (HY-droh-sih-FAL-ik) **hydr/o-** *fluid; water* **cephal/o-** *head* **-ic** *pertaining to*
meningitis	Inflammation and infection of the meninges of the brain or spinal cord caused by a bacterium or virus. There is fever, headache, **nuchal rigidity** (stiff neck with pain and inability to touch the chin to the chest), lethargy, vomiting, irritability, and sensitivity to light (photophobia). Treatment: Vaccination to prevent bacterial meningitis in susceptible groups (particularly college students); antibiotic drug to treat bacterial meningitis; corticosteroid drug to decrease inflammation	**meningitis** (MEN-in-JY-tihs) **mening/o-** *meninges* **-itis** *infection of; inflammation of* **nuchal** (NOO-kal) **nuch/o-** *neck* **-al** *pertaining to*
migraine headache	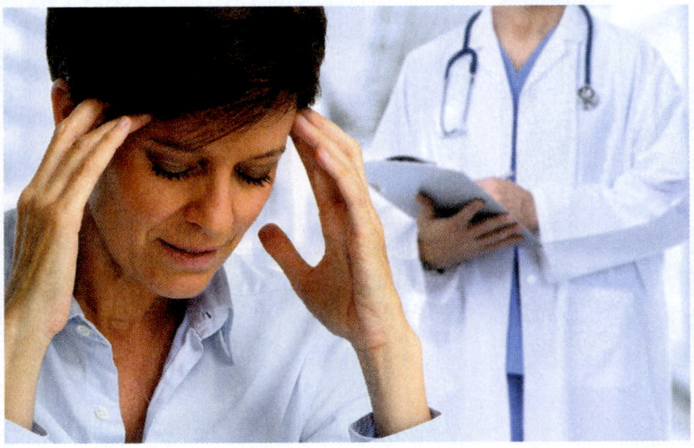 Specific type of recurring headache that has a sudden onset with severe, throbbing pain, often on just one side of the head (see Figure 9-21 ■). Migraines are caused by constriction of the arteries in the brain followed by a sudden dilation (which causes pain), accompanied by the release of substances by the trigeminal nerve (cranial nerve V) that cause inflammation. Migraine pain is often accompanied by nausea and vomiting and sensitivity to light (photophobia) and sound. Prior to a migraine, some patients see a **scintillating scotoma**, a moving line of brilliantly flashing bars in the visual field. Treatment: Drug to keep the blood vessels from dilating to prevent or treat a migraine	**migraine** (MY-grayn) **scintillating** (SIN-tih-LAY-ting) **scintill/o-** *point of light* **-ating** *pertaining to having* **scotoma** (skoh-TOH-mah) **scot/o-** *darkness* **-oma** *mass; tumor* A scotoma is not an actual tumor, but it appears as a mass that blocks the vision.

FIGURE 9-21 ■ Migraine.
Migraine headaches can be caused by foods, food additives, wine, stress, bright lights, smells, changes in the weather, and some drugs. Migraines cause severe pain for hours and sometimes for days, and episodes can occur several times a month.

Word or Phrase	Description	Pronunciation/Word Parts
narcolepsy	Brief, involuntary episodes of falling asleep during the daytime while engaged in activity. The patient is not unconscious and can be aroused, but is unable to keep from falling asleep. There is a hereditary component to narcolepsy, and it may be an autoimmune disorder. There is also an underlying abnormality of **rapid eye movement (REM)** sleep. Treatment: Central nervous system stimulant drug	**narcolepsy** (NAR-koh-LEP-see) **narc/o-** *sleep; stupor* **-lepsy** *seizure*

Word or Phrase	Description	Pronunciation/Word Parts
neurocognitive disorder (NCD)	Disease of the brain in which many neurons in the cerebrum die, the cerebral cortex shrinks in size, and there is progressive deterioration in mental function (see Figure 9-22 ■). Formerly known as **dementia** or **senility**. The most common neurocognitive disorder is **Alzheimer disease**, but NCD also includes **traumatic brain injury (TBI)**, Parkinson disease, **multi-infarct dementia** (the cumulative effect of multiple cerebrovascular accidents), multiple sclerosis, the neurodegenerative effects of alcohol abuse and drug abuse, and other, lesser-known diseases. At first, there is a gradual decline in mental abilities with forgetfulness and difficulty learning new things, focusing on a task, remembering names, performing daily activities, planning, and making decisions. The patient uses the wrong words, is unable to comprehend what others are saying, and speaks or acts inappropriately. The more neurons that are destroyed, the greater the cognitive impairment. Psychiatric symptoms of depression, anxiety, impulsiveness, and combativeness can also occur. The symptoms become more severe over time, culminating in an inability to care for personal needs or recognize friends and family and complete memory loss. Treatment: Drug to inhibit the enzyme that breaks down acetylcholine, although this can only slow the progression of symptoms; there is no cure.	**neurocognitive** (NYOOR-oh-KAWG-nih-tiv) **neur/o-** *nerve* **cognit/o-** *thinking* **-ive** *pertaining to* **dementia** (deh-MEN-shah) **de-** *reversal of; without* **ment/o-** *chin; mind* **-ia** *condition; state; thing* Dementia: *Condition (of being) without (the) mind* **senility** (seh-NIL-ih-tee) **senil/o-** *old age* **-ity** *condition; state* **Alzheimer** (AWLZ-hy-mer)

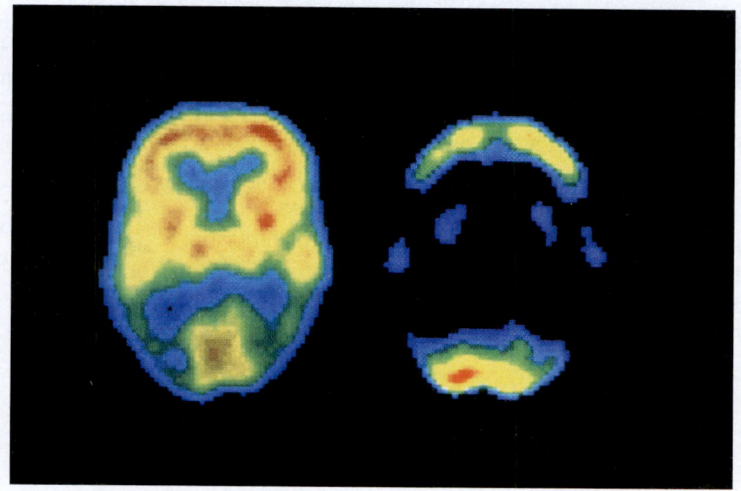

FIGURE 9-22 ■ PET scan of a normal brain and the brain of a patient with Alzheimer disease.
The PET scan on the left shows the metabolic activity of a normal brain. Areas with the highest metabolic activity appear yellow to red. This patient's scan shows large, symmetrical areas of metabolism and brain activity. The PET scan on the right shows the metabolic activity of the brain in a patient with Alzheimer disease. Notice the large, central area that is without any evidence of metabolic brain activity.

Dive Deeper

Alzheimer disease is a hereditary dementia that is known to run in families with inherited mutations on chromosomes 1, 14, and 21. At autopsy, the neurons show characteristic **neurofibrillary tangles** that distort the cells. There are also microscopic **beta amyloid senile plaques**. The brain also has a decreased level of the neurotransmitter acetylcholine. Alzheimer disease that occurs in early middle age is known as *early-onset Alzheimer disease* (formerly known as *presenile dementia*).

neurofibrillary (NYOOR-oh-FIB-rih-LAIR-ee)
neur/o- *nerve*
fibrill/o- *muscle fiber; nerve fiber*
-ary *pertaining to*

beta amyloid (BAY-tah AM-ih-loyd)

senile (SEE-nile)
sen/o- *old age*
-ile *pertaining to*

plaque (PLAK)

Word or Phrase	Description	Pronunciation/Word Parts
Parkinson disease	Chronic, degenerative disease due to an imbalance in the levels of the neurotransmitters dopamine and acetylcholine in the brain. There is muscle rigidity and tremors. In the later stages, the patient has difficulty initiating voluntary movements except with effort and concentration (see Figure 9-23 ■). Other signs include a mask-like facial expression, shuffling gait, or inability to ambulate. Also known as **parkinsonism**. Treatment: Drug that balances the neurotransmitters by increasing the amount of dopamine or inhibiting the action of acetylcholine in the brain, although this can only slow the progression of symptoms; there is no cure.	**Parkinson** (PAR-kin-son) **parkinsonism** (PAR-kin-son-IZM) The suffix **-ism** means *disease from a specific cause; process.*

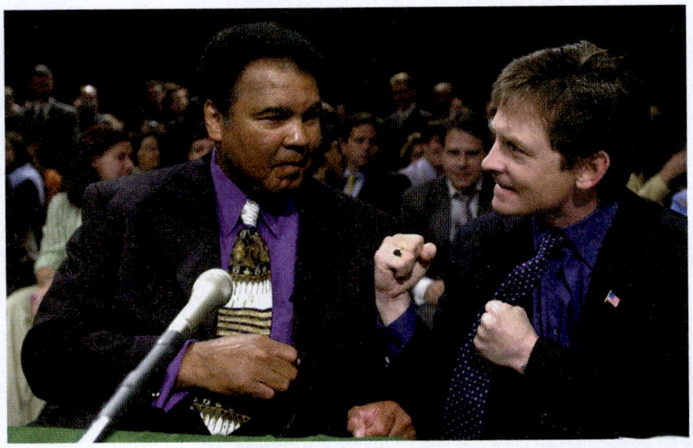

FIGURE 9-23 ■ **Parkinson disease.** Parkinson patients boxing legend Muhammad Ali and actor Michael J. Fox talk with each other before testifying at a Senate hearing on Parkinson disease research. Muhammad Ali shows advanced symptoms of the disease with an expressionless face and difficulty initiating movement of his hands.

Word or Phrase	Description	Pronunciation/Word Parts
syncope	Temporary loss of consciousness. A **syncopal episode** is one in which the patient becomes lightheaded and then faints and briefly remains unconscious. It is most often caused by carotid artery stenosis and plaque that block blood flow to the brain or by a cardiac arrhythmia that decreases blood flow to the brain. Treatment: Correct the underlying cause.	**syncope** (SIN-koh-pee) **syncopal** (SIN-koh-pal) **syncop/o-** *fainting* **-al** *pertaining to*

Word or Phrase	Description	Pronunciation/Word Parts

Spinal Cord

neural tube defect	Congenital abnormality of the neural tube (embryonic structure that becomes the fetal brain and spinal cord). The fetus's vertebrae form incompletely (**spina bifida**), and there is an abnormal opening in the vertebral column that is only covered by meninges and skin. A **meningocele** is a protrusion of the meninges through the skin. A **meningomyelocele** is a protrusion of the meninges and the spinal cord through the skin (see Figure 9-24 ■). Also known as a **myelomeningocele**. Children with this condition may also have hydrocephalus (described previously). The amount of spinal cord involvement determines the degree of impairment of muscle control of the legs and bladder and bowel function. A sample of amniotic fluid taken during the pregnancy shows an elevated level of alpha fetoprotein. Treatment: Surgery to close the defect immediately after birth because of the risk of infection. The surgery is not able to restore impaired function to the muscles. The hydrocephalus, if present, is treated separately.	**neural** (NYOOR-al) 　**neur/o-** *nerve* 　**-al** *pertaining to* **spina bifida** (SPY-nah BIF-ih-dah) **meningocele** (meh-NING-goh-seel) 　**mening/o-** *meninges* 　**-cele** *hernia* **myelomeningocele** (MY-eh-LOH-meh-NING-goh-seel) 　**myel/o-** *bone marrow; myelin; spinal cord* 　**mening/o-** *meninges* 　**-cele** *hernia* **meningomyelocele** (meh-NING-goh-MY-eh-loh-SEEL) 　**mening/o-** *meninges* 　**myel/o-** *bone marrow; myelin; spinal cord* 　**-cele** *hernia* Meningomyelocele: *Hernia (of the) meninges (and) spinal cord*

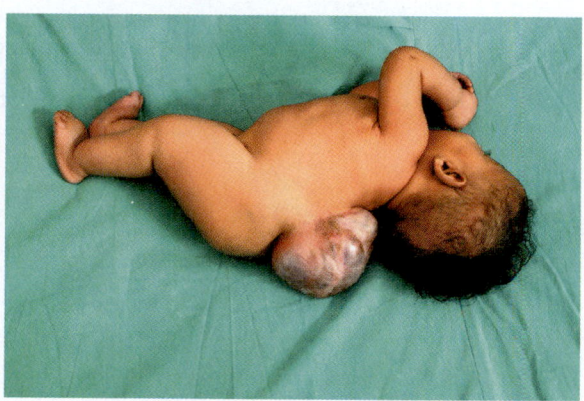

FIGURE 9-24 ■ Meningomyelocele.
This newborn has a meningomyelocele with part of the meninges and spinal cord in a hernia sac outside the body. These delicate tissues are easily traumatized, allowing infection to enter and affect the brain, so surgery is done shortly after birth to close the defect.

Clinical Connections

Dietetics. A folic acid supplement taken during pregnancy greatly reduces the risk of a neural tube defect. Folic acid is present in prenatal vitamins and in enriched cereals and breads.

Word or Phrase	Description	Pronunciation/Word Parts

radiculopathy	Acute or chronic condition that occurs because of a tumor, arthritis, or a **herniated nucleus pulposus (HNP)** (when the contents of an interverte-bral disk are forced out through a weak area in the disk wall). Also known as a **slipped disk**. Any of these conditions can result in pressure on nearby spinal nerve roots (see Figure 9-25 ■). An HNP usually involves a lumbar disk and is often caused by heavy lifting and poor body mechanics. It is known as **sciatica** when the disk presses on branches of the sciatic nerve whose nerve roots are between the L4 and L5 vertebrae. The sciatic nerve is a combined sensory and motor nerve, and, depending on where it is compressed, there is pain and tingling (paresthesias) or numbness and muscle weakness.
	
	Treatment: Anti-inflammatory drug; bedrest; traction to the spine; physical therapy; injection into the nerve root of a corticosteroid drug to decrease inflammation
	Surgery: Rhizotomy, diskectomy, or laminectomy
		radiculopathy
		(rah-DIH-kyoo-LAW-pah-thee)
		  radicul/o- *spinal nerve root*
		  -pathy *disease*
		
		herniated (HER-nee-AA-ted)
		  herni/o- *hernia*
		  -ated *composed of; pertaining to a condition*
		
		nucleus pulposus (NOO-klee-uhs pul-POH-suhs)
		
		sciatica (sy-AT-ih-kah)

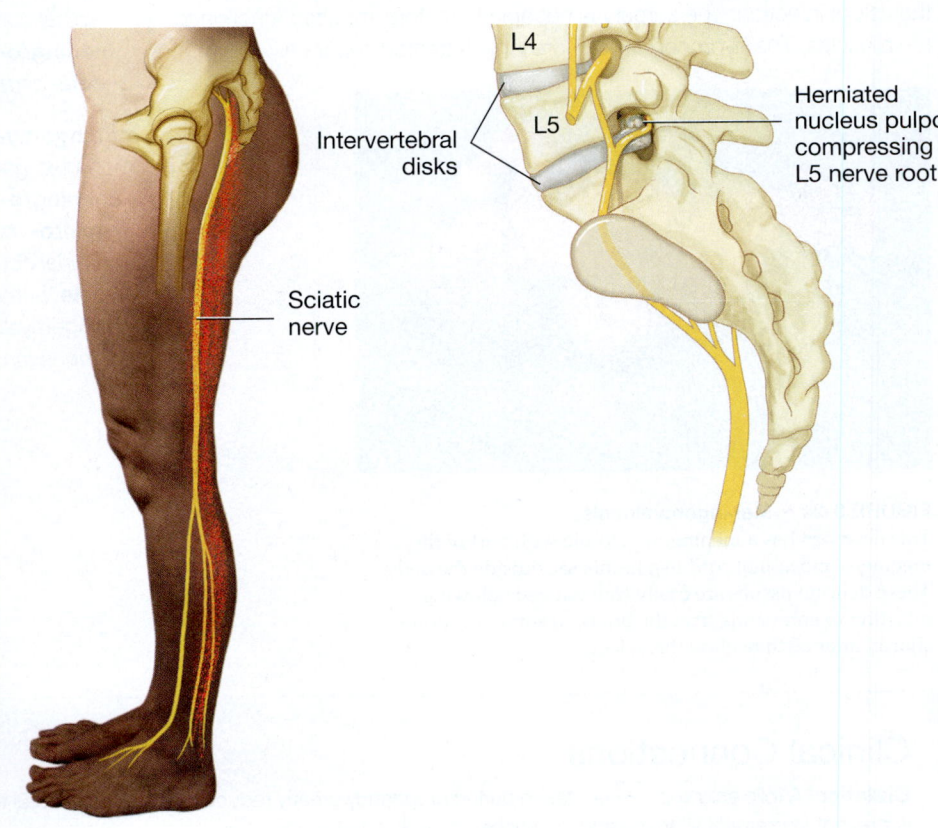

A.   **B.**

FIGURE 9-25 ■ Radiculopathy.
A. The path of the sciatic nerve in the leg. **B.** A herniated nucleus pulposus or slipped disk in the lumbar area (L4–L5) presses on either the dorsal or ventral nerve roots of the sciatic nerve. This causes either pain and tingling or numbness and weakness in the areas shown in red.

Word or Phrase	Description	Pronunciation/Word Parts

spinal cord injury (SCI)	Trauma to the spinal cord with partial or complete **transection** of the cord. This interrupts nerve impulses to particular dermatomes, causing partial or complete anesthesia (loss of sensation) and **paralysis** (an inability to voluntarily move the muscles). An injury to the lower spinal cord causes **paraplegia** with paralysis of the legs (see Figure 9-26 ■). A patient with paraplegia is a **paraplegic**. An injury to the upper spinal cord causes **quadriplegia** with paralysis of all four extremities. A patient with quadriplegia is a **quadriplegic**. Also known as **tetraplegia.** Without nerve impulses, the muscles lose their tone and eventually atrophy. This is known as **flaccid paralysis**. However, the reflex arc of the lower spinal cord often remains intact and, in response to pain or a full bladder, the spinal cord will send nerve impulses that cause the muscles to spasm. This is known as **spastic paralysis**. The bladder may also contract spontaneously, causing incontinence.
	
	Treatment: Traction with weights is applied to the skull to align the vertebrae; surgery may be needed to fuse damaged vertebrae; corticosteroid drug to decrease spinal cord inflammation; muscle relaxant drug; passive range-of-motion exercises and splints
		transection (tran-SEK-shun)
		  trans- *across; through*
		  sect/o- *cut*
		  -ion *action; condition*
		The duplicate *s* is omitted.
		
		paralysis (pah-RAL-ih-sihs)
		  para- *abnormal; apart from; beside; two parts of a pair*
		  ly/o- *break down; destroy*
		  -sis *abnormal condition; process*
		Paralysis: *Abnormal condition (of) two parts of a pair (arms or legs) break down (being paralyzed)*
		
		paraplegia (PAIR-ah-PLEE-jah)
		  para- *abnormal; apart from; beside; two parts of a pair*
		  pleg/o- *paralysis*
		  -ia *condition; state; thing*
		
		paraplegic (PAIR-ah-PLEE-jik)
		  para- *abnormal; apart from; beside; two parts of a pair*
		  pleg/o- *paralysis*
		  -ic *pertaining to*
		
		quadriplegia
		(KWAH-drih-PLEE-jah)
		  quadri- *four*
		  pleg/o- *paralysis*
		  -ia *condition; state; thing*
		Quadriplegia: *Condition (in which all) four (extremities have) paralysis*
		
		quadriplegic (KWAH-drih-PLEE-jik)
		  quadri- *four*
		  pleg/o- *paralysis*
		  -ic *pertaining to*
		
		tetraplegia (TEH-trah-PLEE-jah)
		The combining form **tetr/a-** means *four*.
		
		flaccid (FLAS-id)
		
		spastic (SPAS-tik)
		  spast/o- *spasm*
		  -ic *pertaining to*

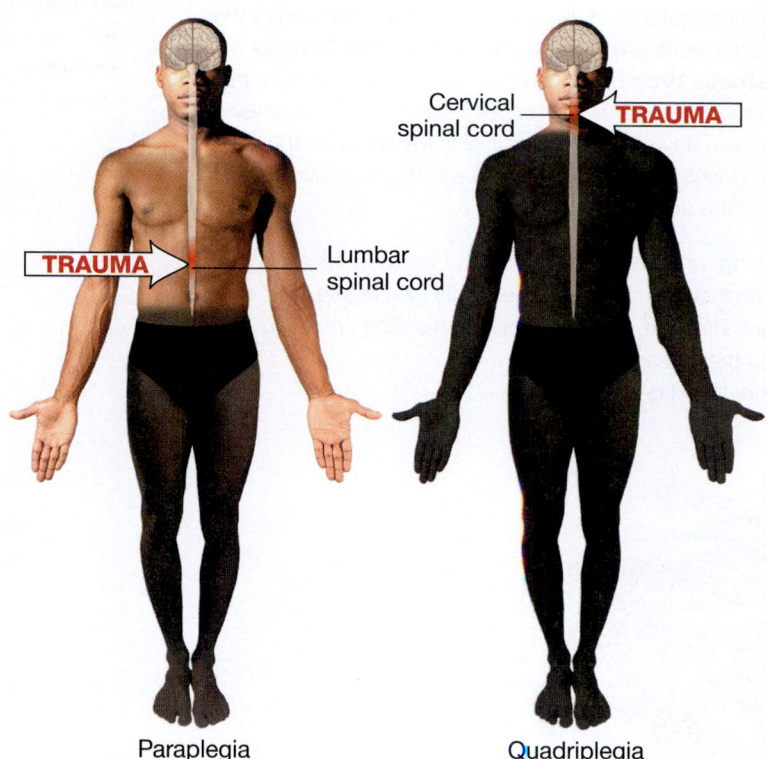

Cervical spinal cord · TRAUMA

TRAUMA · Lumbar spinal cord

Paraplegia   Quadriplegia

FIGURE 9-26 ■ Spinal cord injury.
The level of the spinal cord where an injury occurs and whether the spinal cord was partially or completely transected determines how much of the body is affected and to what extent. Paraplegia affects the lower body and the legs. Quadriplegia affects the body from the neck down, all four extremities, and even the breathing.

Word or Phrase	Description	Pronunciation/Word Parts

Nerves

amyotrophic lateral sclerosis (ALS)	Chronic, progressive disease of the motor nerves coming from the spinal cord to the body. This causes muscle wasting and spasms, with eventual paralysis of all the muscles, including swallowing and respiratory muscles. There is no damage to the sensory nerves and so sensation remains intact, and cognitive abilities are not affected. Some cases of ALS are caused by the lack of an enzyme, which is an inherited defect, but in most cases the cause is not known. Also known as **Lou Gehrig disease** after the famous baseball player who developed the disease in the late 1930s. Treatment: Supportive care	**amyotrophic** (ah-MY-oh-TROH-fik) **a-** *away from; without* **my/o-** *muscle* **troph/o-** *development* **-ic** *pertaining to* **sclerosis** (skleh-ROH-sihs) **scler/o-** *hard; sclera* **-osis** *abnormal condition; process*
anesthesia	Condition in which sensation of any type—including touch, pressure, proprioception, or pain—is absent. Local areas of anesthesia can occur temporarily; example: when your hand goes numb from pressing on a nerve in your arm as you sleep. Third-degree burns cause permanent anesthesia of the damaged skin. A spinal cord injury causes permanent anesthesia along a dermatome at the level of the injury. Temporary therapeutic anesthesia to relieve pain can be produced in specific regions by injecting an **anesthetic drug** under the skin, near a nerve root, or into the epidural space in the spinal canal. Unconsciousness is accompanied by an inability to perceive any sensation, and this is the basis for the use of drugs that induce general anesthesia prior to a surgical procedure. Treatment: Correct the underlying cause.	**anesthesia** (AN-es-THEE-zha) **an-** *not; without* **esthes/o-** *feeling; sensation* **-ia** *condition; state; thing* **anesthetic** (AN-es-THEH-tik) **an-** *not; without* **esthet/o-** *feeling; sensation* **-ic** *pertaining to*
Bell palsy	Weakness, drooping, or paralysis of one side of the face because of inflammation of the facial nerve (cranial nerve VII) (see Figure 9-27 ■). It is caused by a viral infection, possibly herpes virus. The condition usually lasts a month and then disappears. Treatment: Corticosteroid drug	**palsy** (PAWL-zee)

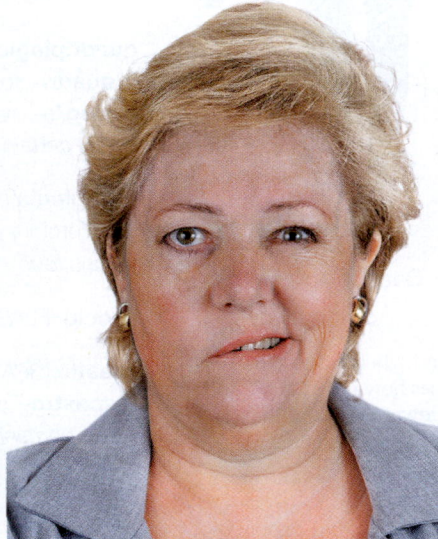

FIGURE 9-27 ■ Bell palsy.
This patient with Bell palsy has paralysis of the facial nerve on the right side of her face, as shown by the drooping of her right lower eyelid, cheek, and right corner of her mouth.

Word or Phrase	Description	Pronunciation/Word Parts

carpal tunnel syndrome (CTS)	Chronic condition caused by repetitive motions of the hand and wrist, often from constant typing. There is tingling in the hand because of inflammation with swelling of the tendons from the forearm muscles whose tendons go through the carpal tunnel of the wrist bones to reach the hand. This swelling compresses the median nerve. Bending or extending the wrist for 60 seconds (Phalen's maneuver) aggravates the pain and is a positive diagnostic test.
	Treatment: Rest; splinting the wrist; using a split keyboard to correctly position the wrists; physical therapy; injection of a corticosteroid drug; surgery, if needed
		carpal (KAR-pal)
		  carp/o- *wrist*
		  -al *pertaining to*

Guillain-Barré syndrome	Autoimmune disorder in which the body makes antibodies against myelin. There is acute inflammation of the peripheral nerves, destruction of myelin with interruption of nerve conduction, muscle weakness, and changes in sensation (paresthesias). This disease is caused by a triggering event such as an infection (often a viral respiratory illness), stress, or trauma. The muscle weakness begins in the legs and then rapidly involves the entire body. The patient may even temporarily require respiratory support until the inflammation subsides. Guillain-Barré does not recur, and the patient recovers some or all neurologic function over a period of days to months. Treatment: Corticosteroid drug to treat inflammation	**Guillain-Barré** (GEE-yah bah-RAY)

hyperesthesia	Condition in which there is a heightened awareness and sensitivity to touch and increased response to painful stimuli.
	Treatment: Antidepressant drug or tranquilizer drug
		hyperesthesia (HY-per-es-THEE-zha)
		  hyper- *above; more than normal*
		  esthes/o- *feeling; sensation*
		  -ia *condition; state; thing*

multiple sclerosis (MS)	Chronic, progressive, degenerative autoimmune disorder in which the body makes antibodies against myelin. There is acute inflammation of the nerves and destruction of myelin (**demyelination**) with interruption of nerve conduction in the brain and spinal cord. The areas of demyelination eventually become scar tissue that hardens (sclerosis). These areas are known as *plaque* and can be seen on MRI scans of the brain. MS can be caused by a triggering event such as a viral infection. Patients are typically in their 20s to early middle age. There is double vision, nystagmus, large muscle weakness, uncoordinated gait, spasticity, early fatigue after repeated muscle contractions, tremors, paresthesias, inability to walk, and sometimes dementia. Heat, stress, and fatigue temporarily worsen the symptoms. There can be remissions in which there is some improvement, followed by exacerbations or flare-ups, but always with worsening of the condition over time.
	Treatment: Physical therapy; corticosteroid drug; muscle relaxant drug
		sclerosis (skleh-ROH-sihs)
		  scler/o- *hard; sclera*
		  -osis *abnormal condition; process*
		Sclerosis: *Abnormal condition (of) hard(ness)*
		
		demyelination (dee-MY-eh-lih-NAY-shun)
		  de- *reversal of; without*
		  myelin/o- *myelin*
		  -ation *being; having; process*

Word or Phrase	Description	Pronunciation/Word Parts
neuralgia	Pain along the path of a nerve and its branches that is caused by an injury. Neuralgia can cause mild-to-severe pain. **Trigeminal neuralgia**, also known as **tic douloureux**, is characterized by episodes of brief but severe, stabbing pain (like an electrical shock) on one or both sides of the face or jaw along the distribution of the trigeminal nerve (cranial nerve V). **Causalgia** is severe, burning pain along a nerve and its branches. **Complex regional pain syndrome (CRPS)** occurs after an injury to one body part; its symptoms include causalgia that is chronic and is coupled with changes in skin color and temperature, and swelling. Treatment: Anti-inflammatory drug; topical anesthetic drug; corticosteroid drug; antidepressant drug; anticonvulsant drug; skeletal muscle relaxant drug; nerve block; TENS unit; and physical therapy	**neuralgia** (nyoor-AL-jah) **neur/o-** *nerve* **alg/o-** *pain* **-ia** *condition; state; thing* **trigeminal** (try-JEM-ih-nal) **tri-** *three* **gemin/o-** *group; set* **-al** *pertaining to* **tic douloureux** (TIK doo-loo-ROO) **causalgia** (kawz-AL-jah) **caus/o-** *burning* **alg/o-** *pain* **-ia** *condition; state; thing*

Clinical Connections

Dermatology. Shingles is a painful skin condition that is caused by the herpes zoster virus, the virus that causes chickenpox in children. The virus remains dormant in the body until later in life when stress triggers it to erupt. It affects nerves and the skin of the dermatomes, causing redness, pain, and vesicles (see Figure 2-14). Lingering, chronic pain from shingles is **postherpetic neuralgia**.
Treatment: Antiviral drug

Word or Phrase	Description	Pronunciation/Word Parts
neuritis	Inflammation or infection of a nerve. **Polyneuritis** is a generalized inflammation of many nerves in one part of the body or all the nerves in the body. Treatment: Correct the underlying cause; analgesic drug; anti-inflammatory drug; corticosteroid drug; or antibiotic drug	**neuritis** (nyoor-EYE-tihs) **neur/o-** *nerve* **-itis** *infection of; inflammation of* **polyneuritis** (PAW-lee-nyoor-EYE-tihs) **poly-** *many; much* **neur/o-** *nerve* **-itis** *infection of; inflammation of*
neurofibroma-tosis	Hereditary disease with multiple benign fibrous tumors (**neurofibromata**) that grow on the peripheral nerves. These are most noticeable on the skin, but they can be anywhere in the body—on the internal organs or even in the eye. They range in size from small nodules to large tumors. Treatment: Surgical removal of large tumors that cause pain or disability	**neurofibromatosis** (NYOOR-oh-fy-BROH-mah-TOH-sihs) **neur/o-** *nerve* **fibr/o-** *fiber* **-omatosis** *condition of masses; condition of tumors* **neurofibroma** (NYOOR-oh-fy-BROH-mah) **neur/o-** *nerve* **fibr/o-** *fiber* **-oma** *mass; tumor* Greek singular noun: Form the plural by changing the singular ending *-oma* to *-omata*.
neuroma	Benign tumor of a nerve. A **Morton neuroma** specifically forms from repetitive damage to the nerve that is near the metatarsophalangeal joints between the ball of the foot and the toes. Treatment: Surgical removal	**neuroma** (nyoor-OH-mah) **neur/o-** *nerve* **-oma** *mass; tumor*

Word or Phrase	Description	Pronunciation/Word Parts
neuropathy	General category for any type of disease or injury to a nerve. Treatment: Correct the underlying cause.	**neuropathy** (nyoor-AW-pah-thee) **neur/o-** *nerve* **-pathy** *disease*

Clinical Connections

Endocrinology. Diabetic neuropathy is a chronic, slowly progressive condition that affects the peripheral nerves in diabetic patients. It is caused by a lack of blood flow (arteriosclerosis) to the nerves. There is severe pain and a loss of sensation and sense of position, particularly in the feet. Treatment: Manage the diabetes mellitus.

diabetic (DY-ah-BET-ik)
diabet/o- *diabetes*
-ic *pertaining to*

neuropathy (nyoor-AW-pah-thee)
neur/o- *nerve*
-pathy *disease*

Word or Phrase	Description	Pronunciation/Word Parts
paresthesia	Condition in which abnormal sensations, such as tingling, burning, or pinpricks, are felt on the skin (see Figure 9-28 ■). Paresthesias are often the result of chronic nerve damage from a pinched nerve or diabetic neuropathy. Treatment: Correct the underlying cause; anticonvulsant drug; antianxiety drug; or antidepressant drug	**paresthesia** (PAIR-es-THEE-zha) **para-** *abnormal; apart from; beside; two parts of a pair* **esthes/o-** *feeling; sensation* **-ia** *condition; state; thing* The final *a* in the prefix **para-** is deleted. Paresthesia: *Condition (of) abnormal feeling or sensation*

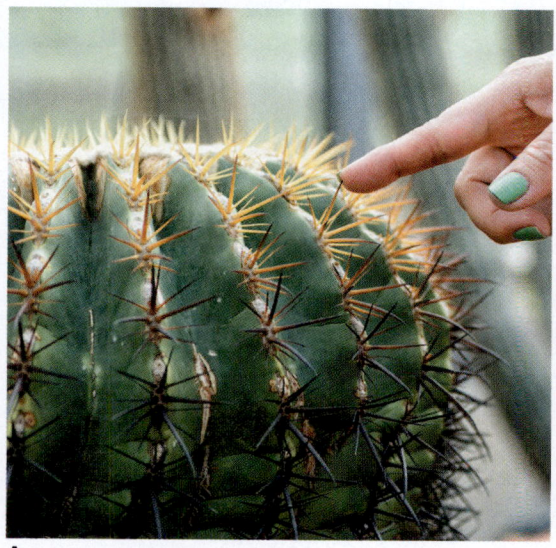 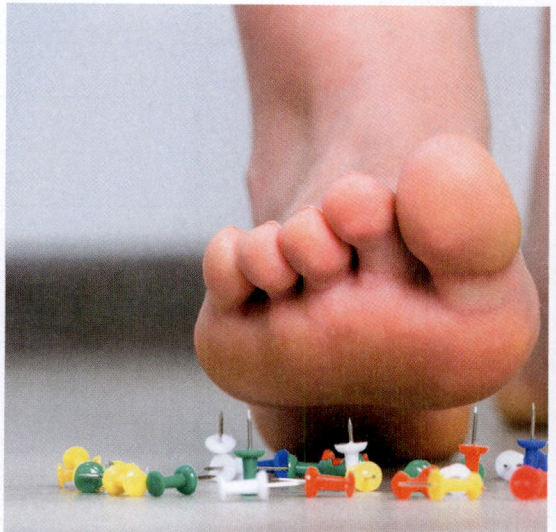

A.   **B.**

FIGURE 9-28 ■ Paresthesias.
Some patients with paresthesias have shooting or stabbing pain. Others experience burning, tingling, numbness, or a feeling of ants crawling on the skin.

9.3 PRACTICE LAPS

Use the Answer Key at the end of the book to check your answers.

A. Give the Meaning of Combining Forms

Next to each combining form, write its meaning. The first one has been done for you.

Combining Form	Meaning	Combining Form	Meaning
1. **fibr/o-**	*fiber*	28. ict/o-	
2. alg/o-		29. isch/o-	
3. amnes/o-		30. lex/o-	
4. arteri/o-		31. ly/o-	
5. athet/o-		32. malign/o-	
6. carp/o-		33. mening/o-	
7. cephal/o-		34. ment/o-	
8. cerebr/o-		35. myelin/o-	
9. cognit/o-		36. my/o-	
10. comat/o-		37. narc/o-	
11. concuss/o-		38. neur/o-	
12. contus/o-		39. nuch/o-	
13. convuls/o-		40. phas/o-	
14. crani/o-		41. phob/o-	
15. caus/o-		42. phot/o-	
16. diabet/o-		43. pleg/o-	
17. dur/o-		44. radicul/o-	
18. encephal/o-		45. scintill/o-	
19. epilept/o-		46. scler/o-	
20. esthes/o-		47. scot/o-	
21. esthet/o-		48. sect/o-	
22. express/o-		49. senil/o-	
23. format/o-		50. spast/o-	
24. glob/o-		51. syncop/o-	
25. hemat/o-		52. troph/o-	
26. herni/o-		53. ven/o-	
27. hydr/o-		54. ventricul/o-	

B. Build Words

Read the definition of the medical word. Look at the combining form that is given. Select the correct suffix from the Suffix List, and write it on the blank line. Then build the medical word, and write it on the line. (Remember: You may need to remove the combining vowel. Always remove the hyphens and slash.) Be sure to check your spelling.

Suffix List

-al (pertaining to)	-ic (pertaining to)	-ity (condition; state)	-oma (mass; tumor)
-ant (pertaining to)	-ion (action; condition)	-lepsy (seizure)	-ose (full of)
-cele (hernia)	-itis (infection of;	-oid (resembling)	-pathy (disease)
-ia (condition; state; thing)	inflammation of)		

Definition of the Medical Word	Combining Form	Suffix	Build the Medical Word
Example: Condition (of) bruising	**contus/o-**	*-ion*	*contusion*

[You think condition *(-ion) +* bruising *(contus/o-). You change the order of the word parts to put the suffix last. You write* contusion*.]*

1. Infection of (or) inflammation of (a) nerve	neur/o-		
2. Pertaining to cancer	malign/o-		
3. Hernia (of the) meninges	mening/o-		
4. Condition (of a) seizure	convuls/o-		
5. Tumor (of) blood	hemat/o-		
6. Condition (of) memory loss	amnes/o-		
7. Pertaining to (a) seizure	epilept/o-		
8. Condition (of a) small area of dead tissue	infarct/o-		
9. Tumor (of a) nerve	neur/o-		
10. Disease (of the) spinal nerve root	radicul/o-		
11. State (of) old age	senil/o-		
12. Pertaining to (a) spasm	spast/o-		
13. Pertaining to fainting	syncop/o-		
14. Seizure (like the state during) sleep	narc/o-		
15. Condition (from a) violent impact	concuss/o-		
16. Full of unconsciousness	comat/o-		
17. (Movement) resembling (being) without position or purpose	athet/o-		
18. Inflammation (or) infection (of the) brain	encephal/o-		
19. Disease (of a) nerve	neur/o-		
20. Pertaining to (the) neck	nuch/o-		
21. Inflammation (or) infection (of the) meninges	mening/o-		
22. Pertaining to diabetes	diabet/o-		
23. Tumor (of) darkness (in the visual field)	scot/o-		

C. Define Abbreviations

1. ALS _____
2. AVM _____
3. CP _____
4. CRPS _____
5. CTS _____
6. CVA _____
7. DT _____
8. HNP _____
9. ICP _____

10. LOC _____
11. MS _____
12. NCD _____
13. REM _____
14. RIND _____
15. SCI _____
16. TBI _____
17. TIA _____

9.4 Laboratory, Diagnostic, and Radiologic Procedures

Word or Phrase	Description	Pronunciation/Word Parts

Laboratory Tests

Word or Phrase	Description	Pronunciation/Word Parts
alpha fetoprotein (AFP)	Test of a sample of amniotic fluid taken from the uterus by amniocentesis during pregnancy (described in Chapter 12, Gynecology and Obstetrics). It is used to diagnose a neural tube defect in the fetus before birth. The fetal liver makes alpha fetoprotein, and small amounts are normally present in the amniotic fluid. However, an increased level indicates that alpha fetoprotein is leaking into the amniotic fluid through a meningocele or meningomyelocele.	**alpha fetoprotein** (AL-fah FEE-toh-PROH-teen)
cerebrospinal fluid (CSF) examination	Test that visually examines the CSF for clarity and color, microscopically for cells, and chemically for proteins and other substances. Normal CSF is clear and colorless. CSF with a pink or reddish tint contains a large number of red blood cells, and this indicates bleeding in the brain or spinal cord from a stroke or trauma. Cloudy CSF contains a large number of white blood cells from a bacterial infection such as encephalitis or meningitis. An elevated level of protein indicates infection or the presence of a tumor. The presence of oligoclonal bands points to multiple sclerosis. Myelin-basic protein is elevated in multiple sclerosis and amyotrophic lateral sclerosis.	**cerebrospinal** (seh-REE-broh-SPY-nal) **cerebr/o-** cerebrum **spin/o-** backbone; spine **-al** pertaining to

Word or Phrase	Description	Pronunciation/Word Parts

Radiologic and Nuclear Medicine Procedures

Word or Phrase	Description	Pronunciation/Word Parts
cerebral angiography	Radiologic procedure in which radiopaque contrast dye is injected into a large artery in the arm or leg. The dye travels to the carotid artery and an x-ray is taken to visualize the arterial circulation in the brain (see Figure 9-29 ■). This is done to show an aneurysm, stenosis, plaque in the arteries, or a tumor. A tumor is seen as an interwoven collection of new blood vessels, or it can be seen indirectly when it forces the arteries into abnormal positions. Also known as **arteriography**. The x-ray image is an **angiogram** or an **arteriogram**.	**angiography** (AN-jee-AW-grah-fee) **angi/o-** *blood vessel; lymphatic vessel* **-graphy** *process of recording* **angiogram** (AN-jee-oh-GRAM) **angi/o-** *blood vessel; lymphatic vessel* **-gram** *picture; record* **arteriography** (ar-TEER-ee-AW-grah-fee) **arteri/o-** *artery* **-graphy** *process of recording* **arteriogram** (ar-TEER-ee-oh-GRAM) **arteri/o-** *artery* **-gram** *picture; record*

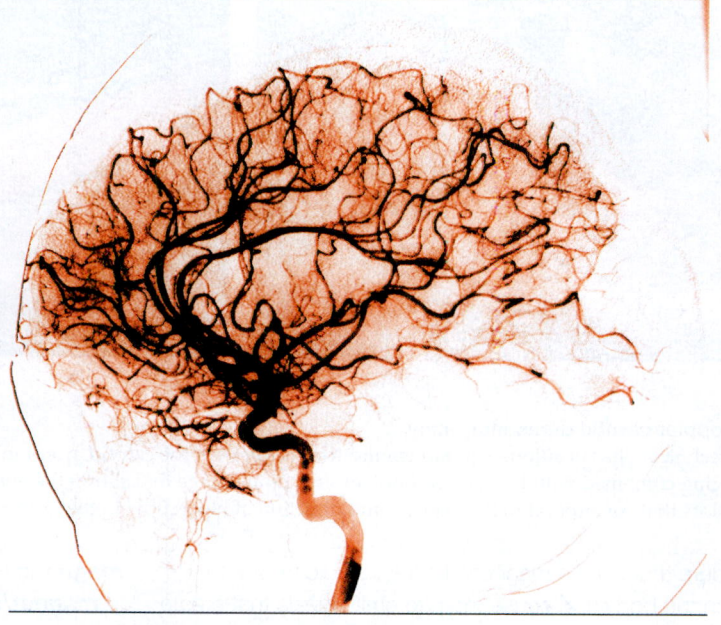

FIGURE 9-29 ■ Arteriogram.
The injected dye clearly outlines the patient's large carotid artery in the neck and its many smaller branches within the cerebrum. There is no evidence of carotid artery plaques or cerebral aneurysm.

Word or Phrase	Description	Pronunciation/Word Parts
computerized axial tomography (CAT, CT)	Radiologic procedure that uses x-rays to create many individual, closely spaced images ("slices"). CT scans are used to view the cranium, brain, vertebral column, and spinal cord. Radiopaque contrast dye can be injected to provide more detail.	**axial** (AK-see-al) **axi/o-** *axis* **-al** *pertaining to* **tomography** (toh-MAW-grah-fee) **tom/o-** *cut; layer; slice* **-graphy** *process of recording*

Word or Phrase	Description	Pronunciation/Word Parts
Doppler ultrasonography	Ultrasound procedure that uses ultra high-frequency sound waves to produce a two-dimensional image to visualize areas of stenosis and plaque as well as turbulence in the blood flow in the carotid arteries (see Figure 9-30 ■). Also known as a **carotid duplex scan**.	**ultrasonography** (UL-trah-soh-NAW-grah-fee) **ultra-** *beyond; higher* **son/o-** *sound* **-graphy** *process of recording* **carotid** (kah-RAW-tid) **duplex** (DOO-pleks)

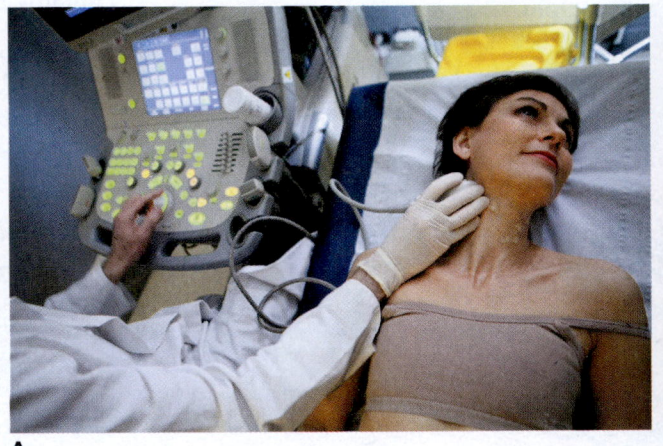 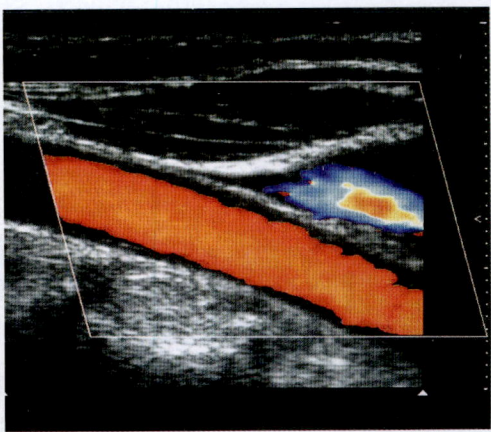

A.   B.

FIGURE 9-30 ■ Doppler carotid ultrasonography.
A. An ultrasound technician has positioned an ultrasound transducer over the carotid artery in the patient's neck.
B. Ultrasound imaging combined with Doppler technology creates an image that shows the anatomy of the carotid artery as well as colors that correspond to the velocity and direction of blood flow in that artery.

Word or Phrase	Description	Pronunciation/Word Parts
magnetic resonance imaging (MRI)	Radiologic procedure that uses a magnetic field and radio waves to align the protons in the body and cause them to emit signals that create an image. Magnetic resonance imaging is a type of tomography that creates images as many individual "slices." MRI scans are used to view the cranium, brain, vertebral column, and spinal cord (see Figure 9-13). Radiopaque contrast dye can be injected to provide more detail.	**magnetic** (mag-NET-ik) **magnet/o-** *magnet* **-ic** *pertaining to* **resonance** (REZ-oh-nans)
myelography	Radiologic procedure in which a radiopaque contrast dye is injected into the subarachnoid space at the level of the L3 and L4 vertebrae. The contrast dye outlines the spinal canal and shows spinal nerves, nerve roots, and intervertebral disks, as well as tumors, herniated disks, or obstructions within the cavity. The x-ray image is a **myelogram**. Because a myelogram can cause the side effect of a severe headache, an MRI scan of the spine is more often done.	**myelography** (MY-eh-LAW-grah-fee) **myel/o-** *bone marrow; myelin; spinal cord* **-graphy** *process of recording* **myelogram** (MY-eh-loh-GRAM) **myel/o-** *bone marrow; myelin; spinal cord* **-gram** *picture; record*
positron emission tomography (PET) scan	Nuclear medicine procedure that uses a radioactive substance (combined with glucose molecules) injected intravenously. As the glucose is metabolized, the radioactive substance emits positrons, and these form gamma rays that are detected by a gamma camera. The camera produces an image that reflects the amount of cellular metabolism in that area (see Figure 9-17). An area of increased metabolism can be due to a cancerous tumor. Areas of decreased metabolism can be due to dementia, Parkinson disease, or epilepsy.	**positron** (PAW-zih-trawn) **emission** (ee-MIH-shun) **emiss/o-** *send out* **-ion** *action; condition* **tomography** (toh-MAW-grah-fee) **tom/o-** *cut; layer; slice* **-graphy** *process of recording*

Word or Phrase	Description	Pronunciation/Word Parts
skull x-ray	Radiologic procedure in which a plain film (without contrast dye) is taken of the skull. An x-ray can show fractures of the bones of the skull but cannot clearly show the soft tissues of the brain or the blood vessels.	

Other Diagnostic Tests

electroencephalography (EEG)	Procedure to record the electrical activity of the brain (see Figure 9-31 ■). Multiple electrodes are placed on the scalp overlying specific lobes of the brain. The electrodes are attached by lead wires to an **electroencephalograph**, a machine that records brain waves. The computerized recording of the brain waves is an **electroencephalogram**. There are four types of normal brain waves (named for letters of the Greek alphabet): alpha, beta, delta, and theta. The patterns of brain waves in the right and left hemispheres of the cerebrum should be the same. A difference between the two hemispheres suggests a tumor or injury. The presence of abnormal waves suggests encephalopathy or dementia. Brain waves during an epileptic seizure show specific patterns that are used to diagnose the particular type of epilepsy (see Figure 9-20). In order to induce an epileptic seizure during an EEG, the patient may be asked to look at flashing lights or have a sleep-deprived EEG recording. An EEG is also done as part of a polysomnography procedure to diagnose sleep disorders and also as part of evoked potential testing.	**electroencephalography** (ee-LEK-troh-en-SEF-ah-LAW-grah-fee) **electr/o-** *electricity* **encephal/o-** *brain* **-graphy** *process of recording* **electroencephalograph** (ee-LEK-troh-en-SEF-ah-loh-GRAF) **electr/o-** *electricity* **encephal/o-** *brain* **-graph** *instrument used to record* **electroencephalogram** (ee-LEK-troh-en-SEF-ah-loh-GRAM) **electr/o-** *electricity* **encephal/o-** *brain* **-gram** *picture; record*

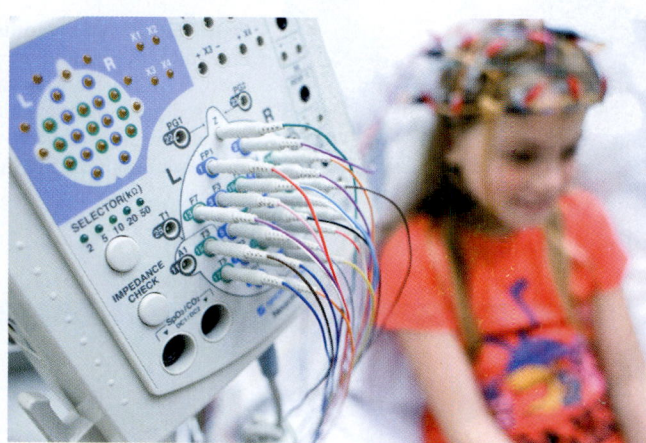

FIGURE 9-31 ■ Electroencephalography (EEG). This young patient is having an EEG to diagnose what type of epileptic seizures she is having. The electrodes are placed on her scalp in a specific pattern, as shown in the diagram on the upper left of the EEG machine. The electrodes pick up the electrical impulses of brain waves and display them on a computer screen.

evoked potential testing	Procedure in which an EEG is used to record changes in brain waves that occur following various stimuli. It is used to evaluate the potential ability of a particular nervous pathway to conduct nerve impulses. A stimulus is presented to evoke (stimulate) a response. Also known as **evoked response testing**. For a **visual evoked potential (VEP)** or **visual evoked response (VER)**, the patient watches a computer monitor that displays rapidly alternating checkerboard patterns. This evaluates nerve pathways from the eye to the cerebrum. For a **brainstem auditory evoked potential (BAEP)** or **brainstem auditory evoked response (BAER)**, the patient wears headphones and listens to a series of clicks in one ear and then the other. This evaluates nerve pathways from the ears to the cerebrum. For a **somatosensory evoked potential (SSEP)** or **somatosensory evoked response (SSER)**, a small electrical impulse is administered to the arm or leg. This evaluates nerve pathways from the extremities to the cerebrum. These tests are also used to detect subtle abnormalities in patients with multiple sclerosis, head trauma, or spinal cord injury. The patient cannot voluntarily alter the results of these tests. Evoked potential testing is particularly helpful with patients who are very young or are unable to respond to standard vision and hearing tests.	**evoked** (ee-VOKED) **potential** (poh-TEN-shal) **potent/o-** *capable of doing* **-ial** *pertaining to* **somatosensory** (soh-MAH-toh-SEN-soh-ree) **somat/o-** *body* **sens/o-** *feeling* **-ory** *having the function of*

Word or Phrase	Description	Pronunciation/Word Parts
nerve conduction study	Procedure to measure the speed at which an electrical impulse travels along a nerve. An electrode applied to the skin delivers an electrical impulse to stimulate a peripheral nerve. Another electrode a measured distance away records how long it takes for the electrical impulse to reach it. This test is usually performed in conjunction with electromyography to help differentiate between weakness due to nerve disorders versus weakness due to muscle disorders.	**conduction** (con-DUK-shun) **conduct/o-** *carrying; conveying* **-ion** *action; condition*
polysomnography	Procedure to diagnose what is causing insomnia, sleep disruption, sleep apnea, or narcolepsy (see Figure 9-32 ■). Also known as a **sleep study**.	**polysomnography** (PAW-lee-sawm-NAW-grah-fee) **poly-** *many; much* **somn/o-** *sleep* **-graphy** *process of recording* Polysomnography: *Process of recording many (of the body's activities during) sleep*

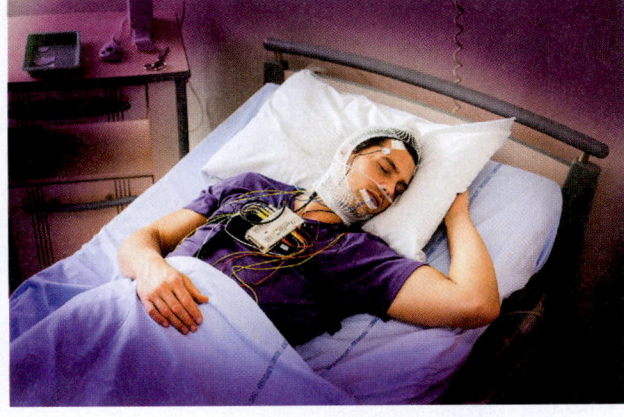

FIGURE 9-32 ■ Polysomnography.
Electrodes placed on the patient's face and head, as well as various other monitors, are used to record the patient's EEG, eye movements, muscle activity, heartbeat, and respirations during sleep.

9.4 PRACTICE LAPS

Use the Answer Key at the end of the book to check your answers.

A. Give the Meaning of Combining Forms

Next to each combining form, write its meaning. The first one has been done for you.

Combining Form	Meaning	Combining Form	Meaning
1. **axi/o-**	*axis*	9. myel/o-	
2. angi/o-		10. potent/o-	
3. arteri/o-		11. sens/o-	
4. cerebr/o-		12. somat/o-	
5. electr/o-		13. somn/o-	
6. emiss/o-		14. son/o-	
7. encephal/o-		15. spin/o-	
8. magnet/o-		16. tom/o-	

B. Build Words

Read the definition of the medical word. Look at the combining form that is given. Select the correct suffix from the Suffix List, and write it on the blank line. Then build the medical word, and write it on the line. (Remember: You may need to remove the combining vowel. Always remove the hyphens and slash.) Be sure to check your spelling.

Suffix List

-al (pertaining to)   -graphy (process of recording)
-gram (picture; record)   -ion (action; condition)

Definition of the Medical Word	Combining Form	Suffix	Build the Medical Word
Example: Pertaining to (an) axis	**axi/o-**	*-al*	*axial*

[*You think* pertaining to (-al) + axis (axi/o-). You change the order of the word parts to put the suffix last. You write axial.]

1. Process of recording (an image as a) cut, slice, or layer	tom/o-	_____	_____
2. Picture (or) record (of an) artery	arteri/o-	_____	_____
3. Action (of) carrying (or) conveying	conduct/o-	_____	_____
4. Process of recording (a) blood vessel	angi/o-	_____	_____
5. Process of recording (the) spinal cord	myel/o-	_____	_____

C. Define Abbreviations

1. AFP   _____
2. BAEP _____
4. CSF   _____
5. CT   _____

6. EEG   _____
7. MRI   _____
8. PET   _____
9. SSEP _____

9.5 Medical Procedures, Drugs, and Surgical Procedures

Word or Phrase	Description	Pronunciation/Word Parts

Medical Procedures

Word or Phrase	Description	Pronunciation/Word Parts
Babinski sign	Neurologic test in which the end of the metal handle of a percussion hammer is used to firmly stroke the lateral sole of the foot from the heel to the toes. A normal test (negative Babinski) produces a downward curling of the toes. An abnormal test (positive Babinski) produces extension of the great toe and fanning out of the other toes (see Figure 9-33 ■). A positive Babinski indicates injury to the parietal lobe of the cerebrum or to the spinal nerves.	**Babinski** (bah-BIN-skee)

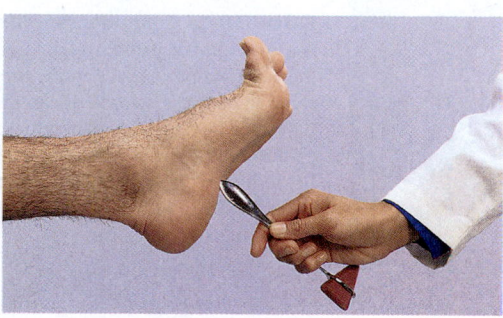

FIGURE 9-33 ■ Positive Babinski sign.
This patient has a positive (abnormal) Babinski sign with extension of the great toe and fanning out of the other toes laterally.

Word or Phrase	Description	Pronunciation/Word Parts
Glasgow Coma Scale (GCS)	Numerical scale that measures the depth of a coma. The total score ranges from 1 to 15 and is the sum of individual scores for eye opening, motor response, and verbal response following a painful stimulus (such as pressure on the nail bed or on the bony ridge over the eye).	**Glasgow** (GLAS-goh)
lumbar puncture (LP)	Procedure to obtain cerebrospinal fluid (CSF) for testing. Also known as a **spinal tap**. The patient is positioned with the upper legs flexed toward the chest. This curves the spine and widens the space between the spinous processes of two vertebrae, allowing accurate positioning of a spinal needle (see Figure 9-34 ■). The needle is inserted in the space between the L3–4 or L4–5 vertebrae and into the subarachnoid space. Cerebrospinal fluid flows through the needle and is collected and sent to a laboratory. Before the spinal needle is removed, a calibrated **manometer** (a thin tube) can be attached to measure the intracranial pressure as the CSF rises in the manometer.	**lumbar** (LUM-bar) 　**lumb/o-** *lower back* 　**-ar** *pertaining to* **puncture** (PUNGK-chur) 　**punct/o-** *hole; perforation* 　**-ure** *result of; system* **manometer** (mah-NAW-meh-ter) 　**man/o-** *frenzy; thin* 　**-meter** *instrument used to measure* Manometer: *Instrument used to measure (that is a) thin (tube)*

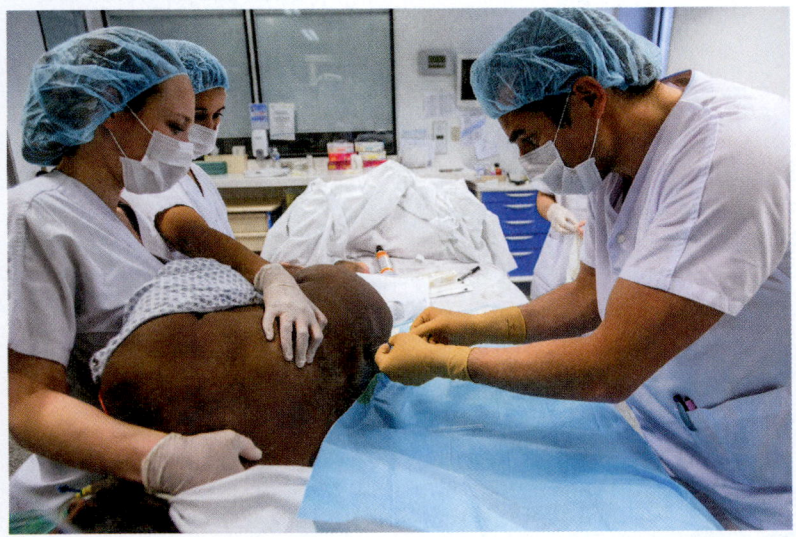

A.

Cauda equina
L4 vertebra spinous process
Dura mater
Cerebrospinal fluid in subarachnoid space
Spinal needle
L5 vertebra spinous process

L4
L5

B.

FIGURE 9-34 ■ Lumbar puncture.
A. For a lumbar puncture, the needle is inserted into the subarachnoid space in the lumbar area of the spinal canal to obtain a sample of cerebrospinal fluid. **B.** This patient is having a lumbar puncture. He is correctly positioned on his side, but he does not have much flexibility of the spine, and so a nurse is helping the patient to maintain this position while the physician inserts the spinal needle.

Word or Phrase	Description	Pronunciation/Word Parts
Mini-Mental State Examination (MMSE)	Tests the patient's concrete and abstract thought processes and long- and short-term memory. The patient is asked to state his or her name, the date, and where he or she is. If the answers are all correct, the patient is said to be oriented to person, time, and place (oriented x3). The patient is asked to perform simple mental arithmetic, recall objects or words, name the current president and recent past presidents, spell a word backward, and give the meaning of a proverb.	**mental** (MEN-tal) **ment/o-** *chin; mind* **-al** *pertaining to*
neurologic examination	Tests coordination, sensation, balance, and gait (see Table 9-6 ■)	
spinal traction	Procedure in which a fracture of the vertebra is immobilized while it heals. Two metal pins are surgically inserted into the cranium and attached to a set of tongs with a rope and pulley and 7–10 pounds of weight. This keeps the vertebral fracture in alignment while it heals. A patient with a partially healed fracture of the vertebra can be fitted for a halo vest with pins in the cranium attached to a metal ring (halo). This allows the patient to be ambulatory.	**traction** (TRAK-shun) **tract/o-** *pulling* **-ion** *action; condition*

Table 9-6   Tests Included in a Neurologic Examination

Category	Tests	Pronunciation/Word Parts
Coordination tests	• Rapid alternating movements: The patient taps the tip of the index finger against the thumb as rapidly as possible. • Finger-to-nose test: With eyes closed, the patient touches the tip of the index finger to the nose. • The patient touches the nose, then touches the physician's finger as it moves to various locations, then touches the nose again. • Heel-to-shin test: The patient puts the heel of one foot onto the opposite leg and then runs it from the knee down the shin to the toes.	
Sensation tests	• With the patient's eyes closed, the skin is touched in various places with a cotton swab (to test light touch), a vibrating tuning fork (to test vibration), and the point of a pin (pinprick to test pain). One or two pins are used to see if the patient can distinguish the number of things touching the skin (two-point discrimination). • The patient's toe or finger is moved up and down, and the patient is asked to identify the direction (to test body position and **proprioception**).	**proprioception** (PROH-pree-oh-SEP-shun) **propri/o-** *one's own body* **-ception** *having a receptor*
Balance test	• **Romberg test**. The patient stands with the feet together and the eyes closed. In a normal test, the patient does not sway excessively or lose balance. The Romberg test is also known as the **station test**.	**Romberg** (RAWM-berg)
Gait tests	• The manner of walking is assessed for a normal arm swing and stride. • The patient is asked to walk across the room in a heel-to-toe fashion. The patient is asked to walk on the toes, on the heels, and then hop in place on each foot.	

Word or Phrase	Description	Pronunciation/Word Parts
transcutaneous electrical nerve stimulation (TENS)	Procedure that uses an electrical device (a TENS unit) to control chronic pain (see Figure 9-35 ■). Its battery produces regular, preset electrical impulses that travel through wires to electrodes on the skin. These impulses block the transmission of pain sensations to the brain. The impulses also stimulate the body to produce its own natural pain-relieving endorphins.	**transcutaneous** (TRANS-kyoo-TAY-nee-us) **trans-** *across; through* **cutane/o-** *skin* **-ous** *pertaining to*

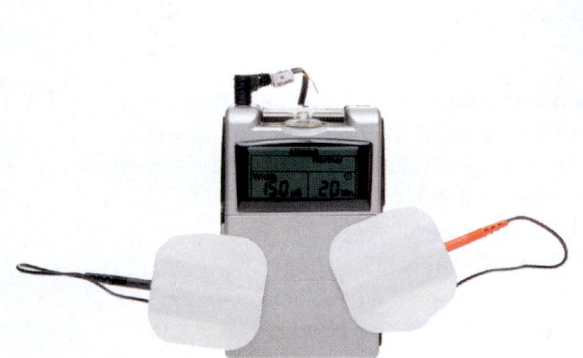

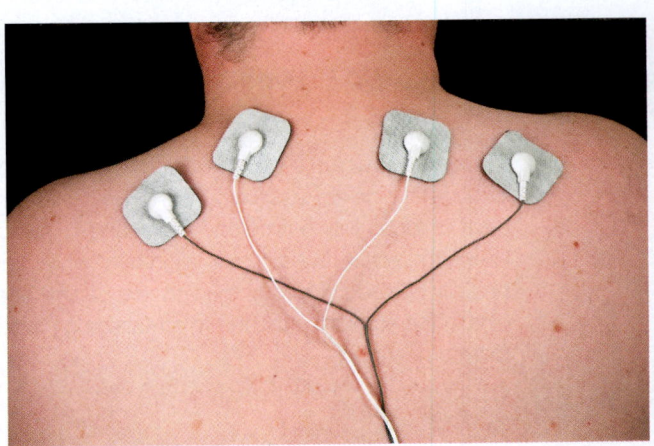

A.

B.

FIGURE 9-35 ■ Transcutaneous electrical nerve stimulation (TENS) unit.
A. A TENS unit consists of a battery pack and electrode patches. **B.** The patches are placed on the skin in the area of the pain. The TENS unit releases electrical impulses at regular, preset intervals.

Category	Indication	Pronunciation/Word Parts

Drugs

Category	Indication	Pronunciation/Word Parts
analgesic drug	Treats mild-to-moderate pain as an over-the-counter drug (aspirin, acetaminophen, and nonsteroidal anti-inflammatory drug). **Narcotic** drugs are used to treat severe, chronic pain.	**analgesic** (AN-al-JEE-zik) **an-** *not; without* **alges/o-** *sensation of pain* **-ic** *pertaining to* **narcotic** (nar-KAW-tik) **narc/o-** *sleep; stupor* **-tic** *pertaining to*
antiepileptic drug	Prevents the seizures of epilepsy. Also known as an **anticonvulsant drug**.	**antiepileptic** (AN-tee-EP-ih-LEP-tik) **anti-** *against* **epilept/o-** *seizure* **-ic** *pertaining to* **anticonvulsant** (AN-tee-con-VUL-sant) **anti-** *against* **convuls/o-** *seizure* **-ant** *pertaining to*
corticosteroid drug	Treats inflammation from chronic pain and multiple sclerosis. Also used to treat swelling and edema in the brain or spinal cord following traumatic injury or stroke.	**corticosteroid** (KOR-tih-koh-STAIR-oyd) **cortic/o-** *cortex; outer region* **-steroid** *steroid*
drug for Alzheimer disease	Inhibits an enzyme that breaks down acetylcholine	

Category	Indication	Pronunciation/Word Parts
drug for neuralgia and neuropathy	Works in various ways to treat the many different causes of neuralgia and neuropathy. These drugs include anticonvulsant drugs, antianxiety drugs, and antidepressant drugs.	
drug for Parkinson disease	Stimulates dopamine receptors or inhibits the action of acetylcholine to allow more dopamine to reach the brain	

Word or Phrase	Description	Pronunciation/Word Parts

Surgical Procedures

Word or Phrase	Description	Pronunciation/Word Parts
aneurysmectomy	Procedure to remove an aneurysm and repair the artery	**aneurysmectomy** (AN-yoor-iz-MEK-toh-mee) **aneurysm/o-** *aneurysm; dilation* **-ectomy** *surgical removal*
biopsy	Procedure to remove a tumor or mass from the brain or other part of the nervous system. In an **excisional biopsy**, the entire tumor or mass is removed and sent to a laboratory for microscopic examination to determine if it is benign or malignant. Even a benign brain tumor must be totally removed because it causes increasing intracranial pressure within the inflexible bony cranium or compresses nerves.	**biopsy** (BY-awp-see) **bi/o-** *living organism; living tissue* **-opsy** *process of viewing* **excisional** (ek-SIH-zhun-al) **ex-** *away from; out* **cis/o-** *cut* **-ion** *action; condition* **-al** *pertaining to*
carotid endarterectomy	Procedure to remove plaque from the carotid artery. This opens up the lumen of the artery, restores blood flow to the brain, and decreases the possibility of a stroke.	**endarterectomy** (END-ar-ter-EK-toh-mee) **endo-** *innermost; within* **arter/o-** *artery* **-ectomy** *surgical removal*
craniotomy	Incision into the cranium to expose the brain tissue. A craniotomy is the first phase of any type of brain surgery, such as removing a subdural hematoma or excising a brain tumor.	**craniotomy** (KRAY-nee-AW-toh-mee) **crani/o-** *cranium; top part of the skull* **-tomy** *process of cutting; process of making an incision*
diskectomy	Procedure to remove part or all of a herniated nucleus pulposus from an intervertebral disk. This relieves pressure on the adjacent dorsal nerve roots and relieves the pain.	**diskectomy** (dis-KEK-toh-mee) **disk/o-** *disk* **-ectomy** *surgical removal*
laminectomy	Procedure to remove the lamina (the flat area of the arch of the vertebra). Removal of this bony segment relieves pressure on the dorsal nerve roots and relieves pain from a herniated nucleus pulposus.	**laminectomy** (LAM-ih-NEK-toh-mee) **lamin/o-** *flat area on a vertebra* **-ectomy** *surgical removal*

Clinical Connections

Pain Management. This subspecialty for treating chronic or severe pain is shared by both neurology and anesthesiology. Pain management procedures include a dorsal nerve root injection into an area where a nerve is compressed. Surgical treatment includes a **rhizotomy**, an incision to cut the spinal nerve roots. The dorsal (sensory) nerve roots can be cut to relieve severe pain. The ventral (motor) nerve roots can be cut to relieve severe muscle spasticity and spasm.

rhizotomy (ry-ZAW-toh-mee)
rhiz/o- *spinal nerve root*
-tomy *process of cutting; process of making an incision*

Word or Phrase	Description	Pronunciation/Word Parts
stereotactic neurosurgery	Procedure to remove a tumor deep within the cerebrum. A CT or MRI scan is used to show the tumor in three dimensions and give its precise coordinates. The patient's head is fixed in a stereotactic apparatus that guides the position of a probe as it is inserted into the brain. Then heat, cold, or high-energy gamma rays are used to destroy the tumor.	**stereotactic** (STAIR-ee-oh-TAK-tik) **stere/o-** *three dimensions* **tact/o-** *touch* **-ic** *pertaining to* **neurosurgery** (NYOOR-oh-SER-jer-ee) **neur/o-** *nerve* **surg/o-** *operative procedure* **-ery** *process*
ventriculoperito-neal shunt	Procedure to insert a plastic tube to connect the ventricles of the brain to the peritoneal cavity. The shunt continuously removes excess cerebrospinal fluid associated with hydrocephalus.	**ventriculoperitoneal** (ven-TRIH-kyoo-loh-PAIR-ih-toh-NEE-al) **ventricul/o-** *chamber that is filled; ventricle* **peritone/o-** *peritoneum* **-al** *pertaining to*

9.5 PRACTICE LAPS

Use the Answer Key at the end of the book to check your answers.

A. Give the Meaning of Combining Forms

Next to each combining form, write its meaning. The first one has been done for you.

Combining Form	Meaning	Combining Form	Meaning
1. **cortic/o-**	*cortex; outer region*	14. ment/o-	
2. alges/o-		15. narc/o-	
3. aneurysm/o-		16. neur/o-	
4. arter/o-		17. peritone/o-	
5. bi/o-		18. propri/o-	
6. cis/o-		19. punct/o-	
7. cutane/o-		20. rhiz/o-	
8. disk/o-		21. stere/o-	
9. epilept/o-		22. surg/o-	
10. lamin/o-		23. tact/o-	
11. log/o-		24. tract/o-	
12. lumb/o-		25. ventricul/o-	
13. man/o-			

B. Build Words

Read the definition of the medical word. Look at the combining form that is given. Select the correct suffix from the Suffix List, and write it on the blank line. Then build the medical word, and write it on the line. (Remember: You may need to remove the combining vowel. Always remove the hyphens and slash.) Be sure to check your spelling.

Suffix List

-al (pertaining to)	-ion (action; condition)	-tomy (process of cutting; process of making an incision)
-ar (pertaining to)	-meter (instrument used to measure)	
-ectomy (surgical removal)	-opsy (process of viewing)	-ure (result of; system)

Definition of the Medical Word	Combining Form	Suffix	Build the Medical Word
Example: Result of (a) hole (or) perforation	**punct/o-**	*-ure*	*puncture*

[*You think result of (-ure) + hole; perforation (punct/o-). You change the order of the word parts to put the suffix last. You write puncture.*]

1. Process of cutting or making an incision (in the) spinal nerve root	rhiz/o-	_____	_____
2. Pertaining to (the) mind	ment/o-	_____	_____
3. Pertaining to (the) lower back	lumb/o-	_____	_____
4. Surgical removal (of the) flat area on a vertebra	lamin/o-	_____	_____
5. Process of viewing living tissue	bi/o-	_____	_____
6. Instrument used to measure (that is a) thin (tube)	man/o-	_____	_____
7. Action (of) pulling	tract/o-	_____	_____
8. Process of cutting or making an incision (in the) cranium	crani/o-	_____	_____
9. Surgical removal (of an) aneurysm	aneurysm/o-	_____	_____

C. Define Abbreviations

1. GCS _____

2. LP _____

3. MMSE _____

4. TENS _____

Abbreviations Summary

AFP	alpha fetoprotein		**LP**	lumbar puncture
ALS	amyotrophic lateral sclerosis		**MMSE**	Mini-Mental State Examination
AVM	arteriovenous malformation		**MRI**	magnetic resonance imaging
BAEP	brainstem auditory evoked potential		**MS**	multiple sclerosis
BAER	brainstem auditory evoked response		**NCD**	neurocognitive disorder
CAT, CT	computerized axial tomography		**NICU**	neurologic intensive care unit (pronounced "NIK-yoo")
CNS	central nervous system			
CP	cerebral palsy		**PET**	positron emission tomography
CRPS	complex regional pain syndrome		**REM**	rapid eye movement
CSF	cerebrospinal fluid		**RIND**	reversible ischemic neurologic deficit
CTS	carpal tunnel syndrome		**SCI**	spinal cord injury
CVA	cerebrovascular accident		**SSEP**	somatosensory evoked potential
DT	delirium tremens		**SSER**	somatosensory evoked response
EEG	electroencephalogram; electroencephalography		**TBI**	traumatic brain injury
GCS	Glasgow Coma Scale (or Score)		**TENS**	transcutaneous electrical nerve stimulation
HNP	herniated nucleus pulposus		**TIA**	transient ischemic attack
ICP	intracranial pressure		**VEP**	visual evoked potential
LOC	loss of consciousness		**VER**	visual evoked response

Word Alert

Abbreviations. Abbreviations are commonly used in all types of medical documents; however, they can mean different things to different people and their meanings can be misinterpreted. Always verify the meaning of an abbreviation.

- *CP* means *cerebral palsy*, but it also means *cardiopulmonary*.
- *CNS* means *central nervous system*, but it can be confused with the sound-alike abbreviation *C&S*, which means *culture and sensitivity*.
- *HNP* means *herniated nucleus pulposus*, but it can be confused with the sound-alike abbreviation *H&P*, which means *history and physical (examination)*.
- *NICU* means *neurologic intensive care unit*, but it also means *neonatal intensive care unit*.

It's Greek To Me! Did you notice that some words have two different combining forms? Combining forms from both Greek and Latin remain a part of medical language today.

Word	Greek	Latin	Medical Word Examples
mind	psych/o-	ment/o-	psychomotor; dementia
nerve	neur/o-	nerv/o-	neuron; nervous
seizure	epilept/o-	convuls/o-, ict/o-	epileptic; convulsion, postictal
feeling or sensation	esthes/o-, esthet/o-	sens/o-	paresthesia, anesthetic; sensory
spinal nerve root	rhiz/o-	radicul/o-	rhizotomy; radiculopathy

Career Focus

Meet Amelia, a pharmacy technician

"Here in the hospital pharmacy, I have the responsibility of making IVs and filling orders. I deliver med carts; I deliver patient meds. I do expiration dates—pulling all expired drugs off the shelf. I also get to work with wonderful pharmacists. Even though I initial all the drug orders that I fill, they cannot leave the pharmacy until the pharmacist has checked off on them. The best part of my job is meeting different people. I enjoy helping people and making someone's day a little better."

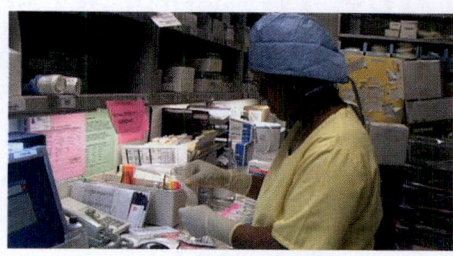

- **Pharmacy technicians** are allied health professionals who assist pharmacists in their work. Pharmacy technicians provide pharmacy services to home health, long-term care, outpatient facilities, and hospitals. They also work in retail pharmacies (drug stores).

- **Neurologists** are physicians who practice in the medical specialty of neurology. They diagnose and treat patients with diseases of the nervous system. Physicians can take additional training and become board certified in the subspecialty of pediatric neurology.

- **Neurosurgeons** perform surgery on the brain, spinal cord, and nerves. Malignancies of the nervous system are treated medically by an **oncologist** or surgically by a neurosurgeon.

---

pharmacy (FAR-mah-see)

---

technician (tek-NIH-shun)
  techn/o- *technical skill*
  -ician *skilled expert; skilled professional*

---

neurologist (nyoor-AW-loh-jist)
  neur/o- *nerve*
  log/o- *study of; word*
  -ist *person who specializes in; thing that specializes in*

---

neurosurgeon (NYOOR-oh-SER-jun)
  neur/o- *nerve*
  surg/o- *operative procedure*
  -eon *person who performs*

---

oncologist (ong-KAW-loh-jist)
  onc/o- *mass; tumor*
  log/o- *study of; word*
  -ist *person who specializes in; thing that specializes in*

Chapter Review Exercises

Dive In: Medical Language Exercises

Test your knowledge of the chapter by completing these review exercises. Use the Answer Key at the end of the book to check your answers. Note: Each of the numbered exercise headers corresponds to a numbered learning outcome at the beginning of the chapter.

9.1 Anatomy

MATCHING EXERCISE

Match each word or phrase to its location or description.

1. cauda equina	_____ hormone that prepares the body for "fight or flight"
2. corpus callosum	_____ four hollow areas within the cerebrum that contain CSF
3. cranial nerves	_____ between the pons and the spinal cord
4. cranium	_____ cells that make myelin around the larger axons of cranial nerves and spinal nerves
5. dermatome	_____ rapid, involuntary muscle reaction controlled by the spinal cord
6. frontal	_____ largest of the cerebral lobes
7. epinephrine	_____ there are 12 pairs of them
8. gustatory cortex	_____ group of nerve roots at the inferior end of the spinal cord
9. medulla oblongata	_____ perform specialized tasks that assist neurons in their work
10. neuroglia	_____ area in the meninges that contains cerebrospinal fluid
11. olfactory cranial nerve	_____ area of the frontal lobe that receives sensory impulses from the taste receptors
12. reflex	_____ area of the skin that supplies sensory information to a specific spinal nerve
13. Schwann	_____ dome-shaped bone at the top of the skull
14. subarachnoid space	_____ band of nerve fibers that connects the two hemispheres of the cerebrum
15. ventricles	_____ sense of smell

CIRCLE EXERCISE

Circle the correct word from the choices given.

1. The (**cerebellum, cerebrum, ventricle**) is divided into two hemispheres.

2. The olfactory cortex receives sensory impulses from the (**ears, eyes, nose**).

3. The most delicate of the meninges and the one that is closest to the brain is the (**arachnoid, dura mater, pia mater**).

4. The functional unit of the nervous system is the (**nerve, neuron, neurotransmitter**).

5. In the majority of people, the (**cerebellum, gyrus, left hemisphere of the cerebrum**) performs math, analysis, and logical thinking.

6. The hypothalamus is located (**above, below, beside**) the thalamus.

7. The (**auditory, oculomotor, trigeminal**) cranial nerve controls eye movements.

8. Which of the following is *not* a structure in the cerebrum? (**dorsal nerve roots, parietal lobe, sulci**)

9. Cerebrospinal fluid is produced by (**astrocytes, ependymal cells, ventricles**).

10. Sensory information consists of all of the following *except* (**motor commands, pain, sensations**).

11. (**Axons, Cerebrospinal fluid, Microglia**) are cells that engulf and destroy dead tissue and pathogens.

12. The part of the nervous system that is active in the "fight-or-flight" response is the (**central nervous system, limbic system, sympathetic division**).

TRUE OR FALSE EXERCISE

*Indicate whether each statement is true or false by writing **T** or **F** on the line.*

1. _____ The cerebral cortex is made up of gray matter.
2. _____ The arachnoid is the outermost membrane of the meninges.
3. _____ The amygdaloid body causes short-term memories to become long-term memories.
4. _____ The brainstem is composed of the midbrain, pons, and medulla oblongata.
5. _____ The epidural space around the spinal cord is filled with fatty tissue.
6. _____ Gyri are elevated folds on the surface of the cerebrum.
7. _____ The autonomic nervous system is composed of the central nervous system and the peripheral nervous system.
8. _____ Efferent nerves carry nerve impulses from the spinal cord to the body.
9. _____ The occipital lobe of the cerebellum is next to the occipital bone of the cranium.
10. _____ The peripheral nervous system consists of the cranial nerves and spinal nerves.
11. _____ The hypothalamus functions as part of the nervous system and endocrine system.
12. _____ Cranial nerve X (vagus nerve) is the only cranial nerve that goes into the thoracic and abdominal cavities.

PLURAL NOUN AND ADJECTIVE EXERCISE

Read the noun and write its plural form and/or adjective form on the line. Only write in the plural noun form if there is a blank line there for it. Be sure to check your spelling. The first one has been done for you.

Singular Noun	Plural Noun	Adjective	Singular Noun	Plural Noun	Adjective
1. **nerve**	*nerves*	*neural*	6. meninges		_____
2. cerebrum		_____	7. spine		_____
3. cerebellum		_____	8. sulcus	_____	
4. cranium		_____	9. thalamus		_____
5. gyrus	_____		10. ventricle	_____	_____

DIVIDING WORDS EXERCISE

Separate these words into their component parts (prefix, combining form, suffix). Some words do not contain all three word parts. The first one has been done for you.

Medical Word	Prefix	Combining Form	Suffix	Medical Word	Prefix	Combining Form	Suffix
1. **nervous**		*nerv/o-*	*-ous*	7. hypothalamic	_____	_____	_____
2. amygdaloid		_____	_____	8. meningeal		_____	_____
3. arachnoid		_____	_____	9. neuroglia		_____	_____
4. cranial		_____	_____	10. olfactory		_____	_____
5. epidural	_____	_____	_____	11. parietal		_____	_____
6. gustatory		_____	_____	12. sensory		_____	_____

SPELLING EXERCISE

Read each medical word pronunciation and write the medical word that it represents. Be sure to check your spelling. The first one has been done for you.

1. **(seh-REE-brum)** _____*cerebrum*_____
2. (soh-MAH-toh-SEN-soh-ree) _____
3. (awk-SIP-ih-tal) _____
4. (HEM-ih-sfeer) _____
5. (SUB-ah-RAK-noyd) _____
6. (seh-REE-broh-SPY-nal) _____

9.2 Physiology

MATCHING EXERCISE

Match each word to its description.

1. axon   _____ directs cellular activities of a neuron
2. cytoplasm   _____ contains structures that produce neurotransmitters
3. neurotransmitter   _____ part of the neuron that may be myelinated
4. nucleus   _____ space between two neurons
5. synapse   _____ chemical messenger between neurons

CIRCLE EXERCISE

Circle the correct answer from the choices given.

1. The neurotransmitter that goes between a motor neuron and a voluntary skeletal muscle is (**acetylcholine, dopamine, endorphins**).
2. A/An (**axon, dendrite, neuron**) is the functional unit of the nervous system.
3. All of the following are true about myelin *except* (**it is a fatty, white insulating layer; it increases the speed of electrical impulses; it provides structural support for neurons**).

TRUE OR FALSE EXERCISE

*Indicate whether each statement is true or false by writing **T** or **F** on the line.*

1. _____ After a nerve impulse passes through the cell body of a neuron, it then goes to the dendrites.
2. _____ Endorphins are the body's own natural pain relievers.
3. _____ Oligodendroglia produce the myelin that surrounds the axons of larger neurons in the brain and spinal cord.
4. _____ The axon of one neuron connects directly to the dendrites of the next neuron.
5. _____ A neurotransmitter binds to a receptor on a dendrite.

DIVIDING WORDS EXERCISE

Separate these words into their component parts (combining form, suffix). The first one has been done for you.

Medical Word	Combining Form	Suffix
1. **neuron**	*neur/o-*	*-on*
2. dendrite		
3. cytoplasm		
4. receptor		
5. myelinated		

SPELLING EXERCISE

Read each medical word pronunciation and write the medical word that it represents. Be sure to check your spelling. The first one has been done for you.

1. **(NYOOR-on)**   *neuron*
2. (SY-toh-plazm)   _____
3. (NYOOR-oh-TRANS-mih-ter)   _____

9.3 Diseases

MATCHING EXERCISE

Match each word or phrase to its description.

1. amnesia	_____ Down syndrome
2. aphasia	_____ temporary loss of consciousness with fainting
3. concussion	_____ continuous seizure activity
4. hydrocephalus	_____ involuntary falling asleep during the day
5. intellectual disability	_____ inability to communicate verbally
6. multiple sclerosis	_____ stiff neck associated with meningitis
7. narcolepsy	_____ radiculopathy in the lumbar area
8. nuchal rigidity	_____ head trauma with loss of consciousness
9. sciatica	_____ symptoms caused by progressive demyelination
10. status epilepticus	_____ partial or total loss of memory
11. syncope	_____ enlarged head in infants and children because of excess CSF

TRUE OR FALSE EXERCISE

*Indicate whether each statement is true or false by writing **T** or **F** on the line.*

1. _____ Causalgia is a severe, burning type of neuralgia along a nerve and its branches.

2. _____ A neural tube defect can result in multiple sclerosis.

3. _____ A hematoma is a type of brain tumor.

4. _____ The most common neurocognitive disorder is Alzheimer disease.

5. _____ Photophobia and throbbing pain are symptoms of a migraine headache.

6. _____ A TIA and a RIND are types of cerebrovascular accidents.

7. _____ Mad cow disease can be transmitted to humans as new variant Creutzfeldt-Jakob disease.

8. _____ The incidence of myelomeningocele can be greatly decreased if the mother takes a folic acid supplement while she is pregnant.

CIRCLE EXERCISE

Circle the correct word from the choices given.

1. (**Amnesia, Myelomeningocele, Shingles**) is a painful skin condition caused by herpes zoster infection of a nerve.

2. Prior to the onset of a seizure, a patient may experience a/an (**aura, coma, polyneuritis**).

3. (**Dyslexia, Status epilepticus, Subdural hematoma**) is caused by trauma to the head.

4. An imbalance of dopamine and acetylcholine in the brain is associated with (**Down syndrome, multiple sclerosis, Parkinson disease**).

5. Abnormal burning or tingling sensations on the skin are (**neuritis, paralysis, paresthesias**).

6. Which of the following is *not* a congenital disorder? (**cerebral palsy, hemiplegia, myelomeningocele**)

7. Neurocognitive disorder includes all of the following *except* (**Alzheimer disease, delirium tremens, traumatic brain injury**).

DIVIDING WORDS EXERCISE

Separate these words into their component parts (prefix, combining form, suffix). Some words do not contain all three word parts. The first one has been done for you.

Medical Word	Prefix	Combining Form	Suffix	Medical Word	Prefix	Combining Form	Suffix
1. **malformation**	*mal-*	*format/o-*	*-ion*	9. intracranial	___	___	___
2. amnesia		___	___	10. malignant		___	___
3. anesthesia	___	___	___	11. meningocele		___	___
4. comatose		___	___	12. postictal	___	___	___
5. dysphagia	___	___	___	13. radiculopathy		___	___
6. dyslexic	___	___	___	14. paraplegia	___	___	___
7. hemiplegic	___	___	___	15. trigeminal	___	___	___
8. infarction		___	___				

SPELLING EXERCISE

Read each medical word pronunciation and write the medical word that it represents. Be sure to check your spelling. The first one has been done for you.

1. **(is-KEE-mee-ah)** _____*ischemia*_____
2. (am-NEE-zha) _____
3. (SEF-al-AL-jah) _____
4. (AWLZ-hy-mer) _____

5. (dis-LEK-see-ah) _____
6. (EP-ih-LEP-see) _____
7. (SPY-nah BIF-ih-dah) _____
8. (KWAH-drih-PLEE-jah) _____

9.4 Laboratory, Diagnostic, and Radiologic Procedures

MATCHING EXERCISE

Match each word, abbreviation, or phrase to its description.

1. alpha fetoprotein
2. EEG
3. myelography
4. PET scan
5. polysomnography
6. cerebral angiography

_____ used to diagnose the type of epilepsy
_____ visualizes blood flow to the brain
_____ shows patterns of metabolism in the brain
_____ indicates the presence of a neural tube defect in a fetus
_____ uses dye to outline the spinal cord and nerves
_____ sleep study

TRUE OR FALSE EXERCISE

*Indicate whether each statement is true or false by writing **T** or **F** on the line.*

1. _____ An electroencephalography records brain-wave patterns.
2. _____ A skull x-ray can show a fractured skull as well as blood flow to the brain.
3. _____ Cerebrospinal fluid is normally clear and colorless.
4. _____ A carotid duplex scan uses Doppler ultrasonography to create an image.
5. _____ A PET scan is a nuclear medicine procedure that uses a gamma camera.
6. _____ There are six types of brain-wave patterns.
7. _____ A nerve conduction study measures the speed of an electrical impulse traveling along a nerve.

CIRCLE EXERCISE

Circle the correct answer from the choices given.

1. All of these procedures take images in thin slices *except* (**carotid duplex scan, computerized axial tomography, magnetic resonance imaging**).
2. Electroencephalography uses (**electrodes, ultrasonic waves, x-rays**).
3. All of these procedures use contrast dye *except* (**cerebral angiography, myelography, positron emission tomography**).
4. Which of the following is a type of evoked potential testing? (**AFP, MRI, VER**)

9.5 Medical Procedures, Drugs, and Surgical Procedures

MATCHING EXERCISE

Match each word or phrase to its description.

1. vision test
2. hearing test
3. Babinski sign
4. oriented x3
5. lumbar puncture
6. Mini-Mental State Examination
7. gait
8. pinprick
9. Romberg test
10. corticosteroid drug
11. rhizotomy

_____ tests patient's balance with the eyes closed

_____ passing this test shows normal function of cranial nerve II (optic nerve)

_____ patient's manner of walking

_____ passing this test shows normal function of cranial nerve VIII (vestibulocochlear nerve)

_____ surgical procedure to cut spinal nerve roots

_____ abnormal upward extension of big toe and fanning out of other toes

_____ patient can state his or her name, date, and location

_____ test to detect numbness on the skin

_____ proverbs, counting backward, recall of objects, names of presidents

_____ spinal tap

_____ used to treat edema of the brain or spinal cord

TRUE OR FALSE EXERCISE

*Indicate whether each statement is true or false by writing **T** or **F** on the line.*

1. _____ Antiepileptic drugs are also known as *anticonvulsant drugs*.
2. _____ A patient with a partially healed vertebral fracture can be fitted for a halo vest to provide spinal traction.
3. _____ A laminectomy is a surgical procedure to remove myelin from a neuron.
4. _____ A TENS unit is used during a sleep study.
5. _____ Testing a patient's proprioception is testing an awareness of body position.

CIRCLE EXERCISE

Circle the correct word from the choices given.

1. All of the following are coordination tests *except* (**diskectomy, heel-to-shin test, rapid alternating movements**).
2. Drugs for Alzheimer disease inhibit an enzyme that breaks down (**acetylcholine, cerebrospinal fluid, red blood cells**).
3. A (**manometer, Mini-Mental State Examination, station test**) is used to measure the pressure of cerebrospinal fluid.
4. A (**biopsy, carotid endarterectomy, ventriculoperitoneal shunt**) is used to remove plaque from an artery to the brain.
5. A (**craniotomy, diskectomy, laminectomy**) is the first phase of surgery to remove a brain tumor.

DIVIDING WORDS EXERCISE

Separate these words into their component parts (prefix, combining form, suffix). Some words do not contain all three word parts. The first one has been done for you.

Medical Word	Prefix	Combining Form	Suffix	Medical Word	Prefix	Combining Form	Suffix
1. **corticosteroid**		*cortic/o-*	*-steroid*	6. craniotomy			
2. analgesic				7. endarterectomy			
3. aneurysmectomy				8. manometer			
4. antiepileptic				9. transcutaneous			
5. biopsy							

SPELLING EXERCISE

Read each medical word pronunciation and write the medical word that it represents. Be sure to check your spelling. The first one has been done for you.

1. (bah-BIN-skee) _____ *Babinski* _____
2. (TRANS-kyoo-TAY-nee-uhs) _____
3. (AN-tee-con-VUL-sant) _____
4. (AN-yoor-iz-MEK-toh-mee) _____
5. (KRAY-nee-AW-toh-mee) _____
6. (NYOOR-oh-SER-jer-ee) _____

RELATED COMBINING FORMS EXERCISE

Write the combining forms on the lines provided. (Hint: See the It's Greek to Me! feature box.)

1. Two combining forms that mean *mind*. _____ _____
2. Two combining forms that mean *nerve*. _____ _____
3. Two combining forms that mean *spinal nerve root*. _____ _____
4. Three combining forms that mean *sensation*. _____ _____ _____
5. Three combining forms that mean *seizure*. _____ _____ _____

PROOFREADING AND SPELLING EXERCISE

Read the following paragraph. Identify each misspelled medical word and write the correct spelling of it on the line provided.

A patient might need nurosurgery because of a subdural hematomma or a tumor such as a menengioma. A cerebrohvascular accident is a stroke or brain attack and is from an infarkt. An ordinary headache is cephalalga, while having half of the body paralysed from a stroke is called hemeplegia. A seizure or a convulsion is known as epilepsee. Inflammation of many individual nerves is polyneuritus. The study of the brain, spinal cord, and nerves is neurology.

1. _____
2. _____
3. _____
4. _____
5. _____
6. _____
7. _____
8. _____
9. _____
10. _____

Immerse Yourself: Analyze Medical Reports

Electronic Patient Record #1

This is an office visit in the format of a SOAP note. Read the note and answer the questions.

PEARSON PEDIATRIC ASSOCIATES

Task Edit View Time Scale Options Help

OFFICE VISIT SOAP NOTE

PATIENT NAME:	JOHNSON, Clarissa
HEALTH RECORD NUMBER:	10-35-67
DATE OF VISIT:	11/19/20xx

SUBJECTIVE: This is a follow-up visit for this 10-year-old female who recently presented with an initial seizure that happened during school hours. The patient was reported to have vacant staring, was unresponsive to the teacher's voice, and had facial tics. She was sent for a neurologic consult. An EEG showed that she had absence seizures.

OBJECTIVE: Today, the patient is alert and oriented x3. Her vital signs are all within normal limits. Her mother reports that she has not had any convulsions since beginning her antiseizure medication.

ASSESSMENT: Epilepsy, characterized by absence seizures, controlled on medication.

PLAN: Continue taking her anticonvulsant medication at the dose prescribed by the neurologist. Call this office in the event of any seizure activity.

1. What is the name of the overall disease category for absence seizures?

2. During this type of seizure, would you expect that the patient would have fallen down at school?

3. What does the abbreviation *EEG* stand for and how is one performed?

4. What does the phrase *oriented x3* mean?

Electronic Patient Record #2

This is a neurologic consultation. Read the report and answer the questions.

CONSULTATION REPORT

Task   Edit   View   Time Scale   Options   Help   ✉ ⤺ ⓘ

📂 📄 📑 📋 ↰ ⧖ ⌨ ▢ ↙ √ 📁

PATIENT NAME:	JENCKS, Justine
PATIENT NUMBER:	12798
DATE OF CONSULTATION:	November 19, 20xx

PEARSON NEUROLOGIC ASSOCIATES

Centennial Medical Building, Suite 312

5005 Frankstown Road

Pittsburgh, PA 15237

November 19, 20xx
Marshall Gibbons, M.D.
Primary Care Associates
19 Walker Avenue
Middletown, PA 15222

Re: JENCKS, Justine

Dear Dr. Gibbons:

I saw your patient, Justine Jencks, in neurologic consultation on November 19, 20xx. She is a 38-year-old, right-handed female who has complained of intermittent dizziness and other symptoms for the past year. She reports temporary dizziness with hyperextension of the neck when raising her hands above her head to reach a high shelf or hang drapes. Two months ago, the patient had an acute episode in which she awoke with a sense of doom, headache, profuse perspiration, nausea, paresthesias of the fingers, dizziness, tachycardia, and felt the room was spinning. On the way to the emergency room, her husband commented about their dogs, but she could only remember her older dog and had no recollection of having another dog. In the emergency room, she said to the nurse that she felt like her "blood pressure was zero." When asked about her last menstrual period, she felt that she might be pregnant but could not explain why she felt this way. On the Mini-Mental State Examination, she could not name the current and most recent presidents but was otherwise oriented x3. She was able to count backward by serial 7s. The physical examination in the emergency room was essentially negative. Her blood pressure and blood sugar results were normal.

The patient has a past history that is significant for possible MS. This was tentatively diagnosed 10 years ago. At that time, laboratory test results were inconclusive: visual evoked responses were abnormal, but the CSF showed no oligoclonal bands, and an MRI scan of the brain was read as negative. At that time, her symptoms included extreme muscle weakness. She could only walk a short distance by using a wide-based gait for stability. This initial episode lasted 2 months and then the symptoms gradually resolved.

She does not routinely have headaches. She denies ever having had seizures. She denies any smell or taste disturbances. She denies difficulty swallowing. She has no speech difficulties and is able to relate her medical history easily.

Examination of cranial nerves V through XII was normal. Examination of the motor system revealed normal muscle strength. Babinski was negative. Sensory examination to light touch, pinprick, vibration, position, and 2-point discrimination was normal. Cerebellar functions in the form of finger-to-nose and heel-to-shin tests were normal. Gait was normal. Romberg sign was negative. There was marked muscle spasm of the trapezius muscles bilaterally and limitation of neck motion laterally to the right and rotationally to the left.

Several of the patient's complaints could be due to a vestibular migraine, but the episode with the 2-hour alteration in memory is problematic and may suggest a TIA. She has some typical migraine symptoms, but the dizziness points to a vestibular focus to the migraine. Because of the past history of possible MS, I will have her undergo an MRI scan with contrast to pinpoint any demyelination that has occurred since her last MRI. I have also ordered a carotid arteriography to rule out blockage of the carotid arteries.

After these tests are obtained, I will follow up with her in about 3 weeks to review the test results.

Thank you for referring this interesting and delightful patient to me.

Sincerely yours,

Adam R. Kimball, M.D.
_____
Adam R. Kimball, M.D.

ARK: smt
D: 11/19/xx
T: 11/19/xx

---

1. Divide *neurologic* into its three word parts and give the meaning of each word part.

   Word Part   **Meaning**

   _____   _____

   _____   _____

   _____   _____

2. Divide *paresthesia* into its three word parts and give the meaning of each word part.

   Word Part   **Meaning**

   _____   _____

   _____   _____

   _____   _____

3. What is the abbreviation for *visual evoked response*? _____

4. Divide *arteriography* into its two word parts and give the meaning of each word part.

   Word Part   **Meaning**

   _____   _____

   _____   _____

5. Two months ago, what symptom did the patient experience in her fingers? _____

6. Define these neurologic abbreviations.

   MS _____

   TIA _____

   CSF _____

7. The sensory examination consisted of five separate tests. Name them.

    a. _____

    b. _____

    c. _____

    d. _____

    e. _____

8. The Mini-Mental State Examination done 2 months ago in the emergency room mentions what three mental status tests?

    a. _____

    b. _____

    c. _____

9. Which test showed that the patient's balance was intact? (**Babinski, Romberg, serial 7s**)

10. Which of the patient's symptoms is directly related to the nervous system? (**nausea, paresthesias, tachycardia**)

11. The carotid arteriography will be done to look for evidence of what disease? (**blockage of the artery, demyelination, muscle weakness**)

12. If present, oligoclonal bands are found in what body fluid? _____

13. When the patient could remember the name of her older dog but not the name of her newest dog, this would be described as which of the following? Circle the correct answer.

    Impairment of both remote and recent memory

    Impairment of remote memory; recent memory intact

    Remote memory intact; impairment of recent memory

14. A specimen of the patient's CSF was tested in the laboratory. What medical procedure was done to obtain that specimen?

    _____

15. The finger-to-nose and heel-to-shin tests for cerebellar function were related to: (**coordination, eyesight, memory**).

16. If the carotid arteriography showed a blockage of those arteries, this would relate to which of the patient's symptoms? (**alteration in memory, multiple sclerosis, wide-based gait**)

17. If the MRI with contrast does show areas of demyelination, what diagnosis would that confirm?

    _____

MyLab Medical Terminology™

MyLab Medical Terminology is a premium online homework management system that includes a host of features to help you study. Registered users will find:

- A multitude of quizzes and activities built within the MyLab platform

- Powerful tools that track and analyze your results—allowing you to create a personalized learning experience

- Videos and audio pronunciations to help enrich your progress

- Streaming lesson presentations (guided lectures) and self-paced learning modules

- A space where you and your instructor can check your progress and manage your assignments

10 Urology
Urinary System

Urology (yoor-AW-loh-jee) is the medical specialty that studies the anatomy and physiology of the urinary system; uses laboratory, diagnostic, and radiologic procedures to diagnose urinary diseases; and uses medical procedures, drugs, and surgical procedures to treat urinary diseases.

⋁ Chapter Overview and Learning Outcomes

After you study this chapter, you should be able to demonstrate mastery of the outcomes by successfully completing the exercises.

10.1 Anatomy
Identify the structures of the urinary system.
Demonstrate proficiency in medical language.
10.1 Practice Laps

10.2 Physiology
Describe the functions of the urinary system.
Demonstrate proficiency in medical language.
10.2 Practice Laps
Vocabulary Review

10.3 Diseases
Describe common urinary diseases.
Demonstrate proficiency in medical language.
10.3 Practice Laps

10.4 Laboratory, Diagnostic, and Radiologic Procedures
Describe common urinary laboratory tests, diagnostic procedures, and radiologic procedures.
Demonstrate proficiency in medical language.
10.4 Practice Laps

10.5 Medical Procedures, Drugs, and Surgical Procedures
Describe common urinary medical procedures, drugs, and surgical procedures.
Demonstrate proficiency in medical language.
10.5 Practice Laps
Abbreviations Summary
Career Focus

Chapter Review Exercises
Dive In: Medical Language Exercises
(Learning Outcomes 10.1–10.5)
Immerse Yourself: Analyze Medical Reports

Medical Language Key

To unlock the definition of a medical word, first break it into word parts. Then give the meaning of each word part. Put the meanings of the word parts in order, beginning with the meaning of the suffix, then the meaning of the prefix (if there is one), then the meaning of the combining form.

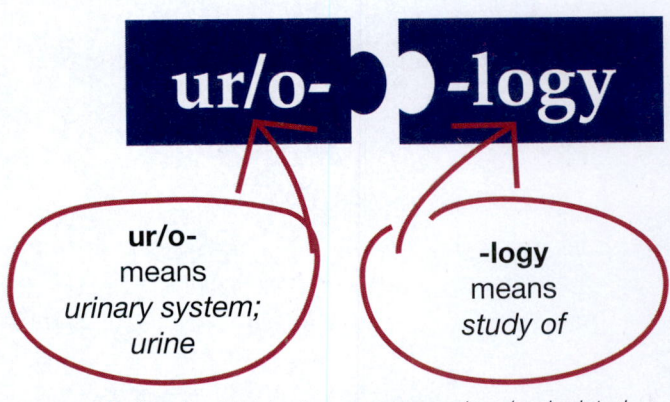

ur/o-
means
urinary system; urine

-logy
means
study of

Urology: ▶ *Study of (the) urinary system, urine, (and related structures).*

The **urinary system** consists of a pathway that begins with the kidneys and ends with the urethra (see Figure 10-1 ■). The urinary system is also known as the **urinary tract**, as a tract is a pathway. It is also known as the **genitourinary (GU) system** or **urogenital system** because the genital system and the urinary system are located near each other and in males share some of the same structures and functions (described in Chapter 11, Male Reproductive Medicine). The urinary system consists of two main structures—the kidneys and the bladder—and the connecting tubes of the ureters and urethra.

The functions of the urinary system are to remove the waste products of cellular metabolism from the blood by producing, transporting, storing, and excreting urine. Because of this last function, it is also known as the **excretory system**. In addition, the urinary system complements the work of the cardiovascular system by helping to maintain the blood pressure and the composition of the blood (pH and the number of red blood cells).

10.1 Anatomy

Kidneys

The **kidneys** are located in the **retroperitoneal space**, a small area behind the peritoneum, the membrane that lines the abdominal cavity. Each kidney sits in a cushion of fatty tissue. The kidney is reddish-brown in color and shaped like (of all things!) a kidney bean. Each kidney measures 4 inches long and 2 inches wide and weighs less than ½ pound (see Figure 10-2 ■). The kidney is positioned at the lower edge of the rib cage in the **flank** area of the back (between the ribs and the hip bone). The **hilum** is an indentation in the medial surface of the kidney where the renal artery enters and the renal vein and ureter exit.

A protective fibrous capsule surrounds each kidney. Just beneath that is the **cortex** tissue layer (see Figure 10-3 ■). Beneath the cortex is the layer of the **medulla**. Each tip of its tissue connects to a **minor calyx**, an area that collects urine. Several minor calices drain into a larger **major calyx**. Major calices drain into the **renal pelvis**, a large, funnel-shaped area that narrows to become the ureter. Urine flows continuously through the minor calices, major calices, renal pelvis, and into the ureter.

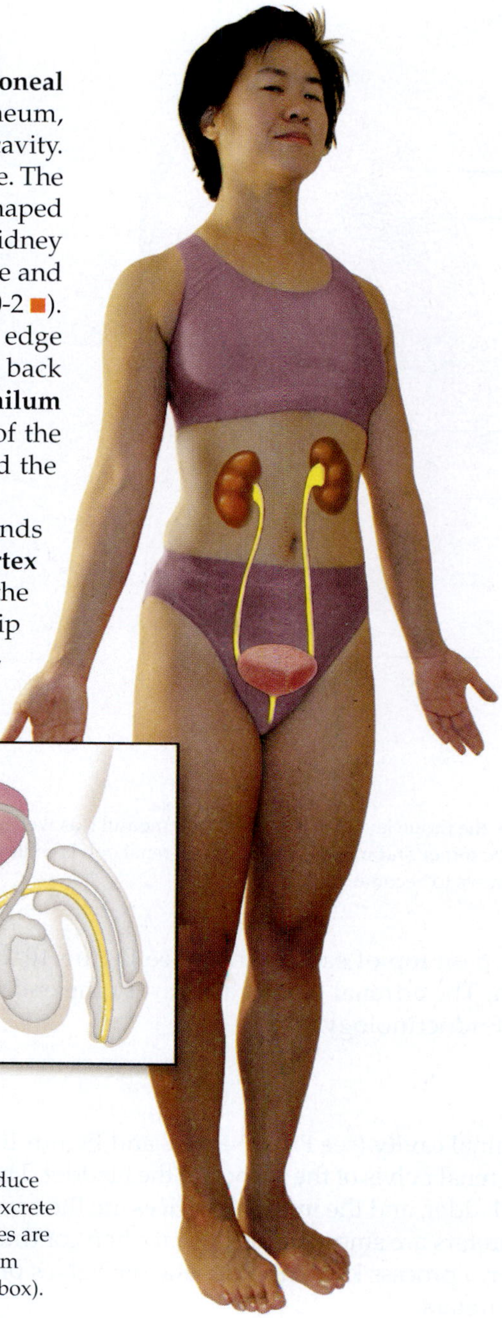

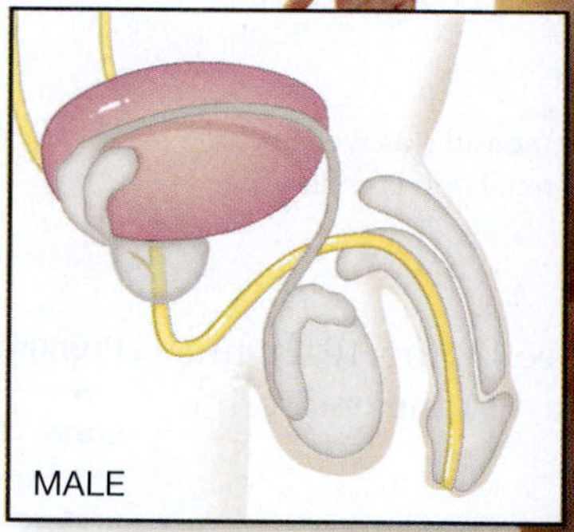

MALE

FIGURE 10-1 ■ **Urinary system.**
The urinary system consists of the kidneys that produce urine, and other structures that transport, store, or excrete urine. In a female, all of the urinary system structures are located within the body. In a male, the urinary system continues outside the body into the penis (see inset box).

Pronunciation/Word Parts

urinary (YOOR-ih-NAIR-ee)
  urin/o- *urinary system; urine*
  -ary *pertaining to*

genitourinary (JEN-ih-toh-YOOR-ih-NAIR-ee)
  genit/o- *genitalia*
  urin/o- *urinary system; urine*
  -ary *pertaining to*

urogenital (YOOR-oh-JEN-ih-tal)
  ur/o- *urinary system; urine*
  genit/o- *genitalia*
  -al *pertaining to*

excretory (EKS-kreh-TOR-ee)
  excret/o- *removing from the body*
  -ory *having the function of*

kidney (KID-nee)

retroperitoneal
(REH-troh-PAIR-ih-toh-NEE-al)
  retro- *backward; behind*
  peritone/o- *peritoneum*
  -al *pertaining to*

flank (FLANK)

hilum (HY-lum)

hilar (HY-lar)
  hil/o- *indentation*
  -ar *pertaining to*

cortex (KOR-teks)

cortical (KOR-tih-kal)
  cortic/o- *cortex; outer region*
  -al *pertaining to*

medulla (meh-DUL-ah)

calyx (KAY-liks)

calices (KAL-ih-seez)
Latin plural noun: Change the singular ending *-yx* to *-ices.*

caliceal (KAL-ih-SEE-al)
  calic/o- *calyx*
  -eal *pertaining to*
The combining form **cali/o-** also means *calyx.*

renal (REE-nal)
  ren/o- *kidney*
  -al *pertaining to*
Renal is the adjective for *kidney.*
The combining form **nephr/o-** means *kidney; nephron.*

pelvis (PEL-vihs)

pelves (PEL-veez)
Latin plural noun: Change the singular ending *-is* to *-es.*

pelvic (PEL-vik)
  pelv/o- *hip bone; pelvis; renal pelvis*
  -ic *pertaining to*
The combining form **pyel/o-** means *renal pelvis.*

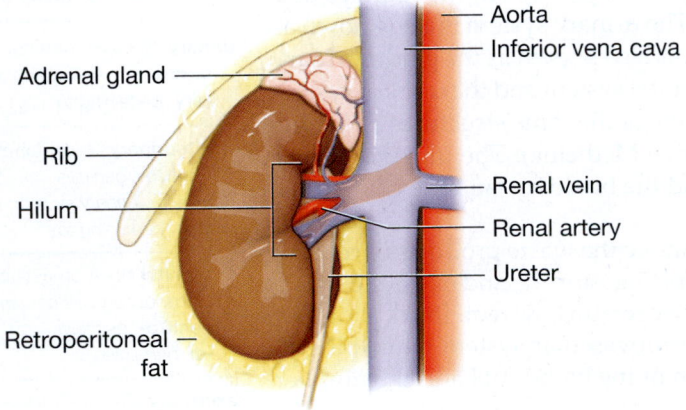

FIGURE 10-2 ■ Kidney.
The kidney is shaped and colored like a kidney bean. The adrenal gland of the endocrine system sits on top of the kidney but is not part of the urinary system. Notice the hilum of the kidney where the renal artery enters and the renal veins and ureter exit.

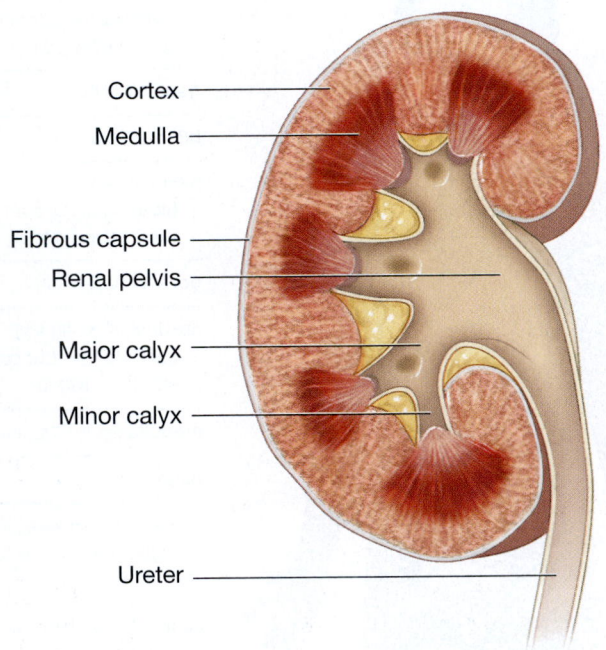

FIGURE 10-3 ■ Cut section of a kidney.
The internal structures of the kidney include the tissue layers of the cortex and medulla, as well as the open areas of the calices and renal pelvis. The minor and major calices and the renal pelvis collect the urine as it is produced. The renal pelvis narrows to become the ureter.

An adrenal gland sits like a cap on top of each kidney (see Figure 10-2), but it is not part of the urinary system. The adrenal glands are part of the endocrine system (described in Chapter 13, Endocrinology).

Ureters

Each **ureter** is located in the abdominal cavity (see Figure 10-4 ■ and Figure 10-5 ■). It is a 12-inch tube that connects the renal pelvis of the kidney to the bladder. The ureters enter the posterior side of the bladder, and the **ureteral orifices** are the openings into the bladder. The walls of the ureters are smooth muscle that often contract and relax to move urine into the bladder, a process known as **peristalsis**. Valves prevent urine from going back up into the ureters.

Pronunciation/Word Parts

ureter (YOOR-eh-ter)

ureteral (yoor-EE-ter-al)
   ureter/o- *ureter*
   -al *pertaining to*

orifice (OR-ih-fihs)

peristalsis (PAIR-ih-STAL-sihs)
The prefix **peri-** means *around*. The suffix **-stalsis** means *process of contraction*.

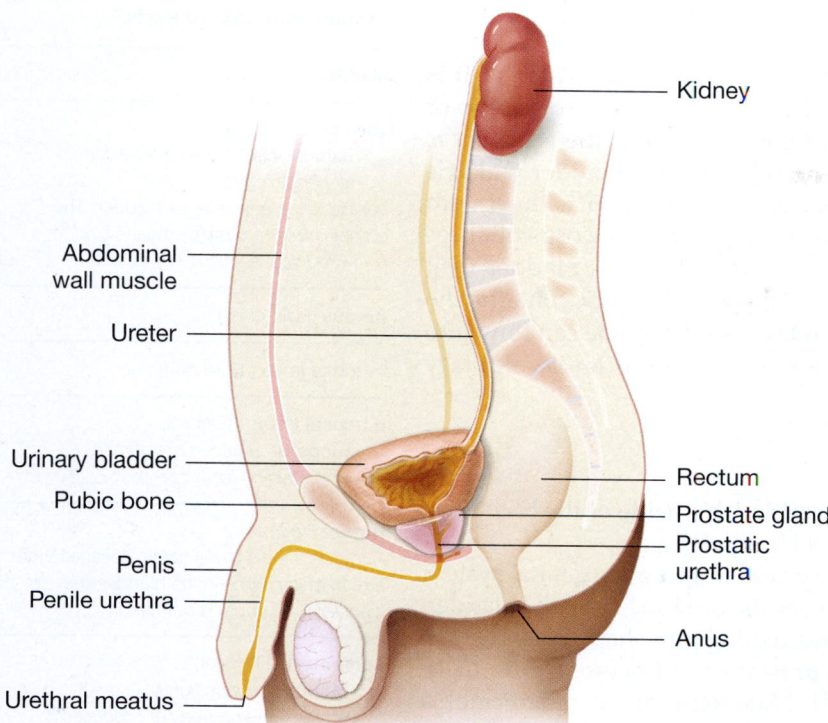

Kidney

Abdominal wall muscle

Ureter

Urinary bladder

Pubic bone

Penis

Penile urethra

Urethral meatus

Rectum

Prostate gland

Prostatic urethra

Anus

FIGURE 10-4 ■ Male urinary system.
The male urethra is long and travels through the prostate gland and along the length of the penis before reaching the outside of the body.

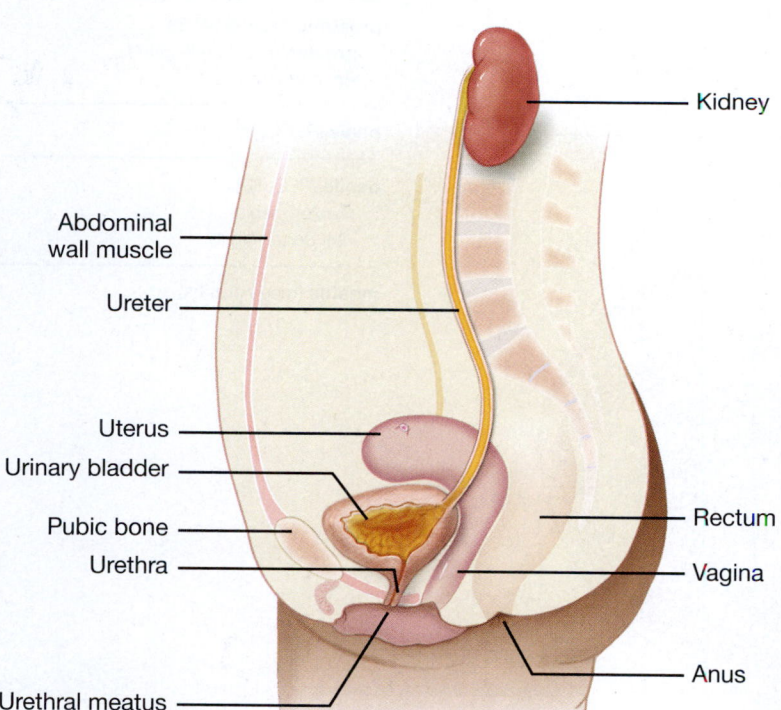

Kidney

Abdominal wall muscle

Ureter

Uterus

Urinary bladder

Pubic bone

Urethra

Urethral meatus

Rectum

Vagina

Anus

FIGURE 10-5 ■ Female urinary system.
The female urethra is short and straight. Notice how the bladder is beneath the uterus. During pregnancy, the bladder is often compressed by the expanding uterus and growing fetus.

Bladder

The **bladder** is an expandable reservoir for holding urine (see Figure 10-6 ■). It is located in the pelvic cavity, where it is held in place by ligaments. The round top of the bladder is the dome or **fundus**. The fundus of any structure is the area that is farthest from the opening, and that describes the round top of the bladder which is farthest from the opening into the urethra. The inside of the bladder is lined with **mucosa**, a mucous membrane. When the bladder is empty, the mucosa collapses into folds or **rugae**. When the bladder is full, smooth muscle in the bladder wall contracts to expel urine. At the base of the bladder, the bladder neck contains the **internal urethral sphincter**, a muscular ring that relaxes so that urine can flow into the urethra. The opening and closing of this internal sphincter is an involuntary reflex that cannot be consciously controlled.

Urethra

The **urethra** is a tube that carries urine from the bladder to outside of the body. The structure of the urethra differs in males and females.

In a male, the urethra is part of both the urinary system and male genital system because it transports both urine and semen. In men, as the urethra leaves the bladder, it first travels though the center of the **prostate gland**, a doughnut-shaped gland at the base of the bladder. This part of the urethra is the **prostatic urethra** (see Figure 10-4). (*Note*: The prostate gland [described in Chapter 11, Male Reproductive Medicine] is not part of the urinary system; however, enlargement of the prostate gland can affect the urinary system by pressing on and narrowing the prostatic urethra.) The **external urethral sphincter**, a muscular ring that can be consciously controlled to release or hold back urine, is located just below the prostate gland. The urethra travels the length of the **penis** (see Figure 10-4). This part is known as the **penile urethra**. In men, the **urethral meatus**, where the urethra ends, is located at the tip of the penis. If the male is uncircumcised, the urethral meatus is covered by the foreskin of the penis.

Pronunciation/Word Parts

bladder (BLAD-er)

vesical (VES-ih-kal)
  vesic/o- *bladder; fluid-filled sac*
  -al *pertaining to*
Vesical is the adjective for *bladder*. The combining form **cyst/o-** means *bladder; fluid-filled sac; semisolid cyst.*

fundus (FUN-duhs)

mucosa (myoo-KOH-sah)

mucosal (myoo-KOH-sal)
  mucos/o- *mucous membrane*
  -al *pertaining to*

rugae (ROO-jee)
Rugae is a Latin plural noun. Because there are so many rugae in the bladder, the singular form (*ruga*) is not used.

sphincter (SFINK-ter)
  sphinct/o- *close tightly*
  -er *person who does or produces; thing that does or produces*

urethra (yoor-EE-thrah)

urethral (yoor-EE-thrawl)
  urethr/o- *urethra*
  -al *pertaining to*

prostate (PRAW-stayt)

prostatic (praw-STAT-ik)
  prostat/o- *prostate gland*
  -ic *pertaining to*

penis (PEE-nihs)

penile (PEE-nile)
  pen/o- *penis*
  -ile *pertaining to*

meatus (mee-AA-tuhs)

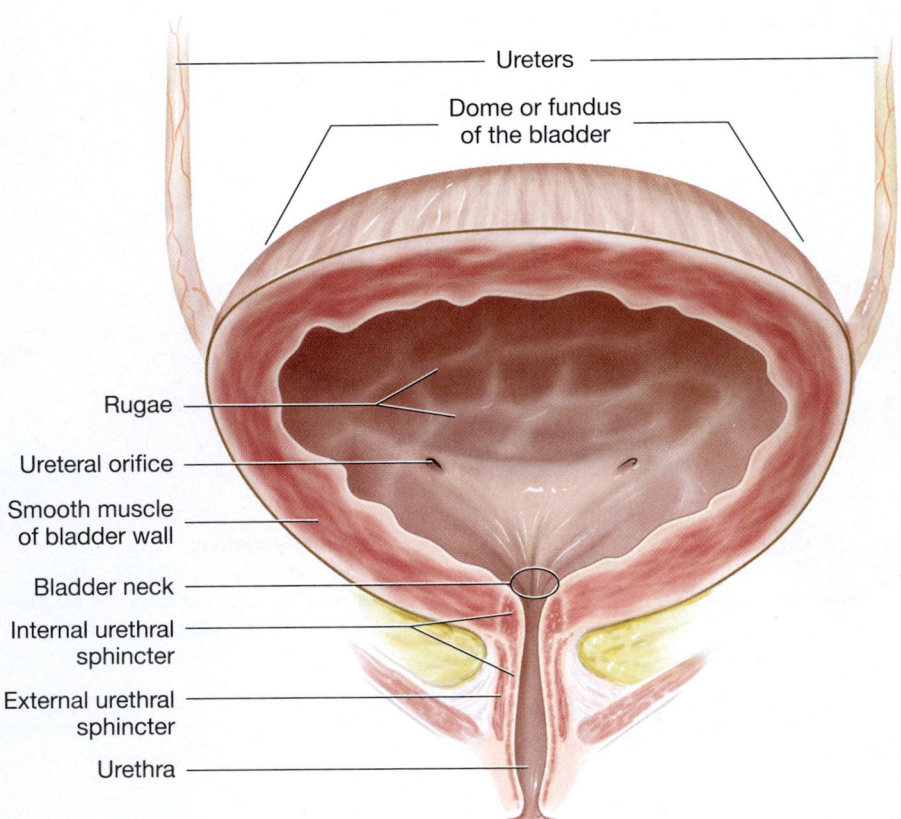

Ureters

Dome or fundus of the bladder

Rugae

Ureteral orifice

Smooth muscle of bladder wall

Bladder neck

Internal urethral sphincter

External urethral sphincter

Urethra

FIGURE 10-6 ■ Bladder.
The bladder is a hollow cavity that collects and temporarily stores urine. Rugae are mucous membrane folds in the bladder wall that allow it to expand as it fills. The ureteral orifices are in the posterior wall of the bladder.

In a female, the urethra is shorter, traveling only 1–2 inches from the bladder to the external surface of the body (see Figure 10-5). The external urethral sphincter is near the very end of the urethra. The urethral meatus is located just anterior to the external opening of the vagina.

Word Alert
Sound-Alike Words

ureter (YOOR-eh-ter)	(noun)	tube that connects the kidney to the bladder
		Example: The ureter is in the abdominal cavity.
ureteral (yoor-EE-ter-al)	(adjective)	pertaining to the ureter
		Example: The ureteral orifice is the opening of the ureter into the bladder.
urethra (yoor-EE-thrah)	(noun)	tube that connects the bladder to the outside of the body
		Example: The male urethra is longer than the female urethra.
urethral (yoor-EE-thrawl)	(adjective)	pertaining to the urethra
		Example: The urethral meatus opens to the outside of the body.
vesical (VES-ih-kal)	(adjective)	pertaining to the bladder
		Example: Intravesical chemotherapy drugs are put into the bladder to treat bladder cancer.
vesicle (VES-ih-kul)	(noun)	small fluid-filled blister on the skin (described in Chapter 2, Dermatology)
		Example: Some viral infections cause vesicles on the skin.

10.1 PRACTICE LAPS

Use the Answer Key at the end of the book to check your answers.

A. Label Structures

Write each anatomy word or phrase in the correct numbered box. Be sure to check your spelling.

cortex	major calyx	minor calyx	ureter
fibrous capsule	medulla	renal pelvis	

1.

2.

3.

4.

5.

6.

7.

kidney	penis	ureter	urinary bladder
penile urethra	prostatic urethra	urethral meatus	

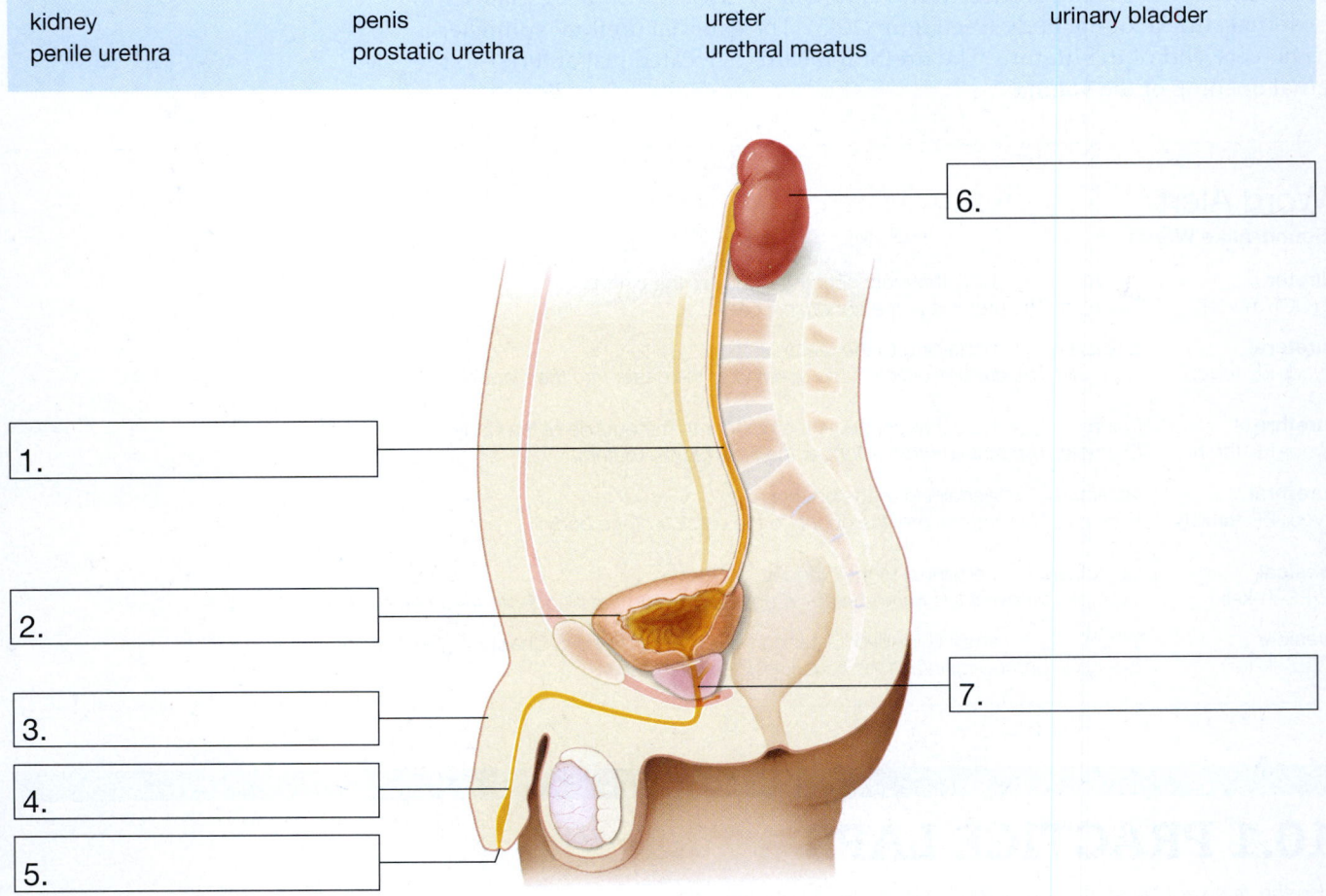

B. Give the Meaning of Combining Forms

Next to each combining form, write its meaning. The first one has been done for you.

Combining Form	Meaning	Combining Form	Meaning
1. **cortic/o-**	*cortex; outer region*	12. peritone/o-	_____
2. calic/o-	_____	13. prostat/o-	_____
3. cali/o-	_____	14. pyel/o-	_____
4. cyst/o-	_____	15. ren/o-	_____
5. excret/o-	_____	16. sphinct/o-	_____
6. genit/o-	_____	17. ureter/o-	_____
7. hil/o-	_____	18. urethr/o-	_____
8. mucos/o-	_____	19. urin/o-	_____
9. nephr/o-	_____	20. ur/o-	_____
10. pelv/o-	_____	21. vesic/o-	_____
11. pen/o-	_____		

C. Build Words

Read the definition of the medical word. Look at the combining form that is given. Select the correct suffix from the Suffix List, and write it on the blank line. Then build the medical word, and write it on the line. (Remember: You may need to remove the combining vowel. Always remove the hyphens and slash.) Be sure to check your spelling.

Suffix List

-al (pertaining to)	-eal (pertaining to)	-ile (pertaining to)
-ar (pertaining to)	-er (thing that does or produces)	-ory (having the function of)
-ary (pertaining to)	-ic (pertaining to)	

Definition of the Medical Word	Combining Form	Suffix	Build the Medical Word
Example: Pertaining to (the) cortex	cortic/o-	*-al*	*cortical*

[*You think pertaining to (-al) + cortex (cortic/o-). You change the order of the word parts to put the suffix last. You combine the word parts and write* cortical.]

1. Having the function of removing from the body	excret/o-		
2. Pertaining to (the) mucosa	mucos/o-		
3. Pertaining to (the) hilum	hil/o-		
4. Pertaining to (the) urine	urin/o-		
5. Pertaining to (the) calyx	calic/o-		
6. Pertaining to (the) ureter	ureter/o-		
7. Pertaining to (the) pelvis	pelv/o-		
8. Pertaining to (the) kidney	ren/o-		
9. Thing that does close tightly	sphinct/o-		
10. Pertaining to (the) penis	pen/o-		
11. Pertaining to (the) prostate gland	prostat/o-		

10.2 Physiology

The function of urine production occurs in the kidneys. By producing urine, the kidneys help to maintain a normal and constant internal environment known as **homeostasis**.

Before urine production begins, the body must already recognize the distinction between essential blood cells (red blood cells, white blood cells, platelets) and nutritional substances that the body needs versus the waste products of metabolism that must be excreted. The circulating blood contains all of these things.

Nutritional substances include glucose (sugar for cellular energy), albumin (protein for building tissues), vitamins, and electrolytes. **Electrolytes** are chemical

Pronunciation/Word Parts

homeostasis (HOH-mee-oh-STAY-sihs)
  home/o- *same*
  -stasis *standing still; staying in one place*

electrolyte (ee-LEK-troh-lite)
  electr/o- *electricity*
  -lyte *dissolved substance*
Electrolyte: *Dissolved substance (that can conduct) electricity (in a solution)*

elements that have a positive or negative electrical charge and conduct electricity when dissolved in a solution; they include:

- Sodium (Na^+)
- Potassium (K^+)
- Chloride (Cl^-)
- Bicarbonate (HCO_3^-).

Nutritional substances are essential to the health of the body, and they must not be excreted in the urine unless there is an excess amount in the blood. *Note:* Albumin is never excreted in the urine unless the glomerulus is damaged.

Waste products that need to be excreted include:

- **Urea** (from protein metabolism)
- **Creatinine** (from muscle contractions)
- **Uric acid** (from the construction of cellular DNA and RNA)
- Drugs and products of drug metabolism.

These waste products must be continually excreted in the urine or they will quickly reach a toxic level in the body.

The **parenchyma** is the functional or working tissue of the kidney (as opposed to its structural framework). The parenchyma is made up of nephrons that are in the tissue layers of the cortex and medulla. A **nephron** is the microscopic, functional unit of the kidney and the site of urine production. Each kidney contains more than 1 million nephrons that, if laid end to end, would be 80 miles in length, about the distance between New York City and Philadelphia!

To start the process of urine production, circulating blood flowing through the renal artery enters the kidney; the renal artery then divides into smaller arterioles. A single arteriole enters each nephron (see Figure 10-7 ■). The first part of the nephron is the **glomerular capsule**. Within this cup-shaped structure, the arteriole becomes the **glomerulus**, a network of intertwining capillaries.

Blood flowing through the glomerular capillaries contains nutritional substances that need to be retained by the body and waste products that need to be excreted, and so it is here that the process of separating those substances begins; that process is known as **filtration**. The capillaries in the glomerulus have special pores in their walls that are not found in other capillaries in the body. Blood cells are too large to pass through these pores, and so they remain in the capillary blood (as they should). But water, waste products, and most nutritional substances are pushed through the capillary pores and into the cup-shaped glomerular capsule by the pressure of the blood. Filtration is the first step in the formation of urine. The capillaries of the glomerulus then combine into a single arteriole that leaves the glomerulus and travels alongside the tubules of the nephron (see Figure 10-7).

Then the **filtrate** (water, waste products, and nutritional substances) in the glomerular capsule flows into the next part of the nephron, the **proximal convoluted tubule**. There, most of the water and nutritional substances move out of the proximal convoluted tubule and return to the blood. This essential process is known as **reabsorption**, the second step in the formation of urine.

The proximal convoluted tubule then becomes a U-shaped tubule known as the **nephron loop**. There, more water and nutritional substances are reabsorbed back into the blood. The nephron loop then becomes the **distal convoluted tubule**, where even more water and nutritional substances are reabsorbed back into the blood. The distal convoluted tubules of many nephrons empty into a common **collecting duct**. Then, specific substances (such as creatinine and metabolized drugs) move from the blood into the collecting duct. This is known as **secretion**, the third and final step in the formation of urine. The fluid that remains is **urine**.

Pronunciation/Word Parts

urea (yoor-EE-ah)

creatinine (kree-AT-ih-neen)

uric acid (YOOR-ik AS-id)

parenchyma (pah-RENG-kih-mah)

nephron (NEH-frawn)
The combining form **nephr/o-** means *kidney; nephron.*

glomerular (gloh-MAIR-yoo-lar)
   glomerul/o- *glomerulus*
   -ar *pertaining to*

glomerulus (gloh-MAIR-yoo-luhs)

glomeruli (gloh-MAIR-yoo-lie)
Latin plural noun: Change the singular ending *-us* to *-i.*

filtration (fil-TRAY-shun)
   filtrat/o- *filtering; straining*
   -ion *action; condition*

filtrate (FIL-trayt)
   filtr/o- *filter*
   -ate *composed of; pertaining to*

proximal (PRAWK-sih-mal)
   proxim/o- *near the center or point of origin*
   -al *pertaining to*

convoluted (CON-voh-LOO-ted)
   convolut/o- *coiled*
   -ed *pertaining to*

tubule (TOO-byool)
   tub/o- *tube*
   -ule *small thing*

tubular (TOO-byoo-lar)
   tubul/o- *small tube*
   -ar *pertaining to*

reabsorption (REE-ab-SORP-shun)
   re- *again and again; backward; unable to*
   absorpt/o- *absorb; take in*
   -ion *action; condition*

distal (DIS-tal)
   dist/o- *away from the center or point of origin*
   -al *pertaining to*

secretion (seh-KREE-shun)
   secret/o- *produce; secrete*
   -ion *action; condition*

urine (YOOR-in)
   ur/o- *urinary system; urine*
   -ine *pertaining to*

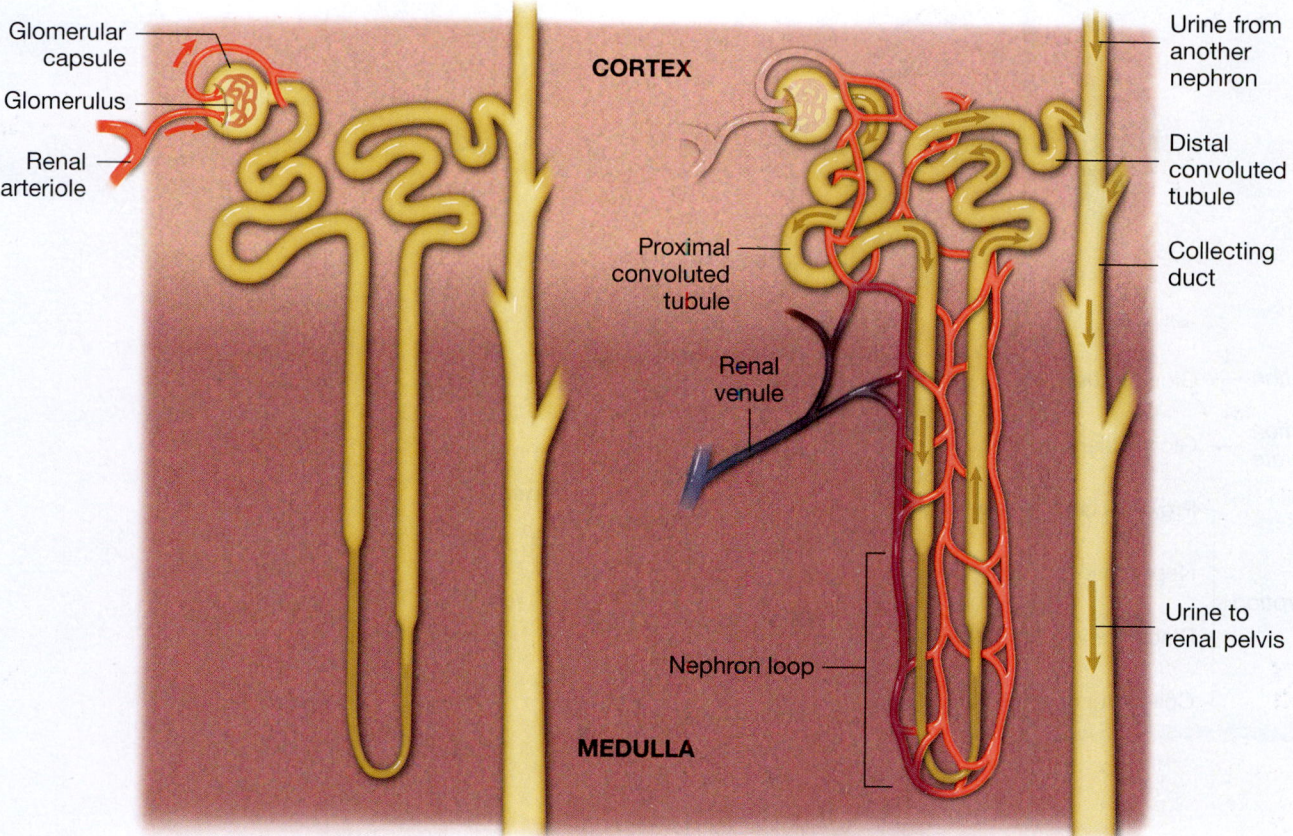

FIGURE 10-7 ■ Nephron.
The functional unit of the kidney is the nephron. It filters the blood, keeping most nutritional substances and returning them to the blood, and sending water and waste substances as urine to the ureter and bladder.

Urine is produced continuously by nephrons in the kidneys (see Figure 10-8 ■). The process of eliminating urine from the body is described in several ways: **urination**, **micturition**, or **voiding**.

Pronunciation/Word Parts

urination (YOOR-ih-NAY-shun)
  urin/o- urinary system; urine
  -ation being; having; process

micturition (MIK-tyoor-IH-shun)
  mictur/o- making urine
  -ition process of making
The combining form **enur/o-** means urinate.

voiding (VOY-ding)

Clinical Connections

Endocrinology. If the blood contains an increased level of glucose (from eating a sugary food or because of the disease of uncontrolled diabetes mellitus), it cannot reabsorb additional glucose, and so that glucose remains in the proximal convoluted tubule and is excreted in the urine.

Across the Life Span

Pediatrics. The kidneys of a fetus begin to produce urine by about the 12th week of life. The urine is excreted and becomes part of the amniotic fluid around the fetus. Children ages 1 to 3 produce about 400–600 mL (about a pint) of urine each day. Children ages 3 to 8 produce about 600–1000 mL (about a quart) of urine daily.

Geriatrics. Adults produce about 1200–1500 mL (1–3 quarts) of urine each day. As a person ages, some nephrons die. Because the body does not repair or replace nephrons, the total number of nephrons in the kidneys continues to decline with age, and kidney function also decreases. Poor renal function can significantly prolong the effects of some drugs. Patients with renal disease and older adults are prescribed lower doses of drugs to prevent toxic symptoms due to decreased excretion of drugs.

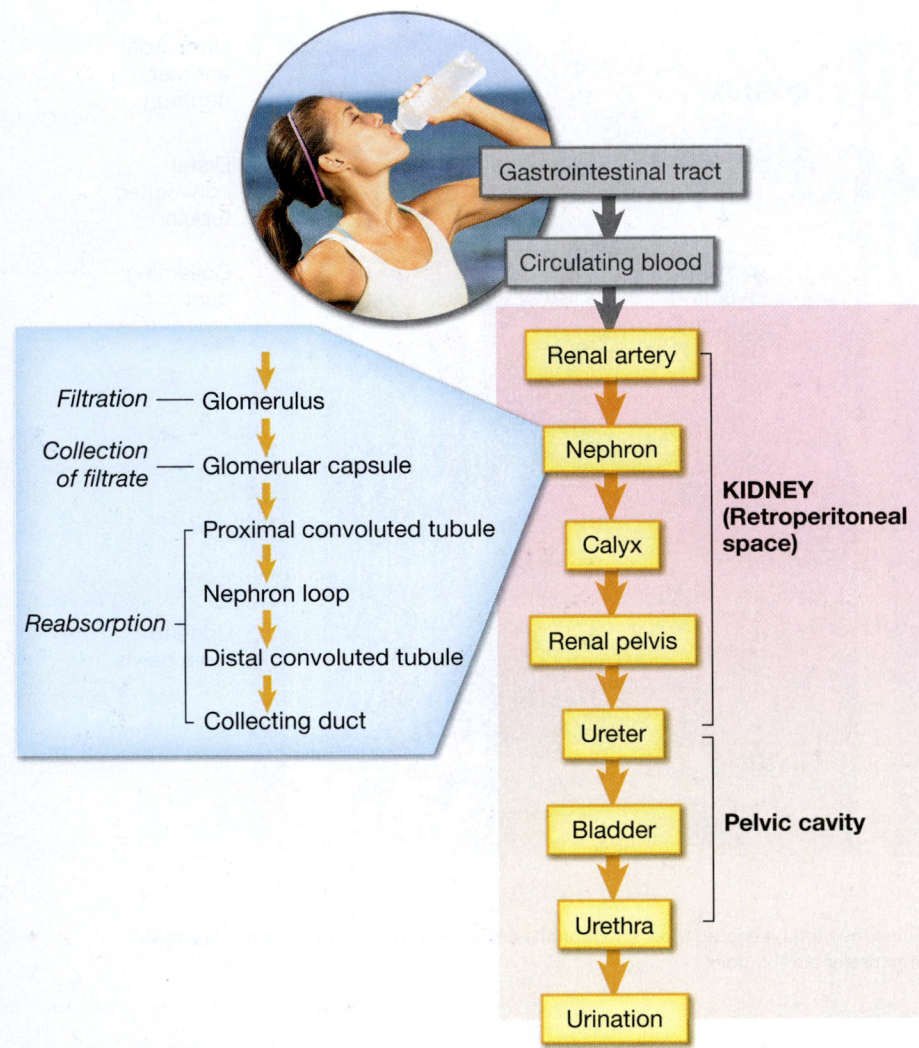

FIGURE 10-8 ■ Pathway of urine production and urination.

In addition to urine production, the kidneys work in conjunction with other body systems to maintain homeostasis.

Cardiovascular System

If the blood pressure in the cardiovascular system decreases, the kidneys will help in two different ways to restore normal blood pressure.

- The kidneys will produce concentrated urine with less water in it. The hormone aldosterone (from the adrenal gland) and antidiuretic hormone (from the posterior pituitary gland in the brain) act on the distal convoluted tubule and collecting duct to cause more sodium and water to be reabsorbed, so less is lost in the urine. This increases the blood volume and the blood pressure.

- The kidneys will release the enzyme **renin** into the blood. Renin is a vasoconstrictor that constricts the arteries in the body and this increases the blood pressure. Renin also stimulates the production of a substance (angiotensin), which, in turn, causes the production of another substance (aldosterone) that causes sodium and water to be reabsorbed from the tubule into the blood, and this also increases the blood pressure.

Blood

The kidneys help in two different ways to maintain the normal composition of the blood.

- If the pH of the blood decreases, the electrolyte bicarbonate (HCO_3^-) moves from the tubules back into the blood, and this increases the pH.

- If the number of red blood cells decreases, the kidneys secrete the hormone **erythropoietin**, which stimulates the bone marrow to produce more red blood cells.

Pronunciation/Word Parts

renin (REE-nin)
  ren/o- *kidney*
  -in *substance*

erythropoietin (eh-RITH-roh-POY-eh-tin)
  erythr/o- *red*
  -poietin *substance that forms*

10.2 PRACTICE LAPS

Use the Answer Key at the end of the book to check your answers.

A. Label Functions

Write each physiology word or phrase in the correct numbered box. Be sure to check your spelling.

collecting duct	glomerular capsule	nephron loop	renal arteriole
distal convoluted tubule	glomerulus	proximal convoluted tubule	renal venule

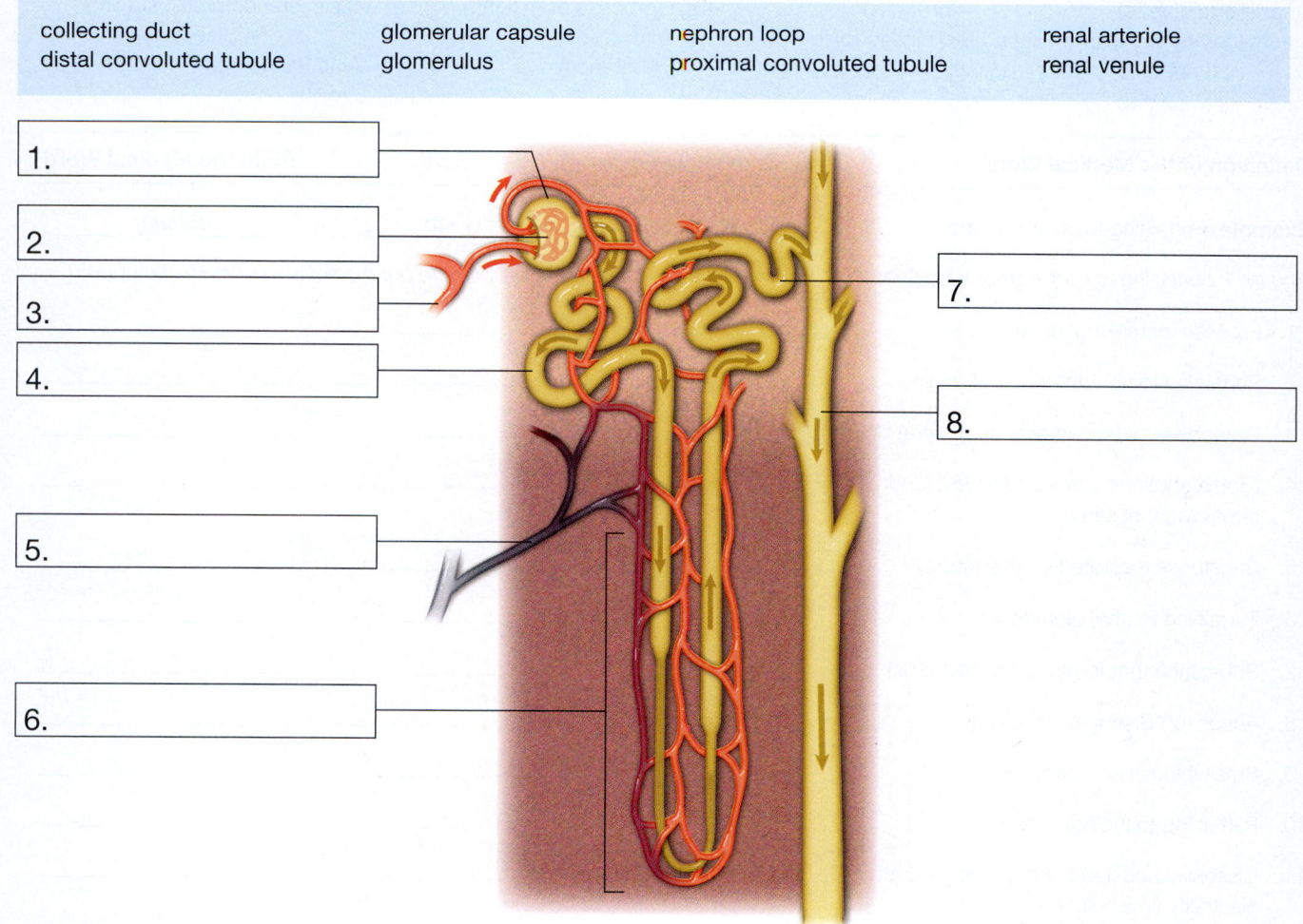

1.

2.

3.

4.

5.

6.

7.

8.

B. Give the Meaning of Combining Forms

Next to each combining form, write its meaning. The first one has been done for you.

Combining Form	Meaning	Combining Form	Meaning
1. **absorpt/o-**	*absorb; take in*	11. nephr/o-	
2. convolut/o-		12. mictur/o-	
3. dist/o-		13. proxim/o-	
4. electr/o-		14. ren/o-	
5. enur/o-		15. secret/o-	
6. erythr/o-		16. tub/o-	
7. filtrat/o-		17. tubul/o-	
8. filtr/o-		18. urin/o-	
9. glomerul/o-		19. ur/o-	
10. home/o-			

C. Build Words

Read the definition of the medical word. Look at the combining form that is given. Select the correct suffix from the Suffix List, and write it on the blank line. Then build the medical word, and write it on the line. (Remember: You may need to remove the combining vowel. Always remove the hyphens and slash.) Be sure to check your spelling. The first one has been done for you.

Suffix List

-al (pertaining to)	-ation (being; having;	-ion (action; condition)	-poietin (substance that forms)
-ar (pertaining to)	process)	-ition (process of making)	-stasis (standing still; staying
-ate (composed of;	-ed (pertaining to)	-lyte (dissolved	in one place)
pertaining to)	-in (substance)	substance)	-ule (small thing)

Definition of the Medical Word	Combining Form	Suffix	Build the Medical Word
Example: Pertaining to (a) small tube	**tubul/o-**	*-ar*	*tubular*

[*You think* pertaining to *(-ar) +* small tube *(tubul/o-). You change the order of the word parts to put the suffix last. You write* tubular.]

1. Process (of making) urine	urin/o-	_____	_____
2. Pertaining to near the point of origin	proxim/o-	_____	_____
3. Composed of (substances that were) filter(ed)	filtr/o-	_____	_____
4. (Body functions are) standing still (and remaining the) same	home/o-	_____	_____
5. Substance (secreted by the) kidney	ren/o-	_____	_____
6. Pertaining to (the) glomerulus	glomerul/o-	_____	_____
7. Substance that forms red (blood cells)	erythr/o-	_____	_____
8. Action (of) filtering or straining	filtrat/o-	_____	_____
9. Small thing (that is a) tube	tub/o-	_____	_____
10. Pertaining to (being) coiled	convolut/o-	_____	_____
11. Dissolved substance (that can conduct) electricity (in a solution)	electr/o-	_____	_____
12. Process of making urine	mictur/o-	_____	_____
13. Action (to) produce (or) secrete	secret/o-	_____	_____

Vocabulary Review

Word or Phrase	Description	Combining Forms
Overview		
urinary system	The structures of the urinary system include the kidneys, ureters, bladder, and urethra. This body system is also known as the **urinary tract**, **genitourinary system**, **urogenital system**, and the **excretory system**. Its functions are to remove the waste products of cellular metabolism by producing, transporting, storing, and excreting urine. It also helps maintain the internal environment of the body—the blood pressure, pH, and the number of red blood cells.	**urin/o-** *urinary system; urine* **genit/o-** *genitalia* **ur/o-** *urinary system; urine* **excret/o-** *removing from the body*

Word or Phrase	Description	Combining Forms
Anatomy of the Urinary System		
Kidneys		
calyx	Collecting area at each tip of medulla that collects urine. Several minor calices drain into a larger major calyx.	**calic/o-** *calyx* **cali/o-** *calyx*
cortex	Layer of tissue beneath the fibrous capsule of the kidney	**cortic/o-** *cortex; outer region*
flank	Area on the back (between the ribs and the hip bone) that overlies the kidneys	
hilum	Indentation in the medial side of each kidney where the renal artery enters and the renal vein and ureter exit	**hil/o-** *indentation*
kidney	Organ of the urinary system that produces urine	**ren/o-** *kidney* **nephr/o-** *kidney; nephron*
medulla	Layer of tissue beneath the cortex of the kidney. Each tip of medulla connects to a minor calyx.	
renal pelvis	Large, funnel-shaped area within the kidney. It collects urine from the major calices. The renal pelvis narrows to become the ureter.	**pelv/o-** *hip bone; pelvis; renal pelvis* **pyel/o-** *renal pelvis*
retroperitoneal space	Area behind the peritoneum, the membrane that lines the abdominal cavity. The kidneys are located there, surrounded by fatty tissue.	**peritone/o-** *peritoneum*
Ureters		
peristalsis	Process of smooth muscle contractions that move urine through the ureter	
ureter	Tube that carries urine from the kidney to the bladder. It is located in the abdominal cavity.	**ureter/o-** *ureter*
ureteral orifice	Opening at the end of the ureter as it enters the bladder	**ureter/o-** *ureter*
Bladder		
bladder	Expandable reservoir for holding urine. It is located in the pelvic cavity.	**cyst/o-** *bladder; fluid-filled sac; semisolid cyst* **vesic/o-** *bladder; fluid-filled sac*
fundus	Round top or dome of the bladder	
internal urethral sphincter	Muscular ring in the bladder neck. It relaxes when the bladder is full so that urine can flow into the urethra. This sphincter is not under conscious control.	**sphinct/o-** *close tightly* **-er** *person who does or produces; thing that does or produces*
mucosa	Mucous membrane that lines the bladder	**mucos/o-** *mucous membrane*
rugae	Folds in the mucosa of the bladder that disappear as the bladder fills with urine	
Urethra		
external urethral sphincter	Muscular ring in the urethra that can be consciously controlled to release or hold back urine. In a male, it is located below the prostate gland. In a female, it is located near the end of the urethra.	**urethr/o-** *urethra* **sphinct/o-** *close tightly* **-er** *person who does or produces; thing that does or produces*
penis	Structure that is part of the male reproductive system. In a male, the urethra passes through the length of the penis as the **penile urethra**.	**pen/o-** *penis*
prostate gland	Gland that is part of the male reproductive system. In a male, the urethra passes through the center of the prostate gland as the **prostatic urethra**.	**prostat/o-** *prostate gland*
urethra	Tube that carries urine from the bladder to the outside of the body. In a male, it goes through the prostate gland and down the length of the penis. In a female, it is a short tube, ending near the external opening of the vagina.	**urethr/o-** *urethra*

Word or Phrase	Description	Combining Forms
urethral meatus	Opening at the end of the urethra that leads to the outside of the body. In a male, it is located at the tip of the penis. In a female, it is located just anterior to the external opening of the vagina.	**urethr/o-** *urethra*

Physiology of the Urinary System

Word or Phrase	Description	Combining Forms
electrolytes	Chemical elements that have a positive or negative electrical charge and conduct electricity when dissolved in a solution. They include sodium (Na^+), potassium (K^+), chloride (Cl^-), and bicarbonate (HCO_3^-).	**electr/o-** *electricity*
erythropoietin	Hormone secreted by the kidneys when the number of red blood cells in the blood decreases. It stimulates the bone marrow to produce more red blood cells.	**erythr/o-** *red*
homeostasis	Normal and constant internal environment of the body. The kidneys help maintain this.	**home/o-** *same*
nutritional substances	Include glucose (sugar for cellular energy), albumin (protein for building tissues), vitamins, and electrolytes. These must not be excreted in the urine unless there is an excessive amount in the blood. Albumin is never excreted unless the glomerulus is damaged.	
parenchyma	Functional or working tissue of the kidney	
renin	Enzyme secreted by the kidneys when the blood pressure is low. It stimulates the production of another substance (angiotensin), which, in turn, produces another substance (aldosterone) that causes sodium and water to be reabsorbed into the blood, thus increasing the blood pressure.	**ren/o-** *kidney*
nutritional substances	Include glucose (sugar for cellular energy), albumin (protein for building tissues), vitamins, and electrolytes. These must not be excreted in the urine unless there is an excessive amount in the blood. Albumin is never excreted unless the glomerulus is damaged.	
urination	Process of excreting urine from the body. Also known as **voiding** or **micturition**.	**urin/o-** *urinary system; urine* **mictur/o-** *making urine* **enur/o-** *urinate*
urine	Water, waste products, and other substances excreted by the kidneys	**ur/o-** *urinary system; urine*
waste products of metabolism	Include **urea** (from protein metabolism), **creatinine** (from muscle contractions), **uric acid** (from the construction of cellular DNA and RNA), and the products of drug metabolism. These must be excreted in the urine.	

Nephron

Word or Phrase	Description	Combining Forms
collecting duct	Large duct that collects fluid from the distal convoluted tubules of many nephrons. The final step of secretion takes place there, and the fluid that remains is urine.	
distal convoluted tubule	Tubule of the nephron that begins at the nephron loop and ends at the collecting duct. Reabsorption takes place there.	**dist/o-** *away from the center or point of origin* **tub/o-** *tube* **tubul/o-** *small tube*
filtration	First step in the formation of urine. Process in which water, some nutritional substances, and wastes in the blood are pushed through pores in the capillaries of the glomerulus. The resulting fluid is **filtrate**.	**filtrat/o-** *filtering; straining* **filtr/o-** *filter*
glomerular capsule	First part of a nephron. It is a cup-shaped structure that surrounds the glomerulus and collects filtrate.	**glomerul/o-** *glomerulus*
glomerulus	Network of intertwining capillaries within the glomerular capsule. Filtration takes place there.	**glomerul/o-** *glomerulus*
nephron	Microscopic, functional unit of the kidney and the site of urine production. Located in the cortex and medulla layers of the kidneys. All of the nephrons together make up the parenchyma.	**nephr/o-** *kidney; nephron*

Word or Phrase	Description	Combining Forms
nephron loop	U-shaped tubule of the nephron that begins at the proximal convoluted tubule and ends at the distal convoluted tubule. Reabsorption takes place there.	
proximal convoluted tubule	Coiled tubule that receives filtrate from the glomerular capsule. Reabsorption takes place there.	**convolut/o-** *coiled* **tub/o-** *tube* **tubul/o-** *small tube*
reabsorption	Second step in the formation of urine. Process by which most of the water and nutritional substances in the filtrate move out of the tubule and return to the blood in a nearby capillary.	**absorpt/o-** *absorb; take in*
secretion	Third and final step in the formation of urine. Process by which specific substances (creatinine, metabolized drugs) move from the blood into the collecting duct.	

Abbreviation Review

Cl⁻	chloride		**K⁺**	potassium
GU	genitourinary		**Na⁺**	sodium
HCO₃⁻	bicarbonate			

10.3 Diseases

Word or Phrase	Description	Pronunciation/Word Parts

Kidneys and Ureters

Word or Phrase	Description	Pronunciation/Word Parts
glomerulonephritis	Infection and inflammation of the glomeruli. This complication develops after an acute infection caused by streptococcal bacteria or by viruses. The original infection, which is often a strep throat, causes the immune system to produce antibodies. These combine with the bacteria or viruses to form antigen–antibody complexes that clog the pores of the capillaries of the glomerulus, and urine production decreases. Treatment: Antibiotic drug for a bacterial infection; corticosteroid drug to decrease inflammation; renal dialysis, if necessary	**glomerulonephritis** (gloh-MAIR-yoo-LOH-neh-FRY-tihs) **glomerul/o-** *glomerulus* **nephr/o-** *kidney; nephron* **-itis** *infection of; inflammation of*
hydronephrosis	Condition in which urine distends the renal pelvis and calices or ureter. This happens when a blood clot, infection, or a kidney stone blocks the flow of urine. In **caliectasis**, the calices of the kidney are enlarged. In **hydroureter**, only the ureter is enlarged. Treatment: Treat the underlying cause.	**hydronephrosis** (HY-droh-neh-FROH-sihs) **hydr/o-** *fluid; water* **nephr/o-** *kidney; nephron* **-osis** *abnormal condition; process* Hydronephrosis: *Abnormal condition (in which the) fluid (of urine distends part of the) kidney* **caliectasis** (KAY-lee-EK-tah-sihs) **cali/o-** *calyx* **-ectasis** *condition of dilation* **hydroureter** (HY-droh-YOOR-eh-ter) *Hydroureter* is a combination of the combining form **hydr/o-** (fluid; water) and the word *ureter*.

Word or Phrase	Description	Pronunciation/Word Parts

nephrolithiasis	Formation of a kidney stone (also known as a **calculus**) in the urinary system. Kidney stones can vary in size from microscopic (often referred to as *sand* or *gravel*) to large (see Figure 10-9 ■) and can be numerous or large enough to fill the renal pelvis or block the ureter (see Figure 10-10 ■). Also known as **calculogenesis**. Kidney stones are composed of magnesium, calcium, or uric acid crystals. **Renal colic** is a spasm of smooth muscle of the ureter or bladder as the kidney stone's jagged edges scrape the mucosa. This causes severe pain, nausea and vomiting, and hematuria.
	
	Treatment: Many stones reach the bladder and are eliminated spontaneously during urination. Stones that do not pass spontaneously can be destroyed (by lithotripsy) or removed surgically (by stone basketing or nephrolithotomy), depending on the size and location of the stone.
		nephrolithiasis
		(NEH-froh-lith-EYE-ah-sihs)
		  nephr/o- *kidney; nephron*
		  lith/o- *stone*
		  -iasis *abnormal condition; process*
		
		calculus (KAL-kyoo-luhs)
		
		calculi (KAL-kyoo-lie)
		Latin plural noun: Change the singular ending *-us* to *-i*.
		
		calculogenesis
		(KAL-kyoo-loh-JEN-eh-sihs)
		  calcul/o- *stone*
		  gen/o- *arising from; produced by*
		  -esis *abnormal condition; process*
		
		colic (KAW-lik)
		  col/o- *colon*
		  -ic *pertaining to*

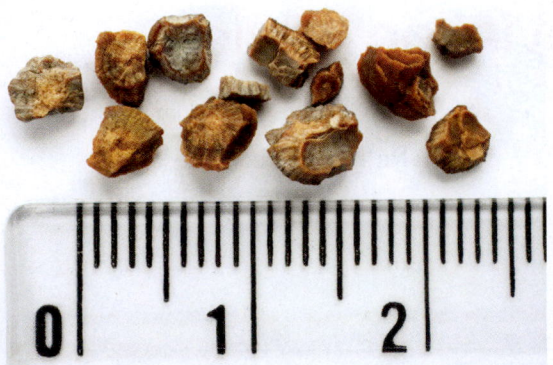

FIGURE 10-9 ■ Kidney stone.
The many sharp, jagged edges of a kidney stone cause hematuria, vomiting, renal colic, and severe pain.

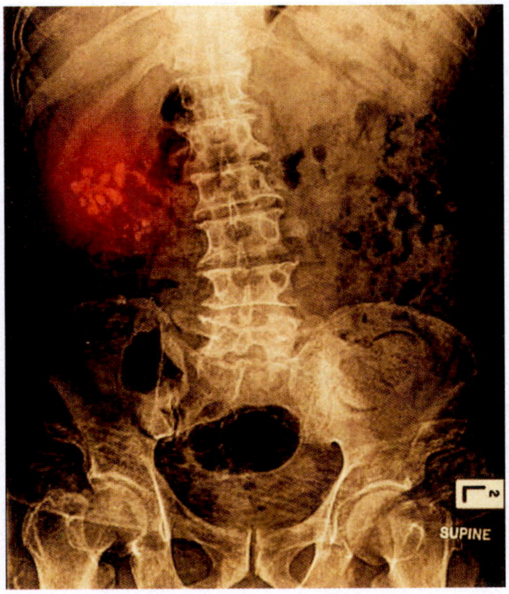

FIGURE 10-10 ■ Nephrolithiasis.
This x-ray shows multiple kidney stones in the right kidney that have become so large that they cannot pass spontaneously. They leave little room in the renal pelvis for urine to collect. *Note*: Remember that when you view an x-ray, the patient's right side corresponds to your left side.

Word Alert
Words with Two Different Meanings

calculus	A kidney stone The name of an advanced branch of mathematics
colic	Spasm of the smooth muscle around the ureters and bladder Spasm of the smooth muscle around the intestines
pelvis	Funnel-shaped area in the kidney that collects urine Hip bones, sacrum, and coccyx that form the bony pelvis

Word or Phrase	Description	Pronunciation/Word Parts
nephropathy	Any disease of the kidney • Diabetic nephropathy involves progressive damage caused by uncontrolled diabetes mellitus. • Kidney infection can cause the capillaries of the glomerulus to harden (**glomerulosclerosis**). Treatment: Correct the underlying cause.	**nephropathy** (neh-FRAW-pah-thee) **nephr/o-** *kidney; nephron* **-pathy** *disease* **glomerulosclerosis** (gloh-MAIR-yoo-LOH-skleh-ROH-sihs) **glomerul/o-** *glomerulus* **scler/o-** *hard; sclera* **-osis** *abnormal condition; process* Glomerulosclerosis: *Condition (of the) glomerulus (becoming) hard*
nephroptosis	Abnormally low position of a kidney Treatment: It sometimes requires surgery, but more often is mentioned as an incidental finding seen on an x-ray.	**nephroptosis** (NEH-frawp-TOH-sihs) **nephr/o-** *kidney; nephron* **-ptosis** *state of drooping; state of falling*
nephrotic syndrome	Damage to the pores of the capillaries of the glomerulus. This allows large amounts of albumin (protein) to leak into the urine, decreasing the amount of protein in the blood. This changes the osmotic pressure of the blood and allows fluid to go into the tissues, producing edema in the extremities; fluid also goes into the abdominal cavity, producing **ascites** (a grossly enlarged, fluid-distended abdomen). Treatment: Diuretic drug to decrease edema; correct the underlying cause.	**nephrotic** (neh-FRAW-tik) **nephr/o-** *kidney; nephron* **-tic** *pertaining to* **ascites** (ah-SY-teez)
polycystic kidney disease	Hereditary disease characterized by cysts in the kidney. This progressive degenerative disease eventually destroys the nephrons, causing kidney failure (see Figure 10-11 ■ and also Figure 10-12 ■). The early stage shows few symptoms; often it is not detected until enlarged kidneys are found during a physical examination. Treatment: Dialysis or kidney transplantation	**polycystic** (PAW-lee-SIS-tik) **poly-** *many; much* **cyst/o-** *bladder; fluid-filled sac; semisolid cyst* **-ic** *pertaining to* Polycystic: *Pertaining to many semisolid cysts*

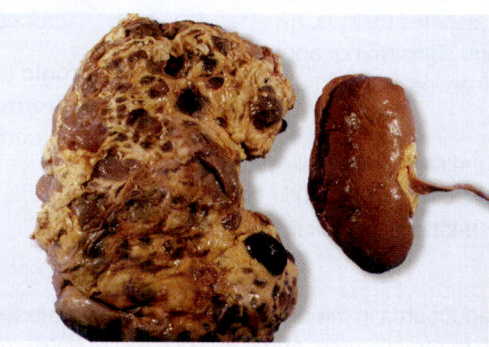

FIGURE 10-11 ■ Polycystic kidney disease.
As nonfunctioning cysts replace large numbers of nephrons, the kidney enlarges but the patient's kidney function progressively decreases. For comparison, the kidney on the right is normal in shape and size.

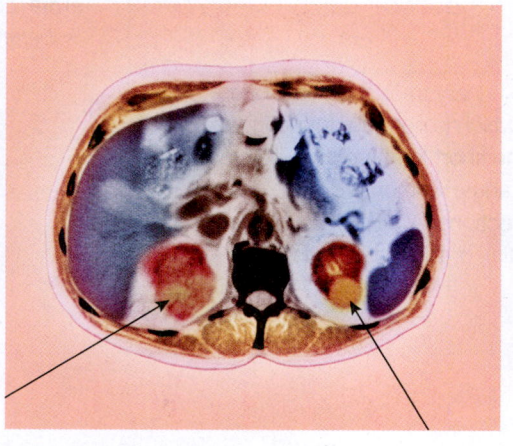

FIGURE 10-12 ■ CT scan of the kidneys.
This colorized computerized tomography (CT) scan shows the abdominal organs and the kidneys. The bottom center of the image shows the patient's vertebral column in black. Small black areas around both sides are the patient's ribs. The top of the image is the patient's abdomen. *Note:* A CT scan is read as if you were at the patient's feet and looking up. Therefore, the patient's liver (light and dark blue) is along the left-hand side of the image. The patient's right kidney (bottom left, see arrow) is enlarged from a cancerous tumor. The patient's left kidney (bottom right, see arrow) has a large cyst.

Word or Phrase	Description	Pronunciation/Word Parts
pyelonephritis	Infection and inflammation of the renal pelvis of the kidney. It is caused by a bacterial infection of the bladder that ascends the ureters and goes into the kidneys. Treatment: Antibiotic drug	**pyelonephritis** (PY-eh-LOH-neh-FRY-tihs) **pyel/o-** *renal pelvis* **nephr/o-** *kidney; nephron* **-itis** *infection of; inflammation of*
renal cell cancer	**Cancerous** tumor (**carcinoma**) that begins in the epithelial cells that line the tubules of the nephron (see Figure 10-12). **Wilms tumor** is cancer of embryonal cells that still remain in the kidney. It occurs in children; also known as **nephroblastoma**. Treatment: Surgery to remove the kidney (nephrectomy); radiation therapy; chemotherapy drug	**cancer** (KAN-ser) **cancerous** (KAN-ser-uhs) **cancer/o-** *cancer* **-ous** *pertaining to* **carcinoma** (KAR-sih-NOH-mah) **carcin/o-** *cancer* **-oma** *mass; tumor* **Wilms** (WILMZ) **nephroblastoma** (NEH-froh-blas-TOH-mah) **nephr/o-** *kidney; nephron* **blast/o-** *embryonic; immature* **-oma** *mass; tumor*
renal failure	Disease in which the kidneys decrease and then stop producing urine. This is due to an acute or chronic disease process. • **Acute kidney injury (AKI)** occurs suddenly and is usually due to trauma, severe blood loss, or overwhelming infection. It is caused by **acute tubular necrosis**, the sudden destruction of large numbers of nephrons and their tubules. Previously known as **acute renal failure (ARF)**. • **Chronic kidney disease (CKD)** begins with **renal insufficiency**, followed by gradual worsening with progressive damage to the kidneys from chronic, uncontrolled diabetes mellitus, hypertension, or glomerulonephritis. Symptoms and signs do not appear until 80 percent of kidney function has been lost. Previously known as **chronic renal failure (CRF)**. **End-stage renal disease (ESRD)** is the final, irreversible stage of chronic renal failure in which there is little or no remaining kidney function. Treatment: Treat the underlying cause; treat end-stage failure with renal dialysis or kidney transplantation.	**acute** (ah-KYOOT) **tubular** (TOO-byoo-lar) **tubul/o-** *small tube* **-ar** *pertaining to* **necrosis** (neh-KROH-sihs) **necr/o-** *dead body; dead tissue* **-osis** *abnormal condition; process* **chronic** (KRAW-nik) **chron/o-** *time* **-ic** *pertaining to*
uremia	An excessive amount of the waste product urea in the blood because of renal failure. The kidneys are unable to remove urea, and it reaches a toxic level in the blood. Treatment: Renal dialysis	**uremia** (yoor-EE-mee-ah) **ur/o-** *urinary system; urine* **-emia** *condition of the blood; substance in the blood*
urinary tract infection (UTI)	Bacterial infection somewhere in the urinary tract. It is most often caused by *Escherichia coli* (*E. coli*), which is normally found in the intestines and rectum. Because of the short length of the urethra in women and its location close to the anus, women are more prone than men to develop urinary tract infections. A UTI can involve just the urethra (urethritis), the bladder (cystitis), or the renal pelvis of the kidney (pyelonephritis). Treatment: Antibiotic drug	

Word or Phrase	Description	Pronunciation/Word Parts

Bladder

| **bladder cancer** | Cancerous tumor (carcinoma) of the epithelial cells lining the bladder, most commonly seen in men over age 60. Hematuria is often the first symptom.
Treatment: Transurethral resection of the bladder tumor; surgery to remove the bladder (cystectomy); radiation therapy; **intravesical** insertion of a chemotherapy drug through a catheter into the bladder | **intravesical** (IN-trah-VES-ih-kal)
intra- *within*
vesic/o- *bladder; fluid-filled sac*
-al *pertaining to* |

Clinical Connections

Oncology. Transitional cell carcinoma occurs in the epithelial cells lining the bladder. Transitional cells are unique in that their shape changes (transitions) each time the bladder fills with urine and empties.

| **cystitis** | Infection or inflammation of the bladder (see Figure 10-13 ■).
It is often caused by bacteria in the urethra that ascend into the bladder, particularly in women because of the short length of the urethra.
• **Interstitial cystitis** is a chronic, progressive infection in which the bladder mucosa becomes extremely irritated and red, with bleeding.
• **Radiation cystitis** is caused by the irritating effects of radiation therapy given to treat bladder cancer.
Treatment: Correct the underlying cause; analgesic drug and antispasmodic drug | **cystitis** (sihs-TY-tihs)
cyst/o- *bladder; fluid-filled sac; semisolid cyst*
-itis *infection of; inflammation of*
Cystitis: *Infection or inflammation of the bladder*

interstitial (IN-ter-STIH-shal)
interstiti/o- *spaces between tissues*
-al *pertaining to*

radiation (RAY-dee-AA-shun)
radi/o- *forearm bone; radius; x-rays*
-ation *being; having; process*
Radiation: *Process (of being exposed to) x-rays* |

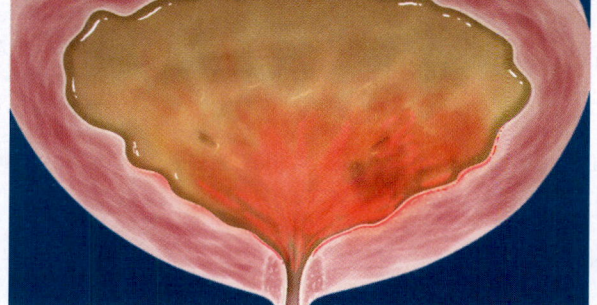

FIGURE 10-13 ■ Acute cystitis.
This bladder shows severe irritation and inflammation of the mucosa with areas of hemorrhage.

| **cystocele** | Hernia in which the bladder bulges through a weakness in the muscular wall of the vagina or rectum. This causes retention of the urine that is within the hernia. Also known as a **vesicocele**.
Treatment: Surgical repair of the hernia, if needed | **cystocele** (SIHS-toh-seel)
cyst/o- *bladder; fluid-filled sac; semisolid cyst*
-cele *hernia*

vesicocele (VES-ih-koh-SEEL)
vesic/o- *bladder; fluid-filled sac*
-cele *hernia* |

Word or Phrase	Description	Pronunciation/Word Parts

incontinence	Inability to voluntarily keep urine in the bladder. It can be due to a spinal cord injury, surgery on the prostate gland, unconsciousness, or a mental condition such as dementia. It can also be due to **stress urinary incontinence (SUI)**, which is caused by weak pelvic floor muscles from childbirth or menopause.
	Treatment: Correct the underlying cause. In a female, muscle tone can be improved by doing Kegel exercises (the perineum is alternately tensed and relaxed); behavioral modification such as bladder training; vaginal sling surgery.
		incontinence (in-CON-tih-nens)
		  in- *in; not; within*
		  contin/o- *hold together*
		  -ence *state*
		Incontinence: *State (of) not (being able to) hold together (urine in the bladder)*

Across the Life Span

Pediatrics. Incontinence of urine is normal in babies because the nerve connections to the external urethral sphincter do not develop until about 2 years of age—about the time that parents begin toilet training.

Middle Age. Incontinence can begin as early as middle age. In a female, the muscles of the pelvic floor begin to relax, and when the patient laughs, coughs, or sneezes, increased intra-abdominal pressure causes urine to pass.

Geriatrics. Dementia often results in incontinence.

Word or Phrase	Description	Pronunciation/Word Parts

neurogenic bladder	Urinary retention due to a lack of innervation of the nerves to the bladder. This can be due to a spinal cord injury, spina bifida, multiple sclerosis, or Parkinson disease.
	Treatment: The bladder must be catheterized often because it does not contract to expel urine.
		neurogenic (NYOOR-oh-JEN-ik)
		  neur/o- *nerve*
		  gen/o- *arising from; produced by*
		  -ic *pertaining to*

overactive bladder	Urinary urgency and frequency due to involuntary contractions of the bladder wall as the bladder fills with urine. Also known as **urge incontinence**. Treatment: Drug for overactive bladder	

urinary retention	Inability to empty the bladder because of an obstruction (enlargement of the prostate gland or a kidney stone), nerve damage (neurogenic bladder), or as a side effect of certain drugs. Even when the bladder contracts, a large amount of **postvoid residual** urine remains in the bladder.
	Treatment: Correct the underlying cause.
		retention (ree-TEN-shun)
		  retent/o- *hold back; keep*
		  -ion *action; condition*
		
		postvoid (POST-voyd)
		Postvoid is a combination of the prefix **post-** (after; behind) and the word *void* (urinate).

vesicovaginal fistula	Formation of an abnormal passageway (fistula) connecting the bladder to the vagina. Urine flows into the vagina and leaks continually to the outside of the body.
	Treatment: Surgical correction
		vesicovaginal (VES-ih-koh-VAJ-ih-nal)
		  vesic/o- *bladder; fluid-filled sac*
		  vagin/o- *vagina*
		  -al *pertaining to*
		
		fistula (FIS-tyoo-lah)

Urethra

Word or Phrase	Description	Pronunciation/Word Parts

urethritis	Infection or inflammation of the urethra
	
	• Gonococcal urethritis is a symptom of the sexually transmitted disease gonorrhea caused by the bacterium *Neisseria gonorrhoeae*.
	• Nongonococcal urethritis is a symptom of the sexually transmitted disease chlamydia caused by the bacterium *Chlamydia trachomatis*.
	• Nonspecific urethritis is an infection or inflammation caused by bacteria, chemicals, or trauma.
	
	Treatment: Treat the underlying cause; antibiotic drug for a bacterial infection
		urethritis (YOOR-ee-THRY-tihs)
		  urethr/o- *urethra*
		  -itis *infection of; inflammation of*

Word or Phrase	Description	Pronunciation/Word Parts

Urine and Urination

Word or Phrase	Description	Pronunciation/Word Parts
albuminuria	Presence of albumin in the urine. Albumin is the major protein in the blood, and so this is also called **proteinuria**. Normally there is no protein in the urine because albumin molecules are too large to pass through pores in the capillaries of the glomerulus; but when there is kidney disease, albumin passes through the damaged pores and is excreted in the urine. Albuminuria is an important first sign of kidney disease. It is also present in pregnant women who are developing preeclampsia (described in Chapter 12, Gynecology and Obstetrics). Treatment: Correct the underlying cause.	**albuminuria** (AL-byoo-mih-NYOOR-ee-ah) **albumin/o-** *albumin* **ur/o-** *urinary system; urine* **-ia** *condition; state; thing* **proteinuria** (PROH-tih-NYOOR-ee-ah) **protein/o-** *protein* **ur/o-** *urinary system; urine* **-ia** *condition; state; thing*
anuria	Absence of urine production by the kidneys because of acute or chronic renal failure. Treatment: Diuretic drug; renal dialysis; kidney transplantation	**anuria** (an-YOOR-ee-ah) **an-** *not; without* **ur/o-** *urinary system; urine* **-ia** *condition; state; thing*
bacteriuria	Presence of bacteria in the urine. Normally, urine is sterile. Bacteria indicate an infection somewhere in the urinary tract. *Note:* A urine specimen that is not collected properly can be contaminated with bacteria when there is no infection. Treatment: Antibiotic drug	**bacteriuria** (BAK-teer-ih-YOOR-ee-ah) **bacteri/o-** *bacterium* **ur/o-** *urinary system; urine* **-ia** *condition; state; thing*
dysuria	Difficult or painful urination. It can be due to many factors (kidney stone, cystitis, etc.). Treatment: Correct the underlying cause.	**dysuria** (dis-YOOR-ee-ah) **dys-** *abnormal; difficult; painful* **ur/o-** *urinary system; urine* **-ia** *condition; state; thing*
enuresis	Involuntary release of urine in an otherwise normal person who should have bladder control. Nocturnal enuresis is involuntary urination during sleep. Laypersons call this *childhood bedwetting*. Treatment: Antidiuretic hormone, a pituitary gland hormone drug; behavioral therapy; biofeedback; acupuncture	**enuresis** (EN-yoor-EE-sihs) **enur/o-** *urinate* **-esis** *abnormal condition; process* Enuresis: *Abnormal condition (that causes the patient to) urinate (involuntarily)*
frequency	Urinating often, usually in small amounts. This can be due to a kidney stone or an enlarged prostate gland that partially blocks the flow of urine from the bladder. It can also be due to a urinary tract infection or over-active bladder. *Note:* Frequency is normally present during pregnancy when the enlarging uterus limits the capacity of the bladder; this is not a disease. Treatment: Correct the underlying cause.	
glycosuria	Glucose in the urine. This is an indication of an elevated blood sugar level that "spills over" into the urine, as seen in uncontrolled diabetes mellitus. Treatment: Correct the underlying cause.	**glycosuria** (GLY-kohs-YOOR-ee-ah) **glycos/o-** *glucose; sugar* **ur/o-** *urinary system; urine* **-ia** *condition; state; thing*

Word or Phrase	Description	Pronunciation/Word Parts
hematuria	Blood in the urine. Hematuria can be gross or frank blood (easily seen with the naked eye) (see Figure 10-14 ■), or it can be microscopic hematuria that can only be detected with urine testing. Hematuria can be caused by a kidney stone, cystitis, or bladder cancer. *Note:* It can also be due to menstrual blood that contaminates a urine specimen. Treatment: Correct the underlying cause. 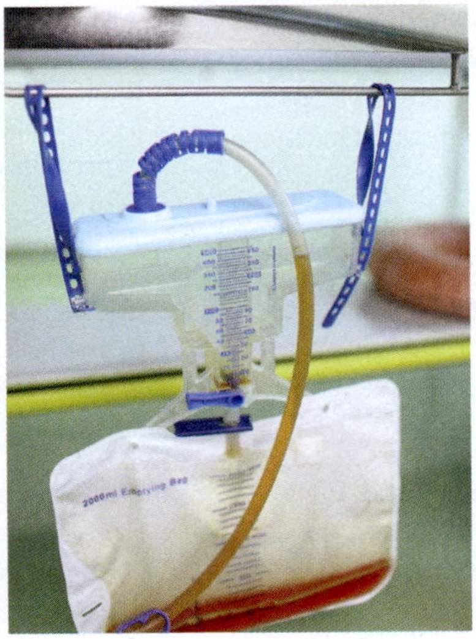 **FIGURE 10-14 ■ Hematuria.** This patient has a catheter in place in the bladder, and the urine is being collected in a bag so that the urine output can be measured. The urine shows the presence of gross blood that can be easily seen with the naked eye.	**hematuria** (HEE-mah-TYOOR-ee-ah) **hemat/o-** *blood* **ur/o-** *urinary system; urine* **-ia** *condition; state; thing*
hesitancy	Inability to initiate a normal stream of urine. There is dribbling, and the urinary stream has a decreased **caliber**. The volume of urine passed is less, and residual urine may remain in the bladder. It can be caused by blockage of the urethra by a kidney stone, a urinary tract infection, or an enlarged prostate gland. Treatment: Correct the underlying cause.	**caliber** (KAL-ih-ber)
hypokalemia	A decreased amount of potassium in the blood. It is usually due to a diuretic drug that causes the kidneys to excrete an excessive amount of urine (and potassium). Treatment: Adjust the dose of the diuretic drug.	**hypokalemia** (HY-poh-kay-LEE-mee-ah) **hypo-** *below; deficient* **kal/i-** *potassium* **-emia** *condition of the blood; substance in the blood*
ketonuria	Ketones in the urine. Ketones are waste products produced when fat is metabolized. Ketonuria is seen in patients with uncontrolled diabetes mellitus who metabolize fat for energy because they cannot metabolize glucose. It is also seen in malnourished patients who do not have enough glucose in the blood and must metabolize their own body fat. Treatment: Correct the underlying cause.	**ketonuria** (KEE-toh-NYOOR-ee-ah) **keton/o-** *ketones* **ur/o-** *urinary system; urine* **-ia** *condition; state; thing*
nocturia	Increased frequency and urgency of urination during the night. It can be due to cystitis, an enlarged prostate gland, or decreased capacity of the bladder in older adults. Nocturia is expressed as the number of times the patient urinates each night (e.g., nocturia x3). Treatment: Correct the underlying cause.	**nocturia** (nawk-TYOOR-ee-ah) **noct/o-** *night* **ur/o-** *urinary system; urine* **-ia** *condition; state; thing*
oliguria	Decreased production of urine due to kidney failure. Dehydration can cause temporary oliguria. Treatment: Correct the underlying cause.	**oliguria** (OH-lih-GYOOR-ee-ah) **olig/o-** *few; scanty* **ur/o-** *urinary system; urine* **-ia** *condition; state; thing*

Word or Phrase	Description	Pronunciation/Word Parts
polyuria	Excessive production of urine due to uncontrolled diabetes mellitus or diabetes insipidus. Treatment: Correct the underlying cause.	**polyuria** (PAW-lee-YOOR-ee-ah) **poly-** *many; much* **ur/o-** *urinary system; urine* **-ia** *condition; state; thing*
pyuria	White blood cells in the urine, indicating a urinary tract infection. Severe pyuria can cause the urine to be cloudy or milky, or the number of white blood cells may be so few that they can be detected only by microscopic examination of a urine specimen. Treatment: Antibiotic drug	**pyuria** (py-YOOR-ee-ah) **py/o-** *pus* **ur/o-** *urinary system; urine* **-ia** *condition; state; thing*
urgency	Strong urge to urinate and a sense of pressure in the bladder as the bladder contracts repeatedly. It is caused by obstruction from an enlarged prostate gland, a kidney stone, or inflammation from a urinary tract infection. Treatment: Correct the underlying cause.	

10.3 PRACTICE LAPS

Use the Answer Key at the end of the book to check your answers.

A. Give the Meaning of Combining Forms

Next to each combining form, write its meaning. The first one has been done for you.

Combining Form	Meaning	Combining Form	Meaning
1. **albumin/o-**	*albumin*	19. lith/o-	
2. bacteri/o-		20. necr/o-	
3. blast/o-		21. nephr/o-	
4. cancer/o-		22. neur/o-	
5. carcin/o-		23. noct/o-	
6. chron/o-		24. olig/o-	
7. col/o-		25. protein/o-	
8. cali/o-		26. pyel/o-	
9. contin/o-		27. py/o-	
10. cyst/o-		28. radi/o-	
11. enur/o-		29. retent/o-	
12. gen/o-		30. scler/o-	
13. glomerul/o-		31. tubul/o-	
14. glycos/o-		32. urethr/o-	
15. hemat/o-		33. ur/o-	
16. hydr/o-		34. vagin/o-	
17. kal/i-		35. vesic/o-	
18. keton/o-			

B. Build Words

Read the definition of the medical word. Look at the combining form that is given. Select the correct suffix from the Suffix List, and write it on the blank line. Then build the medical word, and write it on the line. (Remember: You may need to remove the combining vowel. Always remove the hyphens and slash.) Be sure to check your spelling.

Suffix List

-cele (hernia)	-ic (pertaining to)	-ous (pertaining to)
-ectasis (condition of dilation)	-ion (action; condition)	-pathy (disease)
-emia (condition of the blood; substance in the blood)	-itis (infection of; inflammation of)	-ptosis (state of drooping; state of falling)
-esis (abnormal condition; process)	-oma (mass; tumor)	
	-osis (abnormal condition; process)	

Definition of the Medical Word	Combining Form	Suffix	Build the Medical Word
Example: Pertaining to cancer	**cancer/o-**	*-ous*	*cancerous*

[*You think* pertaining to (-ous) + cancer (cancer/o-). You change the order of the word parts to put the suffix last. You write cancerous.]

1. Infection of (or) inflammation of (the) urethra	urethr/o-		
2. Condition of dilation (of the) calyx	cali/o-		
3. Abnormal condition (of) dead tissue	necr/o-		
4. Disease (of the) kidney	nephr/o-		
5. Action (to) hold back (urine)	retent/o-		
6. Condition of the blood (with) urine (waste products)	ur/o-		
7. State of drooping (of the) kidney	nephr/o-		
8. Hernia (of the) bladder	cyst/o-		
9. Infection of (or) inflammation of (the) bladder	cyst/o-		
10. Mass (or) tumor (that is) cancer	carcin/o-		
11. Pertaining to time	chron/o-		
12. Process (that causes the patient to) urinate (involuntarily)	enur/o-		

C. Define Abbreviations

1. AKI _____

2. CKD _____

3. ESRD _____

4. SUI _____

5. UTI _____

10.4 Laboratory, Diagnostic, and Radiologic Procedures

Word or Phrase	Description	Pronunciation/Word Parts

Laboratory Tests and Diagnostic Procedures

Word or Phrase	Description	Pronunciation/Word Parts
blood urea nitrogen (BUN)	Blood test that measures the amount of the waste product urea in the blood. It is used to monitor kidney function and the progression of kidney disease.	
creatinine	Blood test that measures the amount of the waste product creatinine in the blood. It is used to monitor kidney function and the progression of kidney disease. Together, the creatinine and BUN tests give a comprehensive picture of kidney function. A 24-hour creatinine clearance collects all urine for 24 hours to measure the total amount of creatinine "cleared" (excreted) by the kidneys. The result is compared to the level of creatinine in the blood.	
culture and sensitivity (C&S)	Urine test in which some urine is swabbed onto a culture medium in a Petri dish. This is done to identify the cause of a urinary tract infection (see Figure 10-15 ■). Microorganisms in the urine grow into colonies. The specific disease-causing microorganism is identified and tested to determine its sensitivity to various antibiotic drugs.	**culture** (KUL-chur) **sensitivity** (SEN-sih-TIV-ih-tee) **sensitiv/o-** *affected by; sensitive to* **-ity** *condition; state*

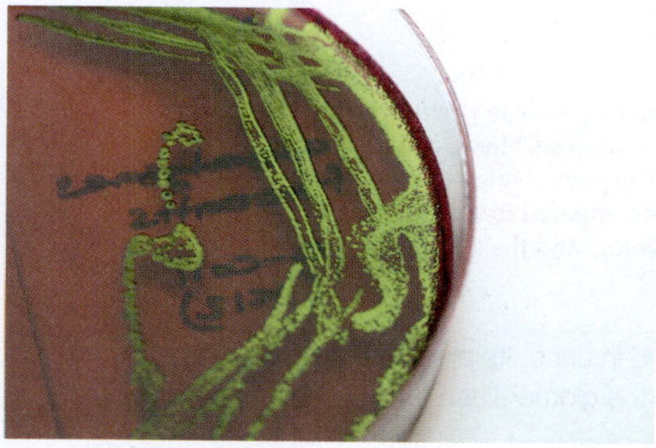

FIGURE 10-15 ■ Culture and sensitivity testing.
This Petri dish grew colonies of the bacterium *E. coli*, the most common cause of a urinary tract infection. Now that the bacterium has been identified by culture, the next step will be to do the sensitivity testing to see which antibiotic drugs the bacterium is sensitive to. One of those antibiotic drugs will then be prescribed to treat this patient's urinary tract infection.

Word or Phrase	Description	Pronunciation/Word Parts
cystometry	Diagnostic procedure that evaluates the function of the nerves to the bladder. A catheter is used to inflate the bladder with liquid (or gas). A **cystometer** is attached to the catheter to measure the pressure in the bladder. The patient indicates when he or she first feels the first urge to urinate. At that time, the cystometer makes a graphic recording known as a **cystometrogram (CMG)**.	**cystometry** (sis-TAW-meh-tree) **cyst/o-** *bladder; fluid-filled sac; semisolid cyst* **-metry** *process of measuring* **cystometer** (sis-TAW-meh-ter) **cyst/o-** *bladder; fluid-filled sac; semisolid cyst* **-meter** *instrument used to measure* **cystometrogram** (sis-toh-MEH-troh-gram) **cyst/o-** *bladder; fluid-filled sac; semisolid cyst* **metr/o-** *measurement; uterus; womb* **-gram** *picture; record*
drug screening	Urine test done to detect an individual who is using illegal, addictive, or performance-enhancing drugs	

Word or Phrase	Description	Pronunciation/Word Parts
leukocyte esterase	Urine test that detects an enzyme (esterase) associated with leukocytes (white blood cells) that are present with a urinary tract infection. This is a urine dipstick test that gives a quick result so that an antibiotic drug can be started immediately. At the same time, a urine specimen is also sent to the laboratory for C&S.	**leukocyte** (LOO-koh-site) **leuk/o-** *white* **-cyte** *cell* **esterase** (ES-ter-ays) The suffix *-ase* means *enzyme*.
urinalysis (UA)	Urine test that describes the color and characteristics of the urine and detects substances in it. A quick urinalysis can be performed in the physician's office by using a dipstick (see Figure 10-16 ■), or the urine specimen can be sent to a laboratory for a full automated analysis. A urinalysis includes the following tests. A. B. **FIGURE 10-16 ■ Urine dipstick.** **A.** This plastic strip with chemical-impregnated pads can perform several different urine tests at one time (pH, protein, glucose, blood, and ketones). The strip is dipped into a urine specimen. The pads change color over time. **B.** The final color of each pad on the strip is compared to a chart on the back of the container; the chart gives a range of colors and the associated test result numbers.	**urinalysis** (YOOR-ih-NAL-ih-sihs) *Urinalysis* contains the combining form **urin/o-** (urinary system; urine) plus a shortened form of *analysis*.
albumin	Albumin (or protein) is not normally found in urine. Its presence (albuminuria or proteinuria) indicates damage to the glomerulus.	**albumin** (al-BYOO-min)
color	Normal urine is light yellow to amber in color, depending on its concentration. Pink or reddish urine indicates red blood cells from bleeding somewhere in the urinary tract. **Turbid** (cloudy or milky) urine indicates white blood cells and a urinary tract infection.	**turbid** (TUR-bid)
glucose	Glucose is not normally found in the urine. Its presence (glycosuria) indicates uncontrolled diabetes mellitus, with excess glucose in the blood "spilling" over from the blood into the urine.	**glucose** (GLOO-kohs)
ketones	Ketones are not normally found in the urine. They are produced when the body cannot use glucose for energy or does not have enough glucose to use. Instead, the body metabolizes fat. The by-product of fat metabolism is ketones. Ketones in the urine are seen in patients with uncontrolled diabetes mellitus or malnutrition or in marathon runners.	**ketones** (KEE-tohnz)
odor	Urine has a faint odor due to the waste products in it. The urine of a patient with uncontrolled diabetes mellitus has a fruity smell because of the glucose in it. When urine stands at room temperature, bacteria from the air grow in it, breaking down the urea into ammonia; this gives old urine its characteristic smell.	

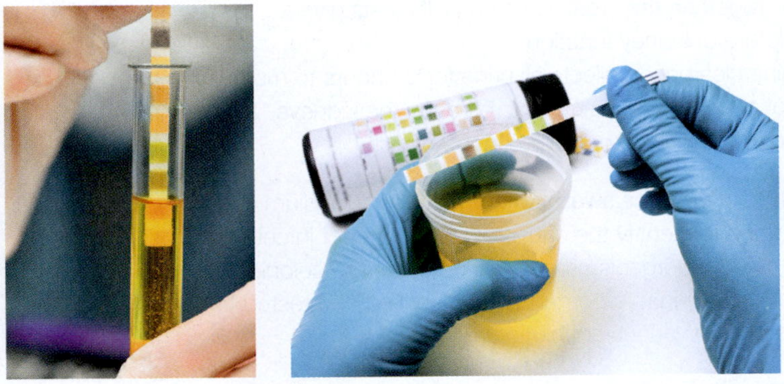

Word or Phrase	Description	Pronunciation/Word Parts

pH	The pH is a measure of how **acidic** or **alkaline** the urine is. Urine normally has a slightly alkaline pH. Acidic urine has a pH lower than 7. Alkaline urine has a pH higher than 7.	**pH** (pee-H)
		
		acidic (ah-SID-ik)
		  acid/o- *acid; low pH*
		  -ic *pertaining to*
		
		alkaline (AL-kah-line)
		  alkal/o- *base; high pH*
		  -ine *pertaining to*

red blood cells (RBCs)	Microscopic examination of the urine is done under a microscope to count the number of **erythrocytes** (red blood cells). Even clear urine can contain **occult** (hidden) blood. Microscopic hematuria is reported as the number of RBCs per **high-power field (hpf).** If the urine specimen has visible blood, the red blood cell count is reported as **TNTC (too numerous to count).** Menstrual blood can give a false-positive result of blood in the urine.	**erythrocyte** (eh-RITH-roh-site)
		  erythr/o- *red*
		  -cyte *cell*
		
		occult (oh-KULT)

sediment	There are several types of sediment in the urine. Crystals (calcium oxalate, uric acid, etc.) can form a kidney stone. **Hyaline casts** are seen with dehydration; under a microscope, they are long, clear structures. Epithelial cells (epi's) are normally present in urine sediment because they are shed continuously from the lining of the urinary tract.	**hyaline** (HY-ah-lin)
		  hyal/o- *clear, glass-like substance*
		  -ine *pertaining to*

specific gravity (SG, sp gr)	Measurement of the concentration of the urine as compared to that of water. The specific gravity of water is 1.000. Concentrated urine has a specific gravity of 1.030 or more, which means the patient has **dehydration**. A urine dipstick is commonly used to determine the specific gravity. A **refractometer** is a handheld instrument that performs a quick measurement of urine specific gravity; it uses light rays that are bent (refracted) by a thin layer of urine spread on glass.	**dehydration** (DEE-hy-DRAY-shun)
		  de- *reversal of; without*
		  hydr/o- *fluid; water*
		  -ation *being; having; process*
		
		refractometer
		(REE-frak-TAW-meh-ter)
		  re- *again and again; backward; unable to*
		  fract/o- *bend; break up*
		  -meter *instrument used to measure*
		Refractometer: *Instrument used to measure again and again (the) bend(ing of light rays in urine)*

white blood cells (WBCs)	Microscopic examination of the urine is done with a microscope to count the number of **leukocytes** (white blood cells) and identify a urinary tract infection. If the urine specimen itself is milky or cloudy, the white blood cell count is reported as TNTC (too numerous to count).	**leukocyte** (LOO-koh-site)
		  leuk/o- *white*
		  -cyte *cell*

urine protein electrophoresis (UPEP)	Urine test to detect an abnormal protein. Some urine is placed in a gel with an electrical current. Substances become charged and move toward the positive or negative electrodes. This test is used to detect Bence-Jones protein, an abnormal protein in the urine of patients with multiple myeloma (a type of cancer).	**electrophoresis**
		(ee-LEK-troh-foh-REE-sihs)
		  electr/o- *electricity*
		  phor/o- *bear; carry; range*
		  -esis *abnormal condition; process*
		Electrophoresis: *Process (of using) electricity (to) carry (substances toward a positive or negative electrode)*

Word or Phrase	Description	Pronunciation/Word Parts

Radiologic and Nuclear Medicine Procedures

Word or Phrase	Description	Pronunciation/Word Parts
intravenous pyelography (IVP)	Radiologic procedure that uses x-rays and contrast dye to visualize the urinary system (see Figure 10-17 ■). The dye is injected intravenously and flows through the blood into the renal artery and kidney. It outlines the renal pelvis, ureters, bladder, and urethra. It shows any blockage, kidney stone, or abnormal anatomy. Also known as an **excretory urography**. The x-ray image is known as a **pyelogram** or **urogram**. Alternately, a **retrograde pyelography** can be done in which a cystoscopy is performed, and a catheter is advanced up into the ureter and dye is injected. The dye outlines the ureter, as well as the renal pelvis and calices. 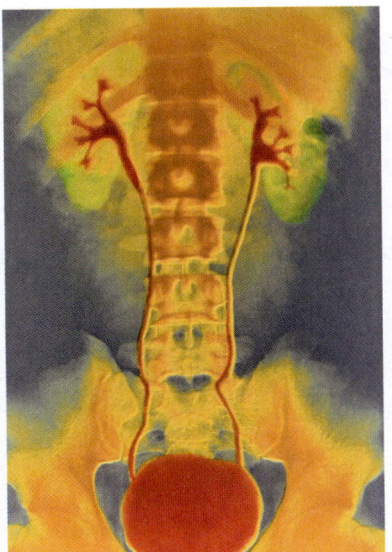 **FIGURE 10-17** ■ **Intravenous pyelogram.** In this color-enhanced image, contrast dye outlines the calices and renal pelvis of each kidney and ureters and bladder. This is a normal pyelogram with no evidence of tumor, obstruction, or kidney stone.	**intravenous** (IN-trah-VEE-nuhs) **intra-** *within* **ven/o-** *vein* **-ous** *pertaining to* **pyelography** (PY-eh-LAW-grah-fee) **pyel/o-** *renal pelvis* **-graphy** *process of recording* **excretory** (EKS-kreh-TOR-ee) **excret/o-** *removing from the body* **-ory** *having the function of* **urography** (yoor-AW-grah-fee) **ur/o-** *urinary system; urine* **-graphy** *process of recording* **pyelogram** (PY-eh-loh-GRAM) **pyel/o-** *renal pelvis* **-gram** *picture; record* **urogram** (YOOR-oh-gram) **ur/o-** *urinary system; urine* **-gram** *picture; record* **retrograde** (REH-troh-grayd) The prefix **retro-** means *backward; behind.* The suffix **-grade** means *state of going.*
kidneys, ureters, bladder (KUB) x-ray	Radiologic procedure that uses x-rays but no contrast dye to visualize the urinary system. It is used to find kidney stones or as a preliminary x-ray (scout film) before performing intravenous pyelography.	
nephro-tomography	Radiologic procedure that uses a computerized tomography (CT) scan and contrast dye injected intravenously. It takes x-ray images as multiple "slices" through the kidneys. The images can be examined layer by layer to show the exact location of tumors.	**nephrotomography** (NEH-froh-toh-MAW-grah-fee) **nephr/o-** *kidney; nephron* **tom/o-** *cut; layer; slice* **-graphy** *process of recording*

Word or Phrase	Description	Pronunciation/Word Parts
renal angiography	Radiologic procedure that uses x-rays and radiopaque contrast dye. The dye is injected intravenously and flows through the blood into the renal artery. It outlines the renal artery and shows any obstruction or blockage. It is also known as **renal arteriography**. The x-ray image is known as a **renal angiogram** or **renal arteriogram**.	**angiography** (AN-jee-AW-grah-fee) **angi/o-** *blood vessel; lymphatic vessel* **-graphy** *process of recording* **arteriography** (ar-TEER-ee-AW-grah-fee) **arteri/o-** *artery* **-graphy** *process of recording* **angiogram** (AN-jee-oh-GRAM) **angi/o-** *blood vessel; lymphatic vessel* **-gram** *picture; record* **arteriogram** (ar-TEER-ee-oh-GRAM) **arteri/o-** *artery* **-gram** *picture; record*
renal scan	Radiologic procedure that uses a radioactive substance injected intravenously. It is taken up by the kidney and emits radioactive particles that are captured by a scanner and made into an image. This procedure is done after a kidney transplantation to look for signs of organ rejection.	
ultrasonography	Radiologic procedure that uses ultrahigh-frequency sound waves emitted by a transducer or probe to produce an image of the urinary system. It is done to look for kidney stones, cysts, tumors, blockages, or infection. The ultrasound image is known as a **sonogram** (see Figure 10-18 ▪). **FIGURE 10-18 ▪ Sonogram of the kidney.** The ultrasound image on the left shows a kidney stone, as designated by the arrow. The image on the right has no stone.	**ultrasonography** (UL-trah-soh-NAW-grah-fee) **ultra-** *beyond; higher* **son/o-** *sound* **-graphy** *process of recording* **sonogram** (SAW-noh-gram) **son/o-** *sound* **-gram** *picture; record*
voiding cysto-urethrography (VCUG)	Radiologic procedure that uses x-rays and contrast dye. The dye is inserted into the bladder through a catheter and outlines the bladder and urethra. The x-ray image, taken while the patient is urinating, is known as a **voiding cystourethrogram**.	**cystourethrography** (SIS-toh-YOOR-eh-THRAW-grah-fee) **cyst/o-** *bladder; fluid-filled sac; semisolid cyst* **urethr/o-** *urethra* **-graphy** *process of recording* **cystourethrogram** (SIS-toh-yoor-EE-throh-gram) **cyst/o-** *bladder; fluid-filled sac; semisolid cyst* **urethr/o-** *urethra* **-gram** *picture; record*

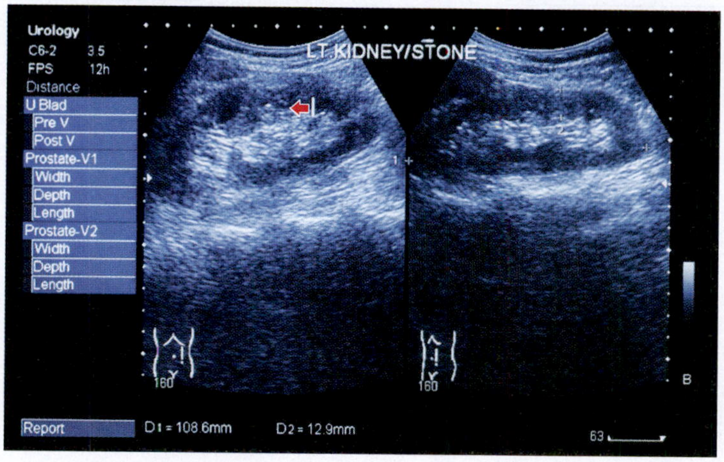

10.4 PRACTICE LAPS

Use the Answer Key at the end of the book to check your answers.

A. Give the Meaning of Combining Forms

Next to each combining form, write its meaning. The first one has been done for you.

Combining Form	Meaning	Combining Form	Meaning
1. **acid/o-**	*acid; low pH*	13. metr/o-	
2. alkal/o-		14. nephr/o-	
3. angi/o-		15. phor/o-	
4. arteri/o-		16. pyel/o-	
5. cyst/o-		17. sensitiv/o-	
6. electr/o-		18. son/o-	
7. erythr/o-		19. tom/o-	
8. excret/o-		20. urethr/o-	
9. fract/o-		21. urin/o-	
10. hyal/o-		22. ur/o-	
11. hydr/o-		23. ven/o-	
12. leuk/o-			

B. Build Words

Read the definition of the medical word. Look at the combining form that is given. Select the correct suffix from the Suffix List, and write it on the blank line. Then build the medical word, and write it on the line. (Remember: You may need to remove the combining vowel. Always remove the hyphens and slash.) Be sure to check your spelling.

Suffix List

-cyte (cell)	-ic (pertaining to)	-metry (process of measuring)
-gram (picture; record)	-ine (pertaining to)	-ory (having the function of)
-graphy (process of recording)	-ity (condition; state)	

Definition of the Medical Word	Combining Form	Suffix	Build the Medical Word
Example: Process of recording (an) artery	**arteri/o-**	*-graphy*	*arteriography*

[You think process of recording (*-graphy*) + artery (*arteri/o-*). You change the order of the word parts to put the suffix last. You write arteriography.]

1. Pertaining to (having a) low pH	acid/o-	_____	_____
2. Process of measuring (the) bladder	cyst/o-	_____	_____
3. Pertaining to (a) clear, glass-like substance (in the urine)	hyal/o-	_____	_____
4. Cell (that is) white	leuk/o-	_____	_____
5. Pertaining to (having a) high pH	alkal/o-	_____	_____
6. Having the function of removing from the body	excret/o-	_____	_____
7. Cell (that is) red	erythr/o-	_____	_____
8. Picture (or) record (of the) renal pelvis	pyel/o-	_____	_____
9. Condition (of being) sensitive to	sensitiv/o-	_____	_____
10. Process of recording urine	ur/o-	_____	_____
11. Picture (or) record (of) sound	son/o-	_____	_____

C. Define Abbreviations

1. BUN _____

2. C&S _____

3. CT _____

4. hpf _____

5. IVP _____

6. KUB _____

7. RBC _____

8. SG _____

9. TNTC _____

10. UPEP _____

11. UA _____

12. VCUG _____

13. WBC _____

10.5 Medical Procedures, Drugs, and Surgical Procedures

Word or Phrase	Description	Pronunciation/Word Parts

Medical Procedures

catheterization	Procedure in which a **catheter** (flexible tube) is inserted through the urethra and into the bladder to drain urine (see Figure 10-19 ■ and Figure 10-14). • A **condom catheter** is shaped like a condom (male contraceptive device). It fits snugly over the penis and collects urine as it leaves the urethral meatus. • A **Foley catheter** is an indwelling tube that drains urine continuously. It has an expandable balloon tip that keeps it positioned in the bladder. The urine is collected in a bag. • A **straight catheter** can be inserted if the bladder becomes full and the patient is unable to urinate, or it can be used to obtain a single sterile urine specimen for testing. • A **suprapubic catheter** is inserted through the abdominal wall (just above the pubic bone) and into the bladder. It is sometimes inserted after bladder or prostate gland surgery.	**catheterization** (KATH-eh-TER-ih-ZAY-shun) **catheter/o-** *catheter* **-ization** *process of creating; process of inserting; process of making* **catheter** (KATH-eh-ter) **condom** (CON-dom) **Foley** (FOH-lee) **suprapubic** (soo-prah-PYOO-bik) **supra-** *above* **pub/o-** *hip bone; pubis* **-ic** *pertaining to*

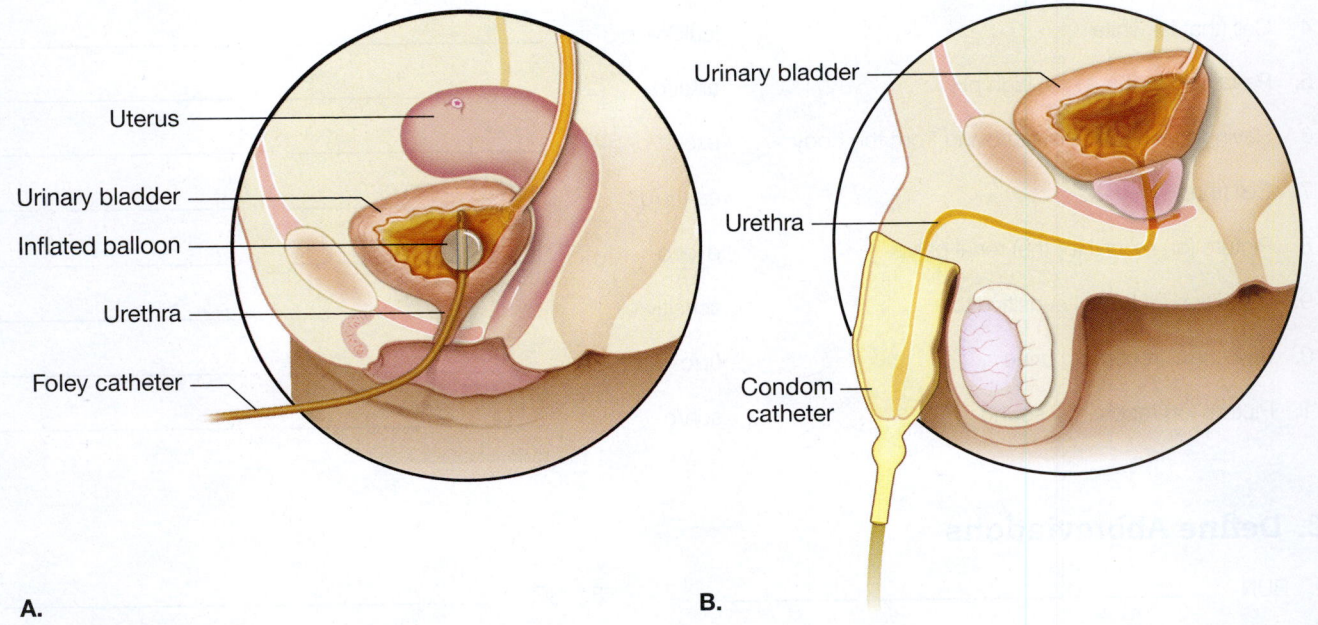

A. | **B.**

FIGURE 10-19 ■ Catheters.
A. This female patient has a Foley catheter inserted in her bladder. The balloon at the tip of the catheter is inflated after it is in the bladder; the balloon holds the catheter in place in the bladder. The catheter continuously drains urine from the bladder, and the urine is collected in a drainage bag. **B.** This male patient has a condom catheter placed over the penis. It also continuously collects urine in a drainage bag.

Word or Phrase	Description	Pronunciation/Word Parts

dialysis	Procedure to remove waste products from the blood of a patient in renal failure. Patients undergo dialysis several times a week (or more often) while waiting for a kidney transplantation. There are two types of dialysis:
	
	 • **Hemodialysis** uses an arteriovenous (AV) fistula to allow easy and reliable access to the blood (see Figure 10-20 ■). An AV fistula is created by surgically joining an artery and vein. After surgery, the fistula enlarges to accommodate two needles, one that removes blood and sends it to the dialysis machine. There the **dialysate fluid** purifies the blood and it is returned to the patient via the other needle.
	
	 • **Peritoneal dialysis** uses a permanent catheter inserted through the abdominal wall. **Dialysate fluid** flows through the catheter and remains in the abdominal cavity for several hours. During that time, the fluid pulls body wastes from the nearby blood vessels. Then the fluid is removed from the abdominal cavity, carrying waste products with it.
	
	 There are two types of peritoneal dialysis:
	
	 • In **continuous ambulatory peritoneal dialysis (CAPD)**, the patient is able to walk around between the three or four daily episodes of dialysis.
	
	 • In **continuous cycling peritoneal dialysis (CCPD)**, a machine inserts and removes dialysate fluid several times a night while the patient sleeps.
		dialysis (dy-AL-ih-sihs)
		 The prefix **dia-** means *complete; through.* The suffix **-lysis** means *process to break down or destroy.*
		
		 hemodialysis
		 (HEE-moh-dy-AL-ih-sihs)
		 The combining form **hem/o-** means *blood.*
		
		 dialysate (dy-AL-ih-sayt)
		   dia- *complete; through*
		   lys/o- *break down; destroy*
		   -ate *composed of; pertaining to*
		
		 peritoneal (PAIR-ih-toh-NEE-al)
		   peritone/o- *peritoneum*
		   -al *pertaining to*
		
		 ambulatory (AM-byoo-lah-TOR-ee)
		   ambulat/o- *walking*
		   -ory *having the function of*

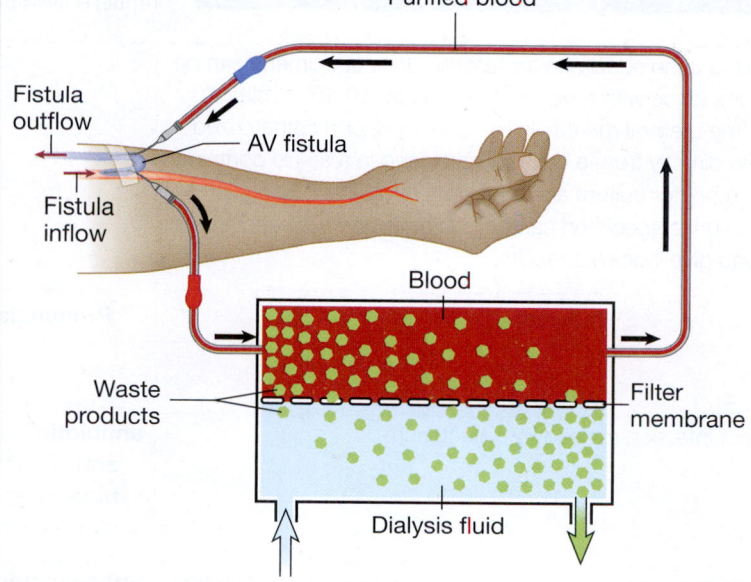

A.

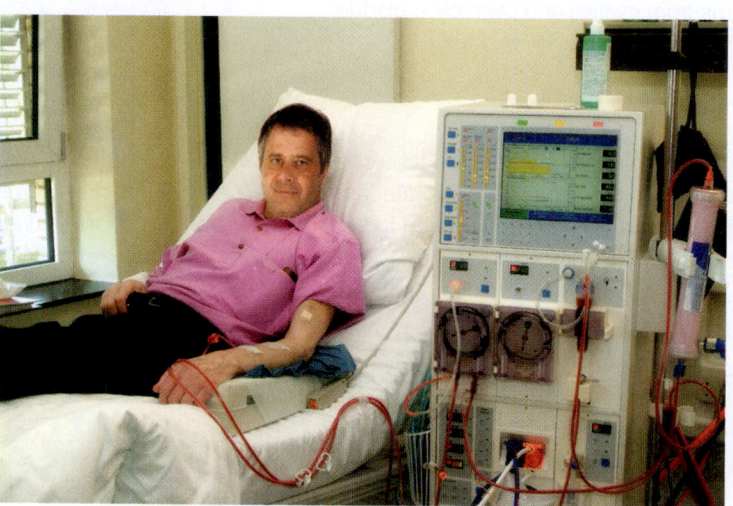

B.

FIGURE 10-20 ■ **Hemodialysis.**
A. Needles inserted into the AV fistula in the patient's arm take blood from the patient to the dialysis machine. In the machine, waste products move from an area of higher concentration (in the blood) to an area of lower concentration (in the dialysate fluid). The cleansed blood is pumped back through the fistula to the patient. **B.** This patient is undergoing hemodialysis. He comes to the dialysis center three times a week, and each session takes 3–5 hours to complete.

Word or Phrase	Description	Pronunciation/Word Parts
intake and output (I&O)	Nursing procedure that documents the total amount of fluid intake (oral, nasogastric tube, intravenous line, etc.) and the total amount of fluid output (urine, wound drainage, etc.) (see Figure 10-21 ■). It is used to monitor the body's fluid balance in patients with renal failure, burns, congestive heart failure, large draining wounds, dehydration, or overdose of diuretic drugs.	

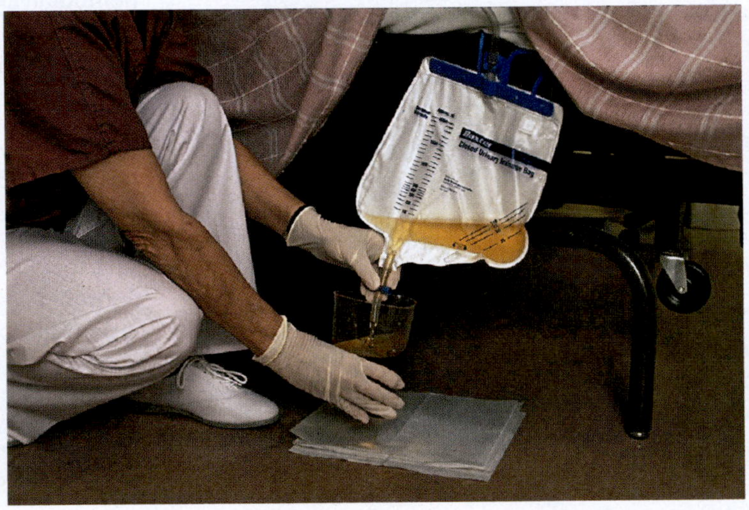

FIGURE 10-21 ■ **Urine output.**
This nurse is measuring the urine output from a patient who has an indwelling Foley catheter that continuously drains urine into a collecting bag. The volume of a liquid (urine) is measured in milliliters (mL).

Word or Phrase	Description	Pronunciation/Word Parts
urine specimen	Procedure to obtain a urine specimen for testing. Urine specimens can be tested in the doctor's office with a dipstick (see Figure 10-16). A clean-caught specimen (the urethral meatus is first cleansed) or a catheterized specimen (obtained directly from a catheter) is placed in a sterile container and sent to a laboratory for culture and sensitivity and other testing. An improperly obtained urine specimen can be contaminated with bacteria or menstrual blood and give incorrect results.	

Category	Indication	Pronunciation/Word Parts

Drugs

Category	Indication	Pronunciation/Word Parts
antibiotic drug	Treats a urinary tract infection caused by a bacterium	**antibiotic** (AN-tee-by-AW-tik) **anti-** *against* **bi/o-** *living organism; living tissue* **-tic** *pertaining to*
antispasmodic drug	Relaxes the smooth muscle in the walls of the ureter, bladder, and urethra. Used to treat spasms from cystitis and overactive bladder.	**antispasmodic** (AN-tee-spaz-MAW-dik) **anti-** *against* **spasmod/o-** *spasm* **-ic** *pertaining to*
diuretic drug	Blocks sodium from being reabsorbed from the tubules into the blood. As the sodium is excreted in the urine, it brings water and potassium with it. This decreases the volume of blood and is used to treat hypertension, congestive heart failure, and nephrotic syndrome.	**diuretic** (DY-yoor-EH-tik) **dia-** *complete; through* **ur/o-** *urinary system; urine* **-etic** *pertaining to* The *a* in *dia-* is deleted when the word is formed.
overactive bladder drug	Decreases contractions of the smooth muscle of the bladder	
potassium supplement drug	Used as a replacement for potassium excreted due to diuretic drugs	

Category	Indication	Pronunciation/Word Parts
urinary analgesic drug	Exerts a pain-relieving effect on the mucosa of the urinary tract	**analgesic** (AN-al-JEE-zik) **an-** *not; without* **alges/o-** *sensation of pain* **-ic** *pertaining to*

Word or Phrase	Description	Pronunciation/Word Parts

Surgical Procedures

Word or Phrase	Description	Pronunciation/Word Parts
bladder neck suspension	Procedure to correct stress urinary incontinence. A supportive sling of muscle tissue or a synthetic mesh is inserted around the bladder neck and the urethra to elevate and suspend them in their normal position within the pelvic cavity. In a female, this procedure is known as a **vaginal sling** when the surgical approach is done through the vagina instead of the abdomen.	**suspension** (sus-PEN-shun) **suspens/o-** *hanging* **-ion** *action; condition*
cystectomy	Procedure to remove the bladder because of bladder cancer. A **radical cystectomy** removes the bladder, surrounding tissues, and lymph nodes.	**cystectomy** (sis-TEK-toh-mee) **cyst/o-** *bladder; fluid-filled sac; semisolid cyst* **-ectomy** *surgical removal* **radical** (RAD-ih-kal) **radic/o-** *root and all parts* **-al** *pertaining to*
cystoscopy	Procedure that uses a **cystoscope** inserted through the urethra in order to examine the inside of the bladder (see Figure 10-22 ■). A wide-angle lens and a light allow a full view of the bladder. A video attachment can create a permanent visual record.	**cystoscopy** (sis-TAW-skoh-pee) **cyst/o-** *bladder; fluid-filled sac; semisolid cyst* **-scopy** *process of using an instrument to examine* **cystoscope** (SIS-toh-skohp) **cyst/o-** *bladder; fluid-filled sac; semisolid cyst* **-scope** *instrument used to examine*

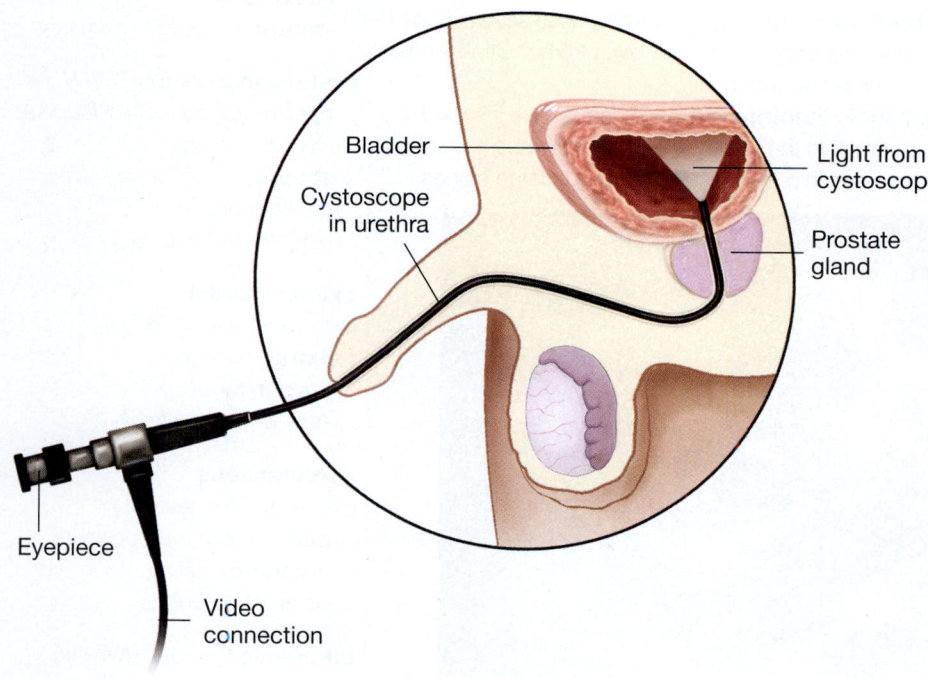

Bladder

Cystoscope in urethra

Light from cystoscope

Prostate gland

Eyepiece

Video connection

FIGURE 10-22 ■ Cystoscopy.
The cystoscope is a flexible tube that is inserted through the urethra and into the bladder. It has a viewing eyepiece and a light to illuminate the inside of the bladder.

Word or Phrase	Description	Pronunciation/Word Parts
kidney transplantation	Procedure to treat a patient in end-stage renal failure by transplanting a new kidney from a **donor** (see Figure 10-23 ■). The patient (the recipient) is matched by blood type and tissue type to the donor. The donor can be living or the kidney can come from a deceased person who has requested to be an organ donor. The patient's diseased kidney is left in place, and the renal artery of the donor kidney is sutured to the patient's iliac artery. Kidney transplantation patients must take an immunosuppressant drug for the rest of their lives to keep their bodies from rejecting their new kidney.	**transplantation** (TRANS-plan-TAY-shun) **transplant/o-** *move and put in another place* **-ation** *being; having; process* **donor** (DOH-nor)

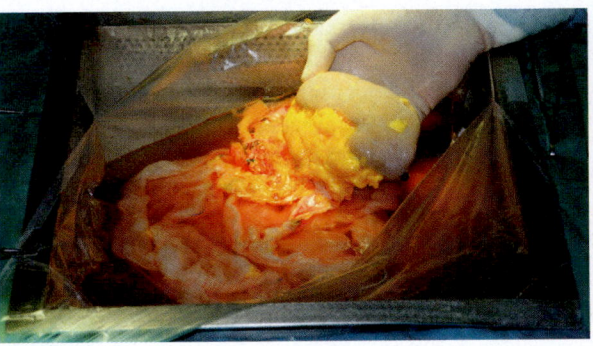 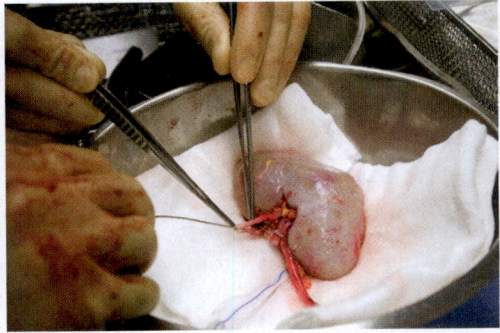

A.   B.

FIGURE 10-23 ■ Kidney transplantation.
A. This functioning kidney is being removed from a living donor. Note the retroperitoneal fat around the kidney. **B.** This donated kidney was flushed with a cold solution and kept on ice to preserve it while it was transported to the patient. Now, it is in a basin, being prepared for transplantation. The surgeons will suture the artery and vein of the donor kidney to the patient's artery and vein. The ureter of the donor kidney will be sutured to the patient's bladder.

Word or Phrase	Description	Pronunciation/Word Parts
lithotripsy	Procedure that uses a laser or sound waves to break up a kidney stone (see Figure 10-24 ■). After an x-ray pinpoints the location of the stone, a **lithotriptor** is used to break up the stone. • **Cystoscopic laser lithotripsy** uses a cystoscope with a holmium laser that is inserted into the bladder to break up a stone. • **Extracorporeal shock wave lithotripsy (ESWL)** uses several hundred pulses of high-energy ultrasonic shock waves from multiple angles outside of the body to break up the stone. • **Percutaneous ultrasonic lithotripsy** uses an endoscope inserted through the flank skin and into the kidney. A lithotriptor probe is inserted through the endoscope and into the kidney to break up large stones.	**lithotripsy** (LITH-oh-TRIP-see) **lith/o-** *stone* **-tripsy** *process of crushing* **lithotriptor** (LITH-oh-TRIP-tor) **lith/o-** *stone* **-triptor** *thing that crushes* **cystoscopic** (SIS-toh-SKAW-pik) **cyst/o-** *bladder; fluid-filled sac; semisolid cyst* **scop/o-** *examine with an instrument* **-ic** *pertaining to* **extracorporeal** (EKS-trah-kor-POR-ee-al) **extra-** *outside* **corpor/o-** *body* **-eal** *pertaining to* **percutaneous** (PER-kyoo-TAY-nee-uhs) **per-** *through; throughout* **cutane/o-** *skin* **-ous** *pertaining to* **ultrasonic** (UL-trah-SAW-nik) **ultra-** *beyond; higher* **son/o-** *sound* **-ic** *pertaining to*

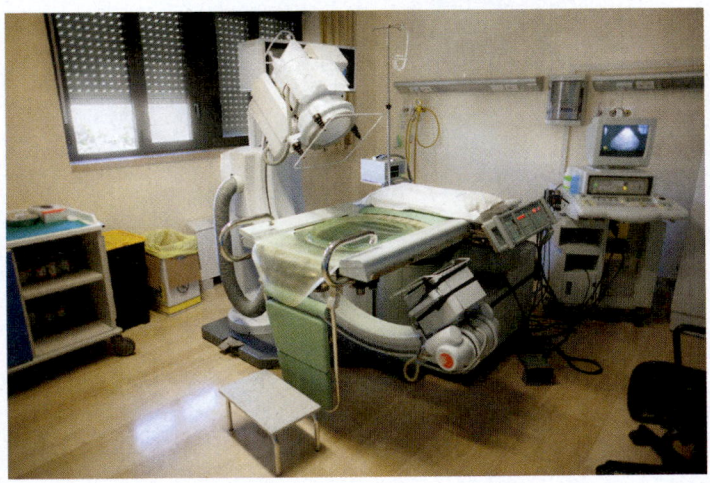

FIGURE 10-24 ■ Lithotripsy.
The patient is immersed in a tank of water. The lithotriptor emits ultrasonic frequencies that create shock waves to break up a kidney stone. The urologist watches the process on a computer screen.

Word or Phrase	Description	Pronunciation/Word Parts
nephrectomy	Procedure to surgically remove a diseased or cancerous kidney. Alternately, a healthy kidney may be removed from a donor so that it can be transplanted into a patient with renal failure.	**nephrectomy** (neh-FREK-toh-mee) **nephr/o-** *kidney; nephron* **-ectomy** *surgical removal*
nephrolithotomy	Procedure in which a small incision is made in the skin and an endoscope is inserted in a percutaneous approach into the kidney to remove a kidney stone that is embedded in the renal pelvis or calices	**nephrolithotomy** (NEH-froh-lith-AW-toh-mee) **nephr/o-** *kidney; nephron* **lith/o-** *stone* **-tomy** *process of cutting; process of making an incision*
nephropexy	Procedure to correct a kidney that is in an abnormally low position (nephroptosis) by suturing it into anatomical position	**nephropexy** (NEH-froh-PEK-see) **nephr/o-** *kidney; nephron* **-pexy** *process of fixing in place*
renal biopsy	Procedure in which a small piece of kidney is removed for microscopic analysis. This is done to confirm or exclude a diagnosis of cancer or kidney disease.	**biopsy** (BY-awp-see) **bi/o-** *living organism; living tissue* **-opsy** *process of viewing*
stone basketing	Procedure in which a cystoscope is inserted into the bladder. A stone basket (a long-handled instrument with several interwoven wires at its end) is then passed through the cystoscope to snare a kidney stone and remove it from the bladder.	
transurethral resection of a bladder tumor (TURBT)	Procedure to remove a tumor from the bladder. A special cystoscope known as a **resectoscope** is inserted through the urethra into the bladder. It has built-in instruments that resect the bladder tumor, cauterize bleeding blood vessels, and use irrigating fluid to flush pieces of tissue out of the bladder.	**transurethral** (TRANS-yoor-EE-thral) **trans-** *across; through* **urethr/o-** *urethra* **-al** *pertaining to* **resection** (ree-SEK-shun) **resect/o-** *cut out; remove* **-ion** *action; condition* **resectoscope** (ree-SEK-toh-skohp) **resect/o-** *cut out; remove* **-scope** *instrument used to examine*
urethroplasty	Procedure that involves plastic surgery to reposition the urethral meatus in a male. It is used to correct congenital hypospadias or epispadias (misplacement of the urethral meatus that is present at birth) (described in Chapter 11, Male Reproductive Medicine).	**urethroplasty** (yoor-EE-throh-PLAS-tee) **urethr/o-** *urethra* **-plasty** *process of reshaping by surgery*

10.5 PRACTICE LAPS

Use the Answer Key at the end of the book to check your answers.

A. Give the Meaning of Combining Forms

Next to each combining form, write its meaning. The first one has been done for you.

Combining Form	Meaning	Combining Form	Meaning
1. **alges/o-**	*sensation of pain*	12. peritone/o-	
2. ambulat/o-		13. pub/o-	
3. bi/o-		14. radic/o-	
4. catheter/o-		15. resect/o-	
5. corpor/o-		16. scop/o-	
6. cutane/o-		17. son/o-	
7. cyst/o-		18. spasmod/o-	
8. hem/o-		19. suspens/o-	
9. lith/o-		20. transplant/o-	
10. lys/o-		21. urethr/o-	
11. nephr/o-			

B. Build Words

Read the definition of the medical word. Look at the combining form that is given. Select the correct suffix from the Suffix List, and write it on the blank line. Then build the medical word, and write it on the line. (Remember: You may need to remove the combining vowel. Always remove the hyphens and slash.) Be sure to check your spelling.

Suffix List

-ation (being; having; process)
-ectomy (surgical removal)
-ization (process of creating; process of inserting)
-opsy (process of viewing)

-ory (having the function of)
-pexy (process of fixing in place)
-plasty (process of reshaping by surgery)
-scope (instrument used to examine)

-scopy (process of using an instrument to examine)
-tripsy (process of crushing)
-triptor (thing that crushes)

Definition of the Medical Word	Combining Form	Suffix	Build the Medical Word
Example: Thing that crushes (a kidney) stone	**lith/o-**	*-triptor*	*lithotripsy*

[*You think* thing that crushes (*-triptor*) + stone (*lith/o-*). You change the order of the word parts to put the suffix last. You write lithotriptor.]

1. Surgical removal (of a) kidney	nephr/o-	_____ _____
2. Process of using an instrument to examine (the) bladder	cyst/o-	_____ _____
3. Process of inserting (a) catheter	catheter/o-	_____ _____
4. Process of viewing living tissue	bi/o-	_____ _____
5. Surgical removal (of the) bladder	cyst/o-	_____ _____
6. Process (to) move and put in another place	transplant/o-	_____ _____
7. Instrument used to examine (the) bladder	cyst/o-	_____ _____
8. Process of crushing (a kidney) stone	lith/o-	_____ _____
9. Having the function of walking	ambulat/o-	_____ _____
10. Process of fixing in place (a) kidney	nephr/o-	_____ _____
11. Instrument used to examine (and) cut out	resect/o-	_____ _____
12. Process of reshaping by surgery (the) urethra	urethr/o-	_____ _____

C. Define Abbreviations

1. CAPD _____

2. CCPD _____

3. ESWL _____

4. I&O _____

5. TURBT _____

Abbreviations Summary

AKI	acute kidney injury		**hpf**	high-power field
ARF	acute renal failure		**I&O**	intake and output
BUN	blood urea nitrogen		**IVP**	intravenous pyelogram; intravenous pyelography
C&S	culture and sensitivity		**K⁺**	potassium
CAPD	continuous ambulatory peritoneal dialysis		**KUB**	kidneys, ureters, bladder
cath	catheterize or catheterization (short form)		**mL**	milliliter (measure of volume)
CCPD	continuous cycling peritoneal dialysis		**Na⁺**	sodium
CKD	chronic kidney disease		**pH**	potential of hydrogen (acid or alkaline)
Cl⁻	chloride		**RBC**	red blood cell
CMG	cystometrogram		**SG; sp gr**	specific gravity
CRF	chronic renal failure		**SUI**	stress urinary incontinence
CT	computerized tomography		**TNTC**	too numerous to count
cysto	cystoscopy (short form)		**TURBT**	transurethral resection of bladder tumor
epi's	epithelial cells (in urine specimen; short form)		**UA**	urinalysis
ESRD	end-stage renal disease		**UPEP**	urine protein electrophoresis (pronounced "U-pep")
ESWL	extracorporeal shock wave lithotripsy		**UTI**	urinary tract infection
GU	genitourinary; gonococcal urethritis		**VCUG**	voiding cystourethrogram; voiding cystourethrography
HCO₃⁻	bicarbonate		**WBC**	white blood cell

Word Alert

Abbreviations. Abbreviations are commonly used in all types of medical documents; however, they can mean different things to different people and their meanings can be misinterpreted. Always verify the meaning of an abbreviation.

- *C&S* means *culture and sensitivity*, but the sound-alike word *CNS* means *central nervous system*.
- *GU* means *genitourinary*, but it also means *gonococcal urethritis*.

It's Greek to Me! Did you notice that some words have two different combining forms? Combining forms from both Greek and Latin remain a part of medical language today.

Word	Greek	Latin	Medical Word Examples
bladder	cyst/o-	vesic/o-	cystitis; vesicovaginal
kidney	nephr/o-	ren/o-	nephritis; renal
(kidney) stone	lith/o-	calcul/o-	lithotripsy; calculogenesis
urinate, making urine, or urine	enur/o-, urin/o-, ur/o-	mictur/o-	enuresis, urination, hematuria; micturition
renal pelvis	pyel/o-	pelv/o-	pyelonephritis; renal pelvis

Career Focus
Meet Cindy, a dialysis nurse

"I came into dialysis because my brother actually was on dialysis for a very long time, and it was something I thought would be interesting. The dialysis center let me come in and observe for a few hours, and I found that was also very fascinating. I had already been a nurse for over 8 years. This dialysis center gave me all the on-the-job training. It was just a whole different field. You really get to know your patients. You do have the time to actually sit down and talk to them. The majority of our patients have hypertension or they have diabetes, so we do a lot of diabetic teaching."

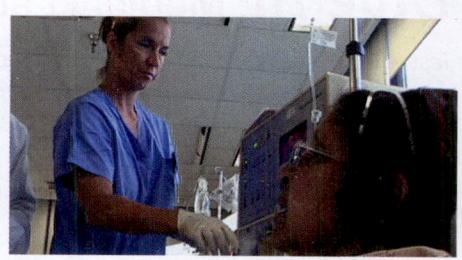

Dialysis nurses are allied health professionals who work in dialysis centers. They specialize in caring for patients with end-stage kidney disease who are receiving dialysis.

- **Urologists** are physicians who practice in the specialty of urology. They diagnose and treat patients with diseases of the urinary system, perform procedures, and do all types of urinary surgeries.

- **Nephrologists** are urologists with further specialized education who only treat patients with long-term chronic kidney disease and dialysis patients. Physicians can take additional training and become board certified in the subspecialty of pediatric nephrology.

- Cancerous tumors of the urinary tract are treated medically by an oncologist or surgically by a urologist or a general surgeon.

---

urologist (yoor-AW-loh-jist)
  ur/o- *urinary system; urine*
  log/o- *study of; word*
  -ist *person who specializes in*

---

nephrologist (neh-FRAW-loh-jist)
  nephr/o- *kidney; nephron*
  log/o- *study of; word*
  -ist *person who specializes in*

Chapter Review Exercises

Dive In: Medical Language Exercises

Test your knowledge of the chapter by completing these review exercises. Use the Answer Key at the end of the book to check your answers. Note: Each of the numbered exercise headers corresponds to a numbered learning outcome at the beginning of the chapter.

10.1 Anatomy

MATCHING EXERCISE

Match each word or phrase to its description.

1. flank   _____ lining of the bladder

2. fundus   _____ renal artery enters the kidney here

3. hilum   _____ travels the length of the penis in a male

4. mucosa   _____ also known as the *genitourinary system*

5. prostate gland   _____ doughnut-shaped gland at the base of the bladder

6. renal pelvis   _____ area of the back that overlies the kidney

7. urethra   _____ funnel-shaped area in the kidney that collects urine

8. urinary system   _____ dome of the bladder

CIRCLE EXERCISE

Circle the correct answer from the choices given.

1. The kidneys are located in the (**glomerular capsule, perineum, retroperitoneal space**).
2. The indentation in the side of the kidney is the (**cortex, hilum, ureter**).
3. The urinary system begins with the kidneys and ends with the (**bladder, prostate gland, urethra**).
4. The ureteral orifices are openings into the (**bladder, fundus, urethra**).
5. One layer of kidney tissue is the (**major calyx, medulla, peristalsis**).

TRUE OR FALSE EXERCISE

*Indicate whether each statement is true or false by writing **T** or **F** on the line.*

1. _____ There is a prostatic urethra and a penile urethra.
2. _____ The male urethra is shorter than the female urethra.
3. _____ Rugae are folds in the bladder mucosa when the bladder is empty.
4. _____ The contraction of smooth muscle to move urine into the bladder is peristalsis.

PLURAL NOUN AND ADJECTIVE EXERCISE

Read the noun and write its plural form and/or adjective form on the line. Only write in the plural noun or adjective if there is a blank line there for it. Be sure to check your spelling. The first one has been done for you.

Singular Noun	Plural Noun	Adjective	Singular Noun	Plural Noun	Adjective
1. **cortex**		*cortical*	6. mucosa		_____
2. bladder		_____	7. pelvis		_____
3. calyx	_____	_____	8. penis		_____
4. hilum		_____	9. ureter	_____	_____
5. kidney	_____	_____	10. urethra		_____

DIVIDING WORDS EXERCISE

Separate these words into their component parts (prefix, combining form, suffix). Some words do not contain all three word parts. The first one has been done for you.

Medical Word	Prefix	Combining Form	Suffix	Medical Word	Prefix	Combining Form	Suffix
1. **urinary**		*urin/o-*	*-ary*	5. ureteral			
2. excretory		_____	_____	6. sphincter		_____	_____
3. renal		_____	_____	7. prostatic		_____	_____
4. retroperitoneal	_____	_____	_____	8. urethral		_____	_____

SPELLING EXERCISE

Read each medical word pronunciation and write the medical word that it represents. Be sure to check your spelling. The first one has been done for you.

1. **(praw-STAT-ik)** _____*prostatic*_____
2. (mee-AA-tuhs) _____
3. (JEN-ih-toh-YOOR-ih-NAIR-ee) _____

4. (KAY-liks) _____
5. (yoor-EE-ter-al) _____

10.2 Physiology

MATCHING EXERCISE

Match each word or phrase to its description.

1. electrolytes
2. erythropoietin
3. filtration
4. homeostasis
5. K+
6. nephron loop
7. parenchyma
8. renin

_____ first step in the production of urine
_____ constant internal environment
_____ hormone that helps produce more red blood cells
_____ the electrolyte potassium
_____ U-shaped tube
_____ chemical elements with a positive or negative charge
_____ vasoconstrictor produced by the kidneys
_____ functional or working tissue of the kidney

CIRCLE EXERCISE

Circle the correct answer from the choices given.

1. Urea is a waste product from (**drug metabolism, muscle contraction, protein metabolism**).
2. The (**glomerular capsule, glomerulus, nephron**) is a network of intertwining capillaries.
3. Nutritional substances return to the blood in the process of (**filtrate, parenchyma, reabsorption**).
4. The hormone from the kidney that stimulates the bone marrow to make more red blood cells is (**erythropoietin, filtrate, renin**).
5. Which of these is a waste product? (**creatinine, electrolyte, sodium**).

TRUE OR FALSE EXERCISE

*Indicate whether each statement is true or false by writing **T** or **F** on the line.*

1. _____ Waste products must be continually excreted in the urine.
2. _____ The first part of a nephron is the collecting duct.
3. _____ Na+ is the electrolyte sodium.
4. _____ The products of drug metabolism are waste products.
5. _____ Blood cells can pass through the pores in the capillaries of the glomerulus.

DIVIDING WORDS EXERCISE

Separate these words into their component parts (prefix, combining form, suffix). Some words do not contain all three word parts. The first one has been done for you.

Medical Word	Prefix	Combining Form	Suffix	Medical Word	Prefix	Combining Form	Suffix
1. **micturition**		*mictur/o-*	*-ition*	6. glomerular		_____	_____
2. convoluted		_____	_____	7. homeostasis		_____	_____
3. electrolyte		_____	_____	8. reabsorption	_____	_____	_____
4. erythropoietin		_____	_____	9. tubule		_____	_____
5. filtrate		_____	_____				

SPELLING EXERCISE

Read each medical word pronunciation and write the medical word that it represents. Be sure to check your spelling. The first one has been done for you.

1. **(NEH-frawn)**   *nephron*
2. (kree-AT-ih-neen)   _____
3. (PRAWK-sih-mal)   _____
4. (HOH-mee-oh-STAY-sihs) _____

10.3 Diseases

MATCHING EXERCISE

Match each word or phrase to its description.

1. albuminuria	_____ any disease of the kidneys
2. anuria	_____ infection of the glomerulus
3. ascites	_____ within the bladder
4. calculus	_____ another name for a kidney stone
5. cystocele	_____ excessive amount of urea in the blood
6. dysuria	_____ low level of potassium in the blood
7. glomerulonephritis	_____ comes from embryonic cells still in the kidney
8. hydroureter	_____ kidneys do not produce any urine
9. hypokalemia	_____ kidney stone blocks urine and distends the ureter
10. intravesical	_____ another name for proteinuria
11. nephropathy	_____ enlarged, fluid-filled abdomen due to loss of protein in the urine
12. Wilms tumor	_____ hernia of the bladder into rectum or vagina
13. uremia	_____ difficult or painful urination

CIRCLE EXERCISE

Circle the correct answer from the choices given.

1. Renal colic is spasm of the smooth muscle because of (**cancer, a kidney stone, over-active bladder**).
2. The final, irreversible stage of renal failure is (**ESRD, SUI, UTI**).
3. Nephroptosis occurs when the kidney is (**diseased, drooping, hard**).
4. A urinary tract infection is caused by (**bacteria, incontinence, no urine production**).
5. With hematuria, there is (**albumin, bacteria, blood**) in the urine.

TRUE OR FALSE EXERCISE

*Indicate whether each statement is true or false by writing **T** or **F** on the line.*

1. _____ Wilms tumor is also known as *nephroblastoma*.
2. _____ Acute renal failure is a gradual worsening with progressive kidney damage.
3. _____ Cystocele is another name for a vesicocele.
4. _____ Incontinence is normal in babies.
5. _____ Stress incontinence in women can be improved by doing Kegel exercises.
6. _____ Pyuria is the presence of protein in the urine.
7. _____ Albumin and protein are normally found in the urine.
8. _____ Pyelonephritis is an infection of the renal pelvis and kidney.
9. _____ A vesicovaginal fistula is an abnormal passageway between the ureter and vagina.
10. _____ Renal colic is caused by a kidney stone in the intestines.
11. _____ Bacteriuria is a symptom of a urinary tract infection.

DIVIDING WORDS EXERCISE

Separate these words into their component parts (prefix, combining form, suffix). Some words do not contain all three word parts. The first one has been done for you.

Medical Word	Prefix	Combining Form	Suffix
1. **cancerous**		*cancer/o-*	*-ous*
2. anuria		_____	_____
3. caliectasis		_____	_____
4. carcinoma		_____	_____
5. cystocele		_____	_____
6. incontinence	_____	_____	_____
7. necrosis		_____	_____
8. nephropathy		_____	_____
9. nephroptosis		_____	_____
10. polycystic	_____	_____	_____
11. uremia		_____	_____

SPELLING EXERCISE

Read each medical word pronunciation and write the medical word that it represents. Be sure to check your spelling. The first one has been done for you.

1. **(KAW-lik)** _____*colic*_____
2. (NEH-froh-lith-EYE-ah-sihs) _____
3. (neh-FRAW-pah-thee) _____
4. (PAW-lee-SIS-tik) _____
5. (neh-KROH-sihs) _____
6. (yoor-EE-mee-ah) _____
7. (sis-TY-tihs) _____
8. (an-YOOR-ee-ah) _____
9. (dis-YOOR-ee-ah) _____
10. (HEE-mah-TYOOR-ee-ah) _____

10.4 Laboratory, Diagnostic, and Radiologic Procedures

MATCHING EXERCISE

Match each word or phrase to its description.

1. creatinine clearance
2. culture and sensitivity
3. cystometry
4. dipstick
5. microscopic examination
6. pH
7. specific gravity
8. urine sediment

_____ does a quick urinalysis

_____ evaluates the function of nerves to the bladder

_____ done using a high-power field

_____ concentration of urine

_____ measure of how acidic or alkaline the urine is

_____ done to identify the cause of a urinary tract infection

_____ crystals, casts, and epithelial cells

_____ often done as a 24-hour urine test

CIRCLE EXERCISE

Circle the correct answer from the choices given.

1. The instrument used to measure pressure in the bladder is a/an (**cystometer, dipstick, drug screening**).
2. A urinalysis describes all of the following *except* the (**color, odor, UPEP**) of the urine.
3. The patient has (**dehydration, kidney stones, occult blood**) if the specific gravity is above 1.030.
4. The substance that "spills over" into the urine of a patient with uncontrolled diabetes mellitus is (**albumin, glucose, sediment**).
5. The (**BUN, KUB, UA**) results show that the urine has TNTC WBC.
6. Intravenous pyelography uses (**a CT scan, contrast dye, sound waves**) to produce an image.
7. Ultrasonography uses (**radiation, sound waves, x-rays**) to produce an image.
8. To detect the presence of a kidney stone, a/an (**cystometrogram, IVP, KUB**) is performed after contrast dye is injected into a vein.

TRUE OR FALSE EXERCISE

*Indicate whether each statement is true or false by writing **T** or **F** on the line.*

1. _____ Drug screening is used to test for illegal, addictive, or performance-enhancing drugs in the urine.
2. _____ An erythrocyte is another name for a WBC.
3. _____ Albumin is usually found in the urine.
4. _____ Ketones in the urine are a by-product of fat metabolism.
5. _____ A cystometer is a handheld instrument used to measure urine specific gravity.

DIVIDING WORDS EXERCISE

Separate these words into their component parts (prefix, combining form, suffix). Some words do not contain all three word parts. The first one has been done for you.

Medical Word	Prefix	Combining Form	Suffix
1. **sensitivity**		*sensitiv/o-*	*-ity*
2. cystometry		_____	_____
3. dehydration	_____	_____	_____
4. leukocyte		_____	_____
5. intravenous	_____	_____	_____
6. pyelogram		_____	_____
7. refractometer	_____	_____	_____
8. ultrasonography	_____	_____	_____

LABORATORY TEST EXERCISE

Review the following form for ordering laboratory tests for a urology patient. Find each of the following tests and put a checkmark next to it.

albumin	creatinine, blood	culture, urine	uric acid
blood urea nitrogen	creatinine clearance	UA	

CPT CODE	LABORATORY TESTS	CPT CODE	LABORATORY TESTS
82040	Albumin	85014	Hematocrit (HCT)
82307	Blood alcohol	83036	Hemoglobin A1c
84520	Blood urea nitrogen (BUN)	84702	Human chorionic gonadotropin (hCG)
82247	Bilirubin, total	82728	Iron, total
87040	Blood culture	84132	Potassium
86900	Blood group	84144	Progesterone
82330	Calcium	85610	Prothrombin time (PT)
82375	Carboxyhemoglobin	84295	Sodium
82378	Carcinoembryonic antigen (CEA)	84403	Testosterone, total
82465	Cholesterol	84443	Thyroid-stimulating hormone (TSH)
85025	Complete blood count (CBC)	84436	Thyroxine (T4), total
82553	Creatine kinase, MB	84478	Triglycerides
82565	Creatinine, blood	84481	Triiodothyronine (T3), free
82575	Creatinine clearance	84550	Uric acid
80051	Electrolyte panel	81001	Urinalysis
82670	Estradiol	87086	Urine culture
82947	Glucose	85048	White blood cell (WBC) count with differential
82951	Glucose tolerance test		

10.5 Medical Procedures, Drugs, and Surgical Procedures

MATCHING EXERCISE

Match each word or phrase to its description.

1. biopsy	_____	has a wide-angle lens and a light to see in the bladder
2. bladder neck suspension	_____	surgery to fix a kidney in its correct position
3. catheter	_____	used to monitor the body's fluid balance
4. cystoscope	_____	also known as a *vaginal sling*
5. diuretic drug	_____	used to treat hypertension and congestive heart failure
6. intake and output	_____	removing a small piece of tissue to look for cancer or kidney disease
7. lithotriptor	_____	used to break up kidney stones
8. nephropexy	_____	flexible tube put in the bladder to drain urine

CIRCLE EXERCISE

Circle the correct answer from the choices given.

1. The nursing procedure that measures the volume of fluid taken in and the urine produced is the (**CCPD, I&O, TURBT**).

2. A kidney donor is matched to the patient needing a kidney transplantation in all of these ways *except* (**blood type, tissue type, urine type**).

3. Ultrasonic lithotripsy uses (**a laser, sound waves, x-rays**) to break up a kidney stone.

4. After the diagnosis of renal cell carcinoma was made, a (**biopsy, nephrectomy, nephropexy**) was performed to remove the entire kidney.

5. A (**catheter, fistula, cystoscope**) is surgically created in the arm in order to perform hemodialysis.

TRUE OR FALSE EXERCISE

*Indicate whether each statement is true or false by writing **T** or **F** on the line.*

1. _____ A urine dipstick test is performed in a hospital laboratory.

2. _____ A radical cystectomy removes the bladder, surrounding tissue, and lymph nodes.

3. _____ A patient taking a diuretic drug might also be taking a potassium supplement.

4. _____ Nephrectomy is surgical removal of the bladder.

DIVIDING WORDS EXERCISE

Separate these words into their component parts (prefix, combining form, suffix). Some words do not contain all three word parts. The first one has been done for you.

Medical Word	Prefix	Combining Form	Suffix
1. **antibiotic**	*anti-*	*bi/o-*	*-tic*
2. catheterization		_____	_____
3. cystectomy		_____	_____
4. dialysate	_____	_____	_____
5. cystoscope		_____	_____
6. nephrectomy		_____	_____
7. percutaneous	_____	_____	_____
8. suprapubic	_____	_____	_____
9. ultrasonic	_____	_____	_____

SPELLING EXERCISE

Read each medical word pronunciation and write the medical word that it represents. Be sure to check your spelling. The first one has been done for you.

1. **(ree-SEK-shun)** _____ *resection* _____

2. (BY-awp-see) _____

3. (sis-TEK-toh-mee) _____

4. (SIS-toh-skohp) _____

5. (DY-yoor-EH-tik) _____

6. (LITH-oh-TRIP-see) _____

7. (NEH-froh-lith-AW-toh-mee) _____

8. (TRANS-plan-TAY-shun) _____

Immerse Yourself: Analyze Medical Reports

Electronic Patient Record

This is an Emergency Department Report. Read the report and answer the questions.

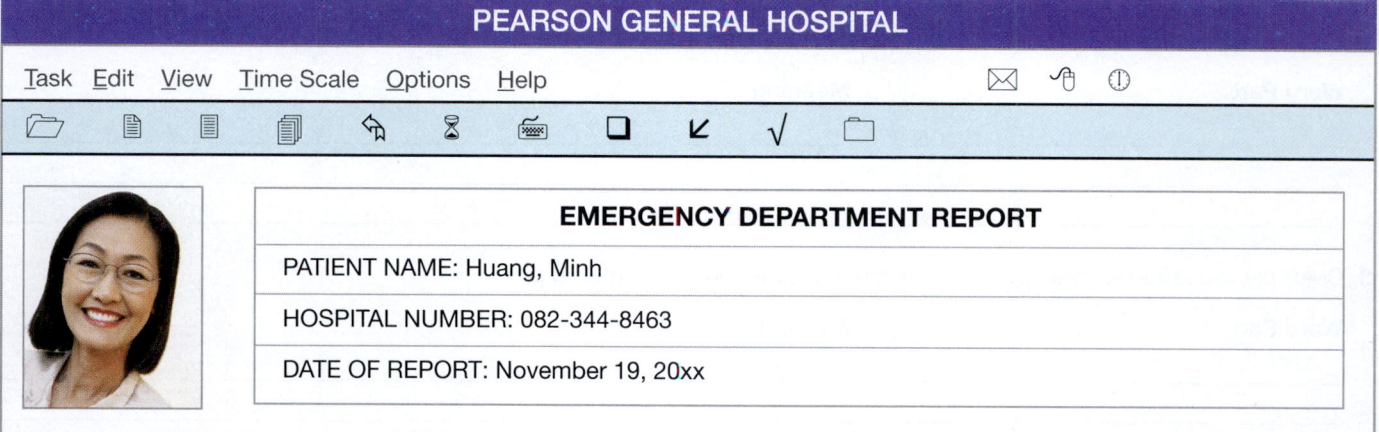

PEARSON GENERAL HOSPITAL

Task Edit View Time Scale Options Help

EMERGENCY DEPARTMENT REPORT

PATIENT NAME: Huang, Minh

HOSPITAL NUMBER: 082-344-8463

DATE OF REPORT: November 19, 20xx

CHIEF COMPLAINT
This 40-year-old female presented to the emergency department with complaints of abdominal pain and nausea and vomiting.

HISTORY OF PRESENT ILLNESS
The patient had been seen 3 days earlier in the office of her primary care physician for a complaint of pressure and pain in the urethra. She was given a tentative diagnosis of urinary tract infection. The physician ordered a clean-catch urine specimen, and the patient provided this to a nearby laboratory. The patient was given a prescription for an antibiotic drug and a urinary analgesic drug. She was told to call the office in 3 days for the result of the urine culture.

The patient states that, even though she was on the antibiotic drug, her symptoms worsened over the next 48 hours. She was drinking fluids, as recommended by her primary care physician.

This evening, when her pain became acute, with pressure in the bladder area, a sense of urgency to urinate, spasm, renal colic, and nausea and vomiting, she presented to the emergency department.

PAST MEDICAL HISTORY
Appendectomy in the remote past. She has a history of kidney stones x2, the last episode being several years ago.

SOCIAL HISTORY
She is married and sexually active in a monogamous relationship. Her husband had a vasectomy several years ago.

PHYSICAL EXAMINATION
Vital signs: Temperature 98.8, pulse 120, respirations 28, blood pressure 140/100; normal blood pressure for her is 116/90. There is tenderness to palpation over the right flank area. There is tenderness to palpation over the suprapubic area. There is no tenderness to palpation elsewhere in the abdomen. Vaginal examination is normal with no vaginal discharge or tenderness. The patient is not currently menstruating.

LABORATORY DATA
A catheterized urine specimen was obtained. It showed no bacteria, no gross blood, and no white blood cells. There was, however, microscopic hematuria. A KUB x-ray revealed no abnormalities. A pregnancy test was negative. However, a CT scan revealed a moderately sized kidney stone located in the bladder neck.

DIAGNOSIS
Solitary kidney stone at the bladder neck.

TREATMENT
In the emergency department, the patient was given pain medication and hydrated with I.V. fluids. The patient was given a urine strainer and will strain all urine. She will call to schedule an appointment with a urologist next week so that these multiple episodes of kidney stones can be investigated. If she passes the stone, the patient will bring it to the hospital laboratory for analysis. When her pain had subsided, she was released. She will follow up as described previously.

Alfred J. Strawberry, M.D.

Alfred J. Strawberry, M.D.

AJS:smt
D: 11/19/xx
T: 11/19/xx

1. Divide *urologist* into its three word parts and give the meaning of each word part.

   Word Part   **Meaning**

   _____   _____

   _____   _____

   _____   _____

2. Divide *suprapubic* into its three word parts and give the meaning of each word part.

   Word Part   **Meaning**

   _____   _____

   _____   _____

   _____   _____

3. Divide *hematuria* into its three word parts and give the meaning of each word part.

   Word Part   **Meaning**

   _____   _____

   _____   _____

   _____   _____

4. What does the abbreviation *KUB* stand for? _____

5. The phrase "tentative diagnosis of a urinary tract infection" could be written with an abbreviation as "tentative diagnosis of a

   _____."

6. What type of urine specimen was obtained by the physician's office lab? _____

7. What type of urine specimen was obtained in the emergency department? _____

8. Why was the patient given a urine strainer?_____

9. Why was it important to know that the patient has already had an appendectomy? _____

10. Why were the patient's pulse, respirations, and blood pressure elevated on admission to the emergency department, but not her temperature? _____

11. Why is it important to know that the patient is not menstruating? _____

12. What is the reason for her microscopic hematuria? _____

13. Why was it important to know that the patient was in a monogamous relationship and that her husband has had a vasectomy? _____

RELATED COMBINING FORMS EXERCISE

Write the combining form on the line provided. (Hint: See the It's Greek to Me! feature box.)

1. Two combining forms that mean *bladder*. _____ _____

2. Two combining forms that mean *kidney*. _____ _____

3. Two combining forms that mean *(kidney) stone*. _____ _____

4. Two combining forms that mean *renal pelvis*. _____ _____

Research Medical Words

ON-THE-JOB CHALLENGE EXERCISE

On the job, you will often encounter new medical words. Practice your medical language skills by researching the medical word in bold and writing its definition on the blank line.

OFFICE CHART NOTE

The patient presented with **strangury** and dysuria. A urinalysis showed both WBCs and RBCs. A diagnosis of cystitis was made, and the patient was given an antibiotic drug.

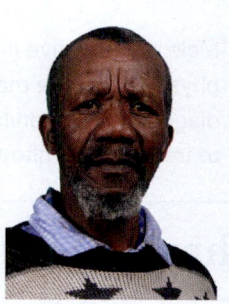

Strangury: _____

SOUND-ALIKE WORDS EXERCISE

Compare and contrast the medical meanings of these sound-alike urology and other words.

1. *calculus* and *calcaneus* (Chapter 7)

_____

2. *vesical* and *vesicle* (Chapter 2)

_____

3. *cortex of the kidney* and *cortex of the adrenal gland* (Chapter 13)

_____

4. *peristalsis* and *peristalsis* (Chapter 3)

_____

MyLab Medical Terminology™

MyLab Medical Terminology is a premium online homework management system that includes a host of features to help you study. Registered users will find:

- A multitude of quizzes and activities built within the MyLab platform

- Powerful tools that track and analyze your results—allowing you to create a personalized learning experience

- Videos and audio pronunciations to help enrich your progress

- Streaming lesson presentations (guided lectures) and self-paced learning modules

- A space where you and your instructor can check your progress and manage your assignments

11 Male Reproductive Medicine
Male Genitourinary System

Male reproductive (REE-proh-DUK-tiv) medicine is the medical specialty that studies the anatomy and physiology of the male genitourinary system; uses laboratory, diagnostic, and radiologic procedures to diagnose male genitourinary diseases; and uses medical procedures, drugs, and surgical procedures to treat male genitourinary diseases.

∨ Chapter Overview and Learning Outcomes

After you study this chapter, you should be able to demonstrate mastery of the outcomes by successfully completing the exercises.

11.1 Anatomy
Identify the structures of the male genitourinary system.
Demonstrate proficiency in medical language.
11.1 Practice Laps

11.2 Physiology
Describe the functions of the male genitourinary system.
Demonstrate proficiency in medical language.
11.2 Practice Laps
Vocabulary Review

11.3 Diseases
Describe common male genitourinary diseases.
Demonstrate proficiency in medical language.
11.3 Practice Laps

11.4 Laboratory, Diagnostic, and Radiologic Procedures
Describe common male genitourinary laboratory tests, diagnostic procedures, and radiologic procedures.
Demonstrate proficiency in medical language.
11.4 Practice Laps

11.5 Medical Procedures, Drugs, and Surgical Procedures
Describe common male genitourinary medical procedures, drugs, and surgical procedures.
Demonstrate proficiency in medical language.
11.5 Practice Laps
Abbreviations Summary
Career Focus

Chapter Review Exercises
Dive In: Medical Language Exercises
(Learning Outcomes 11.1–11.5)
Immerse Yourself: Analyze Medical Reports

Medical Language Key

To unlock the definition of a medical word, first break it into word parts. Then give the meaning of each word part. Put the meanings of the word parts in order, beginning with the meaning of the suffix, then the meaning of the prefix (if there is one), then the meaning of the combining form.

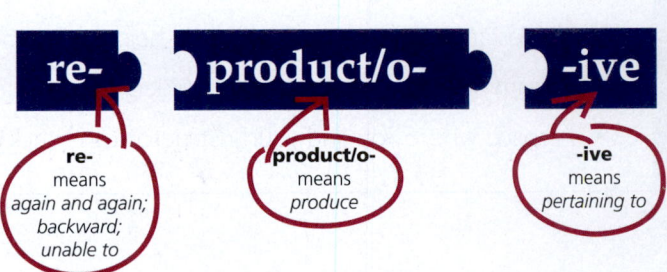

re- means again and again; backward; unable to

product/o- means produce

-ive means pertaining to

Reproductive: ▶ *(Medical specialty) pertaining to again and again produc(ing children).*

The **male genitourinary (GU) system** is a pathway of structures that consists of both the external and internal **genitalia** or **genital organs**. This body system begins outside the body (external), continues within the body (internal), and ends outside the body (external again) (see Figure 11-1 ■). The **external genitalia** include the scrotum, the testes, the epididymides, and part of the vas deferens. Then the pathway transitions to inside the body. The **internal genitalia** are in the pelvic cavity, and they include the rest of the vas deferens, the seminal vesicles, the ejaculatory ducts, the prostate gland, prostatic urethra, and the bulbourethral glands and ducts. Finally, the pathway ends outside the body, where the rest of the external genitalia consists of the penis and penile urethra. The genitourinary system is also known as the **urogenital system** because the male genitalia and the urinary system share some of the same structures and functions.

The function of the male genitourinary system is reproductive, and so it secretes the male hormone testosterone, develops secondary sexual characteristics in the male, produces sperm, and releases semen. In addition, the male genitourinary system complements the work of the urinary system by providing a passageway for urine as it leaves the body.

11.1 Anatomy

External Genitalia

Scrotum

The **scrotum** is a soft pouch of skin behind the penis and in front of the legs (see Figure 11-2 ■). It contains the testes, the epididymides, and part of each vas deferens. Because it is outside the body, the scrotum is always a few degrees cooler than the body's temperature. This temperature difference is necessary for the proper development of sperm. Muscles in the wall of the scrotum contract or relax to move the scrotum closer to or farther away from the body to adjust to temperature changes in the environment. The **perineum** is the area between the posterior scrotum and the anus (which is part of the gastrointestinal system).

Testis

The scrotum contains two **testes** or **testicles**. Each testis is an egg-shaped gland about 2 inches in length (see Figure 11-2). Each testis contains **seminiferous tubules**, small, tightly coiled tubes that produce **spermatozoa** (also known as **sperm**) (see Figure 11-3 ■). Mature spermatozoa are continuously released into the lumen (central opening) of the seminiferous tubules. Each spermatozoon has a head and a tail (flagellum) that propels it forward.

The testes are the **gonads** or sex glands in a male. *Note*: The female gonads are the ovaries, the sex glands that produce an egg (ovum) (described in Chapter 12, Gynecology and Obstetrics).

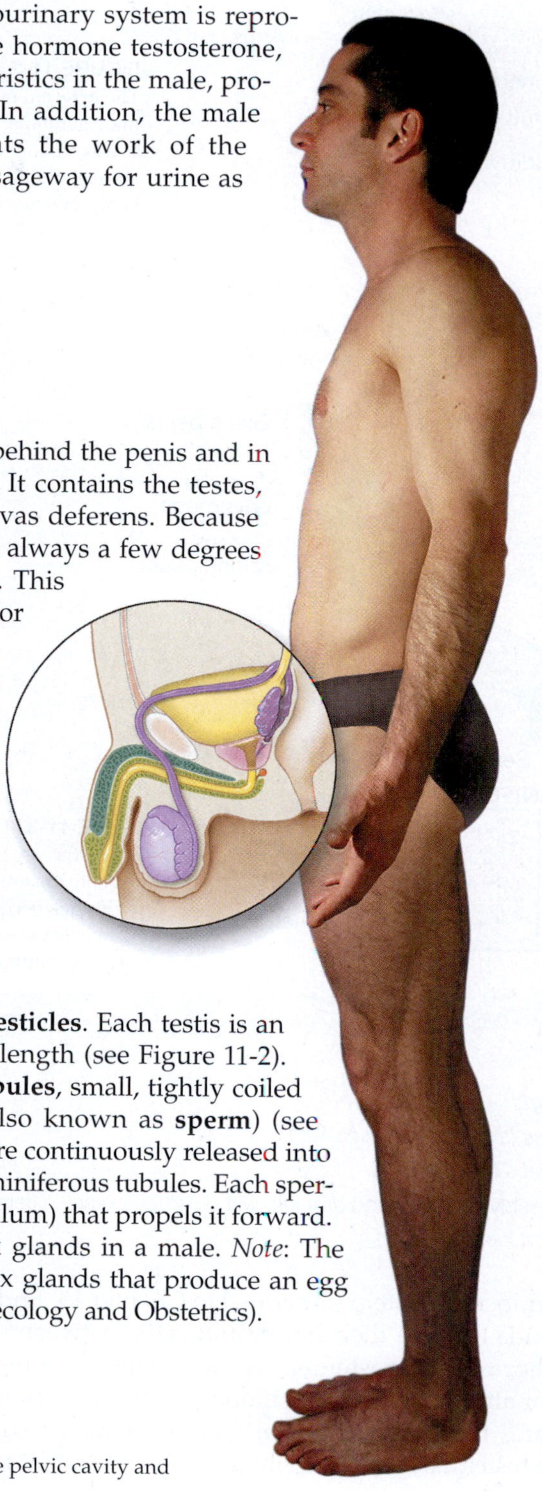

FIGURE 11-1 ■ Male genitourinary system.
The male genitourinary system is located in the pelvic cavity and outside of the body.

Pronunciation/Word Parts

genitourinary (JEN-ih-toh-YOOR-ih-NAIR-ee)
genit/o- *genitalia*
urin/o- *urinary system; urine*
-ary *pertaining to*

genitalia (JEN-ih-TAY-lee-ah)

genital (JEN-ih-tal)
genit/o- *genitalia*
-al *pertaining to*

urogenital (YOOR-oh-JEN-ih-tal)

scrotum (SKROH-tum)

scrotal (SKROH-tal)
scrot/o- *scrotum*
-al *pertaining to*

perineum (PAIR-ih-NEE-um)

perineal (PAIR-ih-NEE-al)
perine/o- *perineum*
-al *pertaining to*

testis (TES-tihs)
The combining forms **didym/o-**, **orchid/o-**, **orchi/o-**, **orch/o-**, **test/i-**, and **test/o-** mean *testis*.

testes (TES-teez)
Latin plural noun: Change the singular ending *-is* to *-es*.

testicle (TES-tih-kul)
test/i- *testis*
-cle *small thing*

testicular (tes-TIH-kyoo-lar)
testicul/o- *testicle; testis*
-ar *pertaining to*

seminiferous (SEM-ih-NIF-er-uhs)
semin/i- *sperm; spermatozoon*
fer/o- *bear*
-ous *pertaining to*

tubule (TOO-byool)
tub/o- *tube*
-ule *small thing*

spermatozoon (SPER-mah-toh-ZOH-on)
spermat/o- *sperm; spermatozoon*
-zoon *animal; living thing*

spermatozoa (SPER-mah-toh-ZOH-ah)
Greek plural noun: Change the singular ending *-on* to *-a*.

sperm (SPERM)
The combining form **sperm/o-** also means *sperm; spermatozoon*.

spermatic (sper-MAT-ik)
spermat/o- *sperm; spermatozoon*
-ic *pertaining to*

gonad (GOH-nad)
gon/o- *ovum; spermatozoon*
-ad *in the direction of; toward*

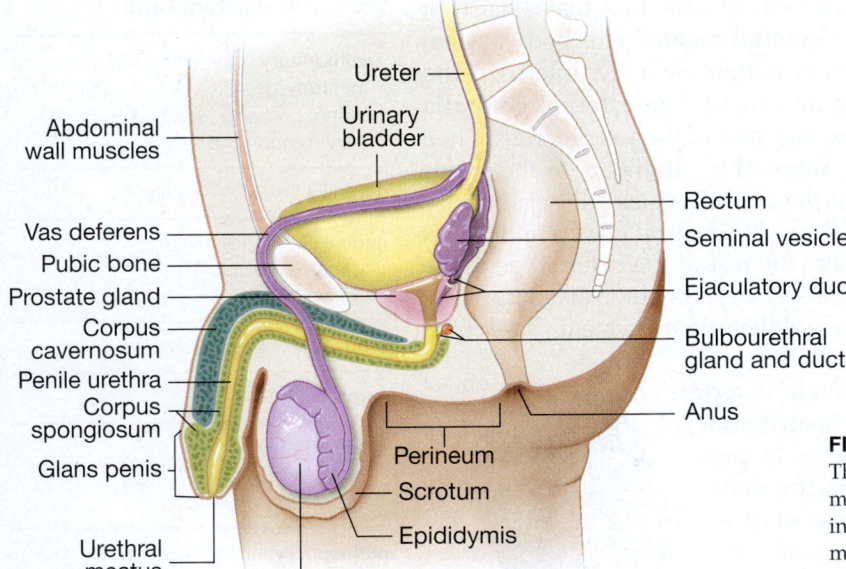

FIGURE 11-2 ■ External and internal male genitalia.
The external male genitalia are connected to the internal male genitalia. Structures of the urinary system are also involved: the urinary bladder is located near the internal male genitalia, and the urethra is shared by both the male genitourinary system and the urinary system.

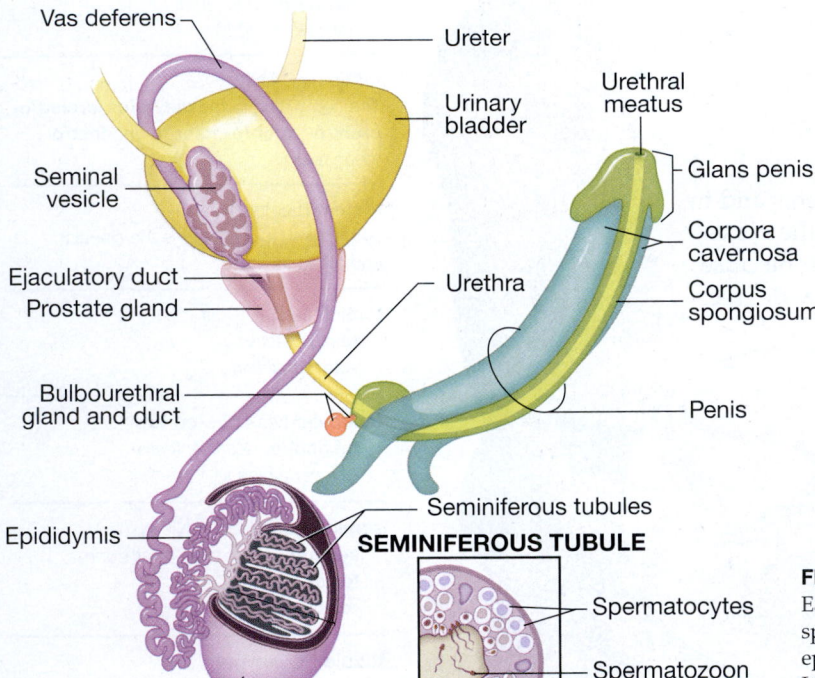

FIGURE 11-3 ■ Structures of the testis and penis.
Each testis contains the seminiferous tubules where spermatozoa are formed. The tightly coiled tube of the epididymis becomes the long, straight duct of the vas deferens. It connects the external genitalia to the internal genitalia. The three columns of erectile tissue in the penis can be seen.

Did You Know?

Scrotum is a Latin word meaning *a bag*.

Testis is a Latin word meaning *a witness (to a man's masculinity)*.

Didymis, the Greek word for *testis*, means *two or twins*.

Testis and *testicle* are used interchangeably (like *drop* and *droplet*), without implying any difference in size.

The testes are also part of the endocrine system (described in Chapter 13, Endocrinology). They are endocrine glands because their **interstitial cells** (between the seminiferous tubules) secrete the hormone testosterone. **Testosterone** is the most abundant and biologically active of all the male sex hormones; it stimulates spermatozoa to mature, and it stimulates the development of male secondary sexual characteristics during puberty. The testes also secrete a small amount of the female hormone estradiol.

Pronunciation/Word Parts

interstitial (IN-ter-STIH-shal)
   interstiti/o- *spaces between tissues*
   -al *pertaining to*

testosterone (tes-TAW-steh-rohn)
Testosterone contains the combining forms **test/o-** (testis) and **steroid/o-** (steroid) and the suffix **-one** (chemical substance).

Epididymis

The **epididymis** is attached to the outer wall of each testis. Each epididymis is a long (20 foot), but tightly coiled, structure (see Figures 11-2 and 11-3). Spermatozoa in the seminiferous tubules are carried by fluid into the epididymis. Within the epididymis, the head of each spermatozoon is given a cap-like layer of enzymes that will eventually help it penetrate and fertilize the egg of the female. Spermatozoa in the epididymis are mature but not yet moving. The epididymis also destroys any defective spermatozoa that are present. The coiled epididymis then becomes the larger, uncoiled duct known as the *vas deferens*.

Vas Deferens

The **vas deferens** is a long duct that receives spermatozoa from the epididymis (see Figures 11-2 and 11-3). Spermatozoa can be stored in the vas deferens for several months in an inactive state. Each vas deferens travels superiorly to become part of the internal genitalia in the pelvic cavity.

Pronunciation/Word Parts

epididymis (EP-ih-DID-ih-mihs)

epididymides (EP-ih-dih-DIM-ih-deez) Greek plural noun: Change the singular ending *-is* to *-ides*. The prefix **epi-** means *above; upon*. The combining form **didym/o-** means *testis*.

vas deferens (VAS DEF-er-enz) The combining form **vas/o-** means *blood vessel; vas deferens*.

Clinical Connections

Neonatology. In the fetus, the testes and vas deferens are not in the scrotum. They develop in the pelvic cavity. Each fetal testis has a **spermatic cord**, a tube that contains the vas deferens, as well as arteries, veins, and nerves. Two months before birth, each testis and its spermatic cord pass through the **inguinal canal** (an opening in the abdominal wall muscle), travel over the pubic bone and through the groin area, to the final permanent location in the scrotum (see Figure 11-4 ■). At that point, the spermatic cord separates into the vas deferens and the other structures. The opening of the inguinal canal usually closes before age 2.

spermatic (sper-MAT-ik)
spermat/o- *sperm; spermatozoon*
-ic *pertaining to*

inguinal (ING-gwih-nal)
inguin/o- *groin*
-al *pertaining to*

canal (kah-NAL)

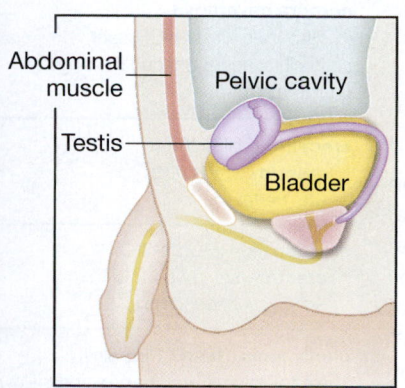
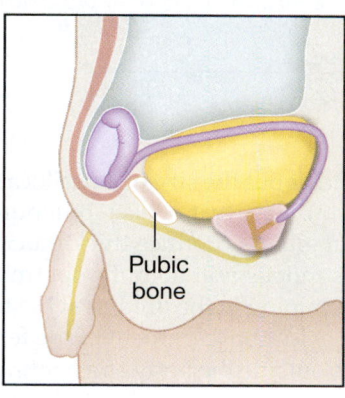
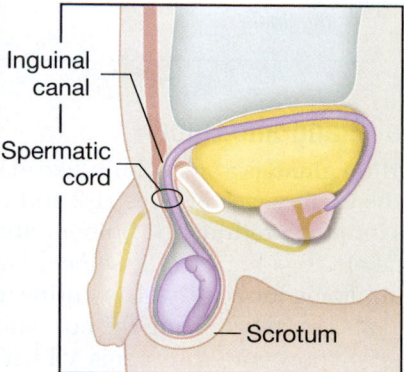

Position of testis in 5-month fetus

Position of testis in 7-month fetus

Position of testis in newborn

FIGURE 11-4 ■ Descent of the testes before birth.
Before birth, the testes and their spermatic cords move from the pelvic cavity, through the inguinal canals, and into the scrotum.

Internal Genitalia

Vas Deferens

Once each **vas deferens** is in the pelvic cavity, it is considered to be part of the internal genitalia. It travels behind the urinary bladder and ends as it merges with the seminal vesicle (see Figures 11-2 and 11-3).

Seminal Vesicle

The **seminal vesicle** is an elongated gland that forms a V-shaped pair along the posterior wall of the urinary bladder (see Figures 11-2 and 11-3). Each seminal gland produces **seminal fluid**, which makes up most of the volume of **semen**. Seminal fluid contains a high level of fructose (a sugar), which is a source of energy for the spermatozoa. The seminal vesicle ends in the ejaculatory duct.

vas deferens (VAS DEF-er-enz) The combining form **vas/o-** means *blood vessel; vas deferens*.

seminal (SEM-ih-nal)
semin/o- *sperm; spermatozoon*
-al *pertaining to*

vesicle (VES-ih-kul)

semen (SEE-men)
Semen is a Latin word meaning seed.

Ejaculatory Duct

The **ejaculatory duct** is a collecting duct (see Figures 11-2 and 11-3). It holds spermatozoa from each vas deferens as well as seminal fluid from the seminal vesicles. Each ejaculatory duct enters the prostate gland and joins with the prostatic urethra from the urinary bladder.

Prostate Gland

The **prostate gland** is a doughnut-shaped gland at the base of the urinary bladder (see Figures 11-2 and 11-3). The urethra from the urinary bladder goes through the center of the prostate gland, and so this part of the urethra is known as the **prostatic urethra**. The prostate gland produces **prostatic fluid**, a milky substance that makes up some of the volume of semen. This fluid contains an antibiotic substance that will kill any bacteria present in the female's vagina. Prostatic fluid also contains a substance that activates enzymes in the head of each spermatozoon so that it can eventually penetrate the female's egg to fertilize it. Prostatic fluid also contains acid phosphatase, an enzyme that will break apart the deposit of semen and release the spermatozoa in the female's vagina. The prostatic urethra becomes the urethra as it leaves the prostate gland.

Word Alert
Sound-Alike Words

prostate	(noun)	gland that surrounds the urethra in men
		Example: When the prostate gland is enlarged, it interferes with urination in men.
prostrate	(adjective)	lying in a face-down position from humility or exhaustion
		Example: After the marathon race, the exhausted winner lay prostrate on the track.

Bulbourethral Gland and Duct

The **bulbourethral gland** is a small, bulb-like gland about the size of a pea located on either side of the urethra (see Figures 11-2 and 11-3). The duct of each bulbourethral gland empties into the urethra. The bulbourethral glands produce thick mucus that makes up some of the volume of the semen. This mucus will help the spermatozoa survive by neutralizing the acidity of any urine remaining in the urethra at the time of ejaculation and also by neutralizing the normally acidic environment of the female's vagina. The urethra now enters the penis, which is outside the body as a continuation of the external genitalia.

External Genitalia

Penis

The rest of the external genitalia consists of the penis and the part of the urethra (penile urethra) that continues within the penis. The **penis** functions as an organ of both the male genital system and the urinary system. As an organ of the male genital system, the penis has an erection to facilitate sexual intercourse. The penis contains three columns of tissue that run its length (see Figures 11-2 and 11-3). One column, the **corpus spongiosum**, is along the underside of the penis. The other two columns, the **corpora cavernosa**, are along the upper surface of the penis. These three columns are composed of **erectile tissue** that fills with blood, causing an **erection** as the penis becomes firm and erect. The penile urethra is the passageway for semen to reach the outside of the body. The **glans penis** is the enlarged tip at the end of the penis. In uncircumcised males, the glans penis is covered by a fold of skin known as the **prepuce** or **foreskin**.

As an organ of the urinary system, the penis contains the penile urethra, which is a passageway for urine to reach the outside of the body. The **urethral meatus** (end opening) is located at the tip of the glans penis (see Figure 11-2 and 11-3).

Pronunciation/Word Parts

ejaculatory (ee-JAH-kyoo-lah-TOR-ee)
  ejaculat/o- *expel suddenly*
  -ory *having the function of*

prostate (PRAW-stayt)

prostatic (praw-STAT-ik)
  prostat/o- *prostate gland*
  -ic *pertaining to*

urethra (yoor-EE-thrah)

urethral (yoor-EE-thral)
  urethr/o- *urethra*
  -al *pertaining to*

bulbourethral (BUL-boh-yoor-EE-thral)
  bulb/o- *bulb-like structure*
  urethr/o- *urethra*
  -al *pertaining to*

penis (PEE-nihs)

penile (PEE-nile)
  pen/o- *penis*
  -ile *pertaining to*

corpus spongiosum
(KOR-puhs SPUN-jee-OH-sum)

corpora cavernosa
(KOR-por-ah KAV-er-NOH-sah)
Latin plural noun: Change the singular ending *-us* to *-a*.

erectile (ee-REK-tile)
  erect/o- *stand up*
  -ile *pertaining to*

erection (ee-REK-shun)
  erect/o- *stand up*
  -ion *action; condition*

glans penis (GLANZ PEE-nihs)
The combining form **balan/o-** means *glans penis*.

prepuce (PREE-poos)

meatus (mee-AA-tuhs)

Word Alert

Sound-Alike Words

gland   (noun)   the prostate gland of the male genitourinary system
a structure of the endocrine system that secretes hormones into the blood
Example: The anterior pituitary gland in the brain secretes hormones that stimulate the testes at the beginning of puberty.

glans   (noun)   enlarged, rounded area
Example: The glans penis is covered by the foreskin in uncircumcised males.

11.1 PRACTICE LAPS

Use the Answer Key at the end of the book to check your answers.

A. Label Structures

Write each anatomy word or phrase in the correct numbered box. Be sure to check your spelling.

bulbourethral gland	epididymis	prostate gland	testis
corpus cavernosum	glans penis	scrotum	vas deferens
ejaculatory duct	penile urethra	seminal vesicle	

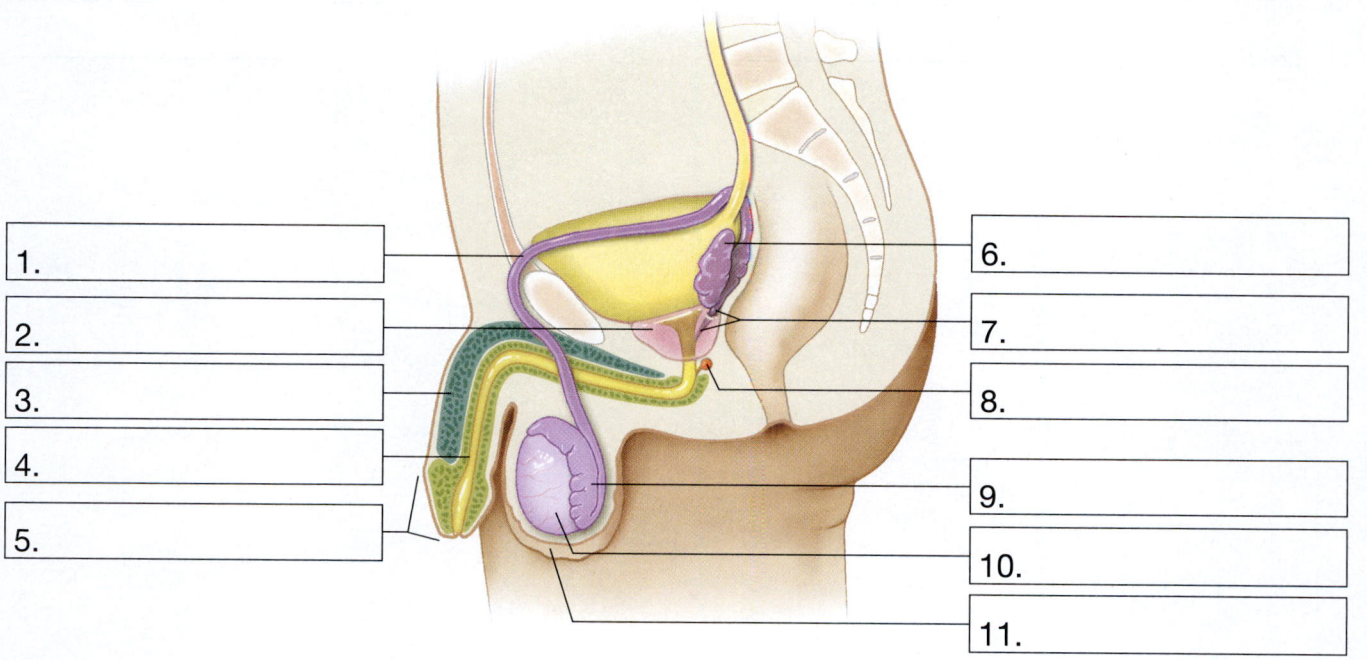

1.

2.

3.

4.

5.

6.

7.

8.

9.

10.

11.

B. Give the Meaning of Combining Forms

Next to each combining form, write its meaning. The first one has been done for you.

Combining Form	Meaning	Combining Form	Meaning
1. **balan/o-**	*glans penis*	15. perine/o-	
2. bulb/o-		16. prostat/o-	
3. didym/o-		17. scrot/o-	
4. ejaculat/o-		18. semin/i-	
5. erect/o-		19. semin/o-	
6. fer/o-		20. spermat/o-	
7. genit/o-		21. sperm/o-	
8. gon/o-		22. test/i-	
9. inguin/o-		23. test/o-	
10. interstiti/o-		24. testicul/o-	
11. orchid/o-		25. tub/o-	
12. orchi/o-		26. urethr/o-	
13. orch/o-		27. urin/o-	
14. pen/o-		28. vas/o-	

C. Build Words

Read the definition of the medical word. Look at the combining form that is given. Select the correct suffix from the Suffix List, and write it on the blank line. Then build the medical word, and write it on the line. (Remember: You may need to remove the combining vowel. Always remove the hyphens and slash.) Be sure to check your spelling.

Suffix List

-ad (in the direction of; toward)	-ar (pertaining to)	-ile (pertaining to)	-ule (small thing)
-al (pertaining to)	-cle (small thing)	-ion (action; condition)	-zoon (animal; living thing)
	-ic (pertaining to)	-ory (having the function of)	

Definition of the Medical Word	Combining Form	Suffix	Build the Medical Word
Example: Small thing (that is a) tube	**tub/o-**	*-ule*	*tubule*

[*You think* small thing (-ule) + tube (tub/o-). You change the order of the word parts to put the suffix last. You write tubule.]

1. Pertaining to (the) genitalia	genit/o-		
2. Pertaining to (the) testicle	testicul/o-		
3. Pertaining to (the) scrotum	scrot/o-		
4. Living thing (that is) sperm	spermat/o-		
5. Pertaining to (an) ovum (or) spermatozoon	gon/o-		
6. Pertaining to (the) genitalia	genit/o-		
7. Pertaining to (the) perineum	perine/o-		
8. Small thing (that is a) testis	test/i-		
9. Pertaining to sperm	spermat/o-		
10. Having the function of (to) expel suddenly	ejaculat/o-		
11. Pertaining to (the) prostate gland	prostat/o-		
12. Pertaining to (the) groin	inguin/o-		
13. Pertaining to (the) penis	pen/o-		
14. Action (of the penis to) stand up	erect/o-		

11.2 Physiology

During **puberty**, the body undergoes rapid changes to reach **sexual maturity** and their is a growth spurt. **Adolescence** is the time period between 11 and 19 years of age during which sexual maturity occurs.

The process of achieving sexual maturity in a male and the ability to father children involves several steps.

Secretion of Hormones

During puberty the anterior pituitary gland in the brain (described in Chapter 13, Endocrinology) begins to secrete two hormones to stimulate the testes. **Follicle-stimulating hormone (FSH)** causes the seminiferous tubules of the testes to enlarge. FSH also stimulates spermatocytes in the seminiferous tubules to begin dividing.

Pronunciation/Word Parts

puberty (PYOO-ber-tee)

sexual (SEK-shoo-al)
  sex/o- *sex*
  -ual *pertaining to*

maturity (mah-TYOOR-ih-tee)
  matur/o- *mature*
  -ity *condition; state*

adolescence (AD-oh-LES-sens)
  adolesc/o- *beginning of being an adult*
  -ence *state*

follicle (FAW-lih-kul)
  folli/o- *sac-like structure*
  -cle *small thing*

hormone (HOR-mohn)

Luteinizing hormone (LH) stimulates the interstitial cells of the testes to begin to secrete the male hormone **testosterone**.

Development of Male Secondary Sexual Characteristics

Primary sexual characteristics are the actual genitalia that a male infant is born with. During puberty, testosterone causes the development of the male **secondary sexual characteristics** (see Figure 11-5 ■). These include enlargement of the external genitalia, development of large body muscles, deepening of the voice (as the larynx grows), the growth of body hair on the face, chest, axillae, and genital area, and development of the sexual drive.

Production of Sperm

Most cells in the body divide by the process of **mitosis**, in which the 46 chromosomes in the cell nucleus duplicate and then divide to create two identical cells, each still with 46 chromosomes. However, the creation of sperm is different from that of other cells in the body. **Spermatogenesis** is the process of producing mature sperm or spermatozoa. The hormones FSH and LH both play a role in spermatogenesis.

The process of spermatogenesis begins during childhood. The seminiferous tubules contain **spermatocytes**. These immature cells are round, and each contains 46 chromosomes. First, the 46 chromosomes duplicate by mitosis, and the duplicating chromosomes exchange genetic material. This creates different combinations of genetic characteristics in the male that can produce different characteristics in his children. Then each spermatocyte divides to produce four individual spermatozoa, each of which contains only 23 chromosomes and is known as a **gamete**. This special process of division is **meiosis**. Meiosis must occur so that a spermatozoon from the

Pronunciation/Word Parts

luteinizing (LOO-tee-ih-NY-zing)

hormone (HOR-mohn)

testosterone (tes-TAW-steh-rohn)

sexual (SEK-shoo-al)
  sex/o- *sex*
  -ual *pertaining to*

mitosis (my-TOH-sihs)
  mit/o- *thread-like strand*
  -osis *abnormal condition; process*

spermatogenesis
(SPER-mah-toh-JEN-eh-sihs)
  spermat/o- *sperm; spermatozoon*
  gen/o- *arising from; produced by*
  -esis *abnormal condition; process*

spermatocyte (sper-MAT-oh-site)
  spermat/o- *sperm; spermatozoon*
  -cyte *cell*

gamete (GAM-eet)

meiosis (my-OH-sihs)
  mei/o- *decrease in number*
  -osis *abnormal condition; process*

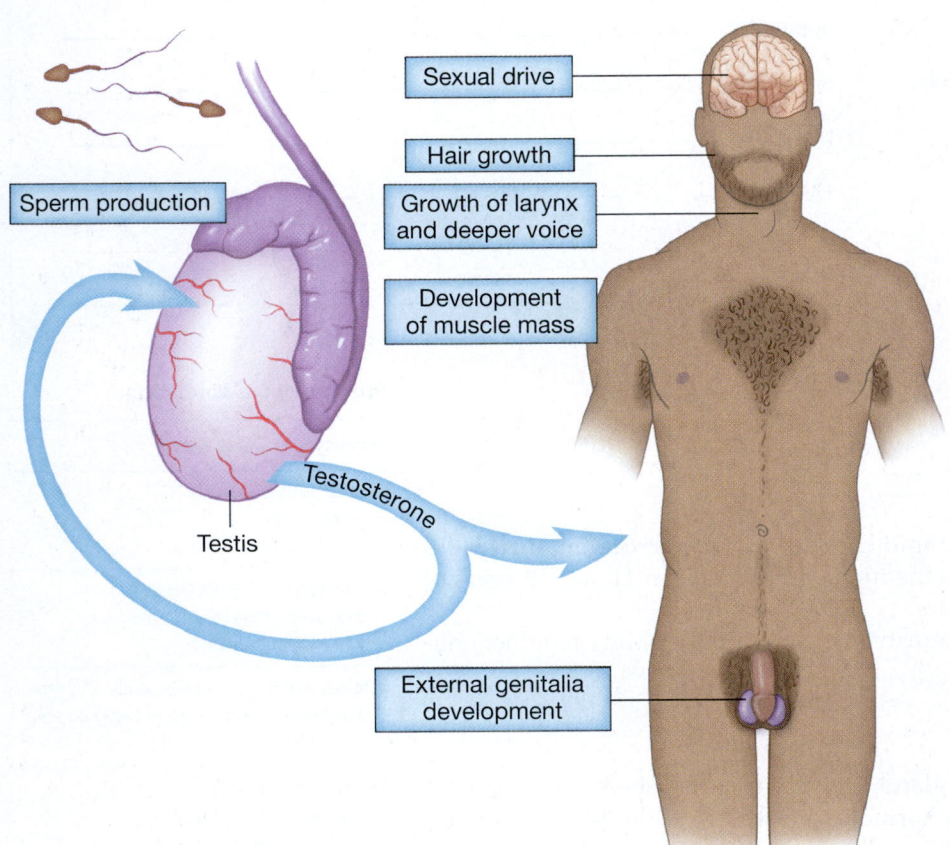

FIGURE 11-5 ■ Testosterone.
Testosterone is a hormone that is secreted by interstitial cells between the seminiferous tubules of the testes. Testosterone causes the development of the male secondary sexual characteristics during puberty. It also causes spermatozoa to develop and mature.

male (with 23 chromosomes) and an egg from the female (with 23 chromosomes), can unite to create a cell with the full number of 46 chromosomes.

The scrotum also plays a role in the production of spermatozoa. The external position of the scrotum means that it is always a few degrees cooler than the body's temperature. This temperature difference is necessary for the proper development of spermatozoa.

Ejaculation

The process of **ejaculation** begins in response to thoughts or sensations that initiate sexual arousal. This relaxes smooth muscles in the walls of arteries in the penis, and the corpora cavernosa and corpus spongiosum become distended with blood and produce an **erection**. Veins in the penis constrict to keep blood in the penis and maintain the erection.

Then impulses from the sympathetic division of the nervous system cause muscles at the base of the penis to contract. Spermatozoa in the vas deferens move into the ejaculatory duct, where they are mixed with fluid from the seminal vesicles. It is at this point that the spermatozoa become active. The spermatozoa then move into the prostatic urethra. The prostate gland contracts, forcing prostatic fluid into the prostatic urethra to mix with the spermatozoa. After the urethra leaves the prostate gland, the spermatozoa are mixed with mucus released from the bulbourethral glands. **Semen** is a combination of spermatozoa and fluids from the seminal vesicles, prostate gland, and the bulbourethral glands. A series of contractions of the smooth muscle of the vas deferens, prostate gland, and urethra cause 2–5 mL of semen to be expelled from the penis through the urethral meatus. This process is ejaculation. Within this small volume of semen are 100–500 million spermatozoa! Sugar and other nutrients in the semen provide energy to keep the spermatozoa swimming strongly as they travel through the female genital tract to fertilize an egg. **Sexual intercourse** of the male with the female deposits the semen in the female's vagina; this is also known as **coitus**.

Pronunciation/Word Parts

ejaculation (ee-JAH-kyoo-LAY-shun)
  ejacul/o- *expel suddenly*
  -ation *being; having; process*

erection (ee-REK-shun)
  erect/o- *stand up*
  -ion *action; condition*

semen (SEE-men)

sexual (SEK-shoo-al)
  sex/o- *sex*
  -ual *pertaining to*

coitus (KOH-ih-tuhs)
The combining forms **coit/o-** and **pareun/o-** mean *sexual intercourse*.

11.2 PRACTICE LAPS

Use the Answer Key at the end of the book to check your answers.

A. Give the Meaning of Combining Forms

Next to each combining form, write its meaning. The first one has been done for you.

Combining Form	Meaning	Combining Form	Meaning
1. **adolesc/o-**	*beginning of being an adult*	7. mei/o-	
2. coit/o-		8. mit/o-	
3. ejacul/o-		9. pareun/o-	
4. erect/o-		10. sex/o-	
5. folli/o-		11. spermat/o-	
6. gen/o-			

B. Build Words

Read the definition of the medical word. Look at the combining form that is given. Select the correct suffix from the Suffix List, and write it on the blank line. Then build the medical word, and write it on the line. (Remember: You may need to remove the combining vowel. Always remove the hyphens and slash.) Be sure to check your spelling.

Suffix List

-ation (being; having; process)	-cyte (cell)	-ence (state)	-ion (action; condition)	-osis (abnormal condition; process)

Definition of the Medical Word	Combining Form	Suffix	Build the Medical Word
Example: Process (of a) thread-like strand	**mit/o-**	*-osis*	*mitosis*

[*You think* process *(-osis)* + thread-like strand *(mit/o-). You change the order of the word parts to put the suffix last. You write* mitosis.]

1. State (of) beginning of being an adult	adolesc/o-	_____	_____
2. Process (to) decrease in number	mei/o-	_____	_____
3. Cell (that is an immature) sperm	spermat/o-	_____	_____
4. Process (to) expel suddenly	ejacul/o-	_____	_____
5. Action (to) stand up	erect/o-	_____	_____

Vocabulary Review

Word or Phrase	Description	Combining Forms
Overview		
genital organs	Male internal and external **genitalia**	**genit/o-** *genitalia*
genitourinary system	The structures of the genitourinary system include the external genitalia (scrotum, testes, epididymides, part of the vas deferens, penis, penile urethra) and the internal genitalia (rest of the vas deferens, seminal vesicles, ejaculatory duct, prostate gland, prostatic urethra, bulbourethral gland and ducts). The genitourinary system shares some structures with the urinary system and is also known as the *urogenital system*. The functions of the genitourinary system are to secrete the male hormone testosterone, develop male secondary sexual characteristics, produce sperm, release semen, and provide a passageway for urine as it leaves the body.	**genit/o-** *genitalia* **urin/o-** *urinary system; urine*
Anatomy of the External Genitalia		
corpora cavernosa	Two columns of erectile tissue along the upper surface of the penis. They fill with blood during sexual arousal.	
corpus spongiosum	Column of erectile tissue along the underside of the penis. It fills with blood during sexual arousal.	

Word or Phrase	Description	Combining Forms
epididymis	Long, coiled structure on the outer wall of each testis. It receives spermatozoa from the seminiferous tubules, adds a cap-like layer of enzymes to them, and destroys defective spermatozoa.	**didym/o-** *testis*
glans penis	Enlarged tip at the end of the penis	**balan/o-** *glans penis*
gonads	The male sex glands (i.e., the testes)	**gon/o-** *ovum; spermatozoon*
inguinal canal	Opening in the abdominal wall muscle of a fetus. Each testis and its spermatic cord pass through the inguinal canal on their way to the scrotum. The opening of the inguinal canal usually closes before age 2.	**inguin/o-** *groin*
interstitial cells	Cells between the seminiferous tubules of the testes. They secrete testosterone when stimulated by luteinizing hormone (LH).	**interstiti/o-** *spaces between tissues*
lumen	Central open area throughout the length of a tube or duct (such as the seminiferous tubule, vas deferens, ejaculatory duct, or urethra)	
penis	Organ that contains three columns of **erectile tissue** that fill with blood during sexual arousal to make an erection. At other times, the penis helps urine to be removed from the body via the penile urethra.	**pen/o-** *penis* **erect/o-** *stand up*
penile urethra	Part of the urethra that is within the penis. It is the passageway for semen and for urine. The **urethral meatus** is at the tip of the glans penis.	**pen/o-** *penis* **urethr/o-** *urethra*
perineum	Area on the outside of the body between the posterior scrotum and the anus	**perine/o-** *perineum*
prepuce	In uncircumcised males, the prepuce is a fold of skin that covers the glans penis. Also known as the **foreskin**.	
scrotum	Pouch of skin behind the penis that holds each testis, epididymis, and part of each vas deferens. Muscles in the wall of the scrotum move it closer to or farther away from the body to control the temperature of the scrotum for sperm production.	**scrot/o-** *scrotum*
seminiferous tubules	Small, tightly coiled tubes within each testis that produce spermatozoa	**semin/i-** *sperm; spermatozoon* **fer/o-** *bear* **tub/o-** *tube*
spermatic cord	A tube that, before birth, contains the vas deferens as well as arteries, veins, and nerves for each testis. In the fetus, each testis and its spermatic cord pass through the inguinal canal and into the scrotum. There the spermatic cord separates into the vas deferens and the other structures.	**spermat/o-** *sperm; spermatozoon*
spermatozoon	An individual mature **sperm**. Each spermatozoon has a head and a tail (flagellum) that propels it forward. A spermatozoon is a gamete because it is a cell whose nucleus of 23 chromosomes can unite with another cell nucleus of 23 chromosomes (the egg of the female) to form a new cell of 46 chromosomes.	**spermat/o-** *sperm; spermatozoon* **sperm/o-** *sperm; spermatozoon*
testis	Egg-shaped gland in each side of the scrotum. Also known as a **testicle**. It contains interstitial cells that secrete testosterone and seminiferous tubules that produce spermatozoa. The testis is an endocrine gland because it secretes testosterone; it also secretes a small amount of the female hormone estradiol.	**test/o-** *testis* **testicul/o-** *testicle; testis* **didym/o-** *testis* **orchid/o-** *testis* **orchi/o-** *testis* **orch/o-** *testis*

Word or Phrase	Description	Combining Forms
testosterone	Most abundant and most biologically active of the male sex hormones. It is secreted by the interstitial cells of the testes. It stimulates spermatozoa to mature. It stimulates the development of secondary sexual characteristics in the male.	**test/o-** *testis*
vas deferens	Long duct that receives spermatozoa from the epididymis and stores them. As each vas deferens travels superiorly, it becomes part of the internal genitalia in the pelvic cavity.	

Anatomy of the Internal Genitalia		
bulbourethral gland	Small, bulb-like gland on the side of the urethra after the urethra leaves the prostate gland. Each gland produces thick mucus that makes up part of the semen. The duct of the gland empties into the urethra.	**bulb/o-** *bulb-like structure* **urethr/o-** *urethra*
ejaculatory duct	Collecting duct that holds spermatozoa from each vas deferens and fluid from each seminal vesicle. The ejaculatory duct enters the prostate gland and joins with the prostatic urethra.	**ejaculat/o-** *expel suddenly*
prostate gland	Doughnut-shaped gland at the base of the bladder. The prostatic urethra goes through its center. The prostate gland produces **prostatic fluid**, a milky fluid that becomes part of the semen.	**prostat/o-** *prostate gland*
prostatic urethra	Part of the urethra that goes through the center of the prostate gland	**urethr/o-** *urethra*
semen	Fluid expelled from the penis during ejaculation. Semen contains spermatozoa, seminal fluid, prostatic fluid, and mucus from the bulbourethral glands.	
seminal vesicle	Elongated gland that forms a V-shaped pair along the posterior wall of the bladder and merges into the ejaculatory duct. Each seminal vesicle produces **seminal fluid**, which makes up most of the volume of semen and contains fructose (sugar) as a source of energy for spermatozoa.	**semin/o-** *sperm; spermatozoon*
vas deferens	Long duct that continues from the external genitalia into the pelvic cavity. Each vas deferens goes behind the urinary bladder and ends as it merges with the seminal vesicle.	**vas/o-** *blood vessel; vas deferens*

Physiology		
coitus	Action in which the male deposits semen in the female's vagina. Also known as **sexual intercourse.**	**coit/o-** *sexual intercourse* **pareun/o-** *sexual intercourse*
ejaculation	Sudden expelling of semen from the penis during sexual arousal of the male	**ejacul/o-** *expel suddenly*
erection	The corpora cavernosa and corpus spongiosum become distended with blood during sexual arousal. Veins constrict to keep the blood in the penis and maintain the erection.	**erect/o-** *stand up*
follicle-stimulating hormone (FSH)	Hormone secreted by the anterior pituitary gland during puberty. It causes the seminiferous tubules of the testes to enlarge during puberty and stimulates spermatocytes in the seminiferous tubules to begin dividing.	**folli/o-** *sac-like structure*
gamete	A cell (male spermatozoon or female egg) that has 23 chromosomes instead of the usual 46 chromosomes like other body cells	
luteinizing hormone (LH)	Hormone secreted by the anterior pituitary gland during puberty. It stimulates the interstitial cells of the testes to begin secreting testosterone.	

Word or Phrase	Description	Combining Forms
meiosis	Process by which a spermatocyte reduces the number of chromosomes in its nucleus to 23, or half the normal number, to create gametes	**mei/o-** *decrease in number*
mitosis	Process by which most body cells divide. The 46 chromosomes in the cell nucleus duplicate and then divide to create two identical cells, each with 46 chromosomes.	**mit/o-** *thread-like strand*
puberty	Beginning of sexual maturity when FSH and LH from the anterior pituitary gland begin to stimulate the testes to produce testosterone. Testosterone stimulates the development of male secondary sexual characteristics, and there is a growth spurt. Also known as **adolescence**, the period of time between 11 and 19 years of age when sexual maturity occurs.	**adolesc/o-** *beginning of being an adult*
semen	A combination of spermatozoa and fluids from the seminal vesicles, prostate gland, and bulbourethral glands. It is expelled through the urethral meatus during ejaculation.	
spermatocyte	Immature, round cell in the seminiferous tubules that contains 46 chromosomes	**spermat/o-** *sperm; spermatozoon*
spermatogenesis	Process of producing mature sperm or spermatozoa	**spermat/o-** *sperm; spermatozoon* **gen/o-** *arising from; produced by*
spermatozoon	An individual mature male gamete. Also known as **sperm**.	**spermat/o-** *sperm; spermatozoon*
testosterone	Causes the development of the **male secondary sexual characteristics**: enlargement of the external genitalia; development of large body muscles; deepening of the voice; growth of body hair on the face, chest, axillae, and genital area; and development of the sexual drive	**test/o-** *testis*

Abbreviation Review

FSH	follicle-stimulating hormone	**LH**	luteinizing hormone
GU	genitourinary		

11.3 Diseases

Word or Phrase	Description	Pronunciation/Word Parts

Male Breast

Word or Phrase	Description	Pronunciation/Word Parts
gynecomastia	Enlargement of the male breast. It is caused by an imbalance of testosterone and estradiol. This occurs during puberty or aging or it can occur because of surgical removal of the testes (and the resulting lack of male hormone) or from a female hormone drug used to treat prostate cancer. Treatment: Androgen (male hormone) drug; plastic surgery to decrease the breast size	**gynecomastia** (GY-neh-koh-MAS-tee-ah) **gynec/o-** *female; woman* **mast/o-** *breast; mastoid process* **-ia** *condition; state; thing* Gynecomastia: *Condition (of enlargement in which the male's breast resembles the) female breast*

Word or Phrase	Description	Pronunciation/Word Parts

Testis and Epididymis

Word or Phrase	Description	Pronunciation/Word Parts
cryptorchidism	Failure of one or both testes to move through the inguinal canal and descend into the scrotum. This causes a low sperm count and male infertility because spermatozoa need the lower temperature of the scrotum to develop properly. Also known as **cryptorchism**. Treatment: Testosterone drug; orchiopexy	**cryptorchidism** (krip-TOR-kih-dizm) **crypt/o-** hidden **orchid/o-** testis **-ism** disease from a specific cause; process
epididymitis	Infection or inflammation of the epididymis. It is caused by a bacterial infection in the urinary tract or by a sexually transmitted disease such as gonorrhea or chlamydia. Treatment: Antibiotic drug	**epididymitis** (EP-ih-DID-ih-MY-tihs) **epi-** above; upon **didym/o-** testis **-itis** infection of; inflammation of
infertility	Inability of a male to impregnate a female after 1 year of regular sexual intercourse. This can be caused by a hormone imbalance of FSH or LH, undescended testes, a varicocele (described later), damage to the testes from a childhood infection of the mumps, infection in the testes, too few spermatozoa (oligospermia), or abnormal spermatozoa. Treatment: Correct the underlying cause.	**infertility** (IN-fer-TIL-ih-tee) **in-** in; not; within **fertil/o-** conceive; form **-ity** condition; state
oligospermia	Fewer than the normal number of spermatozoa are produced by the testes (see Figure 11-6 ■). This is the most common reason for male infertility. It is caused by a hormone imbalance or undescended testes. Treatment: Correct the underlying cause.	**oligospermia** (OH-lih-goh-SPER-mee-ah) **olig/o-** few; scanty **sperm/o-** sperm; spermatozoon **-ia** condition; state; thing

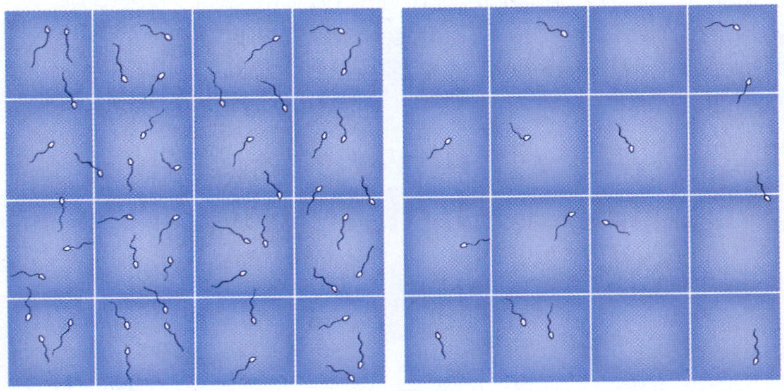

FIGURE 11-6 ■ Oligospermia.
A. This semen specimen shows a normal number of sperm as seen on a counting grid under a microscope. **B.** This semen specimen shows a decreased number of sperm in a patient with oligospermia.

Word or Phrase	Description	Pronunciation/Word Parts
orchitis	Infection or inflammation of the testes. It is caused by a bacterial or viral infection, a childhood infection of the mumps, or trauma to the testes. Treatment: Antibiotic drug for a bacterial infection (an antibiotic drug is not effective against a viral infection)	**orchitis** (or-KY-tihs) **orch/o-** testis **-itis** infection of; inflammation of
testicular cancer	Cancerous tumor of one or both testes. It is the most common cancer in men age 15–35. It arises from immature spermatocytes that are abnormal. Symptoms include a painless lump in a testis. Also known as a **seminoma**. Treatment: Surgery to remove the testis (orchiectomy); radiation therapy or a chemotherapy drug	**seminoma** (SEM-ih-NOH-mah) **semin/o-** sperm; spermatozoon **-oma** mass; tumor
varicocele	Varicose vein in the veins of a testis. The valves in the vein do not close tightly, allowing blood to accumulate. The testis and the scrotum become distended with blood and are painful. A varicocele can cause a low sperm count and infertility. Treatment: Surgical removal of the varicocele	**varicocele** (VAIR-ih-koh-SEEL) **varic/o-** varicose vein **-cele** hernia

Word or Phrase	Description	Pronunciation/Word Parts

Prostate Gland

Word or Phrase	Description	Pronunciation/Word Parts
benign prostatic hyperplasia (BPH)	Benign (not cancerous), gradual enlargement of the prostate gland. This normally occurs as a man ages. The enlarged prostate gland compresses the urethra and causes the bladder to retain urine. There is hesitancy and dribbling of urine on urination and a narrowed urine stream. Treatment: Drug to decrease the size of the prostate gland; minimally invasive procedures such as prostate artery embolization (PAE) or prostate urethral lift (PUL); surgery to reduce the size of the prostate gland by using a laser, microwaves, or radiowaves	**benign** (bee-NINE) **hyperplasia** (HY-per-PLAY-shah) **hyper-** *above; more than normal* **plas/o-** *formation; growth* **-ia** *condition; state; thing*
cancer of the prostate gland	**Cancerous** tumor of the prostate gland. It is categorized as an **adenocarcinoma** because it begins in a gland. This is the most common cancer in men. There are few early symptoms or signs because the cancer grows slowly. Later, the cancer makes the prostate gland feel hard or nodular on digital rectal examination. Treatment: "Watch-and-wait" approach if the cancer is small and the patient is elderly; surgery to remove the prostate gland (prostatectomy); radiation therapy, cryotherapy, or chemotherapy drugs	**adenocarcinoma** (AD-eh-noh-KAR-sih-NOH-mah) **aden/o-** *gland* **carcin/o-** *cancer* **-oma** *mass; tumor*
prostatitis	Acute or chronic bacterial infection and inflammation of the prostate gland. It is caused by a urinary tract infection or a sexually transmitted disease. Treatment: Antibiotic drug	**prostatitis** (PRAW-stah-TY-tihs) **prostat/o-** *prostate gland* **-itis** *infection of; inflammation of*

Clinical Connections

Oncology. There are different types of **cancer** and **cancerous** tumors. A **malignancy** is often named for the site where it begins. A seminoma of the testis begins in immature, abnormal spermatocytes in the testis. (**Semin/o-** means *sperm; spermatozoon*.)

An adenocarcinoma begins in a gland in the body, such as the prostate gland. (**Aden/o-** means *gland*.) The Gleason Score is used to describe how likely the cancer in the prostate gland is to spread. Prostate gland cancer is treated with several types of special radiation therapy that target the cancerous cells and not normal cells. These include external beams of radiation given at multiple angles or an external beam of special proton particles. Another treatment, known as brachytherapy, is described later. Each type of treatment is administered by a radiation **oncologist**, who is an M.D. specializing in cancer therapy.

oncology (ong-KAW-loh-jee)
 onc/o- *mass; tumor*
 -logy *study of*

cancer (KAN-ser)

cancerous (KAN-ser-uhs)
 cancer/o- *cancer*
 -ous *pertaining to*

malignancy (mah-LIG-nan-see)
 malign/o- *cancer*
 -ancy *state*

oncologist (ong-KAW-loh-jist)
 onc/o- *mass; tumor*
 log/o- *study of; word*
 -ist *person who specializes in; thing that specializes in*

Penis

Word or Phrase	Description	Pronunciation/Word Parts
balanitis	Infection and inflammation of the glans penis. It is often associated with phimosis (described later) or with inadequate hygiene of the prepuce. Treatment: Antibiotic drug (for a bacterial infection); antifungal drug (for a yeast or fungal infection)	**balanitis** (BAL-ah-NY-tihs) **balan/o-** *glans penis* **-itis** *infection of; inflammation of* Note: *Balanus* is the Latin name (no longer used) for the glans penis.
chordee	Downward curvature of the penis during an erection. It is caused by a constricting, cord-like band of tissue along the underside of the penis. This is a congenital (present at birth) abnormality that is often associated with hypospadias (described later). Treatment: Surgical correction	**chordee** (kor-DEE)

Word or Phrase	Description	Pronunciation/Word Parts
dyspareunia	Painful or difficult sexual intercourse or **postcoital** pain. It is caused by infection of the penis or prostate gland, chordee of the penis, or phimosis. Treatment: Correct the underlying cause.	**dyspareunia** (DIS-pah-ROO-nee-ah) **dys-** *abnormal; difficult; painful* **pareun/o-** *sexual intercourse* **-ia** *condition; state; thing* **postcoital** (post-KOH-ih-tal) **post-** *after; behind* **coit/o-** *sexual intercourse* **-al** *pertaining to*
epispadias	Congenital condition (present at birth) in which the opening of the urethral meatus is positioned on the top of the glans penis instead of at its tip. Treatment: Surgical correction	**epispadias** (EP-ih-SPAY-dee-as) **epi-** *above; upon* **spad/o-** *opening; tear* **-ias** *condition*
erectile dysfunction (ED)	Inability to achieve or sustain an erection of the penis. It can be caused by hypertension, arteriosclerosis that blocks blood flow into the penis, a neurologic disease (such as a spinal cord injury) that impairs sensory stimuli and nerve transmission, diabetes mellitus, a low level of testosterone, smoking, alcoholism, the side effects of certain drugs, or psychological factors. Also known as **impotence**. Treatment: Drug to stimulate an erection; penile implant	**erectile** (ee-REK-tile) **erect/o-** *stand up* **-ile** *pertaining to* **dysfunction** (dis-FUNK-shun) The prefix **dys-** means *abnormal; difficult; painful.* **impotence** (IM-poh-tens)
hypospadias	Congenital condition (present at birth) in which the opening of the urethral meatus is positioned on the bottom of the glans penis instead of at its tip. Treatment: Surgical correction	**hypospadias** (HY-poh-SPAY-dee-as) **hypo-** *below; deficient* **spad/o-** *opening; tear* **-ias** *condition*
phimosis	Congenital condition in which the opening of the foreskin is too small to allow it to be pulled back from the glans penis. This traps **smegma** (a white, cheesy discharge of skin cells and oil) under the foreskin, which can cause infection. Treatment: Circumcision	**phimosis** (fy-MOH-sihs) **phim/o-** *closed tight* **-osis** *abnormal condition; process* **smegma** (SMEG-mah)
premature ejaculation	Ejaculation of semen that occurs with minimal stimulation and before the penis becomes fully erect. This lessens the enjoyment of sexual intercourse and decreases the chance of conception. It can be caused by a hormone imbalance but is more often caused by stress or a psychological reason. Treatment: Correct the underlying cause.	**ejaculation** (ee-JAH-kyoo-LAY-shun) **ejaculat/o-** *expel suddenly* **-ion** *action; condition*
priapism	Abnormal, continuing erection of the penis with pain and tenderness. It is caused by a spinal cord injury or the side effect of a drug used to treat erectile dysfunction. Treatment: Correct the underlying cause.	**priapism** (PRY-ah-pizm) **priap/o-** *persistent erection* **-ism** *disease from a specific cause; process*
sexually transmitted disease (STD)	Infectious disease that is contracted during sexual intercourse with an infected individual (see Table 11-1). The presence of a sexually transmitted disease means that the patient and all sexual partners need to be treated. Sexually transmitted diseases can also be passed to a fetus (in the uterus or as it is born), causing serious illness, blindness, and even death. Also known as a **sexually transmitted infection (STI)**. Treatment: Antibiotic drug, antiviral drug, or antiretroviral drug	

Table 11-1 Sexually Transmitted Diseases (STDs)

Physicians are required to report all cases of sexually transmitted diseases to the state health department, which, in turn, reports all cases to the national **Centers for Disease Control and Prevention (CDC)**. *Also known as* **sexually transmitted infections (STIs).**

STD	Pronunciation/Word Parts
acquired immunodeficiency syndrome (AIDS) *Note*: This disease and its history, symptoms, diagnosis, and treatment are described in detail in Chapter 6, Hematology and Immunology. Pathogen — Human immunodeficiency virus (HIV), a retrovirus Symptoms — Men: Fever, night sweats, weight loss, fatigue Women: Same Diagnosis — Blood test (ELISA, Western blot, viral RNA load, p24 antigen, CD4 count) or saliva screening test (OraSure) Treatment — Oral antiretroviral drugs taken in combination Other — Treatment can only slow the progress of this disease; there is no cure.	**immunodeficiency** (IH-myoo-NOH-deh-FIH-shun-see) **immun/o-** *immune response* **defici/o-** *inadequate; lacking* **-ency** *condition of being; condition of having*
chlamydia Pathogen — *Chlamydia trachomatis*, a gram-negative coccus (sphere-shaped) bacterium Symptoms — Men: Painful urination with burning and itching. Thin, watery discharge from the urethra. Some men have no symptoms. Women: Frequently have no symptoms or a slight vaginal discharge Diagnosis — Smear of discharge from the urethra (men) or cervix (women) is stained and examined under a microscope Treatment — Oral antibiotic drug Other — Most common sexually transmitted disease. Also known as **nongonococcal urethritis**.	**chlamydia** (klah-MID-ee-ah) **nongonococcal** (non-GAW-noh-KAW-kal) **gon/o-** *ovum; spermatozoon* **cocc/o-** *spherical bacterium* **-al** *pertaining to* **urethritis** (YOOR-ee-THRY-tihs) **urethr/o-** *urethra* **-itis** *infection of; inflammation of*
genital herpes Pathogen — Herpes simplex virus (HSV), type 2 Symptoms — Men: Vesicular lesions (blisters) on the penis, scrotum, perineum, or anus. When the blisters break, they become skin ulcers. There may be flu-like symptoms. Women: Same, with vesicles on the female genitalia or anus Diagnosis — Culture grown from a swab of a lesion, polymerase chain reaction test Treatment — Topical and oral antiviral drugs shorten the duration of each outbreak	**herpes** (HER-peez)
genital warts (condylomata acuminata) (see Figure 11-7 ■) Pathogen — Human papillomavirus (HPV) Certain strains cause genital warts; other strains cause dysplasia of the cervix, which can lead to cervical cancer in women Symptoms — Men: Itching, flesh-colored, irregular lesions that are raised and cauliflower-like Women: Same, with vaginal discharge Diagnosis — Visual examination of the skin of the genital area. In women, a Pap smear of the cervix is examined under a microscope. Treatment — Topical chemicals or cryosurgery, cautery, or laser to remove warts	**condylomata acuminata** (CON-dih-LOH-mah-tah ah-KOO-mih-NAH-tah)

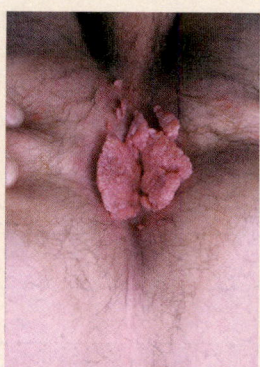

FIGURE 11-7 ■ **Genital warts.**
These raised, irregular, flesh-colored lesions are caused by the human papillomavirus (HPV). In a male, they occur on the penis, scrotum, or perineum. In a female, they occur on the labia or perineum. Some strains of HPV are associated with cancer of the cervix in women.

STD	Pronunciation/Word Parts
gonorrhea Pathogen — *Neisseria gonorrhoeae*, a gram-negative diplococcus (double sphere) bacterium. Also known as **gonococcus (GC)**. Symptoms — Men: Painful urination. Thick yellow discharge from the urethra (gonococcal urethritis). Some men have no symptoms. Women: Painful urination. Thick, yellow vaginal discharge. Half of infected women have no symptoms. Diagnosis — Gram stain of a smear of the discharge shows characteristic gram-negative intracellular diplococci under a microscope Culture grown from a swab of discharge from the urethra (men) or cervix (women) Treatment — Oral antibiotic drug Other — Used to be called "the clap" because of a similar-sounding French word that meant "house of prostitution"	**gonorrhea** (GAW-noh-REE-ah) **gon/o-** *ovum; spermatozoon* **-rrhea** *discharge; flow* **gonococcus** (GAW-noh-KAW-kuhs) **gon/o-** *ovum; spermatozoon* **-coccus** *spherical bacterium*

STD		Pronunciation/Word Parts
syphilis		**syphilis** (SIF-ih-lihs)
Pathogen	*Treponema pallidum*, a spirochete (spiral) bacterium	
Symptoms	Men: Single, painless **chancre** (lesion that ulcerates, forms a crust, and then heals) on the penis. Later, there is fever, rash, and various symptoms that mimic other diseases.	**chancre** (SHANG-ker)
	Women: Same, with chancre on female genitalia	
Diagnosis	Fluid from a lesion viewed with special illumination under darkfield microscopy shows the spiral bacterium; blood tests for antibodies to syphilis (RPR, VDRL, FTA-ABS)	
Treatment	Oral antibiotic drug	
trichomoniasis		**trichomoniasis** (TRIK-oh-moh-NY-ah-sihs)
Pathogen	*Trichomonas vaginalis*, a protozoan with a tail	
Symptoms	Men: Almost no symptoms	
	Women: Greenish-yellow, frothy or bubbly vaginal discharge with a fishy odor. Itching of the vulva and vagina.	
Diagnosis	Wet mount preparation of the vaginal discharge examined under a microscope; culture of the discharge	
Treatment	Oral antiprotozoal drug	

11.3 PRACTICE LAPS

Use the Answer Key at the end of the book to check your answers.

A. Give the Meaning of Combining Forms

Next to each combining form, write its meaning. The first one has been done for you.

Combining Form	Meaning	Combining Form	Meaning
1. **aden/o-**	*gland*	16. mast/o-	
2. balan/o-		17. olig/o-	
3. cancer/o-		18. onc/o-	
4. carcin/o-		19. orchid/o-	
5. cocc/o-		20. orch/o-	
6. coit/o-		21. pareun/o-	
7. crypt/o-		22. phim/o-	
8. defici/o-		23. priap/o-	
9. didym/o-		24. prostat/o-	
10. erect/o-		25. semin/o-	
11. fertil/o-		26. sperm/o-	
12. gon/o-		27. troph/o-	
13. gynec/o-		28. urethr/o-	
14. immun/o-		29. varic/o-	
15. malign/o-		30. venere/o-	

B. Build Words

Read the definition of the medical word. Look at the combining form that is given. Select the correct suffix from the Suffix List, and write it on the blank line. Then build the medical word, and write it on the line. (Remember: You may need to remove the combining vowel. Always remove the hyphens and slash.) Be sure to check your spelling.

Suffix List

-ancy (state)	-itis (infection of; inflammation of)	-ous (pertaining to)
-cele (hernia)	-oma (mass; tumor)	-rrhea (discharge; flow)
-ism (disease from a specific cause; process)	-osis (abnormal condition; process)	

Definition of the Medical Word	Combining Form	Suffix	Build the Medical Word
Example: Pertaining to cancer	**cancer/o-**	*-ous*	*cancerous*

[*You think* pertaining to (*-ous*) + cancer (*cancer/o-*). You change the order of the word parts to put the suffix last. You write cancerous.]

	Definition of the Medical Word	Combining Form	Suffix	Build the Medical Word
1.	Infection (or) inflammation of (the) prostate gland	prostat/o-	_____	_____
2.	Hernia (of a) varicose vein (in the testis)	varic/o-	_____	_____
3.	State (of) cancer	malign/o-	_____	_____
4.	Disease from a specific cause (of a) persistent erection	priap/o-	_____	_____
5.	Abnormal condition (of the foreskin being) closed tight	phim/o-	_____	_____
6.	Infection (or) inflammation of (the) glans penis	balan/o-	_____	_____
7.	Tumor (related to the testes and) sperm	semin/o-	_____	_____
8.	Infection (or) inflammation of (the) testis	orch/o-	_____	_____
9.	Discharge (from a disease related to an organ that produces) ovum or spermatozoon	gon/o-	_____	_____

C. Define Abbreviations

1. AIDS _____

2. BPH _____

3. CDC _____

4. ED _____

5. GC _____

6. HSV _____

7. STD _____

8. STI _____

11.4 Laboratory, Diagnostic, and Radiologic Procedures

Word or Phrase	Description	Pronunciation/Word Parts

Laboratory Tests and Diagnostic Procedures

Word or Phrase	Description	Pronunciation/Word Parts
acid phosphatase	Semen test that detects the presence of acid phosphatase in the vagina and indicates sexual intercourse has occurred because semen contains acid phosphatase. This test is used in rape investigations.	**acid phosphatase** (AS-id FAWS-fah-tays) **phosphat/o-** *phosphate* **-ase** *enzyme*
DNA analysis	Semen test that uses DNA analysis of semen from a crime scene or rape victim that can be compared to samples of known DNA in a criminal database. DNA analysis can also be used to prove paternity (that a particular man is the father of the child being tested).	
herpes simplex virus testing	Test that detects the presence of the DNA of herpes simplex virus type 2 (genital herpes). This test can be performed on blood or on fluid from a skin lesion.	
hormone testing	Blood test that determines the levels of the hormones FSH and LH from the anterior pituitary gland and testosterone from the testes. It is used to diagnose infertility problems.	**hormone** (HOR-mohn)
human immunodeficiency virus (HIV) testing	HIV tests can be performed on blood, urine, or saliva. • ELISA (enzyme-linked immunosorbent assay) is the first screening test; it can be done on blood, urine, or saliva. However, this test can also be positive when the patient has antibodies against some other diseases. • CD4 is a blood test that measures the number of helper T cell lymphocytes (CD4 lymphocytes), the cells that are infected by the HIV retrovirus. • OraSure is a quick screening test that can be done in the doctor's office or clinic; it detects antibodies to HIV in the saliva. • The p24 antigen test is a blood test that detects the actual protein in HIV. It can be positive even before there are any antibodies against HIV in the blood. • The viral RNA load test is a blood test that measures the amount of HIV present; it is used to monitor the patient's response to antiretroviral drugs. • The Western blot test is used to confirm a positive ELISA test result so that a diagnosis of HIV can be made.	
prostate-specific antigen (PSA)	Blood test that detects a glycoprotein in cells of the prostate gland. PSA is increased in men with prostate cancer. The higher the level, the more advanced the cancer. The PSA level falls after successful treatment of the cancer.	**antigen** (AN-tih-jen) *Antigen* is a combination of part of the word *antibody* and the suffix **-gen** (that which produces).
prostatic acid phosphatase (PAP)	Blood test for an enzyme found in the prostate gland. This test measures only acid phosphatase from the prostate gland as opposed to the total acid phosphatase. An increased level indicates cancer of the prostate gland that has metastasized to the body.	

Word or Phrase	Description	Pronunciation/Word Parts
semen analysis	Semen test that is a microscopic examination of the spermatozoa (see Figure 11-8 ■). This test is done as part of a workup for infertility. After not ejaculating for 36 hours, the man gives a semen specimen. A normal **sperm count** is greater than 50 million/mL. The **motility** (forward movement) and **morphology** (normal shape) of the spermatozoa are evaluated. A semen analysis is also done after a vasectomy to verify **aspermia** and a successful sterilization.	**motility** (moh-TIL-ih-tee) **motil/o-** *movement* **-ity** *condition; state* **morphology** (mor-FAW-loh-jee) **morph/o-** *shape* **-logy** *study of* **aspermia** (aa-SPER-mee-ah) **a-** *away from; without* **sperm/o-** *sperm; spermatozoon* **-ia** *condition; state; thing*

FIGURE 11-8 ■ Spermatozoa morphology. The spermatozoon on the right shows normal morphology. Vigorous movement of its tail would indicate normal motility. The spermatozoon on the left has abnormal morphology with a double head and a deformed tail. Abnormal spermatozoa can have enlarged heads, pin heads, or tails that are kinked, doubled, coiled, or missing. All men produce a few abnormal spermatozoa, which are destroyed in the epididymis, but exposure to lead, cigarette smoke, pesticides, or chemicals can increase this number. Large numbers of abnormal spermatozoa cause male infertility.

Word or Phrase	Description	Pronunciation/Word Parts
syphilis testing	Blood tests for syphilis include RPR, VDRL, and FTA-ABS. RPR stands for *rapid plasma reagin*. VDRL stands for *Venereal Disease Research Laboratory*. Venereal disease is an older phrase for the sexually transmitted disease of syphilis. RPR and VDRL tests detect an antibody that is present with syphilis; however, it is also present with other diseases. FTA-ABS stands for *fluorescent treponemal antibody absorption*. This test detects the body's specific antibodies against the bacterium that causes syphilis.	

Radiologic and Nuclear Medicine Procedures

Word or Phrase	Description	Pronunciation/Word Parts
brachytherapy	Type of radiation therapy used to treat prostate cancer. It uses radioactive pellets (known as "seeds") implanted in the prostate gland.	**brachytherapy** (BRAK-ee-THAIR-ah-pee) The prefix **brachy-** means *short (distance away)*.
ProstaScint scan	Radiologic procedure that uses ProstaScint to detect areas of metastasis that have spread from the primary site of prostate gland cancer. ProstaScint is a combination of a radioactive tracer (indium-111) and a monoclonal antibody that binds to receptors on cancer cells in the prostate gland and elsewhere in the body. The radioactive tracer emits gamma rays that are detected by a gamma scintillation camera and made into an image.	

Word or Phrase	Description	Pronunciation/Word Parts
ultrasonography	Radiologic procedure that uses ultra high-frequency sound waves emitted by a transducer or probe to produce an image. Ultrasonography of the testis is used to detect a varicocele or undescended testes. **Transrectal ultrasonography (TRUS)** uses an ultrasound probe inserted into the rectum to obtain an image of the prostate gland or to help guide a needle biopsy of the prostate gland. The **ultrasound** image is a **sonogram**.	**ultrasonography** (UL-trah-soh-NAW-grah-fee) **ultra-** *beyond; higher* **son/o-** *sound* **-graphy** *process of recording* **transrectal** (trans-REK-tal) **trans-** *across; through* **rect/o-** *rectum* **-al** *pertaining to* **ultrasound** (UL-trah-sound) **sonogram** (SAW-noh-gram) **son/o-** *sound* **-gram** *picture; record*

11.4 PRACTICE LAPS

Use the Answer Key at the end of the book to check your answers.

A. Give the Meaning of Combining Forms

Next to each combining form, write its meaning. The first one has been done for you.

Combining Form	Meaning	Combining Form	Meaning
1. **morph/o-**	*shape*	4. rect/o-	
2. motil/o-		5. son/o-	
3. phosphat/o-		6. sperm/o-	

B. Build Words

Read the definition of the medical word. Look at the combining form that is given. Select the correct suffix from the Suffix List, and write it on the blank line. Then build the medical word, and write it on the line. (Remember: You may need to remove the combining vowel. Always remove the hyphens and slash.) Be sure to check your spelling.

Suffix List

-al (pertaining to) -ase (enzyme)	-gram (picture; record) -ity (condition; state)	-logy (study of; word)

Definition of the Medical Word	Combining Form	Suffix	Build the Medical Word
Example: Pertaining to (the) rectum	**rect/o-**	*-al*	*rectal*

[You think pertaining to (-al) + rectum (rect/o-). You change the order of the word parts to put the suffix last. You write rectal.]

1. State (of) movement	motil/o-		
2. Enzyme (that acts on) phosphate	phosphat/o-		
3. Picture (made by) sound	son/o-		
4. Study of (the) shape (of sperm)	morph/o-		

C. Define Abbreviations

1. FTA-ABS _____

2. PAP _____

3. PSA _____

4. RPR _____

5. TRUS _____

6. VDRL _____

11.5 Medical Procedures, Drugs, and Surgical Procedures

Word or Phrase	Description	Pronunciation/Word Parts

Medical Procedures

Word or Phrase	Description	Pronunciation/Word Parts
digital rectal examination (DRE)	Procedure to palpate the prostate gland. A gloved finger inserted into the rectum is used to feel the prostate gland for signs of tenderness, nodules, hardness, or enlargement. This examination should be done yearly in men over age 50.	**digital** (DIJ-ih-tal) **digit/o-** *digit; finger; toe* **-al** *pertaining to*
newborn genital examination	Procedure in which the newborn's external male genitalia are examined for any sign of abnormal positioning of the urethral meatus (epispadias, hypospadias), ambiguous genitalia, or undescended testes (see Figure 11-9 ■). **FIGURE 11-9 ■ Newborn scrotal examination.** The scrotum is palpated as part of the initial genital examination of a newborn. Both testes should be descended and present in the scrotum at birth.	
testicular self-examination (TSE)	Procedure performed by the patient to palpate the testes and scrotum to detect lumps, masses, or enlarged lymph nodes. This should be done monthly to detect early signs of testicular cancer.	

Category	Indication	Pronunciation/Word Parts

Drugs

Category	Indication	Pronunciation/Word Parts
androgen drug	Treats a decreased level of testosterone caused by cryptorchidism, orchiectomy, or decreased LH from the anterior pituitary gland. Also used to treat prostate cancer as a chemotherapy drug. Also used to treat delayed puberty in boys.	**androgen** (AN-droh-jen) **andr/o-** *male* **-gen** *that which produces* *Androgen* is a category that includes testosterone produced by the testes, other testosterone-like hormones, or manufactured testosterone drugs.
antibiotic drug	Treats bacterial infections that cause chlamydia, gonorrhea, and syphilis	**antibiotic** (AN-tee-by-AW-tik) **anti-** *against* **bi/o-** *living organism; living tissue* **-tic** *pertaining to*
antiviral drug	Treats viral infections that cause genital herpes and condylomata acuminata. This drug is applied topically to the affected areas.	**antiviral** (AN-tee-VY-ral) **anti-** *against* **vir/o-** *virus* **-al** *pertaining to*
antiretroviral drug	Treats HIV and AIDS and is given orally.	**antiretroviral** (AN-tee-REH-troh-VY-ral) **anti-** *against* **retro-** *backward; behind* **vir/o-** *virus* **-al** *pertaining to*
benign prostatic hyperplasia drug	Inhibits the male hormone dihydrotestosterone, a hormone that normally causes the prostate gland to enlarge. Other drugs relax the smooth muscle in the prostate gland and urethra to allow urine to flow more freely.	
erectile dysfunction drug	Promotes the release of nitric oxide gas in the penis and inhibits an enzyme; both actions increase blood flow into the penis to create an erection.	

Word or Phrase	Description	Pronunciation/Word Parts

Surgical Procedures

Word or Phrase	Description	Pronunciation/Word Parts
biopsy (Bx)	Procedure to remove tissue from the prostate gland to test for prostatic cancer. A needle is inserted through the rectum or urethra to take a sample of prostatic tissue. **Fine-needle aspiration biopsy** of the testis is performed to investigate a low sperm count or test for cancer. A thin needle is inserted in the testis and a syringe is used to aspirate tissue. An **incisional biopsy** (open biopsy) is performed to remove part of a tumor in the testis.	**biopsy** (BY-awp-see) **bi/o-** *living organism; living tissue* **-opsy** *process of viewing* **aspiration** (AS-pih-RAY-shun) **aspir/o-** *breathe in; suck in* **-ation** *being; having; process* **incisional** (in-SIH-zhun-al) **in-** *in; not; within* **cis/o-** *cut* **-ion** *action; condition* **-al** *pertaining to*

Word or Phrase	Description	Pronunciation/Word Parts
circumcision	Procedure to remove the prepuce (foreskin). This can be done to correct a tight prepuce (phimosis) and allow better hygiene of the glans penis. The foreskin in newborn babies is often removed because of social customs or religious requirements. Circumcision has been found to reduce the risk of penile cancer.	**circumcision** (SER-kum-SIH-zhun) **circum-** *around* **cis/o-** *cut* **-ion** *action; condition*
cryotherapy	Procedure to treat prostate cancer. A needle is inserted through the skin and into the prostate gland. Then a cold gas is injected to freeze cancerous tissues in the prostate gland.	**cryotherapy** (KRY-oh-THAIR-ah-pee) **cry/o-** *cold* **-therapy** *treatment*
orchiectomy	Procedure to remove a testis because of testicular cancer	**orchiectomy** (OR-kee-EK-toh-mee) **orchi/o-** *testis* **-ectomy** *surgical removal*
orchiopexy	Procedure done in an infant to reposition an undescended testis and fix it within the scrotum. Orchiopexy is also used to treat male infertility in an adult.	**orchiopexy** (OR-kee-oh-PEK-see) **orchi/o-** *testis* **-pexy** *process of fixing in place*
penile implant	Procedure to implant an inflatable penile **prosthesis** for patients with erectile dysfunction	**prosthesis** (praws-THEE-sihs)
prostate artery embolization (PAE)	Procedure in which a catheter is inserted in a large artery in the groin and threaded to the prostatic artery. Microscopic beads are injected to decrease blood flow to the prostate gland and decrease the size of the prostate gland. This is a minimally invasive procedure for benign prostatic hyperplasia that some patients prefer over treatment with drugs or surgery.	**embolization** (EM-bol-ih-ZAY-shun) **embol/o-** *embolus; occluding plug* **-ization** *process of creating; process of inserting; process of making*
prostate urethral lift (PUL)	Procedure that uses an endoscope inserted through the urethral meatus of the penis. A stainless steel implant is placed within the urethra to keep enlarged prostatic tissue from narrowing the lumen of the prostatic urethra. This is a minimally invasive procedure for benign prostatic hyperplasia that some patients prefer over treatment with drugs or surgery.	
prostatectomy	Procedure to remove the entire prostate gland, along with the lymph nodes, seminal vesicles, and vas deferens because of prostate cancer (see Figure 11-10 ■).	**prostatectomy** (PRAW-stah-TEK-toh-mee) **prostat/o-** *prostate gland* **-ectomy** *surgical removal*

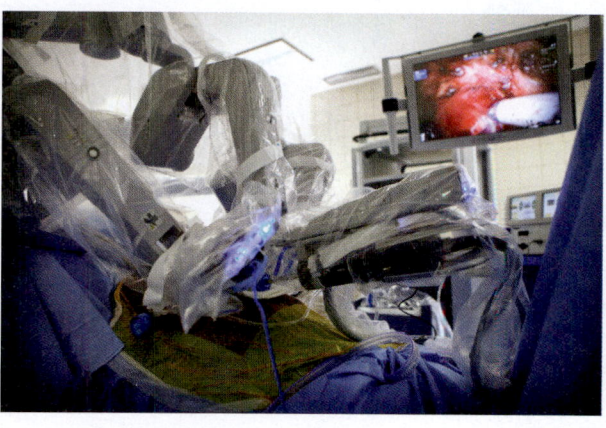

FIGURE 11-10 ■ **Robot-assisted prostatectomy.** Procedure to remove a cancerous prostate gland using robot-assisted surgery. Several portals are placed in the patient's abdomen and robotic instruments are inserted. The robotic 3D camera has 10 times the magnification of the human eye. Robotic instruments allow the surgeon to more precisely remove cancerous tissues while preserving nerves that affect sexual function.

Word or Phrase	Description	Pronunciation/Word Parts

transurethral resection of the prostate (TURP)	Procedure to reduce the size of the prostate gland in patients with benign prostatic hyperplasia. A special cystoscope (a **resectoscope**) is inserted through the urethra. It has built-in cutting instruments and cautery to resect pieces of the prostate gland and cauterize bleeding blood vessels. Chips of prostatic tissue are then irrigated out (see Figure 11-11 ■). Newer techniques vaporize prostatic tissue by using a laser, microwaves and heat, or radio waves and heat. The newer surgeries produce the same results as a TURP, but with less bleeding and a shorter recovery time.
	
	• **Laser**. Holmium laser enucleation of the prostate (**HoLEP**) and photoselective vaporization of the prostate (**PVP**) use a laser to destroy prostatic tissue.
	• **Microwaves and heat**. Transurethral microwave therapy (**TUMT**) uses a microwave antenna on a catheter inserted through the urethra to destroy prostatic tissue.
	• **Radio waves and heat**. Transurethral needle ablation (**TUNA**) uses a resectoscope to place needles in the prostate gland to destroy prostatic tissue with radio waves and heat.
		transurethral
		(TRANS-yoor-EE-thral)
		  trans- *across; through*
		  urethr/o- *urethra*
		  -al *pertaining to*
		
		resection (ree-SEK-shun)
		  resect/o- *cut out; remove*
		  -ion *action; condition*
		
		resectoscope
		(ree-SEK-toh-skohp)
		  resect/o- *cut out; remove*
		  -scope *instrument used to examine*
		
		enucleation
		(ee-NOO-klee-AA-shun)
		  enucle/o- *remove the main part*
		  -ation *being; having; process*

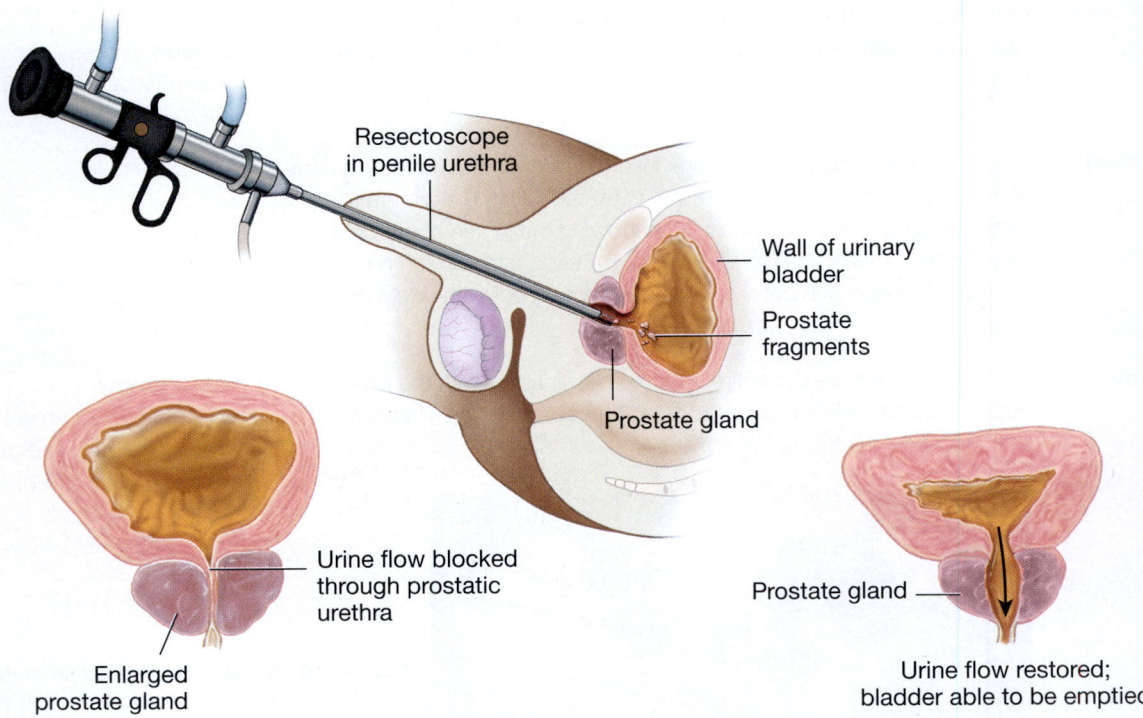

FIGURE 11-11 ■ Transurethral resection of the prostate (TURP).
This surgical procedure used to be the "gold standard" of treatment for benign prostatic hyperplasia. Now, newer techniques use lasers, microwaves, and radio waves to destroy excess tissue.

Word or Phrase	Description	Pronunciation/Word Parts
vasectomy	Procedure in the male to prevent pregnancy in the female. Through a small incision in the scrotum, each vas deferens is identified. A length of each tube is removed, and the cut ends are sutured or destroyed with electrocautery. Spermatozoa continue to be produced by each testis, but they are eventually broken down and absorbed back into the body. A **vasovasostomy** is a reversal of a vasectomy. The cut ends of the vas deferens are rejoined so that spermatozoa are again present in the semen and the male can cause a female to become pregnant.	**vasectomy** (vah-SEK-toh-mee) **vas/o-** *blood vessel; vas deferens* **-ectomy** *surgical removal* **vasovasostomy** (VAY-soh-vah-SAW-stoh-mee) **vas/o-** *blood vessel; vas deferens* **vas/o-** *blood vessel; vas deferens* **-stomy** *surgically created opening* Vasovasotomy: *Surgically created opening (in one part of the) vas deferens (to join another part of the) vas deferens*

11.5 PRACTICE LAPS

Use the Answer Key at the end of the book to check your answers.

A. Give the Meaning of Combining Forms

Next to each combining form, write its meaning. The first one has been done for you.

Combining Form	Meaning	Combining Form	Meaning
1. **andr/o-**	*male*	8. orchi/o-	
2. aspir/o-		9. prostat/o-	
3. bi/o-		10. resect/o-	
4. cis/o-		11. urethr/o-	
5. digit/o-		12. vas/o-	
6. embol/o-		13. vir/o-	
7. enucle/o-			

B. Build Words

Read the definition of the medical word. Look at the combining form that is given. Select the correct suffix from the Suffix List, and write it on the blank line. Then build the medical word, and write it on the line. (Remember: You may need to remove the combining vowel. Always remove the hyphens and slash.) Be sure to check your spelling.

Suffix List

-al (pertaining to)	-ion (action; condition)	-opsy (process of viewing)
-ation (being; having; process)	-ization (process of creating;	-pexy (process of fixing in place)
-ectomy (surgical removal)	process of inserting;	-scope (instrument used to examine)
-gen (that which produces)	process of making)	-therapy (treatment)

Definition of the Medical Word	Combining Form	Suffix	Build the Medical Word
Example: Pertaining to (using a) digit (to do an examination)	**digit/o-**	*-al*	*digital*

[*You think* pertaining to *(-al)* + digit *(digit/o-)*. You change the order of the word parts to put the suffix last. You write digital.]

1. Process of viewing living tissue	bi/o-		
2. That which produces male (characteristics)	andr/o-		
3. Surgical removal (of the) testis	orchi/o-		
4. Process (to) remove the main part	enucle/o-		
5. Surgical removal (of the) vas deferens	vas/o-		
6. Process (to) suck in (tissue)	aspir/o-		
7. Instrument used to examine (and) cut out and remove	resect/o-		
8. Process of fixing in place (a) testis	orchi/o-		
9. Surgical removal (of the) prostate gland	prostat/o-		
10. Process of inserting (an) occluding plug	embol/o-		
11. Treatment (using) cold	cry/o-		
12. Action (to) cut out (and) remove	resect/o-		

C. Define Abbreviations

1. Bx   _____

2. DRE   _____

3. HoLEP   _____

4. PUL   _____

5. PVP   _____

6. TSE   _____

7. TUMT   _____

8. TUNA   _____

9. TURP   _____

Abbreviations Summary

AIDS	acquired immunodeficiency syndrome	**PAE**	prostate artery embolization
BPH	benign prostatic hyperplasia	**PAP**	prostatic acid phosphatase
Bx	biopsy	**PSA**	prostate-specific antigen
CDC	Centers for Disease Control and Prevention	**PUL**	prostate urethral lift
DRE	digital rectal examination	**PVP**	photoselective vaporization of the prostate
ED	erectile dysfunction	**RPR**	rapid plasma reagin (test for syphilis)
FSH	follicle-stimulating hormone	**STD**	sexually transmitted disease
GC	gonococcus (*Neisseria gonorrhoeae*)	**STI**	sexually transmitted infection
GU	genitourinary; gonococcal urethritis	**TRUS**	transrectal ultrasound
HIV	human immunodeficiency virus	**TSE**	testicular self-examination
HoLEP	holmium laser enucleation of the prostate	**TUMT**	transurethral microwave therapy
HPV	human papillomavirus	**TUNA**	transurethral needle ablation
HSV	herpes simplex virus	**TURP**	transurethral resection of the prostate
LH	luteinizing hormone	**VDRL**	Venereal Disease Research Laboratory

Word Alert

Abbreviations. Abbreviations are commonly used in all types of medical documents; however, they can mean different things to different people and their meanings can be misinterpreted. Always verify the meaning of an abbreviation.

- *ED* means *erectile dysfunction*, but it also means *emergency department*.
- *GU* means *genitourinary*, but it also means *gonococcal urethritis*.
- *PAP* means *prostatic acid phosphatase*, but *Pap* is also a short form for *Papanicolaou test*.

It's Greek to Me! Did you notice that some words have two different combining forms? Combining forms from both Greek and Latin remain a part of medical language today.

Word	Greek	Latin	Medical Word Examples
glans penis	balan/o-		balanitis
penis		pen/o-	penile
sexual intercourse	pareun/o-	coit/o-, venere/o-	dyspareunia; postcoital, venereal
testicle; testis	didym/o-, orchid/o-, orchi/o-, orch/o-	test/o-, testicul/o-	epididymitis, cryptorchidism, orchiectomy, orchitis; testosterone, testicular

Career Focus

Meet Mindy, a clinical laboratory scientist and blood bank supervisor

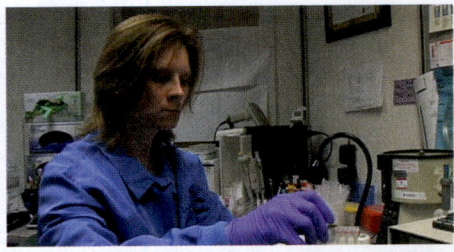

"Clinical laboratory scientist is the newer name, but we know ourselves as medical technologists. In college, I took a microbiology class. I enjoyed it so much that I pursued that as my major. A technologist performs the testing, whether it's hematology, chemistry, blood bank, or microbiology. I have to communicate with the doctors and nurses. I have to have an understanding of medical terminology to be able to communicate clearly with them. When we can interact with the nurses and the doctors to give them the answers they need to care for the patients, that's what's rewarding."

- **Clinical laboratory scientists** are allied health professionals who work in a hospital or a large commercial medical laboratory. They perform all types of laboratory tests on blood, urine, semen, and other body fluids and tissues. They work with microscopes and computerized equipment.

- **Urologists** treat medical conditions of the male genitourinary system.

- **Reproductive medicine physicians** treat male (and female) patients who have difficulty conceiving a child because of infertility.

- **Endocrinologists** treat patients with disorders of the endocrine system, including hormonal disorders that affect men, such as infertility.

- Cancerous tumors of the male genitourinary system are treated medically by an **oncologist** and surgically by a general **surgeon**.

clinical (KLIN-ih-kal)
  clinic/o- *medicine*
  -al *pertaining to*

laboratory (LAB-oh-rah-TOR-ee)
  laborat/o- *testing place*
  -ory *having the function of*

scientist (SY-en-tihst)
  scient/o- *knowledge; science*
  -ist *person who specializes in; thing that specializes in*

urologist (yoor-AW-loh-jist)
  ur/o- *urinary system; urine*
  log/o- *study of; word*
  ist- *person who specializes in*

reproductive (REE-proh-DUK-tiv)
  re- *again and again; backward; unable to*
  product/o- *produce*
  -ive *pertaining to*

endocrinologist
(EN-doh-krih-NAW-loh-jist)
  endo- *innermost; within*
  crin/o- *secrete*
  log/o- *study of; word*
  -ist *person who specializes in; thing that specializes in*

oncologist (ong-KAW-loh-jist)
  onc/o- *mass; tumor*
  log/o- *study of; word*
  -ist *person who specializes in; thing that specializes in*

surgeon (SER-jin)
  surg/o- *operative procedure*
  -eon *person who performs*

Chapter Review Exercises

Dive In: Medical Language Exercises

Test your knowledge of the chapter by completing these review exercises. Use the Answer Key at the end of the book to check your answers. Note: Each of the numbered exercise headers corresponds to a numbered learning outcome at the beginning of the chapter.

11.1 Anatomy

MATCHING EXERCISE

Match each word or phrase to its description.

1. anus
2. bulbourethral gland
3. corpora cavernosa
4. epididymis
5. inguinal canal
6. interstitial cells
7. lumen
8. prostate gland
9. spermatozoon
10. testis
11. urogenital system

_____ central open area through the length of a tube or duct
_____ destroys defective spermatozoa
_____ has a head and a tail
_____ secrete the male hormone testosterone
_____ egg-shaped gland in the scrotum
_____ another name for the genitourinary system
_____ produces thick mucus that is part of the semen
_____ erectile tissue located in the penis
_____ opening in the abdominal wall muscle of a fetus
_____ perineum is the area between the posterior scrotum and this
_____ doughnut-shaped gland

CIRCLE EXERCISE

Circle the correct answer from the choices given.

1. The male sex glands are the (**bulbourethral glands, gonads, prostate gland**).
2. Before birth, the vas deferens is in the (**epididymis, spermatic cord, urethra**).
3. An individual spermatozoon has (**23, 46, 92**) chromosomes.
4. The seminiferous tubules produce (**semen, spermatozoa, testosterone**).
5. The prepuce is also known as the (**epididymis, foreskin, vas deferens**).

TRUE OR FALSE EXERCISE

*Indicate whether each statement is true or false by writing **T** or **F** on the line.*

1. _____ Testosterone is the most abundant and biologically active of the male sex hormones.
2. _____ The word *testicle* shows that it is a smaller size than a *testis*.
3. _____ The corpus spongiosum is a column of erectile tissue on the underside of the penis.
4. _____ The glans penis contains the urethral meatus.

PLURAL NOUN AND ADJECTIVE EXERCISE

Read the noun and write its plural form and/or adjective form on the line. Only write in the plural noun or adjective if there is a blank line there for it. Be sure to check your spelling. The first one has been done for you.

Singular Noun	Plural Noun	Adjective	Singular Noun	Plural Noun	Adjective
1. **corpus cavernosum**	*corpora cavernosa*		7. sperm		_____
2. scrotum		_____	8. epididymis	_____	
3. perineum		_____	9. prostate		_____
4. testis	_____		10. penis		_____
5. testicle	_____	_____	11. urethra		_____
6. spermatozoon	_____				

DIVIDING WORDS EXERCISE

Separate these words into their component parts (prefix, combining form, suffix). Some words do not contain all three word parts. The first one has been done for you.

Medical Word	Prefix	Combining Form	Suffix	Medical Word	Prefix	Combining Form	Suffix
1. **perineal**		*perine/o-*	*-al*	5. gonad		_____	_____
2. testicular		_____	_____	6. inguinal		_____	_____
3. genital		_____	_____	7. seminal		_____	_____
4. spermatozoon		_____	_____	8. ejaculatory		_____	_____

SPELLING EXERCISE

Read each medical word pronunciation and write the medical word that it represents. Be sure to check your spelling. The first one has been done for you.

1. (EP-ih-DID-ih-mihs)   *epididymis*
2. (JEN-ih-toh-YOOR-ih-NAIR-ee)   _____
3. (tes-TIH-kyoo-lar)   _____
4. (ING-gwih-nal)   _____
5. (BUL-boh-yoor-EE-thral)   _____

11.2 Physiology

CIRCLE EXERCISE

Circle the correct answer from the choices given.

1. The final process by which a spermatozoon is created is (**coitus, meiosis, mitosis**).

2. Luteinizing hormone is secreted by the (**anterior pituitary gland, seminal vesicles, prostate gland**).

3. A (**gamete, gonad, spermatocyte**) is a cell that has 23 chromosomes.

4. Testosterone causes all of the following *except* (**enlargement of the external genitalia, sexual drive, stimulation of the interstitial cells**).

5. An immature, round cell in the seminiferous tubules is a (**gamete, spermatocyte, spermatozoon**).

TRUE OR FALSE EXERCISE

Indicate whether each statement is true or false by writing **T** *or* **F** *on the line.*

1. _____ Adolescence is also known as puberty.

2. _____ A spermatozoon is created by meiosis and then mitosis.

3. _____ Ejaculation is the sudden expelling of semen from the prostatic urethra.

4. _____ Follicle-stimulating hormone is another name for testosterone.

DIVIDING WORDS EXERCISE

Separate these words into their component parts (prefix, combining form, suffix). Some words do not contain all three word parts. The first one has been done for you.

Medical Word	Prefix	Combining Form	Suffix	Medical Word	Prefix	Combining Form	Suffix
1. **follicle**		*folli/o-*	*-cle*	4. spermatocyte		_____	_____
2. adolescence		_____	_____	5. ejaculation		_____	_____
3. meiosis		_____	_____				

SPELLING EXERCISE

Read each medical word pronunciation and write the medical word that it represents. Be sure to check your spelling. The first one has been done for you.

1. **(SEK-shoo-al)**   _____*sexual*_____

2. (my-OH-sihs)   _____

3. (SPER-mah-toh-JEN-eh-sihs)   _____

4. (KOH-ih-tuhs)   _____

11.3 Diseases

MATCHING EXERCISE

Match each word or phrase to its description.

1. balanitis
2. cryptorchidism
3. erectile dysfunction
4. gonorrhea
5. gynecomastia
6. postcoital pain
7. priapism
8. seminoma
9. sexually transmitted infection
10. syphilis

_____ undescended testis

_____ caused by a gram-negative diplococcus

_____ persistent erection

_____ also known as an STD

_____ infection of the glans penis

_____ testicular cancer

_____ symptom includes a chancre

_____ enlarged breasts in a male

_____ discomfort after sexual intercourse

_____ can be caused by a spinal cord injury

CIRCLE EXERCISE

Circle the correct answer from the choices given.

1. Infertility is caused by all of the following *except* (**childhood mumps, chordee, undescended testis**).

2. Orchitis is infection or inflammation of the (**glans penis, prostate gland, testes**).

3. A varicocele can cause (**infertility, testicular cancer, a sexually transmitted disease**).

4. The word *adenocarcinoma* tells you that this cancer begins in a (**follicle, gland, tubule**).

5. Erectile dysfunction is also known as (**impotence, priapism, seminoma**).

TRUE OR FALSE EXERCISE

*Indicate whether each statement is true or false by writing **T** or **F** on the line.*

1. _____ Chordee is a downward curvature of the penis during an erection.
2. _____ HIV and AIDS are caused by a retrovirus.
3. _____ Priapism is an abnormal, continuing erection of the penis.
4. _____ Genital warts are also known as *condylomata acuminata*.

DIVIDING WORDS EXERCISE

Separate these words into their component parts (prefix, combining form, suffix). Some words do not contain all three word parts. The first one has been done for you.

Medical Word	Prefix	Combining Form	Suffix
1. **cancerous**		cancer/o-	-ous
2. balanitis			
3. dyspareunia			
4. epididymitis			
5. epispadias			
6. gonorrhea			
7. hyperplasia			
8. infertility			

Medical Word	Prefix	Combining Form	Suffix
9. malignancy			
10. orchitis			
11. phimosis			
12. postcoital			
13. priapism			
14. prostatitis			
15. seminoma			
16. varicocele			

SPELLING EXERCISE

Read each medical word pronunciation and write the medical word that it represents. Be sure to check your spelling. The first one has been done for you.

1. (IN-fer-TIL-ih-tee) _____infertility_____
2. (OH-lih-goh-SPER-mee-ah) _____
3. (VAIR-ih-koh-SEEL) _____
4. (HY-per-PLAY-shah) _____
5. (AD-eh-noh-KAR-sih-NOH-mah) _____
6. (ong-KAW-loh-jist) _____
7. (kor-DEE) _____
8. (DIS-pah-ROO-nee-ah) _____
9. (fy-MOH-sihs) _____
10. (GY-neh-koh-MAS-tee-ah) _____
11. (GAW-noh-REE-ah) _____
12. (SIF-ih-lihs) _____

11.4 Laboratory, Diagnostic, and Radiologic Procedures

MATCHING EXERCISE

Match each word or phrase to its description.

1. acid phosphatase
2. brachytherapy
3. FTA-ABS
4. hormone testing
5. prostate-specific antigen
6. semen analysis
7. ultrasound image

_____ blood test for FSH, LH, or testosterone
_____ also known as a *sonogram*
_____ level is increased in prostate cancer
_____ semen test used in rape investigations
_____ most specific blood test for syphilis
_____ part of an infertility workup
_____ uses radioactive seeds implanted in the prostate gland

CIRCLE EXERCISE

Circle the correct answer from the choices given.

1. The level of (**DNA, PSA, RPR**) is increased with prostatic cancer.
2. The forward movement of sperm is (**antigen, morphology, motility**).
3. Paternity can be proved with a/an (**DNA analysis, ProstaScint scan, ultrasonography**).
4. Transrectal ultrasonography uses sound waves to guide a biopsy of the (**rectum, penis, prostate gland**).
5. Tests for syphilis include all of the following *except* (**FTA-ABS, RPR, TRUS**).

DIVIDING WORDS EXERCISE

Separate these words into their component parts (prefix, combining form, suffix). Some words do not contain all three word parts. The first one has been done for you.

Medical Word	Prefix	Combining Form	Suffix
1. **phosphatase**		*phosphat/o-*	*-ase*
2. transrectal	____	_____	_____
3. ultrasonography	____	_____	_____
4. aspermia	____	_____	_____
5. morphology		_____	_____
6. sonogram		_____	_____

SPELLING EXERCISE

Read each medical word pronunciation and write the medical word that it represents. Be sure to check your spelling. The first one has been done for you.

1. (**HOR-mohn**)   *hormone*
2. (AN-tih-jen)   _____
3. (moh-TIL-ih-tee)   _____
4. (UL-trah-soh-NAW-grah-fee)   _____

11.5 Medical Procedures, Drugs, and Surgical Procedures

MATCHING EXERCISE

Match each word or phrase to its description.

1. antibiotic drug	_____ surgical removal of a testis
2. biopsy	_____ done for social customs or religious requirements
3. circumcision	_____ removal of tissue to test for prostatic cancer
4. DRE	_____ used to treat syphilis
5. holmium laser	_____ feels for nodules or enlargement of the prostate gland
6. orchiectomy	_____ used to destroy enlarged prostate gland tissue

CIRCLE EXERCISE

Circle the correct answer from the choices given.

1. During a circumcision, the (**glans penis, prepuce, prostate gland**) is removed.
2. Surgically fixing a testis in place is a/an (**circumcision, orchiopexy, prosthesis**).
3. A/An (**androgen drug, TURP, vasovasostomy**) is used to reverse a vasectomy.
4. TSE should be performed (**at birth, monthly, yearly**).

TRUE OR FALSE EXERCISE

*Indicate whether each statement is true or false by writing **T** or **F** on the line.*

1. _____ A testicular self-examination is done on a newborn.
2. _____ An antiretroviral drug is used to treat AIDS.
3. _____ A decreased blood level of testosterone can be treated with an androgen drug.
4. _____ An incisional biopsy uses a needle to aspirate tissue.
5. _____ A vasovasostomy is performed to prevent pregnancy in the female.

DIVIDING WORDS EXERCISE

Separate these words into their component parts (prefix, combining form, suffix). Some words do not contain all three word parts. The first one has been done for you.

Medical Word	Prefix	Combining Form	Suffix
1. **antibiotic**	*anti-*	*bi/o-*	*-tic*
2. androgen			
3. biopsy			
4. circumcision			
5. embolization			
6. orchiectomy			
7. transurethral			
8. vasectomy			

SPELLING EXERCISE

Read each medical word pronunciation and write the medical word that it represents. Be sure to check your spelling. The first one has been done for you.

1. (AN-tee-VY-ral)   *antiviral*
2. (BY-awp-see) _____
3. (AS-pih-RAY-shun) _____
4. (OR-kee-oh-PEK-see) _____
5. (vah-SEK-toh-mee) _____

Immerse Yourself: Analyze Medical Reports

Electronic Patient Record #1

This is an Office Visit SOAP Note. Read the note and answer the questions.

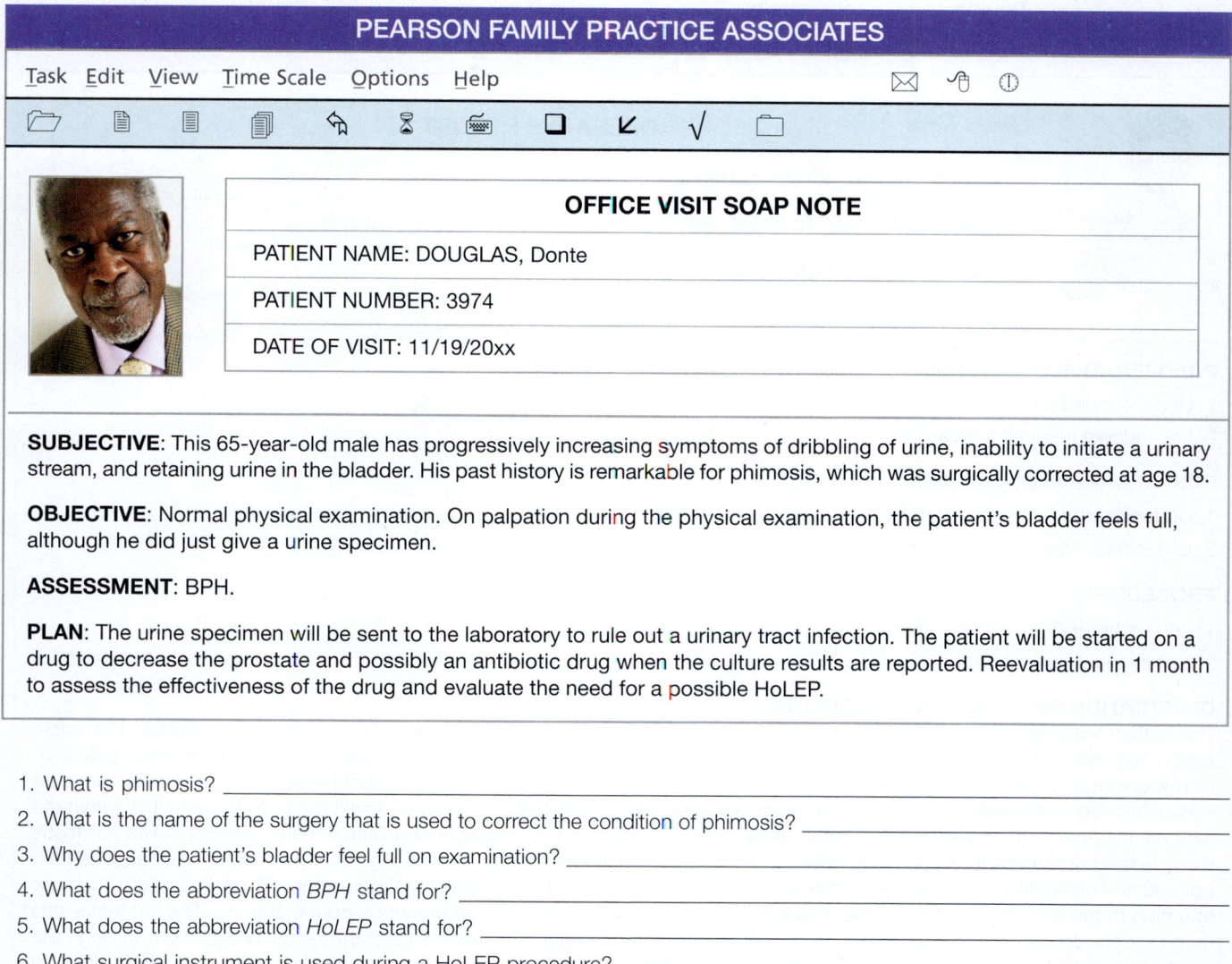

PEARSON FAMILY PRACTICE ASSOCIATES

Task   Edit   View   Time Scale   Options   Help

OFFICE VISIT SOAP NOTE

PATIENT NAME: DOUGLAS, Donte

PATIENT NUMBER: 3974

DATE OF VISIT: 11/19/20xx

SUBJECTIVE: This 65-year-old male has progressively increasing symptoms of dribbling of urine, inability to initiate a urinary stream, and retaining urine in the bladder. His past history is remarkable for phimosis, which was surgically corrected at age 18.

OBJECTIVE: Normal physical examination. On palpation during the physical examination, the patient's bladder feels full, although he did just give a urine specimen.

ASSESSMENT: BPH.

PLAN: The urine specimen will be sent to the laboratory to rule out a urinary tract infection. The patient will be started on a drug to decrease the prostate and possibly an antibiotic drug when the culture results are reported. Reevaluation in 1 month to assess the effectiveness of the drug and evaluate the need for a possible HoLEP.

---

1. What is phimosis? _____

2. What is the name of the surgery that is used to correct the condition of phimosis? _____

3. Why does the patient's bladder feel full on examination? _____

4. What does the abbreviation *BPH* stand for? _____

5. What does the abbreviation *HoLEP* stand for? _____

6. What surgical instrument is used during a HoLEP procedure? _____

Electronic Patient Record #2

This is a hospital Operative Report. Read the report and answer the questions.

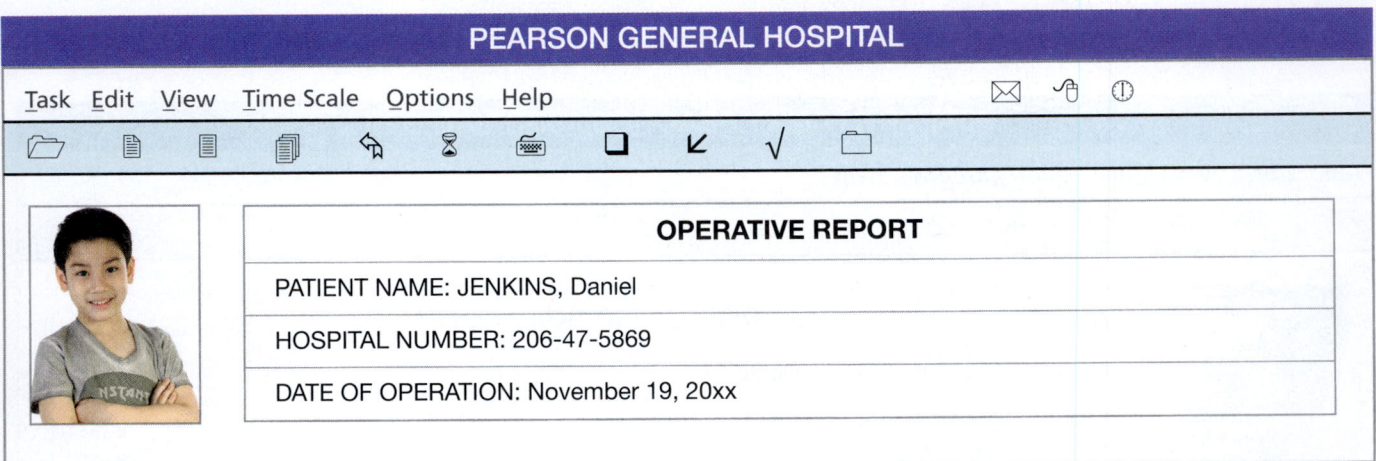

PEARSON GENERAL HOSPITAL

Task Edit View Time Scale Options Help

OPERATIVE REPORT

PATIENT NAME: JENKINS, Daniel

HOSPITAL NUMBER: 206-47-5869

DATE OF OPERATION: November 19, 20xx

PREOPERATIVE DIAGNOSES

1. Undescended left testis
2. Left indirect inguinal hernia

POSTOPERATIVE DIAGNOSES

1. Undescended left testis, corrected
2. Left indirect inguinal hernia, repaired

PROCEDURES

1. Left orchiopexy
2. Left inguinal herniorrhaphy

DESCRIPTION OF OPERATIVE PROCEDURE

The patient was placed in the dorsal supine position, and general anesthesia was induced via mask anesthesia. The pubic region and external genitalia were prepped with antibacterial scrub and draped with sterile surgical drapes. A transverse incision was made in the suprapubic skinfold on the left side. It was carried down through subcutaneous tissue and fat. Bleeding was controlled with electrocautery. The left testis was identified in the operative field and was noted to be lying just within the external inguinal ring. The external oblique fascia was incised with a #15 scalpel and Metzenbaum scissors. The left testis was grasped and freed from its surrounding structures up to the level of the internal inguinal ring. The hernia sac was then opened and dissected up to the level of the inguinal ring, where it was closed with 4-0 Vicryl suture. Then we again turned our attention to the undescended left testis. A scrotal incision was made, and a subcutaneous pouch created. The left testis was then brought down into the pouch, and a 3-0 silk suture was placed in the lower pole of the testis, brought out through the scrotal skin, and tied over a cotton pledget to secure the testis in place. A careful search detected no bleeding in the scrotal or groin incisions. The scrotal incision was closed with 5-0 Vicryl. The external oblique fascia was closed with a running 4-0 Vicryl suture. The subcutaneous tissue was closed with 4-0 Vicryl. The skin was closed with a running subcuticular 3-0 Prolene suture, and the child was discharged from the operating room in satisfactory condition.

James R. Bentley, M.D.

James R. Bentley, M.D.

JRB:btg
D: 11/19/xx
T: 11/19/xx

1. Divide *orchiopexy* into its two word parts and give the meaning of each word part.

   Word Part   **Meaning**

   _____   _____

   _____   _____

2. An incision in the suprapubic skinfold would be located.

   a. below the pubic bone

   b. around the pubic bone

   c. above the pubic bone

3. In the dorsal supine position, the patient is placed on his (**abdomen, back, side**).

4. In a male, the external genitalia include what six structures?

   _____   _____

   _____   _____

   _____   _____

5. Incisions were made in what two areas? _____ _____

6. The hernia sac was closed with sutures. **True   False**

7. *Subcutaneous* means (**around the testis, inside the scrotum, under the skin**).

8. The left testis was not descended. What operative procedure was performed to correct this? _____

9. A preoperative diagnosis represents the patient's condition (**before, during, after**) surgery.

   _____

You Create the Electronic Health Record

Read the patient's words. Then read the partial sentence in the electronic health record and fill in the blank with the correct medical word.

1. Patient's words: "I have had a temperature and I am sweating at night for a while now. Lately, I noticed that I lost a lot of weight and am very tired."

   You type: "Possible diagnosis of infection with human _____ virus (HIV). The _____ screening test Orasure was performed today. Treatment will be started with an oral _____ drug."

2. Patient's words: "My wife and I have been trying for 2 years to have a child. Do you think there could be something wrong with me?"

   You type: "Physical examination revealed that there is an _____ left testicle with the scrotum being empty on the left side. Plan: Order blood tests for the _____ FSH and LH and do a _____ analysis for a sperm count. The patient may need to have surgical correction of the position of the testicle by doing an _____."

MyLab Medical Terminology™

MyLab Medical Terminology is a premium online homework management system that includes a host of features to help you study. Registered users will find:

- A multitude of quizzes and activities built within the MyLab platform

- Powerful tools that track and analyze your results—allowing you to create a personalized learning experience

- Videos and audio pronunciations to help enrich your progress

- Streaming lesson presentations (guided lectures) and self-paced learning modules

- A space where you and your instructor can check your progress and manage your assignments

12 Gynecology and Obstetrics
Female Genital and Reproductive System

Gynecology (GY-neh-KAW-loh-jee) is the medical specialty that studies the anatomy and physiology of the female genital system; uses laboratory, diagnostic, and radiologic procedures to diagnose female genital diseases; and uses medical procedures, drugs, and surgical procedures to treat female genital diseases.

Obstetrics (awb-STEH-triks) is the medical specialty that studies the anatomy and physiology of the female reproductive system; uses laboratory, diagnostic, and radiologic procedures to diagnose female reproductive diseases; and uses medical procedures, drugs, and surgical procedures to monitor pregnancy and childbirth and treat diseases of the reproductive system.

Chapter Overview and Learning Outcomes

After you study this chapter, you should be able to demonstrate mastery of the outcomes by successfully completing the exercises.

12.1 Anatomy

Identify the structures of the female genital and reproductive system.

Demonstrate proficiency in medical language.

12.1 Practice Laps

12.2 Physiology

Describe the functions of the female genital and reproductive system.

Demonstrate proficiency in medical language.

12.2 Practice Laps

Vocabulary Review

12.3 Diseases

Describe common female genital and reproductive diseases.

Demonstrate proficiency in medical language.

12.3 Practice Laps

12.4 Laboratory, Diagnostic, and Radiologic Procedures

Describe common female genital and reproductive system laboratory tests, diagnostic procedures, and radiologic procedures.

Demonstrate proficiency in medical language.

12.4 Practice Laps

12.5 Medical Procedures, Drugs, and Surgical Procedures

Describe common female genital and reproductive system medical procedures, drugs, and surgical procedures.

Demonstrate proficiency in medical language.

12.5 Practice Laps

Abbreviations Summary

Career Focus

Chapter Review Exercises

Dive In: Medical Language Exercises (Learning Outcomes 12.1–12.5)

Immerse Yourself: Analyze Medical Reports

Medical Language Key

To unlock the definition of a medical word, first break it into word parts. Then give the meaning of each word part. Put the meanings of the word parts in order, beginning with the meaning of the suffix, then the meaning of the prefix (if there is one), then the meaning of the combining form.

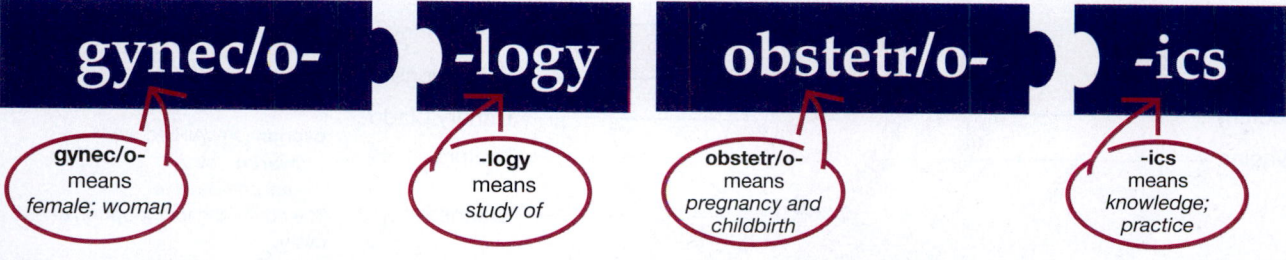

gynec/o-   **-logy**   **obstetr/o-**   **-ics**

gynec/o-
means
female; woman

-logy
means
study of

obstetr/o-
means
*pregnancy and
childbirth*

-ics
means
*knowledge;
practice*

Gynecology (GYN): ▶ *Study of the female (and) woman.*

Obstetrics (OB): ▶ *Knowledge and practice (of treating women during) pregnancy and childbirth.*

The female genital and reproductive system consists of both internal and external structures known as the **genitalia** or **genital organs** (see Figure 12-1■). The **internal genitalia** in the **abdominopelvic cavity** include the ovaries, uterine tubes, uterus, and vagina. The **external genitalia** include the area of the mons pubis, labia majora, labia minora, clitoris, and vaginal introitus. The **breasts** or **mammary glands** are also part of the female genital and reproductive system.

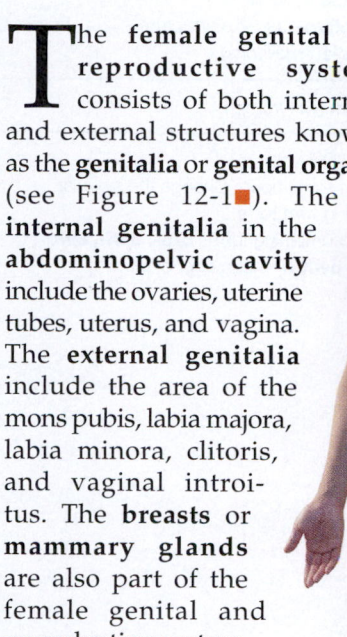

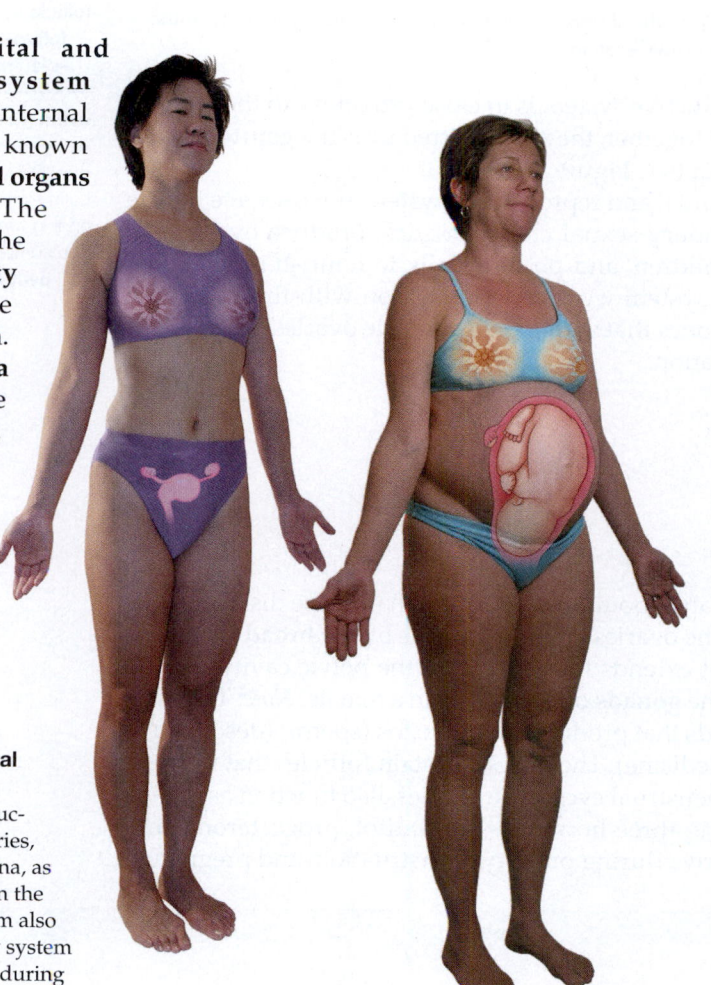

FIGURE 12-1 ■ Female genital and reproductive system.
The female genital and reproductive system consists of the ovaries, uterine tubes, uterus, and vagina, as well as the external genitalia on the outside of the body. This system also includes the breasts. This body system undergoes significant changes during pregnancy and childbirth.

Pronunciation/Word Parts

genital (JEN-ih-tal)
  genit/o- *genitalia*
  -al *pertaining to*

reproductive (REE-proh-DUK-tiv)
  re- *again and again; backward; unable to*
  product/o- *produce*
  -ive *pertaining to*
Reproductive: *Pertaining to again and again produc(ing children)*

genitalia (JEN-ih-TAY-lee-ah)

internal (in-TER-nal)
  intern/o- *inside*
  -al *pertaining to*

abdominopelvic (ab-DAW-mih-noh-PEL-vik)
  abdomin/o- *abdomen*
  pelv/o- *hip bone; pelvis; renal pelvis*
  -ic *pertaining to*

cavity (KAV-ih-tee)
  cav/o- *hollow space*
  -ity *condition; state*

external (EKS-ter-nal)
  extern/o- *outside*
  -al *pertaining to*

mammary (MAM-ah-ree)
  mamm/o- *breast*
  -ary *pertaining to*

Pronunciation/Word Parts

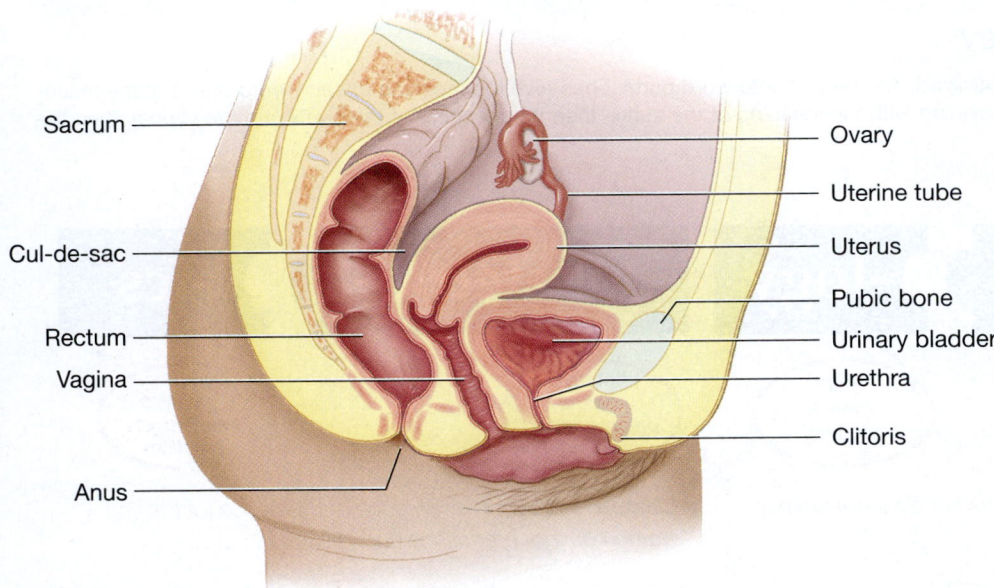

FIGURE 12-2 ■ Abdominopelvic cavity.
The female genital and reproductive organs in the abdominopelvic cavity lie in close proximity to the organs of the urinary system and gastrointestinal system.

The female genital and reproductive system is in close proximity to the urinary system; when they are considered together, they are referred to as the **genitourinary (GU) system** or **urogenital system** (see Figure 12-2 ■).

The functions of the female genital and reproductive system are to secrete female hormones, develop female secondary sexual characteristics, produce ova (eggs), menstruate, conceive and bear children, and produce milk to nourish infants. The female genital and reproductive system works in conjunction with the endocrine system that releases several hormones that stimulate the female ovaries during ovulation and the breasts during lactation.

12.1 Anatomy

Internal Genitalia

Ovaries

An **ovary** is a small egg-shaped gland about 2 inches in length near the distal end of a uterine tube (see Figure 12-3 ■). The ovaries are held in place by the **broad ligament**, a folded sheet of peritoneum that extends to the walls of the pelvic cavity, and by other ligaments. The ovaries are the **gonads** or sex glands in a female. *Note:* The male gonads are the testes, the sex glands that produce spermatozoa (sperm) (described in Chapter 11, Male Reproductive Medicine). The ovaries contain **follicles** that rupture, releasing **ova** (eggs) during the menstrual cycle. The ovaries also function as glands of the endocrine system, secreting three hormones—estradiol, progesterone, and testosterone—each of which is active during puberty, menstruation, and pregnancy.

Did You Know?

Before birth, while a female fetus is still in the mother's uterus, the fetal ovary already has follicles that contain about 2 million **oocytes** (immature ova). These are all the ova that the grown female will ever have, as no more are produced after she is born. By puberty only about 25% of these remain and, of those, only about 400 mature ova are released during all the ovulations throughout her lifetime.

---

genitourinary (JEN-ih-toh-YOOR-ih-NAIR-ee)
  genit/o- *genitalia*
  urin/o- *urinary system; urine*
  -ary *pertaining to*

urogenital (YOOR-oh-JEN-ih-tal)
  ur/o- *urinary system; urine*
  genit/o- *genitalia*
  -al *pertaining to*

ovary (OH-vah-ree)

ovarian (oh-VAIR-ee-an)
  ovari/o- *ovary*
  -an *pertaining to*
The combining form **oophor/o-** also means *ovary.*

ligament (LIG-ah-ment)

gonad (GOH-nad)
  gon/o- *ovum; spermatozoon*
  -ad *in the direction of; toward*

follicle (FAW-lih-kul)
  folli/o- *sac-like structure*
  -cle *small thing*

ovum (OH-vum)

ova (OH-vah)
Latin plural noun: Change the singular ending *-um* to *-a.*
The combining forms **o/o-, ov/i-, ov/o-,** and **ovul/o-** mean *egg; ovum.*

oocyte (OH-oh-site)
  o/o- *egg; ovum*
  -cyte *cell*

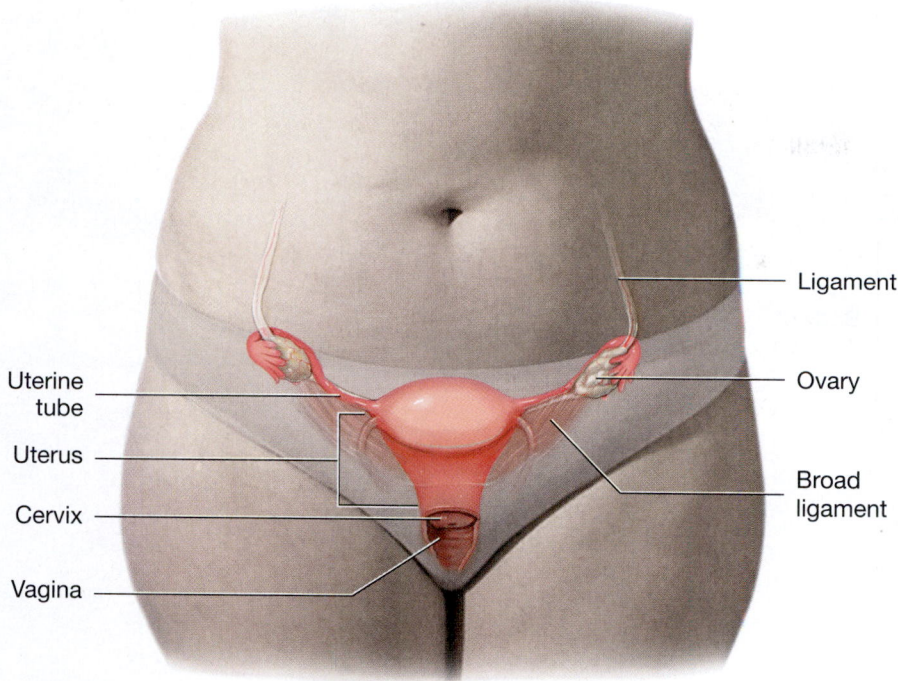

Uterine tube

Uterus

Cervix

Vagina

Ligament

Ovary

Broad ligament

FIGURE 12-3 ■ Ovaries, uterine tubes, and uterus.
The ovaries and uterine tubes lie on either side of the uterus. They are suspended within the abdominopelvic cavity by ligaments. The cervix of the uterus protrudes downward into the vagina.

Uterine Tubes

Each **uterine tube** or **oviduct** is about 5 inches in length and is held in place by the broad ligament. The function of the uterine tube is to transport an ovum from the ovary to the uterus. The proximal end of the uterine tube is connected to the uterus, but its distal end is not directly connected to the ovary (see Figure 12-4 ■). There is an open space (into the abdominopelvic cavity) between each ovary and its uterine tube. The ovary releases an ovum into this open space. **Fimbriae**, the moving, finger-like projections at the end of the uterine tube, create currents that carry the ovum into the **lumen** of the uterine tube. Within the tube, **cilia** (tiny hairs) beat in waves while **peristalsis** (coordinated, wave-like contractions of smooth muscle around the tube) propels the ovum toward the uterus. Fluid inside the uterine tube contains nutrients to nourish the ovum on its 3-day journey to the uterus. Together, the ovaries and the uterine tubes are known as the **adnexa** because they are accessory structures connected to the main organ of the uterus.

Uterus

The **uterus** is an inverted pear-shaped organ about 3 inches in length (see Figure 12-4). The superior portion of the uterus is tipped anteriorly, and part of it rests on the urinary bladder (see Figure 12-2); this normal position is known as **anteflexion**.

The uterus is held in place within the pelvic cavity by the broad ligament and other ligaments that go from the uterus to the sides of the pelvic walls and to the bony sacrum. The broad ligament creates a small pouch, the **cul-de-sac**, between the uterus and the rectum (see Figure 12-2). The **fundus** is the rounded top of the uterus. The body of the uterus, which is its widest part, then narrows to become the **cervix** (neck of the uterus).

The wall of the uterus is composed of three layers: perimetrium, myometrium, and endometrium. The **perimetrium**, the outer layer, is a serous membrane that is part of the peritoneum that lines the abdominopelvic cavity (described in Chapter 3,

Pronunciation/Word Parts

uterine (YOO-teh-rin)
  uter/o- *uterus; womb*
  -ine *pertaining to*

oviduct (OH-vih-dukt)
  ov/i- *egg; ovum*
  -duct *duct; tube*
The combining forms **salping/o-** and **fallopi/o-** mean *uterine tube*. The uterine tube was previously known as the *fallopian tube.*

fimbriae (FIM-bree-ee)
Because there are so many fimbriae, the singular form is seldom used.

lumen (LOO-men)

cilia (SIL-ee-ah)
Because there are so many cilia, the singular form is seldom used.

peristalsis (PAIR-ih-STAL-sihs)
The prefix **peri-** means *around*. The suffix **-stalsis** means *process of contraction.*

adnexa (ad-NEK-sah)

adnexal (ad-NEK-sal)
  adnex/o- *accessory connecting parts*
  -al *pertaining to*

uterus (YOO-ter-us)

uterine (YOO-teh-rin)
  uter/o- *uterus; womb*
  -ine *pertaining to*
The combining forms **hyster/o-**, **metri/o-**, and **metr/o-** also mean *uterus; womb*. Laypersons refer to the uterus as the *womb.*

anteflexion (AN-tee-FLEK-shun)
  ante- *before; forward*
  flex/o- *bending*
  -ion *action; condition*

cul-de-sac (KUL-deh-sak)
The combining form **culd/o-** means *cul-de-sac.*

fundus (FUN-duhs)

fundal (FUN-dal)
  fund/o- *fundus; part farthest from the opening*
  -al *pertaining to*

cervix (SER-viks)

cervical (SER-vih-kal)
  cervic/o- *cervix; neck*
  -al *pertaining to*

perimetrium (PAIR-ih-MEE-tree-um)
  peri- *around*
  metri/o- *uterus; womb*
  -um *period of time; structure*

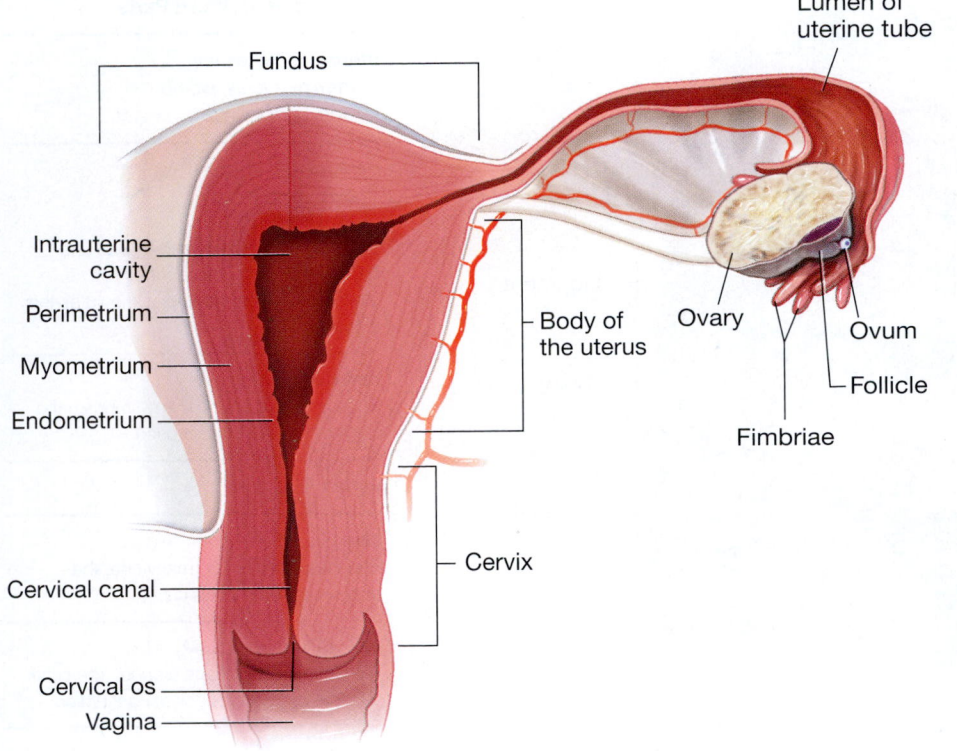

FIGURE 12-4 ■ **Uterus.**
The fundus, body, and cervix are regions of the uterus. The perimetrium is the outer covering of the uterus. The myometrium is the layer of smooth muscle that makes up the uterine wall. The endometrium is the layer of glands and tissue that lines the intrauterine cavity. The ovary contains a follicle that ruptures and releases an ovum. Movements of the fimbriae draw the ovum into the lumen of the uterine tube that goes to the uterus.

Gastroenterology). The **myometrium** (muscle layer) contains smooth muscle fibers that are oriented in different directions. This allows the uterus to contract strongly from all sides to expel the endometrium during menstruation and during labor and the delivery of a baby. Within the uterus is the hollow **intrauterine cavity**, which is lined with **endometrium**, the innermost layer. This is a mucous membrane that contains glands, and this layer thickens during the menstrual cycle. If an ovum is not fertilized, the endometrium is sloughed off and expelled from the body during menstruation, passing through the **cervical canal**. The **cervical os** in the center of the cervix is the opening of the cervical canal. The rounded tip of the cervix projects about ½ inch into the vagina.

Vagina

The **vagina** is a short, tube-like structure about 3 inches in length (see Figures 12-2, 12-3, and 12-4). Within the vagina is the open **vaginal canal**. The cervix of the uterus protrudes into the superior end of the vaginal canal. The **fornix** is the area of the vaginal canal that is behind and around the cervix. At the inferior end of the vaginal canal is the **hymen**, an elastic membrane that partially or completely covers the opening, although it is sometimes absent. The hymen, if present, is easily torn by the insertion of a tampon, a vaginal examination, or sexual intercourse.

The vagina has three functions. During menstruation, it transports the shed endometrium to the outside of the body. During sexual intercourse, it holds the male's penis and collects the ejaculate that contains spermatozoa. During birth, it is part of the birth canal that takes the fetus outside of the mother's body.

Pronunciation/Word Parts

myometrium (MY-oh-MEE-tree-um)
   my/o- *muscle*
   metri/o- *uterus; womb*
   -um *period of time; structure*

intrauterine (IN-trah-YOO-teh-rin)
   intra- *within*
   uter/o- *uterus; womb*
   -ine *pertaining to*

cavity (KAV-ih-tee)
   cav/o- *hollow space*
   -ity *condition; state*

endometrium (EN-doh-MEE-tree-um)

endometrial (EN-doh-MEE-tree-al)
   end/o- *innermost; within*
   metri/o- *uterus; womb*
   -al *pertaining to*

cervical (SER-vih-kal)

canal (kah-NAL)

os (AWS)

vagina (vah-JY-nah)

vaginal (VAJ-ih-nal)
   vagin/o- *vagina*
   -al *pertaining to*
The combining form **colp/o-** also means *vagina*.

fornix (FOR-niks)
The fornix is also known as the *vaginal vault*.

hymen (HY-men)

External Genitalia

Genital Area

The external genitalia consist of the mons pubis, labia majora, labia minora, clitoris, vaginal introitus, and glands that produce lubricating secretions (see Figure 12-5 ■). The **mons pubis** is the rounded, fleshy pad with pubic hair that overlies the pubic bone. The labia consist of two sets of lip-shaped structures that run anteriorly to posteriorly and partially cover the urethral meatus and vaginal introitus. The thicker, outermost lips, the **labia majora**, are fleshy and covered with pubic hair on their surface. The smooth, thin, inner lips, the **labia minora**, lie beneath the labia majora. The **clitoris**, the organ of sexual response in the female, is anterior to the urethral meatus. With sexual stimulation, the clitoris enlarges with blood and becomes firm. The **vaginal introitus** is the vaginal opening on the surface of the body; it is posterior to the urethral meatus. Three sets of glands near the vaginal introitus—**Bartholin glands**, the **urethral glands**, and **Skene glands (BUS)**—secrete mucus during sexual arousal. The **vulva** includes all of these structures, including the mons pubis. The area of skin between the vulva and the anus is the **perineum**.

mons pubis (MAWNZ PYOO-bihs)

labium (LAY-bee-um)

labia majora (LAY-bee-ah mah-JOR-ah)

labia minora (LAY-bee-ah -mih-NOR-ah)
Latin plural noun: Change the singular ending -um to -a.

labial (LAY-bee-al)
 labi/o- *labium; lip*
 -al *pertaining to*

clitoris (KLIT-oh-rihs)

vaginal (VAJ-ih-nal)

introitus (in-TROH-ih-tuhs)

Bartholin (BAR-toh-lin)

urethral (yoor-EE-thral)
 urethr/o- *urethra*
 -al *pertaining to*

Skene (SKEEN)

vulva (VUL-vah)

vulvar (VUL-var)
 vulv/o- *vulva*
 -ar *pertaining to*
The combining form **episi/o-** also means *vulva*.

perineum (PAIR-ih-NEE-um)

perineal (PAIR-ih-NEE-al)
 perine/o- *perineum*
 -al *pertaining to*

Word Alert
Sound-Alike Words

perineum (noun) area of skin between the vulva and the anus
Example: The perineum is an area on the outside of the body.

perimetrium (noun) serous membrane on the outside of the uterus
Example: The perimetrium is the outermost layer of the uterus.

peritoneum (noun) serous membrane that lines the abdominopelvic cavity
Example: The peritoneum secretes peritoneal fluid that fills the spaces between organs in the abdominopelvic cavity.

ANTERIOR / POSTERIOR — Mons pubis, Labia majora, Clitoris, Urethral meatus, Vaginal introitus (entrance), Labia minora, Vulva, Perineum, Anus

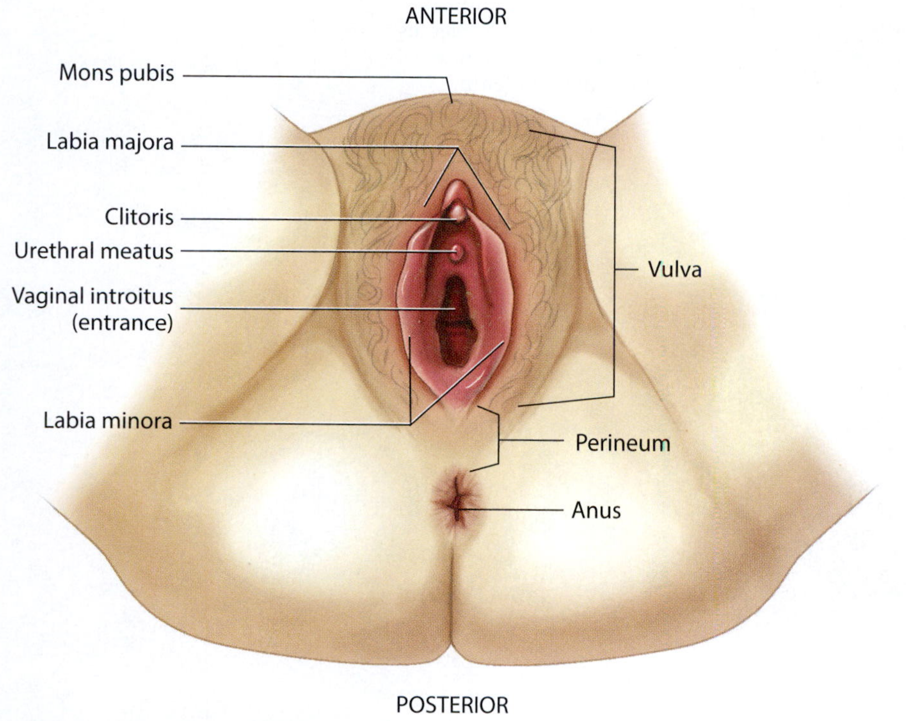

FIGURE 12-5 ■ External female genital area.
The labia majora and labia minora protect and partially cover the urethral meatus and vaginal introitus. The vulva includes all of the structures of the female external genitalia, including the urethral meatus (of the urinary system).

Breasts

The **breasts** or **mammary glands** are located on the chest. They contain adipose (fatty) tissue and glands. The breasts develop at puberty in response to estradiol secreted by the ovaries. They are one of the female secondary sexual characteristics, and they also provide milk to nourish the newborn after birth. The breasts contain **lactiferous lobules** that produce milk that flows through **lactiferous ducts** to the nipple (see Figure 12-6 ■). The **areola** is the pigmented area around the nipple. The surface of the areola is covered with small, elevated areas that secrete oil to protect the nipple when the baby nurses.

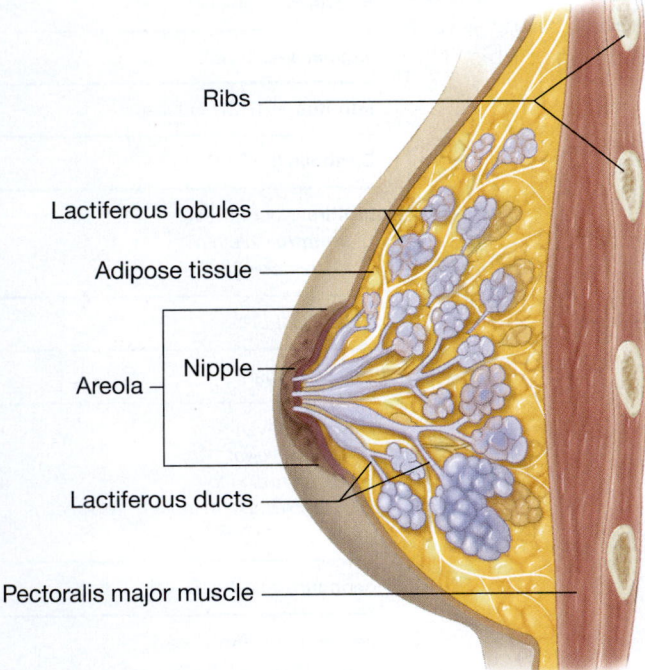

Ribs

Lactiferous lobules

Adipose tissue

Areola

Nipple

Lactiferous ducts

Pectoralis major muscle

FIGURE 12-6 ■ **Breast.**
The breasts or mammary glands develop during puberty, but the lactiferous lobules do not produce milk until after childbirth.

Pronunciation/Word Parts

mammary (MAM-ah-ree)
 mamm/o- *breast*
 -ary *pertaining to*
The combining forms **mamm/a-** and **mast/o-** also mean *breast*.

lactiferous (lak-TIH-fer-uhs)
 lact/i- *milk*
 fer/o- *bear*
 -ous *pertaining to*
The combining forms **galact/o-** and **lact/o-** also mean *milk*.

lobule (LAW-byool)
 lob/o- *lobe of an organ*
 -ule *small thing*

areola (ah-REE-oh-lah)

areolae (ah-REE-oh-lee)
Latin plural noun: Change the singular ending *-a* to *-ae*.

areolar (ah-REE-oh-lar)
 areol/o- *small, circular area*
 -ar *pertaining to*

12.1 PRACTICE LAPS

Use the Answer Key at the end of the book to check your answers.

A. Label Structures

Write each anatomy word or phrase in the correct numbered box. Be sure to check your spelling.

anus   labia minora   urethral meatus
clitoris   mons pubis   vaginal introitus
labia majora   perineum   vulva

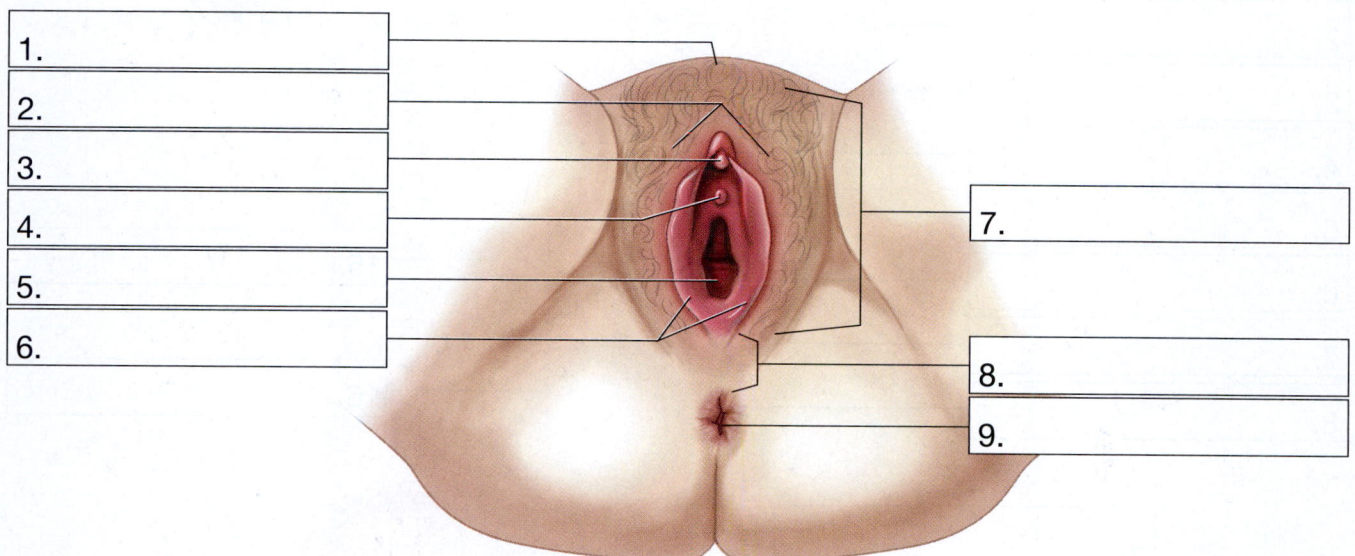

1.

2.

3.

4.

5.

6.

7.

8.

9.

broad ligament
cervical canal
cervical os
endometrium
fimbriae
follicle at time of ovulation

intrauterine cavity
lumen of uterine tube
myometrium
ovary
ovum
perimetrium

uterine cervix
uterine fundus
uterine tube
vagina

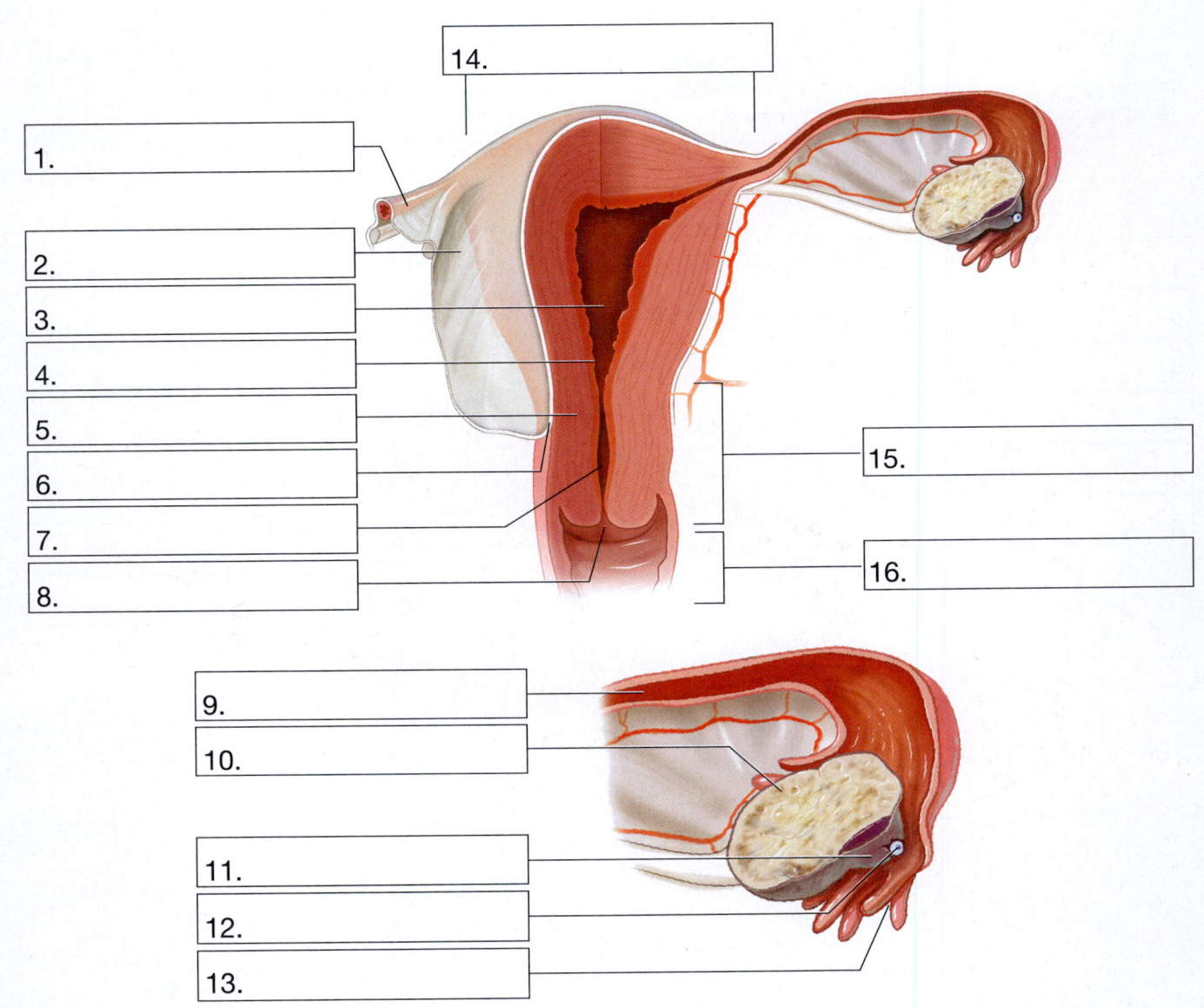

14. _____

1. _____

2. _____

3. _____

4. _____

5. _____

6. _____

7. _____

8. _____

15. _____

16. _____

9. _____

10. _____

11. _____

12. _____

13. _____

B. Give the Meaning of Combining Forms

Next to each combining form, write its meaning. The first one has been done for you.

Combining Form	Meaning	Combining Form	Meaning
1. **cav/o-**	*hollow space*	22. mamm/a-	
2. adnex/o-		23. mamm/o-	
3. areol/o-		24. mast/o-	
4. cervic/o-		25. metri/o-	
5. colp/o-		26. metr/o-	
6. culd/o-		27. my/o-	
7. episi/o-		28. o/o-	
8. extern/o-		29. oophor/o-	
9. fallopi/o-		30. ovari/o-	
10. fer/o-		31. ov/i-	
11. flex/o-		32. ov/o-	
12. fund/o-		33. ovul/o-	
13. galact/o-		34. perine/o-	
14. genit/o-		35. product/o-	
15. gon/o-		36. salping/o-	
16. hyster/o-		37. urethr/o-	
17. intern/o-		38. urin/o-	
18. labi/o-		39. ur/o-	
19. lact/i-		40. uter/o-	
20. lact/o-		41. vagin/o-	
21. lob/o-		42. vulv/o-	

C. Build Words

Read the definition of the medical word. Look at the combining form that is given. Select the correct suffix from the Suffix List, and write it on the blank line. Then build the medical word, and write it on the line. (Remember: You may need to remove the combining vowel. Always remove the hyphens and slash.) Be sure to check your spelling.

Suffix List

-al (pertaining to)	-ary (pertaining to)	-ine (pertaining to)
-an (pertaining to)	-cyte (cell)	-ity (condition; state)
-ar (pertaining to)	-duct (duct; tube)	

Definition of the Medical Word	Combining Form	Suffix	Build the Medical Word
Example: Pertaining to (the) fundus (of the uterus)	**fund/o-**	*-al*	*fundal*

[*You think* pertaining to (-*al*) + fundus (*fund/o-*). You change the order of the word parts to put the suffix last. You write fundal.]

Definition of the Medical Word	Combining Form	Suffix	Build the Medical Word
1. Pertaining to (the) breasts	mamm/o-		
2. Pertaining to (the) uterus	uter/o-		
3. Cell (that is an immature) ovum	o/o-		
4. Pertaining to (the) ovary	ovari/o-		
5. Pertaining to (the) areola	areol/o-		
6. Pertaining to (the) genitalia	genit/o-		
7. State (that is a) hollow space	cav/o-		
8. Tube (that carries) an egg	ov/i-		
9. Pertaining to (the) vulva	vulv/o-		
10. Pertaining to (the) cervix	cervic/o-		
11. Pertaining to accessory connecting parts (the ovary and uterine tube)	adnex/o-		
12. Pertaining to (the) vagina	vagin/o-		
13. Pertaining to (a) lip(-like structure)	labi/o-		
14. Pertaining to (the) perineum	perine/o-		
15. Pertaining to (the) vulva	vulv/o-		

D. Define Abbreviations

1. GU _____

2. GYN _____

3. OB _____

12.2 Physiology

The following processes must be complete in order for a female to reach sexual maturity and have the ability to become pregnant and give birth to a child.

Secretion of Hormones

During **puberty** (or **adolescence**, the time period between 11 and 19 years of age), the body undergoes rapid changes to reach **sexual maturity**. The anterior pituitary gland in the brain (described in Chapter 13, Endocrinology) begins to secrete two hormones to stimulate the ovaries.

- **Follicle-stimulating hormone (FSH)** stimulates a follicle in the ovary to enlarge and produce a mature ovum and to secrete the female hormone estradiol.
- **Luteinizing hormone (LH)** stimulates the follicle to rupture and release its ovum each month during menstruation (described in a later section). Luteinizing hormone also stimulates the ruptured follicle (corpus luteum) to secrete the female hormones estradiol and progesterone.

The ovary itself (its follicle or the cells around the follicle) secretes these three hormones:

- **Estradiol**, which is the most abundant and most biologically active of the female hormones. Estradiol stimulates the development of the female secondary sexual characteristics during puberty. It is secreted by the follicle (and also by the ruptured follicle [corpus luteum] after ovulation). Estradiol causes the endometrium (lining of the uterus) to thicken during the menstrual cycle. Estradiol is also secreted by the placenta during pregnancy.
- **Progesterone**, which is secreted by a ruptured follicle (corpus luteum) after ovulation. Progesterone also causes the endometrium to thicken during the menstrual cycle. It is also secreted by the placenta during pregnancy.
- **Testosterone**, a male hormone secreted by cells around the follicle, plays a role in the female sexual drive.

Development of Female Secondary Sexual Characteristics

Primary sexual characteristics are the actual genitalia that a female infant is born with. During puberty, hormones from the ovary cause the development of the female **secondary sexual characteristics** (see Figure 12-7 ■). Estradiol stimulates the external genitalia, causing enlargement of the genital area and breasts, the growth of body hair in the axillae and genital area, as well as widening of the pelvis and deposition of fat in that area. Estradiol and progesterone stimulate the onset of menstruation and support the development of any pregnancy. Estradiol and testosterone play a role in the female sexual drive.

Production of Ova

Most cells in the body divide by the process of **mitosis**, in which the 46 chromosomes in the cell nucleus duplicate and then divide to create two identical cells, each still with 46 chromosomes. However, the creation of ova is different from that of other cells in the body.

Oogenesis is the process of producing mature ova. Like spermatozoa in the male, a mature ovum is created by mitosis and **meiosis**. Unlike the male, mitosis in the ovary of the female begins before birth as one oocyte (immature ova) divides

Pronunciation/Word Parts

puberty (PYOO-ber-tee)
 puber/o- growing up
 -ty quality; state

adolescence (AD-oh-LES-sens)
 adolesc/o- beginning of being an adult
 -ence state

sexual (SEK-shoo-al)
 sex/o- sex
 -ual pertaining to

maturity (mah-TYOOR-ih-tee)
 matur/o- mature
 -ity condition; state

follicle (FAW-lih-kul)
 folli/o- sac-like structure
 -cle small thing

luteinizing (LOO-tee-ih-NY-zing)

estradiol (ES-trah-DY-awl)
 estr/a- female
 di- two
 -ol chemical substance
The combining form **estr/o-** also means female, and **gynec/o-** means female; woman.

progesterone (proh-JEH-steh-rohn)

testosterone (tes-TAW-steh-rohn)

sexual (SEK-shoo-al)
 sex/o- sex
 -ual pertaining to

mitosis (my-TOH-sihs)
 mit/o- thread-like strand
 -osis abnormal condition; process

oogenesis (OH-oh-JEN-eh-sihs)
 o/o- egg; ovum
 gen/o- arising from; produced by
 -esis abnormal condition; process

meiosis (my-OH-sihs)
 mei/o- decrease in number
 -osis abnormal condition; process

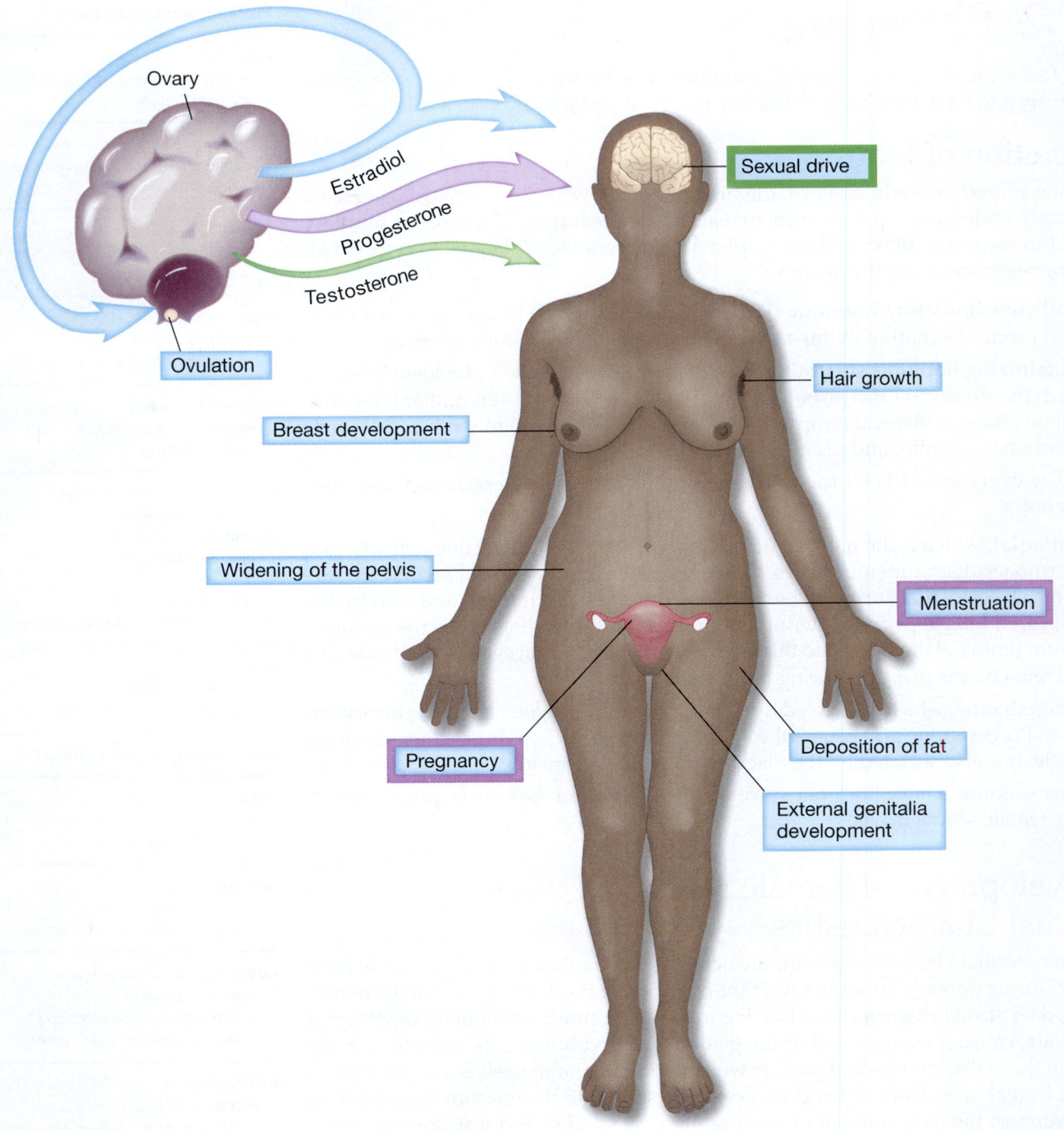

FIGURE 12-7 ■ **Hormones secreted by the ovaries.**
Estradiol produces the female secondary sexual characteristics that occur during puberty. Estradiol and progesterone stimulate the growth of the endometrium prior to menstruation and—if an ovum is fertilized—these hormones stimulate the growth of the endometrium during pregnancy when they are secreted by the placenta. Testosterone plays a role in the female sexual drive.

to become two. Also, the very first step of meiosis occurs there, but then the entire process stops and is put on hold until it begins again when stimulated by hormones during puberty. Meiosis must occur so that an ovum (with 23 chromosomes) from the female and a spermatozoon (with 23 chromosomes) from the male can unite to create a cell with the full number of 46 chromosomes. During puberty, the final step of meiosis occurs as each **oocyte** divides again but divides unevenly, producing an ovum that has 23 chromosomes and a large amount of cytoplasm as well as two or three small, nonfunctioning packets of cytoplasm known as *polar bodies*. Like a spermatozoon, the mature ovum is known as a **gamete**.

Pronunciation/Word Parts

oocyte (OH-oh-site)
  o/o- *ovum*
  -cyte *cell*

gamete (GAM-eet)

The Menstrual Cycle

With the onset of puberty, the female begins to ovulate and menstruate. **Menarche** is the beginning of **menstruation**, which occurs with the first **menstrual period** or **menses**.

Each **menstrual cycle**, on average, lasts 28 days and includes four phases: the menstrual phase, the proliferative phase (followed by ovulation), the secretory phase, and the ischemic phase (see Figure 12-8 ■).

Pronunciation/Word Parts

menarche (meh-NAR-kee)
  men/o- *month*
  -arche *beginning*

menstruation (MEN-stroo-AA-shun)
  menstru/o- *monthly discharge of blood*
  -ation *being; having; process*

menstrual (MEN-stroo-al)
  menstru/o- *monthly discharge of blood*
  -al *pertaining to*

menses (MEN-seez)

THE MENSTRUAL CYCLE

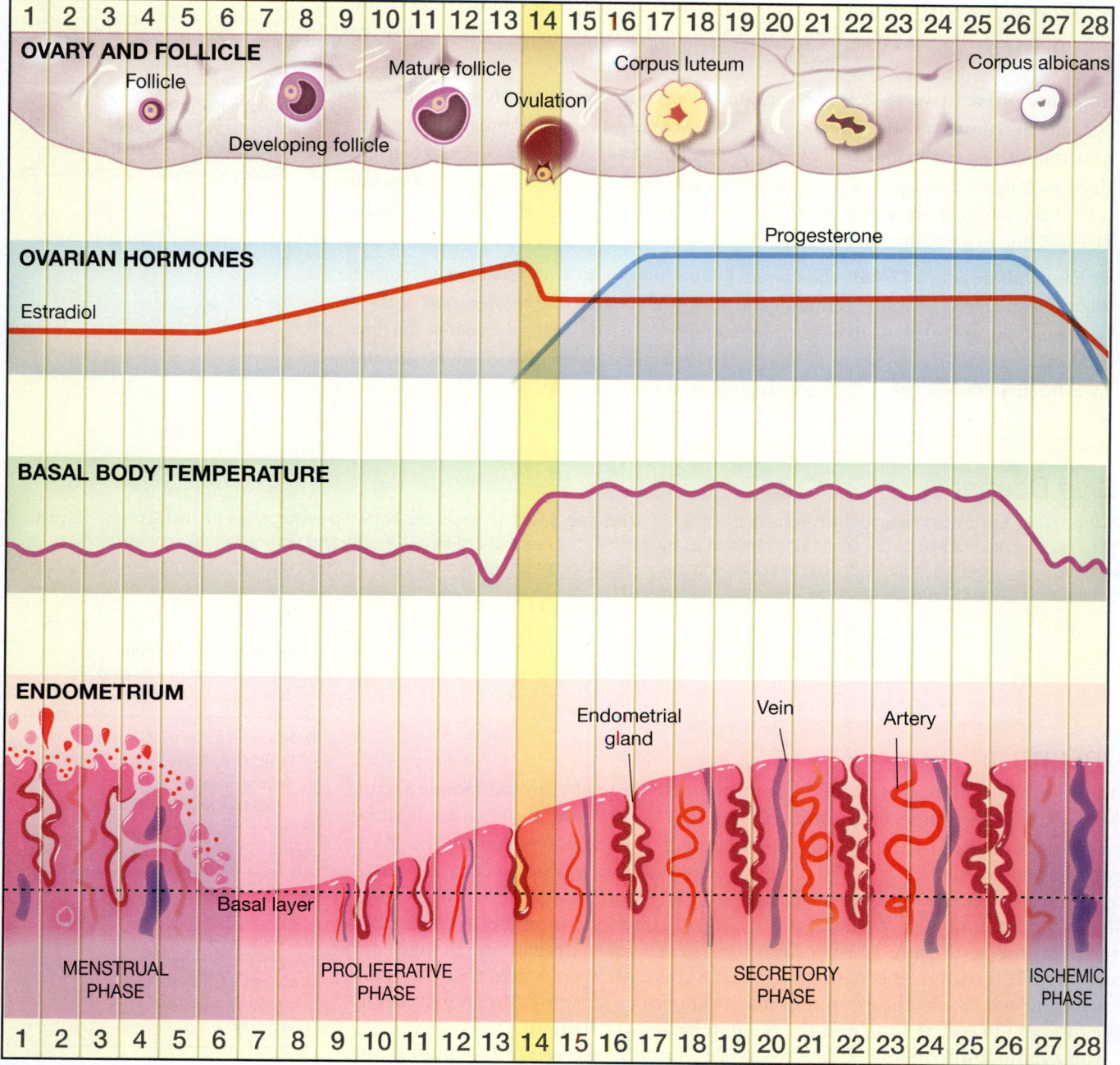

FIGURE 12-8 ■ Menstrual cycle.
Activities in the ovary are related to those in the uterus during the menstrual cycle. Hormones (estradiol and progesterone) produced by the follicle (and then by the corpus luteum) of the ovary cause the endometrium of the uterus to proliferate and thicken. If the ovum is not fertilized, the declining levels of these hormones cause the endometrium to slough off in menstruation.

1. **Menstrual phase (days 1–6).** Menstruation begins. Approximately 30 mL of blood, endometrial tissue, and mucus is sloughed off from the uterus and passes through the vagina and cervical os to the outside of the body. All that remains of the endometrium is a thin layer of glands. During that same period of time, several follicles in the ovary are enlarging and their ova are maturing in preparation for one of them to be released during ovulation on day 14 (see Figure 12-8).

2. **Proliferative phase (days 7–13).** FSH from the anterior pituitary gland stimulates the ovarian follicles to secrete estradiol. One follicle becomes greatly enlarged and produces a mature ovum. The thickness of the endometrium in the uterus increases (proliferates). At the end of the proliferative phase, mucus in the cervical canal thins to allow spermatozoa from the male to swim through it.

   Ovulation (day 14). LH from the anterior pituitary gland causes the enlarged ovarian follicle to rupture, releasing a mature ovum. The **basal (baseline) body temperature** rises about 0.4 degrees at the time of ovulation and stays elevated until the onset of menstruation.

3. **Secretory phase (days 15–26).** The ruptured ovarian follicle fills with yellow fat and becomes the **corpus luteum**. The corpus luteum secretes estradiol and progesterone. Progesterone causes the endometrial glands of the uterus to enlarge, and the endometrium thickens. Small arteries grow to the innermost edge of the endometrium, ready to nourish a fertilized ovum, if one enters the uterus. The basal body temperature continues to be elevated due to progesterone.

4. **Ischemic phase (days 27–28).** The corpus luteum turns into white scar tissue (corpus albicans) and stops secreting estradiol and progesterone. The abrupt decrease in these hormones causes the small arteries in the endometrium to constrict, which stops the flow of blood and causes ischemia of the tissue. The endometrium begins to slough off, and menstruation (the first phase of the menstrual cycle) begins again.

Dive Deeper

In the 1800s, the average age for menarche (the onset of menstruation) was 18 years old. Now the average age for menarche is 12 years old. Researchers point to better health and nutrition as the reason, but feel that childhood obesity and environmental contaminants (such as hormones in animal feed, crop fertilizers and pesticides, and industrial chemicals—all of which have an estrogen-like effect) are contributing to the decrease in the age.

Conception

Of the 100–500 million spermatozoa from the male deposited in the female vagina during sexual intercourse, only some are able to reach the ovum in the uterine tube; this occurs 24–48 hours after sexual intercourse. Substances secreted by the ovum attract the spermatozoa. A cap-like layer of enzymes on the head of each spermatozoon begins to dissolve the layer of cells around the ovum. Many spermatozoa attach to the ovum, but only one penetrates its surface. This is the moment of **conception** or **fertilization** (see Figure 12-9 ■). After that, the surface of the ovum changes and actually repels the other spermatozoa. When a spermatozoon unites with an ovum, the resulting cell has 46 chromosomes and is known as a **zygote**. **Pregnancy** begins at the moment of conception, and the woman becomes **pregnant**.

The zygote immediately begins to divide as it moves through the uterine tube toward the uterus (see Figure 12-10 ■). Within the intrauterine cavity, the zygote sinks into the thickened endometrium. After 4 days of development, the zygote is known as an **embryo**. At this point, it is a hollow ball with an inner mass of cells and an outer layer.

Pronunciation/Word Parts

proliferative (proh-LIH-fer-ah-TIV)
   prolifer/o- *production of more of the same*
   -ative *pertaining to*

ovulation (AW-vyoo-LAY-shun)
   ovul/o- *egg; ovum*
   -ation *being; having; process*

basal (BAY-sal)
   bas/o- *alkaline; base of a structure*
   -al *pertaining to*

secretory (SEE-kreh-TOR-ee)
   secret/o- *produce; secrete*
   -ory *having the function of*

corpus luteum (KOR-puhs LOO-tee-um)

ischemic (is-KEE-mik)
   isch/o- *block; keep back*
   -emic *pertaining to a condition of the blood; pertaining to a substance in the blood*

conception (con-SEP-shun)
   concept/o- *conceive; form*
   -ion *action; condition*

fertilization (FER-til-ih-ZAY-shun)
   fertil/o- *conceive; form*
   -ization *process of creating; process of inserting; process of making*

zygote (ZY-goht)

pregnancy (PREG-nan-see)
   pregn/o- *being with child*
   -ancy *state*

pregnant (PREG-nant)
   pregn/o- *being with child*
   -ant *pertaining to*

embryo (EM-bree-oh)

embryonic (EM-bree-AW-nik)
   embryon/o- *embryo; immature form*
   -ic *pertaining to*

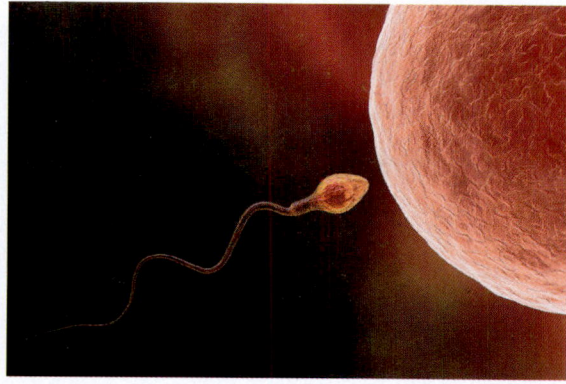

FIGURE 12-9 ■ An ovum and spermatozoon.
An ovum is nearly 100,000 times larger than a spermatozoon. An ovum and a spermatozoon are gametes, and each contains only 23 chromosomes. A fertilized ovum contains 46 chromosomes and is known as a *zygote*.

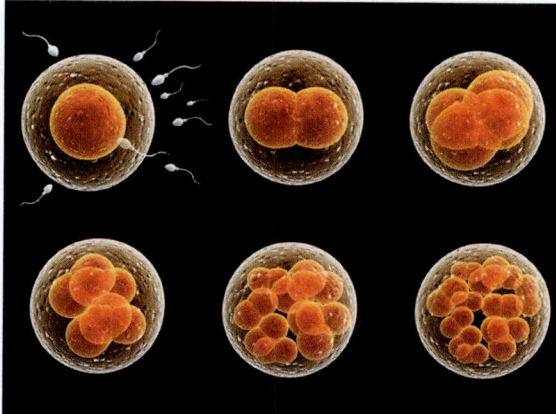

FIGURE 12-10 ■ Zygote.
The zygote (the fertilized ovum) immediately begins to divide, becoming a hollow ball with an inner mass of cells that is known as an *embryo*.

Pronunciation/Word Parts

amnion (AM-nee-on)

amniotic (AM-nee-AW-tik)
   amni/o- *amnion*
   -tic *pertaining to*

chorion (KOR-ee-awn)

chorionic (KOR-ee-AW-nik)
   chorion/o- *chorion*
   -ic *pertaining to*

gonadotropin (GOH-nah-doh-TROH-pin)
   gonad/o- *gonad; ovary; testis*
   trop/o- *having an affinity for; stimulating; turning*
   -in *substance*

fetus (FEE-tuhs)
Fetus is a Latin singular noun. Its plural form *fetuses* does not follow the rule for Latin nouns ending in *-us*.

fetal (FEE-tal)
   fet/o- *fetus*
   -al *pertaining to*

placenta (plah-SEN-tah)

placental (plah-SEN-tal)
   placent/o- *placenta*
   -al *pertaining to*

The inner mass of cells becomes the amnion and the embryo. The **amnion** (or "bag of waters") is a membrane sac that surrounds the embryo and holds **amniotic fluid**. The amniotic fluid comes from water in the mother's blood and later from urine excreted by the fetus. The developing embryo floats in, and is cushioned by, the amniotic fluid.

The outer layer of the zygote becomes the **chorion**. It sends finger-like projections (villi) into the endometrium to absorb nutrients and oxygen. The chorion itself produces the hormone **human chorionic gonadotropin (HCG)** that stimulates the corpus luteum to keep producing estradiol and progesterone. This maintains the thickened endometrium to support the developing embryo and prevents menstruation from occurring during the rest of the pregnancy.

From 9 weeks until delivery, the embryo is known as a **fetus** (see Figure 12-11 ■). The chorion eventually becomes the **placenta**, a pancake-like structure about 7 inches

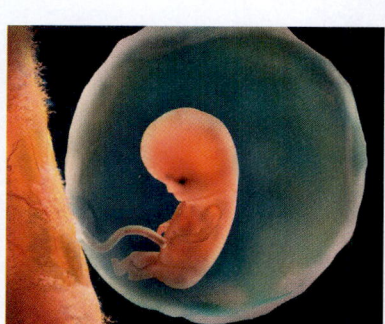

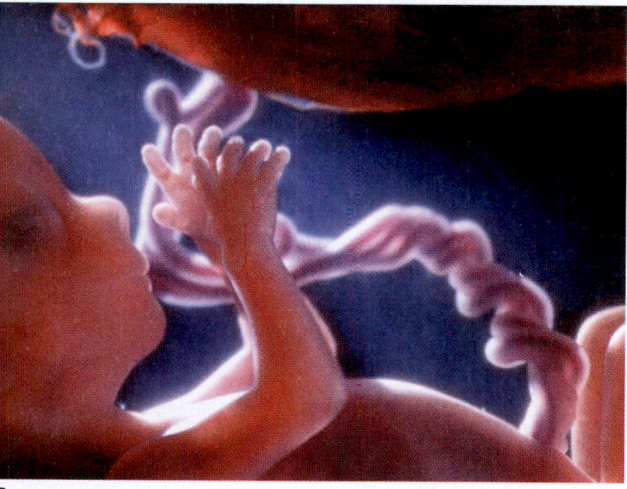

FIGURE 12-11 ■ Fetuses at 9 and 16 weeks' gestation.
A. This fetus at 9 weeks is not quite an inch long and weighs less than 1 ounce. It is floating in amniotic fluid. The face is developing first. The umbilical cord is bringing oxygenated blood to the fetus from the placenta. **B.** This fetus at 16 weeks is 5 inches long from head to buttocks and weighs 3½ ounces. The face, hands, and feet are developed, and the face can have expressions of squinting or frowning. The arteries bringing red, oxygenated blood to the fetus are visible in the umbilical cord.

A.   B.

in diameter and 1–2 inches thick. By the end of the first trimester of pregnancy, the placenta begins to secrete estradiol and progesterone and takes over the job of the corpus luteum. Other structures in the chorion form the rubbery, flexible **umbilical cord** (with its two arteries and one vein) that connects the placenta to the fetus. The umbilical cord and placenta bring oxygen, nutrients, and antibodies from the mother to the fetus and remove carbon dioxide and waste products.

The fetus, placenta, and all fluids and tissue in the pregnant uterus are known as the **products of conception**.

Pronunciation/Word Parts

umbilicus (um-BIL-ih-kuhs)

umbilical (um-BIL-ih-kal)
  umbilic/o- navel; umbilicus
  -al pertaining to

Clinical Connections

Genetics. The sex chromosomes (X and Y) are one of the chromosome pairs that are in the nucleus of every cell in the body. In a female, every cell contains two X chromosomes. In a male, every cell contains an X chromosome and a Y chromosome.

The ovum always contains an X chromosome. A spermatozoon contains either an X chromosome or a Y chromosome. An X chromosome from the ovum and an X chromosome from the spermatozoon unite to create a female infant (XX). An X chromosome from the ovum and a Y chromosome from the spermatozoon unite to create a male infant (XY). **Identical twins** occur when one already developing zygote splits to create two separate but identical zygotes. **Fraternal twins** occur when the ovary releases two ova that are fertilized by different spermatozoa. Multiple zygotes can develop if the ovary releases multiple ova that are all fertilized; this can occur in patients taking ovulation-stimulating drugs for infertility.

fraternal (frah-TER-nal)
  fratern/o- close relationship
  -al pertaining to

Gestation is the period of time that begins at the moment of conception and continues until the moment of birth. The gestational period is approximately 9 months (38–42 weeks), the average being 40 weeks (see Figure 12-12 ■). Gestation can be divided into three time periods, or **trimesters**. Each trimester is 3 months long. For the fetus, the period of time from conception to birth is the **prenatal period**. For the mother, the period of time from conception to labor and delivery and the birth of the baby is known as **antepartum**.

gestation (jes-TAY-shun)
  gestat/o- conception to birth
  -ion action; condition

trimester (TRY-mehs-ter)

prenatal (pree-NAY-tal)
  pre- before; in front of
  nat/o- birth
  -al pertaining to

antepartum (AN-tee-PAR-tum)
  ante- before; forward
  part/o- childbirth; labor
  -um period of time; structure
The combining form par/o- means giving birth.

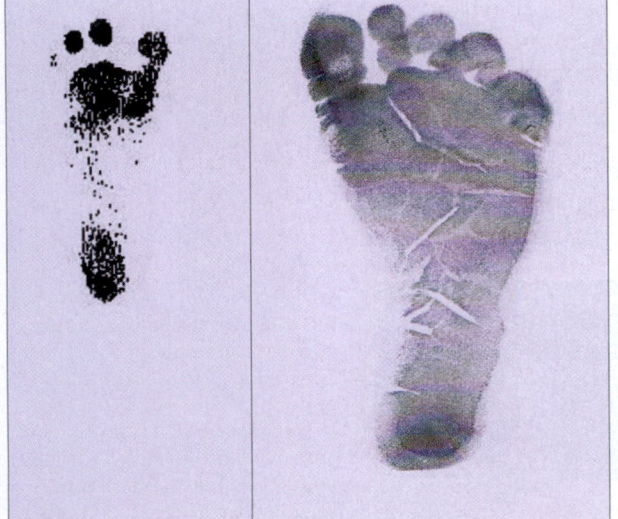

A.   B.

FIGURE 12-12 ■ Newborn footprints.
A. This is the actual footprint on the delivery room record of a fetus who was born prematurely at 23 weeks' gestation. **B.** Here is the footprint of a term neonate.

Dive Deeper

In the uterus, the fetus swallows amniotic fluid each day. The fetal kidneys excrete urine into the amniotic fluid. The amniotic fluid contains urea and creatinine (waste products in the urine), skin cells and hair shed by the fetus, and two important substances (lecithin and sphingomyelin) that can be used to determine the maturity of the fetal lungs when the amniotic fluid is tested before birth.

Labor and Delivery (L&D)

As the fetus grows, the uterus expands, taking up space in the mother's abdominal cavity and displacing her abdominal organs. This causes constipation, urinary frequency, and shortness of breath in the mother. During the last trimester of pregnancy, the uterus contracts irregularly to strengthen itself in preparation for childbirth. These are known as **Braxton Hicks contractions** or "false labor." Progesterone from the placenta keeps these contractions from becoming labor contractions. The cervical os remains closed (not dilated), and the wall of the cervix remains thick (not effaced). A mucous plug in the cervical os keeps out microorganisms. Late in the pregnancy, the head of the fetus drops into the birth position within the mother's pelvis. This process is known as **engagement**. (It is also known as **lightening** because it eases the mother's shortness of breath.) The fetus usually assumes a head-down position. The head becomes the presenting part (the part of the body that will go first through the birth canal). This is a **cephalic presentation**. Any part of the head can be the presenting part, but most commonly it is the top of the head, and this is a **vertex presentation** (see Figure 12-13 ■).

Sometime between 38 and 42 weeks' gestation, labor begins. The weight of the fetus presses on the cervix and vagina. This causes the cervix to begin to dilate and stimulates the release of oxytocin from the posterior pituitary gland in the brain. The uterus itself also produces oxytocin. **Oxytocin** causes the uterus to contract regularly and with increasing strength. The cervix softens as collagen fibers in its wall break down. This is known as **cervical ripening**.

The process of labor and childbirth is known as **parturition**, and it is divided into three stages:

1. **First stage of labor.** Uterine contractions occur about every 30 minutes, increasing in intensity and duration. **Cervical dilation** (widening of the cervical os) progresses from 0 cm to 5 cm, and **effacement** (thinning of the cervical wall) progresses from 0 percent to 50 percent. **Rupture of the membranes (ROM)** occurs, and this releases amniotic fluid. As the

Pronunciation/Word Parts

Braxton Hicks (BRAK-ston HIKS)

contraction (con-TRAK-shun)
  contract/o- *pull together*
  -ion *action; condition*

engagement (en-GAYJ-ment)

cephalic (seh-FAL-ik)
  cephal/o- *head*
  -ic *pertaining to*

vertex (VER-teks)

oxytocin (AWK-see-TOH-sihn)
  ox/y- *oxygen; quick*
  toc/o- *childbirth; labor*
  -in *substance*
Oxytocin: *Substance (that causes) quick childbirth and labor*

parturition (PAR-tyoor-IH-shun)
  parturit/o- *childbirth; labor*
  -ion *action; condition*

dilation (dy-LAY-shun)
  dilat/o- *dilate; widen*
  -ion *action; condition*

effacement (eh-FAYS-ment)
  efface/o- *do away with; obliterate*
  -ment *action; state*

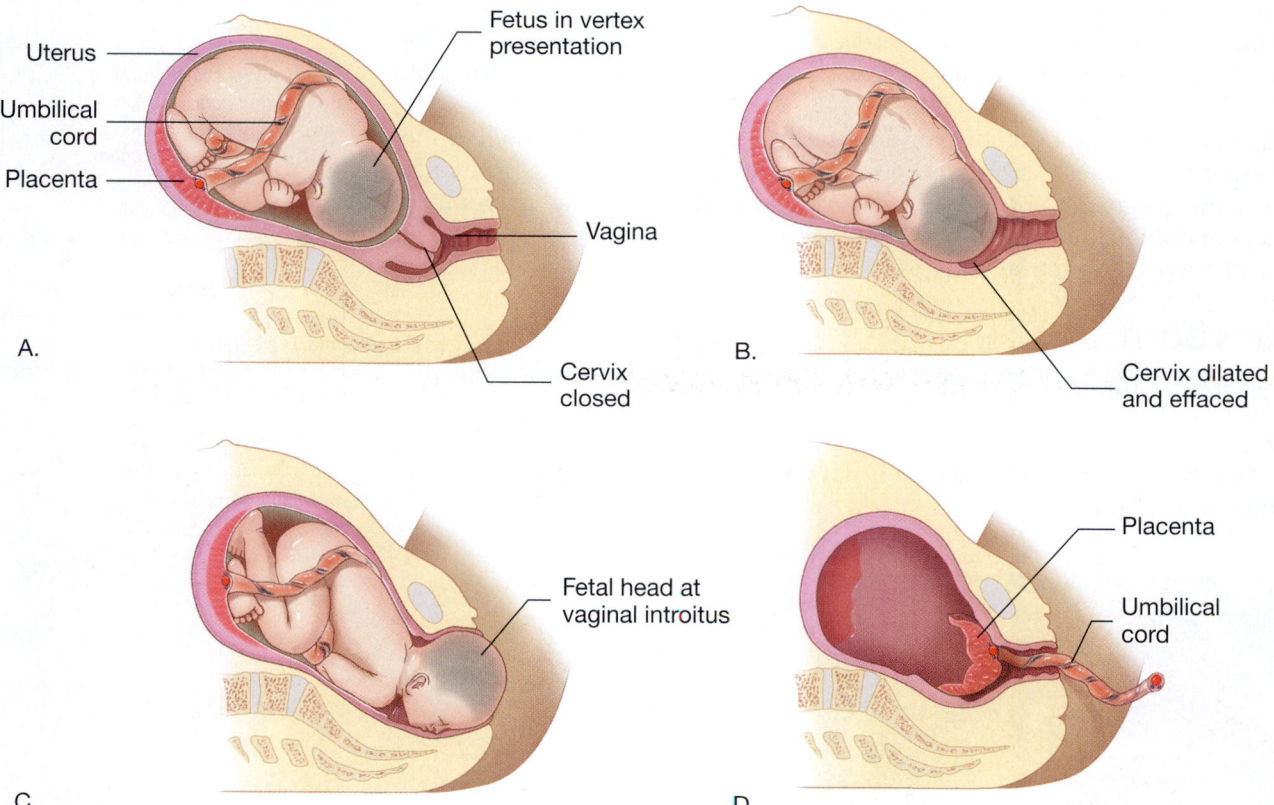

Uterus
Umbilical cord
Placenta

Fetus in vertex presentation

Vagina

Cervix closed

A.

Cervix dilated and effaced

B.

Fetal head at vaginal introitus

C.

Placenta

Umbilical cord

D.

FIGURE 12-13 ■ Labor and delivery.
A. This fetus is in a vertex presentation with the head as the presenting part. The cervical os is closed at the beginning of labor. **B.** Gradually, the cervix dilates to 10 cm, and its wall thins until it is 100% effaced. **C.** The head of the fetus moves through the cervical canal and vagina until the top of the head is visible at the vaginal introitus. This is known as *crowning*. **D.** After birth, the placenta and umbilical cord are expelled.

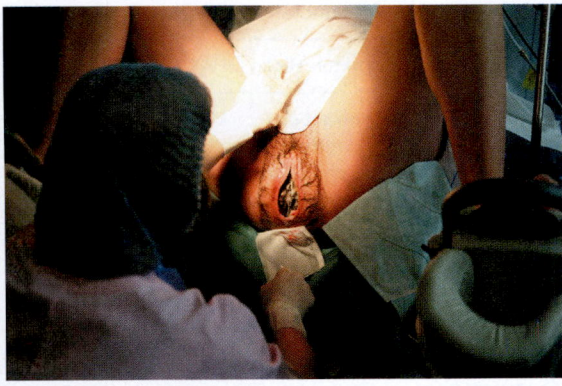

FIGURE 12-14 ■ **Crowning of the head.**
The hair on the baby's head is visible. The top of the head bulges outwardly from the vaginal canal with each contraction.

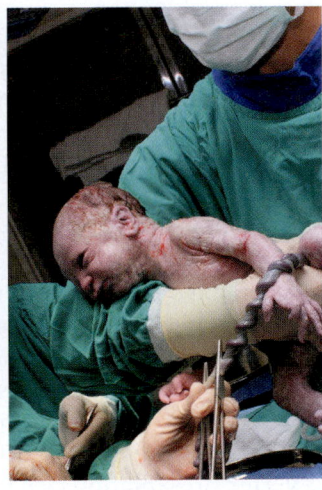

FIGURE 12-15 ■ **Cutting the umbilical cord.**
The obstetrician is using forceps to cut the umbilical cord after delivery. Notice the length of the umbilical cord! This newborn's skin shows the characteristic acrocyanosis that is to be expected right after birth; it disappears in 24 to 48 hours.

uterine contractions intensify, the mother may receive epidural anesthesia (described in a later section) to help control the pain. After 8 to 20 hours of labor, the cervix is completely dilated at 10 cm and 100% effaced (see Figure 12-13), and the mother is ready to deliver.

2. **Second stage of labor.** The head of the fetus is in the vaginal canal. The mother is encouraged to push by holding her breath to raise the intra-abdominal pressure. **Crowning** occurs when the top of the fetal head (crown) is visible at the **vaginal introitus** (see Figure 12-13 and Figure 12-14 ■). The head is delivered and, after several more uterine contractions, the shoulders and the rest of the body are delivered. The umbilical cord is cut and clamped (see Figure 12-15 ■), and the newborn is placed on the mother's abdomen.

3. **Third stage of labor.** The **placenta** is delivered about 30 minutes after the birth. The placenta is also known as the "afterbirth" (see Figure 12-13). Oxytocin causes the uterus to contract to stop blood flow from the surfaces where the placenta pulled away. The obstetrician sutures up the episiotomy, if one was performed (described in a later section).

For the newborn, the period of time after birth is the **postnatal period**. For the mother, the period of time after birth is known as **postpartum**. The uterus gradually returns to its pre-pregnancy size, a process known as **involution**. Small amounts of blood, tissue, and fluid, known as **lochia**, continue to flow from the uterus for a week or so until all of the endometrial lining is shed.

The Newborn

A newborn who is between 38 and 42 weeks' gestation is a **term neonate** (see Figure 12-16 ■). A newborn between 28 and 37 weeks' gestation is **preterm** or **premature**, a reference to the maturity of the internal organs and their ability to function. Because the date of conception is not always known, the gestational age of a newborn is an estimate.

Pronunciation/Word Parts

introitus (in-TROY-tuhs)
Introitus is the Latin word that means entrance.

placenta (plah-SEN-tah)

placental (plah-SEN-tal)
 placent/o- *placenta*
 -al *pertaining to*

postnatal (post-NAY-tal)
 post- *after; behind*
 nat/o- *birth*
 -al *pertaining to*

postpartum (post-PAR-tum)
 post- *after; behind*
 part/o- *childbirth; labor*
 -um *period of time; structure*

involution (IN-voh-LOO-shun)
 involut/o- *enlarged organ returns to normal size*
 -ion *action; condition*

lochia (LOH-kee-ah)

neonate (NEE-oh-nayt)
 ne/o- *new*
 -nate *thing that is born*

neonatal (NEE-oh-NAY-tal)
 ne/o- *new*
 nat/o- *birth*
 -al *pertaining to*

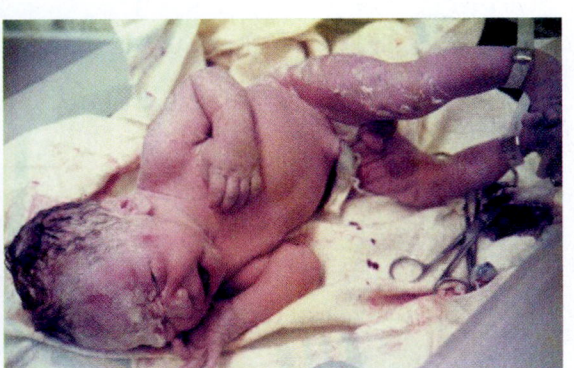

FIGURE 12-16 ■ **Term neonate.**
This male newborn is on the warming table in the delivery room. The vernix caseosa is still visible on his head and legs. His eyes are swollen from the pressure of the birth canal. He is crying vigorously, and his skin still shows some acrocyanosis. There is a plastic clamp where his umbilical cord has been cut. There are identification bracelets on both of his legs.

Clinical Connections

Dermatology. The skin of a newborn is partly covered with **vernix caseosa**, a thick, white, cheesy substance that protects the skin from bacteria present in the mother's vagina during birth. The newborn's face, hands, and feet are often bluish, a temporary condition known as **acrocyanosis**.

Immunology. Blood in the umbilical cord is rich in stem cells and can be used for stem cell transplantation, if needed.

Colostrum is rich in nutrients and contains antibodies from the mother. For the first few days of life, the newborn's intestinal tract is permeable, and this allows the maternal antibodies to be absorbed into the newborn's blood. Maternal antibodies provide passive immunity to common diseases that the mother has already had. This immunity lasts until the newborn begins to make its own antibodies at about 18 months of age.

Orthopedics. The head of a newborn can exhibit **molding**, a temporary elongated reshaping of the fetal cranial bones that occurs as the head passes through the mother's bony pelvis. On the top of the head, the anterior **fontanel** or "soft spot" is a soft area that bulges when the newborn cries because it is only covered by a layer of fibrous connective tissue, not by bone (see Figure 7-4 in Chapter 7). There is also a smaller posterior fontanel at the back of the head. The fontanels allow the brain to grow before the cranial bones fuse together.

Gastroenterology. The first bowel movement is **meconium**, a thick, greenish-black, tar-like substance. It contains mucus and bile (from the fetal digestive tract) and skin cells (that were in amniotic fluid swallowed by the fetus).

vernix caseosa (VER-niks KAY-see-OH-sah)

acrocyanosis (AK-roh-SY-ah-NOH-sihs)
  acr/o- extremity; highest point
  cyan/o- blue
  -osis abnormal condition; process

fontanel (FAWN-tah-NEL)

meconium (meh-KOH-nee-um)

Lactation

Lactation is the production of milk by the mother's breasts when stimulated by the hormone prolactin from the anterior pituitary gland in the brain. After birth, when the newborn cries or sucks, oxytocin secreted by the posterior pituitary gland causes smooth muscles around the lactiferous lobules to contract and expel milk for breastfeeding. This is known as the **let-down reflex**. The first milk, **colostrum**, is a thick, yellowish fluid. By the third day, the colostrum is replaced by regular breast milk that is thin and white.

Pronunciation/Word Parts

lactation (lak-TAY-shun)
  lact/o- milk
  -ation being; having; process

colostrum (koh-LAW-strum)

12.2 PRACTICE LAPS

Use the Answer Key at the end of the book to check your answers.

A. Give the Meaning of Combining Forms

Next to each combining form, write its meaning. The first one has been done for you.

Combining Form	Meaning	Combining Form	Meaning
1. **sex/o-**	*sex*	7. concept/o-	
2. acr/o-		8. contract/o-	
3. adolesc/o-		9. cyan/o-	
4. amni/o-		10. dilat/o-	
5. cephal/o-		11. embryon/o-	
6. chorion/o-		12. estr/a-	

Combining Form	Meaning	Combining Form	Meaning
13. estr/o-	_____	29. nat/o-	_____
14. fertil/o-	_____	30. ne/o-	_____
15. fet/o-	_____	31. o/o-	_____
16. folli/o-	_____	32. ovul/o-	_____
17. fratern/o-	_____	33. ox/y-	_____
18. gen/o-	_____	34. par/o-	_____
19. gestat/o-	_____	35. part/o-	_____
20. gonad/o-	_____	36. parturit/o-	_____
21. gynec/o-	_____	37. placent/o-	_____
22. involut/o-	_____	38. pregn/o-	_____
23. isch/o-	_____	39. puber/o-	_____
24. lact/o-	_____	40. secret/o-	_____
25. mei/o-	_____	41. toc/o-	_____
26. men/o-	_____	42. trop/o-	_____
27. menstru/o-	_____	43. umbilic/o-	_____
28. mit/o-	_____		

B. Build Words

Read the definition of the medical word. Look at the combining form that is given. Select the correct suffix from the Suffix List, and write it on the blank line. Then build the medical word, and write it on the line. (Remember: You may need to remove the combining vowel. Always remove the hyphens and slash.) Be sure to check your spelling.

Suffix List

-al (pertaining to)	-cyte (cell)	-nate (thing that is born)
-ancy (state)	-ence (state)	-osis (abnormal condition;
-ant (pertaining to)	-ic (pertaining to)	process)
-arche (beginning)	-ion (action; condition)	-tic (pertaining to)
-ation (being; having; process)	-ization (process of inserting)	-ual (pertaining to)
-cle (small thing)	-ment (action; state)	

Definition of the Medical Word	Combining Form	Suffix	Build the Medical Word
Example: Pertaining to sex	**sex/o-**	*-ual*	*sexual*

[*You think* pertaining to *(-ual)* + sex *(sex/o-)*. You change the order of the word parts to put the suffix last. You write sexual.]

1. Process (of having an) ovum (released from the follicle)	ovul/o-	_____	_____
2. Beginning (of) month(ly periods)	men/o-	_____	_____

Definition of the Medical Word	Combining Form	Suffix	Build the Medical Word
3. Process (of having) monthly discharge of blood	menstru/o-	_____	_____
4. Pertaining to (the) amnion	amni/o-	_____	_____
5. Process (of having) milk	lact/o-	_____	_____
6. Pertaining to (the) fetus	fet/o-	_____	_____
7. Action (to) conceive (or) form (a child)	concept/o-	_____	_____
8. Pertaining to being with child	pregn/o-	_____	_____
9. Pertaining to (the) embryo	embryon/o-	_____	_____
10. State (of) being with child	pregn/o-	_____	_____
11. Process of inserting (sperm into an ovum to) conceive (a child)	fertil/o-	_____	_____
12. Thing (baby) that is born new	ne/o-	_____	_____
13. Pertaining to (the) placenta	placent/o-	_____	_____
14. Action (when an) enlarged organ (the uterus) returns to normal size	involut/o-	_____	_____
15. Action (to) do away with (or) obliterate (the thick wall of the cervix)	efface/o-	_____	_____
16. Cell (that is an) egg	o/o-	_____	_____
17. Condition (from) conception to birth	gestat/o-	_____	_____
18. State (of) beginning of being an adult	adolesc/o-	_____	_____
19. Small thing (that is a) sac-like structure	folli/o-	_____	_____
20. Process (to) decrease in number (the chromosomes)	mei/o-	_____	_____
21. Action (to) conceive	concept/o-	_____	_____
22. Pertaining to (the) umbilicus	umbilic/o-	_____	_____
23. Action (to) widen	dilat/o-	_____	_____

C. Define Abbreviations

1. FHS   _____

2. LH   _____

3. HCG   _____

4. ROM   _____

Vocabulary Review

Word or Phrase	Description	Combining Forms
Overview		
abdominopelvic cavity	Hollow space in the abdomen and pelvis that contains the internal female genitalia	**abdomin/o-** *abdomen* **pelv/o-** *hip bone; pelvis; renal pelvis* **cav/o-** *hollow space*
external genitalia	Structures on the outside of the female body that include the mons pubis, labia majora, labia minora, clitoris, vaginal introitus, Bartholin glands, urethral glands, and Skene glands	**extern/o-** *outside* **genit/o-** *genitalia*
female genital system	Body system that consists of the structures of the internal and external genitalia. Its functions are to secrete female hormones, develop female secondary sexual characteristics, produce ova, menstruate, conceive and bear children, and produce milk to feed infants.	**genit/o-** *genitalia*
genitalia	Internal and external organs and structures of the female genital and reproductive system. Also known as the **genital organs**.	**genit/o-** *genitalia*
genitourinary system	The combined female genital and reproductive body system and the urinary body system. These two body systems are in close proximity to each other and are often considered together. Also known as the **urogenital system**.	**genit/o-** *genitalia* **urin/o-** *urinary system; urine* **ur/o-** *urinary system; urine*
internal genitalia	Structures in the abdominopelvic cavity that include the ovaries, uterine tubes, uterus, and vagina	**intern/o-** *inside* **genit/o-** *genitalia*
mammary glands	Part of the female reproductive system. Also known as the **breasts**.	**mamm/o-** *breast*
reproductive system	The function of the female genital system is conceiving and bearing children and producing milk to nourish infants	**product/o-** *produce*
Anatomy		
Internal Genitalia		
Ovaries		
adnexa	Accessory organs (the ovaries and uterine tubes) connected to the main organ (the uterus)	**adnex/o-** *accessory connecting parts*
follicle	Small area in the ovary that holds oocytes before puberty and maturing ova after puberty. A follicle ruptures during the menstrual cycle, releasing an ovum, and then becomes the corpus luteum.	**folli/o-** *sac-like structure*
gonads	The sex glands in a female, which are the ovaries	**gon/o-** *ovum; spermatozoon*
oocyte	Immature egg in the follicle of the ovary	**o/o-** *egg; ovum*
ovary	Small, egg-shaped gland near the distal end of the uterine tube. The ovary is held in place by the **broad ligament** and other ligaments. The follicles of the ovary secrete estradiol. The corpus luteum of the ovary secretes estradiol and progesterone. The cells around the follicles secrete testosterone. The ovary is a gonad.	**ovari/o-** *ovary* **oophor/o-** *ovary*

Word or Phrase	Description	Combining Forms
ovum	A mature egg within a follicle in the ovary. It is released during ovulation in the menstrual cycle. The plural is **ova**.	**o/o-** *egg; ovum* **ov/i-** *egg; ovum* **ov/o-** *egg; ovum* **ovul/o-** *egg; ovum*

Uterine Tubes

Word or Phrase	Description	Combining Forms
cilia	Tiny hairs within the uterine tube. They beat in waves to propel an ovum toward the uterus.	
fimbriae	Finger-like projections at the distal end of the uterine tube. They create currents that carry the ovum into the lumen of the uterine tube.	
peristalsis	Smooth wave-like muscle contractions of the uterine tube that move the ovum toward the uterus	
uterine tube	Narrow tube that is connected at its proximal end to the uterus. The distal end is funnel shaped; it is open to the pelvic cavity and is not directly connected to the ovary. It has a long central opening or **lumen**. Also known as an **oviduct**. Formerly known as the **fallopian tube**.	**uter/o-** *uterus; womb* **ov/i-** *egg; ovum* **salping/o-** *uterine tube* **fallopi/o-** *uterine tube*

Uterus

Word or Phrase	Description	Combining Forms
anteflexion	Normal position of the uterus in which the superior portion is tipped anteriorly on top of the bladder	**flex/o-** *bending*
cervix	Narrow, most inferior part of the uterus. It contains the **cervical canal**. Part of the cervix protrudes into the vagina. The **cervical os** is the small central opening in the cervix.	**cervic/o-** *cervix; neck*
cul-de-sac	Small pouch in the broad ligament that is between the uterus and rectum	**culd/o-** *cul-de-sac*
fundus	Rounded top of the uterus	**fund/o-** *fundus; part farthest from the opening*
endometrium	Innermost layer of the uterus that lines the intrauterine cavity. It is a mucous membrane that contains many glands. It thickens and then is shed during the menstrual cycle.	**end/o-** *innermost; within* **metri/o-** *uterus; womb*
intrauterine cavity	Hollow area within the uterus. It is lined with endometrium.	**uter/o-** *uterus; womb* **cav/o-** *hollow space*
myometrium	Smooth muscle layer of the uterine wall. It contracts during menstruation to expel the endometrial lining and during labor and the delivery of a baby.	**my/o-** *muscle* **metri/o-** *uterus; womb*
perimetrium	Serous membrane that is the outer layer of the uterus. It is part of the peritoneum that lines the abdominopelvic cavity.	**metri/o-** *uterus; womb*
uterus	Internal female organ of menstruation and pregnancy. Also known as the **womb**. The uterus is held in place by the **broad ligament** and other ligaments. The parts of the uterus include the fundus, cervix, perimetrium, myometrium, endometrium, and intrauterine cavity. The normal position of the uterus is anteflexion, tipped anteriorly.	**uter/o-** *uterus; womb* **hyster/o-** *uterus; womb* **metri/o-** *uterus; womb* **metr/o-** *measurement; uterus; womb*

Vagina

Word or Phrase	Description	Combining Forms
fornix	Area of the vaginal canal that is behind and around the cervix. Also known as the *vaginal vault*.	
hymen	Elastic membrane that, if present, partially or completely covers the end of the vaginal canal	

Word or Phrase	Description	Combining Forms
vagina	Short, tubular structure connected at its superior end to the cervix and at its inferior end to the outside of the body. It contains the **vaginal canal** and the **vaginal introitus**, the opening to the outside of the body.	**vagin/o-** *vagina* **colp/o-** *vagina*
External Genitalia		
BUS	**Bartholin glands**, **urethral glands**, and **Skene glands** near the vaginal introitus. They secrete mucus during sexual arousal.	**urethr/o-** *urethra*
clitoris	Organ of sexual response in the female that enlarges with blood and becomes firm	
labia	Two sets of lip-shaped structures that partially cover the urethral meatus and the vaginal introitus. The **labia majora**, the thicker, outermost lips, are covered with pubic hair. The **labia minora**, the smooth, thin, inner lips, are beneath the labia majora.	**labi/o-** *labium; lip*
mons pubis	Rounded, fatty pad of tissue covered with pubic hair that lies on top of the pubis (anterior hip bone)	
perineum	Area of skin between the vulva and the anus	**perine/o-** *perineum*
vaginal introitus	Opening of the vagina to the outside of the body	**vagin/o-** *vagina*
vulva	Area that includes the external genitalia as well as the mons pubis (but not the mammary glands)	**vulv/o-** *vulva* **episi/o-** *vulva*

Mammary Glands

areola	Pigmented area around the nipple of the breast	**areol/o-** *small, circular area*
lactiferous lobules	Site of milk production in the mammary glands. The milk flows through the **lactiferous ducts** to the nipple.	**lact/i-** *milk* **fer/o-** *bear* **lact/o-** *milk* **galact/o-** *milk*
mammary glands	Two structures that contain adipose (fatty) tissue and lactiferous lobules. The nipple is the projecting point of the breast where the lactiferous ducts converge. The breasts produce milk to nourish the baby after birth. Also known as the **breasts**.	**mamm/o-** *breast* **mamm/a-** *breast* **mast/o-** *breast; mastoid process*
Physiology		
Secretion of Hormones		
estradiol	Most abundant and biologically active of the female hormones. During puberty, it causes the development of the female sexual characteristics. It is secreted by the follicles of the ovary and the corpus luteum (after ovulation). It causes the endometrium to thicken during the menstrual cycle. During pregnancy, estradiol is also secreted by the placenta.	**estr/a-** *female* **estr/o-** *female* **gynec/o-** *female; woman*
follicle-stimulating hormone (FSH)	Hormone secreted by the anterior pituitary gland in the brain. It stimulates a follicle in the ovary to enlarge and produce a mature ovum. FSH also stimulates the follicles to secrete estradiol.	**folli/o-** *sac-like structure*
gamete	An ovum or spermatozoon. It has 23 chromosomes instead of the usual 46 chromosomes found in other cells in the body.	
luteinizing hormone (LH)	Hormone secreted by the anterior pituitary gland in the brain. It stimulates a follicle in the ovary to rupture and release a mature ovum. LH also stimulates the corpus luteum to secrete estradiol and progesterone.	

Word or Phrase	Description	Combining Forms
oogenesis	Production of a mature ovum from an oocyte through the processes of mitosis and then meiosis	**o/o-** *egg; ovum* **gen/o-** *arising from; produced by*
progesterone	Hormone secreted by the corpus luteum of the ovary after ovulation. It causes the uterine lining to thicken during the menstrual cycle. During pregnancy, it is secreted by the placenta.	
puberty	Rapid physical changes that the female body undergoes to reach sexual maturity with the development of the female secondary sexual characteristics. This is stimulated by hormones from the anterior pituitary gland and the ovary. This period of time is known as **adolescence**.	**puber/o-** *growing up* **adolesc/o-** *beginning of being an adult*
testosterone	Male hormone secreted by cells around the follicles in the ovary. It plays a role in the female sexual drive.	

Female Secondary Sexual Characteristics		
female secondary sexual characteristics	Physical features that develop during puberty because of stimulation by hormones. They include enlargement of the external genitalia (genital area and breasts), the growth of body hair in the axillae and genital area, and widening of the pelvis.	**sex/o-** *sex*

Production of Ova		
gamete	A mature ovum that contains 23 chromosomes	
meiosis	Begins in the fetal ovary before birth. It resumes during puberty to produce a mature ovum with 23 chromosomes and two or three nonfunctioning polar bodies (packets of chromosomes).	**mei/o-** *decrease in number*
mitosis	Process in which a cell with 46 chromosomes divides to produce two identical cells, each with 46 chromosomes. It is the first step in oogenesis, and it occurs in the fetal ovary before birth.	**mit/o-** *thread-like strand*
oocyte	Immature ovum in the fetal ovary before birth	**o/o-** *egg; ovum*
oogenesis	Process of producing a mature ovum. It involves both meiosis and mitosis.	**o/o-** *egg; ovum* **gen/o-** *arising from; produced by*

Menstrual Cycle		
corpus luteum	Remnants of a ruptured follicle in the ovary. The corpus luteum secretes estradiol and progesterone during the menstrual cycle. If the ovum is fertilized, the placenta begins to secrete these hormones, and the corpus luteum becomes white scar tissue (corpus albicans).	
ischemic phase	Days 27–28 of the menstrual cycle. The corpus luteum degenerates into white scar tissue and stops producing estradiol and progesterone. The endometrium sloughs off, and menstruation begins.	**isch/o-** *block; keep back*
menarche	The first cycle of menstruation at the onset of puberty. This is the first **menstrual period** or **menses**.	**men/o-** *month* **menstru/o-** *monthly discharge of blood*
menstrual cycle	A 28-day cycle that consists of the menstrual phase, proliferative phase (followed by ovulation), secretory phase, and ischemic phase	**menstru/o-** *monthly discharge of blood*
menstrual phase	Days 1–6 of the menstrual cycle. The endometrial lining of the uterus is shed.	**menstru/o-** *monthly discharge of blood*

Word or Phrase	Description	Combining Forms
menstruation	Process in which the endometrium of the uterus is shed each month, causing a flow of blood and tissue through the vagina. Under the influence of estradiol, the endometrium thickens in preparation to receive a fertilized ovum. If the ovum is not fertilized, the endometrium is shed to begin another menstrual cycle.	**menstru/o-** *monthly discharge of blood*
ovulation	Day 14 of the menstrual cycle. Luteinizing hormone from the anterior pituitary gland causes the ovarian follicle to rupture, releasing the mature ovum. The **basal (baseline) body temperature** rises during ovulation.	**ovul/o-** *egg; ovum* **bas/o-** *alkaline; base of a structure*
proliferative phase	Days 7–13 of the menstrual cycle. Follicle-stimulating hormone stimulates the follicle to secrete estradiol. A follicle produces a mature ovum, and the thickness of the endometrium increases (proliferates).	**prolifer/o-** *production of more of the same*
secretory phase	Days 15–26 of the menstrual cycle. A ruptured follicle becomes the corpus luteum and secretes estradiol and progesterone. The thickness of the endometrium increases.	**secret/o-** *produce; secrete*
Conception		
amnion	Membrane sac that holds the **amniotic fluid** that surrounds and cushions the developing embryo and fetus. Also known as the "bag of waters."	**amni/o-** *amnion*
antepartum	From the mother's standpoint, the period of time from conception until labor and delivery with the birth of the baby	**part/o-** *childbirth; labor*
chorion	Outer layer of a zygote that sends out finger-like projections (villi) into the endometrium to bring nutrients and oxygen to the embryo. It produces human chorionic gonadotropin. It later develops into the placenta.	**chorion/o-** *chorion*
embryo	A fertilized ovum (zygote) from 4 days after fertilization through 8 weeks of gestation	**embryon/o-** *embryo; immature form*
fertilization	The act of a spermatozoon uniting with an ovum. Also known as **conception**.	**fertil/o-** *conceive; form* **concept/o-** *conceive; form*
fetus	An embryo becomes a fetus beginning at 9 weeks of gestation. It is called a fetus until the moment of birth.	**fet/o-** *fetus*
fraternal twins	The ovary releases two ova that are both fertilized but by different spermatozoa	**fratern/o-** *close relationship*
gestation	Period of time from the moment of conception until birth, approximately 9 months (38–42 weeks), divided into three trimesters	**gestat/o-** *conception to birth*
human chorionic gonadotropin (HCG)	Hormone secreted by the chorion of the zygote. It stimulates the corpus luteum of the ovary to keep producing estradiol and progesterone to maintain the endometrium and prevent menstruation during the pregnancy.	**chorion/o-** *chorion* **gonad/o-** *gonad; ovary; testis* **trop/o-** *having an affinity for; stimulating; turning*
identical twins	An already developing zygote splits in two. This creates two separate but identical zygotes.	
placenta	Large, pancake-like structure that develops from the chorion. It provides nutrients and oxygen to the developing fetus and removes carbon dioxide and waste products. It secretes estradiol and progesterone to maintain the endometrium during pregnancy. Also known as the "afterbirth."	**placent/o-** *placenta*
pregnancy	State of being with child. It begins at the moment of conception and ends with delivery of the newborn.	**pregn/o-** *being with child*

Word or Phrase	Description	Combining Forms
prenatal period	From the fetus's standpoint, the period of time from conception to birth	**nat/o-** *birth*
products of conception	The fetus, placenta, and all fluids and tissue in the pregnant uterus	**concept/o-** *conceive; form*
trimester	A period of 3 months. The time of gestation is divided into three trimesters.	
umbilical cord	Rubbery, flexible cord that connects the placenta to the **umbilicus** (navel) of the fetus. It contains two arteries and one vein.	**umbilic/o-** *navel; umbilicus*
zygote	Cell that is the union of a spermatozoon and an ovum. A zygote has 46 chromosomes.	
Labor and Delivery		
Braxton Hicks contractions	Irregular uterine contractions during the last trimester. These strengthen the uterine muscle in preparation for labor. Also known as *false labor*.	**contract/o-** *pull together*
cephalic presentation	Position of the fetus in which the head is the presenting part that is first to go through the birth canal. **Vertex presentation** is a type of cephalic presentation in which the top of the head is the presenting part.	**cephal/o-** *head*
cervical dilation	Widening of the cervical os from 0 to 5 cm during the first stage of labor	**cervic/o-** *cervix; neck* **dilat/o-** *dilate; widen*
cervical ripening	Softening of the cervix as collagen fibers in its wall break down prior to the onset of labor	**cervic/o-** *cervix; neck*
crowning	The top of the fetal head (crown) is visible at the vaginal introitus during the second stage of labor	
effacement	Thinning of the cervical wall, measured as a percentage from 0 percent to 100 percent, during the first stage of labor	**efface/o-** *do away with; obliterate*
engagement	The fetal head drops into position within the mother's pelvis in anticipation of birth. Also known as "lightening."	
involution	Process by which the uterus gradually returns to a normal size after childbirth	**involut/o-** *enlarged organ returns to normal size*
lochia	Small amounts of blood, tissue, and fluid that flow from the uterus after childbirth	
oxytocin	Hormone produced by the uterus and by the posterior pituitary gland in the brain. It stimulates the uterus to contract and begin labor. After delivery, it stimulates the uterus to contract to stop bleeding. It stimulates the letdown reflex to get milk flowing for breastfeeding.	**ox/y-** *oxygen; quick* **toc/o-** *childbirth; labor*
parturition	The process of labor and delivery. There are three stages: dilation and effacement of the cervix, delivery of the newborn, and delivery of the placenta.	**parturit/o-** *childbirth; labor*
placenta	Delivered during the third stage of labor. Also known as the "afterbirth."	**placent/o-** *placenta*
postnatal period	From the newborn's standpoint, the period of time after birth	**nat/o-** *birth*
postpartum	From the mother's standpoint, the period of time after delivery	**part/o-** *childbirth; labor* **par/o-** *giving birth*
rupture of the membranes (ROM)	Rupture of the amniotic sac during the first stage of labor, with the release of amniotic fluid that flows out of the vagina	

Word or Phrase	Description	Combining Forms
The Newborn		
acrocyanosis	Temporary bluish coloration of the skin of the newborn's face, hands, and feet	**acr/o-** *extremity; highest point* **cyan/o-** *blue*
fontanels	Soft areas on the head between the bones of the cranium in a newborn. In these areas, the brain is only covered with fibrous connective tissue. The largest is the anterior fontanel on the top of the head. There is a smaller posterior fontanel on the back of the head. Fontanels allow the brain to grow before the cranial bones fuse together. Also known as the "soft spots."	
meconium	First bowel movement passed by a newborn. It is a greenish-black, thick, tar-like substance.	
molding	Temporary, elongated reshaping of the fetal cranium as it passes through the mother's bony pelvis	
neonate	A newborn from the time of birth until 1 year of age. A **term neonate** is born between 38 and 42 weeks' gestational age. A **preterm** or **premature neonate** is born between 28 and 37 weeks' gestational age.	**ne/o-** *new* **nat/o-** *birth*
vernix caseosa	Thick, white, cheesy substance that covers some of the skin of the fetus and helps protect it from bacteria present in the mother's vagina during birth	
Lactation		
colostrum	First milk from the breasts. It is a thick, yellowish fluid that is rich in nutrients and contains maternal antibodies to give the newborn passive immunity to common diseases.	
lactation	Production of colostrum and then breast milk by the mammary glands after childbirth when stimulated by prolactin from the posterior pituitary gland	**lact/o-** *milk* **lact/i-** *milk* **galact/o-** *milk*
let-down reflex	Occurs when the newborn cries or sucks. Oxytocin from the posterior pituitary gland causes the lactiferous lobules to contract and expel milk.	

12.3 Diseases

Word or Phrase	Description	Pronunciation/Word Parts

Ovaries and Uterine Tubes

Word or Phrase	Description	Pronunciation/Word Parts
anovulation	Failure of the ovaries to release a mature ovum at the time of ovulation, although the menstrual cycle is normal. This results in infertility. (*Note*: Anovulation is normal before puberty, during pregnancy, and after menopause.) Treatment: Hormone drug to stimulate ovulation	**anovulation** (AN-aw-vyoo-LAY-shun) **an-** *not; without* **ovul/o-** *egg; ovum* **-ation** *being; having; process*

Word or Phrase	Description	Pronunciation/Word Parts

ovarian cancer	**Cancerous** tumor of an ovary. This **malignancy** often does not cause symptoms until it is quite large and has already metastasized (spread to other areas).
	Treatment: Oophorectomy to remove the ovary, possible hysterectomy; chemotherapy drugs
		cancer (KAN-ser)
		
		cancerous (KAN-ser-us)
		  cancer/o- *cancer*
		  -ous *pertaining to*
		
		malignancy (mah-LIG-nan-see)
		  malign/o- *cancer*
		  -ancy *state*

polycystic ovary syndrome	The ovaries contain multiple cysts (see Figure 12-17 ■). When a follicle enlarges and matures but fails to rupture and release an ovum, it then becomes a cyst. With each menstrual cycle, the cysts enlarge, causing pain. This happens month after month until the ovaries are filled with cysts. This syndrome is associated with amenorrhea or menometrorrhagia, infertility, obesity, and insulin resistance syndrome with the development of type 2 diabetes mellitus.
	Treatment: Oral contraceptive drug (to correct hormone levels); weight control; oral antidiabetic drug
	
	FIGURE 12-17 ■ **Polycystic ovary syndrome.**
	The ovary is filled with both small and large cysts. Some of the cysts contain blood.
		polycystic (PAW-lee-SIS-tik)
		  poly- *many; much*
		  cyst/o- *bladder; fluid-filled sac;*
		    semisolid cyst
		  -ic *pertaining to*

salpingitis	Inflammation or infection of the uterine tube. It is due to endometriosis or pelvic inflammatory disease that narrows or blocks the lumen of the tube. This can lead to an ectopic pregnancy (described in a later section). With **hydrosalpinx**, inflammation fills the tube with fluid. With **pyosalpinx**, infection fills the tube with pus.
	Treatment: Treat the underlying cause.
		salpingitis (SAL-ping-JY-tihs)
		  salping/o- *uterine tube*
		  -itis *infection of;*
		    inflammation of
		
		hydrosalpinx (HY-droh-SAL-pinks)
		  hydr/o- *fluid; water*
		  -salpinx *uterine tube*
		
		pyosalpinx (PY-oh-SAL-pinks)
		  py/o- *pus*
		  -salpinx *uterine tube*

Uterus

Word or Phrase	Description	Pronunciation/Word Parts

endometrial cancer	Cancerous tumor of the endometrium of the uterus. The earliest sign is abnormal bleeding. Also known as **uterine cancer**.
	Treatment: Hysterectomy; chemotherapy drugs
		endometrial
		(EN-doh-MEE-tree-al)
		  end/o- *innermost; within*
		  metri/o- *uterus; womb*
		  -al *pertaining to*

Word or Phrase	Description	Pronunciation/Word Parts
endometriosis	Endometrial tissue in abnormal places outside of the uterus. The exact cause is unknown, but it tends to run in families. The endometrium separates (sloughs off) from the uterine wall during each menstrual cycle, but then the blood and tissue go in an abnormal **retrograde** direction up into the uterine tubes and other structures, and implant there. The implanted tissue remains alive, and it is sensitive to hormones during the menstrual cycle that cause it to enlarge and then slough off again. Endometrial tissue that implants in the uterine tubes causes blockage, scarring, and infertility. Endometrial tissue that implants on the outside of the ovary forms "chocolate cysts" that contain old, dark blood. Endometrial tissue can implant on the wall of the abdominopelvic cavity (see Figure 12-18 ■), and these implants can form adhesions between the internal organs. Endometriosis causes pelvic inflammation, pelvic pain, and pain during sexual intercourse. Treatment: Hormone drug to suppress the menstrual cycle (to make the tissue implants become inactive); laparoscopic surgery to destroy the implants 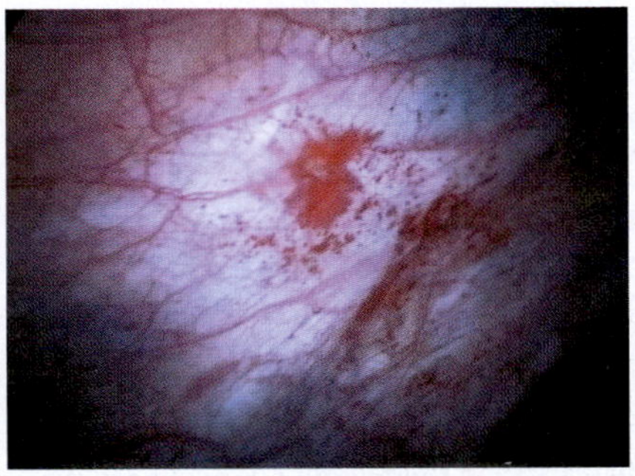 **FIGURE 12-18 ■ Endometriosis.** This area on the outside of the uterus, as seen through a laparoscope inserted through the abdominal wall, shows many endometrial implants with evidence of old blood.	**endometriosis** (EN-doh-MEE-tree-OH-sihs) **end/o-** *innermost; within* **metri/o-** *uterus; womb* **-osis** *abnormal condition; process* **retrograde** (REH-troh-grayd) The prefix **retro-** means *backward; behind.*
leiomyoma	Benign, fibrous tumor in the smooth muscle of the myometrium (see Figure 12-19 ■). It can be small or as large as a soccer ball. Several tumors are **leiomyomata**; also known as **uterine fibroids**. There is pelvic pain, excessive uterine bleeding, and painful sexual intercourse. Treatment: Uterine artery embolization; myomectomy (to remove the tumor); or hysterectomy, depending on the size of the tumor 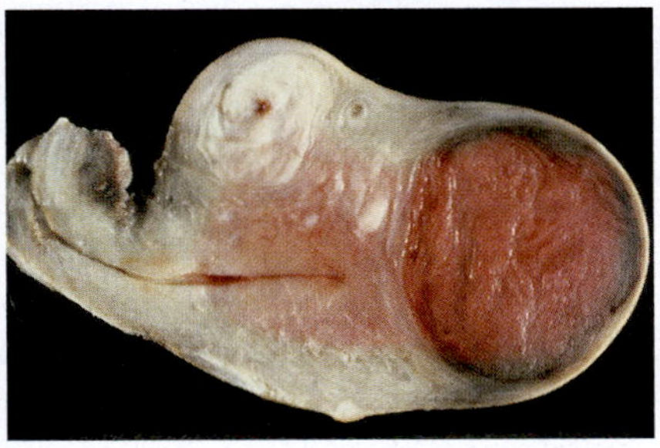 **FIGURE 12-19 ■ Leiomyoma.** This pathology specimen of the cut section of a uterus contains a large, benign, red leiomyoma.	**leiomyoma** (LIE-oh-my-OH-mah) **lei/o-** *smooth* **my/o-** *muscle* **-oma** *mass; tumor* **leiomyomata** (LIE-oh-my-OH-mah-tah) Greek plural noun: Change the singular ending *-oma* to *-omata.* **fibroid** (FY-broyd) **fibr/o-** *fiber* **-oid** *resembling*
leiomyosarcoma	Cancerous tumor of the smooth muscle of the myometrium Treatment: Hysterectomy; chemotherapy drug; radiation therapy	**leiomyosarcoma** (LIE-oh-MY-oh-sar-KOH-mah) **lei/o-** *smooth* **my/o-** *muscle* **sarc/o-** *connective tissue* **-oma** *mass; tumor*

Word or Phrase	Description	Pronunciation/Word Parts

myometritis	Inflammation or infection of the myometrium. It is associated with pelvic inflammatory disease. **Pyometritis** is a bacterial infection of the myometrium that creates pus in the intrauterine cavity.
	Treatment: Antibiotic drug
		myometritis (MY-oh-mee-TRY-tihs)
		  my/o- *muscle*
		  metr/o- *measurement; uterus; womb*
		  -itis *infection of; inflammation of*
		
		pyometritis (PY-oh-mee-TRY-tihs)
		  py/o- *pus*
		  metr/o- *measurement; uterus; womb*
		  -itis *infection of; inflammation of*

pelvic inflammatory disease (PID)	Infection of the cervix that ascends to the uterus, uterine tubes, and ovaries. It is often caused by a sexually transmitted disease. There is pelvic pain, fever, and vaginal discharge. If untreated, it can create scars that block the uterine tubes and cause infertility.
	Treatment: Antibiotic drug
		inflammatory (in-FLAM-ah-TOR-ee)
		  inflammat/o- *redness and warmth*
		  -ory *having the function of*

uterine prolapse	Descent of the uterus from its normal position. This is caused by stretching of the ligaments that support the uterus within the abdominopelvic cavity and/or weakness in the muscles of the floor of the pelvic cavity. Prolapse occurs after childbirth or because of age. The uterus can be so prolapsed that the cervix is visible in the vaginal introitus. Also known as **uterine descensus**. Severe prolapse affects urination and bowel movements. Treatment: Molded plastic form (a pessary) inserted in the vagina to help return the uterus to its normal position; hysterectomy or uterine suspension	**prolapse** (PROH-laps) **descensus** (dee-SEN-suhs)

Menstrual Disorders

Word or Phrase	Description	Pronunciation/Word Parts
abnormal uterine bleeding (AUB)	Sporadic menstrual bleeding without a true menstrual period. It is related to anovulation. The endometrium sloughs off from time to time, but never reaches a full thickness because there is no ovulation and no corpus luteum to secrete progesterone. Also known as **dysfunctional uterine bleeding (DUB)**. Treatment: Hormone drug therapy to restore normal ovulation and menstruation	**dysfunctional** (dis-FUNK-shun-al) The prefix **dys-** means *abnormal; difficult; painful.*

amenorrhea	Absence of monthly menstrual periods. It is caused by a hormone imbalance, thyroid disease, or a tumor of the uterus or ovary. Poor nutrition, stress, chronic disease, intense exercise, or the psychiatric illness of anorexia nervosa can also cause amenorrhea. (*Note:* Amenorrhea is normal before puberty, during pregnancy, and after menopause.)
	Treatment: Correct the underlying cause
		amenorrhea (AA-men-oh-REE-ah)
		  a- *away from; without*
		  men/o- *month*
		  -rrhea *discharge; flow*

dysmenorrhea	Painful menstruation. During menstruation, the uterus releases **prostaglandin** to constrict blood vessels in the uterine wall and prevent excessive bleeding. A high level of prostaglandin causes cramping and temporary ischemia of the myometrium, both of which cause pain. There is also nausea, dizziness, backache, and diarrhea. Pelvic inflammatory disease, endometriosis, or uterine fibroids can also cause dysmenorrhea.
	Treatment: Nonsteroidal anti-inflammatory drug to block the production of prostaglandin; correct the underlying cause
		dysmenorrhea (DIS-men-oh-REE-ah)
		  dys- *abnormal; difficult; painful*
		  men/o- *month*
		  -rrhea *discharge; flow*
		
		prostaglandin (PRAW-stah-GLAN-din)

Word or Phrase	Description	Pronunciation/Word Parts
menopause	Normal cessation of menstrual periods, occurring around middle age. **Perimenopause** is the time around menopause when menstrual periods first become irregular and menstrual flow is lighter. Menopause is also known as **climacteric** or the "change of life." Treatment: Hormone replacement therapy drugs; bioidentical hormone creams; natural estrogen supplements from soy	**menopause** (MEN-oh-pawz) **men/o-** *month* **-pause** *cessation* **perimenopausal** (PAIR-ee-MEN-oh-PAW-zal) **peri-** *around* **men/o-** *month* **paus/o-** *cessation* **-al** *pertaining to* **climacteric** (kly-MAK-ter-ik)

Dive Deeper

As a woman ages, the ovarian follicles deteriorate and stop secreting estradiol. Ovulation and menstruation cease. Decreased estradiol causes vaginal dryness, vaginal atrophy, and dryness of the skin. The breasts decrease in size. The anterior pituitary gland responds to a low blood level of estradiol by secreting more follicle-stimulating hormone (FSH). This causes occasional ovulation and menstruation during perimenopause. These bursts of FSH (which often occur at night) produce vasodilation, and the patient experiences hot flashes with perspiration and flushing. Frequent hot flashes throughout the night can cause sleeplessness and fatigue.

Word or Phrase	Description	Pronunciation/Word Parts
menorrhagia	A menstrual period with excessively heavy flow or a menstrual period that lasts longer than 7 days. It is caused by a hormone imbalance, uterine fibroids, or endometriosis. **Menometrorrhagia** is excessively heavy menstrual flow during menstruation or at other times of the month. **Metrorrhagia** is excessively heavy bleeding at a time other than menstruation. This can be caused by a tubal pregnancy or uterine cancer. Heavy uterine bleeding of any type can cause anemia. Treatment: Hormone drug therapy or correct the underlying cause	**menorrhagia** (MEN-oh-RAY-jah) **men/o-** *month* **rrhag/o-** *excessive discharge; excessive flow* **-ia** *condition; state; thing*
oligomenorrhea	A menstrual period with very light flow or infrequent menstrual cycles (longer than 35 days before the next cycle begins) in a woman who previously had normal menstruation. It is caused by a hormone imbalance. Treatment: Hormone drug therapy	**oligomenorrhea** (OH-lih-goh-MEN-oh-REE-ah) **olig/o-** *few; scanty* **men/o-** *month* **-rrhea** *discharge; flow*
premenstrual syndrome (PMS)	Premenstrual syndrome is caused by high levels of estradiol and progesterone just prior to menstruation. This causes breast tenderness, fluid retention, bloating, and mild mood changes (irritability, anger, sadness) a few days before the onset of menstruation. Treatment: Over-the-counter drug that relieves pain and fluid retention	**premenstrual** (pree-MEN-stroo-al) **pre-** *before; in front of* **menstru/o-** *monthly discharge of blood* **-al** *pertaining to*

Clinical Connections

Psychiatry. Premenstrual dysphoric disorder (PMDD) includes symptoms of PMS plus feelings of depression, anxiety, tearfulness, mood shifts, difficulty concentrating, sleeping and eating disturbances, and breast, joint, and muscle pain. It is a psychiatric mood disorder caused by an alteration in the levels of the neurotransmitters serotonin and norepinephrine in the brain.
Treatment: Antianxiety drug; antidepressant drug; analgesic drug for pain

dysphoric (dis-FOR-ik)
dys- *abnormal; difficult; painful*
phor/o- *bear; carry; range*
-ic *pertaining to*

Word or Phrase	Description	Pronunciation/Word Parts

Cervix

cervical cancer	Cancerous tumor of the cervix. If the cancer is still localized in one site, it is known as **carcinoma *in situ* (CIS)**. There is severe dysplasia of the cells as seen on a Pap test. Later there is ulceration and bleeding. Infection with **human papillomavirus (HPV)**, also known as **genital warts** (a sexually transmitted disease), predisposes to the development of cervical cancer. Treatment: Conization of the cervix or surgery to remove the uterus (hysterectomy)	**carcinoma** (KAR-sih-NOH-mah)
		  carcin/o- *cancer*
		  -oma *mass; tumor*
		
		in situ (IN SY-too)

cervical dysplasia	Abnormal growth of squamous cells in the surface layer of the cervix (see Figure 12-20 ■). It can be caused by infection with the human papillomavirus. Cervical dysplasia is seen on an abnormal Pap test. Severe dysplasia is a precancerous or cancerous condition.
	Treatment: Treat the underlying infection or cancer.
		dysplasia (dis-PLAY-zha)
		  dys- *abnormal; difficult; painful*
		  plas/o- *formation; growth*
		  -ia *condition; state; thing*
		Dysplasia: *Condition (of) abnormal growth*

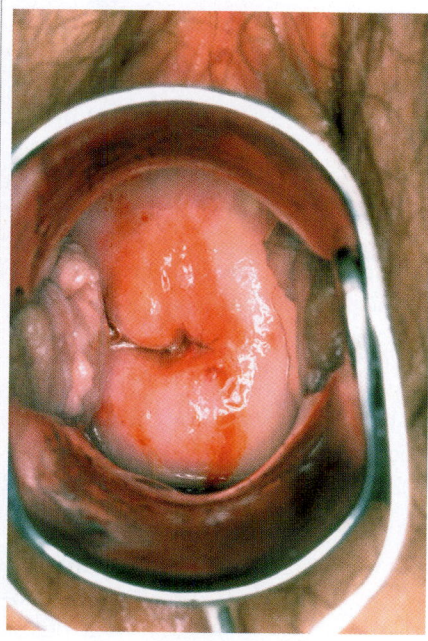

FIGURE 12-20 ■ Cervical dysplasia.
A metal speculum is inserted into the vagina and is used to visualize the cervix. The cervix shows a high degree of cervical dysplasia. These areas of redness are abnormal cells that may develop into cancer.

Vagina

bacterial vaginosis	Bacterial infection of the vagina due to *Gardnerella vaginalis*. There is a white or grayish vaginal discharge that has a fishy odor. This infection is not a sexually transmitted disease.
	Treatment: Antibiotic drug
		vaginosis (VAJ-ih-NOH-sihs)
		  vagin/o- *vagina*
		  -osis *abnormal condition; process*

candidiasis	Yeast infection of the vagina due to *Candida albicans*. There is vaginal itching and **leukorrhea**, a cheesy, white discharge. Candidiasis can occur after taking an antibiotic drug for a bacterial infection. The antibiotic drug kills the disease-causing bacteria, but yeast (which is always present to some degree in the vagina) is not affected by the antibiotic drug, and so it multiplies and causes an infection.
	Treatment: Antiyeast drug applied topically in the vagina
		candidiasis (KAN-dih-DY-ah-sihs)
		  candid/o- *Candida; yeast*
		  -iasis *process; state*
		
		leukorrhea (LOO-koh-REE-ah)
		  leuk/o- *white*
		  -rrhea *discharge; flow*

Word or Phrase	Description	Pronunciation/Word Parts

cystocele	Herniation of the bladder into the vagina because of a weakness in the vaginal wall. It is caused by childbirth or age. It can result in urinary retention.
	Treatment: Colporrhaphy
		cystocele (SIS-toh-seel)
		  cyst/o- *bladder; fluid-filled sac; semisolid cyst*
		  -cele *hernia*

dyspareunia	Painful or difficult sexual intercourse with **postcoital** pain. This can happen when the hymen is across the vaginal introitus or because of infection (of the vagina, cervix, or uterus), pelvic inflammatory disease, or endometriosis. **Retroversion** of the uterus (a backwards tipping of the uterus from its normal position of being tipped anteriorly over the bladder) can also cause dyspareunia.
	Treatment: Correct the underlying cause.
		dyspareunia
		(DIS-pah-ROO-nee-ah)
		  dys- *abnormal; difficult; painful*
		  pareun/o- *sexual intercourse*
		  -ia *condition; state; thing*
		
		postcoital (post-KOY-eh-tal)
		  post- *after; behind*
		  coit/o- *sexual intercourse*
		  -al *pertaining to*
		
		retroversion (REH-troh-VER-zhun)
		  retro- *backward; behind*
		  vers/o- *travel; turn*
		  -ion *action; condition*

rectocele	Herniation of the rectum into the vagina because of weakness in the vaginal wall. It is caused by childbirth or age. It can interfere with bowel movements.
	Treatment: Colporrhaphy
		rectocele (REK-toh-seel)
		  rect/o- *rectum*
		  -cele *hernia*

vaginitis	Vaginal inflammation or infection. Inflammation can be caused by irritation from chemicals in spermicidal jelly or douches. Infection can be caused by candidiasis (yeast infection) or a bacterial or viral sexually transmitted disease (**venereal disease**).
	Treatment: Treat the underlying cause.
		vaginitis (VAJ-ih-NY-tihs)
		  vagin/o- *vagina*
		  -itis *infection of; inflammation of*
		
		venereal (veh-NEER-ee-al)
		  venere/o- *sexual intercourse*
		  -al *pertaining to*

Clinical Connections

Public Health. The first cases of **toxic shock syndrome** were seen in women in 1980. Symptoms included a high fever, vomiting, diarrhea, and hypotension (shock). Physicians interviewed patients and family members to discover a common link. All of the patients had used super-absorbent **tampons** during their menstrual period. The super-absorbent tampons held the menstrual blood over an extended period of time until the normally harmless vaginal bacterium *Staphylococcus aureus* multiplied in the old blood and released toxins. Also, the larger size of the tampon caused tears in the vaginal wall that allowed the toxins to enter the blood and cause severe symptoms throughout the body.

toxic (TAWK-sik)
  tox/o- *poison*
  -ic *pertaining to*

tampon (TAM-pawn)

Word or Phrase	Description	Pronunciation/Word Parts

Breasts

breast cancer	Cancerous tumor, usually an **adenocarcinoma** of the lactiferous lobules of the breast (see Figure 12-21 ■). A lump is detected during mammography or breast self-examination. There can be swelling in the area, enlarged lymph nodes, and nipple discharge. Advanced breast cancer has **peau d'orange** (a dimpling of the skin—that looks like the pores in an orange peel—as the tumor pulls on structures inside the breast) and nipple retraction. Long-term hormone replacement therapy with an estrogen drug after menopause increases the risk of breast cancer. Inherited mutations in the *BRCA1* or *BRCA2* gene increase the risk of developing breast cancer. Breast cancer is categorized as **estrogen receptor positive (ER⁺)** or negative, **progesterone receptor positive (PR⁺)** or negative, and **human epidermal growth factor receptor 2 (HER2)** positive or negative. Treatment: Lumpectomy to remove the tumor or mastectomy to remove the breast; chemotherapy drugs; radiation therapy	**adenocarcinoma** (AD-eh-noh-KAR-sih-NOH-mah) **aden/o-** *gland* **carcin/o-** *cancer* **-oma** *mass; tumor* **peau d'orange** (poh deh-RAHNJ)

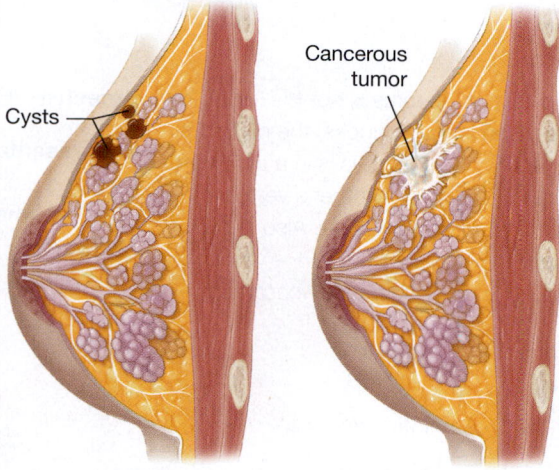

Cysts

Cancerous tumor

FIGURE 12-21 ■ Breast with cysts; breast with cancer.
A lump in the breast can be a benign cyst (fibrocystic disease) or it can be cancer. The presence of many cysts can make it difficult to detect a cancerous tumor on mammography.

Clinical Connections

Public Health. A woman born today has a 1 in 8 chance of developing breast cancer sometime in her life. Breast cancer is the most common type of cancer in women, but men can also develop breast cancer. October is National Breast Cancer Awareness Month. Women are encouraged to do monthly breast self-examinations and have annual mammography to detect early breast cancer (see Figure 12-22 ■).

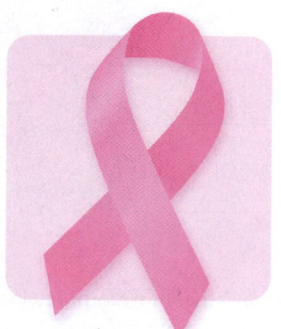

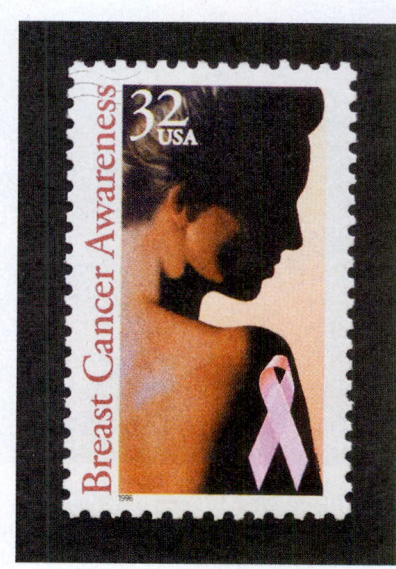

FIGURE 12-22 ■ Breast cancer awareness.
A pink ribbon is the universal symbol for breast cancer awareness.

Word or Phrase	Description	Pronunciation/Word Parts
failure of lactation	Lack of production of milk from the breasts after childbirth. It is caused by hyposecretion of prolactin from the anterior pituitary gland. The breasts do not produce milk or produce an insufficient amount of milk to breastfeed the baby. Treatment: There is no treatment for the mother; switch to bottle feeding	**lactation** (lak-TAY-shun) **lact/o-** *milk* **-ation** *being; having; process*
fibrocystic breasts	Benign condition in which numerous fibrous and fluid-filled cysts form in one or both breasts (see Figure 12-21). The sizes of the cysts can change in response to hormone levels. The cysts can be painful and tender. Severe fibrocystic breasts make it difficult to detect a cancerous tumor on mammography, and so the physician may order an MRI scan instead. Treatment: Hormone therapy; elimination of certain foods (chocolate, caffeine) from the diet sometimes helps	**fibrocystic** (FY-broh-SIS-tik) **fibr/o-** *fiber* **cyst/o-** *bladder; fluid-filled sac; semisolid cyst* **-ic** *pertaining to*
galactorrhea	Discharge of milk from the breasts when the patient is not pregnant or breastfeeding. It is caused by an increased level of prolactin from an adenoma (benign tumor) in the anterior pituitary gland. Treatment: Drug to decrease prolactin production; surgery to remove the adenoma from the anterior pituitary gland in the brain	**galactorrhea** (gah-LAK-toh-REE-ah) **galact/o-** *milk* **-rrhea** *discharge; flow*

Pregnancy and Labor and Delivery

abnormal presentation	Birth position in which the presenting part of the fetus is not the head. In a **breech** presentation, the presenting part is the buttocks, the buttocks and feet, or just the feet (see Figure 12-23 ■). If the fetus is in a transverse lie (the fetal vertebral column is perpendicular to the mother's vertebral column), the shoulder or arm becomes the presenting part. Also known as **malpresentation** of the fetus (see Figure 12-24 ■). Treatment: Version maneuver to turn the fetus or delivery by cesarean section	**breech** (BREECH) **malpresentation** (MAL-pree-sen-TAY-shun) The prefix **mal-** means *bad; inadequate.*

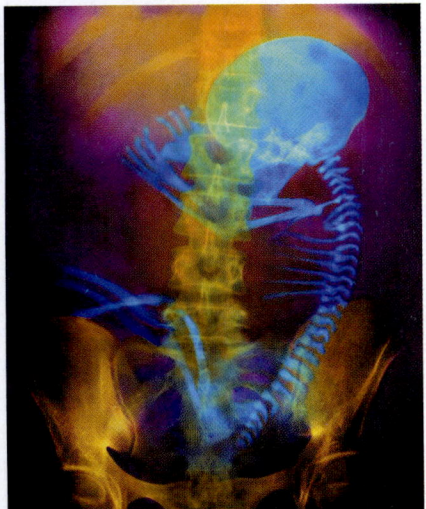

FIGURE 12-23 ■ Breech position.
This colorized x-ray shows a full-term fetus in breech presentation. The fetal skull is at the top, the spine is along the right side of the image, and the presenting part is the buttocks.

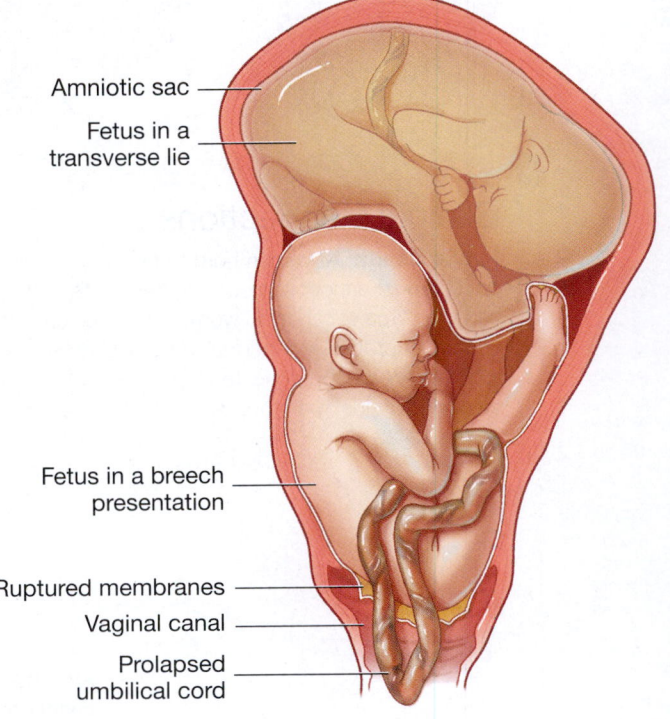

Amniotic sac

Fetus in a transverse lie

Fetus in a breech presentation

Ruptured membranes

Vaginal canal

Prolapsed umbilical cord

FIGURE 12-24 ■ Malpresentation of fraternal twins.
One twin is in the breech position with the buttocks as the presenting part. The amniotic sac around this fetus has already ruptured, and the umbilical cord has prolapsed into the vaginal canal. The second twin, still in its amniotic sac, is in a transverse lie position.

Word or Phrase	Description	Pronunciation/Word Parts
abruptio placentae	Complete or partial separation of the placenta from the uterine wall before the third stage of labor. This results in uterine hemorrhage that threatens the life of the mother as well as disruption of blood flow and oxygen through the umbilical cord, which threatens the life of the fetus. Treatment: Emergency cesarean section	**abruptio placentae** (ab-RUP-shee-oh plah-SEN-tee)
cephalopelvic disproportion (CPD)	The size of the fetal head exceeds the size of the opening in the mother's pelvic bones, and the fetus cannot be born vaginally. Treatment: Cesarean section	**cephalopelvic** (SEF-ah-loh-PEL-vik) **cephal/o-** *head* **pelv/o-** *hip bone; pelvis; renal pelvis* **-ic** *pertaining to* **disproportion** (DIS-proh-POR-shun)

Dive Deeper

Skeletons of prehistoric women have been discovered that show cephalopelvic disproportion, with the skull of the baby still tightly wedged in the mother's pelvic bones at the time of death.

Word or Phrase	Description	Pronunciation/Word Parts
dystocia	Any type of difficult or abnormal labor and delivery Treatment: Correct the underlying cause.	**dystocia** (dis-TOH-shah) **dys-** *abnormal; difficult; painful* **toc/o-** *childbirth; labor* **-ia** *condition; state; thing*
ectopic pregnancy	Implantation of a fertilized ovum somewhere other than in the uterus. It can implant in the cervix, the ovary, or in the abdominopelvic cavity, but most commonly implants in the uterine tube (a **tubal pregnancy**). This occurs more often if the uterine tube has scar tissue or a blockage in it. The patient has a positive pregnancy test, but there is abdominal tenderness as the uterine tube swells from the developing embryo. The tube can bleed, a condition known as **hemosalpinx**, or can suddenly rupture, causing severe blood loss and shock. Treatment: Salpingectomy to remove the embryo and uterine tube	**ectopic** (ek-TAW-pik) **ectop/o-** *outside* **-ic** *pertaining to* **tubal** (TOO-bal) **tub/o-** *tube* **-al** *pertaining to* **hemosalpinx** (HEE-moh-SAL-pinks) **hem/o-** *blood* **-salpinx** *uterine tube*
gestational diabetes mellitus	Temporary disorder of glucose metabolism that occurs only during pregnancy. Increased levels of estradiol and progesterone during pregnancy block the action of insulin from the pancreas. The function of insulin is to metabolize glucose. A decreased action of insulin leads to a high level of unmetabolized glucose in the mother's blood. Excess glucose crosses the placenta and causes the fetus to grow too rapidly (because the fetal pancreas produces insulin that metabolizes the glucose). Treatment: Dietary management; oral antidiabetic drug during pregnancy. This condition ceases with childbirth, but the mother often develops type 2 diabetes mellitus later in life.	**gestational** (jes-TAY-shun-al) **gestat/o-** *conception to birth* **-ion** *action; condition* **-al** *pertaining to* **diabetes** (DY-ah-BEE-teez) **mellitus** (MEL-ih-tuhs)
hydatidiform mole	Abnormal union of an ovum and spermatozoon. It produces hundreds of small, fluid-filled sacs but no embryo. The chorion produces HCG, so the patient has early signs of pregnancy. However, the hydatidiform mole grows more rapidly than a normal pregnancy, and the uterus is much larger than expected for the gestational age. Treatment: Surgery to remove the hydatidiform mole or hysterectomy	**hydatidiform** (HY-dah-TIH-dih-form) **hydatidi/o-** *fluid-filled sacs* **-form** *having the form of* **mole** (MOHL)

Word or Phrase	Description	Pronunciation/Word Parts
incompetent cervix	Spontaneous, premature dilation of the cervix during the second trimester of pregnancy. This can result in spontaneous abortion of the fetus. Treatment: Bed rest and placement of a cerclage (described later) to prevent further dilation until the pregnancy reaches full term	**incompetent** (in-COM-peh-tent)
mastitis	Inflammation or infection of the breast. It is caused by milk engorgement in the breast or by an infection due to the bacterium *Staphylococcus aureus* from the nursing infant's mouth or on the mother's skin. The affected breast is red and swollen, and the mother has a fever. Treatment: Pumping of breast milk; antibiotic drug to treat the infection	**mastitis** (mas-TY-tihs) **mast/o-** breast; mastoid process **-itis** infection of; inflammation of
morning sickness	Nausea and vomiting that is a common, but temporary, condition during the first trimester of pregnancy. It is thought to be due to elevated estradiol and progesterone levels. **Hyperemesis gravidarum** is excessive vomiting that causes weakness, dehydration, and fluid and electrolyte imbalance. Treatment: Intravenous fluids for severe hyperemesis gravidarum	**hyperemesis** (HY-per-EM-eh-sihs) The prefix **hyper-** means *above; more than normal,* and the suffix **-emesis** means *abnormal condition of vomiting.* **gravidarum** (GRAV-ih-DAIR-um)
oligohydramnios	Decreased volume of amniotic fluid. The fetus swallows amniotic fluid but does not excrete a similar volume in its urine because of a congenital abnormality of the fetal kidneys. Oligohydramnios is identified during a routine prenatal ultrasound test. Treatment: Surgery to the fetus while *in utero* or after birth	**oligohydramnios** (OH-lih-GOH-hy-DRAM-nee-ohs) **olig/o-** few; scanty **hydr/o-** fluid; water **-amnios** amniotic fluid ***in utero*** (IN YOO-ter-oh)
placenta previa	Incorrect position of the placenta with its edge partially or completely covering the cervical canal (see Figure 12-25 ■). During labor when the cervix dilates, the connection between the placenta and uterus is suddenly disrupted. This causes moderate-to-severe bleeding in the mother and disrupts the flow of blood from the placenta to the fetus. Treatment: Cesarean section	**placenta previa** (plah-SEN-tah PREE-vee-ah)

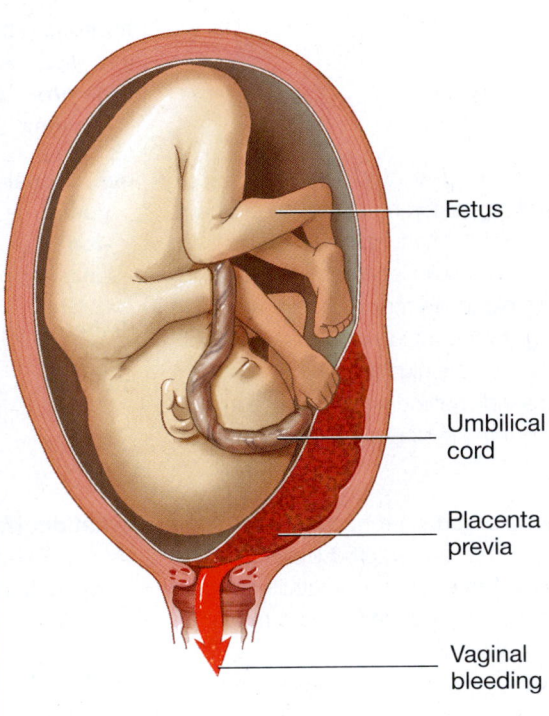

Fetus

Umbilical cord

Placenta previa

Vaginal bleeding

FIGURE 12-25 ■ Placenta previa.
An abnormally low position of the placenta within the uterus can cause bleeding when the cervix dilates during labor and delivery.

Word or Phrase	Description	Pronunciation/Word Parts

polyhydramnios	Increased volume of amniotic fluid. It is caused by maternal diabetes mellitus, twin gestation, or abnormalities in the fetus.
	Treatment: Correct the underlying cause.
		polyhydramnios
		(PAW-lee-hy-DRAM-nee-ohs)
		  poly- _many; much_
		  hydr/o- _fluid; water_
		  -amnios _amniotic fluid_

postpartum hemorrhage	Continual bleeding after delivery from the site where the placenta separated from the uterine wall. The uterus is boggy (soft) and the myometrium does not contract to become firm as it should. This is caused by hyposecretion of oxytocin from the posterior pituitary gland in the brain.
	Treatment: Manual massage of the uterus; intravenous oxytocin drug
		hemorrhage (HEM-oh-rij)
		  hem/o- _blood_
		  -rrhage _excessive discharge; excessive flow_

preeclampsia	Hypertensive disorder of pregnancy with increased blood pressure, edema, weight gain, and protein in the urine (proteinuria). The kidneys allow protein from the blood to be lost in the urine. Low levels of blood proteins change the osmotic pressure of the blood and allow fluid to move into the tissues and cause edema. Preeclampsia can progress to **eclampsia** in which the woman has seizures and the fetus is endangered.
	Treatment: Bed rest; antihypertensive and antiseizure drugs
		preeclampsia
		(PREE-ee-KLAMP-see-ah)
		  pre- _before; in front of_
		  eclamps/o- _seizure_
		  -ia _condition; state; thing_
		
		eclampsia (ee-KLAMP-see-ah)

premature labor	Regular uterine contractions that occur before the fetus is mature. The cervix can dilate, and small amounts of blood or amniotic fluid can leak out. Treatment: Bed rest; tocolytic drug to stop labor	
premature rupture of membranes (PROM)	Spontaneous rupture of the amniotic sac and loss of amniotic fluid before labor begins. The woman must deliver within 24 hours or risk developing a uterine infection. Treatment: Induction of labor	
prolapsed cord	A loop of umbilical cord slips down (prolapses) and becomes caught between the presenting part of the fetus and the opening to the vagina (birth canal) (see Figure 12-24). This occurs if the membranes rupture before the fetal head (or other presenting part) is fully engaged in the woman's pelvis. With each uterine contraction, the umbilical cord is compressed, causing decreased blood flow to the fetus and fetal distress with a decreased heart rate. Treatment: Change the woman's position to move the umbilical cord; give oxygen to the mother; cesarean section	**prolapse** (PROH-laps)

spontaneous abortion (SAB)	Loss of a pregnancy. An early spontaneous abortion usually occurs because of a genetic abnormality or poor implantation of the embryo in the endometrium. A late spontaneous abortion can occur because of preterm labor or an incompetent cervix. In an incomplete abortion, the embryo or fetus is expelled but the placenta and other tissues remain in the uterus. Also known as a **miscarriage**. During a spontaneous abortion, the fetus can be born alive or can be a **stillborn**.
	Treatment: D&C if some of the products of conception are retained
		abortion (ah-BOR-shun)
		  abort/o- _stop prematurely_
		  -ion _action; condition_

uterine inertia	Weak or uncoordinated contractions during a long and nonproductive labor. It is caused by (1) a decreased level of oxytocin secreted by the posterior pituitary gland; (2) the uterus being distended with multiple fetuses and unable to contract normally; or (3) cephalopelvic disproportion or malpresentation of the fetus. A related condition is **arrest of labor** in which uterine contractions have ceased. Also known as **failure to progress**, as the cervix does not progressively dilate and efface. Treatment: Intravenous oxytocin drug; cesarean section for cephalopelvic disproportion; version or cesarean section for malpresentation	**inertia** (in-ER-shah)

Word or Phrase	Description	Pronunciation/Word Parts

	## Clinical Connections
	
	Psychiatry. Postpartum depression is a mood disorder with symptoms of mild-to-moderate depression, anxiousness, irritability, tearfulness, and fatigue. It is caused by hormonal changes after birth and by feelings of overwhelming responsibility and fatigue.
	
	Dietetics. A lack of folic acid during pregnancy can cause a neural tube defect in the fetus (described in Chapter 9, Neurology). Prenatal vitamins for pregnant women and enrichment of cereals and other grain products with added folic acid have greatly decreased the incidence of neural tube defects.
	
	There are many stories about the food cravings of pregnant women: pickles, ice cream, and so forth. Some pregnant women experience **pica**, an unnatural craving for, and compulsive eating of, substances with no nutritional value, such as clay, chalk, starch, or dirt.
		depression (dee-PREH-shun)
		  depress/o- *press down*
		  -ion *action; condition*
		
		pica (PY-kah)

Fetus and Neonate

Word or Phrase	Description	Pronunciation/Word Parts

apnea	Temporary or permanent cessation of breathing in the newborn after birth. The newborn is said to be **apneic**. The immature central nervous system of a newborn fails to maintain a consistent respiratory rate, and there are occasional long pauses between periods of regular breathing.
	Treatment: Apnea monitor in the hospital and at home that sounds an alarm if the newborn stops breathing
		apnea (AP-nee-ah)
		
		apneic (AP-nee-ik)
		  a- *away from; without*
		  pne/o- *breathing*
		  -ic *pertaining to*

fetal distress	Lack of oxygen to the fetus because of decreased blood flow through the placenta or umbilical cord. The fetus has a decreased heart rate and passes meconium because of the stress of a decreased level of oxygen. Treatment: Mother is given oxygen; possible cesarean section	

growth abnormalities	Maternal illness, malnutrition, and smoking can make the fetus **small for gestational age (SGA)**. This is known as **intrauterine growth retardation (IUGR)**. Diabetes mellitus in the mother can make the fetus **large for gestational age (LGA)**. A fetus within the normal growth range for weight and length is said to be **appropriate for gestational age (AGA)**.
	Treatment: Correct the underlying cause.
		intrauterine (IN-trah-YOO-teh-rin)
		  intra- *within*
		  uter/o- *uterus; womb*
		  -ine *pertaining to*

infant respiratory distress syndrome (IRDS)	Difficulty inflating the lungs to breathe because of a lack of surfactant. This occurs mainly in premature newborns.
	Treatment: Oxygen and the use of a respirator; surfactant drug given through the endotracheal tube
		respiratory (RES-pih-rah-TOR-ee)
		  re- *again and again; backward; unable to*
		  spir/o- *breathe; coil*
		  -atory *pertaining to*

jaundice	Yellowish discoloration of the skin in a newborn. During gestation, the fetus has extra red blood cells that are no longer needed after birth. The destruction of those red blood cells releases hemoglobin, which is converted into unconjugated bilirubin. The immature newborn liver is not able to process this much unconjugated bilirubin, and it builds up in the blood (**hyperbilirubinemia**), moves into the tissues, and causes jaundice. The more premature the newborn, the greater the chance of developing jaundice.
	Treatment: **Phototherapy** with bililights (special fluorescent lights that break down bilirubin in the skin to make it water soluble so it can be excreted by the newborn's kidneys)
		jaundice (JAWN-dihs)
		
		hyperbilirubinemia (HY-per-BIL-ee-ROO-bih-NEE-mee-ah)
		  hyper- *above; more than normal*
		  bilirubin/o- *bilirubin*
		  -emia *condition of the blood; substance in the blood*
		
		phototherapy (FOH-toh-THAIR-ah-pee)
		  phot/o- *light*
		  -therapy *treatment*

Word or Phrase	Description	Pronunciation/Word Parts
meconium aspiration	Fetal distress causes the fetus to pass meconium into the amniotic fluid. This can enter the mouth and nose of the fetus/newborn, and, if inhaled with the first breath, it blocks the airway and causes severe respiratory distress. Treatment: Suctioning of the newborn's nose and mouth; use of oxygen and a ventilator after birth, if needed	**aspiration** (AS-pih-RAY-shun) **aspir/o-** *breathe in; suck in* **-ation** *being; having; process*
nuchal cord	Umbilical cord is wrapped around the neck of the fetus. A loose nuchal cord can be present without causing a problem. A tight nuchal cord with one or more loops around the neck can impair blood flow to the brain, causing brain damage or fetal death. Treatment: Emergency cesarean section	**nuchal** (NOO-kal) **nuch/o-** *neck* **-al** *pertaining to*

12.3 PRACTICE LAPS

Use the Answer Key at the end of the book to check your answers.

A. Give the Meaning of Combining Forms

Next to each combining form, write its meaning. The first one has been done for you.

Combining Form	Meaning	Combining Form	Meaning
1. **vagin/o-**	*vagina*	19. hydatidi/o-	
2. abort/o-		20. hydr/o-	
3. aden/o-		21. inflammat/o-	
4. aspir/o-		22. lact/o-	
5. bilirubin/o-		23. lei/o-	
6. cancer/o-		24. leuk/o-	
7. candid/o-		25. malign/o-	
8. carcin/o-		26. mast/o-	
9. cephal/o-		27. melan/o-	
10. cyst/o-		28. men/o-	
11. depress/o-		29. menstru/o-	
12. eclamps/o-		30. metri/o-	
13. ectop/o-		31. metr/o-	
14. end/o-		32. my/o-	
15. fibr/o-		33. nuch/o-	
16. galact/o-		34. olig/o-	
17. gestat/o-		35. ovul/o-	
18. hem/o-		36. pareun/o-	

continued on next page

Combining Form	Meaning	Combining Form	Meaning
37. paus/o-		45. rrhag/o-	
38. pelv/o-		46. salping/o-	
39. phor/o-		47. sarc/o-	
40. phot/o-		48. spir/o-	
41. plas/o-		49. toc/o-	
42. pne/o-		50. tox/o-	
43. py/o-		51. tub/o-	
44. rect/o-		52. uter/o-	

B. Build Words

Read the definition of the medical word. Look at the combining form that is given. Select the correct suffix from the Suffix List, and write it on the blank line. Then build the medical word, and write it on the line. (Remember: You may need to remove the combining vowel. Always remove the hyphens and slash.) Be sure to check your spelling.

Suffix List

-al (pertaining to)	-ic (pertaining to)	-ory (having the function of)
-ant (pertaining to)	-ion (action; condition)	-osis (abnormal condition; process)
-ation (being; having; process)	-itis (infection of; inflammation of)	-pause (cessation)
-cele (hernia)	-oid (resembling)	-rrhea (discharge; flow)
-form (having the form of)	-oma (mass; tumor)	-salpinx (uterine tube)

Definition of the Medical Word	Combining Form	Suffix	Build the Medical Word
Example: Pertaining to (a) tube	**tub/o-**	_-al_	_tubal_

[You think pertaining to (-al) + tube (tub/o-). You change the order of the word parts to put the suffix last. You write tubal.]

Definition of the Medical Word	Combining Form	Suffix	Build the Medical Word
1. Infection of (or) inflammation of (the) vagina	vagin/o-		
2. Cessation (of) month(ly periods)	men/o-		
3. Fluid (in the) uterine tube	hydr/o-		
4. Discharge (from the vagina that is) white	leuk/o-		
5. Pertaining to cancer	malign/o-		
6. Hernia (of the) rectum (into the vagina)	rect/o-		
7. Inflammation of (or) infection of (the) uterine tube	salping/o-		
8. Abnormal condition (of the) vagina	vagin/o-		
9. Having the form of fluid-filled sacs	hydatidi/o-		

Definition of the Medical Word	Combining Form	Suffix	Build the Medical Word
10. Having milk	lact/o-	_____	_____
11. Uterine tube (that contains) blood	hem/o-	_____	_____
12. Flow (of) milk (when not pregnant)	galact/o-	_____	_____
13. Tumor (that is a) cancer	carcin/o-	_____	_____
14. Pertaining to (a pregnancy that is) outside (the uterus)	ectop/o-	_____	_____
15. Hernia (of the) bladder (into the vagina)	cyst/o-	_____	_____
16. (Abnormal structure) resembling fiber	fibr/o-	_____	_____
17. Having the function of redness and warmth	inflammat/o-	_____	_____
18. Uterine tube (that contains) pus	py/o-	_____	_____
19. Action (to) stop prematurely (a pregnancy)	abort/o-	_____	_____

C. Define Abbreviations

1. AGA _____

2. *BRCA* _____

3. CIS _____

4. CPD _____

5. DUB _____

6. ER$^+$ _____

7. HER2 _____

8. HPV _____

9. IRDS _____

10. IUGRf _____

11. LGA _____

12. PID _____

13. PMDD _____

14. PMS _____

15. PR$^+$ _____

16. PROM _____

17. SAB _____

18. SGA _____

12.4 Laboratory, Diagnostic, and Radiologic Procedures

Word or Phrase	Description	Pronunciation/Word Parts

Gynecologic Tests and Procedures

Word or Phrase	Description	Pronunciation/Word Parts
acid phosphatase	Test for an enzyme from the prostate gland that is found in the semen. The presence of acid phosphatase in the vagina indicates sexual intercourse has occurred, and this can be used in rape investigations.	**acid phosphatase** (AS-id FAWS-fah-tays)
BRCA1 or **BRCA2 gene**	Blood test that shows if a patient has inherited the *BRCA1* or *BRCA2* gene mutation, **genetic** mutations that significantly increase the risk of developing breast or ovarian cancer. BRCA stands for *breast cancer*.	**gene** (JEEN) **genetic** (jeh-NEH-tik) **gene/o-** *gene* **-tic** *pertaining to*
estrogen and progesterone receptor assay	**Cytology** test performed on breast tissue that has already been diagnosed as malignant. This test looks for a large number of estrogen and progesterone receptors on the tumor cells. If present, this means that the tumor requires the hormones estrogen (estradiol) and progesterone in order to grow and that chemotherapy drugs that block estrogen and progesterone would be effective in treating this cancer.	**receptor** (ree-SEP-tor) **recept/o-** *receive* **-or** *person who does or produces; thing that does or produces* **assay** (AS-say) **cytology** (sy-TAW-loh-jee) **cyt/o-** *cell* **-logy** *study of*
HER2 status	Cytology test performed on breast tissue that has already been diagnosed as malignant. This test measures the amount of HER2 protein in the cancer cells or the number of *HER2* genes in the cancer cells.	
Pap test	Screening cytology test used to detect abnormal cells (dysplasia) or **carcinoma *in situ* (CIS)** of the cervix. Also known as a **Pap smear**. *Pap* is a shortened version of *Papanicolaou*, the name of the doctor who developed the test. This is an **exfoliative cytology** test because it examines cells that have been scraped off the cervix. A small plastic or wooden spatula is used to scrape off **ectocervical cells** from the outside wall of the cervix. Then a **cytobrush** is inserted into the cervical os to obtain **endocervical cells** (see Figure 12-26 ■). A cervical broom (Papette®) can obtain both types of cells at the same time and also test for the sexually transmitted disease of human papillomavirus (HPV). The cell specimen is transferred to a glass slide and sprayed with a fixative. Alternatively, with **liquid cytology**, the specimen is rinsed in a vial of fixative. This captures all the cells, prevents cell drying, and gives a more accurate result. The slides or vials are sent to the laboratory where the cells are examined under a microscope for abnormalities (see Figure 12-27 ■). The Bethesda System is used to report Pap test results.	**Pap test** **exfoliative** (eks-FOH-lee-ah-TIV) **cytology** (sy-TAW-loh-jee) **cyt/o-** *cell* **-logy** *study of* **ectocervical** (EK-toh-SER-vih-kal) **ecto-** *outermost; outside* **cervic/o-** *cervix; neck* **-al** *pertaining to* **endocervical** (EN-doh-SER-vih-kal) **end/o-** *innermost; within* **cervic/o-** *cervix; neck* **-al** *pertaining to*

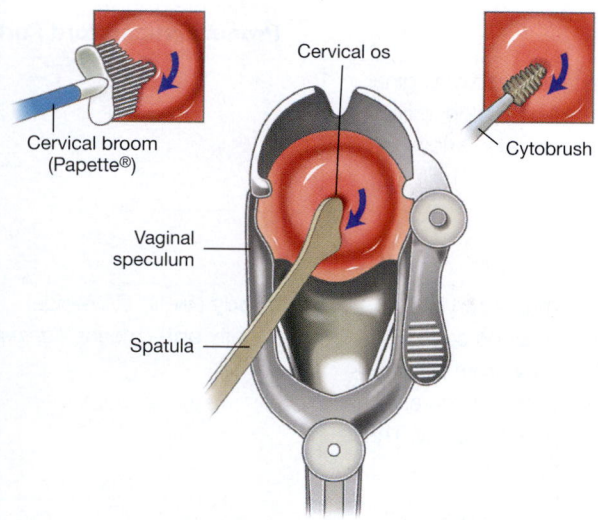

FIGURE 12-26 ■ **Taking a Pap test.**
A metal vaginal speculum is used to spread the vaginal walls apart to reveal the cervix. Cells from the cervix are obtained using a wooden spatula and a cytobrush or a cervical broom (Papette®). A microscope is used to examine the cells and detect cells that are precancerous or cancerous.

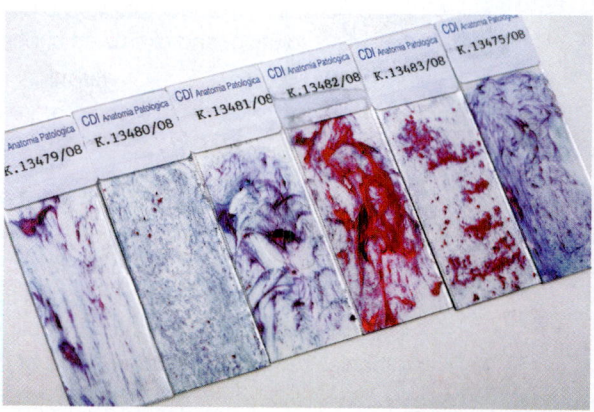

FIGURE 12-27 ■ **Pap tests.**
These stained slides from Pap tests from different women will be examined under a microscope by a pathologist.

Dive Deeper

Pap Test Terminology. From the Bethesda System Guidelines.

Specimen Adequacy.

- Satisfactory (enough cells were collected; cell quality was sufficient for diagnosis)
- Unsatisfactory (enough cells were not collected; cell quality was poor)

Normal Pap Test. Findings are reported as:

- Negative for intraepithelial lesion or malignancy
- The presence of infectious organisms [*Trichomonas*, herpes, HPV] is also reported.

Abnormal Pap Test. Findings are reported as one of the following:

ASC	Atypical **squamous** cells
LSIL	Low-grade squamous intraepithelial lesion
HSIL	High-grade squamous intraepithelial lesion
CIN	cervical intraepithelial **neoplasia**
SCC	Squamous cell **carcinoma**

squamous (SKWAY-muhs)
  squam/o- *scale-like cell*
  -ous *pertaining to*

neoplasia (NEE-oh-PLAY-shah)
  ne/o- *new*
  plas/o- *formation; growth*
  -ia *condition; state; thing*

carcinoma (KAR-sih-NOH-mah)
  carcin/o- *cancer*
  -oma *mass; tumor*

Word or Phrase	Description	Pronunciation/Word Parts
wet mount	Cytology test to detect yeasts, parasites, or bacteria. A swab of vaginal discharge is sent to a laboratory. The cells are placed on a slide, mixed with saline solution, and examined under a microscope. Also known as a **wet prep**.	

Infertility Diagnostic Tests

antisperm antibody test	Test that detects antibodies against sperm in the woman's cervical mucus. Some antibodies attack the tail of the spermatozoon so that it cannot swim; other antibodies prevent the spermatozoon from penetrating the ovum. Men produce antibodies to their own spermatozoa after a vasectomy when the spermatozoa must be absorbed by the body. These antibodies remain even after reversal of the vasectomy.	**antibody** (AN-tih-BAW-dee) The prefix **anti-** means *against*.
hormone testing	Blood test to determine the levels of FSH and LH from the anterior pituitary gland and estradiol and progesterone from the ovaries. It is used to diagnose menstruation and infertility problems.	

Pregnancy and Prenatal Diagnostic Tests

amniocentesis	Procedure to test the amniotic fluid. Using ultrasound guidance, a needle is inserted through the pregnant woman's abdomen and into the uterus to obtain a sample of amniotic fluid (see Figure 12-28 ■). This is done between 15 and 18 weeks' gestation when there is a sufficient amount of amniotic fluid. The following tests are performed:
	
	• **Chromosome studies** of fetal skin cells can determine the sex of the fetus and identify genetic abnormalities such as Down syndrome.
	• **Alpha fetoprotein (AFP)**. An increased level indicates a neural tube defect (myelomeningocele).
	• **L/S ratio** (lecithin/sphingomyelin) test for fetal lung maturity. **Lecithin** is a component of surfactant that keeps the alveoli from collapsing with each exhalation. **Sphingomyelin** is also a component of surfactant, and its level is higher when the fetal lungs are immature; when the lungs are mature, the lecithin level is higher.
		amniocentesis (AM-nee-OH-sen-TEE-sihs)
		  amni/o- *amnion*
		  -centesis *procedure to puncture*
		
		chromosome (KROH-moh-sohm)
		  chrom/o- *color*
		  -some *body*
		Chromosome: *Body (within the nucleus that takes on) color (when stained)*
		
		alpha fetoprotein (AL-fah FEE-toh-PROH-teen)
		
		lecithin (LES-ih-thin)
		
		sphingomyelin (SFING-goh-MY-eh-lin)

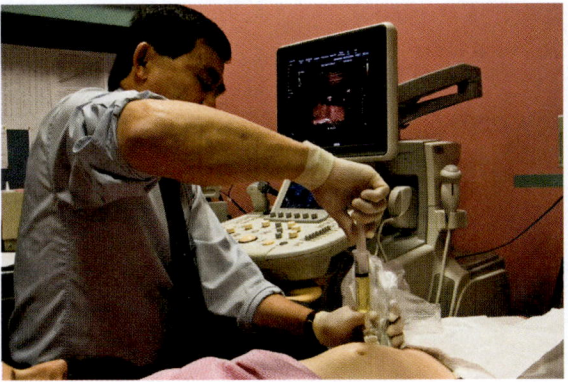

FIGURE 12-28 ■ Amniocentesis.
The obstetrician is withdrawing amniotic fluid through a needle inserted into the intrauterine cavity. The ultrasound machine produced sound waves and an ultrasound transducer (the plastic-covered instrument in his left hand) was used to bounce the sound waves off the uterus and create an image on the computer screen. The sound waves generated by the ultrasound machine do not injure the developing fetus, and the image helps the obstetrician locate a pocket of amniotic fluid.

chorionic villus sampling (CVS)	Genetic test of the chorionic villi of the placenta. A needle is inserted through the pregnant woman's abdomen or a catheter is inserted through the cervix to aspirate some of the chorionic villi from the placenta. This test is performed when a fetal genetic defect is suspected. It can be performed at 12 weeks, which is earlier than an amniocentesis.	**chorionic** (KOR-ee-AW-nik)
		  chorion/o- *chorion*
		  -ic *pertaining to*
		
		villus (VIL-uhs)
		Latin plural noun: Change the singular ending *-us* to *-i*.

Word or Phrase	Description	Pronunciation/Word Parts
pregnancy test	Blood test to detect human chorionic gonadotropin (HCG) secreted by the fertilized ovum. Serum HCG is positive just 9 days after conception. Home pregnancy tests that detect HCG in the urine are easy to use but are not always accurate. Only a positive blood test (serum beta HCG) is diagnostic of pregnancy. The presence of HCG does not indicate that the pregnancy is normal because HCG is also produced when there is an ectopic pregnancy or a hydatidiform mole.	

Radiologic Procedures

hystero-salpingography	Procedure in which radiopaque contrast dye is injected through the cervix and into the uterus. It coats and outlines the uterus and uterine tubes and shows narrowing, scarring, and blockage. The x-ray image is a **hysterosalpingogram**. This test is done as part of an infertility workup.	**hysterosalpingography** (HIS-ter-oh-SAL-ping-GAW-grah-fee) **hyster/o-** *uterus; womb* **salping/o-** *uterine tube* **-graphy** *process of recording* **hysterosalpingogram** (HIS-ter-OH-sal-PING-goh-gram) **hyster/o-** *uterus; womb* **salping/o-** *uterine tube* **-gram** *picture; record*
mammography	Procedure that uses x-rays to create an image of the breast. The breast is compressed and slightly flattened (see Figure 12-29 ■). Mammography is used to detect areas of microcalcification, infection, cysts, and tumors, many of which cannot be felt on a breast examination. The x-ray image is a **mammogram**. Alternatives to mammography include the following. • **Xeromammography** uses a photon beam and a dry chemical developer. The image is a **xeromammogram**. • A **magnetic resonance image (MRI)** scan produces a clearer image than mammography in patients who have multiple cysts in the breasts.	**mammography** (mah-MAW-grah-fee) **mamm/o-** *breast* **-graphy** *process of recording* **mammogram** (MAM-oh-gram) **mamm/o-** *breast* **-gram** *picture; record* **xeromammography** (ZEER-oh-mah-MAW-grah-fee) **xer/o-** *dry* **mamm/o-** *breast* **-graphy** *process of recording* **xeromammogram** (ZEER-oh-MAM-oh-gram) **xer/o-** *dry* **mamm/o-** *breast* **-gram** *picture; record*

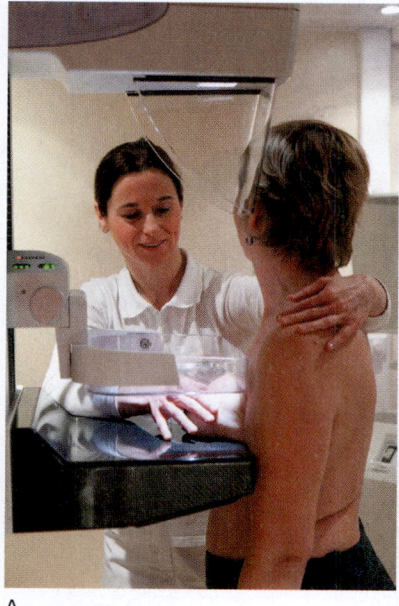

A.

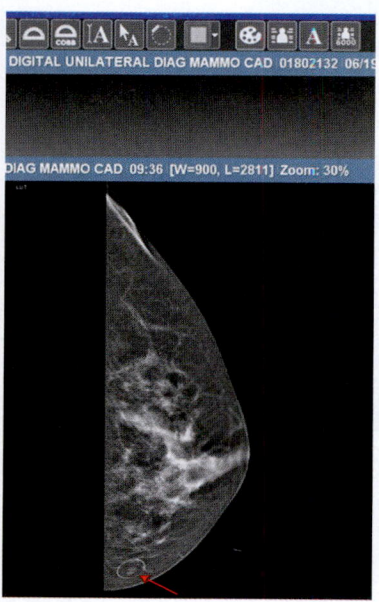

B.

FIGURE 12-29 ■ **Mammography.**
A. A radiologic technician positions the patient for mammography. The breast is compressed because, the less distance the x-ray travels, the sharper the image that is obtained. **B.** This mammogram shows dense, fibrous tissue and some cysts in the breast, but no evidence of cancer. An ultrasound was then performed to further examine the suspicious, circled area near the bottom of the mammogram image.

Word or Phrase	Description	Pronunciation/Word Parts

ultrasonography	Procedure that uses ultra high-frequency sound waves emitted by a transducer or probe to produce an image on a computer screen. Three-dimensional ultrasonography couples the ultrasound with a position sensor to generate a high-resolution image in three dimensions (see Figure 12-30 ■). The **ultrasound** image is a **sonogram**. Ultrasonography of the breast or uterus can differentiate between benign, fluid-filled cysts and solid tumors that need to be biopsied. A pelvic ultrasound can be used to diagnose a normal pregnancy versus a hydatidiform mole or ectopic pregnancy. In early pregnancy, the beating heart is seen. The image can show multiple fetuses and the sex of the fetus. An ultrasound is done routinely at 16–20 weeks in a normal pregnancy to estimate the gestational age. Serial ultrasounds can be done over time if there is a question of intrauterine growth retardation. The length of the femur of the fetus, its **biparietal diameter (BPD)** (distance between the two parietal bones of the cranium), and the crown-to-rump length are used to calculate the gestational age of the fetus. Ultrasound can show the position of the placenta to diagnose placenta previa. Pelvic ultrasound is used during amniocentesis to locate a large area of amniotic fluid in which to insert the needle. A **transvaginal ultrasound** uses an ultrasound probe inserted into the vagina to determine the thickness of the endometrium in patients with abnormal uterine bleeding.	**ultrasonography** (UL-trah-soh-NAW-grah-fee)
		  ultra- *beyond; higher*
		  son/o- *sound*
		  -graphy *process of recording*
		
		ultrasound (UL-trah-sound)
		
		sonogram (SAW-noh-gram)
		  son/o- *sound*
		  -gram *picture; record*
		
		biparietal (BY-pah-RY-eh-tal)
		  bi- *two*
		  pariet/o- *wall of a cavity*
		  -al *pertaining to*
		
		transvaginal (trans-VAJ-ih-nal)
		  trans- *across; through*
		  vagin/o- *vagina*
		  -al *pertaining to*

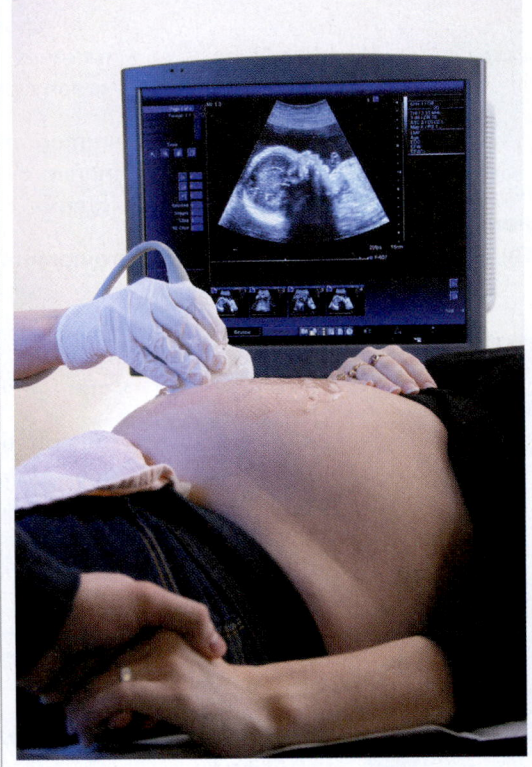

FIGURE 12-30 ■ Three-dimensional ultrasonography. Sound waves generated by a transducer pass through the abdominal wall of the pregnant female, bounce off the fetus, and are used to create a computer image. Details of the fetus are clearly visible in this type of ultrasound. Sound waves, rather than x-rays, are used so that the fetus is not exposed to any radiation.

12.4 PRACTICE LAPS

Use the Answer Key at the end of the book to check your answers.

A. Give the Meaning of Combining Forms

Next to each combining form, write its meaning. The first one has been done for you.

Combining Form	Meaning	Combining Form	Meaning
1. **pariet/o-**	*wall of a cavity*	10. mamm/o-	
2. amni/o-		11. ne/o-	
3. carcin/o-		12. plas/o-	
4. cervic/o-		13. recept/o-	
5. chrom/o-		14. salping/o-	
6. chorion/o-		15. son/o-	
7. cyt/o-		16. vagin/o-	
8. gene/o-		17. xer/o-	
9. hyster/o-			

B. Build Words

Read the definition of the medical word. Look at the combining form that is given. Select the correct suffix from the Suffix List, and write it on the blank line. Then build the medical word, and write it on the line. (Remember: You may need to remove the combining vowel. Always remove the hyphens and slash.) Be sure to check your spelling.

Suffix List

-centesis (procedure to puncture)   -ic (pertaining to)   -some (body)
-gram (picture; record)   -logy (study of)   -tic (pertaining to)
-graphy (process of recording)   -or (thing that does or produces)

Definition of the Medical Word	Combining Form	Suffix	Build the Medical Word
Example: Body (in the nucleus that takes on) color (when stained)	**chrom/o-**	*-some*	*chromosome*

[You think body (-some) + color (chrom/o-). You change the order of the word parts to put the suffix last. You write chromosome.]

Definition of the Medical Word	Combining Form	Suffix	Build the Medical Word
1. Process of recording (the) breast	mamm/o-		
2. Thing that does receive	recept/o-		
3. Procedure to puncture (the) amnion	amni/o-		
4. Pertaining to (the) chorion	chorion/o-		
5. (The) study of cell(s)	cyt/o-		
6. Picture (or) record (of) sound	son/o-		
7. Pertaining to gene(s)	gene/o-		
8. Picture (or) record (of the) breast	mamm/o-		

C. Define Abbreviations

1. AFP _____
2. ASC _____
3. BPD _____
4. BRCA _____
5. CIN _____
6. CIS _____
7. CVS _____
8. HSIL _____
9. L/S _____
10. LSIL _____
11. MRI _____
12. SCC _____

12.5 Medical Procedures, Drugs, and Surgical Procedures

Word or Phrase	Description	Pronunciation/Word Parts

Medical Procedures of the External and Internal Genitalia

Word or Phrase	Description	Pronunciation/Word Parts
colposcopy	Procedure that uses a magnifying, lighted scope to visually examine the vagina and cervix	**colposcopy** (kol-PAW-skoh-pee) **colp/o-** *vagina* **-scopy** *process of using an instrument to examine*
gynecologic examination	Procedure to physically examine the external and internal genitalia. This is performed with the patient supine in the **dorsal lithotomy position**. The hips and knees are flexed, and the feet are elevated in stirrups. The external genitalia are examined visually for any skin lesions, rashes, or discharge from the vagina. The internal genitalia are first examined using a **bimanual examination** (see Figure 12-31 ■). A mass, cystocele, rectocele, or any enlargement of the uterus can be palpated with the gloved hands. Tenderness to palpation can indicate infection or endometriosis. Then a vaginal **speculum** (see Figure 12-32 ■) is inserted into the vagina to visually examine the cervix for abnormalities, and a Pap test is performed.	**gynecologic** (GY-neh-koh-LAW-jik) **gynec/o-** *female; woman* **log/o-** *study of; word* **-ic** *pertaining to* **dorsal** (DOR-sal) **dors/o-** *back; dorsum* **-al** *pertaining to* **lithotomy** (lith-AW-toh-mee) **lith/o-** *stone* **-tomy** *process of cutting; process of making an incision* *Note*: This is the same body position that was used in the past to treat patients with kidney stones (**lith/o-**). **bimanual** (by-MAN-yoo-al) **bi-** *two* **manu/o-** *hand* **-al** *pertaining to* **speculum** (SPEH-kyoo-lum)

Word or Phrase	Description	Pronunciation/Word Parts

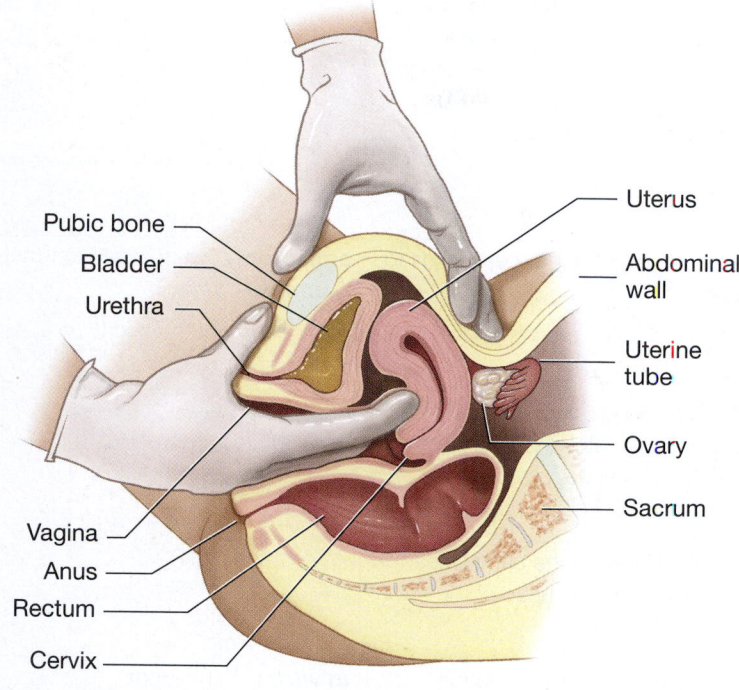

FIGURE 12-31 ■ Bimanual examination.
By using both hands, the gynecologist is able to examine the shape of the non-pregnant uterus and detect tenderness and masses.

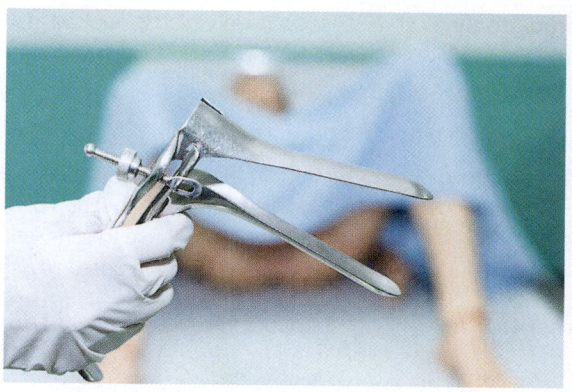

FIGURE 12-32 ■ Vaginal speculum.
A speculum (metal or plastic) has two blades that are closed together as the speculum is inserted into the vagina and then moved apart to separate the walls of the vagina so that the cervix can be seen.

Medical Procedures of the Breast

breast self-examination (BSE)	Procedure to systematically palpate all areas of the breast (starting with the nipple and moving outward in concentric circles to include under the arm) to detect lumps, masses, or enlarged lymph nodes (see Figure 12-33 ■). BSE should be done monthly to detect early signs of breast cancer.	

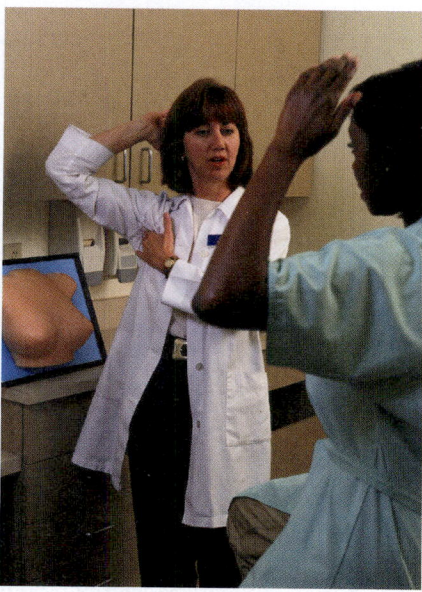

FIGURE 12-33 ■ Breast self-examination.
This nurse is instructing the patient on how to perform self-examination of the breasts to feel for masses or lumps. All areas of both breasts are palpated in a consistent way. The lymph nodes under the arms are also palpated for any sign of enlargement.

Word or Phrase	Description	Pronunciation/Word Parts
Tanner staging	System used to describe the development of the female breasts from childhood through puberty. There are five different stages, from Tanner stage 1 (nipple and areola are flat against the chest wall) to Tanner stage 5 (enlargement of the entire breast). The Tanner system is also used to describe the development of the female external genitalia.	

Medical Procedures for Obstetrics

amniotomy	Procedure in which a hooked instrument is inserted into the cervical os to rupture the amniotic sac and induce labor	**amniotomy** (AM-nee-AW-toh-mee) **amni/o-** *amnion* **-tomy** *process of cutting;* *process of making an incision*
Apgar score	Procedure that assigns a score to a newborn at 1 and 5 minutes after birth. Points (0–2) are given for each of the following: heart rate, respiratory rate, muscle tone, response to stimulation, and skin color, for a total possible score of 10. Normally, one point is always taken off because of acrocyanosis.	**Apgar** (AP-gar)
assisted delivery	Procedure in which a vacuum extractor (cup applied to the baby's head) is used to exert gentle suction to facilitate delivery of the head of the newborn during a vaginal delivery	

assisted reproductive technology (ART)	Procedures that use technology to assist the process of conception. When the man's sperm count is low or the woman's cervical mucus contains antibodies against spermatozoa, the man's semen is collected, concentrated, and inserted into the uterus, a procedure known as **intrauterine insemination**. In men with a very low sperm count, sperm can be taken directly from the testis or epididymis. Then, under a microscope, a micropipette is used to inject a single sperm into the cytoplasm of one ovum, a procedure known as **intracytoplasmic sperm injection (ICSI)** (see Figure 12-34 ■).
	When the man's sperm count is normal, the following ART procedures can be performed.
	
	• **In vitro fertilization (IVF)**. The woman receives ovulation-stimulating drugs. Then mature ova are harvested with a needle inserted into the ovary. Some of the ova are combined with spermatozoa and allowed to grow from 2 to 5 days in a culture medium. Then one fertilized ovum (or more) is inserted into the uterus. A newborn conceived by IVF was previously known as a "test tube baby."
	• **Zygote intrafallopian transfer (ZIFT)**. The same procedure is followed but the fertilized ovum (zygote) is inserted into the uterine tube.
	• **Gamete intrafallopian transfer (GIFT)**. The ova and spermatozoa (gametes) are collected, and both are immediately inserted into the uterine (fallopian) tube.
		in vitro (IN VEE-troh)
		
		intrafallopian
		(IN-trah-fah-LOH-pee-an)
		  intra- *within*
		  fallopi/o- *uterine tube*
		  -an *pertaining to*
		
		insemination
		(in-SEM-ih-NAY-shun)
		  in- *in; not; within*
		  semin/o- *sperm; spermatozoa*
		  -ation *being; having; process*
		
		intracytoplasmic
		(IN-trah-SY-toh-PLAS-mik)
		  intra- *within*
		  cyt/o- *cell*
		  plasm/o- *plasma*
		  -ic *pertaining to*
		
		injection (in-JEK-shun)
		  inject/o- *insert; put in*
		  -ion *action; condition*

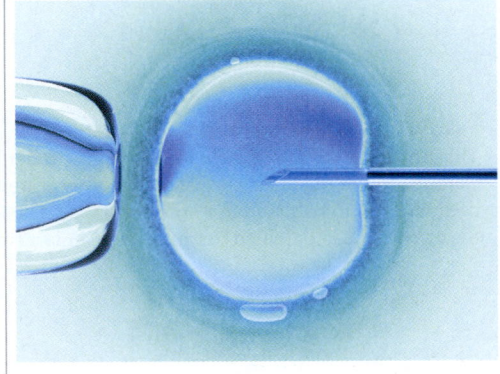

FIGURE 12-34 ■ Intracytoplasmic sperm injection (ICSI).
A type of assisted reproductive technology. Under a microscope, a micropipette (on the right) is used to penetrate the cytoplasm of an ovum and insert a single spermatozoon to fertilize it. A glass rod on the left holds the ovum in place during this procedure.

Word or Phrase	Description	Pronunciation/Word Parts
epidural anesthesia	Procedure to produce local anesthesia by injecting an anesthetic drug into the epidural space between vertebrae in the woman's lower back. This blocks pain and sensation in the abdomen, perineum, and legs during labor and delivery. Epidural anesthesia is not given until the cervix is more than 4 cm dilated; otherwise, it can prolong labor.	**epidural** (EP-ih-DOOR-al) **epi-** *above; upon* **dur/o-** *dura mater* **-al** *pertaining to* **anesthesia** (AN-es-THEE-zhah) **an-** *not; without* **esthes/o-** *feeling; sensation* **-ia** *condition; state; thing*
fundal height	Procedure to measure the height of the uterine fundus during each prenatal visit. The fundus of the uterus moves superiorly as pregnancy progresses. The distance in centimeters from the top of the woman's symphysis pubis (anterior pubic bone) to the top of the uterine fundus is measured in centimeters to provide a general indication of fetal growth.	**fundal** (FUN-dal) **fund/o-** *fundus; part farthest from the opening* **-al** *pertaining to*
induction of labor	Procedure that uses an oxytocin drug to induce (cause) labor to begin. This is done when the woman is past her estimated due date or when the health of the woman or fetus necessitates delivery.	**induction** (in-DUK-shun) **induct/o-** *leading in* **-ion** *action; condition*
Nägele rule	Procedure used to calculate the **estimated date of birth (EDB)**, also known as the **estimated date of delivery (EDD)** or "due date." This is done by adding 9 months and 7 days to the date of the first day of the woman's **last menstrual period (LMP)**. Often the patient does not remember the first day of her last menstrual period, and so the EDB is just an approximate date. **Estimated date of confinement (EDC)** is an older phrase that indicated when a woman was to be confined to her home around her due date.	**Nägele** (NAY-gul)
nonstress test (NST)	Procedure that uses an external monitor on the woman's abdomen to display and monitor the **fetal heart rate (FHR)**. A normal test (reactive test) will show at least two increases in the fetal heart rate associated with fetal movement as felt by the woman. A nonreactive test, which is abnormal, is followed up by performing a **biophysical profile (BPP)** that combines a nonstress test with ultrasonography that shows fetal movement, fetal heart rate, and the amniotic fluid volume.	**biophysical** (BY-oh-FIZ-ih-kal) **bi/o-** *living organism; living tissue* **physic/o-** *body* **-al** *pertaining to*
obstetrical history	Procedure to document past pregnancies and deliveries, which is a standard of good prenatal care. A **nulligravida** is a woman who has never been pregnant and is not pregnant now. A **primigravida** is a woman who is pregnant for the first time. She is primiparous ("primip" for short). A **multigravida** is a woman who has been pregnant more than once. If she has given birth many times, she is said to be **multiparous**. In the past, the obstetrical history was documented as **gravida (G)** (the number of pregnancies), **para (P)** (the number of deliveries), and **abortion (Ab)** (the number of abortions). The **G/TPAL system** provides even more details. **G**ravida: Number of times pregnant **T**erm: Number of term births **P**remature: Number of premature births **A**bortions: Number of abortions (spontaneous or therapeutic) **L**iving: Number of living children	**nulligravida** (NUL-ih-GRAV-ih-dah) **null/i-** *none* **-gravida** *pregnancy* **primigravida** (PREE-mih-GRAV-ih-dah) **prim/i-** *first* **-gravida** *pregnancy* **multigravida** (MUL-tih-GRAV-ih-dah) **mult/i-** *many* **-gravida** *pregnancy* **multiparous** (mul-TIH-pah-ruhs) **mult/i-** *many* **par/o-** *giving birth* **-ous** *pertaining to* **gravida** (GRAV-ih-dah) **para** (PAIR-ah)

Word or Phrase	Description	Pronunciation/Word Parts
version	Procedure to manually correct a breech or other malpresentation of the fetus prior to delivery. The obstetrician puts his or her hands on the woman's abdominal wall and manipulates the uterus until the fetus is in a cephalic presentation.	**version** (VER-zhun) **vers/o-** *travel; turn* **-ion** *action; condition*

Category	Indication	Pronunciation/Word Parts

Drugs

Category	Indication	Pronunciation/Word Parts
antiyeast drug	Applied topically to treat *Candida albicans* infection of the vagina	**antiyeast** (AN-tee-YEEST)
drug for amenorrhea and abnormal uterine bleeding	Corrects the lack of hormones	
drug for contraception to prevent pregnancy	Suppresses the release of FSH and LH from the anterior pituitary gland. Other drugs kill sperm or keep them from reaching the uterus.	**contraception** (CON-trah-SEP-shun) *Contraception* is a combination of the prefix **contra-** that means *against* and a shortened form of the word *conception*.
drug for endometriosis	Suppresses the menstrual cycle for several months and causes endometrial implants in the pelvic cavity to atrophy	
drug used to dilate the cervix	Applied topically to the cervix to cause dilation and effacement	
drug used to induce labor	Stimulates the uterus and increases the strength and frequency of contractions of the smooth muscle of the uterine wall	
hormone replacement therapy (HRT) drug	Treats the symptoms and consequences of menopause (hot flashes, vaginal dryness, osteoporosis) caused by a decreased level of estradiol.	**estrogen** (ES-troh-jen) **estr/o-** *female* **-gen** *that which produces* Estrogen is the drug form of the female hormone estradiol.

Clinical Connections

Pharmacology. The long-term use of the drug estrogen has been associated with an increased risk of breast cancer, endometrial cancer, and thrombophlebitis. Instead, **bioidentical hormone** creams (estradiol, progesterone, testosterone) can be prescribed; these are applied topically.

The combining form **bi/o-** means *living organism; living tissue.*

Category	Indication	Pronunciation/Word Parts
nonsteroidal anti-inflammatory drug (NSAID)	Treats the pain associated with dysmenorrhea	**nonsteroidal** (NON-steh-ROY-dal)
ovulation-stimulating drug	Stimulates the anterior pituitary gland to secrete FSH and LH to stimulate ovulation and treat infertility. These drugs cause several mature ova to be released at the same time for *in vitro* fertilization.	

Category	Indication	Pronunciation/Word Parts
tocolytic drug	Suppresses uterine contractions to prevent premature labor and delivery	**tocolytic** (TOH-koh-LIH-tik) **toc/o-** *childbirth; labor* **lyt/o-** *break down; destroy* **-ic** *pertaining to*

Word or Phrase	Description	Pronunciation/Word Parts

Surgical Procedures of the Uterus, Uterine Tubes, and Ovaries

Word or Phrase	Description	Pronunciation/Word Parts
biopsy (Bx)	Procedure used to diagnose abnormal uterine bleeding and uterine cancer. An endometrial biopsy uses a speculum to visualize the cervix and a dilator to expand the cervical os. A pipette or catheter is inserted into the uterus and rotated while suction pulls in tissue. For larger biopsy specimens, an abdominal surgical procedure is performed.	**biopsy** (BY-awp-see) **bi/o-** *living organism; living tissue* **-opsy** *process of viewing*
cryosurgery	Procedure to destroy small areas of abnormal tissue on the cervix. Colposcopy is used to visualize the cervical lesions. Then a **cryoprobe** containing extremely cold liquid nitrogen is touched to the areas to freeze and destroy the abnormal tissues.	**cryosurgery** (KRY-oh-SER-jer-ee) **cry/o-** *cold* **surg/o-** *operative procedure* **-ery** *process* **cryoprobe** (KRY-oh-prohb) **cry/o-** *cold* **-probe** *rod-ike instrument*
dilation and curettage (D&C)	Procedure to remove abnormal tissue from inside the uterus for the purpose of treating abnormal uterine bleeding, diagnosing uterine cancer, performing a therapeutic abortion, or removing the products of conception following a spontaneous but incomplete abortion. The cervix is dilated with progressively larger dilators inserted into the cervical os. A **tenaculum** (long, scissors-like instrument with two curved, pointed ends) is used to grasp and hold the cervix. Then a **curet** (instrument with a sharp-edged circular or oval ring at one end) is inserted to scrape the endometrium. Alternatively, a vacuum aspirator is inserted to suction out pieces of endometrium.	**dilation** (dy-LAY-shun) **dilat/o-** *dilate; widen* **-ion** *action; condition* **curettage** (KYOOR-eh-TAWZH) **tenaculum** (teh-NAH-kyoo-lum) **curet** (kyoor-ET)
endometrial ablation	Procedure that uses heat or cold to destroy the endometrium to treat abnormal uterine bleeding. A laser, hot fluid in a balloon, or an electrode with electrical current is inserted into the uterus. Alternatively, a cryoprobe is inserted to freeze the endometrium.	**ablation** (ah-BLAY-shun) **ablat/o-** *destroy; take away* **-ion** *action; condition*
hysterectomy	Procedure to remove the uterus because of uterine fibroids, endometriosis, uterine prolapse, abnormal uterine bleeding, or uterine or cervical cancer. An abdominal hysterectomy is performed with a laparoscope through an abdominal incision. A **total vaginal hysterectomy (TVH)** is performed through the vagina. A total hysterectomy involves removing both the uterus and cervix. **TAH-BSO** is a total abdominal hysterectomy and bilateral salpingo-oophorectomy (removal of both uterine tubes and ovaries). A **radical hysterectomy** to treat cancer of the uterus involves removal of the uterus, cervix, upper vagina, and pelvic lymph nodes.	**hysterectomy** (HIS-ter-EK-toh-mee) **hyster/o-** *uterus; womb* **-ectomy** *surgical removal* **radical** (RAD-ih-kal) **radic/o-** *root and all parts* **-al** *pertaining to*

Word or Phrase	Description	Pronunciation/Word Parts
laparoscopy	Procedure to visualize the abdominopelvic cavity, uterus, uterine tubes, and ovaries. **Laparoscopic** surgery begins with a small incision near the umbilicus, and carbon dioxide gas is used to inflate the abdominal cavity. Then a **laparoscope**, which is a fiberoptic **endoscope**, is inserted through the incision (see Figure 12-35 ■). Grasping and cutting instruments are inserted through other abdominal incisions. Pelvic adhesions, pelvic inflammatory disease, and endometriosis can be treated, a biopsy taken, or a hysterectomy performed laparoscopically.	**laparoscopy** (LAP-ar-AW-skoh-pee) **lapar/o-** *abdomen* **-scopy** *process of using an instrument to examine* **laparoscopic** (LAP-ar-oh-SKAW-pik) **lapar/o-** *abdomen* **scop/o-** *examine with an instrument* **-ic** *pertaining to* **laparoscope** (LAP-ar-oh-SKOHP) **lapar/o-** *abdomen* **-scope** *instrument used to examine* **endoscope** (EN-doh-skohp) **end/o-** *innermost; within* **-scope** *instrument used to examine*

Scope — Video connection

Instrument sleeve

A.

B.

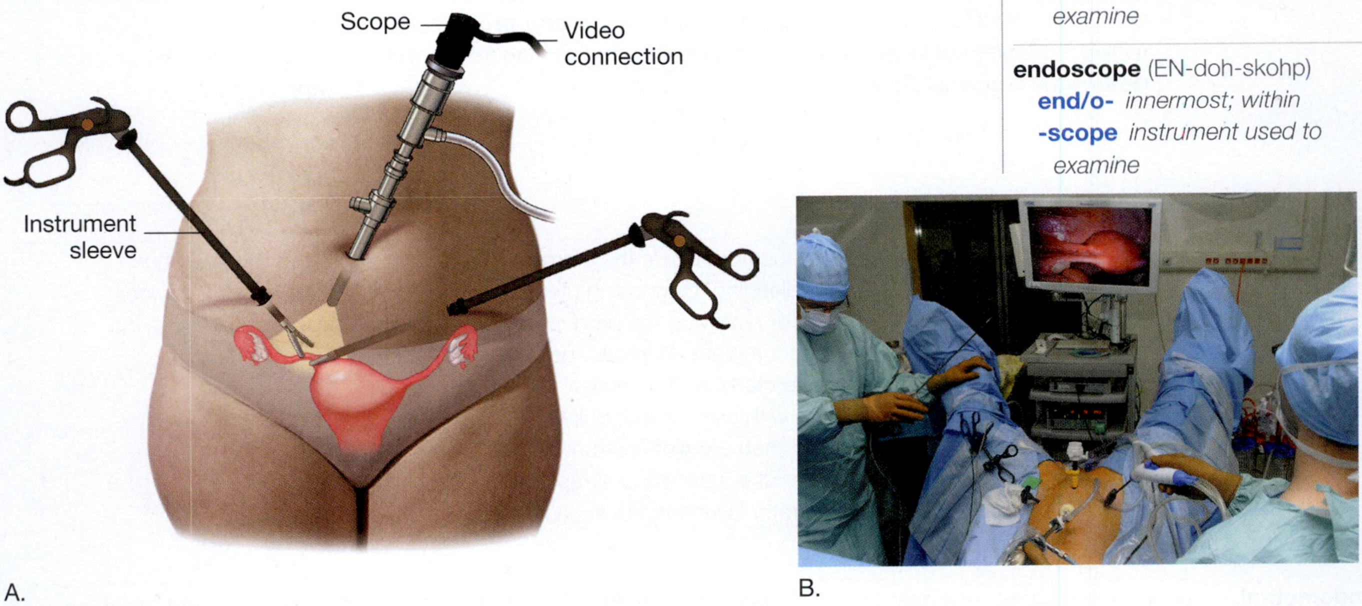

FIGURE 12-35 ■ Laparoscopic surgery.
A. Small incisions in the abdomen allow visualization of the uterus, uterine tubes, and ovaries with a lighted scope. **B.** This patient is having a hysterectomy. The image from the laparoscope can be seen on the computer screen in the operating room. The surgeon watches the image on the screen as he manipulates the grasping and cutting instruments that are within the patient's abdominal cavity.

myomectomy	Procedure to remove leiomyomata (uterine fibroids) from the uterus. This procedure can be done vaginally or through a laparoscope inserted into the abdominal cavity. The removal of large fibroids requires a hysterectomy.	**myomectomy** (MY-oh-MEK-toh-mee) **my/o-** *muscle* **om/o-** *mass; tumor* **-ectomy** *surgical removal*
oophorectomy	Procedure to remove an ovary because of large ovarian cysts or ovarian cancer. A **bilateral oophorectomy** removes both ovaries.	**oophorectomy** (OH-oh-for-EK-toh-mee) **oophor/o-** *ovary* **-ectomy** *surgical removal* **bilateral** (by-LAT-er-al) **bi-** *two* **later/o-** *side* **-al** *pertaining to*

Word or Phrase	Description	Pronunciation/Word Parts
salpingectomy	Procedure to remove the uterine tube because of ovarian cancer or an ectopic pregnancy in the tube. A bilateral salpingectomy removes both uterine tubes. A **bilateral salpingo-oophorectomy (BSO)** removes both uterine tubes and both ovaries.	**salpingectomy** (SAL-pin-JEK-toh-mee) **salping/o-** *uterine tube* **-ectomy** *surgical removal* **salpingo-oophorectomy** (sal-PING-goh-OH-oh-for-EK-toh-mee) **salping/o-** *uterine tube* **oophor/o-** *ovary* **-ectomy** *surgical removal*
therapeutic abortion (TAB)	Procedure for planned termination of a pregnancy at any time during gestation. It is performed because the fetus is abnormal or because the pregnancy is unwanted. All products of conception are removed from the uterus with suction. Also known as an **elective abortion**.	**therapeutic** (THAIR-ah-PYOO-tik) **therapeut/o-** *therapy; treatment* **-ic** *pertaining to* **abortion** (ah-BOR-shun) **abort/o-** *stop prematurely* **-ion** *action; condition* **elective** (ee-LEK-tiv)
tubal ligation	Procedure to prevent pregnancy. A short segment of each uterine tube is removed. The cut ends are sutured and then crushed or cauterized. The woman continues to ovulate, but the ovum released from the ovary cannot travel to the uterus and sperm deposited in the vagina cannot reach the ovum. Also known as "getting your tubes tied." A **tubal anastomosis** is a procedure to rejoin the uterine tube segments so that the woman can again become pregnant.	**tubal** (TOO-bal) **tub/o-** *tube* **-al** *pertaining to* **ligation** (ly-GAY-shun) **ligat/o-** *bind; tie up* **-ion** *action; condition* **anastomosis** (ah-NAS-toh-MOH-sihs) **anastom/o-** *create an opening between two structures* **-osis** *abnormal condition; process*
uterine artery embolization	Procedure used to treat uterine fibroids. A catheter is inserted into the femoral artery in the groin and threaded to the uterine artery. Radiopaque contrast dye is injected to identify the arteriole that supplies blood to a large fibroid. Tiny particles are injected to block the arteriole. Without a blood supply, the fibroid shrinks in size.	**embolization** (EM-bol-ih-ZAY-shun) **embol/o-** *embolus; occluding plug* **-ization** *process of creating; process of inserting; process of making*
uterine suspension	Procedure to suspend and fix the uterus in an anatomically correct position. It is used to correct a retroverted uterus or uterine prolapse. The ligaments that support the uterus are shortened, which pulls the uterus up into a normal position, or surgical mesh (sling) or surgical tape are used to reposition the uterus. Also known as a **hysteropexy**.	**suspension** (sus-PEN-shun) **suspens/o-** *hanging* **-ion** *action; condition* **hysteropexy** (HIS-ter-oh-PEK-see) **hyster/o-** *uterus; womb* **-pexy** *process of fixing in place*

Word or Phrase	Description	Pronunciation/Word Parts

Surgical Procedures of the Cervix and Vagina

Word or Phrase	Description	Pronunciation/Word Parts
colporrhaphy	Procedure to suture a weakness in the vaginal wall. This procedure is done to correct a cystocele or a rectocele that is bulging into the vaginal canal.	**colporrhaphy** (kol-POR-ah-fee) **colp/o-** *vagina* **-rrhaphy** *procedure of suturing*
conization	Procedure to remove a large, cone-shaped section of tissue that includes the cervical os and part of the cervical canal. It is used to excise an abnormal area identified by a Pap test. A laser knife or a **loop electrosurgical excision procedure (LEEP)** with a hot wire loop is used to burn and cut away the tissue. Alternately, a scalpel (cold knife conization) can be used so that no cells are damaged by heat.	**conization** (KOH-nih-ZAY-shun) **con/o-** *cone* **-ization** *process of creating; process of inserting; process of making*
culdoscopy	Procedure that begins in the vagina and cul-de-sac but whose ultimate purpose is to examine the abdominopelvic cavity and the external surfaces of the uterus, uterine tubes, and ovaries for signs of endometriosis or adhesions. An endoscope is inserted into the vagina and then pushed through the posterior wall of the vagina (into the area of the cul-de-sac behind the cervix) (see Figure 12-2) and then into the abdominopelvic cavity. This procedure is performed under local anesthesia and leaves no abdominal scars.	**culdoscopy** (kul-DAW-skoh-pee) **culd/o-** *cul-de-sac* **-scopy** *process of using an instrument to examine*

Surgical Procedures of the Breast

Word or Phrase	Description	Pronunciation/Word Parts
biopsy (Bx)	Procedure to remove a small piece of tissue for examination under a microscope to look for abnormal or cancerous cells. A breast biopsy can be done by **fine-needle aspiration** (a very fine needle is inserted into the mass and a syringe is used to aspirate tissue) or by **vacuum-assisted biopsy** (a probe with a cutting device is inserted through the skin and rotated to suck in multiple specimens). First, mammography or ultrasound is used to identify the location of the mass, and a needle or wire marker is inserted to pinpoint the site. A **stereotactic biopsy** uses three different angles of mammography to precisely locate the mass that is to be biopsied. For an **incisional biopsy**, an incision is made in the skin overlying the mass and a large part (but not all) of the mass is removed. For an **excisional biopsy**, the entire mass is removed along with a surrounding margin of normal tissue.	**biopsy** (BY-awp-see) **bi/o-** *living organism; living tissue* **-opsy** *process of viewing* **aspiration** (AS-pih-RAY-shun) **aspir/o-** *breathe in; suck in* **-ation** *being; having; process* **stereotactic** (STAIR-ee-oh-TAK-tik) **stere/o-** *three dimensions* **tact/o-** *touch* **-ic** *pertaining to* **incisional** (in-SIH-zhun-al) **in-** *in; not; within* **cis/o-** *cut* **-ion** *action; condition* **-al** *pertaining to* **excisional** (ek-SIH-zhun-al) **ex-** *away from; out* **cis/o-** *cut* **-ion** *action; condition* **-al** *pertaining to*
lumpectomy	Procedure to excise a small malignant tumor of the breast. Adjacent normal breast tissue and the axillary lymph nodes are also removed in case any cancerous cells have already spread to them. The rest of the breast is left intact.	**lumpectomy** (lum-PEK-toh-mee)

Word or Phrase	Description	Pronunciation/Word Parts

mammaplasty	Procedure to change the size, shape, or position of the breast. Also known as a **mammoplasty**. An **augmentation mammaplasty** augments (enlarges) the size of a small breast by inserting a breast **prosthesis** (implant) under the skin or chest muscles (see Figure 12-36 ■). A **reduction mammaplasty** reduces the size of a large, **pendulous** breast. The procedure can be performed in conjunction with a **mastopexy** (breast lift) to reposition a sagging breast. A **reconstructive mammaplasty** is done to reconstruct a breast after a mastectomy.
	
	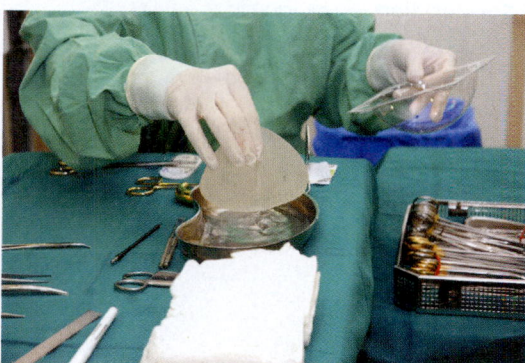
	
	FIGURE 12-36 ■ **Breast implant.**
	A breast prosthesis or implant is a soft-walled container filled with silicone gel or saline (salt water). It is placed beneath the skin of the breast or beneath the pectoralis major muscle of the chest during augmentation mammaplasty or reconstructive breast surgery.
		mammaplasty
		(MAM-ah-PLAS-tee)
		  mamm/a- *breast*
		  -plasty *process of reshaping by surgery*
		
		mammoplasty
		(MAM-oh-PLAS-tee)
		  mamm/o- *breast*
		  -plasty *process of reshaping by surgery*
		
		augmentation
		(AWG-men-TAY-shun)
		  augment/o- *increase in degree or size*
		  -ation *being; having; process*
		
		prosthesis (praws-THEE-sihs)
		
		reduction (ree-DUK-shun)
		  reduct/o- *bring back; decrease*
		  -ion *action; condition*
		
		pendulous (PEN-dyoo-luhs)
		  pendul/o- *hanging down*
		  -ous *pertaining to*
		
		mastopexy (MAS-toh-PEK-see)
		  mast/o- *breast; mastoid process*
		  -pexy *process of fixing in place*
		
		reconstructive
		(REE-con-STRUK-tiv)
		  re- *again and again; backward; unable to*
		  construct/o- *build*
		  -ive *pertaining to*

mastectomy	Procedure to surgically remove part or all of the breast to excise a malignant tumor. In a **simple** or **total mastectomy**, the entire breast, the overlying skin, and the nipple are removed, but not the chest muscle or axillary (underarm) lymph nodes. In a **modified radical mastectomy**, an **axillary node dissection** is also performed and some of the axillary lymph nodes are removed. In a **radical mastectomy**, the pectoralis major and minor muscles of the chest wall are also removed; this procedure is performed infrequently. A **prophylactic mastectomy** can be performed to prevent breast cancer from occurring in a woman who has a strong family history of breast cancer or has the *BRCA1* or *BRCA2* gene mutation. A mastectomy is often followed by a mammaplasty to reconstruct the breast or reconstructive breast surgery.	**mastectomy** (mas-TEK-toh-mee)
		  mast/o- *breast; mastoid process*
		  -ectomy *surgical removal*
		
		radical (RAD-ih-kal)
		  radic/o- *root and all parts*
		  -al *pertaining to*
		
		dissection (dih-SEK-shun)
		  dissect/o- *cut apart*
		  -ion *action; condition*
		
		prophylactic (PROH-fih-LAK-tik)
		  pro- *before*
		  phylact/o- *guarding; protecting*
		  -ic *pertaining to*

Word or Phrase	Description	Pronunciation/Word Parts
reconstructive breast surgery	Procedure to rebuild a breast after a mastectomy. This can be done at the same time as the mastectomy or as a later operative procedure. Also known as a reconstructive mammaplasty. During the mastectomy, a silicone or saline-filled breast implant prosthesis is inserted under the skin to recreate the fullness of the breast. After surgery, a tattoo can be done on the skin to mimic the pigmented area of the areola. Alternately, the woman's own tissue can be used to recreate the fullness of the breast by using a DIEP flap or a TRAM flap. • **DIEP (deep inferior epigastric perforator) flap**. An incision is made in the lower abdomen, and the skin and fat are excised as a flap. The blood vessels in the flap are reattached to blood vessels in the chest wall. • **TRAM (transverse rectus abdominis muscle) flap** (see Figure 12-37 ■). A transverse incision is made around an area in the abdomen. Skin, fat, and muscle are excised, except for one end that is left attached to the blood vessels there (pedicle graft); the other end is sutured to the area of the mastectomy. 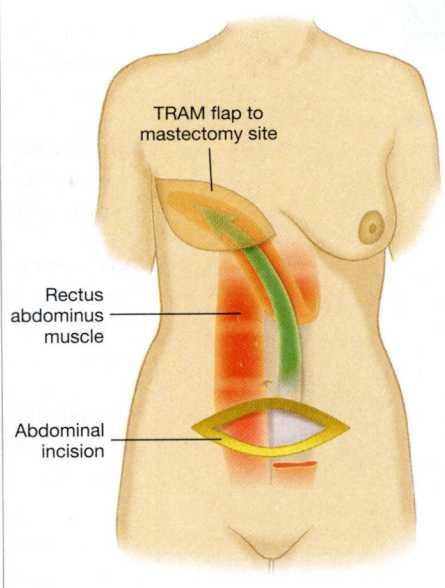 Rectus abdominus muscle Abdominal incision TRAM flap to mastectomy site **FIGURE 12-37 ■ TRAM flap reconstruction.** This older technique of breast reconstructive surgery uses a skin, fat, and muscle flap from the abdomen to reconstruct the breast following a mastectomy. This provides a natural feel to the reconstructed breast and takes the place of a synthetic breast implant.	**reconstructive** (REE-con-STRUK-tiv) **re-** *again and again; backward; unable to* **construct/o-** *build* **-ive** *pertaining to* Reconstructive: *Pertaining to again build(ing the breast)* **transverse** (trans-VERS) The prefix **trans-** means *across; through,* and the suffix **-verse** means *travel; turn.*

Surgical Procedures for Obstetrics

cerclage	Procedure to place a purse-string suture around the cervix to prevent it from dilating prematurely. The suture is removed prior to delivery.	**cerclage** (sir-CLAWJ)
cesarean section	Procedure to deliver a fetus. It is done because of cephalopelvic disproportion, failure to progress during labor, the mother being past the due date, or medical problems in the mother or fetus. The fetus is delivered through an incision in the abdominal wall and uterus. Also known as a *C-section*. A woman can still have a **vaginal birth after cesarean section (VBAC)**.	**cesarean** (seh-SAIR-ee-an)
episiotomy	Procedure that makes an incision in the posterior edge of the vagina and into the perineum to prevent a spontaneous tear of those tissues during delivery of the baby's head. Spontaneous vaginal tears can have ragged tissue edges that are difficult to suture and can extend into the rectum, causing incontinence.	**episiotomy** (eh-PIZ-ee-AW-toh-mee) **episi/o-** *vulva* **-tomy** *process of cutting; process of making an incision*

12.5 PRACTICE LAPS

Use the Answer Key at the end of the book to check your answers.

A. Give the Meaning of Combining Forms

Next to each combining form, write its meaning. The first one has been done for you.

Combining Form	Meaning	Combining Form	Meaning
1. **reduct/o-**	*bring back; decrease*	28. induct/o-	
2. ablat/o-		29. inject/o-	
3. abort/o-		30. insemin/o-	
4. amni/o-		31. lapar/o-	
5. anastom/o-		32. later/o-	
6. aspir/o-		33. ligat/o-	
7. augment/o-		34. lith/o-	
8. bi/o-		35. log/o-	
9. cis/o-		36. lyt/o-	
10. colp/o-		37. mamm/a-	
11. construct/o-		38. mamm/o-	
12. con/o-		39. manu/o-	
13. cry/o-		40. mast/o-	
14. culd/o-		41. mult/i-	
15. cyt/o-		42. my/o-	
16. dilat/o-		43. null/i-	
17. dissect/o-		44. om/o-	
18. dors/o-		45. oophor/o-	
19. embol/o-		46. par/o-	
20. end/o-		47. pendul/o-	
21. episi/o-		48. phylact/o-	
22. esthes/o-		49. physic/o-	
23. estr/o-		50. plasm/o-	
24. fallopi/o-		51. prim/i-	
25. fund/o-		52. radic/o-	
26. gynec/o-		53. salping/o-	
27. hyster/o-		54. scop/o-	

continued on next page

Combining Form	Meaning	Combining Form	Meaning
55. stere/o-	_____	59. therapeut/o-	_____
56. surg/o-	_____	60. toc/o-	_____
57. suspens/o-	_____	61. tub/o-	_____
58. tact/o-	_____	62. vers/o-	_____

B. Build Words

Read the definition of the medical word. Look at the combining form that is given. Select the correct suffix from the Suffix List, and write it on the blank line. Then build the medical word, and write it on the line. (Remember: You may need to remove the combining vowel. Always remove the hyphens and slash.) Be sure to check your spelling.

Suffix List

-ation (being; having; process)
-ectomy (surgical removal)
-gen (that which produces)
-gravida (pregnancy)
-ic (pertaining to)
-ion (action; condition)

-ization (process of inserting)
-opsy (process of viewing)
-osis (abnormal condition; process)
-pexy (process of fixing in place)
-plasty (process of reshaping by surgery)
-rrhaphy (procedure of suturing)

-scope (instrument used to examine)
-scopy (process of using an instrument to examine)
-tomy (process of cutting; process of making an incision)

Definition of the Medical Word	Combining Form	Suffix	Build the Medical Word
Example: Action (to) destroy or take away (tissue)	**ablat/o-**	*-ion*	*ablation*

[*You think* action (*-ion*) + take away (or) destroy (*ablat/o-*). You change the order of the word parts to put the suffix last. You write ablation.]

1. Process of cutting (the) amnion	amni/o-	_____	_____
2. Process of viewing living tissue	bi/o-	_____	_____
3. Process (to) create an opening between two structures	anastom/o-	_____	_____
4. Instrument used to examine within	end/o-	_____	_____
5. That (a drug) which produces female (characteristics)	estr/o-	_____	_____
6. Pregnancy (that is one of) many	mult/i-	_____	_____
7. Surgical removal (of the) uterine tube	salping/o-	_____	_____
8. Pertaining to therapy (or) treatment	therapeut/o-	_____	_____
9. Process of using an instrument to examine (the) abdomen	lapar/o-	_____	_____
10. Action (to) bind (or) tie up	ligat/o-	_____	_____
11. Surgical removal (of the) ovary	oophor/o-	_____	_____
12. Pregnancy none	null/i-	_____	_____

Definition of the Medical Word	Combining Form	Suffix	Build the Medical Word
13. Process of using an instrument to examine (the) vagina	colp/o-	_____	_____
14. Surgical removal (of the) uterus	hyster/o-	_____	_____
15. Procedure of suturing (the) vagina	colp/o-	_____	_____
16. Process of inserting (an) occluding plug	embol/o-	_____	_____
17. Process of making an incision (in the) vulva	episi/o-	_____	_____
18. Process of fixing in place (the) uterus	hyster/o-	_____	_____
19. Process of using an instrument to examine (the) cul-de-sac	culd/o-	_____	_____
20. Action (to) cut apart	dissect/o-	_____	_____
21. Process of reshaping by surgery (on the) breast	mamm/o-	_____	_____
22. Surgical removal (of the) breast	mast/o-	_____	_____
23. Process (to) increase in degree or size	augment/o-	_____	_____
24. Process of fixing in place (the) breast	mast/o-	_____	_____

C. Define Abbreviations

1. AB, Ab _____

2. ART _____

3. BPP _____

4. BSE _____

5. BSO _____

6. Bx _____

7. DIEP _____

8. D&C _____

9. EDB _____

10. EDC _____

11. EDD _____

12. G _____

13. GIFT _____

14. HRT _____

15. ICSI _____

16. IVF _____

17. LEEP _____

18. LMP _____

19. NSAID _____

20. P _____

21. TAB _____

22. TAH-BSO _____

23. TRAM _____

24. VBAC _____

25. ZIFT _____

Abbreviations Summary

AB, Ab	abortion		**IUGR**	intrauterine growth retardation
AFP	alpha fetoprotein		**IVF**	*in vitro* fertilization
AGA	appropriate for gestational age		**L&D**	labor and delivery
ART	assisted reproductive technology		**LEEP**	loop electrosurgical excision procedure
ASC	atypical squamous cells		**LGA**	large for gestational age
AUB	abnormal uterine bleeding		**LH**	luteinizing hormone
BPD	biparietal diameter (of the fetal head)		**LMP**	last menstrual period
BPP	biophysical profile		**L/S**	lecithin/sphingomyelin (ratio)
BRCA	breast cancer (gene)		**LSIL**	low-grade squamous intraepithelial lesion
BSE	breast self-examination		**MRI**	magnetic resonance imaging
BSO	bilateral salpingo-oophorectomy		**NB**	newborn
Bx	biopsy		**NICU**	neonatal intensive care unit (pronounced "NIK-yoo")
Ca	cancer; carcinoma (pronounced "c-a")		**NST**	nonstress test
CIN	cervical intraepithelial neoplasia		**NSAID**	nonsteroidal anti-inflammatory drug
CIS	carcinoma *in situ*		**OB**	obstetrics
CNM	certified nurse midwife		**OB/GYN**	obstetrics and gynecology
CPD	cephalopelvic disproportion		**P**	para
CVS	chorionic villus sampling		**Pap**	Papanicolaou (test or smear) (short form)
D&C	dilation and curettage		**PID**	pelvic inflammatory disease
DIEP	deep inferior epigastric perforator (flap)		**PMDD**	premenstrual dysphoric disorder
DUB	dysfunctional uterine bleeding		**PMS**	premenstrual syndrome
EDB	estimated date of birth		**PR$^+$**	progesterone receptor positive
EDC	estimated date of confinement		**PROM**	premature rupture of membranes
EDD	estimated date of delivery		**ROM**	rupture of membranes
ER$^+$	estrogen receptor positive		**SAB**	spontaneous abortion
FHR	fetal heart rate		**SCC**	squamous cell carcinoma
FSH	follicle-stimulating hormone		**SGA**	small for gestational age
G	gravida		**TAB**	therapeutic abortion
GIFT	gamete intrafallopian transfer		**TAH-BSO**	total abdominal hysterectomy and bilateral salpingo-oophorectomy
G/TPAL	see *G* and *TPAL*			
GU	genitourinary		**TPAL**	term newborns, premature newborns, abortions, living children
GYN	gynecology			
HCG	human chorionic gonadotropin		**TRAM**	transverse rectus abdominis muscle (flap) (pronounced "tram")
HER2	human epidermal growth factor receptor 2			
HPV	human papillomavirus		**TVH**	total vaginal hysterectomy
HRT	hormone replacement therapy		**VBAC**	vaginal birth after cesarean section (pronounced "V-back")
HSIL	high-grade squamous intraepithelial lesion			
ICSI	intracytoplasmic sperm injection		**ZIFT**	zygote intrafallopian transfer
IRDS	infant respiratory distress syndrome			

Word Alert

Abbreviations. Abbreviations are commonly used in all types of medical documents; however, they can mean different things to different people and their meanings can be misinterpreted. Always verify the meaning of an abbreviation.

- *AI* means *artificial insemination*, but it also means *aortic insufficiency*, *apical impulse*, and *artificial intelligence*.

- *Ca* means *cancer*, but it also means the mineral *calcium*.

- *D&C* means *dilation and curettage*, but it can be confused with *D/C* (*discontinue* or *discharge*).

- *EDC* means *estimated date of confinement*, but it also means *extensor digitorum communis* (a muscle).

- *G* means *gravida*, but it also means *gauge (of a needle)*.

- *NICU* means *neonatal intensive care unit*, but it also means *neurologic intensive care unit*.

- *P* means *para*, but it also means the mineral *phosphorus* and *pulse (rate)*.

- *ROM* means *rupture of membranes*, but it also means *range of motion*.

It's Greek to Me! Did you notice that some words have two different combining forms? Combining forms from both Greek and Latin remain a part of medical language today.

Word	Greek	Latin	Medical Word Examples
breast	mast/o-	mamm/a-, mamm/o-	mastitis; mammaplasty, mammography
childbirth; labor	toc/o-	part/o-, parturit/o-	oxytocin; postpartum, parturition
egg; ovum	o/o-	ov/i-, ov/o-, ovul/o-	oocyte; oviduct, ovum, ovulation
female; woman	gynec/o-	estr/a-, estr/o-	gynecology; estradiol, estrogen
birth; giving birth	par/o-	nat/o-	multiparous; prenatal
milk	galact/o-	lact/i-, lact/o-	galactorrhea; lactiferous, lactation
ovary	oophor/o-	ovari/o-	oophorectomy; ovarian
sexual intercourse	pareun/o-	coit/o-, venere/o-	dyspareunia; postcoital, venereal
uterus; womb	hyster/o-, metri/o-, metr/o-	uter/o-	hysterectomy, endometriosis, metrorrhagia; uterine
vagina	colp/o-	vagin/o-	colposcopy; vaginal
vulva	episi/o-	vulv/o-	episiotomy; vulvar

Career Focus

Meet Michele, a nurse midwife

"I think the role of the nurse midwife differs from that of a physician in that you're more holistically focused on the whole person. You look at psychological factors and social factors. You provide more support and more education. I work in an outpatient setting, providing GYN services. I do labor and delivery in the hospital. I have many clients that I'm seeing for their second and third babies. So that's kind of nice to see growing families. It's a very rewarding career because you get to see new families blossoming."

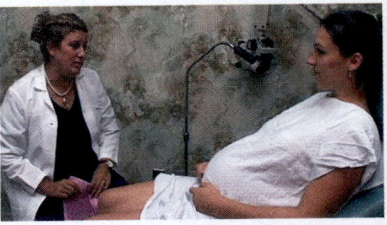

- **Nurse midwives** are allied health professionals who (with the supervision of a physician) manage a patient's prenatal care, delivery, and postpartum care. They are employed in hospitals, obstetricians' offices, and birthing centers. They also manage home births. They can become certified nurse midwives (CNM).

- **Gynecologists** are physicians who practice in the medical specialty of gynecology. They diagnose and treat patients with diseases of the female genital and reproductive system. Most gynecologists are also obstetricians who continue to care for their patients during pregnancy and labor and delivery.

- **Obstetricians** are physicians who practice in the medical specialty of obstetrics. Obstetricians deliver babies and perform cesarean sections.

- **Neonatologists** are physicians who practice in the medical specialty of neonatology. They diagnose and treat the fetus during pregnancy, labor and delivery, and also treat the newborn baby. Most neonatologists work in the **neonatal intensive care unit (NICU)** in a hospital.

- **Pediatricians** are physicians who practice in the medical specialty of pediatrics. They diagnose and treat newborns, infants, children, and adolescents.

- **Endocrinologists** treat female patients with disorders of the endocrine system, including hormonal disorders that affect menstruation and cause infertility.

- Cancerous tumors of the female genital and reproductive system are treated medically by an **oncologist** and surgically by a general **surgeon**.

---

nurse midwife (NURS MID-wyfe)

---

gynecologist (GY-neh-KAW-loh-jist)
  gynec/o- *female; woman*
  log/o- *study of; word*
  -ist *person who specializes in; thing that specializes in*

---

obstetrician (AWB-steh-TRIH-shun)
  obstetr/o- *pregnancy and childbirth*
  -ician *skilled expert; skilled professional*

---

neonatologist (NEE-oh-nay-TAW-loh-jist)
  ne/o- *new*
  nat/o- *birth*
  log/o- *study of; word*
  -ist *person who specializes in; thing that specializes in*

---

pediatrician (PEE-dee-ah-TRIH-shun)
  ped/o- *child*
  iatr/o- *medical treatment; physician*
  -ician *skilled expert; skilled professional*

---

endocrinologist (EN-doh-krih-NAW-loh-jist)
  end/o- *innermost; within*
  crin/o- *secrete*
  log/o- *study of; word*
  -ist *person who specializes in; thing that specializes in*

---

oncologist (ong-KAW-loh-jist)
  onc/o- *mass; tumor*
  log/o- *study of; word*
  -ist *person who specializes in; thing that specializes in*

---

surgeon SER-jen
  surg/o- *operative procedure*
  -eon *person who performs*

Chapter Review Exercises

Dive In: Medical Language Exercises

Test your knowledge of the chapter by completing these review exercises. Use the Answer Key at the end of the book to check your answers. Note: Each of the numbered exercise headers corresponds to a numbered learning outcome at the beginning of the chapter.

12.1 Anatomy

MATCHING EXERCISE

Match each word or phrase to its description. Each word can have more than one matching description.

1. breasts
2. cervix
3. genitalia
4. ovaries
5. labia
6. perineum
7. uterine tube
8. uterus
9. vagina
10. vulva

_____ gonads

_____ parts of this organ are the fundus and the body

_____ follicles in these glands rupture to release a mature ovum

_____ also known as the *mammary glands*

_____ area of skin between the vulva and the anus

_____ has a lumen and a fimbriated end

_____ has a muscular layer known as the *myometrium*

_____ also known as the *oviduct*

_____ contains the fornix

_____ areola is one of its structures

_____ the labia are located within this area

_____ along with the uterine tubes, collectively known as the *adnexa*

_____ structure in which the inferior end is covered by the hymen

_____ contain the lactiferous lobules

_____ contains an os

_____ normal position is anteflexion

_____ includes both external and internal structures

_____ two pairs of lips of tissue

CIRCLE EXERCISE

Circle the correct answer from the choices given.

1. The internal genitalia include the following *except* the (**clitoris, ovary, vagina**).
2. The ovaries are held in place by the (**areola, broad ligament, perimetrium**).
3. The intrauterine cavity is lined with (**cilia, endometrium, follicles**).
4. The neck of the uterus is the (**cervix, fundus, perineum**).
5. The (**Bartholin glands, gonads, mammary glands**) are near the vaginal introitus.
6. The (**cul-de-sac, fimbriae, hymen**) is an elastic membrane across the end of the vaginal canal.

TRUE OR FALSE EXERCISE

*Indicate whether each statement is true or false by writing **T** or **F** on the line.*

1. _____ The cervical canal is a continuation of the intrauterine cavity.
2. _____ The uterus is suspended within the pelvic cavity by the broad ligament and the fimbriae.
3. _____ The internal opening within the uterine tube is known as the *os*.

continued

4. _____ The cilia are moving, finger-like projections at the distal end of the uterine tube.

5. _____ Oocytes are immature ova.

6. _____ The normal position of the uterus is in anteflexion.

7. _____ The area of skin between the vulva and the anus is the perimetrium.

8. _____ The mammary glands contain lactiferous lobules and ducts.

PLURAL NOUN AND ADJECTIVE EXERCISE

Read the noun and write its plural form and/or adjective form on the line. Only write in the plural noun or adjective form if there is a blank line there for it. Be sure to check your spelling. The first one has been done for you.

Singular Noun	Plural Noun	Adjective	Singular Noun	Plural Noun	Adjective
1. **labium**	*labia*	*labial*	6. ovary	_____	_____
2. areola	_____	_____	7. ovum	_____	
3. cervix		_____	8. uterus		_____
4. endometrium		_____	9. vagina		_____
5. fundus		_____	10. vulva		_____

DIVIDING WORDS EXERCISE

Separate these words into their component parts (prefix, combining form, suffix). Some words do not contain all three word parts. The first one has been done for you.

Medical Word	Prefix	Combining Form	Suffix	Medical Word	Prefix	Combining Form	Suffix
1. **vulvar**		*vulv/o-*	*ar*	6. anteflexion	_____	_____	_____
2. reproductive	_____	_____	_____	7. intrauterine	_____	_____	_____
3. genital		_____	_____	8. mammary		_____	_____
4. ovarian		_____	_____	9. lobule		_____	_____
5. oocyte		_____	_____				

SPELLING EXERCISE

Read each medical word pronunciation and write the medical word that it represents. Be sure to check your spelling. The first one has been done for you.

1. **(in-TER-nal)** _____ *internal* _____

2. (JEN-ih-toh-YOOR-ih-NAIR-ee) _____

3. (YOO-teh-rin) _____

4. (MY-oh-MEE-tree-um) _____

5. (PAIR-ih-NEE-um) _____

RELATED COMBINING FORMS EXERCISE

Write the combining forms on the line provided. (Hint: See the It's Greek to Me! feature box.)

1. Three combining forms that mean *breast.* _____ _____ _____

2. Four combining forms that mean *egg; ovum.* _____ _____ _____ _____

3. Three combining forms that mean *female; woman.* _____ _____ _____

4. Three combining forms that mean *milk.* _____ _____ _____

5. Two combining forms that mean *ovary.* _____ _____

6. Four combining forms that mean *uterus; womb.* _____ _____ _____ _____

7. Two combining forms that mean *vagina.* _____ _____

8. Two combining forms that mean *vulva.* _____ _____

12.2 Physiology

MATCHING EXERCISE

Match each word or phrase to its description.

1. amnion
2. embryo
3. engagement
4. false labor
5. fertilization
6. fetus
7. gamete
8. gestation
9. placenta
10. presenting part
11. trimester
12. umbilical cord
13. zygote

_____ fertilized ovum with 46 chromosomes

_____ also known as *conception*

_____ part of the fetus that goes first through the birth canal

_____ membrane that holds fluid around the fetus

_____ spermatozoon or an ovum with 23 chromosomes

_____ source of nutrients and oxygen for the fetus

_____ connects the placenta to the fetus

_____ developmental stage before the fetus

_____ the embryo after week 9

_____ time from conception to birth

_____ equals 3 months' time

_____ fetal head drops into position in the woman's pelvis

_____ also known as Braxton Hicks contractions

MATCHING EXERCISE

Match each word or phrase to its description.

1. colostrum
2. crowning
3. dilation
4. effacement
5. lactation
6. let-down reflex
7. postpartum
8. rupture of membranes

_____ newborn cries and breasts release milk

_____ widening of the diameter of the cervical os

_____ releases amniotic fluid

_____ time period after birth (for the mother)

_____ thinning of the cervical wall

_____ fetal scalp visible at vaginal introitus

_____ production of breast milk after childbirth

_____ first milk from the breast

TRUE OR FALSE EXERCISE

*Indicate whether each statement is true or false by writing **T** or **F** on the line.*

1. _____ A newborn is also known as a *neonate*.
2. _____ Adolescence is another name for puberty.
3. _____ FSH and LH are secreted by the ovary.
4. _____ The onset of menstruation is known as *menarche*.
5. _____ Ovulation occurs on the first day of the menstrual cycle.
6. _____ Human chorionic gonadotropin is secreted by the vagina.
7. _____ The prenatal period is the period of time before conception.
8. _____ Gestation is from the moment of conception until the moment of birth.
9. _____ Oxytocin causes the uterus to contract during labor.
10. _____ Acrocyanosis is a bluish discoloration of a newborn's face and extremities.
11. _____ Crowning is when the top of the fetal head is visible at the vaginal introitus.

CIRCLE EXERCISE

Circle the correct answer from the choices given.

1. (**Corpus luteum, Estradiol, Luteinizing**) is the most abundant and biologically active of the female hormones.
2. (**Conception, Gestation, Oogenesis**) is the process of producing mature ova.
3. Which of the following is associated with the menstrual cycle? (**engagement, dilation, proliferative phase**)
4. At birth, a normal neonate has all of the following visible on its body *except* (**meconium, molding, vernix caseosa**).
5. Most cells in the body divide by (**meiosis, mitosis, oogenesis**).
6. When a spermatozoon fertilizes an ovum, the resulting cell is a/an (**embryo, oocyte, zygote**).
7. The process of labor and childbirth is (**effacement, gestation, parturition**).

DIVIDING WORDS EXERCISE

Separate these words into their component parts (prefix, combining form, suffix). Some words do not contain all three word parts. The first one has been done for you.

Medical Word	Prefix	Combining Form	Suffix	Medical Word	Prefix	Combining Form	Suffix
1. **sexual**		*sex/o-*	*-ual*	7. oocyte		_____	_____
2. puberty		_____	_____	8. menstruation		_____	_____
3. follicle		_____	_____	9. conception		_____	_____
4. adolescence		_____	_____	10. pregnant		_____	_____
5. prenatal	_____	_____	_____	11. postnatal	_____	_____	_____
6. umbilical		_____	_____	12. neonate		_____	_____

SPELLING EXERCISE

Read each medical word pronunciation and write the medical word that it represents. Be sure to check your spelling. The first one has been done for you.

1. (PYOO-ber-tee) _____*puberty*_____
2. (ES-trah-DY-awl) _____
3. (OH-oh-JEN-eh-sihs) _____
4. (EM-bree-AW-nik) _____
5. (FER-til-ih-ZAY-shun) _____

12.3 Diseases

MATCHING EXERCISE

Match each word or phrase to its description.

1. candidiasis	_____ yeast infection of the vagina
2. breast skin	_____ axillary ones can be enlarged from breast cancer
3. endometriosis	_____ discharge of milk from the breast without pregnancy
4. galactorrhea	_____ climacteric
5. hydatidiform mole	_____ scanty amniotic fluid
6. leiomyomata	_____ prolapse of the uterus
7. lymph nodes	_____ where peau d'orange dimpling associated with cancer occurs
8. menopause	_____ many smooth muscle tumors of the uterus
9. oligohydramnios	_____ hypertensive disorder of pregnancy
10. oligomenorrhea	_____ pus in the uterine tube
11. preeclampsia	_____ scanty menstrual flow
12. pyosalpinx	_____ "chocolate cysts" on the ovary
13. uterine descensus	_____ abnormal union of an ovum and spermatozoon

TRUE OR FALSE EXERCISE

Indicate whether each statement is true or false by writing **T** *or* **F** *on the line.*

1. _____ Anovulation is normal prior to menarche, during pregnancy, and after menopause.
2. _____ Polycystic ovary syndrome is associated with insulin resistance and type 2 diabetes mellitus.
3. _____ Infection and pus in the uterine tube is known as *hydrosalpinx*.
4. _____ Endometriosis occurs because of a retrograde flow of menstrual blood and tissue.
5. _____ Leiomyomata are also known as *uterine fibroids*.
6. _____ Uterine prolapse is also known as *uterine descensus*.
7. _____ Amenorrhea is associated with painful menstruation.
8. _____ Menopause is also known as *climacteric*.
9. _____ Premenstrual syndrome (PMS) is a psychiatric disorder.
10. _____ Genital warts can cause cervical cancer.
11. _____ Leukorrhea is a cheesy, white discharge from the breasts.
12. _____ Dyspareunia is difficult or painful sexual intercourse.
13. _____ A rectocele is when the vagina bulges into the rectum.
14. _____ A lack of prolactin from the anterior pituitary gland causes the breasts not to produce milk after the baby is born.
15. _____ Abruptio placentae refers to any type of difficult or abnormal labor and delivery.

CIRCLE EXERCISE

Circle the correct answer from the choices given.

1. Galactorrhea is a disease that affects the (**breasts, perineum, vagina**).
2. (**Amenorrhea, Dysmenorrhea, Menometrorrhagia**) is the complete absence of monthly menstrual periods.
3. (**Cervical, Endometrial, Ovarian**) cancer is the most difficult to detect and is often widespread before symptoms become severe.
4. Dyspareunia and dysmenorrhea are symptoms of (**endometriosis, menopause, pregnancy**).
5. A yeast infection in the vagina is known as (**anovulation, candidiasis, hydrosalpinx**).
6. (**Menometrorrhagia, Metrorrhagia, Myometritis**) is an infection or inflammation in the muscular wall of the uterus.
7. An ectopic pregnancy can result in (**eclampsia, hemosalpinx, involution**).
8. Mastitis is a postpartum inflammation of the (**breast, perineum, uterus**).
9. (**Gestational diabetes mellitus, Prolapsed cord, Salpingitis**) cuts off the supply of oxygen to the fetus.
10. Yellowish discoloration of the skin in the neonate is known as (**acrocyanosis, apnea, jaundice**).
11. Pain during sexual intercourse is known as (**abortion, dyspareunia, eclampsia**).

DIVIDING WORDS EXERCISE

Separate these words into their component parts (prefix, combining form, suffix). Some words do not contain all three word parts. The first one has been done for you.

Medical Word	Prefix	Combining Form	Suffix	Medical Word	Prefix	Combining Form	Suffix
1. **hemorrhage**		*hem/o-*	*-rrhage*	7. premenstrual	_____	_____	_____
2. polyhydramnios	_____	_____	_____	8. cystocele		_____	_____
3. anovulation	_____	_____	_____	9. dyspareunia	_____	_____	_____
4. hydrosalpinx		_____	_____	10. galactorrhea		_____	_____
5. amenorrhea	_____	_____	_____	11. hemosalpinx		_____	_____
6. dysmenorrhea	_____	_____	_____				

SPELLING EXERCISE

Read each medical word pronunciation and write the medical word that it represents. Be sure to check your spelling. The first one has been done for you.

1. (PREE-ee-KLAMP-see-ah)   *preeclampsia*
2. (AN-aw-vyoo-LAY-shun)   _____
3. (DIS-men-oh-REE-ah)   _____
4. (REK-toh-seel)   _____
5. (mas-TY-tihs)   _____

12.4 Laboratory, Diagnostic, and Radiologic Procedures

MATCHING EXERCISE

Match each word or phrase to its description.

1. acid phosphatase
2. alpha fetoprotein
3. chorionic villus sampling
4. cytobrush
5. Down syndrome
6. estrogen receptor assay
7. mammogram
8. pregnancy test
9. ultrasonography

_____ cytology test on breast tissue
_____ done on the placenta
_____ shows the hormone HCG
_____ chromosome abnormality identified on amniocentesis
_____ increased level indicates neural tube defect
_____ used during a Pap test
_____ x-ray image of the breast
_____ enzyme test used in rape investigations
_____ uses sound waves to produce an image

TRUE OR FALSE EXERCISE

*Indicate whether each statement is true or false by writing **T** or **F** on the line.*

1. _____ The presence of the *BRCA1* gene mutation greatly increases the risk of developing fibrocystic disease of the breast.
2. _____ The estrogen receptor assay predicts whether estrogen-blocking drugs will be successful in treating a patient's breast cancer.
3. _____ A Pap test is reported as one of two results, either negative for cancerous cells or positive for cancerous cells.

CIRCLE EXERCISE

Circle the correct answer from the choices given.

1. A wet mount is a cytology test for all of the following *except* (**antibodies, bacteria, parasites, yeasts**).
2. (**BRCA, CVS, SCC**) is a genetic mutation that increases the risk of breast cancer.
3. All of the following are related to a Pap test *except* (**alpha fetoprotein, cytobrush, exfoliative cytology**).
4. The L/S ratio (**confirms pregnancy, is a type of x-ray, shows fetal lung maturity**).
5. An ultrasound of the pregnant uterus can show all of the following *except* (**estradiol hormone level, intrauterine growth retardation, sex of the fetus**).

12.5 Medical Procedures, Drugs, and Surgical Procedures

MATCHING EXERCISE

Match each word or phrase to its description.

1. colposcope
2. cryoprobe
3. dorsal lithotomy
4. epidural anesthesia
5. G/TPAL
6. incisional biopsy
7. laparoscopy
8. mastopexy
9. speculum
10. tenaculum
11. tocolytic
12. tubal ligation

_____ drug used to stop premature labor
_____ instrument used to examine the cervix
_____ procedure to prevent pregnancy
_____ given before delivery of the newborn
_____ low-power microscope used to examine the cervix
_____ instrument used to hold the cervix during a D&C
_____ uses small abdominal incisions and carbon dioxide gas
_____ instrument used to freeze cervical lesions
_____ position used to perform a gynecologic examination
_____ used to report the obstetrical history
_____ only part of a tumor is removed
_____ repositions a sagging breast

TRUE OR FALSE EXERCISE

*Indicate whether each statement is true or false by writing **T** or **F** on the line.*

1. _____ A fine-needle aspiration biopsy uses a thin needle to inject drugs into a cancerous tumor.
2. _____ During a LEEP procedure, a cold knife is used to cut away a cone of tissue from the cervix.
3. _____ A lumpectomy is a more extensive procedure than a mastectomy.
4. _____ A hysteropexy is also known as a *uterine suspension*.
5. _____ Hormone replacement therapy treats the vaginal dryness and hot flashes associated with menopause.
6. _____ A bimanual examination uses two hands to examine the mammary glands.
7. _____ DIEP and TRAM are surgical procedures to recreate a breast after mastectomy.

CIRCLE EXERCISE

Circle the correct answer from the choices given.

1. A (**bioidentical hormone, cryoprobe, speculum**) is used to visually examine the cervix.
2. (**Amniotomy, Breast self-examination, Tanner staging**) should be done monthly.
3. Assisted reproductive technology includes all of the following *except* (**BPP, GIFT, ICSI, ZIFT**).
4. Bioidentical hormones are used to (**produce an abortion, remove biopsy tissue, treat menopause**).
5. A lumpectomy is performed on the (**breast, ovary, uterus**).

DIVIDING WORDS EXERCISE

Separate these words into their component parts (prefix, combining form, suffix). Some words do not contain all three word parts. The first one has been done for you.

Medical Word	Prefix	Combining Form	Suffix	Medical Word	Prefix	Combining Form	Suffix
1. **reconstructive**	*re-*	*construct/o-*	*-ive*	5. dysmenorrhea	_____	_____	_____
2. anovulation	_____	_____	_____	6. polycystic	_____	_____	_____
3. amniotomy		_____	_____	7. retroversion	_____	_____	_____
4. cystocele		_____	_____	8. salpingectomy		_____	_____

SPELLING EXERCISE

Read each medical word pronunciation and write the medical word that it represents. Be sure to check your spelling. The first one has been done for you.

1. **(ah-NAS-toh-MOH-sihs)**   *anastomosis*
2. (HIS-ter-oh-PEK-see)   _____
3. (mas-TEK-toh-mee)   _____
4. (eh-PIZ-ee-AW-toh-mee)   _____
5. (AM-nee-AW-toh-mee)   _____

Immerse Yourself: Analyze Medical Reports

Electronic Patient Record #1

This is an Office Visit SOAP Note. Read the Note and answer the questions.

PEARSON PRIMARY CARE ASSOCIATES

Task   Edit   View   Time Scale   Options   Help

OFFICE VISIT SOAP NOTE

PATIENT NAME: BRADLEY, Emily

MEDICAL RECORD NUMBER: 16-7934

DATE OF VISIT: 11/19/20xx

SUBJECTIVE: The patient comes in today with complaints of menorrhagia during some months of her menstrual cycle and oligomenorrhea during other months. She denies dysmenorrhea or dyspareunia. The patient has a past history of a tubal ligation. She is married and has three children.

OBJECTIVE: With the patient in the dorsal lithotomy position, a colposcopy was performed. There was the presence of old blood in the cervical canal and vagina. Bimanual examination did not show any tenderness or enlargement of the uterus.

ASSESSMENT: Hormone imbalance.

PLAN: The patient will have blood drawn for FSH and LH. Depending on the results, she may need to have an endometrial biopsy done.

---

1. Define these words:

   menorrhagia _____

   oligomenorrhea _____

   dysmenorrhea _____

   dyspareunia _____

2. What surgery did the patient have in the past? _____

3. Could the patient be pregnant? Why not? _____

4. Describe the dorsal lithotomy position. _____

5. What is a colposcopy? _____

6. How is a bimanual examination performed? _____

7. Define FSH and LH. _____   _____

Electronic Patient Record #2

This is an Admission History and Physical Examination done in the neonatal intensive care unit. Read the report and answer the questions.

PEARSON GENERAL HOSPITAL

Task Edit View Time Scale Options Help

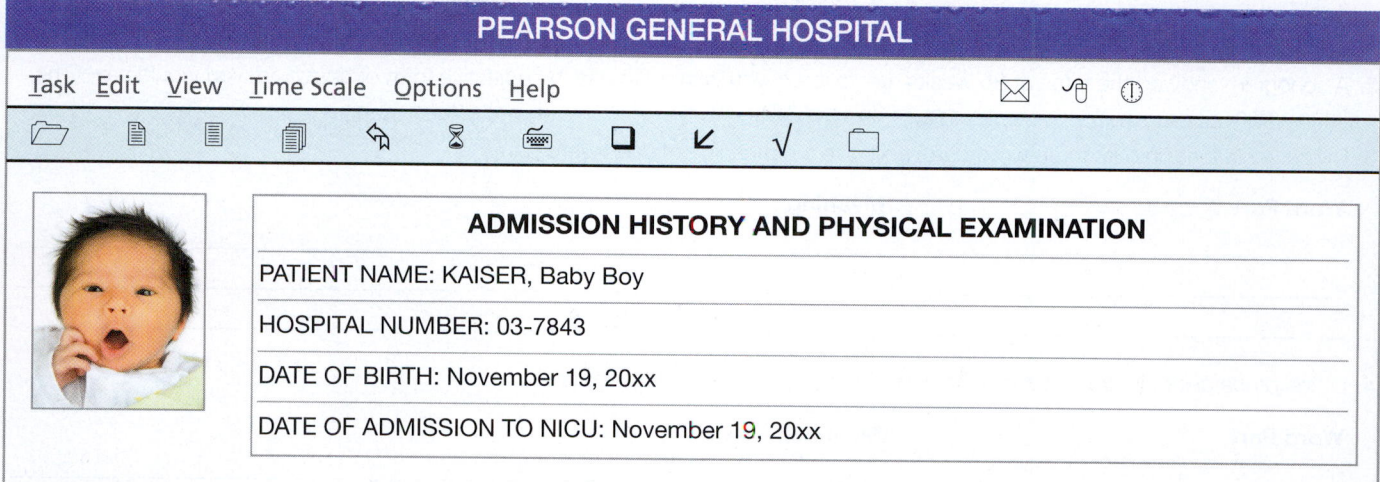

ADMISSION HISTORY AND PHYSICAL EXAMINATION

PATIENT NAME: KAISER, Baby Boy

HOSPITAL NUMBER: 03-7843

DATE OF BIRTH: November 19, 20xx

DATE OF ADMISSION TO NICU: November 19, 20xx

HISTORY
This is a 3360 g, full-term male infant, who was transferred from the delivery room to the NICU after birth because of respiratory distress. The infant was born to a 34-year-old mother with an EDB of 11/22/xx, and he had an EGA of 40 weeks.

MATERNAL HISTORY
The mother was G2, TPAL 0-0-1-0 with a SAB 2 years ago. The mother had prenatal care beginning in the first trimester of this pregnancy. She took prenatal vitamins. She denied smoking or the use of alcohol or drugs. A sonogram on 10/10/xx showed a single fetus in breech presentation at 35 weeks' gestation.

LABOR AND DELIVERY HISTORY
The membranes ruptured spontaneously 14 hours prior to the onset of labor. The mother had a temperature of 103.2 degrees prior to delivery and was started on an antibiotic drug. A version of the breech presentation was performed. Labor was induced and lasted 8 hours.

The baby was born via a normal spontaneous vaginal delivery. Apgars were 8 and 8 at 1 and 5 minutes, respectively. There was no evidence of meconium aspiration on visualization of the mouth, pharynx, and vocal cords. The infant was tachypneic despite suctioning and the administration of blow-by oxygen, and so he was brought to the neonatal intensive care unit.

PHYSICAL EXAMINATION
Heart rate 200 beats/minute, respiratory rate 70/minute, temperature 101.2, weight 3360 g, length 54 cm, head circumference 33.5 cm. General: Full-term, AGA male. Alert, active, responsive. Head: Moderate molding present. Fontanels soft. Palate intact. Eyes: Pupils equal and reactive to light. Chest symmetrical. Now pink in room air with only mild tachypnea and mild sternal retractions. Breath sounds equal bilaterally. Clavicles intact. Abdomen: Bowel sounds present. No hepatosplenomegaly. There is a three-vessel umbilical cord. Genitalia normal. Anus patent. Neurologic: Strong cry, strong suck, normal muscle tone.

IMPRESSION
Term male infant, estimated gestational age of 38.5 weeks, appropriate for gestational age. Rule out pneumonia.

PLAN
Admit to the neonatal intensive care unit. Vital signs every hour until stable. Cardiorespiratory monitor. Intravenous fluids of dextrose 10% in water at 80 cc/kg/day. Hold oral feedings for now. Chest x-ray to rule out pneumonia.

Bonita C. Grant, M.D.

Bonita C. Grant, M.D.

BCG: cgm
D: 11/19/xx
T: 11/19/xx

1. Give the definitions of these abbreviations.

   a. AGA _____

   b. EDB _____

   c. EGA _____

   d. NICU _____

   e. SAB _____

2. A sonogram showed the fetus at 35 weeks' gestation. If you wanted to use the adjective form of *gestation*, you would say, "The fetus had a _____ age of 35 weeks."

3. Divide *gestational* into its three word parts and give the meaning of each word part.

   Word Part   **Meaning**

   _____   _____

   _____   _____

   _____   _____

4. Divide *prenatal* into its three word parts and give the meaning of each word part.

   Word Part   **Meaning**

   _____   _____

   _____   _____

   _____   _____

5. What is the abbreviation for the medical phrase *normal spontaneous vaginal delivery*? _____

6. The sonogram (ultrasound) done on 10/10/xx showed what fetal presentation? _____

7. What procedure was performed to correct this presentation? Circle the correct answer.

   Apgar   repeat sonogram   version   vaginal delivery

8. What does the mother's TPAL score of 0-0-1-0 mean? _____

9. What moderate condition of the head was noted on the physical examination? _____

10. The newborn's estimated gestational age was 38.5 weeks. Is this a term newborn?   **Yes   No**

11. Where are the fontanels located? _____

12. What test was ordered to rule out pneumonia? _____

13. Rupture of the membranes many hours prior to delivery can cause infection in the mother and in the newborn. What information is given in the record that tells you that the mother and newborn did develop an infection? _____

14. Circle the correct answer. If there had been meconium-stained amniotic fluid, we would know that the fetus had experienced (**dysmenorrhea**, **fetal distress**, **premature birth**).

Proofreading and Spelling Exercise

Read the following paragraph. Identify each misspelled medical word and write the correct spelling of it on the line.

A woman may request a gynicologic exam because of pain and dysparunia. When the gynecologist does an examination, the uteris can be felt, but not the uterin tubes. A pregnant woman's obstetical history notes that she is a primogravida. Her doctor might recommend an amniosentesis and a cecarean section. An older woman might need to have a histerectomy and an ophorectomy.

1. _____

2. _____

3. _____

4. _____

5. _____

6. _____

7. _____

8. _____

9. _____

10. _____

You Write the Medical Report

You are a healthcare professional interviewing a patient. Listen to the patient's statements and then enter them in the patient's medical record using medical words and phrases. Be sure to check your spelling. The first one has been done for you.

1. The patient says, "I didn't produce any milk with my last pregnancy."

   You write: The patient has a history of *failure of lactation.*

2. The patient says, "I had my womb taken out, with all my tubes and my ovaries too. That was last year."

   You write: The patient had a _____ and a bilateral _____ last year.

3. The patient says, "I am having itching and a white, cheesy discharge from my vagina because of a yeast infection. I want an antibiotic drug."

   You write: The patient is complaining of _____ coming from the vagina due to an infection with _____. She was prescribed a topical _____ drug.

4. The patient says, "I can finally breathe because the baby's head dropped down yesterday. I am due on January 21."

   You write: Based on my examination and the mother's comments, the mother reports _____, and there is now _____ of the fetal head within the maternal pelvis. Her _____ [abbreviation] is January 21.

5. The patient says, "I had a workup done last month because I couldn't get pregnant. They said I had an infection in my tubes and that my ovaries had lots of cysts in them. I also had pain when I had sexual intercourse with my husband. They took a scope and looked into my abdomen to check this out, and they said that was because of pieces of the lining of the uterus being in the wrong places."

   You write: The patient had an _____ workup last month. She was found to have _____ and _____ ovary syndrome. She also complained of _____ during sexual intercourse with her husband. She had a _____ to investigate this and was diagnosed as having _____.

6. The patient says, "I started my periods when I was 16. I always have pain with my periods. Recently, my periods have changed and are very light. But I am too young to be in the change of life."

   You write: Patient had _____ at age 16. She reports she has always had _____ with her periods. Recently, she has noticed _____. She is only 30, and so this is probably a hormonal imbalance and not the beginning of _____.

MyLab Medical Terminology™

MyLab Medical Terminology is a premium online homework management system that includes a host of features to help you study. Registered users will find:

- A multitude of quizzes and activities built within the MyLab platform
- Powerful tools that track and analyze your results—allowing you to create a personalized learning experience
- Videos and audio pronunciations to help enrich your progress
- Streaming lesson presentations (guided lectures) and self-paced learning modules
- A space where you and your instructor can check your progress and manage your assignments

13 Endocrinology

Endocrine System

Endocrinology (EN-doh-krih-NAW-loh-jee) is the medical specialty that studies the anatomy and physiology of the endocrine system; uses laboratory, diagnostic, and radiologic procedures to diagnose endocrine diseases; and uses medical procedures, drugs, and surgical procedures to treat endocrine diseases.

⌄ Chapter Overview and Learning Outcomes

After you study this chapter, you should be able to demonstrate mastery of the outcomes by successfully completing the exercises.

13.1 Anatomy
Identify the structures of the endocrine system.
Demonstrate proficiency in medical language.
13.1 Practice Laps

13.2 Physiology
Describe the functions of the endocrine system.
Demonstrate proficiency in medical language.
13.2 Practice Laps
Vocabulary Review

13.3 Diseases
Describe common endocrine diseases.
Demonstrate proficiency in medical language.
13.3 Practice Laps

13.4 Laboratory, Diagnostic, and Radiologic Procedures
Describe common endocrine laboratory tests, diagnostic procedures, and radiologic procedures.
Demonstrate proficiency in medical language.
13.4 Practice Laps

13.5 Medical Procedures, Drugs, and Surgical Procedures
Describe common endocrine medical procedures, drugs, and surgical procedures.
Demonstrate proficiency in medical language.
13.5 Practice Laps
Abbreviations Summary
Career Focus

Chapter Review Exercises
Dive In: Medical Language Exercises (Learning Outcomes 13.1–13.5)
Immerse Yourself: Analyze Medical Reports

Medical Language Key

To unlock the definition of a medical word, first break it into word parts. Then give the meaning of each word part. Put the meanings of the word parts in order, beginning with the meaning of the suffix, then the meaning of the prefix (if there is one), then the meaning of the combining form.

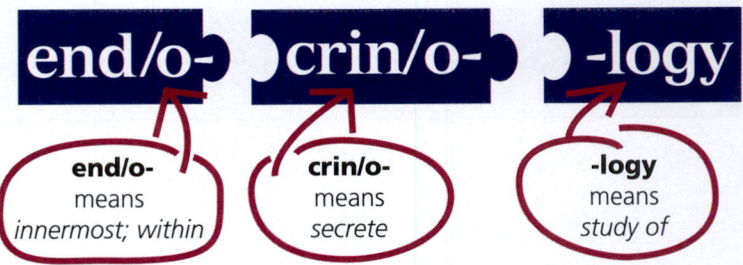

Endocrinology: ▶ *Study of (glands) within (the body that) secrete (hormones).*

The **endocrine system** is different from other body systems in that it is made up of **glands** that are in various locations throughout the body (see Figure 13-1 ■). These glands include the pituitary gland, hypothalamus, pineal gland, thyroid gland, parathyroid glands, thymus, pancreas, adrenal glands, ovaries, and testes. All endocrine glands are alike in the following ways:

1. They secrete substances known as **hormones**. Hormones are the chemical messengers of the endocrine system.

2. They secrete their hormones directly into the blood and not through ducts.

3. Their hormones regulate specific body functions.

The functions of the endocrine system are to use hormones to stimulate specific body organs and to help maintain **homeostasis**, a state of equilibrium of the body's internal environment, so that all body systems can function optimally. The endocrine system does this by using hormones to regulate body fluids, electrolytes, glucose, cellular metabolism, growth, and the sleep–wake cycle.

Word Alert
Sound-Alike Words

endocrine	(adjective)	descriptive word for glands that secrete hormones directly into the blood
		Example: The thyroid gland is one of the glands of the endocrine system.
exocrine	(adjective)	descriptive word for glands that release substances through ducts (not directly into the blood)
		Example: The sebaceous glands in the skin are exocrine glands that produce oil.

Several endocrine glands work in conjunction with other body systems. The anterior pituitary gland secretes hormones that stimulate the development of secondary sexual characteristics in the male and female reproductive systems. A hormone secreted by the posterior pituitary gland stimulates contractions for the birth of a baby (described in Chapter 12, Gynecology and Obstetrics). The hypothalamus in the brain is also part of the central nervous system (described in Chapter 9, Neurology). The thymus plays an active role in the immune response (described in Chapter 6, Hematology and Immunology). The pancreas secretes insulin and is active in the digestive process (described in Chapter 3, Gastroenterology).

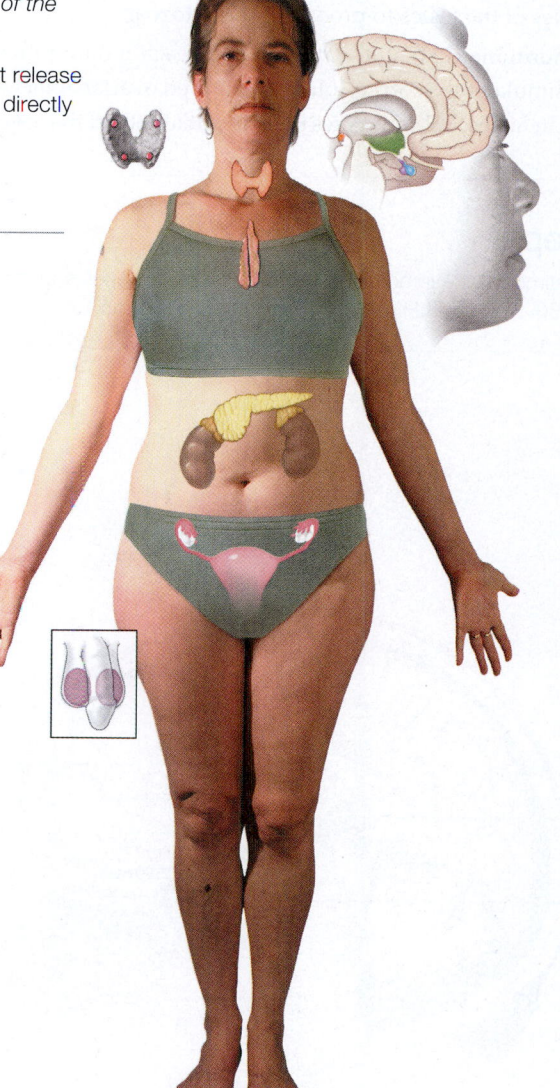

FIGURE 13-1 ■ Endocrine system.
The endocrine system consists of glands that perform very different functions. They are related to each other because they all secrete hormones into the blood.

Pronunciation/Word Parts

endocrine (EN-doh-krin)
   end/o- *innermost; within*
   -crine *pertaining to secreting*

gland (GLAND)

glandular (GLAN-dyoo-lar)
   glandul/o- *gland*
   -ar *pertaining to*
The combining form **aden/o-** also means *gland*.

hormone (HOR-mohn)

hormonal (hor-MOH-nal)
   hormon/o- *hormone*
   -al *pertaining to*

homeostasis (HOH-mee-oh-STAY-sihs)
   home/o- *same*
   -stasis *standing still; staying in one place*

13.1 Anatomy

Pituitary Gland

The **pituitary gland** is located in the brain, just above the sphenoid sinus, and it sits in a bony cup (the **sella turcica**) of the sphenoid bone (see Figure 13-2 ■). The pituitary gland is a bulb-shaped gland at the end of a stalk of tissue from the hypothalamus. Even though it is about the size of a pea, the pituitary gland is the "master gland of the body" because the effects of its hormones are felt throughout the body. The pituitary gland is also known as the **hypophysis**. It consists of an anterior and posterior lobe, each of which has a very different endocrine function.

Anterior Pituitary Gland

The **anterior pituitary gland** (or **adenohypophysis**) is a gland that secretes seven hormones (see Figure 13-3 ■).

1. **Thyroid-stimulating hormone (TSH)** stimulates the thyroid gland to grow and to secrete its own thyroid hormones, T_3 and T_4.

2. **Prolactin (PRL)** stimulates the development of the breasts during puberty and stimulates them to produce milk for breastfeeding.

3. **Follicle-stimulating hormone (FSH)** stimulates **follicles** in the ovaries of females to produce mature ova and to secrete the hormone estradiol. In males, FSH stimulates the seminiferous tubules of the testes to produce spermatozoa.

4. **Luteinizing hormone (LH)** stimulates a follicle each month to release a mature ovum in females and stimulates the corpus luteum (ruptured ovarian follicle) to secrete estradiol and progesterone. In males, LH stimulates the interstitial cells of the testes to secrete testosterone.

Dive Deeper

FSH and LH stimulate the female and male sex glands (ovaries and testes), which are known as the **gonads**. So, FSH and LH are known as **gonadotropins**.

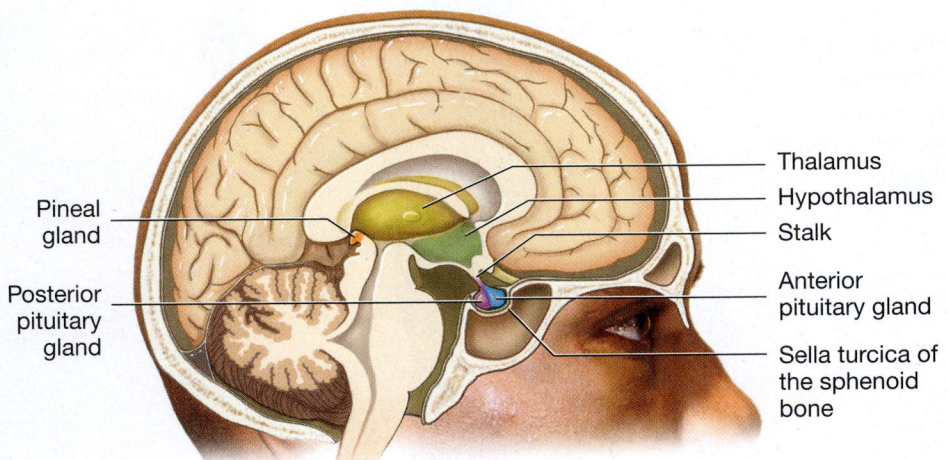

Pineal gland — Posterior pituitary gland

Thalamus — Hypothalamus — Stalk — Anterior pituitary gland — Sella turcica of the sphenoid bone

FIGURE 13-2 ■ Endocrine glands in the brain.
The hypothalamus has a stalk of tissue that goes to the pituitary gland. The pituitary gland sits in a bony cup (the sella turcica) in the sphenoid bone. The pineal gland is located between the two lobes of the thalamus.

5. **Adrenocorticotropic hormone (ACTH)** stimulates the cortex of the adrenal gland to secrete its hormones.

6. **Growth hormone (GH)** stimulates growth and protein synthesis in all cells. It increases height and weight during childhood and puberty.

7. **Melanocyte-stimulating hormone (MSH)** is not normally present in adults. In pregnant women, it stimulates melanocytes in the skin to produce the pigment melanin. This causes a distinctive darkened pigmentation on the face and abdomen of the woman (described in Chapter 2, Dermatology).

Pronunciation/Word Parts

adrenocorticotropic
(ah-DREE-noh-KOR-tih-koh-TROH-pik)
  adren/o- *adrenal gland*
  cortic/o- *cortex; outer region*
  trop/o- *having an affinity for; stimulating; turning*
  -ic *pertaining to*

melanocyte (meh-LAN-oh-site)
  melan/o- *black*
  -cyte *cell*

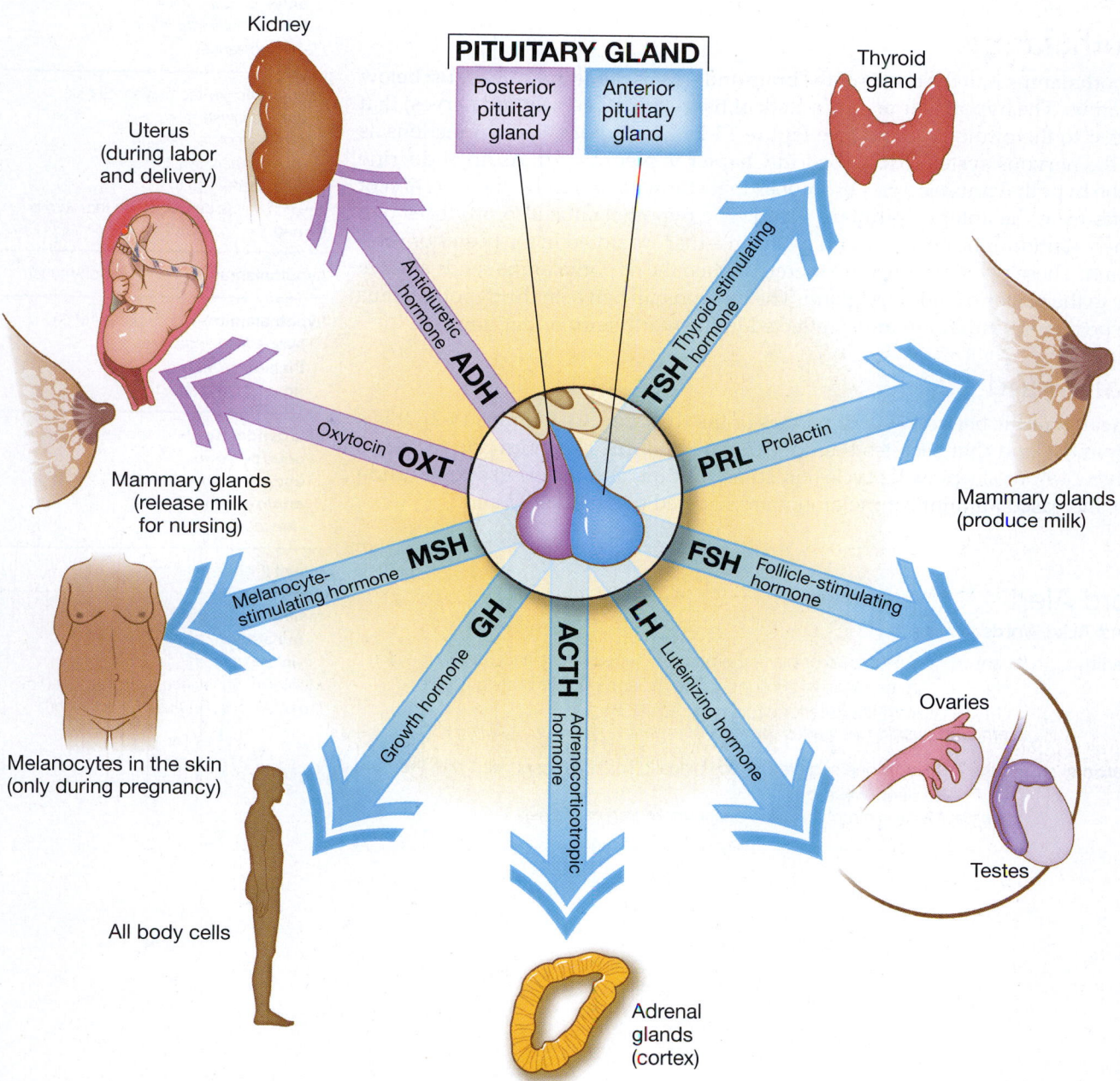

FIGURE 13-3 ■ **Hormones of the anterior and posterior pituitary gland.**
The anterior pituitary gland produces and secretes seven different hormones. The posterior pituitary gland stores and secretes two hormones that are actually produced by the hypothalamus.

Posterior Pituitary Gland

The **posterior pituitary gland** (or **neurohypophysis**) is not so much a gland as it is a structure that stores two hormones that are produced by the hypothalamus (see Figure 13-3); these hormones are secreted in response to a nerve impulse from the hypothalamus (described in the next section).

1. **Oxytocin (OXT)** stimulates the pregnant uterus to contract during labor and delivery. It stimulates the uterus to contract after birth to prevent hemorrhaging. It also stimulates the breasts to release milk for breastfeeding.

2. **Antidiuretic hormone (ADH)** acts on the kidneys to increase the reabsorption of sodium and water from the kidney tubules back into the blood. This decreases urine output (antidiuretic effect) and helps to maintain a normal blood volume and blood pressure.

Hypothalamus

The **hypothalamus** is in the center of the brain and—as its name indicates—just below the thalamus. The hypothalamus has a stalk of tissue (blood vessels and nerves) that connects it to the pituitary gland (see Figure 13-2). The hypothalamus functions as part of the nervous system (described in Chapter 9, Neurology). As an endocrine gland, the hypothalamus secretes hormones that stimulate or inhibit the secretion of hormones from the anterior pituitary gland. The hypothalamus also produces two hormones—antidiuretic hormone and oxytocin—that are stored in the posterior pituitary gland. These two hormones are secreted when the hypothalamus sends a nerve impulse to the posterior pituitary gland. The relationship between the hypothalamus and the posterior pituitary gland is reflected in the word **neuroendocrine**.

Pineal Gland

The **pineal gland** is between the two lobes of the thalamus (see Figure 13-2). It is a small, round gland that secretes the hormone **melatonin**. This hormone regulates the body's 24-hour sleep–wake cycle (circadian rhythm) and the onset and duration of sleep. Increased amounts of melatonin are secreted during the winter.

Word Alert
Sound-Alike Words

melanin	(noun)	dark brown or black pigment produced by melanocytes in the skin in response to sunlight and to melanocyte-stimulating hormone from the anterior pituitary gland
		Example: Sunshine increases the level of melanin in the skin, causing it to tan.
melatonin	(noun)	hormone secreted by the pineal gland; it is associated with the sleep-wake cycle
		Example: Melatonin regulates the onset and duration of sleep.

Pronunciation/Word Parts

posterior (pohs-TEER-ee-or)
  poster/o- *back part*
  -ior *pertaining to*

neurohypophysis
(NYOOR-oh-hy-PAW-fih-sihs)
  neur/o- *nerve*
  -hypophysis *pituitary gland*
The neurohypophysis releases stored hormones when stimulated by a nerve impulse from the hypothalamus.

oxytocin (AWK-see-TOH-sin)
  ox/y- *oxygen; quick*
  toc/o- *childbirth; labor*
  -in *substance*

antidiuretic (AN-tee-DY-yoor-EH-tik)
  anti- *against*
  dia- *complete; through*
  ur/o- *urinary system; urine*
  -etic *pertaining to*
The *a* in *dia-* is deleted when the word is formed.

hypothalamus (HY-poh-THAL-ah-muhs)

hypothalamic (HY-poh-thah-LAM-ik)
  hypo- *below; deficient*
  thalam/o- *thalamus*
  -ic *pertaining to*

neuroendocrine (NYOOR-oh-EN-doh-krin)
  neur/o- *nerve*
  end/o- *innermost; within*
  crin/o- *secrete*
  -ine *pertaining to*

pineal (PIN-ee-al)

melatonin (MEL-ah-TOH-nin)
  melaton/o- *black*
  -in *substance*
Melatonin: *Substance (that is secreted by the pineal gland in the) black (of night)*

Thyroid Gland

The **thyroid gland**, which has two lobes connected by a bridge of tissue (isthmus), is located in the neck across the anterior surface of the trachea (see Figure 13-4 ■). It secretes three hormones when stimulated by TSH from the anterior pituitary gland.

1. **Triiodothyronine (T_3)** increases the rate of cellular metabolism throughout the body.
2. **Thyroxine (T_4)** is secreted, but then most of it is changed by the liver into T_3.
3. **Calcitonin** regulates the amount of calcium in the blood. If the calcium level is too high, calcitonin suppresses the activity of osteoclasts that normally break down bone (this decreases the amount of calcium in the blood), and calcitonin increases the amount of calcium excreted in the urine. Calcitonin has an opposite effect from that of parathyroid hormone secreted by the parathyroid glands.

When the thyroid gland is functioning properly, producing neither too much nor too little of its three hormones, this steady state is known as **euthyroidism**.

Parathyroid Glands

The four **parathyroid glands** are small glands located on the posterior surface of the thyroid gland (see Figure 13-4). Each gland is about the size of a grain of rice. The parathyroid glands secrete **parathyroid hormone**, which regulates the amount of calcium in the blood. If the calcium level is too low, parathyroid hormone stimulates the release of calcium from the bones and into the blood. Parathyroid hormone has an opposite effect from that of calcitonin secreted by the thyroid gland.

Thymus Gland

The **thymus gland** is located posterior to the sternum; it is a pink gland with two lobes. During childhood and puberty, the thymus gland is large, but it shrinks during adulthood. The thymus gland functions as part of the body's immune response (described in Chapter 6, Hematology and Immunology). As an endocrine gland, the thymus secretes **thymosin**, which stimulates immature T cell lymphocytes in the thymus gland to develop and mature.

Pronunciation/Word Parts

thyroid (THY-royd)
  thyr/o- shield-shaped structure; thyroid gland
  -oid resembling
The combining form **thyroid/o-** also means thyroid gland.

triiodothyronine
(try-EYE-oh-doh-THY-roh-neen)
  tri- three
  iod/o- iodine
  thyr/o- shield-shaped structure; thyroid gland
  -nine pertaining to a chemical substance
Each molecule of T_3 contains three iodine atoms.

thyroxine (thy-RAWK-seen)

calcitonin (KAL-sih-TOH-nin)
  calc/i- calcium
  ton/o- pressure; tone
  -in substance
The combining form **calc/o-** also means calcium.

euthyroidism (yoo-THY-royd-izm)
  eu- good; normal
  thyroid/o- thyroid gland
  -ism disease from a specific cause; process

parathyroid (PAIR-ah-THY-royd)
  para- abnormal; apart from; beside; two parts of a pair
  thyr/o- shield-shaped structure; thyroid gland
  -oid resembling
Parathyroid: (Structures) resembling two parts of a pair (on the) thyroid gland

thymus (THY-muhs)

thymic (THY-mik)
  thym/o- rage; thymus
  -ic pertaining to

thymosin (thy-MOH-sin)

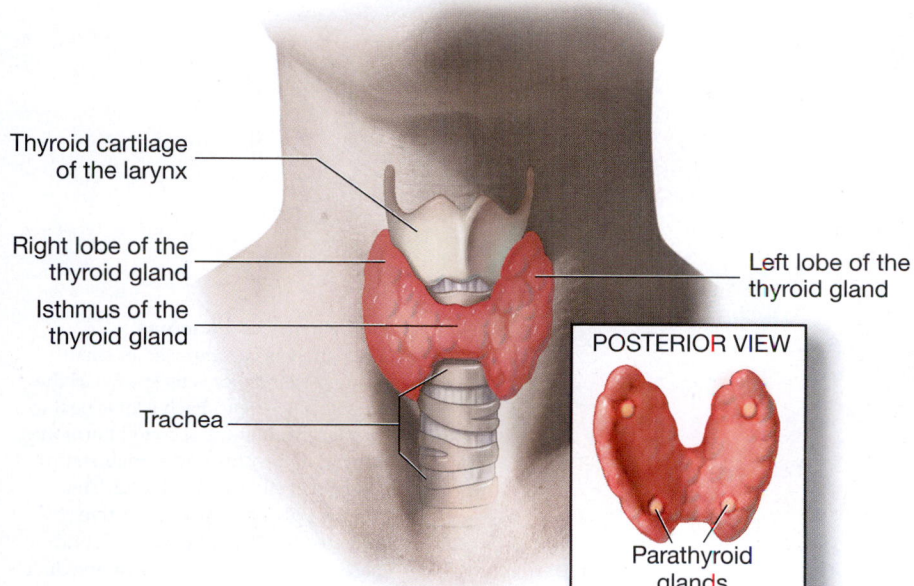

Thyroid cartilage of the larynx

Right lobe of the thyroid gland

Isthmus of the thyroid gland

Trachea

Left lobe of the thyroid gland

POSTERIOR VIEW

Parathyroid glands

FIGURE 13-4 ■ Thyroid gland and parathyroid glands.
This anterior view of the thyroid gland shows its two lobes. The thyroid cartilage of the larynx sounds and looks like it is related to the thyroid gland, but it is part of the respiratory system, not the endocrine system. The parathyroid glands are located on the posterior surface of the thyroid gland.

Pancreas

The **pancreas** is a yellow, elongated, triangular gland that is posterior to the stomach (see Figure 13-5 ■). The pancreas functions as part of the digestive system (described in Chapter 3, Gastroenterology). As an endocrine gland, the pancreas secretes three hormones from a group of cells known as the **islets of Langerhans**.

1. **Glucagon** is secreted by **alpha cells** in the islets of Langerhans. **Glucose** is simple sugar that is the main source of energy for cellular metabolism. When the blood glucose level is too low, glucagon stimulates the liver to convert **glycogen** (glucose stored in the liver) and release it to increase the level of **glucose**.

2. **Insulin** is secreted by **beta cells** in the islets of Langerhans. Insulin transports glucose to a body cell, binds to an insulin receptor on the cell membrane, and transports glucose into the cell. Within the cell, glucose is metabolized to produce energy. Insulin decreases the level of glucose in the blood.

3. **Somatostatin** is secreted by **delta cells** in the islets of Langerhans. Somatostatin inhibits the secretion of glucagon and insulin by the pancreas. It also inhibits the secretion of growth hormone from the anterior pituitary gland.

Clinical Connections

Pathology. The pancreas was first identified as an organ by a Greek anatomist, and so the alpha, beta, and delta cells of the pancreas were named and abbreviated as letters in the Greek alphabet: alpha (α) cells, beta (β) cells, and delta (Δ) cells.

Pronunciation/Word Parts

pancreas (PAN-kree-as)

pancreatic (PAN-kree-AT-ik)
  pancreat/o- *pancreas*
  -ic *pertaining to*

islets of Langerhans (EYE-lets of LANG-ger-hanz)

glucagon (GLOO-kah-gawn)
  gluc/o- *glucose; sugar*
  ag/o- *lead to*
  -on *structure; substance*

alpha (AL-fah)

glycogen (GLY-koh-jen)
  glyc/o- *glucose; sugar*
  -gen *that which produces*

glucose (GLOO-kohs)
  gluc/o- *glucose; sugar*
  -ose *full of*
The combining form **glycos/o-** also means *glucose; sugar*.

insulin (IN-soo-lin)
  insul/o- *island*
  -in *substance*
The combining form **insulin/o-** means *insulin*.

beta (BAY-tah)

somatostatin (SOH-mah-toh-STAT-in)
  somat/o- *body*
  stat/o- *standing still; staying in one place*
  -in *substance*
Somatostatin: *Substance (that makes the) body (to be) standing still (without growth)*

delta (DEL-tah)

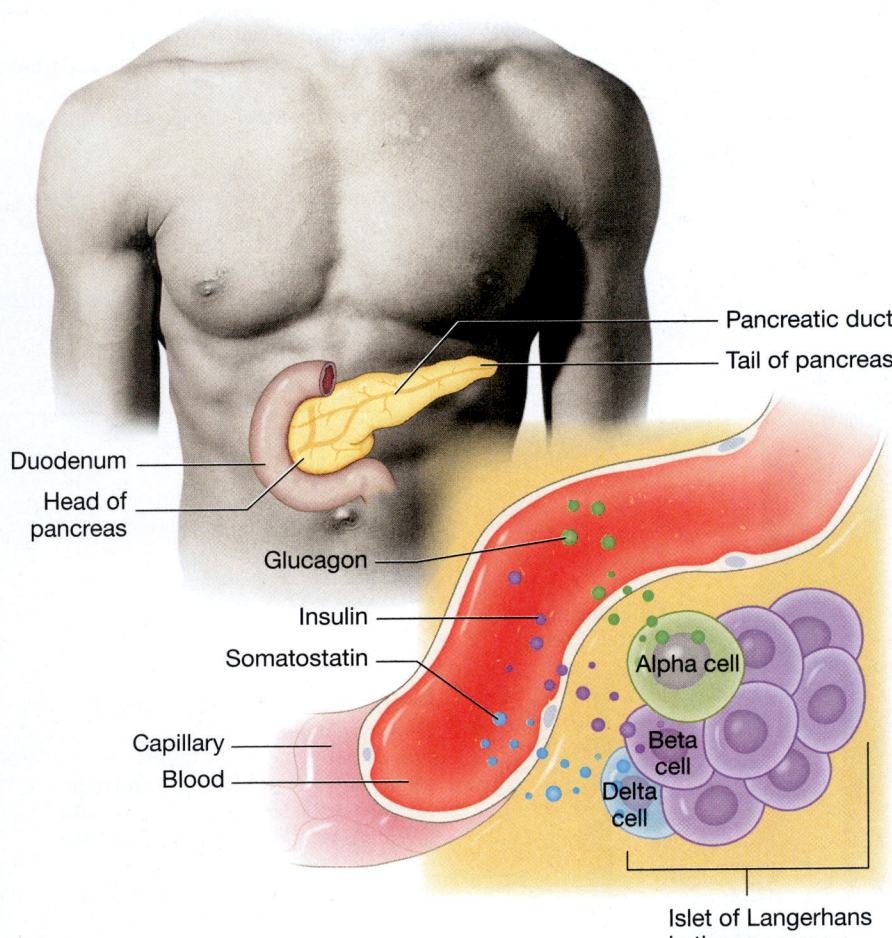

Duodenum
Head of pancreas
Glucagon
Insulin
Somatostatin
Capillary
Blood
Pancreatic duct
Tail of pancreas
Alpha cell
Beta cell
Delta cell
Islet of Langerhans in the pancreas

FIGURE 13-5 ■ **Pancreas.**
The pancreas is composed of small groups (islands) of cells known as the *islets of Langerhans*. Each islet is next to a capillary so that the secreted hormones (glucagon, insulin, and somatostatin) can go directly into the blood. The pancreas also produces digestive enzymes (amylase, lipase, etc.), and these flow through the pancreatic duct that empties into the duodenum.

Adrenal Glands

Each **adrenal gland** is draped over the superior end of a kidney (see Figure 13-6 ■). An adrenal gland consists of two parts: the cortex (an outer layer) and the medulla (an inner layer). Each of these layers functions independently of the other and secretes its own hormones.

Adrenal Cortex

The **adrenal cortex** secretes three groups of hormones: mineralocorticoids, glucocorticoids, and androgens. The adrenal cortex secretes these hormones when stimulated by ACTH from the anterior pituitary gland.

1. **Aldosterone** is the most abundant and biologically active of the **mineralocorticoid** hormones. The adrenal cortex secretes aldosterone when the blood pressure is low. Aldosterone causes reabsorption of sodium and water from tubules in the nephron of the kidney into the blood and causes potassium to be excreted in the urine. This increases the blood volume and thus the blood pressure.

2. **Cortisol** is the most abundant and biologically active of the **glucocorticoid** hormones. It stimulates the liver to convert **glycogen** (glucose stored in the liver) and release it to increase the level of glucose in the blood. Cortisol decreases the formation of proteins and new tissue, and it also exerts a strong anti-inflammatory effect.

3. **Androgens** are male sex hormones. The adrenal cortex secretes androgens, but the testes secrete testosterone, the most abundant and biologically active of the androgens. In the blood, some of the androgens are changed to **estrogens** (female sex hormones).

Adrenal Medulla

The **adrenal medulla** secretes three hormones: norepinephrine, epinephrine, and dopamine. **Norepinephrine** increases the heart rate and raises the blood pressure and blood glucose level during exercise. The release of **epinephrine** is triggered by a nerve impulse from the hypothalamus via the sympathetic nervous system during times of danger or anger. Epinephrine raises the blood pressure even more and prepares the body to either fight or run away from danger (the so-called "fight-or-flight" response). **Dopamine** is secreted into the blood during times of stress.

Clinical Connections

Neurology and Psychiatry. Norepinephrine and dopamine are also neurotransmitters between the brain and spinal cord. An imbalance in the level of dopamine is related to Parkinson disease. Cocaine, narcotic drugs, and alcohol increase the amount of dopamine, and this causes the euphoria and excitement ("high") craved by addicts. A decreased level of dopamine may cause schizophrenia and depression.

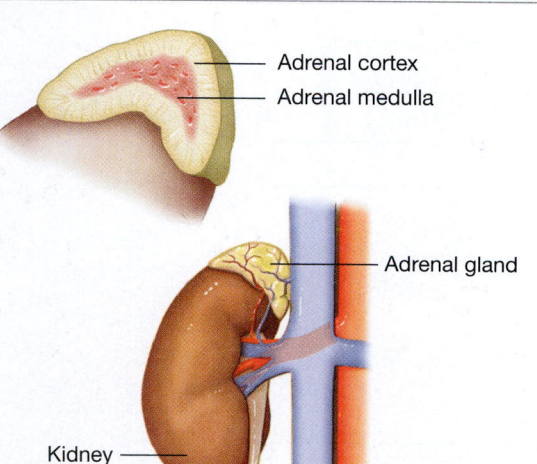

Adrenal cortex
Adrenal medulla

Adrenal gland

Kidney

FIGURE 13-6 ■ Adrenal gland.
The adrenal gland is on top of each kidney but is part of the endocrine system, while the kidney belongs to the urinary system. The two parts of the adrenal gland—the cortex and the medulla—function as two separate endocrine glands.

Ovaries

The **ovaries** are small, egg-shaped glands near the uterus in the pelvic cavity; they are the female sex glands (gonads) (described in Chapter 12, Gynecology and Obstetrics). As an endocrine gland, follicles in the ovary secrete **estradiol** when stimulated by FSH from the anterior pituitary gland. Estradiol is the most abundant and biologically active of the estrogens (female sex hormones). The corpus luteum (ruptured ovarian follicle) secretes estradiol and **progesterone** when stimulated by LH from the anterior pituitary gland. The cells around the follicle secrete testosterone (male sex hormone) when stimulated by LH from the anterior pituitary gland.

Testes

The **testes** or **testicles** are egg-shaped glands in the scrotum, a pouch of skin behind the penis; they are the male sex glands (gonads) (described in Chapter 11, Male Reproductive Medicine). As an endocrine gland, the seminiferous tubules of the testes produce spermatozoa when stimulated by FSH from the anterior pituitary gland. Interstitial cells in the testes secrete testosterone when stimulated by LH from the anterior pituitary gland. **Testosterone** is the most abundant and biologically active of the androgens (male sex hormones).

Pronunciation/Word Parts

ovary (OH-vah-ree)

ovarian (oh-VAIR-ee-an)
  ovari/o- *ovary*
  -an *pertaining to*

estradiol (ES-trah-DY-awl)
  estr/a- *female*
  di- *two*
  -ol *chemical substance*

progesterone (proh-JEH-steh-rohn)

testis (TES-tihs)

testes (TES-teez)
Latin plural noun: Change the singular ending *-is* to *-es.*

testicle (TES-tih-kul)
Testicle is a combination of *testis* and the suffix **-cle** (*small thing*).

testicular (tes-TIH-kyoo-lar)
  testicul/o- *testicle; testis*
  -ar *pertaining to*

testosterone (tes-TAW-steh-rohn)
Testosterone contains the combining form **test/o-** (*testis*), a shortened version of the combining form **steroid/o-** (*steroid*), and the suffix **-one** (*chemical substance*).

13.1 PRACTICE LAPS

Use the Answer Key at the end of the book to check your answers.

A. Label Structures

Write each anatomy word or phrase in the correct numbered box. Be sure to check your spelling.

adrenal gland	parathyroid gland	thymus
hypothalamus	pineal gland	thyroid gland
ovary	pituitary gland	
pancreas	testis	

1.
2.
3.
4.
5.
6.
7.
8.
9.
10.

| isthmus of the thyroid gland | parathyroid glands | thyroid cartilage of larynx |
| left lobe of thyroid gland | right lobe of thyroid gland | trachea |

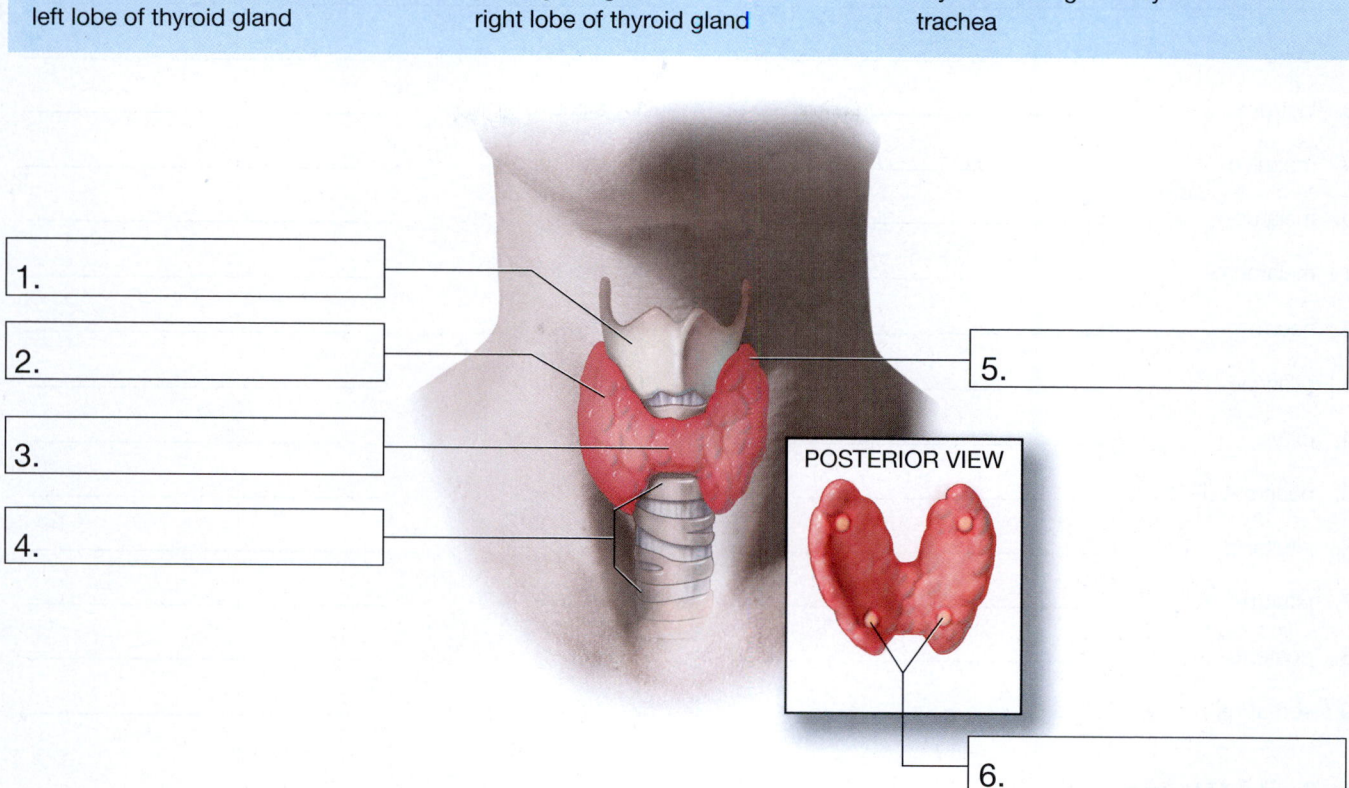

POSTERIOR VIEW

1.

2.

3.

4.

5.

6.

B. Give the Meaning of Combining Forms

Next to each combining form, write its meaning. The first one has been done for you.

Combining Form	Meaning	Combining Form	Meaning
1. **mineral/o-**	*electrolyte; mineral*	14. estr/o-	
2. aden/o-		15. folli/o-	
3. adrenal/o-		16. galact/o-	
4. adren/o-		17. glandul/o-	
5. ag/o-		18. gluc/o-	
6. andr/o-		19. glyc/o-	
7. anter/o-		20. glycos/o-	
8. calc/i-		21. gonad/o-	
9. calc/o-		22. home/o-	
10. cortic/o-		23. hormon/o-	
11. crin/o-		24. hypophys/o-	
12. end/o-		25. insulin/o-	
13. estr/a-		26. insul/o-	

continued on next page

Combining Form	Meaning	Combining Form	Meaning
27. iod/o-		40. stat/o-	
28. lact/o-		41. stimul/o-	
29. medull/o-		42. testicul/o-	
30. melan/o-		43. test/o-	
31. melaton/o-		44. thalam/o-	
32. neur/o-		45. thym/o-	
33. ovari/o-		46. thyroid/o-	
34. ox/y-		47. thyr/o-	
35. pancreat/o-		48. toc/o-	
36. pituitar/o-		49. ton/o-	
37. pituit/o-		50. trop/o-	
38. poster/o-		51. ur/o-	
39. somat/o-		52. viril/o-	

C. Build Words

Read the definition of the medical word. Look at the combining form that is given. Select the correct suffix from the Suffix List, and write it on the blank line. Then build the medical word, and write it on the line. (Remember: You may need to remove the combining vowel. Always remove the hyphens and slash.) Be sure to check your spelling.

Suffix List

-al (pertaining to)	-cle (small thing)	-hypophysis (pituitary gland)	-ose (full of)
-an (pertaining to)	-crine (pertaining to secreting)	-ic (pertaining to)	-stasis (standing still; staying in one place)
-ar (pertaining to)		-in (substance)	
-ary (pertaining to)	-gen (that which produces)	-ior (pertaining to)	

Definition of the Medical Word	Combining Form	Suffix	Build the Medical Word
Example: Pertaining to (the) medulla	**medull/o-**	*-ary*	*medullary*

[*You think* pertaining to *(-ary)* + medulla *(medull/o-)*. You change the order of the word parts to put the suffix last. You write medullary.]

1. Substance (produced by an) island (of cells)	insul/o-		
2. (Thing that is) full of sugar	gluc/o-		
3. Pertaining to secreting within	end/o-		
4. That (hormone) which produces female	estr/o-		
5. Small thing (that is a) sac-like structure	folli/o-		
6. Pertaining to (a) gland	glandul/o-		

Definition of the Medical Word	Combining Form	Suffix	Build the Medical Word
7. Pertaining to (the) pituitary gland	pituit/o-	_____	_____
8. Pertaining to (a) hormone	hormon/o-	_____	_____
9. Staying in one place (and staying the) same	home/o-	_____	_____
10. (Part of the) pituitary gland (that is a) gland	aden/o-	_____	_____
11. That (hormone) which produces male	andr/o-	_____	_____
12. Pertaining to (the) thymus	thym/o-	_____	_____
13. Pertaining to (the) testicle	testicul/o-	_____	_____
14. Substance (that is secreted by the pineal gland in the) black (of night)	melaton/o-	_____	_____
15. Pertaining to (the) pancreas	pancreat/o-	_____	_____
16. Pertaining to (an) ovary	ovari/o-	_____	_____
17. Pertaining to (the) front part	anter/o-	_____	_____

D. Define Abbreviations

1. ACTH _____

2. ADH _____

3. FSH _____

4. GH _____

5. LH _____

6. OXT _____

7. PRL _____

8. T_4 _____

9. TSH _____

13.2 Physiology

Hormone Actions

While the nervous system (described in Chapter 9, Neurology) uses neurotransmitters as chemical messengers that travel between two neurons (or between a neuron and an organ), the endocrine system uses **hormones** as chemical messengers. Hormones are secreted into the blood and travel throughout the body. Some neurotransmitters that are in the brain and spinal cord are also considered to be hormones because they are secreted by an endocrine gland and travel in the blood.

In the blood, a hormone comes in contact with all tissues, but it exerts an effect only on a gland or organ whose cell membrane has a **receptor** where that specific hormone can bind. A hormone is like a key that unlocks a receptor on a gland or organ and produces an effect. Other hormones cannot unlock those receptors.

A unique feature of the endocrine system is the "chain reaction" sequence of effects: A hormone secreted by an endocrine gland can stimulate another endocrine gland to release its hormones and then those hormones stimulate receptors on an organ to produce an effect.

The action of hormones involves **stimulation** or **inhibition**. Some hormones stimulate an endocrine gland to secrete its hormones, or they directly stimulate receptors on an organ or tissue. Other hormones inhibit an endocrine gland from secreting its hormones.

When two hormones, such as T_3 and T_4, work in conjunction with one another to accomplish an enhanced effect, this is known as **synergism**. When two hormones, such as calcitonin and parathyroid hormone, exert opposite effects, this is known as **antagonism** (see Figure 13-7 ■).

The endocrine system maintains body **homeostasis** through the use of hormones and a negative feedback mechanism. For example, after the anterior pituitary gland secretes thyroid-stimulating hormone, it then monitors the blood levels of thyroid hormones. If the levels are still low (negative feedback), the anterior pituitary gland secretes more thyroid-stimulating hormone.

Pronunciation/Word Parts

hormone (HOR-mohn)

hormonal (hor-MOH-nal)
  hormon/o- *hormone*
  -al *pertaining to*

receptor (ree-SEP-ter)
  recept/o- *receive*
  -or *person who does or produces; thing that does or produces*

stimulation (STIM-yoo-LAY-shun)
  stimul/o- *exciting; strengthening*
  -ation *being; having; process*

inhibition (IN-hih-BIH-shun)
  inhibit/o- *block; hold back*
  -ion *action; condition*

synergism (SIN-er-jizm)
  syn- *together*
  erg/o- *activity; work*
  -ism *disease from a specific cause; process*

antagonism (an-TAG-on-izm)
  antagon/o- *opposing effect*
  -ism *disease from a specific cause; process*

homeostasis (HOH-mee-oh-STAY-sihs)
  home/o- *same*
  -stasis *standing still; staying in one place*

	HORMONE	ACTION		SOURCE	
BODY METABOLISM	T_3 and T_4	↑	Increases metabolism	Thyroid	
BLOOD GLUCOSE	Cortisol	↑	Increases blood glucose	Adrenal cortex	
	Epinephrine	↑	Increases blood glucose	Adrenal medulla	
	Glucagon	↑	Increases blood glucose	Pancreas	
	Insulin	↓	Decreases blood glucose (glucose transported into cells to be metabolized)	Pancreas	
BLOOD CALCIUM	Parathyroid hormone	↑	Increases blood calcium	Parathyroid	
	Calcitonin	↓	Decreases blood calcium	Thyroid	
BLOOD SODIUM	Aldosterone	↑	Increases blood sodium	Adrenal cortex	

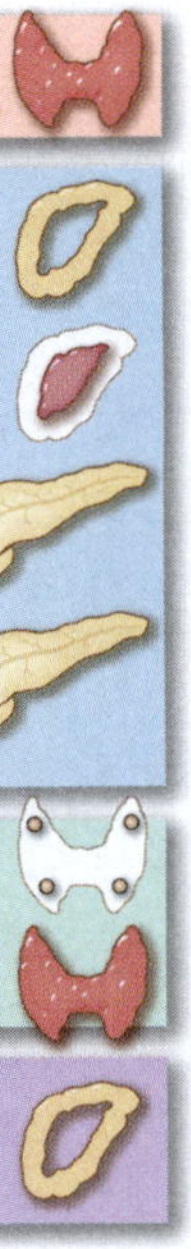

FIGURE 13-7 ■ Effects of hormones. Hormones from various endocrine glands affect body metabolism, blood glucose, blood calcium, and blood sodium in similar (synergism) or opposite (antagonism) ways.

13.2 PRACTICE LAPS

Use the Answer Key at the end of the book to check your answers.

A. Give the Meaning of Combining Forms

Next to each combining form, write its meaning. The first one has been done for you.

Combining Form	Meaning	Combining Form	Meaning
1. **antagon/o-**	*opposing effect*	5. inhibit/o-	
2. erg/o-		6. recept/o-	
3. home/o-		7. stimul/o-	
4. hormon/o-			

B. Build Words

Read the definition of the medical word. Look at the combining form that is given. Select the correct suffix from the Suffix List, and write it on the blank line. Then build the medical word, and write it on the line. (Remember: You may need to remove the combining vowel. Always remove the hyphens and slash.) Be sure to check your spelling.

Suffix List

-al (pertaining to) -ation (being; having; process) -ion (action; condition)	-ism (disease from a specific cause; process) -or (thing that does or produces)	-stasis (standing still; staying in one place)

Definition of the Medical Word	Combining Form	Suffix	Build the Medical Word
Example: Action (to) block (or) hold back	**inhibit/o-**	*-ion*	*inhibition*

[*You think* action (-ion) + block (or) hold back (inhibit/o-). *You change the order of the word parts to put the suffix last. You write* inhibition.]

Definition of the Medical Word	Combining Form	Suffix	Build the Medical Word
1. Thing that does receive	recept/o-		
2. Having (a) strengthening (effect)	stimul/o-		
3. Process (of an) opposing effect	antagon/o-		
4. Pertaining to (a) hormone	hormon/o-		
5. Staying in one place (and staying the) same	home/o-		

Vocabulary Review

Word or Phrase	Description	Combining Forms
Overview		
endocrine system	Body system that includes endocrine glands in various locations in the body that produce and secrete hormones directly into the blood. These glands include the pituitary gland, hypothalamus, pineal gland, thyroid gland, parathyroid glands, thymus, pancreas, adrenal glands, ovaries, and testes.	**end/o-** *innermost; within* **crin/o-** *secrete*
gland	Structure of the endocrine system that produces and secretes one or more hormones into the blood	**glandul/o-** *gland*
homeostasis	State of equilibrium of the internal environment of the body. The endocrine system plays a role in homeostasis by using hormones to regulate body fluids, electrolytes, glucose, cellular metabolism, growth, and the sleep–wake cycle (circadian rhythm).	**home/o-** *same*
hormone	Chemical messenger of the endocrine system that is produced by a gland and secreted into the blood. It exerts an effect on a gland or an organ that has a receptor for that specific hormone to bind to.	**hormon/o-** *hormone*
Pituitary Gland		
pituitary gland	Endocrine gland in the brain that is connected by a stalk of tissue to the hypothalamus. The pituitary gland sits in the bony cup of the sella turcica in the sphenoid bone. It is the "master gland of the body." Also known as the **hypophysis**. It consists of an anterior lobe and posterior lobe, each of which has a different endocrine function.	**pituit/o-** *pituitary gland* **pituitar/o-** *pituitary gland* **hypophys/o-** *pituitary gland*
Anterior Pituitary Gland		
adrenocorticotropic hormone (ACTH)	Hormone produced and secreted by the anterior pituitary gland. It stimulates the cortex of the adrenal gland to secrete its hormones.	**adren/o-** *adrenal gland* **cortic/o-** *cortex; outer region* **trop/o-** *having an affinity for; stimulating; turning*
anterior pituitary gland	Lobe of the pituitary gland that produces and secretes seven hormones: thyroid-stimulating hormone (TSH), prolactin (PRL), follicle-stimulating hormone (FSH), luteinizing hormone (LH), adrenocorticotropic hormone (ACTH), growth hormone (GH), and melanocyte-stimulating hormone (MSH). Also known as the **adenohypophysis** because it is a true gland.	**anter/o-** *front part* **pituit/o-** *pituitary gland* **pituitar/o-** *pituitary gland* **aden/o-** *gland* **hypophys/o-** *pituitary gland*
follicle-stimulating hormone (FSH)	Hormone produced and secreted by the anterior pituitary gland. In females, it stimulates follicles in the ovary to produce mature ova and to secrete the hormone estradiol. In males, it stimulates the seminiferous tubules of the testes to produce spermatozoa.	**folli/o-** *sac-like structure* **stimul/o-** *exciting; strengthening*
gonadotropins	Category of hormones that stimulates the male and female sex glands (gonads). It includes FSH and LH.	**gonad/o-** *gonad; ovary; testis* **trop/o-** *having an affinity for; stimulating; turning*
growth hormone (GH)	Hormone produced and secreted by the anterior pituitary gland. It stimulates growth and protein synthesis in all cells. It increases height and weight during childhood and puberty.	

Word or Phrase	Description	Combining Forms
luteinizing hormone (LH)	Hormone produced and secreted by the anterior pituitary gland. In females, it stimulates a follicle in the ovary to release a mature ovum each month. It stimulates the corpus luteum (ruptured ovarian follicle) to secrete estradiol and progesterone. In males, it stimulates the interstitial cells of the testes to secrete testosterone.	
melanocyte-stimulating hormone (MSH)	Hormone produced and secreted by the anterior pituitary gland. It is secreted in pregnant women and stimulates melanocytes in the skin to produce melanin. This causes a darkened pigmentation on the face and abdomen.	**melan/o-** *black*
prolactin (PRL)	Hormone produced and secreted by the anterior pituitary gland. It stimulates the development of the breasts during puberty and stimulates them to produce milk for breastfeeding.	**lact/o-** *milk* **galact/o-** *milk*
thyroid-stimulating hormone (TSH)	Hormone produced and secreted by the anterior pituitary gland. It stimulates the thyroid gland to grow and to secrete the thyroid hormones T_3 and T_4.	**thyr/o-** *shield-shaped structure; thyroid gland* **stimul/o-** *exciting; strengthening*
Posterior Pituitary Gland		
antidiuretic hormone (ADH)	Hormone produced by the hypothalamus but stored in and secreted by the posterior pituitary gland. ADH acts on the tubules of the kidneys to increase the reabsorption of sodium and water back into the blood. This decreases urine output (antidiuretic effect) and helps to maintain a normal blood volume and blood pressure.	**ur/o-** *urinary system; urine*
oxytocin (OXT)	Hormone produced by the hypothalamus but stored in and secreted by the posterior pituitary gland. It stimulates the pregnant uterus to contract during labor and childbirth and causes the uterus to contract after birth to prevent hemorrhaging. It stimulates the breasts to release milk for breastfeeding.	**ox/y-** *oxygen; quick* **toc/o-** *childbirth; labor*
posterior pituitary gland	Lobe of the pituitary gland that stores and secretes ADH and oxytocin produced by the hypothalamus; it secretes these hormones in response to a nerve impulse from the hypothalamus. Also known as the **neurohypophysis**.	**poster/o-** *back part* **pituit/o-** *pituitary gland* **neur/o-** *nerve*
Hypothalamus		
hypothalamus	Endocrine gland in the brain just below the thalamus. The hypothalamus secretes hormones that stimulate or inhibit the secretion of hormones from the anterior pituitary gland. It also produces oxytocin hormone and antidiuretic hormone that are stored in the posterior pituitary gland.	**thalam/o-** *thalamus*
Pineal Gland		
melatonin	Hormone secreted by the pineal gland. It regulates the 24-hour sleep–wake cycle and the onset and duration of sleep.	**melaton/o-** *black*
pineal gland	Endocrine gland between the two lobes of the thalamus. It secretes the hormone melatonin.	
Thyroid Gland		
calcitonin	Hormone secreted by the thyroid gland. It regulates the amount of calcium in the blood. If the calcium level is too high, calcitonin suppresses bone breakdown (to decrease calcium released into the blood) and increases the excretion of calcium in the urine.	**calc/i-** *calcium* **ton/o-** *pressure; tone* **calc/o-** *calcium*

Word or Phrase	Description	Combining Forms
euthyroidism	Steady state of normal functioning of the thyroid gland producing and secreting its hormones	**thyroid/o-** *thyroid gland*
triiodothyronine (T₃)	Hormone secreted by the thyroid gland. It increases the rate of cellular metabolism.	**iod/o-** *iodine* **thyr/o-** *shield-shaped structure; thyroid gland*
thyroxine (T₄)	Hormone secreted by the thyroid gland. Most of it is changed into T₃ by the liver.	
thyroid gland	Endocrine gland in the neck that secretes the hormones T₃, T₄, and calcitonin when stimulated by TSH from the anterior pituitary gland	**thyr/o-** *shield-shaped structure; thyroid gland* **thyroid/o-** *thyroid gland*

Parathyroid Glands		
parathyroid glands	Four small endocrine glands on the posterior surface of the thyroid gland. They secrete parathyroid hormone.	**thyr/o-** *shield-shaped structure; thyroid gland*
parathyroid hormone	Hormone secreted by the parathyroid glands. It regulates the amount of calcium in the blood. If the calcium level is too low, parathyroid hormone stimulates the release of calcium from the bones and into the blood.	**thyr/o-** *shield-shaped structure; thyroid gland*

Thymus Gland		
thymus	Endocrine gland posterior to the sternum and within the mediastinum. It secretes hormones called **thymosins**.	**thym/o-** *rage; thymus*
thymosin	Secreted by the thymus. It causes immature T cell lymphocytes in the thymus to mature.	**thym/o-** *rage; thymus*

Pancreas		
glucagon	Hormone secreted by **alpha cells** in the islets of Langerhans. It stimulates the liver to convert glycogen (glucose stored in the liver) to glucose and release it into the blood.	**gluc/o-** *glucose; sugar* **ag/o-** *lead to*
glucose	A simple sugar that is the main source of energy for cellular metabolism. Glucose in the blood comes from digested foods and from glycogen (glucose stored in the liver) when it is converted into glucose by the hormone glucagon.	**gluc/o-** *glucose; sugar* **glycos/o-** *glucose; sugar*
glycogen	Glucose stored in the liver. It is converted to glucose by the hormone glucagon from the pancreas and by the hormone cortisol from the adrenal cortex.	**glyc/o-** *glucose; sugar*
insulin	Hormone secreted by **beta cells** in the islets of Langerhans. It transports glucose into the cells where it is metabolized for energy.	**insul/o-** *island* **insulin/o-** *insulin*
pancreas	Endocrine gland posterior to the stomach. It contains the **islets of Langerhans** (alpha, beta, and delta cells) that secrete the hormones glucagon, insulin, and somatostatin.	**pancreat/o-** *pancreas*
somatostatin	Hormone secreted by **delta cells** in the islets of Langerhans. It inhibits the secretion of glucagon and insulin from the pancreas. It inhibits the secretion of growth hormone from the anterior pituitary gland.	**somat/o-** *body* **stat/o-** *standing still; staying in one place*

Word or Phrase	Description	Combining Forms
Adrenal Glands		
adrenal cortex	Outer layer of the adrenal gland. When stimulated by ACTH from the anterior pituitary gland, the adrenal cortex secretes three groups of hormones: mineralocorticoids (primarily aldosterone), glucocorticoids (primarily cortisol), and androgens (male sex hormones).	**adren/o-** *adrenal gland* **cortic/o-** *cortex; outer region*
adrenal glands	Endocrine glands on top of the kidneys. The adrenal gland consists of two parts: the cortex (an outer layer) and the medulla (an inner layer), each of which is a gland that secretes its own hormones.	**adrenal/o-** *adrenal gland* **adren/o-** *adrenal gland* **ren/o-** *kidney*
adrenal medulla	Inner layer of the adrenal gland. It secretes the hormones norepinephrine, epinephrine, and dopamine.	**adren/o-** *adrenal gland* **medull/o-** *inner region; medulla*
aldosterone	Most abundant and biologically active of the mineralocorticoid hormones secreted by the adrenal cortex. When the blood pressure is low, aldosterone causes reabsorption of sodium and water from tubules in the kidney into the blood. This increases the blood volume and the blood pressure.	
androgens	Group of male sex hormones secreted by the adrenal cortex and by the testes. It includes testosterone, the most abundant and biologically active of the androgens.	**andr/o-** *male* **viril/o-** *masculine*
cortisol	Most abundant and biologically active of the glucocorticoid hormones secreted by the adrenal cortex. It stimulates the liver to convert glycogen to glucose to increase the level of glucose in the blood. It decreases the formation of proteins and new tissues, and it has an anti-inflammatory effect.	
dopamine	Hormone secreted by the adrenal medulla during times of stress. It is also a neurotransmitter between the brain and spinal cord of the nervous system.	
epinephrine	Hormone secreted by the adrenal medulla in response to a nerve impulse from the sympathetic division of the nervous system during times of danger or anger. It produces the "fight-or-flight" response.	
glucocorticoids	Group of hormones secreted by the adrenal cortex, of which cortisol is the most abundant and biologically active.	**gluc/o-** *glucose; sugar* **cortic/o-** *cortex; outer region*
mineralocorticoids	Group of hormones secreted by the adrenal cortex, of which aldosterone is the most abundant and biologically active.	**mineral/o-** *electrolyte; mineral* **cortic/o-** *cortex; outer region*
norepinephrine	Hormone secreted by the adrenal medulla. It is also a neurotransmitter between the brain and the spinal cord of the nervous system.	
Ovaries		
estradiol	Most abundant and biologically active of all the female sex hormones. Estradiol is secreted by the follicles and corpus luteum of the ovary when stimulated by FSH from the anterior pituitary gland.	**estr/a-** *female* **estr/o-** *female*
ovaries	Endocrine glands near the uterus; they are the female sex glands (gonads). FSH from the anterior pituitary gland stimulates the follicles of the ovary to secrete estradiol. LH from the anterior pituitary gland stimulates the corpus luteum (ruptured ovarian follicle) to secrete estradiol and progesterone. The cells around the follicles secrete the male sex hormone testosterone.	**ovari/o-** *ovary*

Word or Phrase	Description	Combining Forms
progesterone	Female sex hormone secreted by the corpus luteum of the ovary when stimulated by LH from the anterior pituitary gland	
Testes		
testes	Endocrine glands on either side of the scrotum; they are the male sex glands (gonads). Also known as **testicles**. FSH from the anterior pituitary gland stimulates their seminiferous tubules to produce spermatozoa. LH from the anterior pituitary gland stimulates their interstitial cells to secrete testosterone.	**testicul/o-** *testicle; testis* **test/o-** *testicle; testis*
testosterone	Most abundant and biologically active of the male sex hormones. Testosterone is secreted by the interstitial cells of the testes when stimulated by LH from the anterior pituitary gland.	**test/o-** *testicle; testis*
Hormone Actions		
antagonism	Process in which two hormones exert opposite effects	**antagon/o-** *opposing effect*
inhibition	Action of a hormone that inhibits an endocrine gland from secreting its hormones	**inhibit/o-** *block; hold back*
receptor	Structure on the cell membrane of an organ or gland where a hormone binds and exerts an effect	**recept/o-** *receive*
stimulation	Action of a hormone that stimulates an endocrine gland to secrete its hormones or stimulates a receptor on an organ or tissue	**stimul/o-** *exciting; strengthening*
synergism	Process in which two hormones work together to accomplish an enhanced effect	**erg/o-** *activity; work*

13.3 Diseases

Word or Phrase	Description	Pronunciation/Word Parts

Anterior Pituitary Gland

hyperpituitarism	Hypersecretion of one or all of the hormones of the anterior pituitary gland. It is caused by a benign tumor (**adenoma**) in the anterior pituitary gland. Treatment: Drug therapy to suppress secretion of the hormones or surgery to remove the adenoma, with radiation therapy to destroy any remaining adenoma	**hyperpituitarism** (HY-per-pih-TOO-ih-tair-IZM) **hyper-** *above; more than normal* **pituitar/o-** *pituitary gland* **-ism** *disease from a specific cause; process* **adenoma** (AD-eh-NOH-mah) **aden/o-** *gland* **-oma** *mass; tumor* **adenomata** (AD-eh-NOH-mah-tah) Greek plural noun: Change the singular ending -oma to -omata.

Word or Phrase	Description	Pronunciation/Word Parts
hypopituitarism	Hyposecretion of one or more of the hormones of the anterior pituitary gland. It is caused by an injury or a defect in the anterior pituitary gland. **Panhypopituitarism** is hyposecretion of all of the hormones. Treatment: Drug therapy to replace the hormone(s)	**hypopituitarism** (HY-poh-pih-TOO-ih-tair-IZM) **hypo-** *below; deficient* **pituitar/o-** *pituitary gland* **-ism** *disease from a specific cause; process* **panhypopituitarism** (pan-HY-poh-pih-TOO-ih-tair-IZM) The prefix **pan-** means *all*.

Thyroid-Stimulating Hormone (TSH)

Hypersecretion and hyposecretion of TSH are described in a later section about hypersecretion and hyposecretion of hormones from the thyroid gland.

Prolactin (PRL)

| galactorrhea | Hypersecretion of prolactin. It is caused by an adenoma in the anterior pituitary gland. In women, the high level of prolactin stimulates the breasts to produce milk, even though the patient is not pregnant. It also inhibits the secretion of FSH and LH and this stops menstruation. Galactorrhea can also occur in men who have an adenoma in the anterior pituitary gland. Treatment: Drug therapy to suppress secretion of prolactin or surgery to remove the adenoma, with radiation therapy to destroy any remaining adenoma | **galactorrhea** (gah-LAK-toh-REE-ah) **galact/o-** *milk* **-rrhea** *discharge; flow* |
| failure of lactation | Hyposecretion of prolactin. It is caused by a defect in the anterior pituitary gland. The low level of prolactin prevents the development of the lactiferous lobules (milk glands) in the breasts during puberty, and the breasts do not make enough milk for breastfeeding after the baby is born. Treatment: None | **lactation** (lak-TAY-shun) **lact/o-** *milk* **-ation** *being; having; process* |

Clinical Connections

Pathology. In almost all patients with an endocrine gland tumor, the tumor is a benign (not cancerous) adenoma. A **microadenoma** is a very small benign tumor.

Nuclear Medicine. Radiation therapy uses x-rays delivered in small (fractionated) doses every day for several weeks to destroy any adenoma remaining after surgery.

microadenoma (MY-kroh-AD-eh-NOH-mah) **micr/o-** *one millionth; small* **aden/o-** *gland* **-oma** *mass; tumor*

Follicle-Stimulating Hormone (FSH) and Luteinizing Hormone (LH)

Hypersecretion and hyposecretion of FSH and LH are described in a later section about hypersecretion and hyposecretion of hormones from the ovaries and testes.

Adrenocorticotropic Hormone (ACTH)

Hypersecretion and hyposecretion of ACTH are described in a later section about hypersecretion and hyposecretion of hormones from the adrenal gland.

Word or Phrase	Description	Pronunciation/Word Parts

Growth Hormone (GH)

Word or Phrase	Description	Pronunciation/Word Parts
gigantism	Hypersecretion of growth hormone during childhood and puberty (see Figure 13-8 ■). It is caused by an adenoma in the anterior pituitary gland. The high level of growth hormone stimulates the bones and tissues to grow excessively. Treatment: Drug therapy to suppress secretion of growth hormone or surgery to remove the adenoma, with radiation therapy to destroy any remaining adenoma 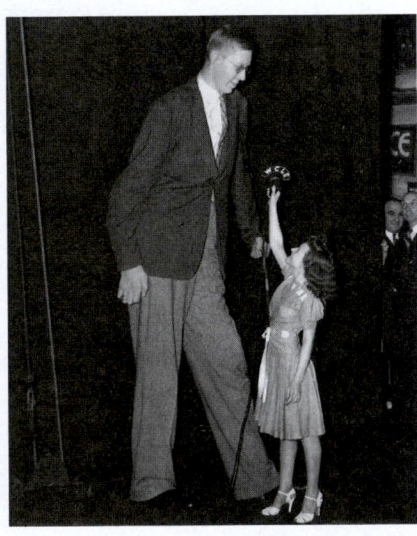 **FIGURE 13-8 ■ Gigantism.** The tallest man who ever lived suffered from gigantism. Robert Wadlow was born in 1918 and was of average weight and length at birth. By the time he was 8 years old, he was taller than his father. As a teenager, he was 8'11" and weighed 490 pounds. He wore size 37AA shoes that were over 18" in length. His height was a curiosity and he was often interviewed and went on tour with the circus. He died at the age of 22. The tallest living man now is Sultan Kosen of Turkey, who was born in 1982 and is 8'2" tall.	**gigantism** (jy-GAN-tizm) **gigant/o-** *giant* **-ism** *disease from a specific cause; process*
acromegaly	Hypersecretion of growth hormone during adulthood. It is caused by an adenoma in the anterior pituitary gland. Because the growth plates at the ends of the long bones have already fused, the patient cannot grow taller. So, the high level of growth hormone causes the facial features, jaw, hands, and feet to widen and enlarge (see Figure 13-9 ■). Treatment: Drug therapy to suppress secretion of growth hormone or surgery to remove the adenoma, with radiation therapy to destroy any remaining adenoma 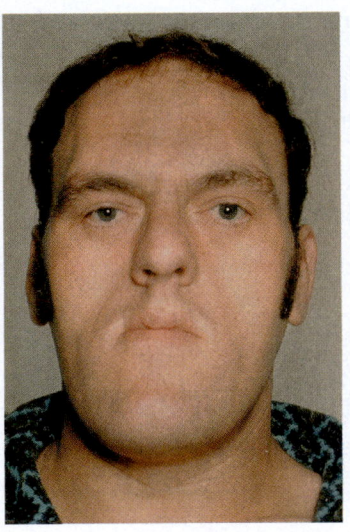 **FIGURE 13-9 ■ Acromegaly.** An increased level of growth hormone in adulthood causes the face and extremities to widen excessively.	**acromegaly** (AK-roh-MEG-ah-lee) **acr/o-** *extremity; highest point* **-megaly** *enlargement*

Word or Phrase	Description	Pronunciation/Word Parts
dwarfism	Hyposecretion of growth hormone during childhood and puberty. It is caused by a defect in the anterior pituitary gland. The low level of growth hormone causes a lack of growth and short stature, but with normal body proportions. Hyposecretion in adults causes decreased muscle mass, fatigue, and other symptoms. Treatment: Drug therapy with growth hormone	**dwarfism** (DWORF-izm) *Dwarfism* is a combination of the word *dwarf* and the suffix **-ism** (*disease from a specific cause; process*).

Clinical Connections

Genetics. Dwarfism has other causes besides hyposecretion of growth hormone. Achondroplasia is a genetic mutation in which cartilage does not convert to bone. This results in an individual with small extremities but a normal-sized trunk. Short stature in an otherwise normal person can also be caused by severe malnutrition, very short parents (heredity), or severe kidney or heart disease as a child.

Posterior Pituitary Gland

Antidiuretic Hormone (ADH)

Word or Phrase	Description	Pronunciation/Word Parts
syndrome of inappropriate ADH (SIADH)	Hypersecretion of ADH. It is caused by an adenoma in the posterior pituitary gland. (It can also be caused by brain infections, multiple sclerosis, or stroke.) The high level of ADH acts on the kidneys to increase reabsorption of excessive amounts of water and some sodium from the kidney tubules back into the blood. This dilutes the blood, creating a low blood level of sodium, and that causes headache, weakness, confusion, and eventually coma. Treatment: Restriction of water intake; surgery to remove the adenoma, with radiation therapy to destroy any remaining adenoma	
diabetes insipidus (DI)	Hyposecretion of ADH. It is caused by a defect in the posterior pituitary gland, a brain infection, head trauma, or heredity. The low level of ADH decreases reabsorption of sodium and water from the kidney tubules and so excessive amounts of water are excreted in the urine (**polyuria**). There is also weakness (due to water loss and dehydration) and thirst, which causes an increased intake of fluids (**polydipsia**). Treatment: Drug therapy with antidiuretic hormone	**diabetes** (DY-ah-BEE-teez) **insipidus** (in-SIP-ih-duhs) **polyuria** (PAW-lee-YOOR-ee-ah) **poly-** *many; much* **ur/o-** *urinary system; urine* **-ia** *condition; state; thing* **polydipsia** (PAW-lee-DIP-see-ah) **poly-** *many; much* **dips/o-** *thirst* **-ia** *condition; state; thing*

Clinical Connections

Urology. The Latin word *insipidus* and the English word *insipid* both mean *lacking a distinctive appearance or taste*. Patients with diabetes insipidus have tasteless, dilute urine (like water) while the urine of patients with diabetes mellitus is sweet. Before there were laboratories, physicians used to taste the patient's urine to make a diagnosis of either diabetes insipidus or diabetes mellitus.

Word or Phrase	Description	Pronunciation/Word Parts

Oxytocin (OXT)

	There is no specific disease associated with hypersecretion of oxytocin.	

uterine inertia	Hyposecretion of oxytocin. It is caused by a defect in the posterior pituitary gland. Before a woman gives birth, the low level of oxytocin in her blood causes weak and uncoordinated contractions of the pregnant uterus. This prolongs labor and delays the birth of the baby. After the birth of the baby, the low blood level of oxytocin causes **postpartum hemorrhage** (the uterus does not contract, and there is hemorrhaging at the site where the placenta separated from the uterus).
	Treatment: Drug therapy with oxytocin hormone
		uterine (YOO-teh-rin)
		    uter/o- *uterus; womb*
		    -ine *pertaining to*
		
		inertia (in-ER-shah)
		
		postpartum (post-PAR-tum)
		    post- *after; behind*
		    part/o- *childbirth; labor*
		    -um *period of time; structure*

Pineal Gland

Melatonin

seasonal affective disorder (SAD)	Hypersecretion of melatonin. The exact cause is not known. Melatonin is normally secreted during the night. The longer nights and decreased hours of sunshine during the winter months may disrupt the body's circadian rhythm (biological clock) and increase the secretion of melatonin. The high level of melatonin causes depression, weight gain, and an increased desire for food and sleep. There is also a decreased level of the neurotransmitter serotonin that affects the mood.
	Treatment: Exposure to sunlight or to bright light from a light box (phototherapy) to suppress melatonin secretion; drug therapy with melatonin and/or an antidepressant drug
		affective (ah-FEK-tiv)
		    affect/o- *have an influence on; mood; state of mind*
		    -ive *pertaining to*

	There is no specific disease associated with hyposecretion of melatonin.	

Thyroid Gland

T$_3$ and T$_4$ Thyroid Hormones

hyperthyroidism	Hypersecretion of T$_3$ and T$_4$ thyroid hormones. It is caused by an adenoma (or **nodule**) in the thyroid gland. (It can also be caused by an adenoma in the anterior pituitary gland that causes hypersecretion of TSH that stimulates the overproduction of T$_3$ and T$_4$.) The high levels of T$_3$ and T$_4$ cause tremors of the hands, tachycardia, palpitations, restlessness, nervousness, diarrhea, insomnia, fatigue, and generalized weight loss. The thyroid gland is enlarged (a **goiter**) and can be felt on palpation of the neck. The eyes are dry and irritated with slow eyelid closing ("lid lag"). The most common type of hyperthyroidism is **Graves disease**. This is an autoimmune disease in which the body produces antibodies that stimulate TSH receptors on the thyroid gland, and this increases the production of thyroid hormones. The entire thyroid gland becomes enlarged (diffuse toxic goiter), and there is **exophthalmos** (see Figure 13-10 ■).
	Treatment: Antithyroid drug to suppress the secretion of T$_3$ and T$_4$ or surgery to remove the thyroid gland (thyroidectomy), with radiation therapy with radioactive iodine to destroy the remaining thyroid gland
		hyperthyroidism
		(HY-per-THY-royd-izm)
		    hyper- *above; more than normal*
		    thyroid/o- *thyroid gland*
		    -ism *disease from a specific cause; process*
		
		nodule (NAW-dyool)
		    nod/o- *knob of tissue; node*
		    -ule *small thing*
		
		goiter (GOY-ter)
		
		exophthalmos
		(EKS-off-THAL-mohs)
		Exophthalmos is a combination of the prefix **ex-** (*away from; out*) and the Greek word *ophthalmos* (*eye*).

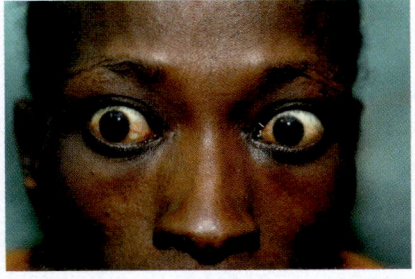

FIGURE 13-10 ■ Exophthalmos.
Exophthalmos is a well-known sign of hyperthyroidism. Edema behind the eyeballs causes them to protrude. This creates a staring expression that shows a large amount of white sclerae.

Word or Phrase	Description	Pronunciation/Word Parts

Dive Deeper

A **goiter** is a chronic and progressive enlargement of the thyroid gland. It is also known as **thyromegaly**. A physician can feel this enlargement during a physical examination (see Figure 13-11 ■) even before it becomes visible. The causes of goiter include:

1. An **adenoma** or nodule growing in the thyroid gland. This is known as an **adenomatous goiter** or **nodular goiter**. If there are many nodules, it is a **multinodular goiter**. An adenoma or nodule is usually benign but can be cancerous.

2. A cancerous tumor growing in the thyroid gland.

3. Chronic inflammation of the thyroid gland as seen in thyroiditis.

4. A lack of iodine in the soil, water, and diet. This causes the thyroid gland to enlarge to help it capture more iodine; this is known as a **simple goiter**, a **nontoxic goiter**, or an **endemic goiter** (because it occurs in people who live in an area where the soil is poor in iodine).

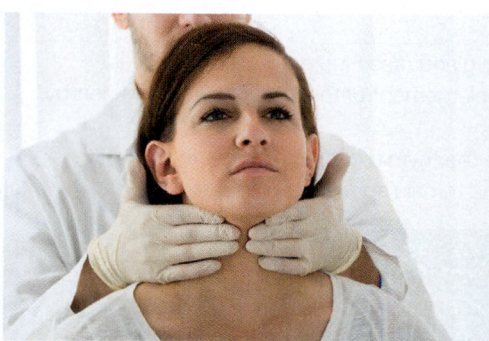
A.

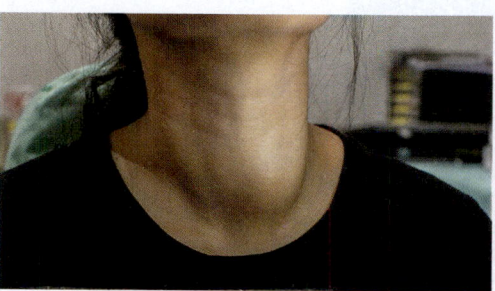
B.

FIGURE 13-11 ■ Physical examination of the thyroid gland.
A. The anterior location of the thyroid gland means that even mild enlargement can be detected. This physician is palpating the edges of the patient's thyroid gland to determine its size. **B.** A large goiter can cause severe swelling of the neck with coughing and difficulty swallowing.

goiter (GOY-ter)

thyromegaly
(THY-roh-MEG-ah-lee)
   thyr/o- *shield-shaped structure;*
   thyroid gland
   -megaly *enlargement*

adenoma (AD-eh-NOH-mah)
   aden/o- *gland*
   -oma *mass; tumor*

adenomatous
(AD-eh-NOH-mah-tuhs)
   aden/o- *gland*
   -oma *mass; tumor*
   -tous *pertaining to*

nodular (NAW-dyoo-lar)
   nodul/o- *small, knobby mass*
   -ar *pertaining to*

multinodular
(MUL-tee-NAW-dyoo-lar)
The combining form **mult/i-**
means *many.*

nontoxic (non-TAWK-sik)
   non- *not*
   tox/o- *poison*
   -ic *pertaining to*

endemic (en-DEM-ik)
   en- *in; inward; within*
   dem/o- *people; population*
   -ic *pertaining to*

Clinical Connections

Dietetics. The production of T₃ is dependent on adequate amounts of the trace mineral iodine in the diet. The ancient Chinese used seaweed to treat goiter because seaweed contains iodine. Iodine can be obtained from eating seafood, from vegetables grown in soil that contains iodine, and from drinking water that contains iodine. In the areas of the Great Lakes and Midwest of the United States, the soil and water are deficient in iodine. This is known as the "goiter belt" because persons living there tend to develop endemic goiters from having too little iodine. Iodine was first added to table salt in 1924, and iodized salt was sold everywhere by 1940. The widespread use of iodized salt has decreased the incidence of this type of goiter.

Word or Phrase	Description	Pronunciation/Word Parts
hypothyroidism	Hyposecretion of T_3 and T_4 thyroid hormones. It is usually caused by an inadequate amount of iodine in the diet. It can also be caused by hyposecretion of TSH from the anterior pituitary gland or by treatments for hyperthyroidism that remove the thyroid gland. Another possible cause is a defect in the thyroid gland at birth that causes **congenital hypothyroidism**. Untreated congenital hypothyroidism results in stunted growth and developmental delay. **Hashimoto thyroiditis** is an autoimmune disorder in which the body makes antibodies against the thyroid gland, causing loss of function and replacement of the thyroid tissue with fibrous tissue. The low levels of T_3 and T_4 cause fatigue, decreased body temperature, dry hair and skin, constipation, and weight gain. Severe hypothyroidism in adults causes **myxedema**, with swelling of the subcutaneous and connective tissues, tingling in the hands and feet because of nerve compression, lack of menstruation, hair loss, an enlarged heart, bradycardia, an enlarged tongue, slow speech, and mental impairment. Treatment: Thyroid hormone supplement drug	**hypothyroidism** (HY-poh-THY-royd-izm) **hypo-** *below; deficient* **thyroid/o-** *thyroid gland* **-ism** *disease from a specific cause; process* **congenital** (con-JEN-ih-tal) **congenit/o-** *present at birth* **-al** *pertaining to* **Hashimoto** (HASH-ee-MOH-toh) **thyroiditis** (THY-roy-DY-tihs) **thyroid/o-** *thyroid gland* **-itis** *infection of; inflammation of* **myxedema** (MIKS-eh-DEE-mah) **myx/o-** *mucus-like substance* **-edema** *swelling*
thyroid carcinoma	Malignant tumor of the thyroid gland (see Figure 13-12 ■). There is hoarseness, neck pain, and enlargement of the thyroid gland and nearby cancerous lymph nodes. Treatment: Surgery to remove the thyroid gland (thyroidectomy), with radiation therapy to destroy the remaining thyroid gland 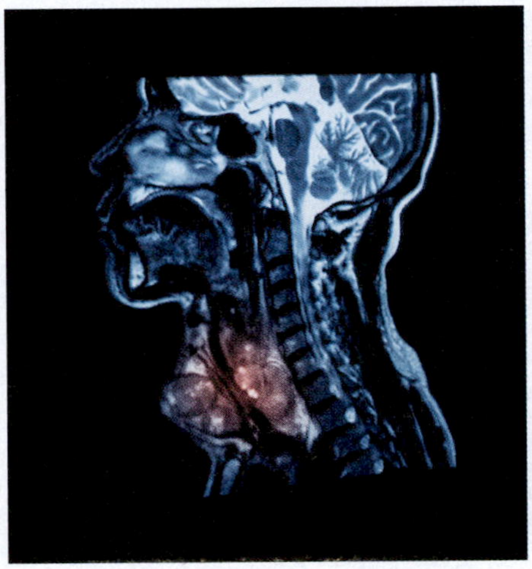 **FIGURE 13-12** ■ **Thyroid carcinoma.** Magnetic resonance imaging shows a large, malignant tumor of the thyroid gland.	**carcinoma** (KAR-sih-NOH-mah) **carcin/o-** *cancer* **-oma** *mass; tumor*

Word or Phrase	Description	Pronunciation/Word Parts

Parathyroid Glands

Parathyroid Hormone

Word or Phrase	Description	Pronunciation/Word Parts
hyperpara-thyroidism	Hypersecretion of parathyroid hormone. It is caused by an adenoma in the parathyroid gland. The high level of parathyroid hormone stimulates the release of too much calcium from the bones, and the calcium level in the blood is too high (**hypercalcemia**). The bones become demineralized and prone to fracture. There is also muscle weakness, fatigue, and depression. Excess calcium is excreted in the urine, and this can form kidney stones. Treatment: Surgery to remove the parathyroid glands	**hyperparathyroidism** (HY-per-PAIR-ah-THY-royd-izm) **hyper-** *above; more than normal* **para-** *abnormal; apart from; beside; two parts of a pair* **thyroid/o-** *thyroid gland* **-ism** *disease from a specific cause; process* **hypercalcemia** (HY-per-kal-SEE-mee-ah) **hyper-** *above; more than normal* **calc/o-** *calcium* **-emia** *condition of the blood; substance in the blood*
hypopara-thyroidism	Hyposecretion of parathyroid hormone. It is caused by the accidental removal of the parathyroid glands during surgery to remove the thyroid gland (thyroidectomy). The low level of parathyroid hormone causes the calcium level in the blood to become very low (**hypocalcemia**). This causes irritability of the nerves, skeletal muscle cramps, or sustained muscle spasm (tetany). Treatment: Parathyroid hormone supplement drug	**hypoparathyroidism** (HY-poh-PAIR-ah-THY-royd-izm) **hypo-** *below; deficient* **para-** *abnormal; apart from; beside; two parts of a pair* **thyroid/o-** *thyroid gland* **-ism** *disease from a specific cause; process* **hypocalcemia** (HY-poh-kal-SEE-mee-ah) **hypo-** *below; deficient* **calc/o-** *calcium* **-emia** *condition of the blood; substance in the blood*

Pancreas

Insulin

Word or Phrase	Description	Pronunciation/Word Parts
hyperinsulinism	Hypersecretion of insulin. It is caused by an adenoma in the pancreas. The high level of insulin causes **hypoglycemia** (a low level of glucose in the blood). There is shakiness, headache, sweating, dizziness, and even fainting. If left untreated, hypoglycemia can progress to insulin shock and then coma as the blood glucose level becomes too low to support brain activity. Treatment: Supplemental sugar drink or dextrose intravenous fluids; surgery to remove the adenoma	**hyperinsulinism** (HY-per-IN-soo-lin-IZM) **hyper-** *above; more than normal* **insulin/o-** *insulin* **-ism** *disease from a specific cause; process* **hypoglycemia** (HY-poh-gly-SEE-mee-ah) **hypo-** *below; deficient* **glyc/o-** *glucose; sugar* **-emia** *condition of the blood; substance in the blood*

Word or Phrase	Description	Pronunciation/Word Parts

Dive Deeper

Persons with a normal level of insulin can also become hypoglycemic when they are dieting or fasting. Diabetic patients can become hypoglycemic when they take an oral antidiabetic drug or inject insulin but then skip a meal.

Clinical Connections

Neonatology. In a mother with uncontrolled gestational diabetes, the fetus is constantly exposed to a high level of glucose in its blood (from the mother via the umbilical cord), and its pancreas constantly secretes large amounts of insulin before birth. This causes the fetus to gain weight, and it becomes large for gestational age. After birth, the newborn drinks small amounts of milk at first, but its pancreas continues to secrete large amounts of insulin. This causes hypoglycemia and sometimes a seizure as the blood sugar quickly falls below normal.
Treatment: Dextrose intravenous fluids

insulin resistance syndrome (IRS)	Hypersecretion of insulin. This is not caused by an adenoma. It occurs when receptors on body cells develop a resistance and do not allow insulin to transport glucose into the cell. There is a high level of glucose remaining in the blood (hyperglycemia), and there is a high level of insulin as the pancreas continues to secrete insulin to try to lower the blood glucose level. Eventually, the pancreas is unable to produce more insulin, and the patient develops diabetes mellitus. Treatment: Treat the diabetes mellitus.	**resistance** (ree-ZIS-tans) **resist/o-** *withstand the effect of* **-ance** *state*

Source: David W. Harbaugh

"Your chart says you have IRS . . . it's either a problem with insulin resistance syndrome or the Internal Revenue Service."

Word or Phrase	Description	Pronunciation/Word Parts

diabetes mellitus (DM)	Hyposecretion of insulin. It is caused by an inability of the beta cells of the pancreas to secrete enough insulin. A person who has diabetes mellitus is a **diabetic**. Laypersons call it "sugar diabetes." The word *mellitus* means *honeyed.* In the past, diabetes mellitus was diagnosed by tasting the urine which had a sweet taste. The different types and names of diabetes mellitus are described in Table 13-1 ■.
	 Treatment: Drug therapy with injections of insulin or an oral antidiabetic drug (depending on the type of diabetes mellitus); diet management, weight control, and exercise; ongoing consultation with a diabetologist physician or a certified diabetes educator (CDE)
		diabetes (DY-ah-BEE-teez)
		
		 mellitus (MEL-ih-tuhs)
		
		 diabetic (DY-ah-BET-ik)
		    diabet/o- *diabetes*
		    -ic *pertaining to*

Table 13-1 Diabetes Mellitus

	Type 1	Type 1.5	Type 2
Other Names	Insulin-dependent diabetes mellitus (IDDM) Juvenile-onset diabetes mellitus	Slow-onset type I Latent autoimmune diabetes in adults (LADA)	Non-insulin-dependent diabetes mellitus (NIDDM) Adult-onset diabetes mellitus (AODM)
Onset	Child, adolescent, young adult	Adult	Adult
Autoimmune disorder	Yes	Yes	No
Antibodies present	Yes	Yes	No
Amount of insulin secreted	None	Too little	Too little
Insulin resistance	No	No	Yes
Body weight	Normal	Normal	Obese
Percentage of all diabetics	10%	15%	75%
Drug therapy	Insulin	Insulin and oral antidiabetic drugs	Oral antidiabetic drugs, occasionally insulin

Dive Deeper

A low level of insulin results in an increased level of glucose in the blood (**hyperglycemia**). Excess glucose in the blood is excreted in the urine (**glycosuria**). As it is excreted, it holds water to it by osmosis, and this increases the amount of urine (**polyuria**). With excessive urination, the patient becomes thirsty and drinks often (**polydipsia**). The patient also feels hungry and eats often (**polyphagia**) because the glucose in the blood cannot be metabolized by the cells.

A "brittle diabetic" has difficulty controlling the blood glucose level, with frequent swings from hyperglycemia to hypoglycemia.

hyperglycemia (HY-per-gly-SEE-mee-ah)
   hyper- *above; more than normal*
   glyc/o- *glucose; sugar*
   -emia *condition of the blood; substance in the blood*

glycosuria (GLY-kohs-YOOR-ee-ah)
   glycos/o- *glucose; sugar*
   ur/o- *urinary system; urine*
   -ia *condition; state; thing*

polyuria (PAW-lee-YOOR-ee-ah)
   poly- *many; much*
   ur/o- *urinary system; urine*
   -ia *condition; state; thing*

polydipsia (PAW-lee-DIP-see-ah)
   poly- *many; much*
   dips/o- *thirst*
   -ia *condition; state; thing*

polyphagia (PAW-lee-FAY-jah)
   poly- *many; much*
   phag/o- *eating; swallowing*
   -ia *condition; state; thing*

Word or Phrase	Description	Pronunciation/Word Parts

Clinical Connections

Obstetrics. Gestational diabetes mellitus (GDM) occurs only during pregnancy, when increased levels of estradiol and progesterone block the action of insulin. The pregnant woman's pancreas is temporarily unable to secrete enough insulin to meet the increased demands from the growing fetus. This type of diabetes mellitus resolves once the baby is delivered; however, many women who had GDM develop type 2 diabetes later in life.

gestational (jes-TAY-shun-al)
  gestat/o- *conception to birth*
  -ion *action; condition*
  -al *pertaining to*

Word Alert
Sound-Alike Words

diabetes insipidus   Caused by hyposecretion of ADH from the posterior pituitary gland

diabetes mellitus   Caused by hyposecretion of insulin or resistance to the insulin that is secreted

Dive Deeper

Excessive urination (polyuria) is a symptom of both diabetes insipidus and diabetes mellitus, but for different reasons. In diabetes insipidus, a lack of ADH causes excessive amounts of water to be excreted in the urine. In diabetes mellitus, excess glucose excreted in the urine holds water to it by osmotic pressure, increasing the volume of urine.

| diabetic ketoacidosis (DKA) | A high level of **ketones** in the blood. This occurs in untreated or uncontrolled diabetes mellitus when there is no insulin to metabolize glucose for cellular energy, and the body turns to other sources of energy such as fat or protein. Body fat contains the most calories per gram, but fat does not metabolize cleanly and leaves ketones, an acidic by-product. The patient's breath has a unique "fruity" or "nail polish" odor from the high level of both glucose and ketones in the blood. A diabetic coma occurs when a very high level of ketones (which are acidic) lowers the pH of the blood to the point that chemical reactions in the body cannot occur and the patient becomes unconscious.
Treatment: Drug therapy with insulin | **ketoacidosis**
(KEE-toh-AS-ih-DOH-sihs)
  ket/o- *ketones*
  acid/o- *acid; low pH*
  -osis *abnormal condition; process*

ketones (KEE-tohnz) |

Dive Deeper

Over time, complications of untreated or uncontrolled diabetes mellitus affect various organs of the body.

1. **Diabetic neuropathy.** Decreased or abnormal sensation in the extremities because of nerve damage due to demyelination of the nerves.

2. **Diabetic nephropathy.** Degenerative changes in the nephrons of the kidneys because of the high levels of glucose and ketones. This causes kidney failure.

3. **Diabetic retinopathy.** Degenerative changes of the retina of the eye because of the local effect of high levels of glucose and ketones. There is formation of new, fragile blood vessels that hemorrhage easily; this causes blindness.

4. **Atherosclerosis.** Fatty deposits and plaque formation with hardening of the arteries, which is accelerated in diabetes mellitus because of abnormalities in fat metabolism.

5. **Impotence.** Nerve damage and atherosclerosis of the arteries to the penis result in difficulty having an erection.

neuropathy (nyoor-AW-pah-thee)
  neur/o- *nerve*
  -pathy *disease*

nephropathy
(neh-FRAW-pah-thee)
  nephr/o- *kidney; nephron*
  -pathy *disease*

retinopathy
(RET-ih-NAW-pah-thee)
  retin/o- *retina*
  -pathy *disease*

Word or Phrase	Description	Pronunciation/Word Parts

Clinical Connections

Podiatry. Patients with diabetes are at high risk for developing gangrene of the feet because of:

- Increased blood sugar that decreases the effectiveness of white blood cells fighting infection. Small cuts do not heal easily and can progress to become an ulcer or gangrene, requiring amputation.
- Decreased sensation in the extremities due to diabetic neuropathy
- Poor eyesight from age and diabetic retinopathy that interferes with proper foot care.

Patients with diabetes are advised to see a podiatrist or physician to have their toenails trimmed.

Adrenal Cortex

Aldosterone		
hyper-aldosteronism	Hypersecretion of aldosterone. It is caused by an adenoma in the adrenal cortex. (It can also be caused by hypersecretion of ACTH from an adenoma in the anterior pituitary gland.) A high level of aldosterone causes the reabsorption of a large amount of sodium and water from the tubules of the kidney into the blood; this causes hypertension, and there is an electrolyte imbalance and weakness as large amounts of potassium are excreted in the urine. Treatment: Surgery to remove the adenoma	**hyperaldosteronism** (HY-per-al-DAW-steh-rohn-IZM) *Hyperaldosteronism* is a combination of the prefix **hyper-** (*above; more than normal*), *aldosterone* (with the -e deleted), and the suffix **-ism** (*disease from a specific cause; process*).
hypo-aldosteronism	Hyposecretion of aldosterone. It is caused by a defect in the adrenal cortex. There is dizziness, a low level of sodium in the blood, weakness, and decreased blood pressure. Treatment: Drug therapy with an aldosterone hormone drug	**hypoaldosteronism** (HY-poh-al-DAW-steh-rohn-IZM)

Word or Phrase	Description	Pronunciation/Word Parts
Cortisol		
Cushing disease and syndrome	Cushing disease is caused by hypersecretion of cortisol from an adenoma in the adrenal cortex. Cushing syndrome occurs in a patient who takes corticosteroid drugs on a long-term basis. The high level of cortisol stimulates the liver to convert too much glycogen to glucose, causing a high level of glucose in the blood. This results in rapid weight gain, with deposits of fat in the face (moon face), upper back (buffalo hump), and abdomen (see Figure 13-13 ■). There is a thinning of connective tissue in the skin of the face that allows the blood vessels to show through, giving a reddened appearance to the cheeks. The thinned connective tissue in the skin across the obese abdomen is stretched, causing small hemorrhages and red and purple striae. There is also a wasted appearance of the muscles in the extremities and muscle weakness because of the lack of protein synthesis. Treatment: Surgery to remove the adenoma; discontinue corticosteroid drugs	**Cushing** (KOOSH-ing) **syndrome** (SIN-drohm) The prefix **syn-** means *together*, and the suffix -**drome** means *a running*.

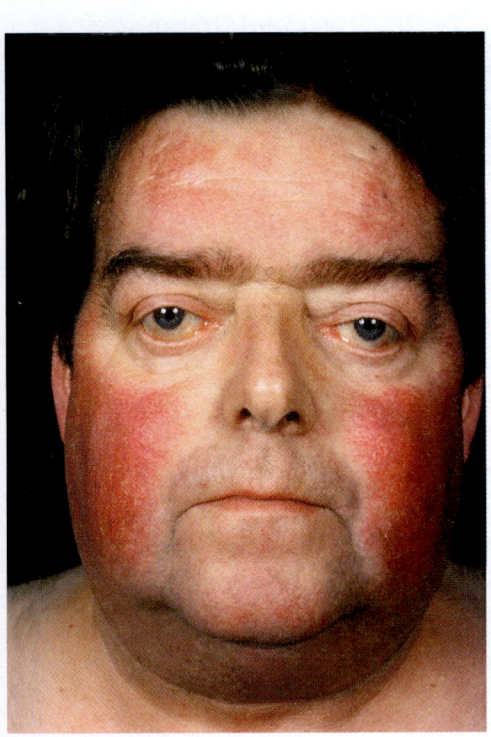

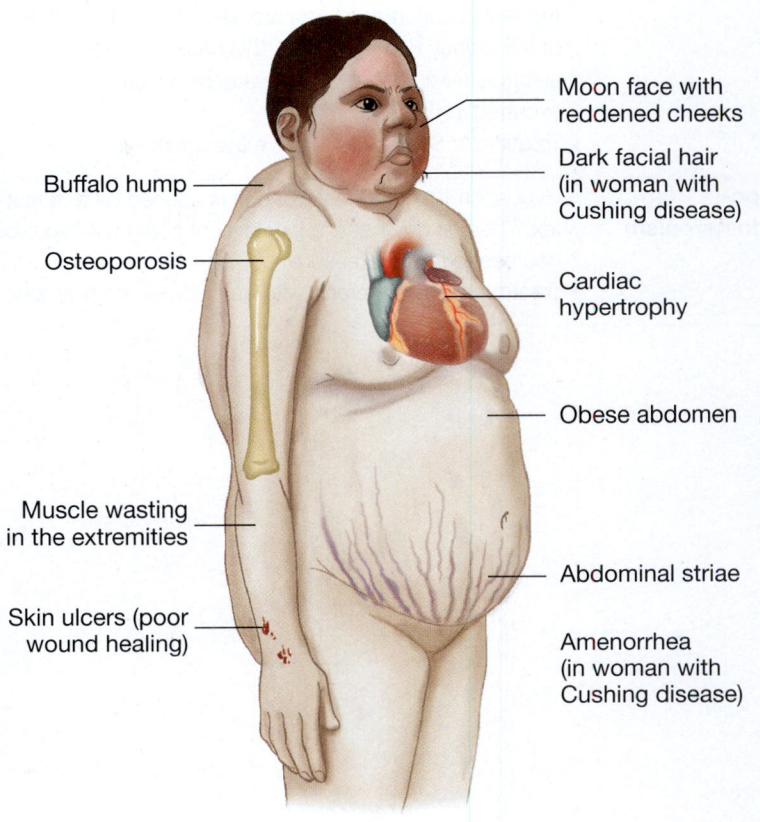

Moon face with reddened cheeks

Dark facial hair (in woman with Cushing disease)

Buffalo hump

Osteoporosis

Cardiac hypertrophy

Obese abdomen

Muscle wasting in the extremities

Abdominal striae

Skin ulcers (poor wound healing)

Amenorrhea (in woman with Cushing disease)

A.   B.

FIGURE 13-13 ■ Cushing disease and syndrome.
A. This patient shows the characteristic signs of Cushing syndrome. Deposits of fat in the cheeks give a moon-face appearance. Breakdown of protein in the connective tissues thins the skin, allowing blood vessels to show through and give the cheeks a reddened appearance. **B.** The abdomen is obese, while the extremities are thin and there is muscle wasting and weakness. In female patients with Cushing disease, there is also dark facial hair and amenorrhea.

Word or Phrase	Description	Pronunciation/Word Parts
Addison disease	Hyposecretion of cortisol. This is an autoimmune disorder in which the body produces antibodies that destroy the adrenal cortex. (It can also be caused by hyposecretion of ACTH from the anterior pituitary gland.) Also known as **adrenal insufficiency**. There is a low level of blood glucose, fatigue, weight loss, and decreased ability to tolerate stress, disease, or surgery. Patients have an unusual bronze color to the skin, even in areas not exposed to the sun. Treatment: Corticosteroid drug	**Addison** (AD-ih-son)

Clinical Connections

Pathology. John F. Kennedy had Addison disease and was given regular doses of cortisone for many years. The allegation that he had Addison disease was denied by his family and doctors during the presidential race in spite of his bronze skin color. President Kennedy was assassinated in 1963, and his autopsy found that his adrenal glands were nonexistent (Addison disease). This information was never made public until 1992 when it was published in the *Journal of the American Medical Association*.

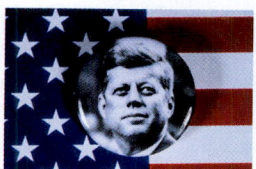

Androgens

Word or Phrase	Description	Pronunciation/Word Parts

adrenogenital syndrome	Hypersecretion of androgens. It is caused by an adenoma in the adrenal gland. In girls, the clitoris and labia enlarge and resemble a penis and scrotum. In boys, it causes precocious puberty. In adult females, it causes **virilism** with masculine facial features and body build, **hirsutism** (excessive, dark hair on the forearms and face), and amenorrhea.
	Treatment: Surgery to remove the adenoma
		adrenogenital
		(ah-DREE-noh-JEN-ih-tal)
		  adren/o- *adrenal gland*
		  genit/o- *genitalia*
		  -al *pertaining to*
		
		virilism (VIR-ih-lizm)
		  viril/o- *masculine*
		  -ism *disease from a specific cause; process*
		
		hirsutism (HER-soo-tizm)
		  hirsut/o- *hairy*
		  -ism *disease from a specific cause; process*

	There is no specific disease associated with hyposecretion of androgens.	

Adrenal Medulla

Epinephrine and Norepinephrine

Word or Phrase	Description	Pronunciation/Word Parts

pheochromocytoma	Hypersecretion of norepinephrine and epinephrine because of an adenoma in the adrenal medulla. This type of adenoma has a characteristic appearance of gray-tan tissue. The high levels of norepinephrine and epinephrine cause heart palpitations, severe sweating, and headaches with severe hypertension that can cause a stroke.
	Treatment: Surgery to remove the pheochromocytoma
		pheochromocytoma
		(FEE-oh-KROH-moh-sy-TOH-mah)
		  phe/o- *gray*
		  chrom/o- *color*
		  cyt/o- *cell*
		  -oma *mass; tumor*
		Pheochromocytoma: *Tumor (with a) gray color (to the) cells (when viewed under a microscope)*

	There is no specific disease associated with hyposecretion of epinephrine and norepinephrine.	

Word or Phrase	Description	Pronunciation/Word Parts

Ovaries

Estradiol and Progesterone

precocious puberty	Hypersecretion of estradiol in a female child. It is caused by an adenoma in the ovary. (It can also be caused by hypersecretion of FSH from an adenoma in the anterior pituitary gland.) The high level of estradiol causes premature development of the breasts and female secondary sexual characteristics and the onset of menstruation and ovulation.
	Treatment: Surgery to remove the adenoma
		precocious (prih-KOH-shuhs)
		
		puberty (PYOO-ber-tee)
		  puber/o- *growing up*
		  -ty *quality; state*

infertility	Hyposecretion of estradiol in an adult female or an imbalance in the amount of estradiol and progesterone. (It can also be caused by a lack of FSH and LH from the anterior pituitary gland.) There is a lack of ovulation, abnormal menstruation, or a history of miscarriages.
	Treatment: Female hormone drug
		infertility (IN-fer-TIL-ih-tee)
		  in- *in; not; within*
		  fertil/o- *conceive; form*
		  -ity *condition; state*

menopause	Hyposecretion of estradiol in an adult female. This is a normal result of the aging process in which the ovaries secrete less and less estradiol. It can also be caused by surgical removal of the ovaries (oophorectomy) due to cancer. The resulting low level of estradiol causes vaginal dryness, thinning of the hair, and lack of sexual drive. As the hypothalamus senses a low estradiol level, it stimulates the anterior pituitary gland to secrete FSH to stimulate the ovary. These bursts of FSH cause hot flashes.
	Treatment: Female hormone replacement therapy, but only for a limited time because these drugs cause an increased risk of breast and endometrial cancer, blood clots, stroke, heart attack, and dementia
		menopause (MEN-oh-pawz)
		  men/o- *month*
		  -pause *cessation*

Testes

Testosterone

precocious puberty	Hypersecretion of testosterone in a male child. It is caused by an adenoma in the testis. (It can also be caused by hypersecretion of LH from an adenoma in the anterior pituitary gland.) The high level of testosterone causes the premature development of the male secondary sexual characteristics, with development of a beard, deepening of the voice, and sperm production.
	Treatment: Surgery to remove the adenoma
		precocious (prih-KOH-shuhs)
		
		puberty (PYOO-ber-tee)
		  puber/o- *growing up*
		  -ty *quality; state*

gynecomastia	Hyposecretion of testosterone in an adult male. This is a normal result of the aging process in which the testes secrete less testosterone. (It can also be caused by surgical removal of the testes due to cancer, by estrogen drug treatment for prostate cancer, by excessive alcohol consumption, or as a side effect of some drugs.) However, androgens continue to be secreted by the adrenal cortex and converted to estradiol in the blood. The low level of testosterone is no longer in balance with the level of estradiol, and this causes enlargement of the male breasts.
	Treatment: Androgen drug; plastic surgery to decrease the breast size
		gynecomastia (GY-neh-koh-MAS-tee-ah)
		  gynec/o- *female; woman*
		  mast/o- *breast; mastoid process*
		  -ia *condition; state; thing*

infertility	Hyposecretion of testosterone in an adult male. It is caused by failure of one or both of the testes to descend into the scrotum before birth. (It can also be caused by surgical removal of the testes due to cancer or by the lack of LH from the anterior pituitary gland.) The low level of testosterone causes too few spermatozoa to be produced.
	Treatment: Surgery as a child to bring the testes into the scrotum to prevent infertility as an adult; androgen drug for an adult
		infertility (IN-fer-TIL-ih-tee)
		  in- *in; not; within*
		  fertil/o- *conceive; form*
		  -ity *condition; state*

13.3 PRACTICE LAPS

Use the Answer Key at the end of the book to check your answers.

A. Give the Meaning of Combining Forms

Next to each combining form, write its meaning. The first one has been done for you.

Combining Form	Meaning	Combining Form	Meaning
1. **resist/o-**	*withstand the effect of*	20. hirsut/o-	
2. acid/o-		21. insulin/o-	
3. acr/o-		22. ket/o-	
4. aden/o-		23. lact/o-	
5. adren/o-		24. mast/o-	
6. affect/o-		25. men/o-	
7. calc/o-		26. micr/o-	
8. carcin/o-		27. myx/o-	
9. chrom/o-		28. nod/o-	
10. congenit/o-		29. part/o-	
11. diabet/o-		30. phag/o-	
12. dips/o-		31. pituitar/o-	
13. fertil/o-		32. puber/o-	
14. galact/o-		33. thyr/o-	
15. genit/o-		34. thyroid/o-	
16. gigant/o-		35. tox/o-	
17. glyc/o-		36. ur/o-	
18. glycos/o-		37. uter/o-	
19. gynec/o-		38. viril/o-	

B. Build Words

Read the definition of the medical word. Look at the combining form that is given. Select the correct suffix from the Suffix List, and write it on the blank line. Then build the medical word, and write it on the line. (Remember: You may need to remove the combining vowel. Always remove the hyphens and slash.) Be sure to check your spelling.

Suffix List

-al (pertaining to)	-ine (pertaining to)	-ive (pertaining to)	-ty (quality; state)
-ance (state)	-ism (disease from a specific	-megaly (enlargement)	-ule (small thing)
-ation (being; having; process)	cause; process)	-oma (mass; tumor)	
	-itis (infection of;	-pause (cessation)	
-ic (pertaining to)	inflammation of)	-rrhea (discharge; flow)	

Definition of the Medical Word	Combining Form	Suffix	Build the Medical Word
Example: State (of being able to) withstand the effect of	**resist/o-**	*-ance*	*resistance*

[*You think* state (*-ance*) + withstand the effect of (*resist/o-*). You change the order of the word parts to put the suffix last. You write resistance.]

#	Definition of the Medical Word	Combining Form	Suffix	Build the Medical Word
1.	Infection of (or) inflammation of (the) thyroid gland	thyroid/o-		
2.	Small thing (that is a) node	nod/o-		
3.	Having milk	lact/o-		
4.	Disease from a specific cause (of being a) giant	gigant/o-		
5.	Discharge (or) flow (of) milk	galact/o-		
6.	Pertaining to diabetes	diabet/o-		
7.	Enlargement (of the) extremities	acr/o-		
8.	Mass (or) tumor (in a) gland	aden/o-		
9.	Pertaining to (being) present at birth	congenit/o-		
10.	Pertaining to mood	affect/o-		
11.	State (of) growing up	puber/o-		
12.	Pertaining to (the) uterus	uter/o-		
13.	Mass (or) tumor (that is) cancer	carcin/o-		
14.	Cessation (of) month(ly periods)	men/o-		

C. Define Abbreviations

1. ACTH _____
2. ADH _____
3. AODM _____
4. DI _____
5. DKA _____
6. DM _____
7. FSH _____
8. GH _____
9. IDDM _____

10. IRS _____
11. LADA _____
12. NIDDM _____
13. LH _____
14. OXT _____
15. PRL _____
16. SAD _____
17. SIADH _____
18. TSH _____

13.4 Laboratory, Diagnostic, and Radiologic Procedures

Word or Phrase	Description	Pronunciation/Word Parts

Blood Tests

Word or Phrase	Description	Pronunciation/Word Parts
antithyroglobulin antibodies	Test that detects antibodies against thyroglobulin (precursor hormone to the thyroid gland hormones T_3 and T_4). A positive test result indicates Hashimoto thyroiditis or Graves disease.	**antithyroglobulin** (AN-tee-THY-roh-GLAW-byoo-lin) **anti-** against **thyr/o-** shield-shaped structure; thyroid gland **globul/o-** shaped like a globe **-in** substance
calcium	Test that measures the level of calcium to determine if the parathyroid gland is secreting a normal amount of parathyroid hormone.	**calcium** (KAL-see-um)
cortisol level	Test that measures the level of cortisol to determine if the adrenal cortex is secreting a normal amount of cortisol. (It also determines if the anterior pituitary gland is secreting ACTH to stimulate the adrenal cortex.) A metabolite of cortisol, **17-hydroxycorticosteroids**, can also be measured in the urine to indirectly measure the level of cortisol in the blood.	**cortisol** (KOR-tih-sawl) **hydroxycorticosteroids** (hy-DRAWK-see-KOR-tih-koh-STAIR-oydz)
fasting blood sugar (FBS)	Test that measures the blood glucose level after the patient has fasted (not eaten) for at least 12 hours. The results indicate if the pancreas is secreting a normal amount of insulin. It is the initial screening test for diabetes mellitus. If the result is abnormal, a glucose tolerance test will be ordered. A fasting blood sugar is also known as a **fasting blood glucose (FBG)**.	
FSH assay and LH assay	Test that measures the levels of FSH and LH to determine if the anterior pituitary gland is secreting a normal amount of these hormones. This is part of an infertility workup for men and women.	**assay** (AS-say)

Word or Phrase	Description	Pronunciation/Word Parts
glucose self-testing	Self-test that measures the level of glucose (blood sugar). Patients with diabetes test their own blood glucose level one or more times each day (see Figure 13-14 ■).	**glucose** (GLOO-kohs) **gluc/o-** *glucose; sugar* **-ose** *full of*

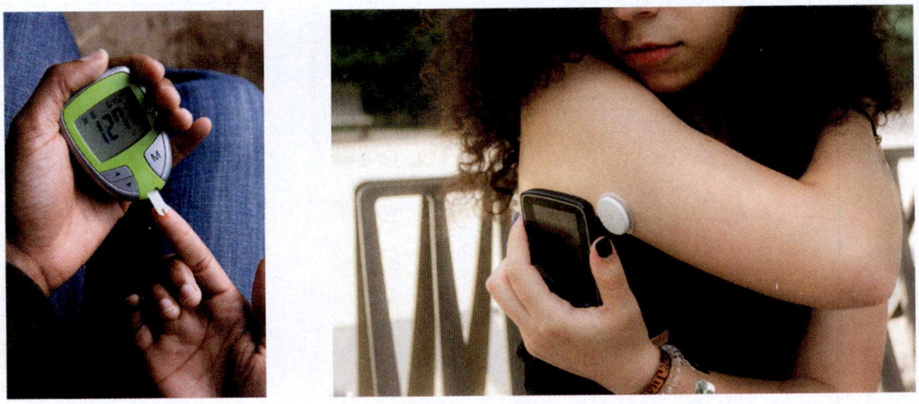

A.   B.

FIGURE 13-14 ■ Blood glucose monitoring.
A. The patient pricks the fingertip; the blood glucose monitor automatically tests the drop of blood and displays the numerical value of the blood glucose level on the monitor screen. The normal range for blood glucose is between 70 and 150 mg/dL in a healthy person or in a patient whose diabetes mellitus is under control. Fingerstick testing must be done several times each day. **B.** Continuous glucose monitoring (CGM) uses a needle attached to an adhesive patch on the skin. It monitors the blood glucose level every 5 minutes. An app loaded onto a cell phone allows the cell phone to display the most recent blood glucose reading as well as a graph of blood glucose readings throughout the day.

Clinical Connections

Technology in Medicine. Personal medical devices can capture blood glucose readings and transmit them electronically or wirelessly to the patient's physician. This type of remote monitoring can help decrease the number of office visits needed by patients with diabetes.

Word or Phrase	Description	Pronunciation/Word Parts
glucose tolerance test (GTT)	Test that measures the level of glucose to determine if the pancreas is secreting a normal amount of insulin. After the patient has fasted for 12 hours, a blood specimen is obtained. Then the patient drinks glucose (in a sugary drink known as **Glucola**) or is given **dextrose** intravenously. A blood specimen is obtained every hour for 4 hours. Normally, the blood glucose returns to a normal level within 1 to 2 hours. A continuing elevated blood glucose level indicates diabetes mellitus. Also known as an **oral glucose tolerance test (OGTT)**.	**Glucola** (gloo-KOH-lah) **dextrose** (DEKS-trohs) **dextr/o-** *right; sugar* **-ose** *full of*
growth hormone (GH)	Test that measures the level of GH to determine if the anterior pituitary gland is secreting a normal amount of growth hormone	
hemoglobin A$_{1c}$ (HbA$_{1c}$)	Test that measures the A$_{1c}$ fraction of hemoglobin in red blood cells. Hemoglobin A$_{1c}$ binds with glucose in the blood. Because red blood cells only live about 12 weeks, the hemoglobin A$_{1c}$ result indicates the average level of blood glucose during the previous 12 weeks. It is used to monitor how well a diabetic patient is controlling the blood glucose level over time with diet and drugs. Also known as **glycohemoglobin** or **glycosylated hemoglobin**.	**hemoglobin A$_{1c}$** (HEE-moh-GLOH-bin AA-one-see) **glycohemoglobin** (GLY-koh-HEE-moh-GLOH-bin) **glycosylated** (gly-KOH-sih-LAY-ted) The combining form **glyc/o-** means *glucose; sugar*.

Word or Phrase	Description	Pronunciation/Word Parts
testosterone	Test that measures the levels of total testosterone and free testosterone to determine if the testes are secreting a normal amount of testosterone. (It also indirectly determines if the anterior pituitary gland is secreting luteinizing hormone to stimulate the testes.) This is part of an infertility workup.	
thyroid function tests (TFTs)	Test that measures the levels of T_3, T_4, and TSH to determine if the thyroid gland is secreting normal amounts of thyroid hormones. (It also determines if the anterior pituitary gland is secreting enough TSH to stimulate the thyroid gland.) Another test value—the **free thyroxine index (FTI)** or **T_7**—can be calculated from this.	

Urine Tests

Word or Phrase	Description	Pronunciation/Word Parts
ADH stimulation test	Test that measures the concentration of urine to determine if the posterior pituitary gland is releasing a normal amount of ADH. The patient does not drink water for 12 hours; then a urine specimen is obtained. Then ADH is given, the patient drinks water, and another urine specimen is obtained. In a patient with diabetes insipidus, the second urine specimen will be more concentrated because of the ADH. Also known as the **water deprivation test**.	
estradiol	Test that measures the level of estradiol to determine if the ovaries are secreting a normal amount. (It also determines if the anterior pituitary gland is secreting FSH to stimulate the ovaries.) This is part of an infertility workup.	
urine dipstick	Test that measures glucose, ketones, and other substances in the urine (see Figure 13-15 ■). This is a rapid screening test used to evaluate diabetic patients.	

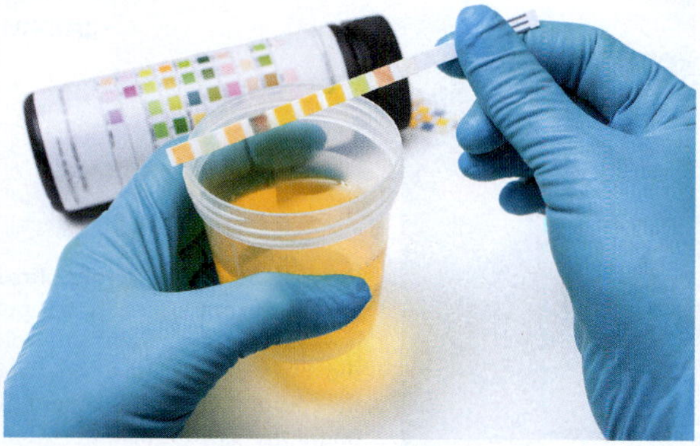

FIGURE 13-15 ■ Urine dipstick.
This plastic strip with chemical-impregnated pads can perform several different laboratory urine tests at one time (pH, protein, glucose, blood, and ketones). The strip is dipped into a urine specimen. The pads change color over a short period of time. The final color of each pad on the strip is compared to a chart on the back of the container; the chart gives a range of colors and the associated test result numbers.

Word or Phrase	Description	Pronunciation/Word Parts
vanillylmandelic acid (VMA)	A 24-hour urine test that measures the levels of epinephrine and norepinephrine to determine if the adrenal medulla is secreting a normal amount of these hormones. VMA, a by-product of these hormones, is measured.	**vanillylmandelic acid** (VAN-ih-LIL-man-DEL-ik AS-id)

Word or Phrase	Description	Pronunciation/Word Parts

Radiologic Procedures

Word or Phrase	Description	Pronunciation/Word Parts
radioactive iodine uptake (RAIU) and thyroid scan	Procedure that combines a thyroid scan with a radioactive iodine uptake procedure. The thyroid scan shows the size and shape of the thyroid gland. The radioactive iodine uptake shows how well the thyroid gland is able to absorb radioactive iodine from the blood. A normal scan will show uniform distribution of radioactive iodine throughout the thyroid gland. An abnormal scan can show an adenoma, cyst, or a cancerous tumor. An adenoma appears as a bright spot ("hot spot") because of its increased uptake of radioactive iodine. A darker area ("cold spot") can be a benign cyst or a cancerous tumor, neither of which absorbs iodine (see Figure 13-16 ■).	**radioactive** (RAY-dee-oh-AK-tiv) **radi/o-** *forearm bone; radius; x-rays* **act/o-** *action* **-ive** *pertaining to* **iodine** (EYE-oh-dine)

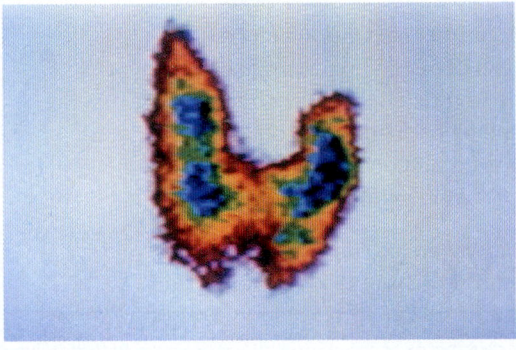

FIGURE 13-16 ■ Thyroid scan.
This patient's thyroid scan shows two dark blue "cold spots" in the right lobe of the thyroid gland and one large dark blue "cold spot" in the left lobe. These are areas of decreased uptake of radioactive iodine. They could be benign cysts or cancerous tumors. A biopsy will be needed to make a diagnosis. (Remember, when you view the image, your right side corresponds to the patient's left side.)

Word or Phrase	Description	Pronunciation/Word Parts
thyroid ultrasonography	Procedure that uses sound waves generated by a transducer that is placed on the neck (see Figure 13-17 ■). It shows thyroid enlargement and thyroid nodules. The image or record is a **thyroid ultrasound**.	**ultrasonography** (UL-trah-soh-NAW-grah-fee) **ultra-** *beyond; higher* **son/o-** *sound* **-graphy** *process of recording*

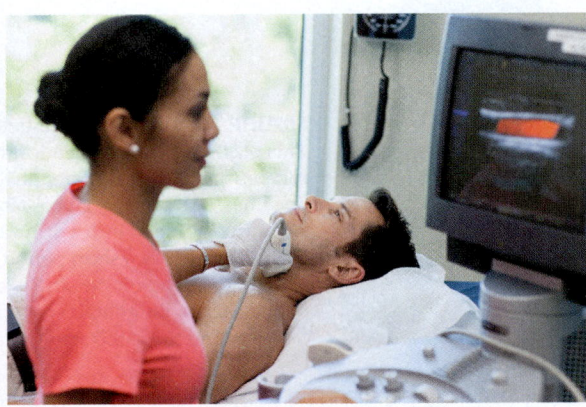

FIGURE 13-17 ■ Thyroid ultrasound.
This ultrasound technician is performing ultrasonography of the patient's thyroid gland. She moves the transducer as she views the ultrasound image on the computer screen to obtain the best view. Ultrasonography uses a transducer that emits sound waves rather than x-rays to create an image of the thyroid gland.

13.4 PRACTICE LAPS

Use the Answer Key at the end of the book to check your answers.

A. Give the Meaning of Combining Forms

Next to each combining form, write its meaning. The first one has been done for you.

Combining Form	Meaning	Combining Form	Meaning
1. **act/o-**	*action*	5. radi/o-	
2. dextr/o-		6. son/o-	
3. globul/o-		7. thyr/o-	
4. gluc/o-			

B. Define Abbreviations

1.	ADH		8. GTT	
2.	CGM		9. LH	
3.	FBG		10. OGTT	
4.	FBS		11. RAIU	
5.	FSH		12. TFTs	
6.	FTI		13. TSH	
7.	GH		14. VMA	

13.5 Medical Procedures, Drugs, and Surgical Procedures

Word or Phrase	Description	Pronunciation/Word Parts

Medical Procedures

Word or Phrase	Description	Pronunciation/Word Parts
ADA diet	Special physician-prescribed diet for diabetic patients that follows the guidelines of the **American Diabetes Association (ADA)**. The amounts of carbohydrate and fat are limited. The physician orders the upper limit for the total daily number of calories for a diabetic patient in the hospital (e.g., 1200-calorie ADA diet). Rather than using the ADA diet, diabetic patients can just count calories. A dietitian or diabetes educator helps the patient plan a menu that fits lifestyle and food preferences.	

Category	Indication	Pronunciation/Word Parts

Drugs

Category	Indication	Pronunciation/Word Parts
antidiabetic drug	Treats type 2 diabetes mellitus by stimulating the pancreas to secrete more insulin or by increasing the number of insulin receptors on cells. These drugs are given orally. They are not insulin and they cannot be used to treat patients with type 1 diabetes mellitus.	**antidiabetic** (AN-tee-DY-ah-BET-ik) **anti-** *against* **diabet/o-** *diabetes* **-ic** *pertaining to*
antithyroid drug	Treats hyperthyroidism by inhibiting the production of T_3 and T_4. Antithyroid drugs are given orally on a continuing basis. Alternately, radioactive sodium iodide 131 (I-131) is given orally, but it acts in an entirely different way. It is taken up by the thyroid gland and emits low-level radiation that destroys thyroid gland cells. It has a short half-life and is excreted in the urine, limiting the number of cells that are destroyed. Some functioning thyroid gland tissue still remains.	**antithyroid** (AN-tee-THY-royd) **anti-** *against* **thyr/o-** *shield-shaped structure; thyroid gland* **-oid** *resembling*
corticosteroid drug	Mimics the action of cortisol from the adrenal cortex. It is used to treat severe inflammation and as hormone replacement therapy for Addison disease.	**corticosteroid** (KOR-tih-koh-STAIR-oyd) **cortic/o-** *cortex; outer region* **-steroid** *steroid*
growth hormone supplement drug	Provides growth hormone	
insulin	Treats type 1 and type 1.5 diabetes mellitus. It can also be used to treat type 2 diabetes mellitus that cannot be controlled with oral antidiabetic drugs. Insulin must be injected from one to several times each day to control the blood glucose level (see Figure 13-18 ■). Insulin is classified according to how quickly it acts (which depends on the size of the insulin crystal) and how many hours its therapeutic effect continues.	**insulin** (IN-soo-lin)

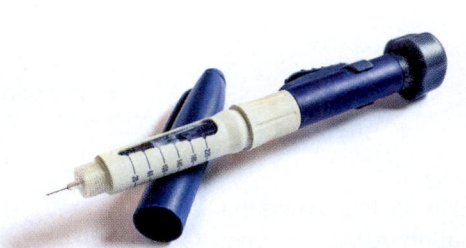

A.

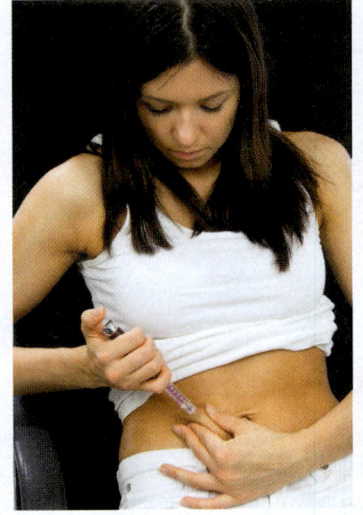

B.

FIGURE 13-18 ■ **Insulin injection.**
A. This device looks like a pen but has a fine needle and a syringe with calibrations to inject a measured dose of insulin. Insulin is measured in units. **B.** This diabetic patient is injecting insulin using an insulin syringe. Insulin is a liquid drug that is injected subcutaneously into the fat layer beneath the skin. The skin is pinched up, and the needle is inserted at an angle so that it does not go into the muscle beneath. The back of the arms, abdomen, and several other sites can be used for insulin injections. A new site must be selected for each injection.

Category	Indication	Pronunciation/Word Parts
thyroid supplement drug	Treats a lack of thyroid hormones and hypothyroidism	

Word or Phrase	Description	Pronunciation/Word Parts

Surgical Procedures

Word or Phrase	Description	Pronunciation/Word Parts
adrenalectomy	Procedure to remove the adrenal gland because of an adenoma or cancerous tumor	**adrenalectomy** (ah-DREE-nal-EK-toh-mee) **adrenal/o-** *adrenal gland* **-ectomy** *surgical removal*
fine-needle biopsy	Procedure that uses a fine needle to take a small sample of tissue from a thyroid nodule. The tissue is sent to the pathology department to determine if the nodule is benign or cancerous.	**biopsy** (BY-awp-see) **bi/o-** *living organism; living tissue* **-opsy** *process of viewing*
parathyroidectomy	Procedure to remove one or more of the parathyroid glands to treat hyperparathyroidism. Also, a parathyroidectomy can occur accidentally when part of the thyroid gland is surgically removed.	**parathyroidectomy** (PAIR-ah-THY-royd-EK-toh-mee) **para-** *abnormal; apart from; beside; two parts of a pair* **thyroid/o-** *thyroid gland* **-ectomy** *surgical removal*
thymectomy	Procedure to remove the thymus in patients with myasthenia gravis, an autoimmune disease	**thymectomy** (thy-MEK-toh-mee) **thym/o-** *rage; thymus* **-ectomy** *surgical removal*
thyroidectomy	Procedure to remove the thyroid gland. All of the thyroid gland can be removed or just one part (**subtotal thyroidectomy**) or just one lobe (**thyroid lobectomy**).	**thyroidectomy** (THY-royd-EK-toh-mee) **thyroid/o-** *thyroid gland* **-ectomy** *surgical removal* **lobectomy** (loh-BEK-toh-mee) **lob/o-** *lobe of an organ* **-ectomy** *surgical removal*
transsphenoidal hypophysectomy	Procedure to remove an adenoma from the pituitary gland (hypophysis). The pituitary gland is difficult to visualize through an incision in the cranium, so the surgical instruments are inserted through the nose and an incision is made in the sphenoid sinus (transsphenoidal).	**transsphenoidal** (TRANS-sfee-NOY-dal) **trans-** *across; through* **sphenoid/o-** *sphenoid bone; sphenoid sinus* **-al** *pertaining to* **hypophysectomy** (HY-paw-fih-SEK-toh-mee) **hypophys/o-** *pituitary gland* **-ectomy** *surgical removal*

13.5 PRACTICE LAPS

Use the Answer Key at the end of the book to check your answers.

A. Give the Meaning of Combining Forms

Next to each combining form, write its meaning. The first one has been done for you.

Combining Form	Meaning	Combining Form	Meaning
1. **cortic/o-**	*cortex; outer region*	6. lob/o-	
2. adrenal/o-		7. sphenoid/o-	
3. bi/o-		8. thym/o-	
4. diabet/o-		9. thyr/o-	
5. hypophys/o-		10. thyroid/o-	

B. Build Words

Read the definition of the medical word. Look at the combining form that is given. Select the correct suffix from the Suffix List, and write it on the blank line. Then build the medical word, and write it on the line. (Remember: You may need to remove the combining vowel. Always remove the hyphens and slash.) Be sure to check your spelling.

Suffix List

-ectomy (surgical removal)	-opsy (process of viewing)	-steroid (steroid)

Definition of the Medical Word	Combining Form	Suffix	Build the Medical Word
Example: Steroid (drug from the) outer region (of the adrenal gland)	**cortic/o-**	*-steroid*	*corticosteroid*

[*You think* steroid (-steroid) + outer region (cortic/o-). You change the order of the word parts to put the suffix last. You write corticosteroid.]

Definition of the Medical Word	Combining Form	Suffix	Build the Medical Word
1. Surgical removal (of the) lobe of an organ	lob/o-		
2. Surgical removal (of the) thymus	thym/o-		
3. Surgical removal (of the) pituitary gland	hypophys/o-		
4. Process of viewing living tissue	bi/o-		
5. Surgical removal (of the) adrenal gland	adrenal/o-		
6. Surgical removal (of the) thyroid gland	thyroid/o-		

Abbreviations Summary

ACTH	adrenocorticotropic hormone		**IRS**	insulin resistance syndrome
ADA	American Diabetes Association, American Dietetic Association		**LADA**	latent autoimmune diabetes in adults
			LH	luteinizing hormone
ADH	antidiuretic hormone		**MSH**	melanocyte-stimulating hormone
AODM	adult-onset diabetes mellitus		**NIDDM**	non-insulin-dependent diabetes mellitus
CDE	certified diabetes educator		**OGTT**	oral glucose tolerance test
CGM	continuous glucose monitoring		**OXT**	oxytocin
DI	diabetes insipidus		**PRL**	prolactin
DKA	diabetic ketoacidosis		**RAIU**	radioactive iodine uptake
DM	diabetes mellitus		**SAD**	seasonal affective disorder
FBG	fasting blood glucose		**SIADH**	syndrome of inappropriate antidiuretic hormone
FBS	fasting blood sugar			
FSH	follicle-stimulating hormone		T_3	triiodothyronine
FTI	free thyroxine index		T_4	thyroxine
GDM	gestational diabetes mellitus		T_7	free thyroxine index (FTI)
GH	growth hormone		**TFTs**	thyroid function tests
GTT	glucose tolerance test		**TSH**	thyroid-stimulating hormone
HbA$_{1c}$	hemoglobin A$_{1c}$		**VMA**	vanillylmandelic acid
IDDM	insulin-dependent diabetes mellitus			

Word Alert

Abbreviations. Abbreviations are commonly used in all types of medical documents; however, they can mean different things to different people and their meanings can be misinterpreted. Always verify the meaning of an abbreviation.

- *ADA* means *American Diabetes Association* and *American Dietetic Association*, but it also means *American Dental Association* and *Americans with Disabilities Act.*

It's Greek to Me! Did you notice that some words have two different combining forms? Combining forms from both Greek and Latin remain a part of medical language today.

Word	Greek	Latin	Medical Word Examples
female	gynec/o-	estr/a-, estr/o-	gynecomastia; estradiol, estrogen
male, masculine	andr/o-	viril/o-	androgen; virilism
milk	galact/o-	lact/o-	galactorrhea; prolactin
pituitary gland	hypophys/o-	pituitar/o-, pituit/o-	adenohypophysis; hypopituitarism, pituitary

Career Focus

Meet Maureen, a diabetes educator

"I work in a large city hospital that has a very large diabetic population, and that's how I got interested in the disease. On a typical day we see patients who have had diabetes anywhere from just a few weeks to years. Diabetic education has really changed a lot because we're really trying to empower the patient. People live with diabetes every day, so they should have the tools to take care of their diabetes. The more information they have, the better choices that they're going to make. What we try and do is teach them how—about their food, how to monitor their blood glucose, what their medications are, how to take them properly and consistently, and what to do if their blood glucose is either too high or too low."

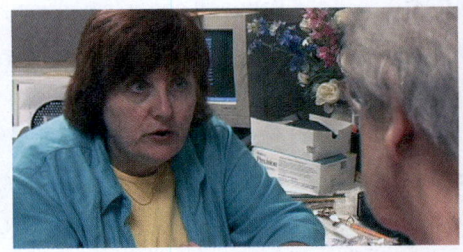

- **Diabetes educators** are allied health professionals who counsel and educate patients with diabetes mellitus and their families. They work in hospitals, clinics, and some physicians' offices. They can be members of the **ADA (American Diabetes Association, American Dietetics Association)** and they can become a **certified diabetes educator (CDE).**

- **Endocrinologists** are physicians who practice in the specialty of endocrinology. They diagnose and treat patients with diseases of the endocrine system. Some endocrinologists specialize and become **diabetologists** who only treat patients with diabetes mellitus. Physicians can take additional training and become board certified in the subspecialties of reproductive endocrinology or pediatric endocrinology. Surgery on the endocrine system is performed by a general surgeon or a neurosurgeon. Cancerous tumors of the endocrine system are treated medically by an oncologist or surgically by a general surgeon or neurosurgeon.

endocrinologist (EN-doh-krih-NAW-loh-jist)
end/o- *innermost; within*
crin/o- *secrete*
log/o- *study of; word*
-ist *person who specializes in; thing that specializes in*

diabetologist (DY-ah-beh-TAW-loh-jist)
diabet/o- *diabetes*
log/o- *study of; word*
-ist *person who specializes in; thing that specializes in*

Chapter Review Exercises

Dive In: Medical Language Exercises

Test your knowledge of the chapter by completing these review exercises. Use the Answer Key at the end of the book to check your answers. Note: Each of the numbered exercise headers corresponds to a numbered learning outcome at the beginning of the chapter.

13.1 Anatomy

MATCHING EXERCISE

Match each word or phrase to its description. A word or phrase can have more than one matching description.

1. hypothalamus
2. pituitary gland
3. pineal gland
4. thyroid gland
5. parathyroid glands
6. thymus
7. oxytocin
8. pancreas
9. adrenal glands
10. ovaries
11. testes

_____ in the center of the brain below the thalamus

_____ secrete estradiol

_____ in the scrotum in a male

_____ causes the pregnant uterus to contract during labor

_____ shield-shaped structure with an isthmus

_____ on top of the kidneys

_____ two of its hormones are stored and released by the posterior pituitary gland

_____ gland that shrinks during adulthood

_____ in the bony cup of the sella turcica

_____ develops T cell lymphocytes for the body's immune response

_____ contains an anterior and a posterior lobe

_____ four small glands on the back of the thyroid gland

_____ secretes insulin

_____ associated with the 24-hour sleep–wake cycle

_____ yellow, triangular gland posterior to the stomach

CIRCLE EXERCISE

Circle the correct answer from the choices given.

1. The (**adrenal medulla, pineal gland, testis**) secretes the hormone norepinephrine.
2. The (**ovary, pituitary gland, thymus**) secretes estradiol and is responsible for the secondary sexual characteristics in the female.
3. The (**ovaries, parathyroid glands, testes**) are four small glands located on a shield-shaped gland.
4. The (**adrenal gland, pancreas, pituitary gland**) contains two layers called the cortex and the medulla, each of which functions separately as a gland.
5. The (**adrenal gland, pituitary gland, thymus**) shrinks in size in adults.
6. Insulin is secreted by the (**alpha, beta, delta**) cells of the pancreas.
7. The pineal gland secretes (**calcitonin, melatonin, oxytocin**).
8. The hormone that affects the blood level of sodium is (**aldosterone, cortisol, insulin**).
9. All of the following are gonadotropins *except* (**FSH, LH, OXT**).

TRUE OR FALSE EXERCISE

*Indicate whether each statement is true or false by writing **T** or **F** on the line.*

1. _____ Insulin is secreted by the delta cells in islets of Langerhans in the pancreas.
2. _____ Melatonin is another name for melanin.
3. _____ Testosterone is the most abundant and biologically active of the male sex hormones.

4. _____ The follicles of the ovary secrete FSH when stimulated by estradiol from the anterior pituitary gland.

5. _____ Epinephrine prepares the body with the so-called "fight-or-flight" response.

6. _____ The hormone insulin lowers the level of glucose in the blood.

PLURAL NOUN AND ADJECTIVE EXERCISE

Read the noun and write its plural form and/or adjective form on the line. Only write in the plural noun form if there is a blank line there for it. Be sure to check your spelling. The first one has been done for you.

Singular Noun	Plural Noun	Adjective
1. **gland**	*glands*	*glandular*
2. hypothalamus		
3. hormone		
4. thymus		
5. pancreas		
6. cortex		
7. medulla		
8. ovary		
9. testis		

DIVIDING WORDS EXERCISE

Separate these words into their component parts (prefix, combining form, suffix). Some words do not contain all three word parts. The first one has been done for you.

Medical Word	Prefix	Combining Form	Suffix
1. **anterior**		*anter/o-*	*-ior*
2. glandular			
3. homeostasis			
4. hypothalamic			
5. hormonal			
6. pituitary			
7. endocrine			
8. adenohypophysis			
9. prolactin			
10. follicle			
11. melatonin			
12. euthyroid			
13. parathyroid			
14. pancreatic			
15. glycogen			
16. insulin			

SPELLING EXERCISE

Read each medical word pronunciation and write the medical word that it represents. Be sure to check your spelling. The first one has been done for you.

1. (pohs-TEER-ee-or)   *posterior*
2. (pih-TOO-eh-TAIR-ee) _____
3. (HOH-mee-oh-STAY-sihs) _____
4. (ES-trah-DY-awl) _____

5. (AWK-see-TOH-sin _____
6. (PAN-kree-AT-ik) _____
7. (EP-ih-NEH-frin) _____
8. (tes-TIH-kyoo-lar) _____

RELATED COMBINING FORMS EXERCISE

Write the combining forms on the line provided. (Hint: See the It's Greek to Me! feature box.)

1. Two combining forms that mean *male, masculine.*   _____ _____
2. Three combining forms that mean *female.*   _____ _____ _____
3. Two combining forms that mean *milk.*   _____ _____
4. Three combining forms that mean *pituitary gland.*   _____ _____ _____

13.2 Physiology

MATCHING EXERCISE

Match each word or phrase to its description.

1. antagonism   _____ structure on an organ or gland that a hormone can bind to
2. hormone   _____ when two hormones exert opposite effects
3. inhibition   _____ when two hormones work in conjunction with each other
4. receptor   _____ secreted through a duct into the blood
5. synergism   _____ stopping an endocrine gland from secreting its hormones

CIRCLE EXERCISE

Circle the correct word from the choices given.

1. A hormone is a key that unlocks a (**cortex, receptor, sella turcica**) on a gland.
2. When two hormones exert opposite effects, that is (**antagonism, inhibition, synergism**).
3. The endocrine system maintains body homeostasis through the use of all of the following *except* (**hormones, negative feedback mechanism, neurotransmitters**).

TRUE OR FALSE EXERCISE

*Indicate whether each statement is true or false by writing **T** or **F** on the line.*

1. _____ The endocrine system uses neurotransmitters as chemical messengers.
2. _____ Some neurotransmitters in the brain and spinal cord are considered to be hormones because they are secreted by an endocrine gland through a duct and into the blood.
3. _____ The actions of hormones involve stimulation or inhibition.

DIVIDING WORDS EXERCISE

Separate these words into their component parts (prefix, combining form, suffix). Some words do not contain all three word parts. The first one has been done for you.

Medical Word	Prefix	Combining Form	Suffix
1. **stimulation**		*stimul/o-*	*-ation*
2. receptor		_____	_____
3. synergism	_____	_____	_____
4. inhibition		_____	_____
5. antagonism		_____	_____

SPELLING EXERCISE

Read each medical word pronunciation and write the medical word that it represents. Be sure to check your spelling. The first one has been done for you.

1. **(an-TAG-on-izm)**   *antagonism*
2. (ree-SEP-ter)   _____
3. (SIN-er-jizm)   _____
4. (STIM-yoo-LAY-shun)   _____

13.3 Diseases

MATCHING EXERCISE

Match each word or phrase to its description.

1. thyromegaly
2. diabetes insipidus
3. myxedema
4. exophthalmos
5. galactorrhea
6. gigantism
7. insulin resistance syndrome
8. menopause
9. microadenoma
10. polydipsia
11. uterine inertia

_____ bulging, staring eyes
_____ excessive thirst
_____ not enough ADH
_____ hyposecretion of estradiol
_____ too little oxytocin
_____ severe hypothyroidism in an adult
_____ milk secretion from breasts of a nonpregnant female
_____ goiter
_____ hypersecretion of growth hormone during childhood
_____ very small benign tumor of an endocrine gland
_____ receptors on body cells do not allow insulin to transport glucose into the cell

TRUE OR FALSE EXERCISE

*Indicate whether each statement is true or false by writing **T** or **F** on the line.*

1. _____ A goiter is also known as *thyromegaly*.
2. _____ Diabetes insipidus is also known as *sugar diabetes*.
3. _____ Addison disease is also known as *hirsutism*.
4. _____ Gestational diabetes only occurs in men.
5. _____ Moon face and buffalo hump are characteristics of Cushing syndrome.
6. _____ Gynecomastia is the overproduction of milk by the breasts during pregnancy.

CIRCLE EXERCISE

Circle the correct answer from the choices given.

1. Diabetic patients are at risk for all of the following *except* (**diabetic neuropathy, gangrene from small skin cuts, hypercalcemia**).
2. Hyposecretion of oxytocin causes (**exophthalmos, postpartum hemorrhage, virilism**).
3. The most common type of hyperthyroidism is (**goiter, Graves disease, seasonal affective disorder**).
4. All of the following types of diabetes mellitus are autoimmune disorders *except* (**juvenile onset, LADA, type 2**).
5. Gestational diabetes is associated with (**acromegaly, Addison disease, pregnancy**).
6. Which disease is associated with the adrenal cortex? (**diabetes, thyroiditis, virilism**).
7. A large volume of urine could indicate (**diabetes insipidus, precocious puberty, thyroiditis**).

DIVIDING WORDS EXERCISE

Separate these words into their component parts (prefix, combining form, suffix). Some words do not contain all three word parts. The first one has been done for you.

Medical Word	Prefix	Combining Form	Suffix
1. **lactation**		*lact/o-*	*-ation*
2. hyperpituitarism			
3. adenoma			
4. galactorrhea			
5. gigantism			
6. acromegaly			
7. polyuria			
8. hyperthyroidism			
9. thyroiditis			
10. hypoglycemia			
11. hirsutism			
12. infertility			

SPELLING EXERCISE

Read each medical word pronunciation and write the medical word that it represents. Be sure to check your spelling. The first one has been done for you.

1. (MY-kroh-AD-eh-NOH-mah)   *microadenoma*
2. (AK-roh-MEG-ah-lee)
3. (PAW-lee-DIP-see-ah)
4. (HY-per-THY-royd-izm)
5. (THY-roy-DY-tihs)
6. (gah-LAK-toh-REE-ah)

13.4 Laboratory, Diagnostic, and Radiologic Procedures

MATCHING EXERCISE

Match each word, phrase, or abbreviation to its description.

1. CGM
2. estradiol
3. FBS
4. glucose tolerance test
5. glycohemoglobin
6. RAIU
7. urine dipstick
8. ultrasound
9. VMA

_____ uses a sugary drink or intravenous dextrose
_____ measured with a 24-hour urine test
_____ rapid screening test that measures glucose and ketones
_____ uses sound waves to generate an image
_____ HbA$_{1c}$
_____ blood level is tested as part of an infertility workup
_____ uses radioactive iodine to show a "hot spot" or "cold spot"
_____ eliminates the need for frequent fingersticks for blood
_____ cannot eat for 12 hours before this test

TRUE OR FALSE EXERCISE

*Indicate whether each statement is true or false by writing **T** or **F** on the line.*

1. _____ A positive antithyroglobulin antibodies test result indicates Hashimoto thyroiditis.

2. _____ A blood test for calcium shows if there is enough parathyroid hormone.

3. _____ HbA$_{1c}$ results show the average level of blood glucose during the preceding 12 months.

4. _____ Free thyroxine index is also known as T$_7$.

CIRCLE EXERCISE

Circle the correct answer from the choices given.

1. A "cold spot" or "hot spot" might be seen on a/an (**ADH stimulation test, fasting blood glucose, thyroid scan**).

2. HbA$_{1c}$ is also known as (**antithyroglobulin antibodies, FSH, glycosylated hemoglobin**).

3. All of the following are laboratory tests for diabetes *except* (**blood calcium, fasting blood glucose, GTT**).

4. Thyroid function tests include all of the following *except* (**estradiol, T$_4$, TSH**).

LABORATORY TEST EXERCISE

Review the form below for ordering laboratory tests for an endocrinology patient. Find each of the following tests related to endocrinology and put a checkmark next to it.

calcium, total blood	metabolic panel, comprehensive	T$_4$, total
electrolyte panel	potassium	testosterone, total
estradiol	progesterone	TSH
glucose, fasting	prolactin	urinalysis, automated
glucose tolerance test (GTT)	sodium	
hemoglobin A$_{1c}$	T$_3$, total	

CPT CODE	PANELS AND PROFILES
80047	Metabolic Panel, Basic
80050	General Health Panel
80051	Electrolyte Panel
80053	Metabolic Panel, Comprehensive
80055	Obstetric Panel
80061	Lipid Panel
80069	Renal Function Panel
80076	Hepatic Function Panel
80100	Drug Screening Panel

CPT CODE	BLOOD TESTS
80162	Digoxin Drug Level
82040	Albumin
82055	Blood Alcohol (ETOH)
82247	Bilirubin, Total
82310	Calcium, Total Blood
82375	Carboxyhemoglobin
82378	Carcinoembryonic Antigen (CEA)
82435	Chloride
82465	Cholesterol
82553	Creatine Kinase, MB

CPT CODE	BLOOD TESTS
82565	Creatinine, Blood
82575	Creatinine Clearance
82670	Estradiol
82947	Glucose, Fasting
82951	Glucose Tolerance Test (GTT)
83036	Hemoglobin A_{1c}
83540	Iron
83550	Iron, TIBC
83718	HDL Lipoprotein
83719	VLDL Lipoprotein
83721	LDL Lipoprotein
84132	Potassium
84144	Progesterone
84146	Prolactin
84155	Protein, Total
84295	Sodium
84403	Testosterone, Total
84443	Thyroid-Stimulating Hormone (TSH)
84436	Thyroxine (T_4), Total
84478	Triglycerides
84480	Triiodothyronine (T_3), Total
84484	Troponin
84520	Blood Urea Nitrogen (BUN)
84550	Uric Acid
85004	White Blood Cell (WBC) Count with Differential
85014	Hematocrit (HCT)
85018	Hemoglobin (Hgb)
85025	Complete Blood Count (CBC)
85049	Platelet Count
85610	Prothrombin Time (PT)
85730	Partial Thromboplastin Time (PTT)
86592	Syphilis Blood Test (VDRL or RPR)
86701	HIV-1 Antibody
86812	Human Leukocyte Antigen (HLA) Typing
86900	Blood Type
86910	Blood Type for Paternity Testing
87340	Hepatitis B Surface Antigen
36415	Venipuncture
81001	Urinalysis, Automated
82270	Stool Occult Blood
87040	Blood Culture
87045	Stool Culture
87086	Urine Culture
87116	Acid-Fast Bacilli Culture
87177	Ova and Parasites
89220	Sputum Analysis
89300	Semen Analysis

13.5 Medical Procedures, Drugs, and Surgical Procedures

MATCHING EXERCISE

Match each word or phrase to its description.

1. antidiabetic drug   _____ surgical treatment for myasthenia gravis

2. corticosteroid drug   _____ removes just part of the thyroid gland

3. insulin   _____ used to treat patients with type 2 diabetes mellitus

4. lobectomy   _____ patients with Addison disease must take these

5. radioactive I-131   _____ this drug is given by subcutaneous injection

6. thymectomy   _____ emits gamma radiation that destroys the thyroid gland

CIRCLE EXERCISE

Circle the correct answer from the choices given.

1. An ADA diet limits all of the following foods *except* (**carbohydrates, fats, iodine**).
2. Insulin is used to treat all of the following types of diabetes mellitus *except* (**1, 1.5, 2**).
3. A thymectomy is used to treat patients with (**diabetes mellitus, hyperthyroidism, myasthenia gravis**).
4. To remove an adenoma from the pituitary gland, the surgeon has to insert surgical instruments through the (**abdomen, brain, nose**).

TRUE OR FALSE EXERCISE

*Indicate whether each statement is true or false by writing **T** or **F** on the line.*

1. _____ Antidiabetic drugs are a form of insulin.
2. _____ An adrenalectomy can be done to remove an adenoma or a cancerous tumor from the adrenal gland.
3. _____ A sample of tissue from a fine-needle biopsy is sent to the pathology department.

DIVIDING WORDS EXERCISE

Separate these words into their component parts (prefix, combining form, suffix). Some words do not contain all three word parts. The first one has been done for you.

Medical Word	Prefix	Combining Form	Suffix
1. **antidiabetic**	*anti-*	*diabet/o-*	*-ic*
2. adrenalectomy		_____	_____
3. biopsy		_____	_____
4. parathyroidectomy	_____	_____	_____
5. thyroidectomy		_____	_____
6. transsphenoidal	_____	_____	_____
7. hypophysectomy		_____	_____

SPELLING EXERCISE

Read each medical word pronunciation and write the medical word that it represents. Be sure to check your spelling. The first one has been done for you.

1. (BY-awp-see)   *biopsy*

2. (KOR-tih-koh-STAIR-oyd)   _____

3. (THY-royd-EK-toh-mee)   _____

4. (AN-tee-DY-ah-BET-ik)   _____

5. (loh-BEK-toh-mee)   _____

Immerse Yourself: Analyze Medical Reports

Electronic Patient Record #1

This is an Office Visit Note. Read the Note and answer the questions.

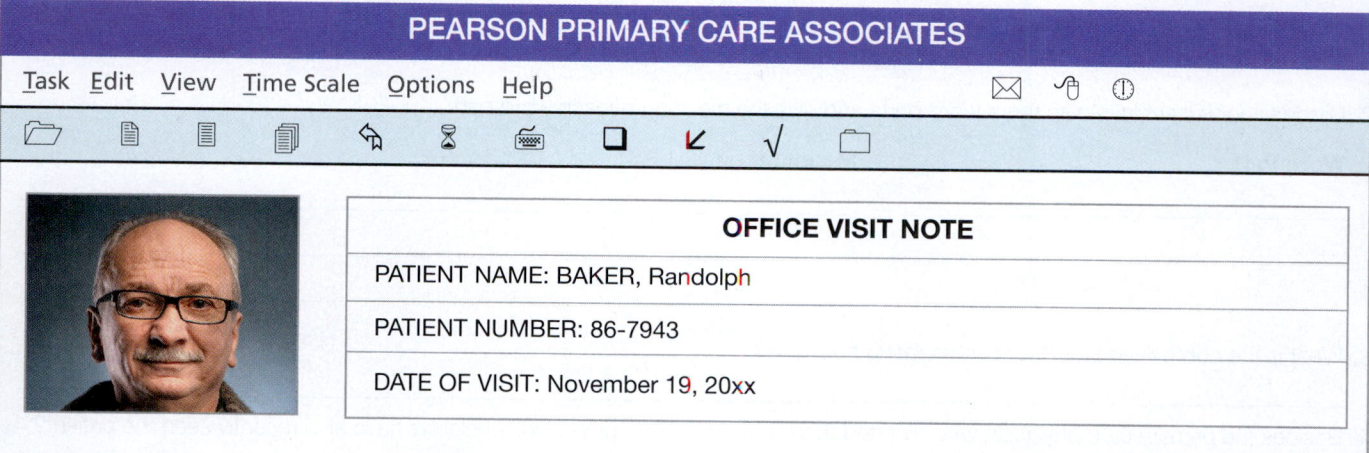

PEARSON PRIMARY CARE ASSOCIATES

Task Edit View Time Scale Options Help

OFFICE VISIT NOTE

PATIENT NAME: BAKER, Randolph

PATIENT NUMBER: 86-7943

DATE OF VISIT: November 19, 20xx

HISTORY
This is a 54-year-old male who presents with fatigue. He also has headaches. Because of a history of some visual field defects during his headaches, his ophthalmologist ordered an MRI of the brain to look for any tumors or masses. I reviewed the scans and did not see anything but the expected postsurgical changes of the brain. Lab tests show that he does have some residual function of the pituitary gland, so his endocrinologist only placed him on testosterone transdermal patches and thyroid hormone replacement. He also has a history of depression, which could explain the fatigue and headache, or they could be due to low thyroid hormone replacement levels.

PHYSICAL EXAMINATION
HEENT: Normal. Lungs: Clear to auscultation. Cardiovascular: Regular rate and rhythm, without murmurs, rubs, or gallops. Abdomen: Nondistended, nontender. Extremities: No edema.

ASSESSMENT

1. Fatigue. Possibly due to hypothyroidism. Will check T_3, T_4, and TSH levels.

2. Headache, possibly within the context of depression. He is on a rather low dose of an antidepressant drug at this time.

3. Hypopituitarism, after surgical removal of an adenoma.

PLAN

1. Will obtain T_3, T_4, and TSH levels, as well as FSH, LH, free and total testosterone, and baseline ACTH.

2. Follow up in 1 week.

Edward Allen Selcher, M.D.

Edward Allen Selcher, M.D.

EAS:blg
D: 11/19/xx
T: 11/19/xx

1. Divide *endocrinologist* into its four word parts and give the meaning of each word part.

   Word Part   **Meaning**

   _____   _____

   _____   _____

   _____   _____

   _____   _____

2. Divide *hypopituitarism* into its three word parts and give the meaning of each word part.

   Word Part   **Meaning**

   _____   _____

   _____   _____

   _____   _____

3. What is the abbreviation for *thyroid-stimulating hormone*?

   _____

4. Besides the primary care physician who dictated this report, what two physician specialists have also recently seen the patient?

   _____   _____

5. What two hormones does the patient already take as drugs for hormone replacement therapy?

   _____   _____

6. What do these abbreviations mean?

   ACTH: _____

   FSH: _____

   LH: _____

7. The patient is taking thyroid hormone replacement for his (**headaches, hypothyroidism, lungs**). Circle the correct answer.

8. The patient's fatigue, headache, and visual field defects could be signs of a recurring tumor in the brain. What test has already been done to look for a tumor?

   _____

9. The patient's MRI of the brain showed postsurgical changes, meaning changes that are present because of a surgery that was done. Which surgery of the brain was performed in the past?

   _____

Proofreading and Spelling Exercise

Read the following paragraph. Identify each misspelled medical word and write the correct spelling of it on the line.

Endocrineology is the study of glands and hormones. The pituraty gland is the master gland. In diabetes mellitis, there is too much glukose and not enough insulin. A tumor in the adrenal medula is a feochromocytoma. If there is an adenoma in the thyroid gland, then a thyroectomy would be done. Graves disease is associated with exofthalmos and a goiter. An enlarged thyroid gland is thyromegalee. Galactorhea is milk production in a woman who is not pregnant.

1. _____
2. _____
3. _____
4. _____
5. _____
6. _____
7. _____
8. _____
9. _____
10. _____

MyLab Medical Terminology™

MyLab Medical Terminology is a premium online homework management system that includes a host of features to help you study. Registered users will find:

- A multitude of quizzes and activities built within the MyLab platform

- Powerful tools that track and analyze your results—allowing you to create a personalized learning experience

- Videos and audio pronunciations to help enrich your progress

- Streaming lesson presentations (guided lectures) and self-paced learning modules

- A space where you and your instructor can check your progress and manage your assignments

14 Ophthalmology

Eye

Ophthalmology (OFF-thal-MAW-loh-jee) is the medical specialty that studies the anatomy and physiology of the eye; uses laboratory, diagnostic, and radiologic procedures to diagnose eye diseases; and uses medical procedures, drugs, and surgical procedures to treat eye diseases.

⌄ Chapter Overview and Learning Outcomes

After you study this chapter, you should be able to demonstrate mastery of the outcomes by successfully completing the exercises.

14.1 Anatomy
Identify the structures of the eye.
Demonstrate proficiency in medical language.
14.1 Practice Laps

14.2 Physiology
Describe the function of the eye.
Demonstrate proficiency in medical language.
14.2 Practice Laps
Vocabulary Review

14.3 Diseases
Describe common eye diseases.
Demonstrate proficiency in medical language.
14.3 Practice Laps

14.4 Laboratory, Diagnostic, and Radiologic Procedures
Describe common eye laboratory tests, diagnostic procedures, and radiologic procedures.
Demonstrate proficiency in medical language.
14.4 Practice Laps

14.5 Medical Procedures, Drugs, and Surgical Procedures
Describe common eye medical procedures, drugs, and surgical procedures.
Demonstrate proficiency in medical language.
14.5 Practice Laps
Abbreviations Summary
Career Focus

Chapter Review Exercises
Dive In: Medical Exercises
(Learning Outcomes 14.1–14.5)
Immerse Yourself: Analyze Medical Reports

Medical Language Key

To unlock the definition of a medical word, first break it into word parts. Then give the meaning of each word part. Put the meanings of the word parts in order, beginning with the meaning of the suffix, then the meaning of the prefix (if there is one), then the meaning of the combining form.

    Ophthalmology has a challenging spelling and pronunciation. Notice the unusual letter combination of "phth." The "ph" is pronounced as an "f."

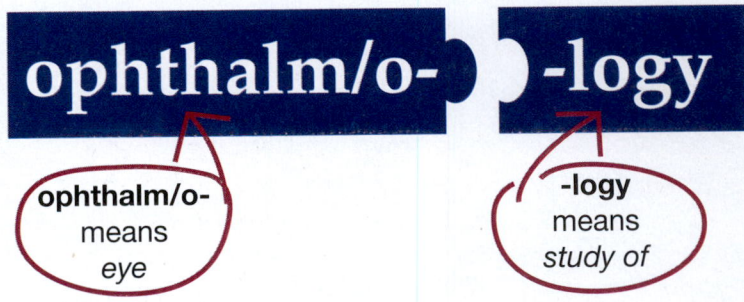

ophthalm/o- means *eye*

-logy means *study of*

Ophthalmology: ▶ *Study of (the) eye (and related structures).*

The **eye** consists of two identical main organs with their associated structures and is categorized as one of the body's special senses rather than as a body system (see Figure 14-1 ■). Each eye is located within an **orbit**, a hollow socket in the anterior skull, and this bony orbit surrounds all but the anterior surface of the eye. The walls of the orbit are made up of several different cranial and facial bones (described in Chapter 7, Orthopedics). The optic nerve, arteries, and veins travel through openings in the posterior bony wall of the orbit to reach the eye. Within the bony orbit, a layer of fat cushions and protects the eye.

The function of the eyes is to provide sensory information of visual images that can be interpreted by the visual cortex in the brain to become the sense of sight. The eyes work in conjunction with the muscular and nervous systems (to move the eyes) and with the inner ear and the nervous system (to help maintain the body's sense of balance).

14.1 Anatomy

Anatomy of the Anterior Eye

Eyelids

The upper and lower **eyelids** are a pair of fleshy structures above and below the eye (Figure 14-2 ■). They protect the delicate tissues of the eye, as they blink involuntarily to prevent foreign substances from touching the eye; they also blink many times a minute to spread a layer of tears that keeps the surface of the eye continually moist. At the edges of the eyelids are sebaceous glands that secrete oil, which acts as a barrier to keep tears on the surface of the eye.

The **eyelashes** in the eyelids and the eyebrows above the eye are hairs that form a protective barrier that extends outward from the eye to keep foreign substances from coming in contact with the eye.

Iris and Pupil

The **iris** is a colored, circular structure (see Figure 14-2). At the center of the iris is the **pupil**, a round opening that allows light rays to enter the eye. The iris of the eye has muscles that can increase or decrease the diameter of the pupil. In dim light, these muscles relax to dilate the pupil, a process known as **mydriasis**. In bright light, these muscles contract to constrict the pupil, a process known as **miosis**.

The pupil itself appears black because very little light is reflected from the back of the eye. However, if you take a picture with flash photography, this flash of intense light does reflect from the back of the eye, and the photograph shows an eye with a red pupil because of blood vessels in the back of the eye.

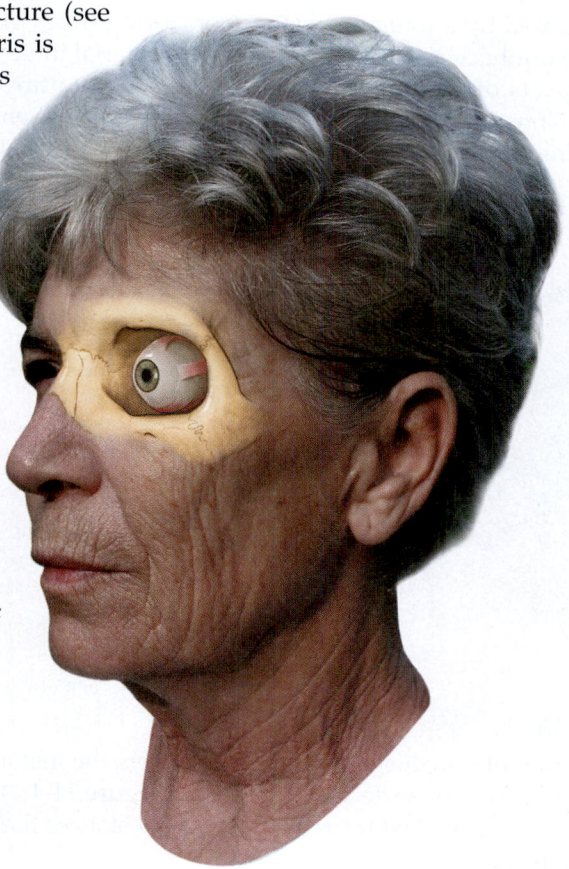

FIGURE 14-1 ■ Eye.
The eyes consist of two identical but individual organs that sit in bony sockets of the cranium. Nerves connect the eyes to the visual cortex in the brain to provide the special sense of sight.

Pronunciation/Word Parts

eye (EYE)
The combining forms **ocul/o-** and **ophthalm/o-** means *eye*. The combining form **opt/o-** means *eye; vision*.

orbit (OR-bit)

eyelid (EYE-lid)
The combining form **blephar/o-** means *eyelid*.

iris (EYE-rihs)

irides (IH-rih-deez)
Greek plural noun: Change the singular ending *-is* to *-ides*.

iridal (IH-rih-dal)
　irid/o- *iris*
　-al *pertaining to*
The combining form **ir/o-** also means *iris*.

pupil (PYOO-pil)

pupillary (PYOO-pih-LAIR-ee)
　pupill/o- *pupil*
　-ary *pertaining to*
The combining form **cor/o-** also means *pupil*.

mydriasis (mih-DRY-eh-sihs)
　mydr/o- *widening*
　-iasis *process; state*

miosis (my-OH-sihs)
　mi/o- *narrowing*
　-osis *abnormal condition; process*
Miosis: *Process (of) narrowing (the size of the pupil)*

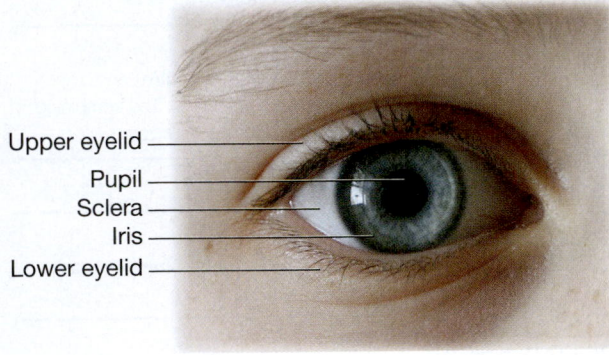

Upper eyelid
Pupil
Sclera
Iris
Lower eyelid

FIGURE 14-2 ■ **Anterior surface of the eye.**
The anterior surface is the only part of the eye that is visible on the surface of the body. The sclera (white of the eye), iris, and pupil are part of this area. The cornea is a transparent layer over the iris and pupil.

Clinical Connections

Genetics. Eye color is a genetically determined trait. In each cell, chromosome 15 contains genes for brown/blue and brown/brown eye colors. Chromosome 19 contains a gene for blue/green eye colors. Both parents contribute combinations of these genes to their baby.

At birth, a baby's irides appear to be slate gray to blue in color because of the lack of the brown pigment melanin in the iris. Exposure to light triggers the production of melanin by melanocytes in the iris. Babies who inherit a brown/brown or brown/blue gene have many melanocytes in their iris, and they develop dark brown or light brown eyes. Babies who inherit a blue/blue or blue/green gene have no melanocytes in the iris, and their eyes are blue, hazel, or green.

Lacrimal Glands

A **lacrimal gland** is located in the superior-lateral aspect of each eye (see Figure 14-3 ■). The lacrimal glands continuously produce and release tears that travel through the **lacrimal ducts**. The lacrimal gland produces tears when stimulated by cranial nerve VII when the eye is irritated or touched by a foreign substance or during times of emotional distress. Tears contain an antibacterial enzyme to prevent bacterial infections in the eye. At the medial aspects of the upper and lower eyelids, two tiny openings drain away excess tears. Those tears flow into the **lacrimal sac** and then into the **nasolacrimal duct** to the inside of the nose. That is why, when your eyes water, your nose also runs!

Pronunciation/Word Parts

lacrimal (LAK-rih-mal)
  lacrim/o- *tears*
  -al *pertaining to*
The combining form **dacry/o-** means *lacrimal sac; tears.*

nasolacrimal (NAY-soh-LAK-rih-mal)
  nas/o- *nose*
  lacrim/o- *tears*
  -al *pertaining to*

conjunctiva (CON-junk-TY-vah)

conjunctivae (CON-junk-TY-vee)
Latin plural noun: Change the singular ending *-a* to *-ae.*

conjunctival (CON-junk-TY-val)
  conjunctiv/o- *conjunctiva*
  -al *pertaining to*

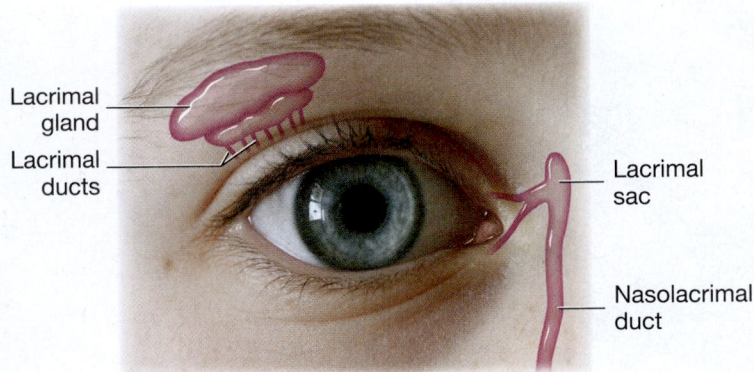

Lacrimal gland
Lacrimal ducts
Lacrimal sac
Nasolacrimal duct

FIGURE 14-3 ■ **Lacrimal glands.**
The lacrimal glands release tears to lubricate the anterior surface of the eye. Excess tears flow into the lacrimal sac, drain into the nasolacrimal duct, and eventually enter the nose.

Conjunctiva, Sclera, and Cornea

The **conjunctiva** is a delicate, transparent mucous membrane that covers the inside of the eyelids and continues across the anterior surface of the eye (see Figure 14-4 ■). The conjunctiva produces watery, clear mucus that traps any foreign substances that come in contact with the surface of the eye.

Pronunciation/Word Parts

sclera (SKLAIR-ah)

sclerae (SKLAIR-ee)
Latin plural noun: Change the singular ending -a to -ae.

scleral (SKLAIR-al)
 scler/o- *hard; sclera*
 -al *pertaining to*

cornea (KOR-nee-ah)

corneae (KOR-nee-ee)
Latin plural noun: Change the singular ending -a to -ae.

corneal (KOR-nee-al)
 corne/o- *cornea*
 -al *pertaining to*
The combining form **kerat/o-** means *cornea; hard, fibrous protein.*

extraocular (EKS-trah-AW-kyoo-lar)
 extra- *outside*
 ocul/o- *eye*
 -ar *pertaining to*

superior (soo-PEER-ee-or)
 super/o- *above*
 -ior *pertaining to*

rectus (REK-tuhs)
Rectus is a Latin word meaning *straight.*

inferior (in-FEER-ee-or)
 infer/o- *below*
 -ior *pertaining to*

medial (MEE-dee-al)
 medi/o- *middle*
 -al *pertaining to*

lateral (LAT-er-al)
 later/o- *side*
 -al *pertaining to*

oblique (oh-BLEEK)
Oblique is an English word that means *on a slant.*

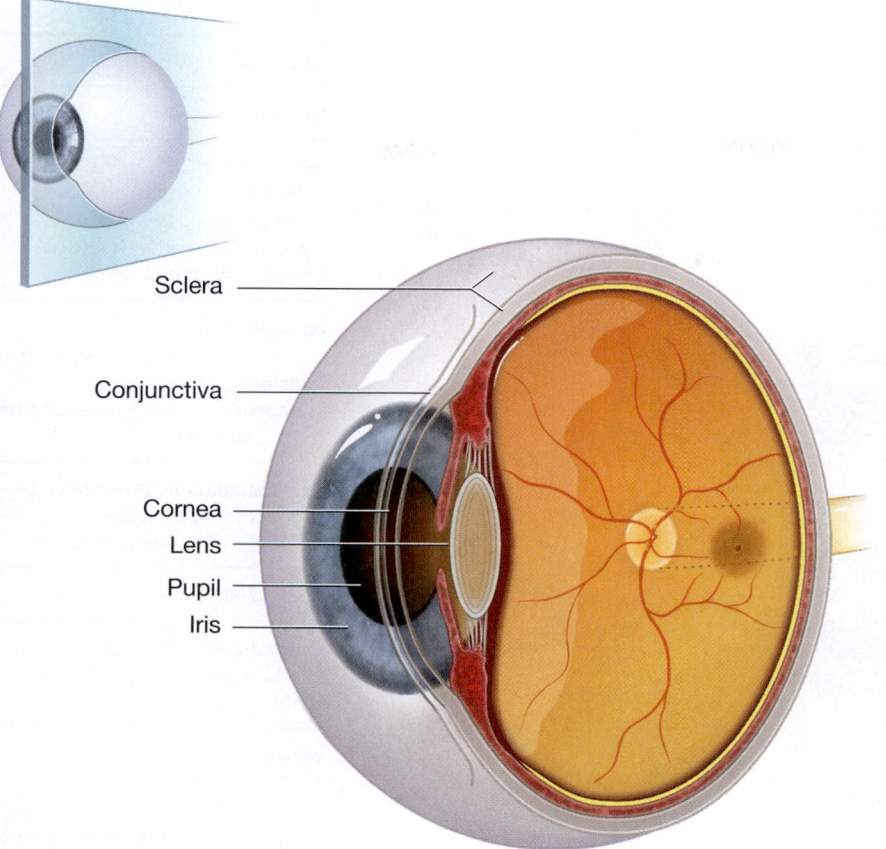

FIGURE 14-4 ■ **External and internal structures at the front of the eye.**
The transparent conjunctiva covers the anterior surface of the eye and also lines the inner eyelid. The white sclera surrounds most of the eye. On the anterior surface of the eye, the sclera changes into the transparent cornea. The colored iris and the pupil can be seen behind the cornea. The lens of the eye is behind the iris.

Beneath the conjunctiva is the **sclera**, a tough, fibrous, connective tissue that forms an outer layer around most of the eye. This tissue is white and opaque and is known as the "white of the eye" (see Figure 14-2 and Figure 14-4). The sclera protects the internal structures of the eye and maintains the shape of the eye. The sclera is the site of attachment for all of the muscles that move the eye (described in the next section).

Across the anterior surface of the eye, the white sclera changes into a transparent layer known as the **cornea** (see Figure 14-4). The iris and pupil can be seen behind the transparent cornea. The cornea allows light to enter the eye, and it bends (refracts) the rays of light. The cornea itself contains no blood vessels. It receives oxygen and nutrients from tears that flow across its surface and from aqueous humor that flows beneath it in the anterior chamber (described later). The cornea does have nerves, however, and it is the most sensitive area on the anterior surface of the eye.

Extraocular Muscles

Six **extraocular muscles (EOM)** are attached to the sclera by tendons. These muscles move the eye in all directions. Four are straight muscles (and have *rectus* in their names). The other two wrap around the eye in a slanted manner (and have *oblique* in their names) (see Figure 14-5 ■).

- **Superior rectus muscle**: Turns the eye superiorly
- **Inferior rectus muscle**: Turns the eye inferiorly
- **Medial rectus muscle**: Turns the eye medially (toward the midline)
- **Lateral rectus muscle**: Turns the eye laterally (away from the midline)
- **Superior oblique muscle**: Turns the eye inferiorly and laterally
- **Inferior oblique muscle**: Turns the eye superiorly and laterally

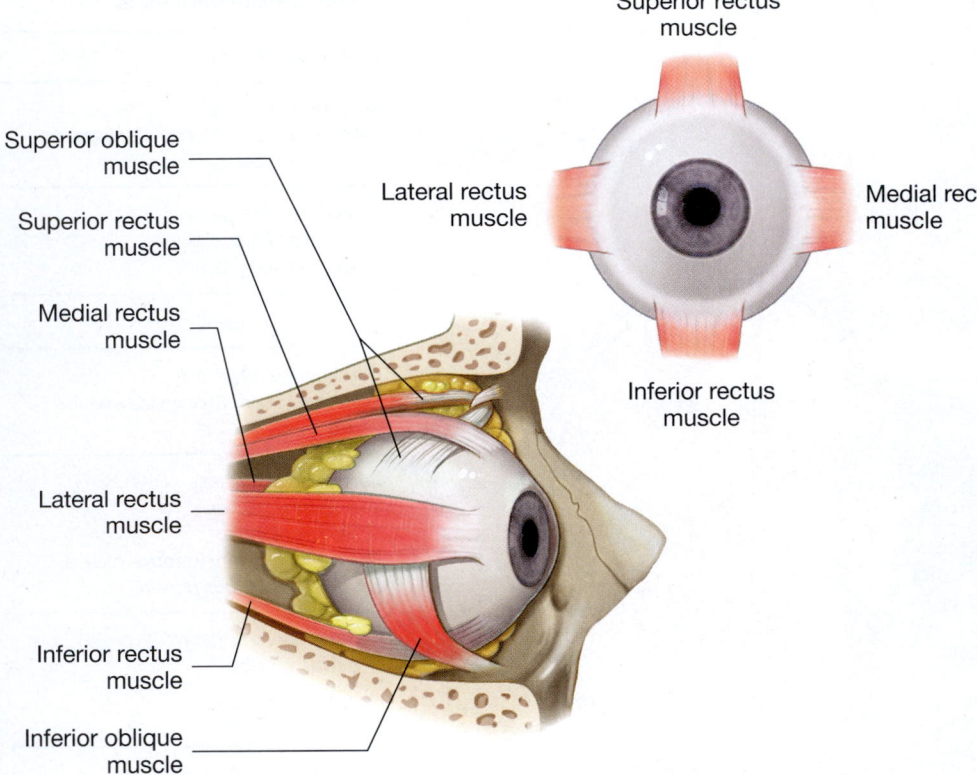

FIGURE 14-5 ■ Extraocular muscles.
The eye can move in all directions because of six different extraocular muscles that are attached by tendons to the sclera.

Lens

The **lens** is a transparent, flexible disk posterior to the pupil (see Figure 14-4). The lens is surrounded by a clear membrane called the **lens capsule**. The lens is able to change shape through the process of **accommodation**, as muscles of the ciliary body contract or relax to move suspensory ligaments that are attached to the lens (described in the next section). The lens accommodates by becoming thicker and more rounded when you look at objects close by (near vision) or by becoming thinner and flatter to focus on objects at a distance (far vision).

Choroid and Ciliary Body

The **choroid** is a spongy membrane of blood vessels that is part of the internal structure of the eye (see Figure 14-6 ■). The choroid begins at the outer edge of the iris and continues around the eye, but it cannot be seen on the anterior surface of the eye because it lies beneath the white sclera. In the posterior cavity, the choroid is the middle layer between the sclera and the retina. The blood vessels of the choroid supply blood to the eye.

The **ciliary body** is an extension of the choroid (see Figure 14-6). It has suspensory ligaments that hold the lens in place behind the iris. The ciliary body contains muscles that contract or relax to change the shape of the lens to focus light rays coming through the pupil. The ciliary body also produces aqueous humor.

The **uvea** or **uveal tract** is a collective word for the iris, choroid, and ciliary body.

Anterior and Posterior Chambers

The **anterior cavity** of the eye consists of two very small chambers. The **anterior chamber** is a very small space between the cornea and the iris (see Figure 14-7 ■). The **posterior chamber** is a very narrow space posterior to the iris. The iris is a dividing structure between the anterior and posterior chambers of the anterior eye. The only opening in this is the pupil. Aqueous humor circulates through both the anterior and posterior chambers.

Pronunciation/Word Parts

lens (LENZ)

lenses (LEN-sehs)

lenticular (len-TIH-kyoo-lar)
  lenticul/o- *lens*
  -ar *pertaining to*
The combining forms **phac/o-** and **phak/o-** also mean *lens*.

capsule (KAP-sool)

capsular (KAP-soo-lar)
  capsul/o- *capsule; enveloping structure*
  -ar *pertaining to*

accommodation (ah-KAW-moh-DAY-shun)
  accommod/o- *adapt*
  -ation *being; having; process*

choroid (KOH-royd)

choroidal (koh-ROY-dal)
  choroid/o- *choroid*
  -al *pertaining to*

ciliary (SIL-ee-AIR-ee)
  cili/o- *hair-like structure*
  -ary *pertaining to*
The combining form **cycl/o-** means *ciliary body; circle; cycle*.

uvea (YOO-vee-ah)

uveal (YOO-vee-al)
  uve/o- *uvea*
  -al *pertaining to*

anterior (an-TEER-ee-or)
  anter/o- *before; front part*
  -ior *pertaining to*

cavity (KAV-ih-tee)
  cav/o- *hollow space*
  -ity *condition; state*

posterior (pos-TEER-ee-or)
  poster/o- *back part*
  -ior *pertaining to*

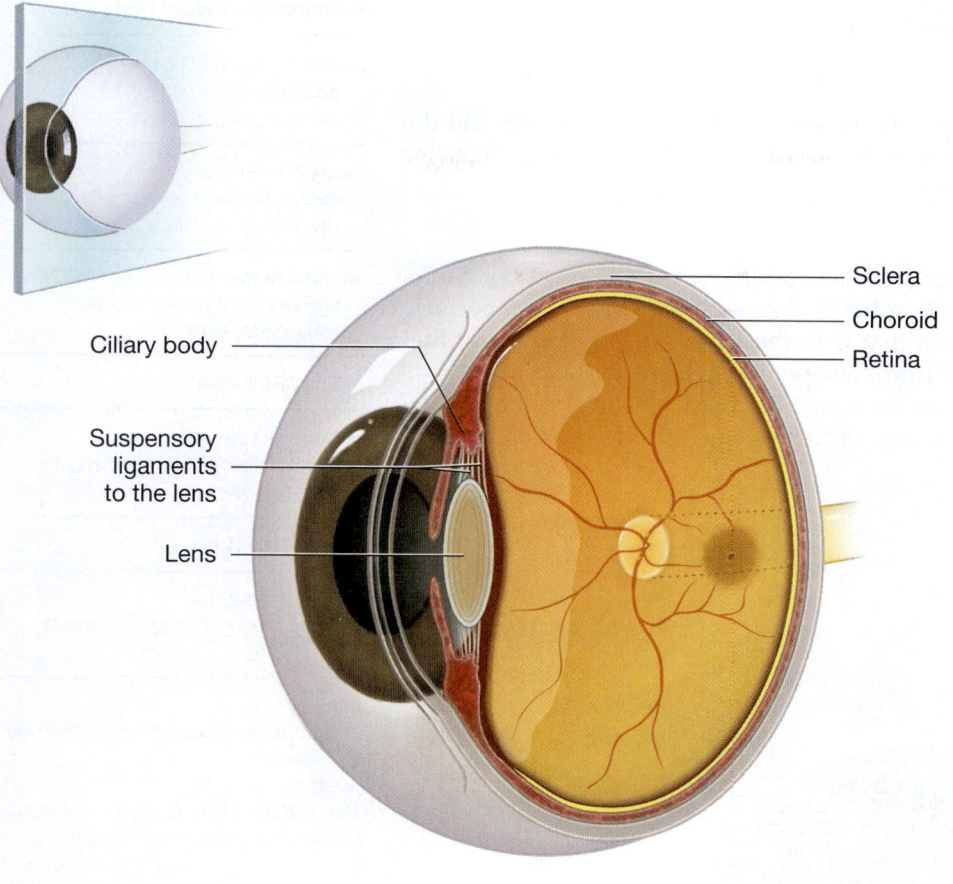

FIGURE 14-6 ■ Tissue layers of the eye.
The white sclera is a tough, fibrous connective tissue layer that helps to maintain the shape of the eyeball. The choroid is a spongy layer beneath the sclera that contains blood vessels. Beneath the choroid, the retina lines the curved wall of the posterior cavity. The choroid also extends anteriorly and becomes the ciliary body. The ciliary body has projections that end in suspensory ligaments that are attached to the lens of the eye.

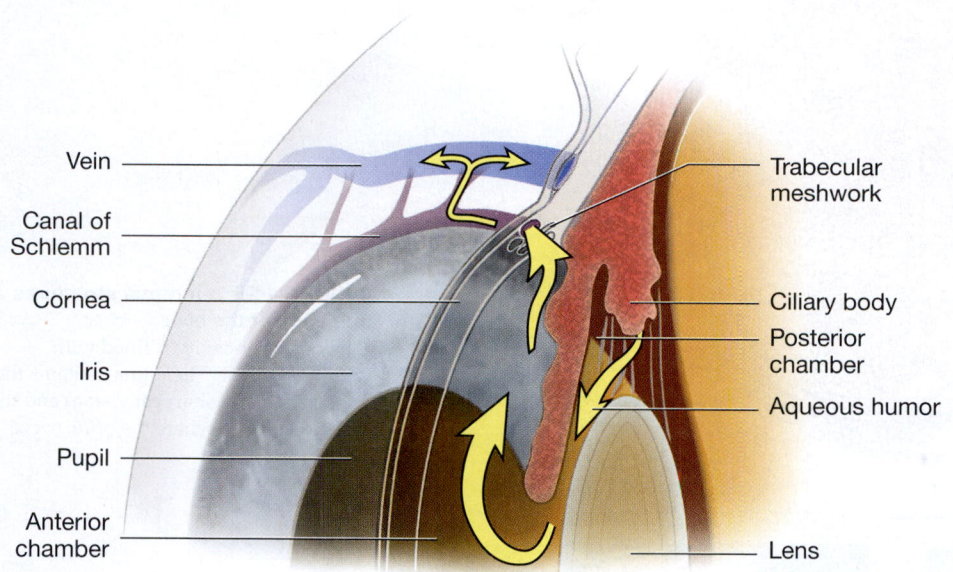

FIGURE 14-7 ■ Aqueous humor.
Aqueous humor produced by the ciliary body circulates throughout the posterior chamber, and then moves anteriorly through the pupil, and into the anterior chamber. It drains through the trabecular meshwork and empties into the canal of Schlemm.

Aqueous humor is a clear, watery fluid that is produced continuously by the ciliary body. Aqueous humor carries nutrients and oxygen to the cornea and lens. Aqueous humor circulates through the posterior chamber, through the pupil, and into the anterior chamber. It then drains through the **trabecular meshwork**, a mesh of interlacing fibers around the edge of the iris, and empties into the **canal of Schlemm**, a circular canal around the iris. From there, the aqueous humor is absorbed into the blood in a nearby vein. The rate of production of aqueous humor normally equals the rate of drainage.

Pronunciation/Word Parts

aqueous humor
(AA-kwee-uhs HYOO-mor)
  aque/o- *clear, watery fluid*
  -ous *pertaining to*

---

trabecular (trah-BEH-kyoo-lar)
  trabecul/o- *mesh*
  -ar *pertaining to*

Schlemm (SHLEM)

Anatomy of the Posterior Eye

Posterior Cavity

The **posterior cavity** is the largest space in the eye. It lies between the lens and the retina (see Figure 14-8 ■). It is filled with **vitreous humor**, a clear, gel-like substance that helps maintain the shape of the eye.

Retina

The **retina** is a thin layer of tissue that lines the curved wall of the posterior cavity (see Figure 14-8 and Figure 14-9 ■). **Fundus** is a general word for *retina* because the fundus of any structure is the area that is farthest from the opening, and that describes the retina, which is farthest from the opening to the eye (the pupil).

There are two distinct landmarks on the retina. The **optic disk** is a bright, yellow-white circle with distinct edges in the area of the retina closest to the nose. This is

Pronunciation/Word Parts

posterior (pos-TEER-ee-or)
  poster/o- back part
  -ior pertaining to

cavity (KAV-ih-tee)
  cav/o- hollow space
  -ity condition; state

vitreous humor (VIT-ree-uhs HYOO-mor)
  vitre/o- clear, gel-like substance
  -ous pertaining to

retina (RET-ih-nah)

retinae (RET-ih-nee)
Latin plural noun: Change the singular ending -a to -ae.

fundus (FUN-duhs)

fundi (FUN-die)
Latin plural noun: Change the singular ending -us to -i.

fundal (FUN-dal)
  fund/o- fundus; part farthest from the opening
  -al pertaining to
The combining form **fundu/o-** also means fundus; part farthest from the opening.

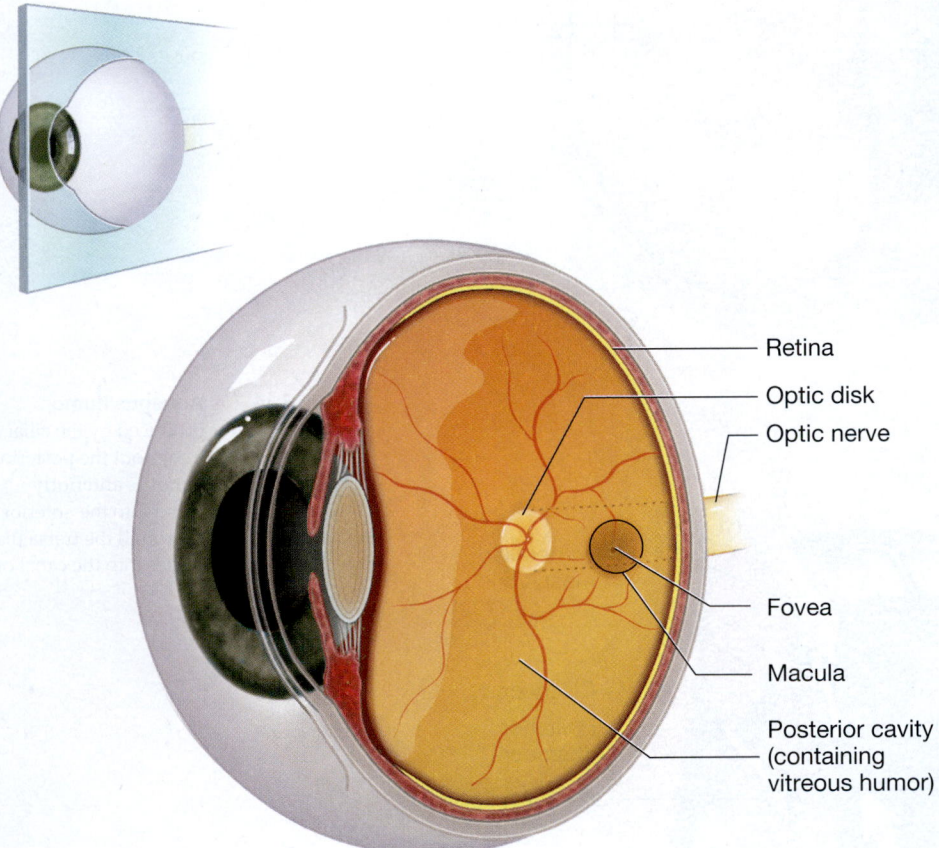

Retina
Optic disk
Optic nerve
Fovea
Macula
Posterior cavity (containing vitreous humor)

FIGURE 14-8 ■ Internal structures at the back of the eye.
The posterior cavity is filled with vitreous humor. The retina contains the macula (area of sharpest vision) and the optic disk (area where the optic nerve enters).

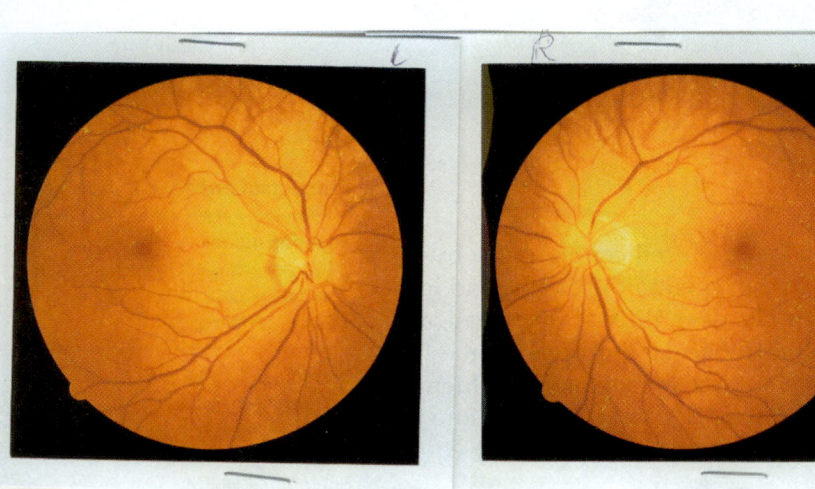

FIGURE 14-9 ■ Retinae of both eyes.
Dilation of the pupil permits visualization of the retina. The structures of the optic disk, retinal blood vessels, and macula can clearly be seen. Note that the size and shape of these structures are not identical in each eye.

where the **optic nerve** (cranial nerve II) enters the eye. The retinal arteries also enter through the optic disk and spread across the retina, and the retinal veins leave the eye at the optic disk. The optic disk is not stimulated by light or color images and is known as "the blind spot." The second landmark is the **macula**, a dark, yellow-orange circular area with indistinct edges. The macula contains the **fovea**, a small central depression. The macula and fovea lie directly opposite the pupil. Light rays entering the pupil fall on the macula, specifically on the fovea, which is the area of sharpest vision. The retina contains special light-sensitive cells: rods that detect black and white and cones that detect color. The optic nerve (cranial nerve II) carries sensory information of visual images from the retina to the optic chiasm in the brain.

Word Alert

Sound-Alike Words

anterior cavity	small cavity at the front of the eye
	Example: The anterior cavity consists of the anterior chamber and the posterior chamber.
anterior chamber	very small space between the cornea and the iris
	Example: Aqueous humor circulates through the anterior chamber.
posterior cavity	large cavity at the back of the eye between the lens and the retina
	Example: The posterior cavity is filled with vitreous humor, a clear, gel-like substance.
posterior chamber	very narrow space behind the iris
	Example: Aqueous humor circulates through the posterior chamber.
macula	area on the retina that is a dark, yellow-orange circular area with indistinct edges
	Example: The macula showed degenerative changes.
macule	small, flat, pigmented spot on the skin
	Example: Sun exposure increases the number of macules (freckles) on the skin.
miosis	decreased diameter of the pupil when the muscles of the iris contract
	Example: Bright light causes miosis, and the size of the pupil decreases.
mitosis	process by which most body cells reproduce
	Example: In mitosis, the dividing cell duplicates and then splits into two cells.

Dive Deeper

The cranial nerves are part of the peripheral nervous system (described in Chapter 9, Neurology). They relay sensory information from the eyes to the brain for the sense of sight; they also relay motor information from the brain to move the extraocular muscles and eyelids, change the size of the pupil, and produce tears.

- **Cranial nerve II (optic nerve)** carries sensory information of visual images from the retina to the optic chiasm in the brain for the sense of sight.

- **Cranial nerve III (oculomotor nerve)** carries motor commands from the brain to four of the six extraocular muscles to move the eye, to muscles that move the eyelids, and to muscles in the iris that change the size of the pupil.

- **Cranial nerve IV (trochlear nerve)** carries motor commands from the brain to one extraocular muscle (superior oblique muscle) to move the eye. The bony socket of the eye has a loop of ligament attached to the bone. When a motor command from the brain travels along the trochlear nerve, the superior oblique muscle contracts, pulling its tendon through the ligament loop like a rope through a pulley.

- **Cranial nerve V** carries sensory information from the eyelids and eyebrows to the brain.

- **Cranial nerve VI** carries motor commands from the brain to one extraocular muscle (lateral rectus muscle) to move the eye.

- **Cranial nerve VII** carries motor commands from the brain to the lacrimal glands to produce tears.

Pronunciation/Word Parts

optic (AWP-tik)
 opt/o- *eye; vision*
 -ic *pertaining to*

macula (MAK-yoo-lah)

maculae (MAK-yoo-lee)
Latin plural noun: Change the singular ending -a to -ae.

macular (MAK-yoo-lar)
 macul/o- *small area; spot*
 -ar *pertaining to*

fovea (FOH-vee-ah)

foveae (FOH-vee-ee)
Latin plural noun: Change the singular ending -a to -ae.

foveal (FOH-vee-al)
 fove/o- *small, depressed area*
 -al *pertaining to*

cranial (KRAY-nee-al)
 crani/o- *cranium; top part of the skull*
 -al *pertaining to*

optic (AWP-tik)
 opt/o- *eye; vision*
 -ic *pertaining to*
The combining form **op/o-** also means *vision*.

oculomotor (AW-kyoo-loh-MOH-tor)
 ocul/o- *eye*
 mot/o- *movement*
 -or *person who does or produces; thing that does or produces*

trochlear (TROH-klee-ar)
 trochle/o- *pulley-shaped structure*
 -ar *pertaining to*

14.1 PRACTICE LAPS

Use the Answer Key at the end of the book to check your answers.

A. Label Structures

Write each anatomy word or phrase in the correct numbered box. Be sure to check your spelling.

iris	lacrimal gland	nasolacrimal duct	sclera
lacrimal ducts	lacrimal sac	pupil	

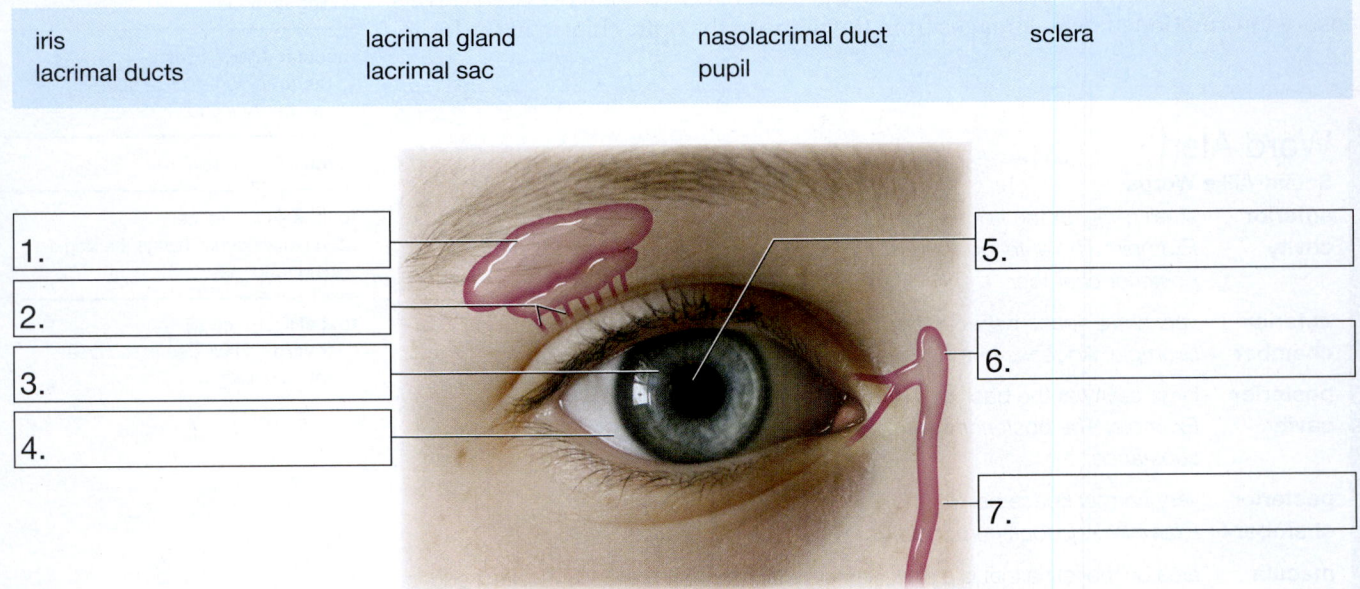

1.
2.
3.
4.
5.
6.
7.

Write each anatomy word or phrase in the correct numbered box. Be sure to check your spelling.

choroid	fovea	optic disk	retina
ciliary body	iris	optic nerve	sclera
conjunctiva	lens	posterior cavity	suspensory ligaments
cornea	macula	pupil	

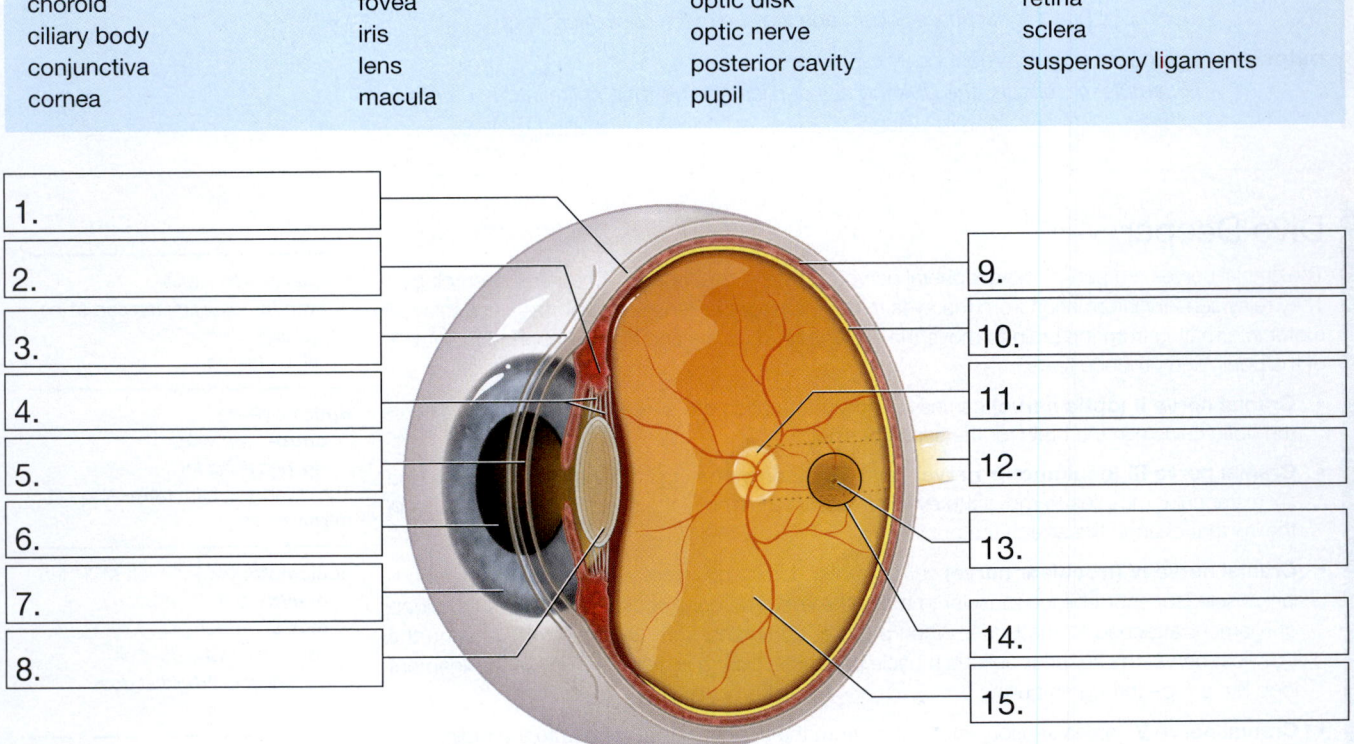

1.
2.
3.
4.
5.
6.
7.
8.
9.
10.
11.
12.
13.
14.
15.

B. Give the Meaning of Combining Forms

Next to each combining form, write its meaning. The first one has been done for you.

Combining Form	Meaning	Combining Form	Meaning
1. **aque/o-**	*clear, watery fluid*	21. macul/o-	
2. accommod/o-		22. medi/o-	
3. anter/o-		23. mi/o-	
4. blephar/o-		24. mot/o-	
5. capsul/o-		25. mydr/o-	
6. cav/o-		26. nas/o-	
7. choroid/o-		27. ocul/o-	
8. cili/o-		28. ophthalm/o-	
9. conjunctiv/o-		29. opt/o-	
10. corne/o-		30. phac/o-	
11. cycl/o-		31. phak/o-	
12. fove/o-		32. poster/o-	
13. fund/o-		33. pupill/o-	
14. fundu/o-		34. scler/o-	
15. infer/o-		35. super/o-	
16. irid/o-		36. trabecul/o-	
17. ir/o-		37. trochle/o-	
18. lacrim/o-		38. uve/o-	
19. later/o-		39. vitre/o-	
20. lenticul/o-			

C. Build Words

Read the definition of the medical word. Look at the combining form that is given. Select the correct suffix from the Suffix List, and write it on the blank line. Then build the medical word, and write it on the line. (Remember: You may need to remove the combining vowel. Always remove the hyphens and slash.) Be sure to check your spelling.

Suffix List

-al (pertaining to)	-iasis (process; state)	-ity (condition; state)
-ar (pertaining to)	-ic (pertaining to)	-osis (abnormal condition; process)
-ary (pertaining to)	-ior (pertaining to)	-ous (pertaining to)
-ation (being; having; process)		

Definition of the Medical Word	Combining Form	Suffix	Build the Medical Word
Example: Pertaining to (the) back part	**poster/o-**	*-ior*	*posterior*

[*You think* pertaining to (*-ior*) + back part (*poster/o-*). You change the order of the word parts to put the suffix last. You write posterior.]

1.	Pertaining to (the) sclera	scler/o-		
2.	Pertaining to (the) clear, gel-like substance (in the eye)	vitre/o-		
3.	Pertaining to (the) pupil	pupill/o-		
4.	Pertaining to (the) eye (and) vision	opt/o-		
5.	Pertaining to (the) lens	lenticul/o-		
6.	Process (of) narrowing (of the pupil)	mi/o-		
7.	Pertaining to (the) tears	lacrim/o-		
8.	Pertaining to (the) front part	anter/o-		
9.	Process (of the lens) adapt(ing)	accommod/o-		
10.	State (of a) hollow space	cav/o-		
11.	Pertaining to (a) hair-like structure	cili/o-		
12.	Pertaining to (the) conjunctiva	conjunctiv/o-		
13.	Pertaining to (the) side	later/o-		
14.	Pertaining to (a) small area	macul/o-		
15.	Process (of) widening (of the pupil)	mydr/o-		
16.	Pertaining to (a structure like) mesh	trabecul/o-		
17.	Pertaining to (the) iris	irid/o-		
18.	Pertaining to (a) pulley-shaped structure	trochle/o-		

14.2 Physiology

The function of the eyes is the special sense of sight or **vision**, a process that involves many structures of the eye and nervous system. Vision begins as light rays from an object pass through the cornea and lens, which bend and focus the light rays through the process of **refraction**. Muscles in the ciliary body contract or relax to change the shape of the lens to further bend and focus the light rays. Light rays from objects directly in the line of vision fall on the fovea of the macula, creating the clearest, sharpest image. The rest of the retina picks up light rays from objects at the edges of the **visual field** for **peripheral vision**.

The retina contains special light-sensitive cells known as rods and cones. **Rods** are sensitive to all levels of light and can detect black and white, but they cannot detect color. Rods function in daytime and nighttime vision. It takes only one photon (light particle) to activate a rod, so rods can detect objects in very low light, but they only produce a somewhat grainy, black-and-white image of that object.

Cones are sensitive only to color. There are three types of cones, each of which responds to only red light, green light, or blue light. The cones are concentrated in the macula. It takes many photons to activate a cone, which is why it is difficult to see colors in dim light. Cones produce a sharp color image that is superimposed on the black-and-white image created by the rods.

When looking at an object, the rods and cones everywhere in the retina respond to the light rays to create an image. At this point, because of the way in which the light rays have been bent by the cornea and the lens, the image of the object is actually upside down and backward on the retina (see Figure 14-10 ■). This upside-down and backward image is then converted to nerve impulses that are transmitted to the **optic nerve**.

The nerve impulses travel on the optic nerve (cranial nerve II) to the **optic chiasm**, a juncture where part of one optic nerve crosses over to join part of the optic nerve from the other side, and vice versa (see Figure 14-11 ■). These combined nerves carry

Pronunciation/Word Parts

vision (VIH-shun)
  vis/o- *sight; vision*
  -ion *action; condition*

refraction (ree-FRAK-shun)
  re- *again and again; backward; unable to*
  fract/o- *bend; break up*
  -ion *action; condition*
  Refraction: *Action (to) again and again bend (light rays)*

visual (VIH-shoo-al)
  vis/o- *sight; vision*
  -ual *pertaining to*

peripheral (peh-RIF-eh-ral)
  peripher/o- *outer aspects*
  -al *pertaining to*

optic (AWP-tik)
  opt/o- *eye; vision*
  -ic *pertaining to*
  The combining form **op/o-** also means *vision*.

chiasm (KY-azm)
  Chiasm is a Greek word meaning *a crosspiece*.

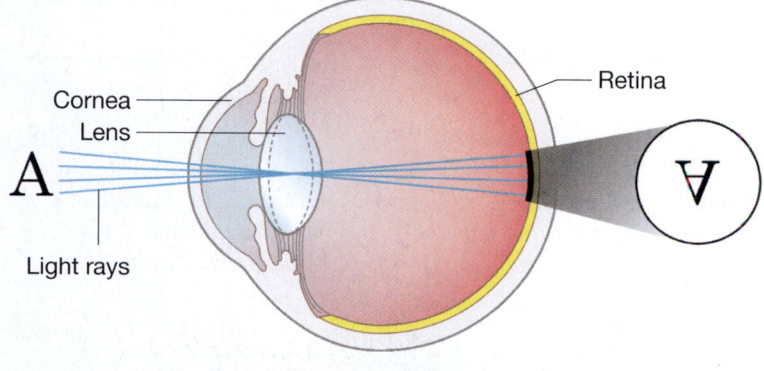

FIGURE 14-10 ■ Light rays coming from an object to the retina.
The cornea and lens focus light rays from an object onto the retina. An object directly in the line of vision produces an image on the macula. This image is sharp and clear, but upside down and backward.

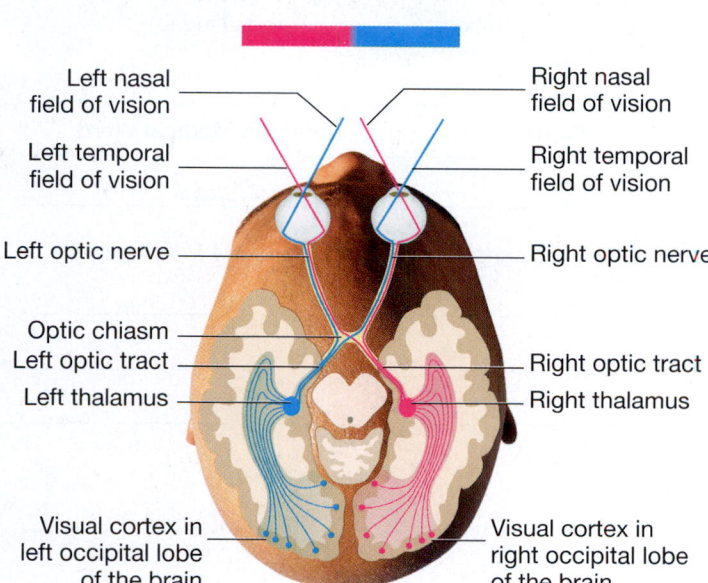

FIGURE 14-11 ■ Optic nerve, optic chiasm, thalamus, and visual cortex.
From the retina, the image of an object travels as sensory information through the optic nerve (cranial nerve II) to the optic chiasm. The optic chiasm is a crossing point where parts of one optic nerve cross over to join the optic nerve on the other side, and vice versa. The combined nerves then go to each side of the thalamus, and then to the visual cortex in each occipital lobe of the brain where the sensory information is interpreted.

images that merge part of the visual field of one eye with part of the visual field of the other eye to create three-dimensional, **stereoscopic vision** with a perception of depth and distance. These combined nerves enter the **thalamus** in the brain. There the sensory images are interpreted so that, if needed, there can be a quick motor reflex to blink or move away from something coming toward the eye. Then the sensory images are sent to the **visual cortex** in the right and left occipital lobes of the brain. The visual cortex merges the images from both eyes to create a single, three-dimensional image that is then turned right side up to face in the direction of the original object. A different area in the occipital lobe associates this visual image with long-term visual memories and communicates with the frontal lobe of the brain where decisions are made about the meaning of what was seen and how to react to it.

Pronunciation/Word Parts

stereoscopic (STAIR-ee-oh-SKAW-pik)
  stere/o- three dimensions
  scop/o- examine with an instrument
  -ic pertaining to

thalamus (THAL-ah-muhs)

cortex (KOR-teks)

cortices (KOR-tih-seez)

14.2 PRACTICE LAPS

Use the Answer Key at the end of the book to check your answers.

A. Give the Meaning of Combining Forms

Next to each combining form, write its meaning. The first one has been done for you.

Combining Form	Meaning	Combining Form	Meaning
1. **fract/o-**	*bend; break up*	4. scop/o-	
2. opt/o-		5. stere/o-	
3. op/o-		6. vis/o-	

B. Build Words

Read the definition of the medical word. Look at the combining form that is given. Select the correct suffix from the Suffix List, and write it on the blank line. Then build the medical word, and write it on the line. (Remember: You may need to remove the combining vowel. Always remove the hyphens and slash.) Be sure to check your spelling. The first one has been done for you.

Suffix List

-al (pertaining to)	-ic (pertaining to)	-ion (action; condition)	-ual (pertaining to)

Definition of the Medical Word	Combining Form	Suffix	Build the Medical Word
Example: Pertaining to (the) fundus	**fund/o-**	*-al*	*fundal*

[You think pertaining to (-al) + fundus (fund/o-). You change the order of the word parts to put the suffix last. You write fundal.]

1. Condition (of) sight	vis/o-		
2. Pertaining to (the) eye (or) vision	opt/o-		
3. Pertaining to sight (or) vision	vis/o-		

Vocabulary Review

Word or Phrase	Description	Combining Forms
Overview		
eye	One of the body's special senses that consists of two identical main organs with their associated structures. The function of the eyes is to provide sensory information of visual images that can be interpreted by the visual cortex in the brain to become the sense of sight.	**ocul/o-** eye **ophthalm/o-** eye **opt/o-** eye; vision
Anatomy of the Anterior Eye		
accommodation	Change in the shape of the lens as the muscles of the ciliary body contract or relax to move the suspensory ligaments to the lens. The lens becomes thicker and more rounded to see objects close by (near vision) or thinner and flatter to see objects at a distance (far vision).	**accommod/o-** adapt
anterior cavity	Area at the front of the eye that consists of the anterior chamber and the posterior chamber	**anter/o-** before; front part
anterior chamber	Very small space between the cornea and the iris. Aqueous humor circulates through it.	**anter/o-** before; front part
aqueous humor	Clear, watery fluid produced continuously by the ciliary body. It circulates through the posterior chamber, pupil, and the anterior chamber, as it carries nutrients and oxygen to the cornea and lens. It drains through the trabecular meshwork, the canal of Schlemm, and is absorbed into the blood in a nearby vein.	**aque/o-** clear, watery fluid
canal of Schlemm	Circular canal around the iris. Aqueous humor from the trabecular meshwork flows through the canal of Schlemm and is absorbed by a nearby vein.	
choroid	Spongy membrane of blood vessels that begins at the iris and continues around the posterior eye. In the posterior cavity, it is the middle layer between the sclera and the retina.	**choroid/o-** choroid
ciliary body	Extension of the choroid. It has suspensory ligaments that hold the lens in place. Muscles in the ciliary body contract or relax to change the shape of the lens. The ciliary body also produces aqueous humor.	**cili/o-** hair-like structure **cycl/o-** ciliary body; circle; cycle
conjunctiva	Delicate, transparent mucous membrane that covers the inside of the eyelids and the anterior surface of the eye. It produces clear, watery mucus.	**conjunctiv/o-** conjunctiva
cornea	Transparent layer over the anterior surface of the eye that allows light to enter the eye and bends the light rays. It is the most sensitive area on the anterior surface of the eye. It contains no blood vessels but receives oxygen and nutrients from tears on its surface and aqueous humor beneath it.	**corne/o-** cornea **kerat/o-** cornea; hard, fibrous protein
cranial nerves of the anterior eye	Cranial nerve III (**oculomotor nerve**) carries motor commands to move four extraocular muscles, move the eyelids, and change the size of the pupil. Cranial nerve IV (**trochlear nerve**) carries motor commands to move the superior oblique extraocular muscle. Cranial nerve V carries sensory information from the eyelids and eyebrows to the brain. Cranial nerve VI carries motor commands to move the lateral rectus extraocular muscle. Cranial nerve VII carries motor commands to the lacrimal glands to produce tears.	**crani/o-** cranium; top part of the skull **ocul/o-** eye **mot/o-** movement **troche/o-** pulley-shaped structure

Word or Phrase	Description	Combining Forms
extraocular muscles	Six muscles that are attached to the sclera by tendons and move the eye in all directions: • **superior rectus muscle** • **inferior rectus muscle** • **medial rectus muscle** • **lateral rectus muscle** • **superior oblique muscle** • **inferior oblique muscle** *Rectus* means *straight,* and *oblique* means *on a slant.* Each rectus muscle is a straight structure, whereas each oblique muscle wraps around the eyeball on a slant.	**ocul/o-** *eye* **super/o-** *above* **infer/o-** *below* **medi/o-** *middle* **later/o-** *side*
eyelashes	Hairs in the eyelids that form a protective barrier that extends outward and keeps foreign substances from coming in contact with the eye	
eyelids	Pair of fleshy structures above and below the eye. They protect the eye as they blink involuntarily to prevent foreign substances from coming in contact with the eye and to spread tears to keep the eye surface moist. The eyelids contain the eyelashes and sebaceous glands that secrete oil to keep tears on the surface of the eye.	**blephar/o-** *eyelid*
iris	Colored, circular structure around the pupil. The color of the iris is determined by genetics. In dim light, muscles in the iris relax to dilate (increase the diameter of) the pupil. In bright light, those muscles constrict (decrease the diameter of) the pupil. The iris is a dividing structure between the anterior chamber and the posterior chamber.	**irid/o-** *iris* **ir/o-** *iris*
lacrimal gland	Gland in the superior-lateral aspect of the eye. It continuously produces and releases tears through the **lacrimal duct.**	**lacrim/o-** *tears* **dacry/o-** *lacrimal sac; tears*
lacrimal sac	Structure that collects tears as they drain from the medial aspect of the eye. The sac empties into the nasolacrimal duct.	**lacrim/o-** *tears* **dacry/o-** *lacrimal sac; tears*
lens	Transparent, flexible disk posterior to the pupil. It is surrounded by the lens capsule. Muscles of the ciliary body change the lens shape (accommodation) to become thicker and more rounded for near vision or thinner and flatter for far vision.	**lenticul/o-** *lens* **phac/o-** *lens* **phak/o-** *lens*
lens capsule	Clear membrane that surrounds the lens	**capsul/o-** *capsule; enveloping structure*
miosis	Contraction of the muscles of the iris to constrict (decrease the diameter of) the pupil and limit the amount of bright light entering the eye	**mi/o-** *narrowing*
mydriasis	Relaxation of the muscles of the iris to dilate (increase the diameter of) the pupil and increase the amount of light entering the eye	**mydr/o-** *widening*
nasolacrimal duct	Structure that carries tears from the lacrimal sac to the inside of the nose	**nas/o-** *nose* **lacrim/o-** *tears*
orbit	Hollow bony socket in the anterior skull. It surrounds all but the anterior part of the eye and contains a layer of fat to cushion and protect the eye.	

Word or Phrase	Description	Combining Forms
posterior chamber	Very narrow space posterior to the iris. Aqueous humor circulates through it.	**poster/o-** *back part*
pupil	Dark, round, central opening in the iris that allows light rays to enter the posterior cavity. In dim light, muscles in the iris relax to dilate the pupil (mydriasis). In bright light, these muscles contract to constrict the pupil (miosis).	**pupill/o-** *pupil* **cor/o-** *pupil*
sclera	White, opaque, tough, fibrous, connective tissue that forms the outer layer around most of the eye, protects the internal structures, and maintains the shape of the eye. Also known as the *white of the eye*. The extraocular muscles are attached to the sclera.	**scler/o-** *hard; sclera*
trabecular meshwork	Interlacing fibers around the edge of the iris. Aqueous humor drains through it and then goes into the canal of Schlemm.	**trabecul/o-** *mesh*
uvea	Collective word for the iris, choroid, and ciliary body. Also known as the **uveal tract**.	**uve/o-** *uvea*

Anatomy of the Posterior Eye

Word or Phrase	Description	Combining Forms
fovea	Small depression in the center of the macula. It is the area of sharpest vision and lies directly opposite the pupil.	**fove/o-** *small, depressed area*
fundus	General word for the retina because it is the area that is farthest from the opening (the pupil).	**fund/o-** *fundus; part farthest from the opening* **fundu/o-** *fundus; part farthest from the opening*
macula	Dark, yellow-orange circular area with indistinct edges located on the retina. It contains the fovea.	**macul/o-** *small area; spot*
optic disk	Bright, yellow-white circle in the retina where the optic nerve and retinal arteries enter, and the retinal veins leave, the posterior cavity. It is not stimulated by light or color images and is known as "the blind spot."	**opt/o-** *eye; vision*
optic nerve	Cranial nerve II. It enters the posterior cavity at the optic disk and carries sensory information of visual images from the retina to the optic chiasm in the brain.	**opt/o-** *eye; vision*
posterior cavity	Large space between the lens and the retina that is filled with vitreous humor	**poster/o-** *back part* **cav/o-** *hollow space*
retina	Thin layer of tissue that lines the posterior cavity. Landmarks on the retina include the optic disk and the macula. The retina is also known as the *fundus*.	**retin/o-** *retina*
vitreous humor	Clear, gel-like substance that fills the posterior cavity and helps maintain the shape of the eye	**vitre/o-** *clear, gel-like substance*

Physiology

Word or Phrase	Description	Combining Forms
cones	Light-sensitive cells concentrated in the macula of the retina that detect color. There are three types of cones, each of which responds only to red, green, or blue light.	
optic chiasm	Area of the brain where part of each optic nerve crosses over to join part of the optic nerve from the other side. These combined nerves carry images that merge part of the visual field of one eye with part of the visual field of the other eye.	**opt/o-** *eye; vision*

Word or Phrase	Description	Combining Forms
optic nerve	Cranial nerve II. It enters the posterior cavity at the optic disk and carries sensory information of visual images from the retina to the optic chiasm in the brain.	**opt/o-** *eye; vision*
refraction	The bending and focusing of light rays as they pass through the cornea and then through the lens	**fract/o-** *bend; break up*
rods	Light-sensitive cells in the retina that detect black and white but not color. Rods function in daytime and nighttime vision. In low light, they produce a grainy, black-and-white image.	
stereoscopic vision	Three-dimensional vision with depth and distance perception	**stere/o-** *three dimensions* **scop/o-** *examine with an instrument*
thalamus	Area in the brain where sensory images can be quickly interpreted so there can be a quick motor reflex to blink or move away	
vision	The special sense of sight	**vis/o-** *sight; vision*
visual cortex	Area in the right and left occipital lobes of the brain. It merges the images from both eyes to create a single image, then turns the image right side up and facing in the direction of the original object.	**vis/o-** *sight; vision*
visual field	The field of vision, including all objects that can be seen, centrally and to the side (**peripheral vision**).	**vis/o-** *sight; vision* **peripher/o-** *outer aspects*

14.3 Diseases

Word or Phrase	Description	Pronunciation/Word Parts

Eyelids

blepharitis	Infection or inflammation of the eyelid with redness, crusts, and scales at the bases of the eyelashes. Acute blepharitis is caused by an infection or an allergy. Chronic blepharitis is caused by rosacea, inflammation of the skin, or microscopic mites that live in the sebaceous glands. Treatment: Antibiotic drug for an infection; corticosteroid drug for inflammation	**blepharitis** (BLEF-ah-RY-tihs) **blephar/o-** *eyelid* **-itis** *infection of; inflammation of*
blepharoptosis	Drooping of the upper eyelid from excessive fat or sagging of the tissues due to age. It can also be from a disease that affects the muscles or nerves (such as a stroke or myasthenia gravis). Treatment: Blepharoplasty or treat the underlying cause	**blepharoptosis** (BLEF-ah-rawp-TOH-sihs) **blephar/o-** *eyelid* **-ptosis** *state of drooping; state of falling*

Word or Phrase	Description	Pronunciation/Word Parts

ectropion	Injury or a growth on the lower eyelid that causes it to turn outward (see Figure 14-12 ■). Ectropion may also be seen as a birth defect in patients with Down syndrome or from nerve damage to the facial muscles in patients with Bell palsy. The outward turning of the lower eyelid exposes the conjunctiva and allows tears to escape, causing chronic dry eye and conjunctivitis.
	Treatment: Artificial tears eye drops or surgical correction
	
	FIGURE 14-12 ■ Ectropion. With the eyelid turned outward, the exposed conjunctiva becomes inflamed. Tears spill out, and the surface of the eye is dry and irritated.
		ectropion (ek-TROH-pee-on)
		  ec- *out; outward*
		  trop/o- *having an affinity for; stimulating; turning*
		  -ion *action; condition*
		Ectropion: *Condition (of) outward turning (of the eyelid)*

entropion	The lower eyelid turns inward because of weakening of the muscles and tendons. This causes the lower eyelashes to touch the eye, causing chronic conjunctivitis and pain.
	Treatment: Artificial tears eye drops or surgical correction
		entropion (en-TROH-pee-on)
		  en- *in; inward; within*
		  trop/o- *having an affinity for; stimulating; turning*
		  -ion *action; condition*

hordeolum	Red, painful swelling or a pimple containing pus on the eyelid. It is caused by a bacterial infection (staphylococcus) in a sebaceous (oil) gland. Also known as a **stye**. Sometimes, when the acute infection subsides, the hordeolum becomes a **chalazion**, a chronically inflamed and granular lump or semisolid cyst. Treatment: Antibiotic drug for a hordeolum; warm compresses or surgical removal for a chalazion	**hordeolum** (hor-DEE-oh-lum) **chalazion** (kah-LAY-zee-on)

Lacrimal Glands

dacryocystitis	Bacterial infection of the lacrimal sac. The sac is painful and contains pus.
	Treatment: Antibiotic drug
		dacryocystitis (DAK-ree-OH-sihs-TY-tihs)
		  dacry/o- *lacrimal sac; tears*
		  cyst/o- *bladder; fluid-filled sac; semisolid cyst*
		  -itis *infection of; inflammation of*

xerophthalmia	Insufficient production of tears resulting in eye irritation. It occurs with aging, because of an ectropion, or as a side effect of certain drugs. Also known as **dry eyes syndrome**.
	Treatment: Artificial tears eye drops; surgery to insert silicone plugs into each opening in the medial aspect of the lower eyelids to keep tears in the eye
		xerophthalmia (ZEER-off-THAL-mee-ah)
		  xer/o- *dry*
		  ophthalm/o- *eye*
		  -ia *condition; state; thing*

Word or Phrase	Description	Pronunciation/Word Parts

Conjunctiva, Sclera, and Cornea

conjunctivitis	Inflamed, reddened, and swollen conjunctiva with dilated blood vessels in the sclera (see Figure 14-13 ■). It may be caused by a foreign substance in the eye, a chemical splashed in the eye, allergens or pollution in the air, chlorinated water in swimming pools, mechanical irritation from eyelashes (entropion), or dryness due to a lack of tears (xerophthalmia). It can also be caused by a bacterial or viral infection. Acute contagious bacterial conjunctivitis with mucus discharge is known as **pinkeye**.
	Treatment: Corticosteroid drug for inflammation; antibiotic drug for a bacterial infection; antiviral drug for a viral infection
		conjunctivitis
		(con-JUNK-tih-VY-tihs)
		conjunctiv/o-
		  conjunctiva
		-itis *infection of;*
		  inflammation of

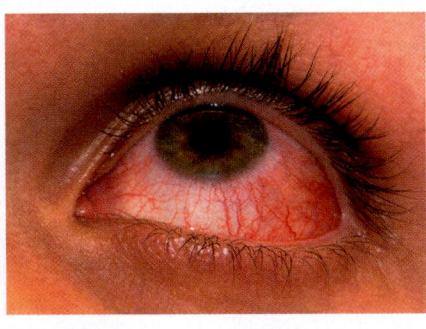

FIGURE 14-13 ■ Conjunctivitis.
Eye strain and hours working at a computer has caused the blood vessels in the conjunctiva to become dilated, giving it a reddened, streaky appearance.

Clinical Connections

Obstetrics. When a woman with the sexually transmitted disease of gonorrhea gives birth, the eyes of the newborn may become infected from the birth canal. A gonorrheal infection of the eye causes conjunctivitis and can cause blindness. By state law, all newborns are given antibiotic eye drops or eye ointment to prevent blindness caused by gonorrhea. *Chlamydia*, another organism that causes a sexually transmitted disease of the genital tract, can also cause conjunctivitis in the newborn.

corneal abrasion	Damage to the cornea due to trauma or repetitive irritation, such as a foreign particle under a contact lens. A chronic bacterial infection in a corneal abrasion can create a **corneal ulcer** with sloughing-off of necrotic tissue. Also known as **ulcerative keratitis**. Treatment: Corticosteroid drug for inflammation; antibiotic drug for infection; surgery of a corneal transplantation	**abrasion** (ah-BRAY-shun) **abras/o-** *scrape off* **-ion** *action; condition* **ulcer** (UL-ser) **ulcerative** (UL-ser-ah-TIV) **ulcerat/o-** *ulcer* **-ive** *pertaining to* **keratitis** (KAIR-ah-TY-tihs) **kerat/o-** *cornea; hard, fibrous protein* **-itis** *infection of; inflammation of*
exophthalmos	Pronounced outward bulging of the anterior surface of the eye with a startled, staring expression. If just one eye is affected, it often has a tumor behind it. If both eyes are affected, the patient usually has hyperthyroidism (see Figure 13-10 in Chapter 13, Endocrinology). Treatment: Correct the underlying cause.	**exophthalmos** (EKS-off-THAL-mohs) The prefix **ex-** means *away from; out*. The Greek word *ophthalmos* means *eye*.

Word or Phrase	Description	Pronunciation/Word Parts
scleral icterus	Yellow discoloration of the conjunctivae, which makes the sclerae also appear yellow. It is caused by **jaundice** due to liver disease (see Figure 14-14 ■). In a patient without jaundice, the normal, white sclerae are said to be **anicteric**. Treatment: Correct the underlying cause. 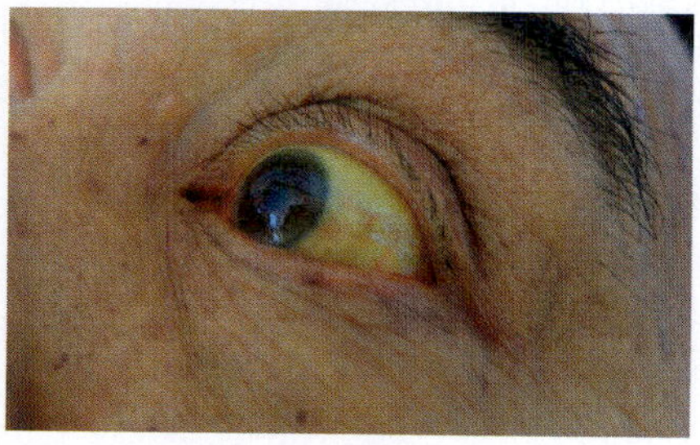	**icterus** (IK-ter-uhs) **icteric** (ik-TAIR-ik) **icter/o-** *jaundice* **-ic** *pertaining to* **jaundice** (JAWN-dihs) **jaund/o-** *yellow* **-ice** *quality; state* **anicteric** (AN-ik-TAIR-ik) **an-** *not; without* **icter/o-** *jaundice* **-ic** *pertaining to*

FIGURE 14-14 ■ Scleral icterus.
This patient's eye has a yellow discoloration. The skin can also take on a yellowish tinge. These changes are due to a high level of bilirubin in the blood that the patient's diseased liver is unable to process.

Extraocular Muscles

Word or Phrase	Description	Pronunciation/Word Parts
nystagmus	Involuntary rhythmic motions of the eye, particularly when looking to the side. Each back-and-forth motion is known as a "beat." Nystagmus can be caused by multiple sclerosis or Ménière disease. Treatment: Correct the underlying cause.	**nystagmus** (nih-STAG-muhs)
strabismus	Deviation of the eye, either medially or laterally. Medial deviation is **esotropia** or **cross-eye** (see Figure 14-15 ■). It is also known as convergent strabismus because the eyes converge (move closer together). Lateral deviation is **exotropia** or **wall-eye**. Strabismus can affect one or both eyes. Treatment: Surgical repositioning of the extraocular muscles, which is done during early childhood 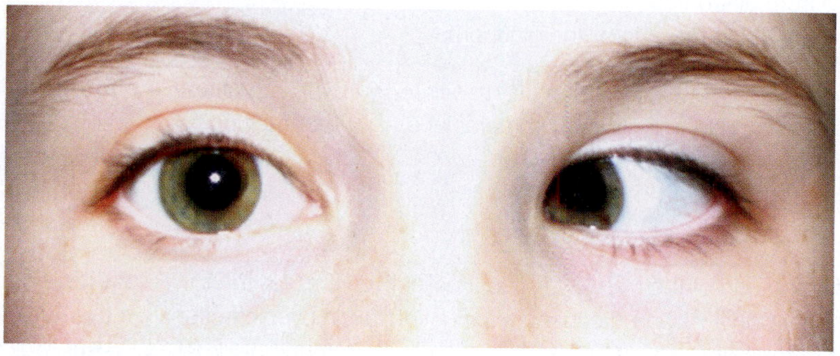	**strabismus** (strah-BIZ-muhs) **esotropia** (EHS-oh-TROH-pee-ah) **es/o-** *inward* **trop/o-** *having an affinity for; stimulating; turning* **-ia** *condition; state; thing* **exotropia** (EKS-oh-TROH-pee-ah) **ex/o-** *away from; external; outward* **trop/o-** *having an affinity for; stimulating; turning* **-ia** *condition; state; thing*

FIGURE 14-15 ■ Esotropia.
In this type of strabismus, one or both eyes deviate medially toward the nose.

Iris, Pupil, and Anterior Chamber

Word or Phrase	Description	Pronunciation/Word Parts
anisocoria	Unequal sizes of the pupils. It is caused by glaucoma, head trauma, stroke, or a tumor that damages the cranial nerve that controls the muscle of the iris (and the size of the pupil). Treatment: Correct the underlying cause.	**anisocoria** (an-EYE-soh-KOR-ee-ah) **anis/o-** *unequal* **cor/o-** *pupil* **-ia** *condition; state; thing*

Word or Phrase	Description	Pronunciation/Word Parts
glaucoma	Increased **intraocular pressure (IOP)** because aqueous humor cannot circulate freely (see Figure 14-16 ■). Glaucoma can progress to blindness. There are two types of glaucoma. • **Open-angle glaucoma**. The angle where the edges of the iris and cornea meet (see Figure 14-7) is normal and open, but the trabecular meshwork is blocked. Open-angle glaucoma is painless, but it destroys peripheral vision, leaving the patient with tunnel vision. • **Closed-angle glaucoma**. The angle itself is too narrow and blocks the flow of aqueous humor. Closed-angle glaucoma causes severe pain, blurred vision, and photophobia. Treatment: Glaucoma drug to lower intraocular pressure; surgery of a laser trabeculoplasty **FIGURE 14-16** ■ **Glaucoma.** This patient's eye shows a silver-gray discoloration because of acute closed-angle glaucoma.	**glaucoma** (glaw-KOH-mah) **glauc/o-** *silver gray* **-oma** *mass; tumor* **intraocular** (IN-trah-AW-kyoo-lar) **intra-** *within* **ocul/o-** *eye* **-ar** *pertaining to*
hyphema	Blood in the anterior chamber. It is caused by trauma or increased intraocular pressure from glaucoma. Treatment: Corticosteroid drug; treat the glaucoma	**hyphema** (hy-FEE-mah)
photophobia	Abnormal sensitivity to bright light. It can be associated with inflammation of the eye, or it can be due to increased intracranial pressure or meningitis in the brain. Treatment: Correct the underlying cause.	**photophobia** (FOH-toh-FOH-bee-ah) **phot/o-** *light* **phob/o-** *avoidance; fear* **-ia** *condition; state; thing*
uveitis	Infection or inflammation of the uvea, which is a collective word for the iris, choroid, and ciliary body. It can be caused by infection in the eye, infection in another part of the body, an allergy, trauma, or an autoimmune disorder. **Iritis** is infection or inflammation that affects the iris. **Choroiditis** is infection or inflammation of the choroid. Treatment: Corticosteroid drug for inflammation; antibiotic drug for infection	**uveitis** (YOO-vee-EYE-tihs) **uve/o-** *uvea* **-itis** *infection of; inflammation of* **iritis** (eye-RY-tihs) **ir/o-** *iris* **-itis** *infection of; inflammation of* **choroiditis** (KOH-royd-EYE-tihs) **choroid/o-** *choroid* **-itis** *infection of; inflammation of*

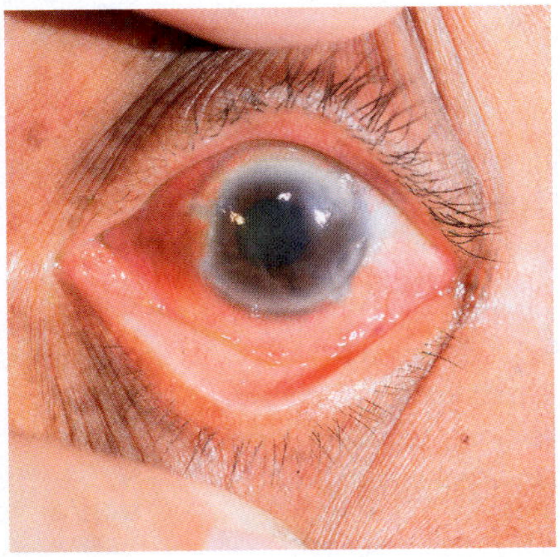

Word or Phrase	Description	Pronunciation/Word Parts

Lens

Word or Phrase	Description	Pronunciation/Word Parts
aphakia	Condition in which the lens of the eye has been surgically removed because of a cataract. Treatment: In most patients, an artificial intraocular lens is put into the eye during cataract surgery. Some cataract patients are not good candidates for an artificial intraocular lens, and so their cataract is removed, but they wear special cataract eyeglasses, and they remain aphakic.	**aphakia** (ah-FAY-kee-ah) **a-** *away from; without* **phak/o-** *lens* **-ia** *condition; state; thing*
cataract	Clouding of the lens (see Figure 14-17 ■). Protein molecules in the lens begin to clump together. This is caused by aging, sun exposure, eye trauma, smoking, and by some drugs. The vision is dull and blurry with faded colors and a yellowish tint around lights. Congenital cataracts are present at birth. Treatment: Cataract surgery	**cataract** (KAT-ah-rakt)

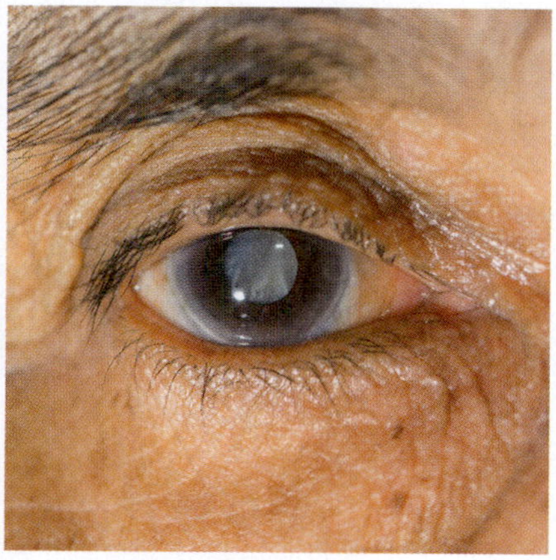

FIGURE 14-17 ■ Cataract.
As a cataract develops, the lens of the eye gradually becomes cloudy and opaque. The vision is blurred, and colors appear faded and yellowed.

Word or Phrase	Description	Pronunciation/Word Parts
presbyopia	Loss of flexibility of the lens with blurry near vision and loss of accommodation. It is caused by aging. Treatment: Corrective lenses	**presbyopia** (PREZ-bee-OH-pee-ah) **presby/o-** *old age* **op/o-** *vision* **-ia** *condition; state; thing*

Word or Phrase	Description	Pronunciation/Word Parts

Posterior Cavity and Retina

color-deficient vision	Genetic condition in which the cones (usually the green or red cones) are absent or do not contain enough visual pigment to respond to the light from colored objects. (see Figure 14-18 ■). Also known as **color blindness**. Treatment: Color blindness glasses and sunglasses correct red-green color-deficient vision with a special lens that filters out specific colors and stimulates the optic nerve to allow correct color perception.	

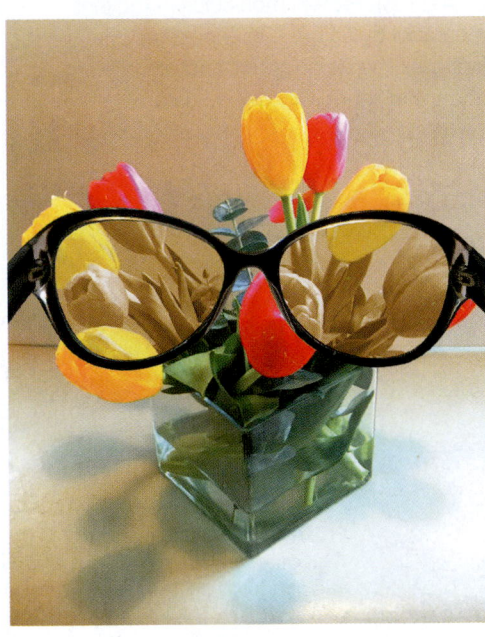

FIGURE 14-18 ■ **Color blindness.**
This is what the world looks like to a person with red-green color-deficient vision.

Clinical Connections

Education. The colors of computer images, textbooks, and other printed materials can be adjusted to accommodate for the disability of color-deficient vision, as they have been in this fifth edition of *Medical Language*.

Disability Accommodations. The Americans with Disabilities Act (ADA) celebrated its 25th anniversary in 2015. Since this law was passed, great strides have been made in making education and employment more accessible to those with disabilities. Extended time on examinations, large-print versions of textbooks, assistive technology that magnifies computer screens, electronic stethoscopes for those with hearing disabilities, and standing wheelchairs for those with spinal cord injuries are among the many technologies used. The concept of universal design seeks to create a learning/living environment that is accessible to all individuals regardless of their disabilities.

Word or Phrase	Description	Pronunciation/Word Parts

diabetic retinopathy	Chronic, progressive condition of the retina in which a large number of new, fragile blood vessels form (**neovascularization**) in patients with uncontrolled diabetes mellitus (see Figure 14-19 ■). These vessels leak, forming exudates (dried fluid deposits) on the retina. They also rupture easily, causing intraocular hemorrhage.
	Treatment: Management of diabetes mellitus; surgery with laser photocoagulation 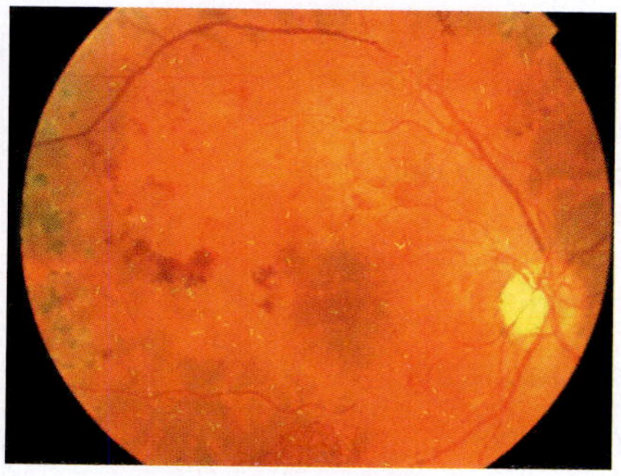
	
	FIGURE 14-19 ■ Diabetic retinopathy.
	This patient's retina shows diabetic retinopathy with neovascularization, the formation of new, fragile blood vessels, as well as some small areas of hemorrhage (center, left) from those new vessels.
		diabetic (DY-ah-BET-ik)
		  diabet/o- diabetes
		  -ic pertaining to
		
		retinopathy
		(RET-ih-NAW-pah-thee)
		  retin/o- retina
		  -pathy disease
		
		neovascularization
		(NEE-oh-VAS-kyoo-LAR-ih-ZAY-shun)
		  ne/o- new
		  vascul/o- blood vessel
		  -ar pertaining to
		  -ization process of creating; process of inserting; process of making

floaters and flashers	Floaters are clumps, dots, or strings of collagen molecules that form in the vitreous humor because of aging and appear as spots in the visual field. Flashers are brief bursts of bright light that occur in the visual field when the vitreous humor pulls on the retina. A sudden increase in the number of floaters and flashers can mean a retinal detachment, which requires surgery. Treatment: None, unless there is a retinal detachment	

macular degeneration	Chronic, progressive loss of central vision as the macula degenerates (see Figure 14-20 ■). In older patients, this is known as **age-related macular degeneration (AMD, ARMD)**.
	 • Dry macular degeneration. The most common type of macular degeneration with thinning and drying-out of the macula.
	Treatment: None
	 • Wet macular degeneration. Abnormal blood vessels grow under the macula. These are fragile and can leak, causing the macula to lift away from the retina.
	Treatment: Photodynamic therapy to destroy abnormal blood vessels; drugs that keep new blood vessels from forming in the retina 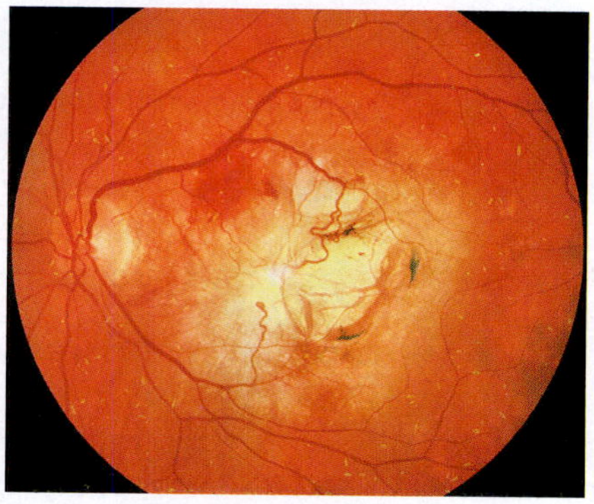
	
	FIGURE 14-20 ■ Macular degeneration.
	This patient's retina shows a large, circular area of macular degeneration (center, right) with smaller areas around it.
		macular (MAK-yoo-lar)
		  macul/o- small area; spot
		  -ar pertaining to
		
		degeneration
		(dee-JEN-er-AA-shun)
		  de- reversal of; without
		  gener/o- creation; production
		  -ation being; having; process

night blindness	Marked decrease in visual acuity at night or in dim light. This occurs with aging or when the diet does not contain enough vitamin A. Treatment: Dietary supplement, if needed	

Word or Phrase	Description	Pronunciation/Word Parts
papilledema	Inflammation and edema of the optic disk. It is caused by increased intra-cranial pressure from a brain tumor or head trauma. Also known as a **choked optic disk**. Treatment: Correct the underlying cause.	**papilledema** (PAP-il-eh-DEE-mah) **papill/o-** *elevated structure* **-edema** *swelling*
retinal detachment	Separation of the retina from the choroid layer beneath it (see Figure 14-21 ■). This can be caused by head trauma or can occur gradually during aging as the vitreous humor changes from a gel-like substance to a watery consistency that flows into small tears in the retina and separates the two layers. In diabetic patients, hemorrhage of the fragile retinal blood vessels can separate the layers. Treatment: Retinopexy with cryotherapy or laser photocoagulation	**retinal** (RET-ih-nal) **retin/o-** *retina* **-al** *pertaining to* **detachment** (dee-TACH-ment)

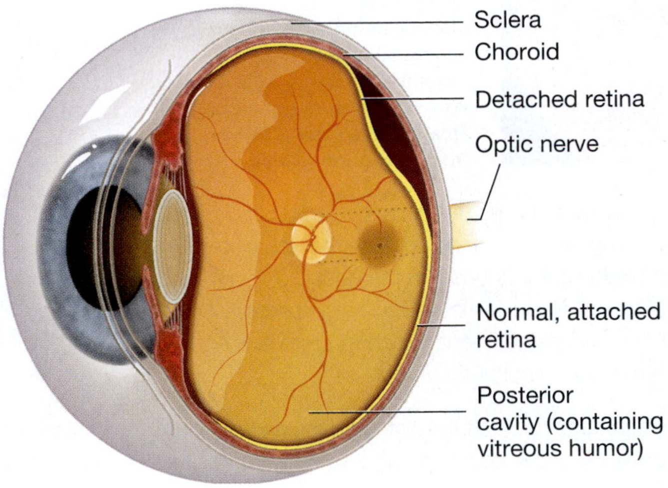

Sclera
Choroid
Detached retina
Optic nerve
Normal, attached retina
Posterior cavity (containing vitreous humor)

FIGURE 14-21 ■ Retinal detachment.
A gradual partial detachment of the retina is painless. The only symptoms are a sudden increase in the number of floaters and brief flashes of light in the visual field. If untreated, however, a partial detachment can become a complete detachment of the retina.

Word or Phrase	Description	Pronunciation/Word Parts
retinitis	Infection or inflammation of the retina. It can also have a genetic cause. • **Cytomegalovirus retinitis** is an opportunistic infection that occurs in patients with AIDS whose immune systems are immunocompromised. Treatment: Antiretroviral drug • **Retinitis pigmentosa (RP)** is a hereditary condition linked to 70 different genes. The retina has abnormal deposits of pigmentation behind the rods and cones, causing loss of night vision or color vision and loss of central or peripheral vision. It can progress to blindness. Treatment: None	**retinitis** (RET-ih-NY-tihs) **retin/o-** *retina* **-itis** *infection of; inflammation of* **cytomegalovirus** (SY-toh-MEG-ah-loh-VY-ruhs) **retinitis pigmentosa** (RET-ih-NY-tihs PIG-men-TOH-sah)
retinoblastoma	Cancerous tumor of the retina in children, arising from abnormal embryonic retinal cells. Treatment: Chemotherapy drug or radiation therapy and surgical removal	**retinoblastoma** (RET-ih-NOH-blas-TOH-mah) **retin/o-** *retina* **blast/o-** *embryonic; immature* **-oma** *mass; tumor*
retinopathy of prematurity	The retina in a premature baby develops abnormal blood vessels that can cause vision loss. If the blood vessel ruptures, it forms a scar that pulls on the retina and can cause a detached retina. Treatment: Laser photocoagulation for a detached retina	**retinopathy** (RET-ih-NAW-pah-thee) **retin/o-** *retina* **-pathy** *disease* **prematurity** (PREE-mah-TYOOR-ih-tee) **pre-** *before; in front of* **matur/o-** *mature* **-ity** *condition; state*

Word or Phrase	Description	Pronunciation/Word Parts

Refractive Disorders of the Eyes

astigmatism	Surface of the cornea is curved more steeply in one area, so there is no single point of focus on the retina. The patient's vision is blurry both near and at a distance. Treatment: Corrective lenses or surgery	**astigmatism** (ah-STIG-mah-tizm) **a-** *away from; without* **stigmat/o-** *mark; point* **-ism** *disease from a specific cause; process*
hyperopia	Light rays from a distant object focus correctly on the retina, and so the patient sees a distant object in sharp focus. However, light rays from a near object come into focus posterior to the retina, and so a near object is blurry (see Figure 14-22 ■). Also known as **farsightedness**. Treatment: Corrective lenses or surgery	**hyperopia** (HY-per-OH-pee-ah) **hyper-** *above; more than normal* **op/o-** *vision* **-ia** *condition; state; thing* Hyperopia: Condition (in which light rays focus on the retina at a) more than normal vision (distance)

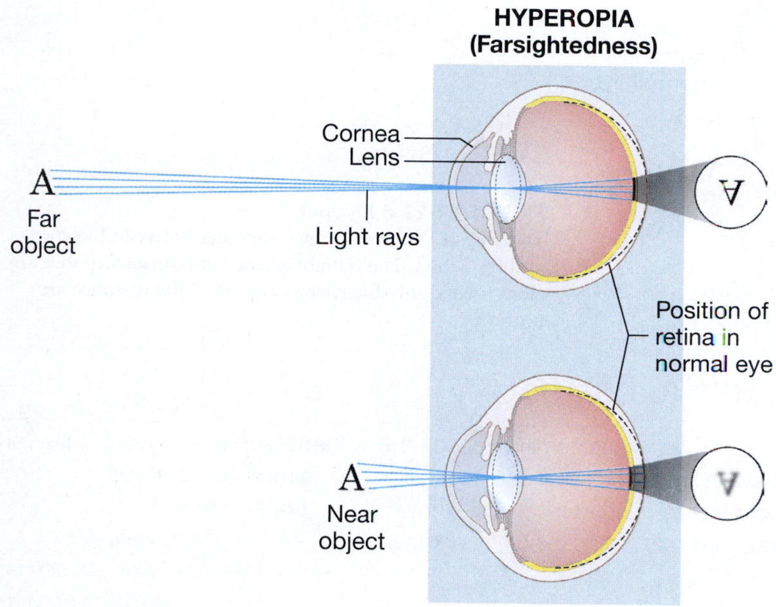

HYPEROPIA
(Farsightedness)

Cornea
Lens

A
Far
object

Light rays

Position of
retina in
normal eye

A
Near
object

FIGURE 14-22 ■ Hyperopia.
There is an abnormally short distance between the cornea and the retina. The patient can see objects clearly in the distance (farsightedness), but close objects are blurry.

Word or Phrase	Description	Pronunciation/Word Parts
myopia	Light rays from a near object focus correctly on the retina, and so the patient sees a near object in sharp focus. However, light rays from a distant object come into focus before the retina, and so a distant object is blurry (see Figure 14-23 ■). Also known as **nearsightedness**. Treatment: Corrective lenses or surgery	**myopia** (my-OH-pee-ah) **myop/o-** *near vision* **-ia** *condition; state; thing*

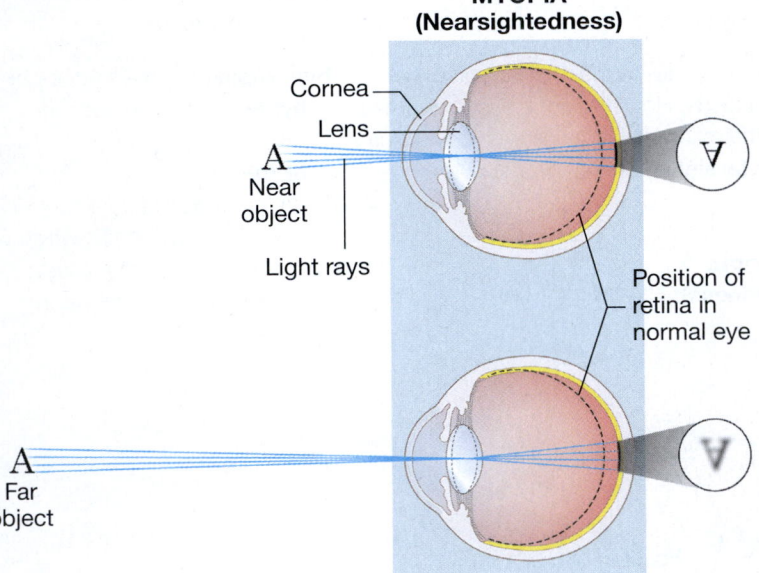

MYOPIA
(Nearsightedness)

Cornea
Lens
A
Near
object
Light rays

Position of
retina in
normal eye

A
Far
object

FIGURE 14-23 ■ Myopia.
There is an abnormally long distance between the cornea and the retina. The patient can see objects clearly that are close (nearsightedness), but objects in the distance are blurry.

Conditions of the Visual Cortex in the Brain

amblyopia	Condition in which the brain ignores the visual image coming from an eye with strabismus or coming from an eye in which the vision is unfocused or cloudy. The brain does this to avoid having double vision. Also known as **lazy eye**. Amblyopia may continue even after the strabismus or other defect is surgically corrected. Treatment: The normal eye is patched until the brain accepts the visual image from the other eye.	**amblyopia** (AM-blee-OH-pee-ah) **ambly/o-** *dimness* **op/o-** *vision* **-ia** *condition; state; thing* Amblyopia: *Condition (of) dimness (because of suppression of) vision (from one eye)*
blindness	Condition of complete or partial severe loss of vision. It is caused by trauma, eye diseases, or defects in the structure of the eye, optic nerve, or visual cortex in the brain. A patient whose best visual acuity is 20/200 even with corrective lenses is legally blind. (*Note*: The vision measurement 20/200 means that a person can only see something at 20 feet that a person with normal vision can see at 200 feet.) Treatment: Correct the underlying cause.	
diplopia	Two visual fields are seen rather than one fused image. It can be caused by amblyopia, by a tumor or trauma that increases intracranial pressure, or by multiple sclerosis that affects nerve conduction to the visual cortex. Treatment: Correct the underlying cause.	**diplopia** (dih-PLOH-pee-ah) **dipl/o-** *double* **op/o-** *vision* **-ia** *condition; state; thing*

Word or Phrase	Description	Pronunciation/Word Parts
scotoma	Temporary or permanent visual field defect in one or both eyes. This is seen as a dark spot, an area, or a curtain in the field of vision. The defect varies in size and can be patchy or solid, stationary or moving. This can be caused by glaucoma, diabetic retinopathy, or macular degeneration when parts of the retina or optic nerve are destroyed. Also, hemorrhage (from a cerebrovascular accident or stroke), a tumor, or trauma in the occipital lobe on one side of the brain can cause a scotoma in the opposite visual field. **Hemianopia** is loss of one-half of the visual field (right or left, top or bottom). Prior to a migraine headache, a patient may see a scintillating scotoma, a temporary moving line of brilliantly flashing bars of light in the visual field. Treatment: Correct the underlying cause.	**scotoma** (skoh-TOH-mah) **scot/o-** *darkness* **-oma** *mass; tumor* *Note:* Although the suffix **-oma** means *mass; tumor*, a scotoma is not an actual tumor, but it appears as a mass in the visual field. **scotomata** (skoh-TOH-mah-tah) Greek plural noun: Change the singular ending *-oma* to *-omata*. **hemianopia** (HEM-ee-ah-NOH-pee-ah) **hemi-** *one-half* **an-** *not; without* **op/o-** *vision* **-ia** *condition; state; thing*

14.3 PRACTICE LAPS

Use the Answer Key at the end of the book to check your answers.

A. Give the Meaning of Combining Forms

Next to each combining form, write its meaning. The first one has been done for you.

Combining Form	Meaning	Combining Form	Meaning
1. **abras/o-**	*scrape off*	20. macul/o-	
2. ambly/o-		21. myop/o-	
3. anis/o-		22. ne/o-	
4. blephar/o-		23. ocul/o-	
5. blast/o-		24. ophthalm/o-	
6. conjunctiv/o-		25. op/o-	
7. cor/o-		26. papill/o-	
8. cyst/o-		27. phak/o-	
9. dacry/o-		28. phob/o-	
10. dipl/o-		29. phot/o-	
11. diabet/o-		30. presby/o-	
12. es/o-		31. retin/o-	
13. ex/o-		32. trop/o-	
14. gener/o-		33. scot/o-	
15. glauc/o-		34. stigmat/o-	
16. icter/o-		35. ulcerat/o-	
17. ir/o-		36. vascul/o-	
18. jaund/o-		37. xer/o-	
19. kerat/o-			

B. Build Words

Read the definition of the medical word. Look at the combining form that is given. Select the correct suffix from the Suffix List, and write it on the blank line. Then build the medical word, and write it on the line. (Remember: You may need to remove the combining vowel. Always remove the hyphens and slash.) Be sure to check your spelling.

Suffix List

-ar (pertaining to)	-ice (quality; state)	-pathy (disease)
-edema (swelling)	-itis (infection of; inflammation of)	-ptosis (state of drooping;
-ia (condition; state; thing)	-ive (pertaining to)	state of falling)
-ic (pertaining to)	-oma (mass; tumor)	

Definition of the Medical Word	Combining Form	Suffix	Build the Medical Word
Example: Pertaining to jaundice	**icter/o-**	*-ic*	*icteric*

[*You think* pertaining to (-ic) + jaundice (icter/o-). You change the order of the word parts to put the suffix last. You write icteric.]

1. Infection of (or) inflammation of (the) iris	ir/o-	_____	_____
2. Disease (of the) retina	retin/o-	_____	_____
3. Mass (of) darkness (in the visual field)	scot/o-	_____	_____
4. Swelling (of an) elevated structure (in the eye)	papill/o-	_____	_____
5. Condition (of) near vision	myop/o-	_____	_____
6. Pertaining to (a) small area (on the retina)	macul/o-	_____	_____
7. Pertaining to (having an) ulcer	ulcerat/o-	_____	_____
8. Infection of (or) inflammation of (the) cornea	kerat/o-	_____	_____
9. State (of the eye being) yellow	jaund/o-	_____	_____
10. Infection of (or) inflammation of (the) eyelid	blephar/o-	_____	_____
11. State of drooping (of the) eyelid	blephar/o-	_____	_____
12. Infection of (or) inflammation of (the) conjunctiva	conjunctiv/o-	_____	_____

C. Define Abbreviations

1. AMD _____

2. IOP _____

3. RP _____

14.4 Laboratory, Diagnostic, and Radiologic Procedures

Word or Phrase	Description	Pronunciation/Word Parts
Laboratory Tests and Diagnostic Procedures		
fluorescein angiography	Procedure in which fluorescein (a fluorescent dye) is injected intravenously. The dye travels to the retinal artery in the eye, where it glows fluorescent yellow-green on flash photography of the retina. The dye reveals retinal leaking and hemorrhages, abnormalities that are common in diabetic patients. The image is an optic **angiogram**.	**fluorescein** (floor-EH-seen) **fluoresce/o-** *emit visible light* **-in** *substance* **angiography** (AN-jee-AW-grah-fee) **angi/o-** *blood vessel; lymphatic vessel* **-graphy** *process of recording* **angiogram** (AN-jee-oh-GRAM) **angi/o-** *blood vessel; lymphatic vessel* **-gram** *picture; record*
Radiologic Procedures		
ultrasonography	Radiologic procedure that uses ultra high-frequency sound waves to create an image of the eye. The ultrasound image is a **sonogram**. • A-scan ultrasound precisely measures the eye prior to the surgical procedure of inserting an intraocular lens. • B-scan ultrasound creates a two-dimensional, cross-sectional image of the inside of the eye to show tumors or hemorrhages.	**ultrasonography** (UL-trah-soh-NAW-grah-fee) **ultra-** *beyond; higher* **son/o-** *sound* **-graphy** *process of recording* **sonogram** (SAW-noh-gram) **son/o-** *sound* **-gram** *picture; record*

14.4 PRACTICE LAPS

Use the Answer Key at the end of the book to check your answers.

A. Give the Meaning of Combining Forms

Next to each combining form, write its meaning. The first one has been done for you.

Combining Form	Meaning
1. **angi/o-**	*blood vessel; lymphatic vessel*
2. fluoresce/o-	
3. son/o-	

B. Build Words

Read the definition of the medical word. Look at the combining form that is given. Select the correct suffix from the Suffix List, and write it on the blank line. Then build the medical word, and write it on the line. (Remember: You may need to remove the combining vowel. Always remove the hyphens and slash.) Be sure to check your spelling.

Suffix List

-gram (picture; record)	-graphy (process of recording)	-in (substance)

Definition of the Medical Word	Combining Form	Suffix	Build the Medical Word
Example: Picture (or) record (of a) blood vessel	**angi/o-**	*-gram*	*angiogram*

[*You think* picture; record *(-gram)* + blood vessel *(angi/o-). You change the order of the word parts to put the suffix last. You write* angiogram.]

1. Substance (that is a dye that) emits visible light	fluoresce/o-	_____	_____
2. Process of recording (a) blood vessel	angi/o-	_____	_____
3. Picture (or) record (of) sound	son/o-	_____	_____

14.5 Medical Procedures, Drugs, and Surgical Procedures

Word or Phrase	Description	Pronunciation/Word Parts
Medical Procedures		
accommodation	Procedure to test the ability of the muscles in the ciliary body to accommodate (contract and flex the lens) as demonstrated on near and distance visual acuity tests	**accommodation** (ah-KAW-moh-DAY-shun) **accommod/o-** *adapt* **-ation** *being; having; process*
color-deficient vision testing	Procedure to determine if the patient has a defect in the red, green, or blue cones in the retina. Each successive color plate requires a higher discrimination of color perception. Color plates that contain numbers are used to test adults (see Figure 14-24 ■), while color plates that contain circles, squares, or animals are used to test children.	

Word or Phrase	Description	Pronunciation/Word Parts

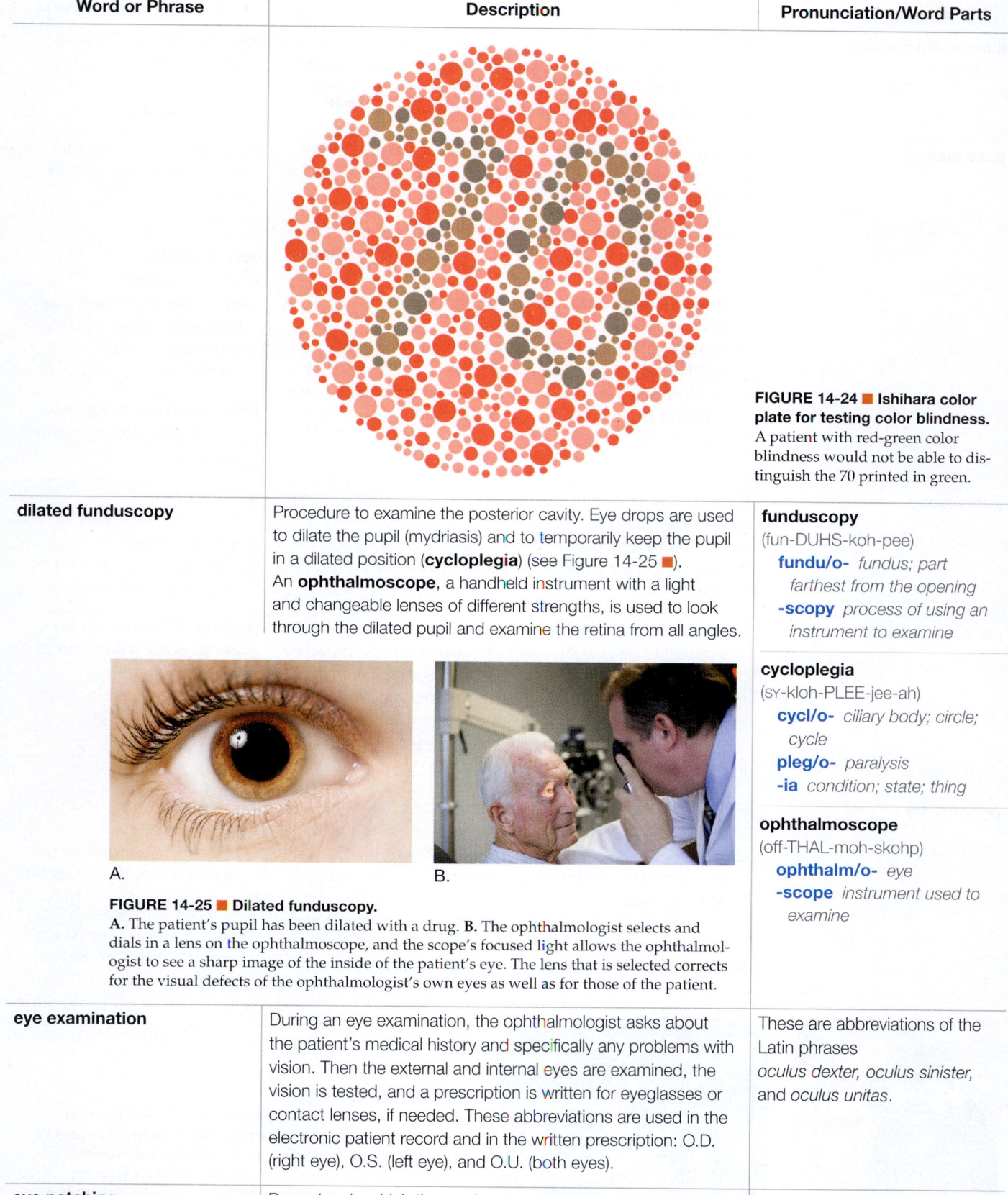

FIGURE 14-24 ■ Ishihara color plate for testing color blindness. A patient with red-green color blindness would not be able to distinguish the 70 printed in green.

Word or Phrase	Description	Pronunciation/Word Parts
dilated funduscopy	Procedure to examine the posterior cavity. Eye drops are used to dilate the pupil (mydriasis) and to temporarily keep the pupil in a dilated position (**cycloplegia**) (see Figure 14-25 ■). An **ophthalmoscope**, a handheld instrument with a light and changeable lenses of different strengths, is used to look through the dilated pupil and examine the retina from all angles.	**funduscopy** (fun-DUHS-koh-pee) **fundu/o-** *fundus; part farthest from the opening* **-scopy** *process of using an instrument to examine* **cycloplegia** (SY-kloh-PLEE-jee-ah) **cycl/o-** *ciliary body; circle; cycle* **pleg/o-** *paralysis* **-ia** *condition; state; thing* **ophthalmoscope** (off-THAL-moh-skohp) **ophthalm/o-** *eye* **-scope** *instrument used to examine*

FIGURE 14-25 ■ Dilated funduscopy.
A. The patient's pupil has been dilated with a drug. **B.** The ophthalmologist selects and dials in a lens on the ophthalmoscope, and the scope's focused light allows the ophthalmologist to see a sharp image of the inside of the patient's eye. The lens that is selected corrects for the visual defects of the ophthalmologist's own eyes as well as for those of the patient.

Word or Phrase	Description	Pronunciation/Word Parts
eye examination	During an eye examination, the ophthalmologist asks about the patient's medical history and specifically any problems with vision. Then the external and internal eyes are examined, the vision is tested, and a prescription is written for eyeglasses or contact lenses, if needed. These abbreviations are used in the electronic patient record and in the written prescription: O.D. (right eye), O.S. (left eye), and O.U. (both eyes).	These are abbreviations of the Latin phrases *oculus dexter, oculus sinister,* and *oculus unitas.*
eye patching	Procedure in which the eye is covered with a soft bandage and a hard outer shield after eye trauma or eye surgery. Also, a normal eye can be patched as a way to treat amblyopia.	

Word or Phrase	Description	Pronunciation/Word Parts
fluorescein staining	Procedure in which a fluorescein (fluorescent dye) strip or drops are applied topically to the cornea to detect corneal abrasions and ulcers. As a light is used to examine the eye, any corneal abrasions or ulcers glow fluorescent yellow-green.	**fluorescein** (floor-EH-seen) **fluoresce/o-** *emit visible light* **-in** *substance*
gaze testing	Procedure to test the extraocular muscles. The patient's eyes follow the healthcare provider's finger from side to side and up and down. • **Conjugate gaze** is when both eyes move together as a unit. This is documented in the patient's record as **EOMI** (*extraocular muscles intact*). • **Dysconjugate gaze** is when the eyes do not move together. • **Convergence** tests the medial rectus muscles. The healthcare provider's finger moves from far away to close to the patient's nose (the *near point*), and the patient's eyes should both move medially to follow the finger.	**conjugate** (CON-joo-gayt) **conjug/o-** *joined together* **-ate** *composed of; pertaining to* **dysconjugate** (dis-CON-joo-gayt) **dys-** *abnormal; difficult; painful* **conjug/o-** *joined together* **-ate** *composed of; pertaining to* **convergence** (con-VER-jenz) **converg/o-** *coming together* **-ence** *state*
gonioscopy	Procedure to look for blockage of the trabecular meshwork in open-angle glaucoma. It uses a slit lamp (see Figure 14-27) with a special lens to illuminate and magnify the tiny trabecular meshwork that is located at the angle between the iris and the cornea.	**gonioscopy** (GOH-nee-AW-skoh-pee) **goni/o-** *angle* **-scopy** *process of using an instrument to examine*
peripheral vision	Procedure to test visual acuity at the edges of the visual field. The patient looks straight ahead while the healthcare provider moves an object toward the edge of the visual field (from the top, bottom, and both sides). The patient indicates when the object is first seen. Alternately, a computer projects dots onto a screen with a grid, and the patient looks straight ahead and indicates when a dot is seen off to the side.	**peripheral** (peh-RIF-eh-ral) **peripher/o-** *outer aspects* **-al** *pertaining to*
phorometry	Procedure to select from many different lenses to find the strength of lens that corrects the patient's refractive error and produces 20/20 vision. A **phoropter** (see Figure 14-26 ■) is an instrument that holds lenses of successive strengths that are dialed into place as the patient looks through each lens at a Snellen chart (described later in this section). Each eye is tested separately. The specifications of that lens are written as a prescription that is duplicated in eyeglasses or contact lenses.	**phorometry** (foh-RAW-meh-tree) **phor/o-** *bear; carry; range* **-metry** *process of measuring* **phoropter** (foh-RAWP-ter) **phor/o-** *bear; carry; range* **-opter** *instrument used to measure vision*

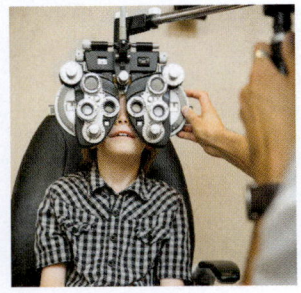

A.

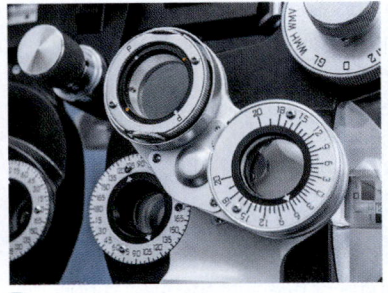

B.

FIGURE 14-26 ■ Phoropter.
A. This instrument helps the ophthalmologist select the most accurate lens to correct the refractive error in each of the patient's eyes. **B.** The ophthalmologist adjusts the dials and changes the lens as the patient looks through the phoropter at an eye chart. From the measurements, the ophthalmologist can write a prescription for eyeglasses that includes specific numbers for the sphere, cylinder, and axis.

Word or Phrase	Description	Pronunciation/Word Parts
pupillary response	Procedure to test that the pupils constrict briskly and equally in response to a bright light. This is documented in the patient's record as **PERRL**: **P**upils **E**qual **R**ound and **R**eactive to **L**ight or **PERRLA** (**P**upils **E**qual, **R**ound, and **R**eactive to **L**ight and **A**ccommodation).	
slit-lamp examination	Procedure to look for abnormalities of the cornea, anterior chamber, trabecular meshwork, iris, or lens. The slit lamp combines a low-power microscope with a high-intensity beam of blue light whose width can be adjusted down to a slit (see Figure 14-27 ■). It is used with fluorescein dye to identify a corneal abrasion. 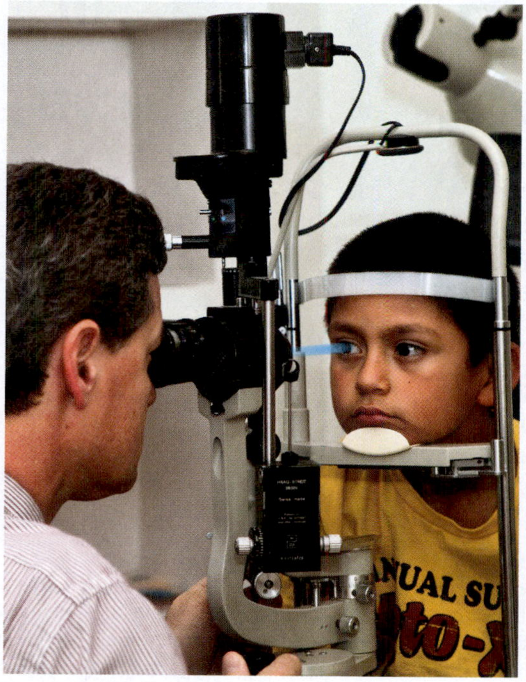 **FIGURE 14-27 ■ Slit-lamp examination.** The patient's chin and forehead are in a fixed position as the ophthalmologist moves the slit lamp from side to side. The slit lamp uses a low-power microscope and a high-intensity, thin beam of light to magnify, illuminate, and view the external and internal eye from different angles.	
tonometry	Procedure to detect increased intraocular pressure and glaucoma. An **air-puff tonometer** is held near but not touching the patient's eye; it emits a short burst of air and measures the pressure of the air as it rebounds from the cornea.	**tonometry** (toh-NAW-meh-tree) **ton/o-** *pressure; tone* **-metry** *process of measuring* **tonometer** (toh-NAW-meh-ter) **ton/o-** *pressure; tone* **-meter** *instrument used to measure*

Word or Phrase	Description	Pronunciation/Word Parts
visual acuity testing	Procedure to test near and distance visual acuity (see Figure 14-28 ■). Each eye is tested separately. A card with typed sentences of decreasing print size is held at a preset distance of 16 inches to test the near vision. The Snellen chart is used to test distance vision from 20 feet away. As an alternative, the Tumbling E chart has capital *E*s facing in various directions, and the patient indicates which way the legs of the *E* are pointing. Children and individuals with limited English proficiency are tested with charts that use pictures. For a patient with a severe vision problem, visual acuity can be measured as the ability to count how many fingers the ophthalmologist holds up or by the ability to perceive light.	**visual** (VIH-shoo-al) **vis/o-** *sight; vision* **-ual** *pertaining to* **acuity** (ah-KYOO-ih-tee) **acu/o-** *needle; sharpness* **-ity** *condition; state*

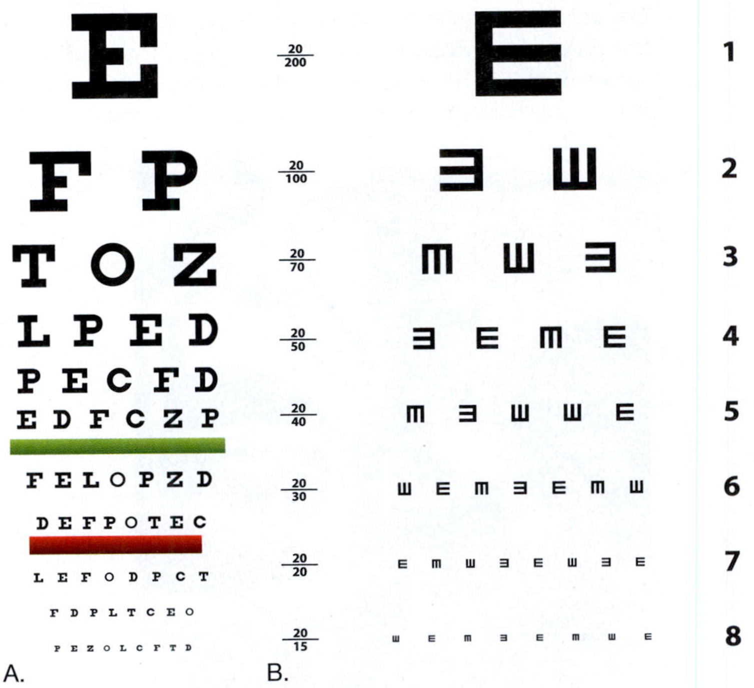

FIGURE 14-28 ■ Snellen and Tumbling E eye charts.
A. Each line on the Snellen chart corresponds to a visual acuity rating. A normal result for this test is 20/20. The first number stands for 20 feet, the distance between the patient and the chart. The second number stands for 20 feet, the distance at which a person with normal vision could see that line. If a patient stands 20 feet from the chart but can only see the top large *E* (a visual acuity of 20/200), that means he/she can only see at 20 feet what a person with normal vision could see from 200 feet away. **B.** Patients who have limited reading ability or English proficiency are shown the Tumbling E chart and are asked to say which way the legs of the *E* are pointing.

Category	Indication	Pronunciation/Word Parts

Drugs

Note: All drugs used topically in the eye are specially formulated to be physiologically similar to the fluids of the eye so as not to damage the delicate tissues of the eye. This includes topical ophthalmic liquid and ointment drugs.

Category	Indication	Pronunciation/Word Parts
antibiotic drug	Treats bacterial infections of the eye. Antibiotic drugs are not effective against viral infections of the eye. Applied topically or given orally.	**antibiotic** (AN-tee-by-AW-tik) **anti-** *against* **bi/o-** *living organism; living tissue* **-tic** *pertaining to*
antiviral drug	Treats viral infections of the eye, specifically herpes simplex virus. Applied topically or given orally.	**antiviral** (AN-tee-VY-ral) **anti-** *against* **vir/o-** *virus* **-al** *pertaining to*
corticosteroid drug	Treats severe inflammation in the eye. Applied topically or given orally.	**corticosteroid** (KOR-tih-koh-STAIR-oyd) **cortic/o-** *cortex; outer region* **-steroid** *steroid*
drug for glaucoma	Lowers the intraocular pressure by decreasing the amount of aqueous humor or by constricting the pupil to open the angle between the iris and the cornea	
mydriatic drug	Dilates the pupil to prepare the eye for an internal examination	**mydriatic** (MIH-dree-AT-ik) **mydr/o-** *widening* **-iatic** *pertaining to a process or a state*

Word or Phrase	Description	Pronunciation/Word Parts

Surgical Procedures

Word or Phrase	Description	Pronunciation/Word Parts
blepharoplasty	Plastic surgery procedure on the eyelids to remove fat and sagging skin. It is often done in conjunction with a facelift. It is also done to correct an ectropion or entropion.	**blepharoplasty** (BLEF-ah-roh-PLAS-tee) **blephar/o-** *eyelid* **-plasty** *process of reshaping by surgery*
capsulotomy	Procedure that is only done during a cataract extraction if the posterior part of the lens capsule is cloudy or wrinkled. A laser is used to make an opening in the posterior part of the capsule to remove the abnormal part.	**capsulotomy** (KAP-soo-LAW-toh-mee) **capsul/o-** *capsule; enveloping structure* **-tomy** *process of cutting; process of making an incision*

Word or Phrase	Description	Pronunciation/Word Parts
cataract surgery	Procedure of **phacoemulsification** to remove a lens affected by a cataract. Preoperatively, a laser is used to measure the length of the eye and the curvature of the cornea so that a customized **intraocular lens (IOL)** can be created before the surgery. During surgery, a small, self-sealing (stitchless) incision is made in the cornea. An ultrasonic probe is inserted, and its sound waves are used to emulsify (break up) the lens (see Figure 14-29 ■). The lens pieces are removed with irrigation and suction, and the intraocular lens is inserted. The IOL folds to pass through the incision and then unfolds inside the capsule. 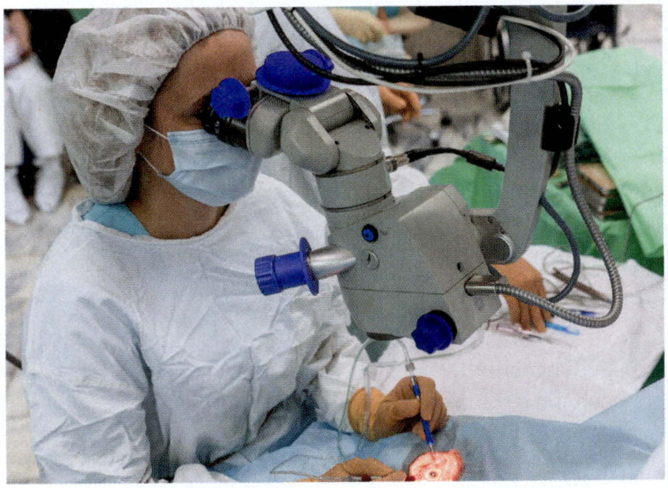 **FIGURE 14-29 ■** **Cataract extraction.** The surgeon looks through an operating microscope that magnifies the small structures of the eye. She inserts a phacoemulsification probe that emits sound waves to break up the lens.	**phacoemulsification** (FAY-koh-ee-MUL-sih-fih-KAY-shun) **phac/o-** *lens* **emulsific/o-** *liquid with suspended particles* **-ation** *being; having; process* **intraocular** (IN-trah-AW-kyoo-lar) **intra-** *within* **ocul/o-** *eye* **-ar** *pertaining to*
corneal transplantation	Procedure to replace a damaged or diseased cornea. The cornea is removed, and a donor cornea is sutured in place. Donor corneae are obtained from people who have died of illness or accident and willed their organs to others.	**transplantation** (TRANS-plan-TAY-shun) **transplant/o-** *move and put in another place* **-ation** *being; having; process*
enucleation	Procedure to remove the entire eye from its bony orbit because of trauma or a tumor	**enucleation** (ee-NOO-klee-AA-shun) **enucle/o-** *remove the main part* **-ation** *being; having; process*
hyperopia surgery	Procedure to correct farsightedness by creating a greater curvature in the cornea, and that corrects the refractive error • **Conductive keratoplasty (CK)** is a noninvasive procedure that uses radio waves delivered by a probe as thin as a hair to spots around the edge of the cornea. • **Laser thermal keratoplasty (LTK)** uses a laser that heats small areas in two concentric rings around the cornea.	**conductive** (con-DUK-tiv) **conduct/o-** *carrying; conveying* **-ive** *pertaining to* **keratoplasty** (KAIR-ah-toh-PLAS-tee) **kerat/o-** *cornea; hard, fibrous protein* **-plasty** *process of reshaping by surgery* **laser** (LAY-zer) **thermal** (THER-mal) **therm/o-** *heat* **-al** *pertaining to*

Word or Phrase	Description	Pronunciation/Word Parts
myopia surgery	Procedure to correct nearsightedness	*in situ* (IN SY-too)
	• **Laser-assisted** *in situ* **keratomileusis (LASIK)**. Preoperatively, a three-dimensional map of the cornea is created and programmed into the laser. A **microkeratome** is used to create a very thin flap on the surface of the cornea. The flap is peeled back, and a cold laser that cuts tissue without heating it is used to reshape the underlying cornea. The surface flap is then put back in place.	**keratomileusis** (KAIR-ah-TOH-my-LOO-sihs) **kerat/o-** *cornea; hard, fibrous protein* **-mileusis** *process of carving*
	• **Photorefractive keratectomy (PRK)**. A very thin outer layer of the cornea is removed and discarded. Then a cold laser is used to reshape the curvature of the remaining cornea. A new outer layer grows back in a few days.	**microkeratome** (MY-kroh-KAIR-ah-tohm) **micr/o-** *one millionth; small* **kerat/o-** *cornea; hard, fibrous protein* **-tome** *area with distinct edges; instrument used to cut*
		photorefractive (FOH-toh-ree-FRAK-tiv) **phot/o-** *light* **re-** *again and again; backward; unable to* **fract/o-** *bend; break up* **-ive** *pertaining to*
		keratectomy (KAIR-ah-TEK-toh-mee) **kerat/o-** *cornea; hard, fibrous protein* **-ectomy** *surgical removal*
photodynamic therapy (PDT)	Procedure to treat wet age-related macular degeneration. A light-sensitive drug is injected into the blood. The drug collects in abnormal vessels under the macula. Laser light then activates the drug and causes it to seal off blood flow through the abnormal blood vessels.	**photodynamic** (FOH-toh-dy-NAM-ik) **phot/o-** *light* **dynam/o-** *movement; power* **-ic** *pertaining to*

Word or Phrase	Description	Pronunciation/Word Parts
retinopexy	Procedure to reattach a detached retina • **Cryopexy** is used to freeze the tissue and fix all three layers (sclera, choroid, retina) together. • **Laser photocoagulation** is used to heat spots on the retina to coagulate and seal the detached retina to the layers beneath it (see Figure 14-30 ■). • **Vitrectomy**. If there is bleeding from the detached retina and the vitreous humor contains blood, the laser's light cannot reach the retina. A vitrectomy must be done first to remove the vitreous humor and replace it with clear, man-made fluid. • **Pneumatic retinopexy (PR)**. A gas bubble is injected into the posterior cavity and positioned against the retinal tear. Then cryopexy or laser photocoagulation is used to seal the tear. This procedure can be done in an ophthalmologist's office. 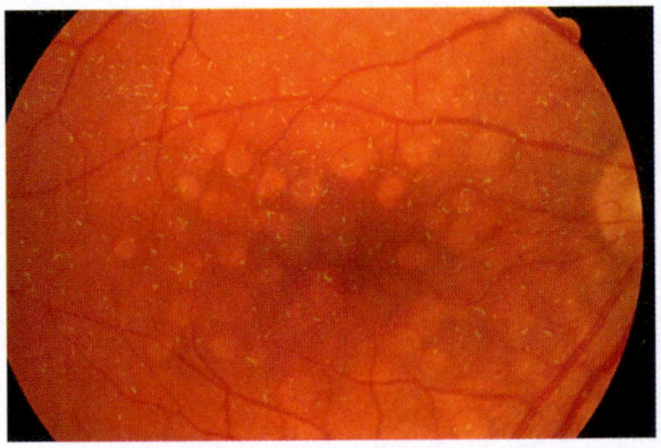 **FIGURE 14-30** ■ **Retinopexy.** This procedure is done to treat a detached retina by using heat or cold to seal the layers (retina, choroid, and sclera) together and prevent further detachment.	**retinopexy** (RET-ih-noh-PEK-see) **retin/o-** *retina* **-pexy** *process of surgically fixing in place* **cryopexy** (KRY-oh-PEK-see) **cry/o-** *cold* **-pexy** *process of surgically fixing in place* **photocoagulation** (FOH-toh-koh-AG-yoo-LAY-shun) **phot/o-** *light* **coagul/o-** *clotting* **-ation** *being; having; process* **vitrectomy** (vih-TREK-toh-mee) **vitre/o-** *clear, gel-like substance* **-ectomy** *surgical removal* **pneumatic** (noo-MAT-ik) **pneum/o-** *air; lung* **-atic** *pertaining to*
strabismus surgery	Procedure to correct esotropia or exotropia. During a **resection**, the extraocular muscle on one side is shortened. During a **recession**, the extraocular muscle on the other side is lengthened and reattached.	**resection** (ree-SEK-shun) **resect/o-** *cut out; remove* **-ion** *action; condition* **recession** (ree-SEH-shun) **recess/o-** *move back* **-ion** *action; condition*
trabeculoplasty	Procedure that uses a laser to treat open-angle glaucoma. The laser creates small holes in half of the trabecular meshwork to increase the flow of aqueous humor.	**trabeculoplasty** (trah-BEH-kyoo-loh-PLAS-tee) **trabecul/o-** *mesh* **-plasty** *process of reshaping by surgery*

14.5 PRACTICE LAPS

Use the Answer Key at the end of the book to check your answers.

A. Give the Meaning of Combining Forms

Next to each combining form, write its meaning. The first one has been done for you.

Combining Form	Meaning	Combining Form	Meaning
1. **accommod/o-**	*adapt*	20. ocul/o-	
2. acu/o-		21. ophthalm/o-	
3. bi/o-		22. peripher/o-	
4. blephar/o-		23. phac/o-	
5. capsul/o-		24. phor/o-	
6. coagul/o-		25. phot/o-	
7. conjug/o-		26. pleg/o-	
8. converg/o-		27. pneum/o-	
9. cortic/o-		28. recess/o-	
10. cry/o-		29. resect/o-	
11. cycl/o-		30. retin/o-	
12. emulsific/o-		31. therm/o-	
13. enucle/o-		32. ton/o-	
14. fluoresce/o-		33. trabecul/o-	
15. fundu/o-		34. transplant/o-	
16. goni/o-		35. vir/o-	
17. kerat/o-		36. vis/o-	
18. micr/o-		37. vitre/o-	
19. mydr/o-			

B. Build Words

Read the definition of the medical word. Look at the combining form that is given. Select the correct suffix from the Suffix List, and write it on the blank line. Then build the medical word, and write it on the line. (Remember: You may need to remove the combining vowel. Always remove the hyphens and slash.) Be sure to check your spelling.

Suffix List

-al (pertaining to)
-atic (pertaining to)
-ectomy (surgical removal)
-iatic (pertaining to a process or a state)
-ion (action; condition)
-ity (condition; state)

-meter (instrument used to measure)
-metry (process of measuring)
-mileusis (process of carving)
-opter (instrument used to measure vision)

-pexy (process of fixing in place)
-plasty (process of reshaping by surgery)
-scope (instrument used to examine)

-scopy (process of using an instrument to examine)
-tomy (process of cutting; process of making an incision)
-ual (pertaining to)

Definition of the Medical Word	Combining Form	Suffix	Build the Medical Word
Example: Pertaining to air (a gas bubble)	**pneum/o-**	*-atic*	*pneumatic*

[*You think* pertaining to (*-atic*) + air (*pneum/o-*). You change the order of the word parts to put the suffix last. You write pneumatic.]

1. Instrument used to measure pressure (in the eye)	ton/o-		
2. Pertaining to sight	vis/o-		
3. Surgical removal (of the) clear, gel-like substance	vitre/o-		
4. Pertaining to a state (of) widening (of the pupil)	mydr/o-		
5. Process of carving (the) cornea	kerat/o-		
6. Process of using an instrument to examine (the) angle (between the iris and cornea)	goni/o-		
7. Process of fixing in place (with) cold	cry/o-		
8. State (of) sharpness (of vision)	acu/o-		
9. Process of reshaping by surgery (on the) eyelid	blephar/o-		
10. Process of measuring (a) range (of vision)	phor/o-		
11. Process of cutting (the) enveloping structure (around the lens)	capsul/o-		

Definition of the Medical Word	Combining Form	Suffix	Build the Medical Word
12. Instrument used to examine (the) eye	ophthalm/o-	_____	_____
13. Pertaining to (the) outer aspects (of vision)	peripher/o-	_____	_____
14. Action (to) move back (a muscle)	recess/o-	_____	_____
15. Instrument used to measure vision range	phor/o-	_____	_____
16. Process of fixing in place (the) retina	retin/o-	_____	_____
17. Process of measuring (the eye) pressure	ton/o-	_____	_____
18. Process of reshaping by surgery (on the) cornea	kerat/o-	_____	_____
19. Process of using an instrument to examine (the) fundus	fund/o-	_____	_____

C. Define Abbreviations

1. CK   _____
2. EOMI   _____
3. IOL   _____
4. LASIK   _____
5. LTK   _____

6. O.D.   _____
7. O.S.   _____
8. PERRL   _____
9. PDT   _____

Abbreviations Summary

AMD	age-related macular degeneration		**O.D.**	Doctor of Optometry
ARMD	age-related macular degeneration		**OS, O.S.**	left eye (Latin, *oculus sinister*)
CK	conductive keratoplasty		**OU, O.U.**	both eyes (Latin, *oculus unitas*); each eye (Latin, *oculus uterque*)
EOM	extraocular muscles			
EOMI	extraocular muscles intact		**PDT**	photodynamic therapy
IOL	intraocular lens		**PERRL**	pupils equal, round, and reactive to light
IOP	intraocular pressure		**PERRLA**	pupils equal, round, and reactive to light and accommodation
LASIK	laser-assisted *in situ* keratomileusis (pronounced LAY-sik)		**PR**	pneumatic retinopexy
LTK	laser thermal keratoplasty		**PRK**	photorefractive keratectomy
OD, O.D.	right eye (Latin, *oculus dexter*)		**RP**	retinitis pigmentosa

Word Alert

Abbreviations. Abbreviations are commonly used in all types of medical documents; however, they can mean different things to different people and their meanings can be misinterpreted. Always verify the meaning of an abbreviation.

- *O.D.* means *right eye* or *Doctor of Optometry*, but it also means *overdose*.

- According to the Institute for Safe Medication Practices (ISMP), the abbreviations for right eye (O.D, O.D.), left eye (OS, O.S.), and both eyes or each eye (OU, O.U.) can be misinterpreted, causing medication errors, and should not be used. However, because they are still used by healthcare professionals, they are included in the Abbreviations Summary.

It's Greek to Me! Did you notice that some words have two different combining forms? Combining forms from both Greek and Latin remain a part of medical language today.

Word	Greek	Latin	Medical Word Examples
cornea	kerat/o-	corne/o-	keratoplasty; corneal
eye	ophthalm/o-	ocul/o-	ophthalmology; ocular
lens	phac/o-, phak/o-	lenticul/o-	phacoemulsification, aphakia; lenticular
pupil	cor/o-	pupill/o-	anisocoria; pupillary
sight, vision	op/o-, opt/o-	vis/o-	hyperopia, optic; visual

Career Focus

Meet Paul, an optician

"I pick up where the optometrist or ophthalmologist leaves off by looking at the prescription and suggesting to the patient the selection of frame styles or lens styles. Either we have the lenses here in stock, or we'll order them from a servicing lab that actually manufactures the lens. We use a lensometer to read the prescription of the lens, and we have to make sure we place the optical center of the lens in front of the patient's pupil. This is a fairly busy practice. From 8:00 A.M. to closing, patients come in to purchase new eyewear or have their old eyewear repaired. I've been dealing with the public all my life. When you dispense a pair of glasses to someone and it puts a new light on everything, it's gratifying; it really is."

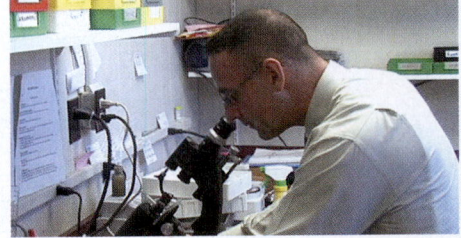

optician (awp-TIH-shun)
  opt/o- *eye; vision*
  -ician *skilled expert; skilled professional*

optometrist (awp-TAW-meh-trist)
  opt/o- *eye; vision*
  metr/o- *measurement; uterus; womb*
  -ist *person who specializes in; thing that specializes in*

optometry (awp-TAW-meh-tree)
  opt/o- *eye; vision*
  -metry *process of measuring*

ophthalmologist (OFF-thal-MAW-loh-jist)
  ophthalm/o- *eye*
  log/o- *study of; word*
  -ist *person who specializes in; thing that specializes in*

- **Opticians** are allied health professionals who use automated equipment to cut, grind, and finish lenses to exact specifications based on a written prescription from an optometrist or ophthalmologist. They also prepare contact lenses and instruct the patient in their care and handling. Opticians work in optical stores or in the office of an optometrist or ophthalmologist.

- **Optometrists** are Doctors of Optometry (O.D.) who have graduated from a school of optometry. They diagnose and treat patients with vision problems and diseases of the eyes. They write prescriptions for eyeglasses and contact lenses. They can administer and prescribe ophthalmic drugs. Optometrists do not perform eye surgery.

- **Ophthalmologists** are physicians (M.D.) who practice in the medical specialty of ophthalmology. They do all of the things an optometrist does, but they also perform surgery on the eye. Cancerous tumors of the eye are treated medically by an oncologist or surgically by an ophthalmologist.

Chapter Review Exercises

Dive In: Medical Language Exercises

Test your knowledge of the chapter by completing these review exercises. Use the Answer Key at the end of the book to check your answers. Note: Each of the numbered exercise headers corresponds to a numbered learning outcome at the beginning of the chapter.

14.1 Anatomy

MATCHING EXERCISE

Match each word or phrase to its description.

1. ciliary body
2. conjunctiva
3. fovea
4. mydriasis
5. orbit
6. superior rectus muscle
7. suspensory ligaments
8. trabecular meshwork
9. uvea
10. canal of Schlemm
11. lacrimal gland

_____ aqueous humor drains through this
_____ turns the eye upward
_____ center of the macula
_____ support the lens
_____ includes the iris, choroid, and ciliary body
_____ increase in the diameter of the pupil
_____ bony socket that holds the eye
_____ interlacing fibers around the edge of the iris
_____ produces tears when stimulated by cranial nerve VII
_____ produces aqueous humor
_____ mucous membrane on the inside of the eyelid

CIRCLE EXERCISE

Circle the correct answer from the choices given.

1. The (**iris, lens, orbit**) is the colored, circular structure around the pupil.
2. The (**cornea, iris, sclera**) is the tough, fibrous, white outer layer of the eye.
3. The "blind spot" on the retina corresponds to the (**fundus, macula, optic disk**).
4. The (**aqueous humor, conjunctiva, vitreous humor**) covers the inside of the eyelids and the anterior surface of the eye.
5. The (**extraocular muscle, fovea, fundus**) is the name of the area that is farthest from the opening (the pupil).

TRUE OR FALSE EXERCISE

*Indicate whether each statement is true or false by writing **T** or **F** on the line.*

1. _____ The nasolacrimal duct carries vitreous humor.
2. _____ The sclera is the clear part of the cornea.
3. _____ The iris is a dividing structure between the anterior and posterior chambers.
4. _____ Eye color is a genetically determined trait.
5. _____ Muscles in the iris contract or relax to constrict or dilate the pupil.
6. _____ At birth, the irides of all babies' eyes appear slate gray to blue in color.
7. _____ Vitreous humor is a clear, watery fluid.
8. _____ The posterior chamber is the largest space in the eye.
9. _____ The trabecular meshwork lies around the edge of the iris.
10. _____ The optic nerve is cranial nerve II.

PLURAL NOUN AND ADJECTIVE EXERCISE

Read the noun and write its plural form and/or adjective form on the line. Only write in the plural noun form if there is a blank line there for it. Be sure to check your spelling. The first one has been done for you.

Singular Noun	Plural Noun	Adjective	Singular Noun	Plural Noun	Adjective
1. **fovea**	*foveae*	*foveal*	6. lens	_____	_____
2. capsule		_____	7. macula	_____	_____
3. conjunctiva	_____	_____	8. retina	_____	_____
4. cornea	_____	_____	9. sclera	_____	_____
5. iris	_____	_____	10. uvea		_____

DIVIDING WORDS EXERCISE

Separate these words into their component parts (prefix, combining form, suffix). Some words do not contain all three word parts. The first one has been done for you.

Medical Word	Prefix	Combining Form	Suffix	Medical Word	Prefix	Combining Form	Suffix
1. **scleral**		*scler/o-*	*-al*	8. lacrimal		_____	_____
2. accommodation		_____	_____	9. lenticular		_____	_____
3. aqueous		_____	_____	10. mydriasis		_____	_____
4. cavity		_____	_____	11. optic		_____	_____
5. ciliary		_____	_____	12. pupillary		_____	_____
6. extraocular		_____	_____	13. superior		_____	_____
7. iridal		_____	_____				

SPELLING EXERCISE

Read each medical word pronunciation and write the medical word that it represents. Be sure to check your spelling. The first one has been done for you.

1. **(mih-DRY-eh-sihs)** _____*mydriasis*_____
2. (PYOO-pih-LAIR-ee) _____
3. (NAY-soh-LAK-rih-mal) _____
4. (EKS-trah-AW-kyoo-lar) _____
5. (SIL-ee-AIR-ee) _____
6. (AWP-tik) _____

14.2 Physiology

MATCHING EXERCISE

Match each word or phrase to its description.

1. refraction — _____ detect red, green, and blue light
2. lens — _____ where parts of each optic nerve cross over to join the other side
3. photon — _____ cornea and lens bend and focus light rays
4. cones — _____ muscles in the ciliary body change the shape of this
5. optic chiasm — _____ light particle

CIRCLE EXERCISE

Circle the correct answer from the choices given.

1. Color vision comes from cells known as (**cones, rods, visual cortices**).
2. Cranial nerve (**II, III, IV, V**) is the optic nerve for vision.
3. Cones are located in the (**lens, macula, optic nerve**).

TRUE OR FALSE EXERCISE

*Indicate whether each statement is true or false by writing **T** or **F** on the line.*

1. _____ Stereoscopic vision is three-dimensional vision.
2. _____ Rods can detect color but not black and white.
3. _____ The image on the retina is upside down and backward.
4. _____ The visual cortex is in the retina.

DIVIDING WORDS EXERCISE

Separate these words into their component parts (prefix, combining form, suffix). Some words do not contain all three word parts. The first one has been done for you.

Medical Word	Prefix	Combining Form	Suffix
1. **vision**		*vis/o-*	*-ion*
2. refraction	_____	_____	_____
3. optic		_____	_____
4. visual		_____	_____

SPELLING EXERCISE

Read each medical word pronunciation and write the medical word that it represents. Be sure to check your spelling. The first one has been done for you.

1. (THAL-ah-muhs)   *thalamus*
2. (AWP-tik)   _____
3. (VIH-shun)   _____
4. (ree-FRAK-shun)   _____
5. (KY-azm)   _____

14.3 Diseases

MATCHING EXERCISE

Match each word or phrase to its description.

1. anisocoria
2. blepharitis
3. cataract
4. entropion
5. exotropia
6. floaters
7. glaucoma
8. macular degeneration
9. myopia
10. retinoblastoma
11. scotoma
12. xerophthalmia

_____ strings of collagen in the vitreous humor
_____ cancerous eye tumor in children
_____ increased IOP
_____ a type of strabismus
_____ clouding of the lens
_____ visual field defect that is solid or patchy
_____ nearsightedness
_____ unequal pupils
_____ dry eyes syndrome
_____ infection or inflammation of the eyelid
_____ loss of central vision
_____ lower eyelid turns inward

TRUE OR FALSE EXERCISE

*Indicate whether each statement is true or false by writing **T** or **F** on the line.*

1. _____ Blepharoptosis is drooping of the upper eyelid from old age.

2. _____ Hordeolum is also known as a *stye*.

3. _____ A newborn baby can get gonorrhea in the eyes, which can cause blindness.

4. _____ Scleral icterus in the eyes is related to jaundice due to liver disease.

5. _____ Esotropia is also known as *cross-eye*.

6. _____ Color-deficient vision is also known as *color blindness*.

7. _____ The two types of macular degeneration are dry and wet.

8. _____ Retinitis pigmentosa is caused by many different genes.

9. _____ Astigmatism is also known as *nearsightedness*.

CIRCLE EXERCISE

Circle the correct answer from the choices given.

1. Involuntary rhythmic motions of the eye when looking to the side are called (**diplopia, nystagmus, strabismus**).

2. A patient with exophthalmos often has (**blindness, glaucoma, hyperthyroidism**).

3. Increased intraocular pressure is related to (**conjunctivitis, glaucoma, presbyopia**).

4. Farsightedness is (**astigmatism, hyperopia, myopia**).

5. Infection of the lacrimal sac is (**blepharitis, conjunctivitis, dacryocystitis**).

6. Abnormal sensitivity to bright light is (**hyphema, photophobia, strabismus**).

7. Neovascularization occurs in patients with (**blindness, diabetes mellitus, presbyopia**).

8. Loss of one-half of the visual field is (**amblyopia, diplopia, hemianopia**).

DIVIDING WORDS EXERCISE

Separate these words into their component parts (prefix, combining form, suffix). Some words do not contain all three word parts. The first one has been done for you.

Medical Word	Prefix	Combining Form	Suffix	Medical Word	Prefix	Combining Form	Suffix
1. **hyperopia**	*hyper-*	*op/o-*	*-ia*	8. glaucoma		_____	_____
2. anicteric	_____	_____	_____	9. hyperopia	_____	_____	_____
3. aphakia	_____	_____	_____	10. intraocular	_____	_____	_____
4. astigmatism	_____	_____	_____	11. keratitis		_____	_____
5. blepharitis		_____	_____	12. papilledema		_____	_____
6. ectropion	_____	_____	_____	13. retinopathy		_____	_____
7. degeneration	_____	_____	_____				

SPELLING EXERCISE

Read each medical word pronunciation and write the medical word that it represents. Be sure to check your spelling. The first one has been done for you.

1. (con-JUNK-tih-VY-tihs)   *conjunctivitis*

2. (BLEF-ah-RY-tihs) _____

3. (ZEER-off-THAL-mee-ah) _____

4. (EKS-off-THAL-mohs) _____

5. (nih-STAG-muhs) _____

6. (strah-BIZ-muhs) _____

7. (KAT-ah-rakt) _____

8. (PREZ-bee-OH-pee-ah) _____

9. (NEE-oh-VAS-kyoo-LAR-ih-ZAY-shun) _____

10. (ah-STIG-mah-tizm) _____

14.4 Laboratory, Diagnostic, and Radiologic Procedures

TRUE OR FALSE EXERCISE

*Indicate whether each statement is true or false by writing **T** or **F** on the line.*

1. _____ Fluorescein dye and an angiogram can reveal retinal leaks and hemorrhages.
2. _____ Ultrasonography uses ultra high-frequency heat waves to create an image.
3. _____ A B-scan can show tumors or hemorrhages inside the eye.
4. _____ Angiography produces an image known as an angiogram.

14.5 Medical Procedures, Drugs, and Surgical Procedures

MATCHING EXERCISE

Match each word or phrase to its description.

1. conjugate gaze
2. corticosteroid drug
3. convergence
4. Ishihara
5. ophthalmoscope
6. peripheral vision
7. PERRL
8. phacoemulsification
9. phoropter
10. retinopexy
11. Snellen chart
12. tonometry
13. trabeculoplasty

_____ used to treat severe eye inflammation
_____ what can be seen at the edge of the visual field
_____ instrument used to do a funduscopic examination
_____ testing how well the eyes move together as a unit
_____ pupillary response
_____ testing how well both eyes focus on the *near point*
_____ procedure for glaucoma to measure intraocular pressure
_____ breaking up the lens during cataract surgery
_____ surgical procedure to reattach a detached retina
_____ instrument that holds lenses of successive strengths to measure the best correction of vision
_____ color-deficient vision test
_____ surgical procedure to treat glaucoma
_____ test for visual acuity at a distance

CIRCLE EXERCISE

Circle the correct answer from the choices given.

1. When the muscles of the ciliary body contract and flex the lens, this is known as (**accommodation, convergence, enucleation**).
2. In order to perform dilated funduscopy, a (**corticosteroid, fluorescein, mydriatic**) drug must first be given.
3. Gonioscopy uses a/an (**ophthalmoscope, phoropter, slit lamp**) to look for a blockage of the trabecular meshwork at the angle of the iris and cornea.
4. Hyperopia surgery includes all of the following *except* (**CK, LASIK, LTK**).
5. A/An (**microkeratome, ophthalmoscope, phoropter**) is used to make a very thin flap on the surface of the cornea.

TRUE OR FALSE EXERCISE

*Indicate whether each statement is true or false by writing **T** or **F** on the line.*

1. _____ A slit lamp uses a high-intensity beam of blue light to look into the eye.
2. _____ A blepharoplasty removes fat and sagging skin from the eyelid.
3. _____ LASIK and PRK are used to surgically correct nearsightedness.
4. _____ Corticosteroid drugs are used to dilate the pupil before an eye exam.
5. _____ A fluorescein dye strip applied to the eye can show corneal ulcers.
6. _____ Dysconjugate gaze is when both eyes do not move together.
7. _____ The Tumbling E chart is used to test visual acuity.

8. _____ Antibiotic drugs can be applied topically to the eye or given orally.

9. _____ A mydriatic drug is used to treat increased eye pressure and glaucoma.

10. _____ Laser photocoagulation is used to heat and seal a detached retina to the layers beneath it.

DIVIDING WORDS EXERCISE

Separate these words into their component parts (prefix, combining form, suffix). Some words do not contain all three word parts. The first one has been done for you.

Medical Word	Prefix	Combining Form	Suffix
1. **antibiotic**	*anti-*	*bi/o-*	*-tic*
2. blepharoplasty		_____	_____
3. dysconjugate	_____	_____	_____
4. funduscopy		_____	_____
5. mydriatic		_____	_____
6. ophthalmoscope		_____	_____
7. phoropter		_____	_____
8. tonometer		_____	_____

SPELLING EXERCISE

Read each medical word pronunciation and write the medical word that it represents. Be sure to check your spelling. The first one has been done for you.

1. **(VIH-shoo-al)**   *visual*
2. (SY-kloh-PLEE-jee-ah)   _____
3. (off-THAL-moh-skohp)   _____
4. (toh-NAW-meh-tree)   _____
5. (BLEF-ah-roh-PLAS-tee)   _____
6. (KAIR-ah-toh-PLAS-tee)   _____
7. (KRY-oh-PEK-see)   _____

PROOFREADING EXERCISE

Read the following paragraph. Identify each misspelled medical word and write the correct spelling of it on the line.

The eye works with the vizual cortex of the brain for the sense of sight. The aquous humor is clear in the anterior chamber. The layers of the eye are the conjuntiva, cornea, and sklera. The retina has the macular where the best vision is. Drops in the eyes cause midriasis so the eyes can be examined. It is not good to have a catarakt or an entropion or blepharotosis. To diagnose eye diseases, a dilated fundoscopic exam is done. The study of the eye is known as ofthalmology.

1. _____   6. _____
2. _____   7. _____
3. _____   8. _____
4. _____   9. _____
5. _____   10. _____

RELATED COMBINING FORMS EXERCISE

Write the combining forms on the line provided. (Hint: See the It's Greek to Me! feature box.)

1. Two combining forms that mean *cornea*. _____ _____

2. Two combining forms that mean *eye*. _____ _____

3. Three combining forms that mean *lens*. _____ _____ _____

4. Two combining forms that mean *pupil*. _____ _____

5. Three combining forms that mean *sight, vision*. _____ _____ _____

Immerse Yourself: Analyze Medical Reports

Electronic Patient Record

This is a Consultation Report by an ophthalmologist. Read the report and answer the questions.

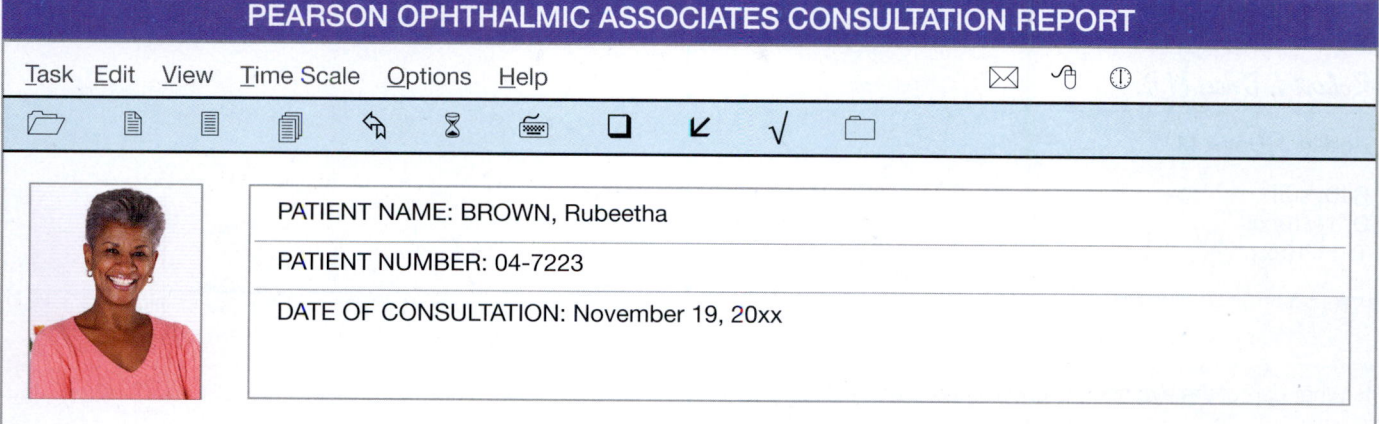

PEARSON OPHTHALMIC ASSOCIATES CONSULTATION REPORT

Task   Edit   View   Time Scale   Options   Help

PATIENT NAME: BROWN, Rubeetha

PATIENT NUMBER: 04-7223

DATE OF CONSULTATION: November 19, 20xx

HISTORY OF PRESENT ILLNESS

This 64-year-old, female comes in today as a referral from her primary care physician. She is complaining of bloodshot eyes, headaches, large floaters in her visual field, and blurred vision at close range.

PAST HISTORY

She has had myopia since childhood (onset at age 12). She was diagnosed by a neurologist as having migraines with an aura of scintillating scotomata followed by a temporary visual field defect of hemianopia, "like a gray curtain" coming down. She denies a history of hyperthyroidism, although she has been tested for this on several occasions. She denies hypertension, heart disease, or diabetes. She has some mild osteoarthritis, particularly in her right knee. Past surgeries include a tonsillectomy and an appendectomy in the remote past.

SOCIAL HISTORY

She is married and has two children, both living away from home. She works in the member services department of an HMO and does paperwork and computer work all day.

PHYSICAL EXAMINATION

The conjunctivae are infected, and the sclerae are anicteric. There is a soft, movable mass in the margin of the right upper eyelid. The patient states that this was from a trauma and has remained unchanged for many years. This is not a chalazion, just scar tissue. There is a moderate amount of crusted exudate on the eyelids. There is mild exophthalmos bilaterally. PERRL. Extraocular movements intact. Dilating drops were instilled in each eye, and a funduscopy was performed. There is evidence of a developing cataract in the right eye. The retinae bilaterally were normal. There was no suggestion of macular degeneration. There were no hemorrhages seen. There were small clumps of vitreous humor visible in the posterior cavity.

VISUAL TESTING

Distance vision without glasses was 20/200 in both eyes. Peripheral vision was normal. Depth perception was normal. Tonometry showed normal intraocular pressures in both eyes.

DIAGNOSES

1. Eye strain and new-onset presbyopia.

2. Severe myopia. Wears corrective lenses for distance vision.

3. Stage I cataract, O.D.

4. Blepharitis.

5. Vitreous floaters. The patient was advised that although these are annoying and appear large, they are actually small and benign and are the result of the aging process.

PLAN

1. The patient has been given a prescription for new eyeglasses. These will be bifocal lenses to correct her myopia and her new-onset presbyopia.
2. The patient was asked to gently cleanse the eyelids and apply an ophthalmic antibiotic ointment twice a day.
3. The patient has been advised of her increased risk of developing glaucoma given her age and race and was advised to have an annual eye examination with tonometry. Follow up in 6 months to evaluate the status of her cataract and do a glaucoma check.

Robert J. Dove, M.D.
_____

Robert J. Dove, M.D.

RJD: smt
D: 11/19/xx
T: 11/19/xx

1. What part of the eye does a funduscopy examine? _____
2. What eye condition has the patient had since childhood? _____
3. What two visual symptoms does the patient have before the onset of a migraine? _____ _____
4. The mass on the patient's eyelid is a chalazion.   True   False
5. What is the meaning of PERRL? _____
6. What abbreviation tells you that the patient's cataract was in the right eye? _____
7. The physical finding of crusted exudates on the eyelids corresponds to which diagnosis? _____
8. Which phrase in the examination of the eye tells you that the patient does not have liver disease? ____
9. A normal tonometry test shows that the patient does not have what disease? _____
10. Why have physicians in the past tested the patient for hyperthyroidism? _____

MyLab Medical Terminology™

MyLab Medical Terminology is a premium online homework management system that includes a host of features to help you study. Registered users will find:

- A multitude of quizzes and activities built within the MyLab platform

- Powerful tools that track and analyze your results—allowing you to create a personalized learning experience

- Videos and audio pronunciations to help enrich your progress

- Streaming lesson presentations (guided lectures) and self-paced learning modules

- A space where you and your instructor can check your progress and manage your assignments

15 Otolaryngology
Ears, Nose, and Throat

Otolaryngology (OH-toh-LAIR-ing-GAW-loh-jee) is the medical specialty that studies the anatomy and physiology of the ears, nose, and throat (ENT); uses laboratory, diagnostic, and radiologic procedures to diagnose ENT diseases; and uses medical procedures, drugs, and surgical procedures to treat ENT diseases.

Chapter Overview and Learning Outcomes

After you study this chapter, you should be able to demonstrate mastery of the outcomes by successfully completing the exercises.

15.1 Anatomy
Identify the structures of the ears, nose, and throat.
Demonstrate proficiency in medical language.
15.1 Practice Laps

15.2 Physiology
Describe the functions of the ears, nose, and throat.
Demonstrate proficiency in medical language.
15.2 Practice Laps
Vocabulary Review

15.3 Diseases
Describe common ENT diseases.
Demonstrate proficiency in medical language.
15.3 Practice Laps

15.4 Laboratory, Diagnostic, and Radiologic Procedures
Describe common ENT laboratory tests, diagnostic procedures, and radiologic procedures.
Demonstrate proficiency in medical language.
15.4 Practice Laps

15.5 Medical Procedures, Drugs, and Surgical Procedures
Describe common ENT medical procedures, drugs, and surgical procedures.
Demonstrate proficiency in medical language.
15.5 Practice Laps
Abbreviations Summary
Career Focus

Chapter Review Exercises
Dive In: Medical Language Exercises
(Learning Outcomes 15.1–15.5)

Immerse Yourself: Analyze Medical Reports

Medical Language Key

To unlock the definition of a medical word, first break it into word parts. Then give the meaning of each word part. Put the meanings of the word parts in order, beginning with the meaning of the suffix, then the meaning of the prefix (if there is one), then the meaning of the combining form.

Although the word *otolaryngology* does not contain combining forms for the words *nose* or *throat*, it is understood that these structures are included in this medical specialty. The word *otorhinolaryngology* does include the combining form *rhin/o-*, which means *nose*.

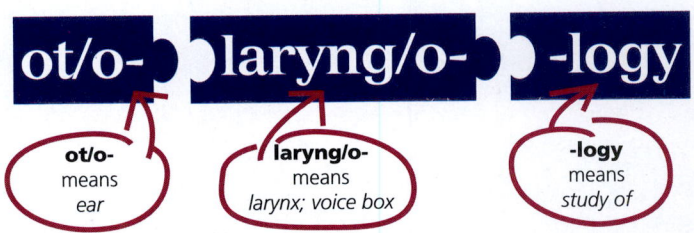

ot/o-
means
ear

laryng/o-
means
larynx; voice box

-logy
means
study of

Otolaryngology: ▶ *Study of (the) ears, (nose, throat), larynx, (and related structures).*

The ears, nose, and throat (ENT) are an interrelated group of anatomic structures that are considered together in the medical specialty of otolaryngology. These structures are located in the head and neck and consist of both external and internal anatomy (see Figure 15-1 ■). The external structures consist of the external ears, nose, and mouth; the internal structures consist of the middle and inner ears, nasal cavity and sinuses, oral cavity, pharynx (throat), and larynx (voice box). The ears, nose, and throat share some structures with the gastrointestinal system (mouth, oral cavity, pharynx) and the respiratory system (nose, nasal cavity, pharynx, larynx) (described in Chapter 3, Gastroenterology, and Chapter 4, Pulmonology). The ears and nose and their special senses of hearing and smell are often presented in conjunction with the nervous system. Otolaryngology includes the interrelated structures and functions of the ears, nose, and throat as the basis of this medical specialty.

The function of the ears is to provide sensory information that can be interpreted by the brain to become the sense of hearing. The inner ears function in conjunction with the eyes, muscular system, and nervous system to maintain the body's sense of balance. The function of the nose is to provide sensory information that can be interpreted by the brain to become the sense of smell. The structures of the nose, mouth, and throat work in conjunction with the respiratory system to produce speech. The oral cavity and pharynx contain lymph nodes and lymphoid tissues that function as part of the body's immune response (described in Chapter 6, Hematology and Immunology).

15.1 Anatomy

Ear

The ear consists of external, middle, and inner parts, each of which contains a number of anatomic structures.

External Ear

The visible external ear is the **auricle** (or **pinna**) (see Figure 15-2 ■). The **helix** is the outer rim of tissue and cartilage that forms the C shape of the external ear and ends at the earlobe. Just behind the external ear is the **mastoid process**, a bony projection of the temporal bone of the cranium. The mastoid process is not solid bone; it contains tiny air cells that have a connection to the middle ear and to the eustachian tube (described in the next section).

The **tragus** is the triangular cartilage that is anterior to the **external auditory meatus**, the opening that leads into the **external auditory canal (EAC)**.

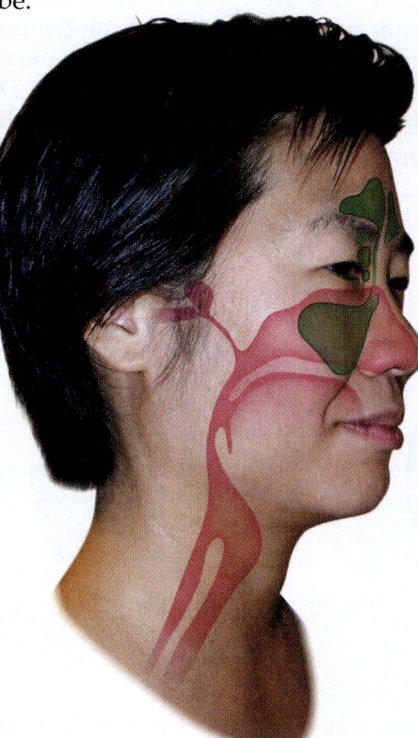

FIGURE 15-1 ■ Ears, nose, and throat (ENT).
The ears, nose, and throat are located in the head and neck. Each of these individual structures is interrelated and connected to the others.

Pronunciation/Word Parts

ear (EER)

otic (OH-tik)
  ot/o- ear
  -ic pertaining to

nose (NOHS)

nasal (NAY-zal)
  nas/o- nose
  -al pertaining to

throat (THROHT)

pharynx (FAIR-ingks)
Pharynx is the medical name for throat.

pharyngeal (fah-RIN-jee-al)
  pharyng/o- pharynx; throat
  -eal pertaining to

external (eks-TER-nal)
  extern/o- outside
  -al pertaining to

auricle (AW-rih-kul)
  aur/i- ear
  -cle small thing

auricular (aw-RIH-kyoo-lar)
  auricul/o- ear
  -ar pertaining to
Auricle refers to the external ear as well as to an ear-shaped structure on the atrium of the heart.

pinna (PIN-ah)
Pinna means a wing or fin.

helix (HEE-liks)

mastoid (MAS-toyd)
  mast/o- breast; mastoid process
  -oid resembling
The combining form **mastoid/o-** also means mastoid process.

process (PRAW-sehs)

tragus (TRAY-guhs)

auditory (AW-dih-TOR-ee)
  audit/o- sense of hearing
  -ory having the function of
The combining form **acous/o-** means hearing; sound, and **audi/o-** means hearing.

meatus (mee-AA-tuhs)

meati (mee-AA-tie)
Latin plural noun: Change the singular ending -us to -i.

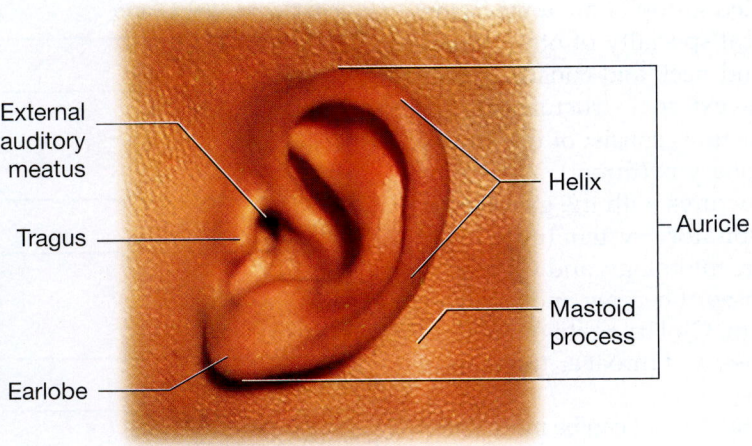

FIGURE 15-2 ■ **External ear.**
The external ear is composed of several types and shapes of tissue and cartilage. The external ear also includes the external auditory canal and the tympanic membrane within the temporal bone of the cranium.

The canal is a passageway that extends from the external ear to the tympanic membrane. The canal has glands that secrete **cerumen**, a waxy, sticky substance that traps dirt and has an antibiotic action against microorganisms that enter the canal. The final structure of the external ear is the **tympanic membrane (TM)** or **eardrum**, a thin, pearly gray membrane at the end of the external auditory canal; it divides the external ear from the middle ear (see Figure 15-3 ■).

Middle Ear

The middle ear is a cavity (hollow area) within the temporal bone of the cranium (see Figure 15-4 ■). The middle ear contains three tiny bones: the malleus, incus, and stapes (known as the "hammer," "anvil," and "stirrup" because of their shapes). Collectively, they are known as the **ossicles**. These bones are connected to each other by ligaments to form the **ossicular chain**. The first bone, the **malleus**, is shaped like a hammer and is connected to the tympanic membrane. Because the tympanic membrane is nearly transparent, the malleus can be seen behind the tympanic membrane when the ear is examined with a lighted instrument (see Figure 15-3). The second bone, the **incus**, is shaped like an anvil. The third bone, the **stapes**, is shaped like a stirrup. The stapes fits into a membrane-covered opening in the temporal bone known as the oval window.

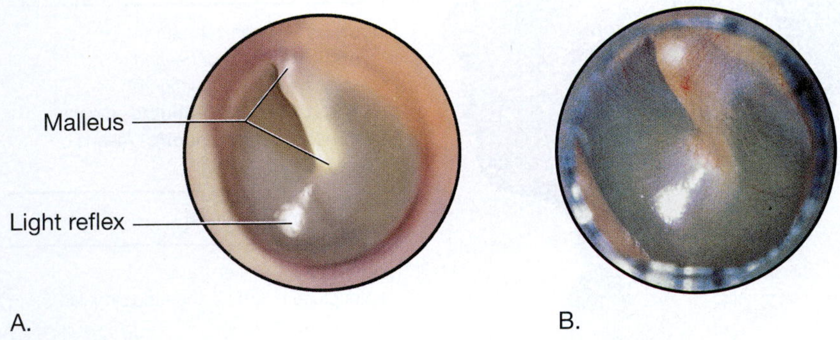

Malleus ——

Light reflex ——

A.

B.

FIGURE 15-3 ■ **Tympanic membrane.**
A. A normal tympanic membrane has a pearly gray color and is so thin that the malleus can be seen behind it. **B.** In this photograph taken during an ear examination, a shiny strip (reflected light from an otoscope) is seen; this is known as the *light reflex*.

Pronunciation/Word Parts

cerumen (seh-ROO-men)

tympanic (tim-PAN-ik)
　tympan/o- *eardrum; tympanic membrane*
　-ic *pertaining to*
The combining form **myring/o-** also means *eardrum; tympanic membrane.*

ossicle (AW-sih-kul)
　oss/i- *bone*
　-cle *small thing*

ossicular (aw-SIH-kyoo-lar)
　ossicul/o- *ossicle; small bone*
　-ar *pertaining to*

malleus (MAL-ee-uhs)

mallei (MAL-ee-eye)
Latin plural noun: Change the singular ending *-us* to *-i.*

mallear (MAL-ee-ar)
　malle/o- *hammer-shaped bone; malleus*
　-ar *pertaining to*

incus (ING-kuhs)

incudes (in-KYOO-deez)

incudal (IN-kyoo-dal)
　incud/o- *anvil-shaped bone; incus*
　-al *pertaining to*

stapes (STAY-peez)

stapedes (STAY-peh-deez)

stapedial (stay-PEE-dee-al)
　staped/o- *stapes; stirrup-shaped bone*
　-ial *pertaining to*

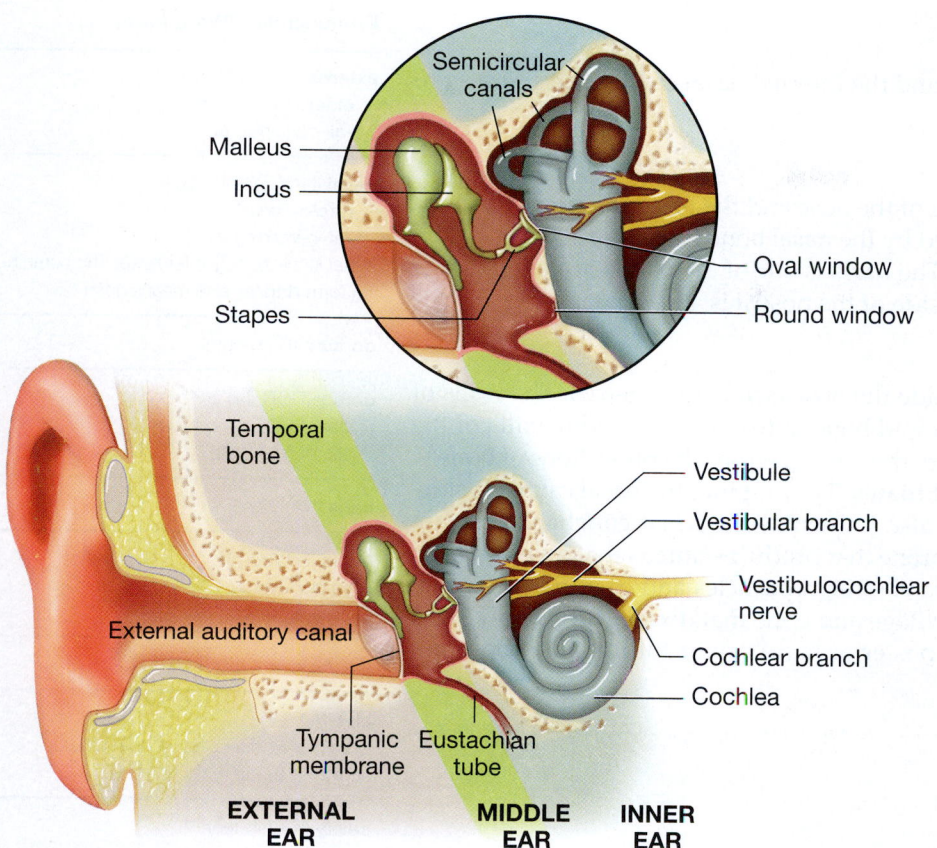

Semicircular canals

Malleus

Incus

Stapes

Oval window

Round window

Temporal bone

Vestibule

Vestibular branch

Vestibulocochlear nerve

External auditory canal

Cochlear branch

Cochlea

Tympanic membrane

Eustachian tube

EXTERNAL EAR

MIDDLE EAR

INNER EAR

FIGURE 15-4 ■ **Structures of the middle ear and inner ear.**
Notice the shapes of the malleus, incus, and stapes in the middle ear (see the inset). Do they look like a hammer, anvil, and stirrup to you? The structures of the inner ear send information about balance and hearing to the brain via the vestibulocochlear nerve.

The middle ear is connected to the air cells of the mastoid process and to the nasopharynx by the **eustachian tube** (see Figure 15-4). The eustachian tube allows air pressure in the middle ear and in mastoid air cells to equalize with air pressure in the nose, throat, and outside the body.

Word Alert

Sound-Alike Words

malleus	(noun)	first bone of the middle ear
		Example: An infection in the middle ear caused scar tissue around the malleus.
malleolus	(noun)	bony projections on the tibia and fibula of the lower leg near the ankle
		Example: The lateral malleolus is a bony projection on the distal end of the fibula.

Inner Ear

Part of the temporal bone of the cranium divides the middle ear from the inner ear. Within this bone are two small, membrane-covered openings that connect the two ear cavities: the **oval window** and the **round window**. The inner ear cavity is filled with fluid and contains three structures: the vestibule, the semicircular canals, and the cochlea (see Figure 15-4). The **vestibule** is the entrance to the inner ear. The superior part of the vestibule becomes the **semicircular canals**, three separate but intertwined fluid-filled canals that are each oriented in a different plane—horizontally, vertically, and obliquely; these send sensory information to the brain about the position of the head. The inferior part of the vestibule becomes the spiral-shaped cochlea. The **cochlea** sends sensory information to the brain about sound waves that enter the ear. Together, all of the structures of the inner ear are known as the **labyrinth**.

Pronunciation/Word Parts

eustachian (yoo-STAY-shun)

vestibule (VES-tih-byool)

vestibular (ves-TIH-byoo-lar)
 vestibul/o- *entrance; vestibule*
 -ar *pertaining to*

semicircular (SEM-ee-SIR-kyoo-lar)
 semi- *half; partly*
 circul/o- *circle*
 -ar *pertaining to*

cochlea (KOH-klee-ah)

cochleae (KOH-klee-ee)
Latin plural noun: Change the singular ending *-a* to *-ae*.

cochlear (KOH-klee-ar)
 cochle/o- *cochlea; spiral-shaped structure*
 -ar *pertaining to*

labyrinth (LAB-ih-rinth)
The combining form **labyrinth/o-** means *labyrinth*.

Nose and Sinuses

The nose consists of the external nose and the internal nasal cavity. The sinuses are connected to the nasal cavity.

External Nose

The external nose consists of the bridge of the nose and the **nasal dorsum** (the vertical ridge in the middle that is supported by the nasal bone (see Figure 15-5 ■). At its tip, the nasal bone becomes cartilage. The **naris** is one of the two external openings or nostrils. The flared cartilage on the side of the nostril is a nasal **ala**.

Nasal Cavity

The **nasal cavity** is the hollow area inside the nose (see Figure 15-6 ■). The walls of the nasal cavity are formed by the ethmoid bone of the cranium and maxilla of the upper jaw. Along these interior walls are three long, scroll-like projections of bone—the **superior**, **middle**, and **inferior turbinates**. They jut into the nasal cavity to slow down inhaled air. The turbinates are also known as the **nasal conchae**. They are covered with **mucosa**, a mucous membrane that produces **mucus** that gives warmth and moisture to the inhaled air and traps foreign particles and bacteria. The **nasal septum** is a central, vertical wall of cartilage and bone that divides the hollow nasal cavity into right and left sides. In the posterior nasal cavity, this cartilage becomes the ethmoid bone of the cranium.

Word Alert
Sound-Alike Words

mucosa   (noun)   a Latin word that means *mucous membrane*
(myoo-KOH-sah)   *Example: The nasal mucosa warms and moistens inhaled air.*

mucous   (adjective)   pertaining to a membrane (the mucosa) that secretes mucus
(MYOO-kuhs)   *Example: Allergies make the mucous membranes of the nose become
                    swollen and inflamed.*

mucus   (noun)   a secretion from a mucous membrane
(MYOO-kuhs)   *Example: A chronic smoker coughs and produces a significant amount
                    of mucus.*

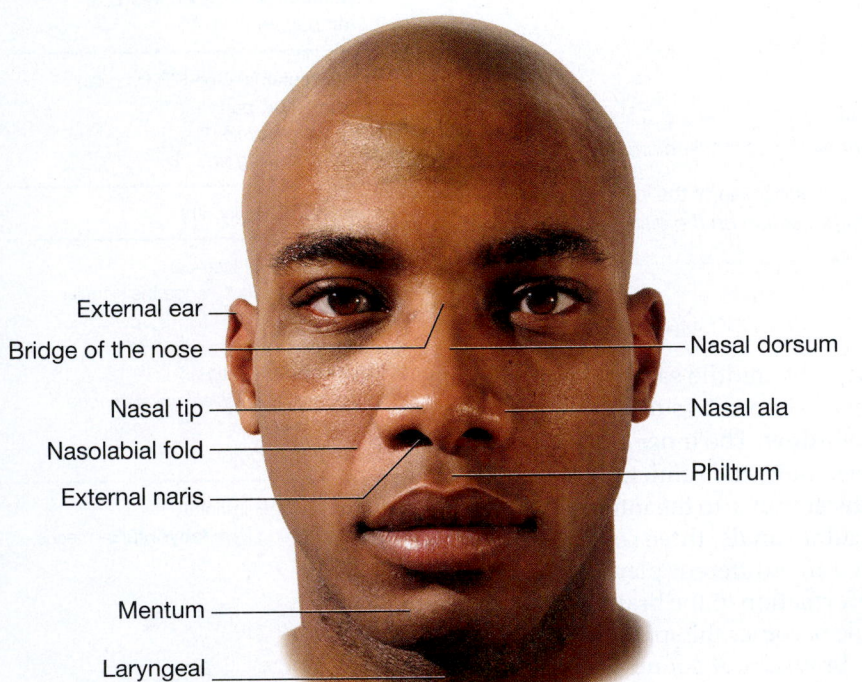

External ear
Bridge of the nose
Nasal tip
Nasolabial fold
External naris
Mentum
Laryngeal prominence

Nasal dorsum
Nasal ala
Philtrum

Pronunciation/Word Parts

external (eks-TER-nal)
  extern/o- *outside*
  -al *pertaining to*

nasal (NAY-zal)
  nas/o- *nose*
  -al *pertaining to*
Nasal is the adjective for *nose*. The combining form **rhin/o-** also means *nose*.

dorsum (DOR-sum)

dorsal (DOR-sal)
  dors/o- *back; dorsum*
  -al *pertaining to*

naris (NAY-rihs)

nares (NAY-reez)
Latin plural noun: Change the singular ending *-is* to *-es*.

ala (AA-lah)

alae (AA-lee)
Latin plural noun: Change the singular ending *-a* to *-ae*.

cavity (KAV-ih-tee)
  cav/o- *hollow space*
  -ity *condition; state*

superior (soo-PEER-ee-or)
  super/o- *above*
  -ior *pertaining to*

inferior (in-FEER-ee-or)
  infer/o- *below*
  -ior *pertaining to*

turbinate (TER-bih-nayt)
  turbin/o- *scroll-like structure*
  -ate *composed of; pertaining to*

conchae (CON-kee)

mucosa (myoo-KOH-sah)

mucosal (myoo-KOH-sal)
  mucos/o- *mucous membrane*
  -al *pertaining to*

mucus (MYOO-kuhs)

septum (SEP-tum)

septal (SEP-tal)
  sept/o- *dividing wall; septum*
  -al *pertaining to*

FIGURE 15-5 ■ External nose, mouth, and neck.
The external nose is supported by the nasal bone, which transitions to cartilage at the tip of the nose. The tissues of the lips, mouth, and chin are supported by the maxilla and mandible bones. The laryngeal prominence in the neck is composed of cartilage around the larynx (voice box).

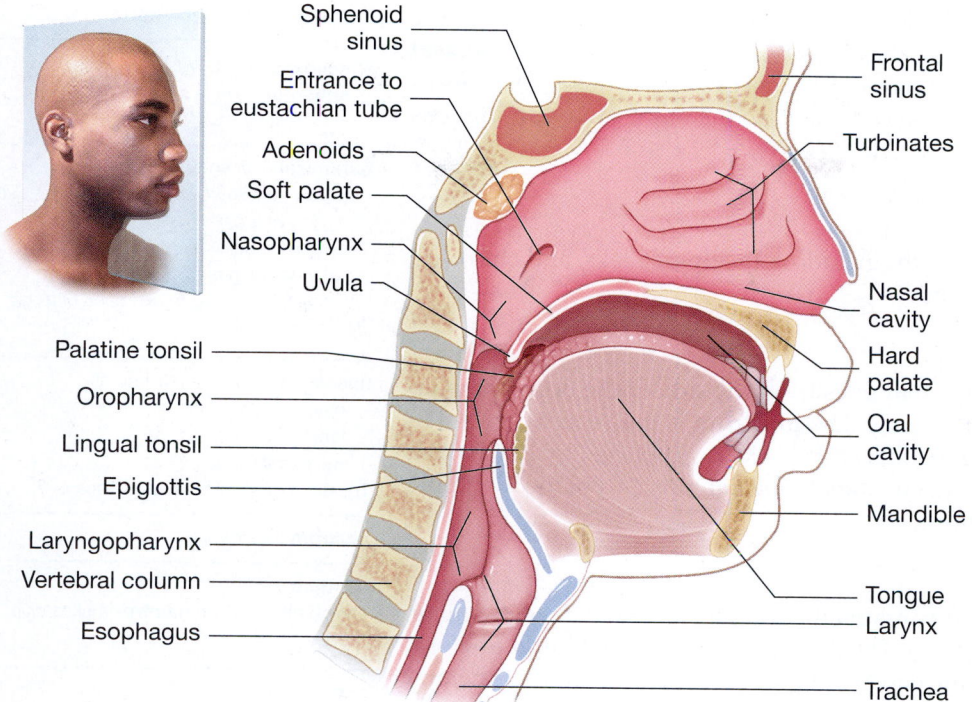

FIGURE 15-6 ■ **Structures of the internal nose, mouth, and throat.**
This midsagittal section of the head and neck shows the turbinates in the nasal cavity, the structures of the oral cavity, the tonsils and adenoids, and the three parts of the pharynx—the nasopharynx, oropharynx, and laryngopharynx. Note how anatomically close the area of the pharynx is to the bones of the vertebral column.

Sinuses

A **sinus** is a hollow, air-filled cavity within a bone that is lined with a mucous membrane that produces mucus. There are four pairs of sinuses, each located in the cranial or facial bone for which it is named (see Figure 15-6 and Figure 15-7 ■). The **frontal sinuses** are located in the frontal bone, just superior and medial to each eyebrow. The **maxillary sinuses**, the largest of the sinuses, are in the maxilla (upper jaw bone) on either side of the nose. The **ethmoid sinuses**, which are groups of small air cells rather than a hollow cavity, are in the ethmoid bone, between the nose and

Pronunciation/Word Parts

sinus (SY-nuhs)
Sinus is a Latin singular noun that has no plural form. The English plural is *sinuses*. The combining form **sinus/o-** means *sinus*.

frontal (FRUN-tal)
  front/o- *front*
  -al *pertaining to*

maxillary (MAK-sih-LAIR-ee)
  maxill/o- *maxilla; upper jaw*
  -ary *pertaining to*

ethmoid (ETH-moyd)
  ethm/o- *sieve*
  -oid *resembling*

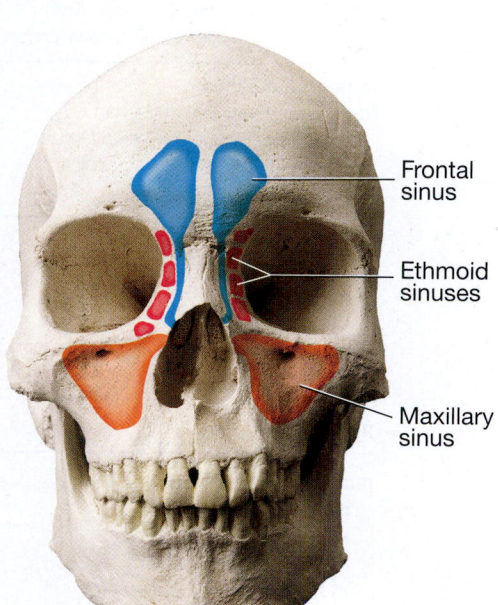

Frontal sinus

Ethmoid sinuses

Maxillary sinus

FIGURE 15-7 ■ **Sinuses.**
The sinuses are hollow cavities or small areas lined with mucosa within the frontal, maxillary, ethmoid, and sphenoid bones of the cranium and face. (The sphenoid sinuses are not seen on this view.)

the eyes. The **sphenoid sinuses** are in the sphenoid bone, which is posterior to the nasal cavity (see Figure 15-6). Together, these sinuses are known as the **paranasal sinuses** because they are two parts of a pair in the area beside the nose. The sinuses are connected to each other; they are also connected to the nasal cavity, and mucus from the sinuses drains into the nasal cavity.

Mouth

The mouth consists of the external mouth (including the lips, cheeks, and chin) and the oral cavity and its internal structures.

External Mouth

The **nasolabial fold** is the skin crease that goes from the side of the nose to the lip at the corner of the mouth (see Figure 15-5). The **philtrum** is the vertical groove in the skin of the upper lip. The skin of the lips and cheeks is supported by the maxilla (upper jaw bone) and mandible (lower jaw bone). The anterior part of the mandible is the chin, also known as the **mentum**.

Oral Cavity

The **oral cavity** is a hollow area that contains the tongue, hard palate, soft palate, uvula, teeth, and gums (see Figure 15-6). The oral cavity is lined with **oral mucosa**; this is known as **buccal mucosa** in the cheek area. The **hard palate** divides the oral cavity from the nasal cavity. The hard palate is made up of three bones: the maxilla (at the front of the mouth), the palatine, and the vomer. The hard palate transitions to the tissue of the **soft palate** and the **uvula**, the fleshy part of the soft palate that hangs down in the posterior oral cavity. The hard and soft palates form the roof of the mouth. The mandible forms the floor of the mouth, where the base of the **tongue** is attached. Each side of the mandible is attached to the temporal bone of the cranium at the movable **temporomandibular joint (TMJ)**. The salivary glands secrete saliva into the oral cavity (described in Chapter 3, Gastroenterology). **Submental lymph nodes** beneath the chin contain special cells that attack bacteria and viruses in the oral cavity as part of the immune response (described in Chapter 6, Hematology and Immunology).

Pharynx

The **pharynx** (throat) is a shared passageway for both food and air. It is divided into three areas: the nasopharynx, the oropharynx, and the laryngopharynx (see Figure 15-6).

Pronunciation/Word Parts

sphenoid (SFEE-noyd)
  sphen/o- *wedge shaped*
  -oid *resembling*

paranasal (PAIR-ah-NAY-zal)
  para- *abnormal; apart from; beside; two parts of a pair*
  nas/o- *nose*
  -al *pertaining to*
Paranasal: *Pertaining to two parts of a pair (beside the) nose.*

nasolabial (NAY-zoh-LAY-bee-al)
  nas/o- *nose*
  labi/o- *labium; lip*
  -al *pertaining to*
The combining form **cheil/o-** means *lip*.

philtrum (FIL-trum)

mentum (MEN-tum)
The combining form **ment/o-** means *chin; mind*.

oral (OR-al)
  or/o- *mouth*
  -al *pertaining to*
Oral is the adjective for *mouth*.

cavity (KAV-ih-tee)
  cav/o- *hollow space*
  -ity *condition; state*

mucosa (myoo-KOH-sah)

buccal (BUK-al)
  bucc/o- *cheek*
  -al *pertaining to*

palate (PAL-at)

uvula (YOO-vyoo-lah)

glossal (GLAW-sal)
  gloss/o- *tongue*
  -al *pertaining to*
Glossal is the adjective for *tongue*. The combining form **lingu/o-** also means *tongue*.

temporomandibular
(TEM-poh-ROH-man-DIH-byoo-lar)
  tempor/o- *side of the head; temple*
  mandibul/o- *lower jaw; mandible*
  -ar *pertaining to*

submental (sub-MEN-tal)
  sub- *below; underneath; less than*
  ment/o- *chin; mind*
  -al *pertaining to*
Submental: *Pertaining to underneath (the) chin*

pharynx (FAIR-ingks)

pharyngeal (fah-RIN-jee-al)
  pharyng/o- *pharynx; throat*
  -eal *pertaining to*

- The **nasopharynx** is posterior to the nasal cavity. The roof and walls of the nasopharynx contain the lymphoid tissue of the **adenoids**. The nasopharynx is connected to the middle ear by the eustachian tube (described previously).
- The **oropharynx** is posterior to the oral cavity. The oropharynx contains the lymphoid tissue of the **palatine tonsils** on either side of the soft palate (see Figure 15-8 ■).
- The **laryngopharynx** is posterior to the larynx. The laryngopharynx extends from the base of the tongue to the entrances to the esophagus and larynx. The laryngopharynx contains the lymphoid tissue of the **lingual tonsils** on either side of the base of the tongue.

The adenoids and tonsils are part of the lymphatic system, and they function in the immune response by producing lymphocytes and macrophages that attack bacteria and viruses in the oral cavity and throat.

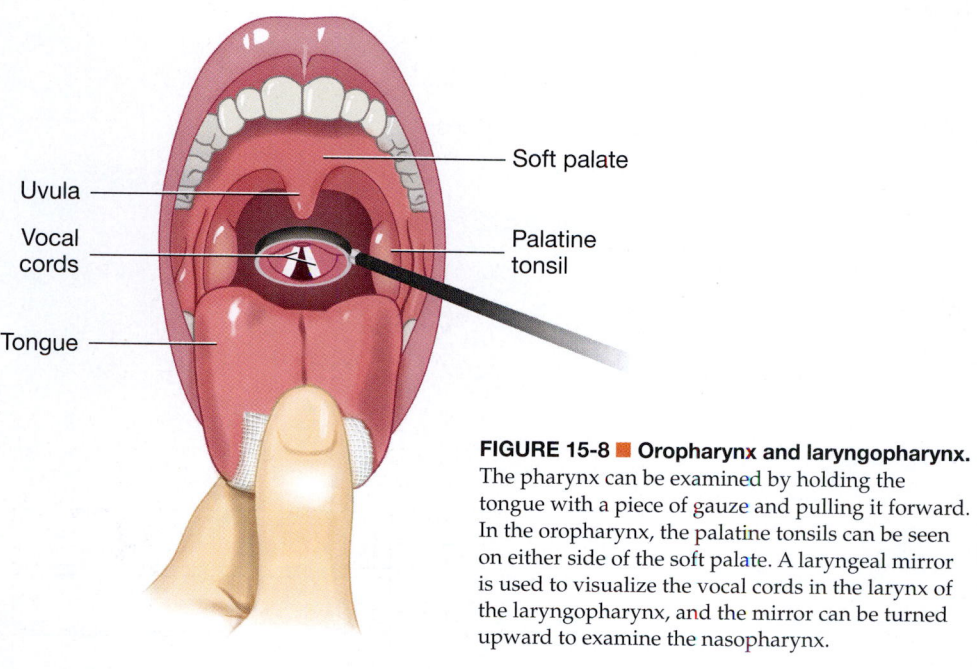

Uvula

Vocal cords

Tongue

Soft palate

Palatine tonsil

FIGURE 15-8 ■ Oropharynx and laryngopharynx. The pharynx can be examined by holding the tongue with a piece of gauze and pulling it forward. In the oropharynx, the palatine tonsils can be seen on either side of the soft palate. A laryngeal mirror is used to visualize the vocal cords in the larynx of the laryngopharynx, and the mirror can be turned upward to examine the nasopharynx.

Larynx

The larynx can be seen on the anterior surface of the neck as the **laryngeal prominence** (Adam's apple) (see Figure 15-5). Internally, the **larynx** (voice box) is a short, triangular structure that remains open during breathing and speaking, allowing air to pass through the vocal cords. During swallowing, muscles in the neck pull the larynx up to the **epiglottis**, a lid-like structure that seals the larynx so that swallowed food goes into the esophagus and not into the trachea and lungs. In the middle of the larynx is the **glottis**, a V-shaped structure of cartilage, ligaments, and the vocal cords (see Figure 15-8). The **vocal cords** are bands of connective tissue that vibrate (up to 100 times per second) to produce sounds during speaking and singing.

Pronunciation/Word Parts

nasopharynx (NAY-zoh-FAIR-ingks)
  nas/o- *nose*
  -pharynx *pharynx; throat*

adenoids (AD-eh-noydz)
  aden/o- *gland*
  -oid *resembling*
The combining form **adenoid/o-** means *structure resembling a gland.*

oropharynx (OR-oh-FAIR-ingks)
  or/o- *mouth*
  -pharynx *pharynx; throat*

palatine (PAL-ah-teen)
  palat/o- *palate*
  -ine *pertaining to*
Palatine and *palatal* are both adjectives for *palate.*

tonsil (TAWN-sil)

tonsillar (TAWN-sih-lar)
  tonsill/o- *tonsil*
  -ar *pertaining to*

laryngopharynx (lah-RING-goh-FAIR-ingks)
  laryng/o- *larynx; voice box*
  -pharynx *pharynx; throat*

lingual (LING-gwal)
  lingu/o- *tongue*
  -al *pertaining to*

larynx (LAIR-ingks)

laryngeal (lah-RIN-jee-al)
  laryng/o- *larynx; voice box*
  -eal *pertaining to*

epiglottis (EP-ih-GLAW-tihs)

epiglottic (EP-ih-GLAW-tik)
  epi- *above; upon*
  glott/o- *glottis of the larynx*
  -ic *pertaining to*

glottis (GLAW-tihs)

vocal (VOH-kal)
  voc/o- *voice*
  -al *pertaining to*

Dive Deeper

The vocal cords relax to lower the pitch of the voice or tighten to raise the pitch. Men have a large larynx and long vocal cords that vibrate at a slow frequency and produce a lower-pitched voice. Women have shorter vocal cords and a higher-pitched voice. The volume of air from the lungs affects how loud or soft the voice is. The voice also resonates in the sinuses, adding fullness to the sound. As sound waves travel from the vocal cords, they are shaped by the soft palate, tongue, and lips into spoken words.

15.1 PRACTICE LAPS

Use the Answer Key at the end of the book to check your answers.

A. Label Structures

Write each anatomy word or phrase in the correct numbered box. Be sure to check your spelling.

cochlea	malleus	temporal bone
cochlear branch of the vestibulocochlear nerve	mastoid bone	tympanic membrane
	oval window	vestibular branch of the vestibulocochlear nerve
eustachian tube	round window	
external auditory canal	semicircular canals	vestibule
incus	stapes	vestibulocochlear nerve

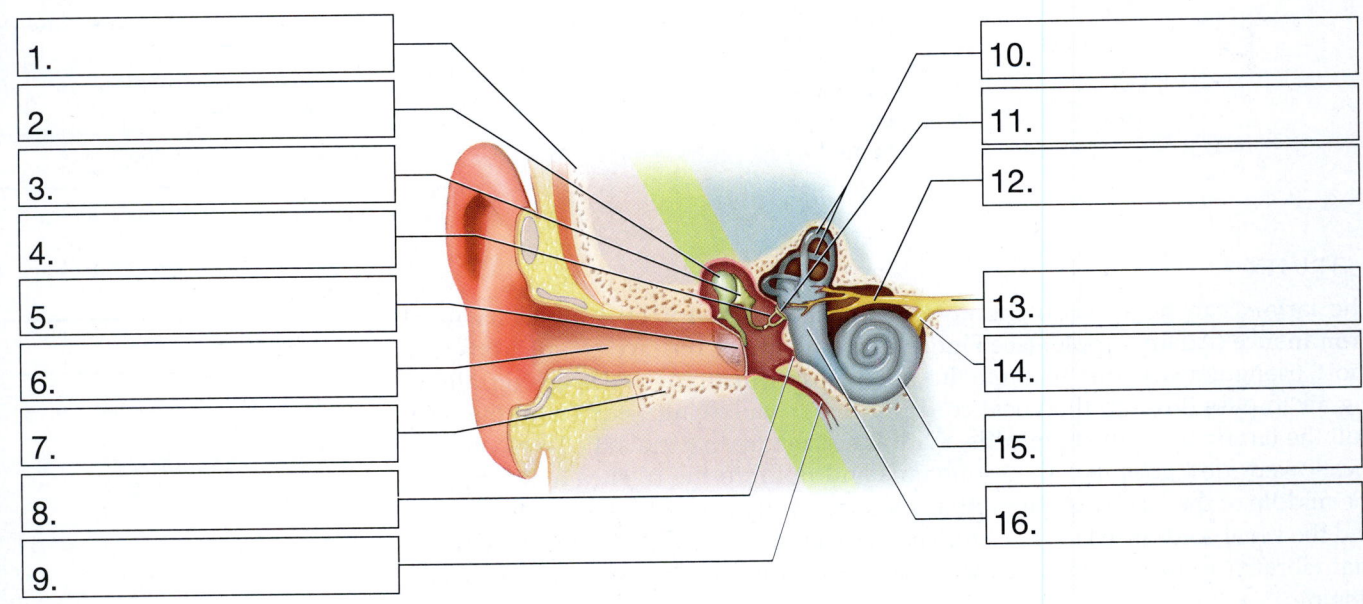

1.

2.

3.

4.

5.

6.

7.

8.

9.

10.

11.

12.

13.

14.

15.

16.

adenoids
entrance to eustachian tube
epiglottis
esophagus
frontal sinus
hard palate
laryngopharynx

larynx
lingual tonsil
mandible
nasal cavity
nasopharynx
oral cavity
oropharynx

palatine tonsil
soft palate
sphenoid sinus
tongue
trachea
turbinates
uvula

1.

2.

3.

4.

5.

6.

7.

8.

9.

10.

11.

12.

13.

14.

15.

16.

17.

18.

19.

20.

21.

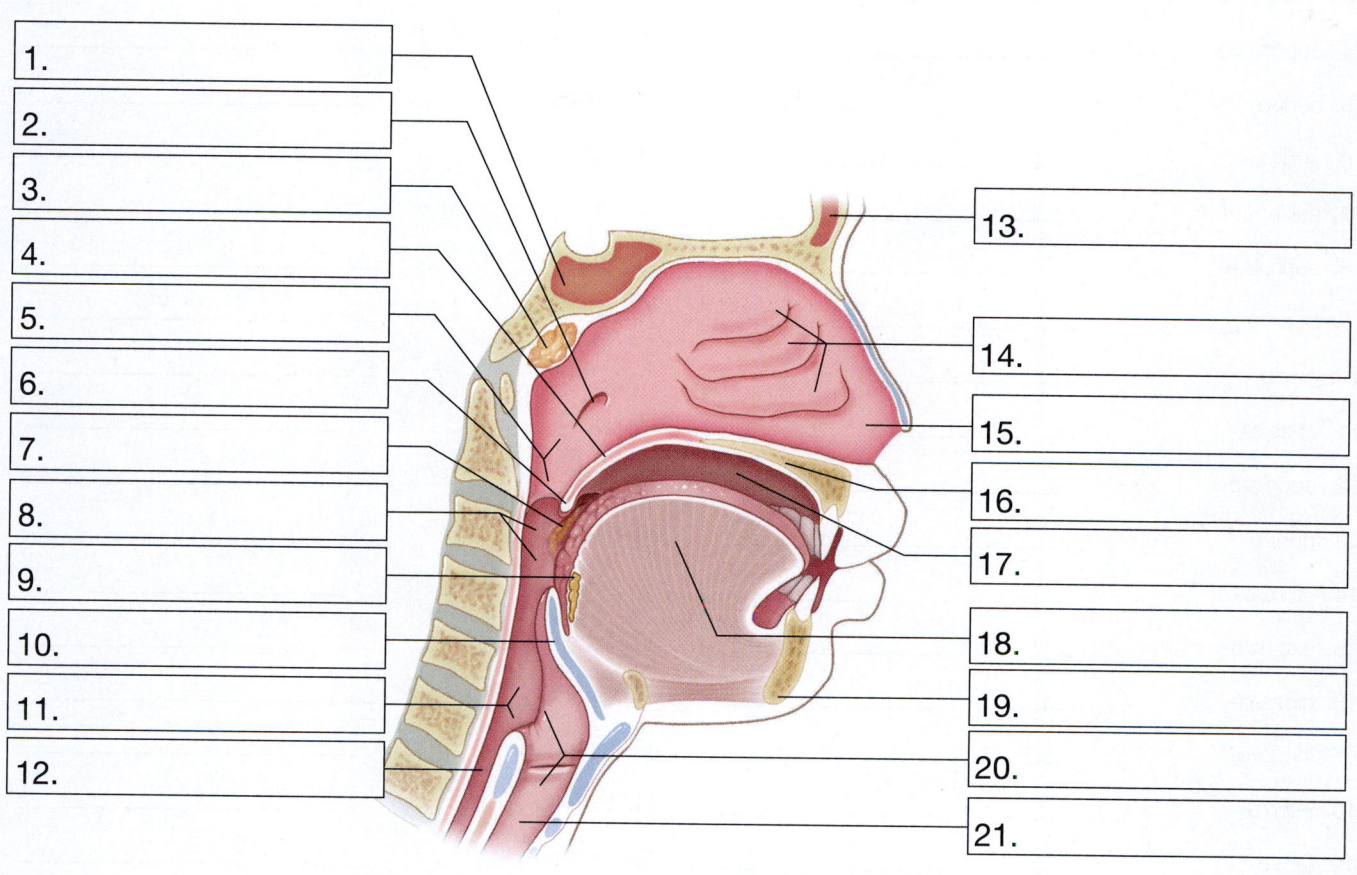

B. Give the Meaning of Combining Forms

Next to each combining form, write its meaning. The first one has been done for you.

Combining Form	Meaning	Combining Form	Meaning
1. **front/o-**	*front*	24. mast/o-	
2. acous/o-		25. mastoid/o-	
3. aden/o-		26. maxill/o-	
4. adenoid/o-		27. ment/o-	
5. audi/o-		28. mucos/o-	
6. audit/o-		29. myring/o-	
7. aur/i-		30. nas/o-	
8. auricul/o-		31. or/o-	
9. bucc/o-		32. oss/i-	
10. cav/o-		33. ossicul/o-	
11. cheil/o-		34. ot/o-	
12. cochle/o-		35. rhin/o-	
13. dors/o-		36. sept/o-	
14. ethm/o-		37. sinus/o-	
15. extern/o-		38. sphen/o-	
16. gloss/o-		39. staped/o-	
17. incud/o-		40. tempor/o-	
18. infer/o-		41. tonsill/o-	
19. labi/o-		42. turbin/o-	
20. labyrinth/o-		43. tympan/o-	
21. lingu/o-		44. vestibul/o-	
22. malle/o-		45. voc/o-	
23. mandibul/o-			

C. Build Words

Read the definition of the medical word. Look at the combining form that is given. Select the correct suffix from the Suffix List, and write it on the blank line. Then build the medical word, and write it on the line. (Remember: You may need to remove the combining vowel. Always remove the hyphens and slash.) Be sure to check your spelling.

Suffix List

-al (pertaining to)	-cle (small thing)	-ity (condition; state)
-ar (pertaining to)	-ial (pertaining to)	-ory (having the function of)
-ate (composed of; pertaining to)	-ic (pertaining to)	

Definition of the Medical Word	Combining Form	Suffix	Build the Medical Word
Example: Pertaining to (the) back (or) dorsum	**dors/o-**	*-al*	*dorsal*

[*You think* pertaining to (*-al*) + back or dorsum (*dors/o-*). You change the order of the word parts to put the suffix last. You write dorsal.]

1. Pertaining to (the) nose	nas/o-		
2. Pertaining to (the) tongue	gloss/o-		
3. Pertaining to (a) hammer-shaped bone	malle/o-		
4. Small thing (that is a) bone (in the ear)	oss/i-		
5. Pertaining to (an) entrance	vestibul/o-		
6. Composed of (a) scroll-like structure	turbin/o-		
7. Pertaining to (the) eardrum	tympan/o-		
8. State (of having a) hollow space	cav/o-		
9. Pertaining to (a) spiral-shaped structure	cochle/o-		
10. Pertaining to (the) cheek	bucc/o-		
11. Having the function of (the) sense of hearing	audit/o-		
12. Small thing (that is the) ear	aur/i-		
13. Pertaining to (an) anvil-shaped bone	incud/o-		
14. Pertaining to (the) mouth	or/o-		
15. Pertaining to (the) ear	ot/o-		
16. Pertaining to (a) stirrup-shaped bone	staped/o-		

D. Define Abbreviations

1. EAC
2. ENT
3. TM
4. TMJ

15.2 Physiology

Hearing

The sense of hearing is made possible by structures that begin with the external ear and end in the auditory cortex of the brain. The position of an **external ear** on each side of the head (1) allows more sounds to be heard and (2) lets each ear hear sounds at a slightly different time so that the source of the sound can be accurately determined. The shape of the external ear efficiently captures sound waves and funnels them into the external auditory canal, where they travel to the **tympanic membrane** (see Figure 15-9 ■).

The tympanic membrane changes the sound waves into vibrations that cause movements of the malleus, the incus, and then the stapes of the middle ear. The vibrations of the stapes are transmitted through the small, membrane-covered **oval window** between the middle and inner ear. This causes the fluid in the vestibule of the inner ear to vibrate, and these vibrations are transmitted to the **cochlea**. Within the cochlea, hair cells (sensory receptors) detect these vibrations as loudness (intensity) and pitch (frequency). The loudness of the sound corresponds to the number of hair cells that are moved. The pitch of the sound corresponds to the location of the stimulated hair cells. The hair cells change this vibration into nerve impulses that travel through the **cochlear branch** of the **vestibulocochlear nerve** (cranial nerve VIII) (see Figure 15-4) to the medulla oblongata in the brainstem. From there, the impulses travel to the **auditory cortex** in each temporal lobe of the brain to be interpreted for the sense of hearing. When the vibration has traveled through the cochlea, it returns to the vestibule where it causes the small, membrane-covered round window to bulge. The **round window** acts as a "safety valve" in the bone around the inner ear, allowing vibrations in the vestibule to decrease as they cause the membrane to bulge into the middle ear cavity.

Pronunciation/Word Parts

tympanic (tim-PAN-ik)
  tympan/o- *eardrum; tympanic membrane*
  -ic *pertaining to*

cochlea (KOH-klee-ah)

cochlear (KOH-klee-ar)
  cochle/o- *cochlea; spiral-shaped structure*
  -ar *pertaining to*

vestibulocochlear
(ves-TIH-byoo-loh-KOH-klee-ar)
  vestibul/o- *entrance; vestibule*
  cochle/o- *cochlea; spiral-shaped structure*
  -ar *pertaining to*

auditory (AW-dih-TOR-ee)
  audit/o- *sense of hearing*
  -ory *having the function of*
The combining form **audi/o-** means *hearing*. The combining form **acous/o-** means *hearing; sound*.

cortex (KOR-teks)

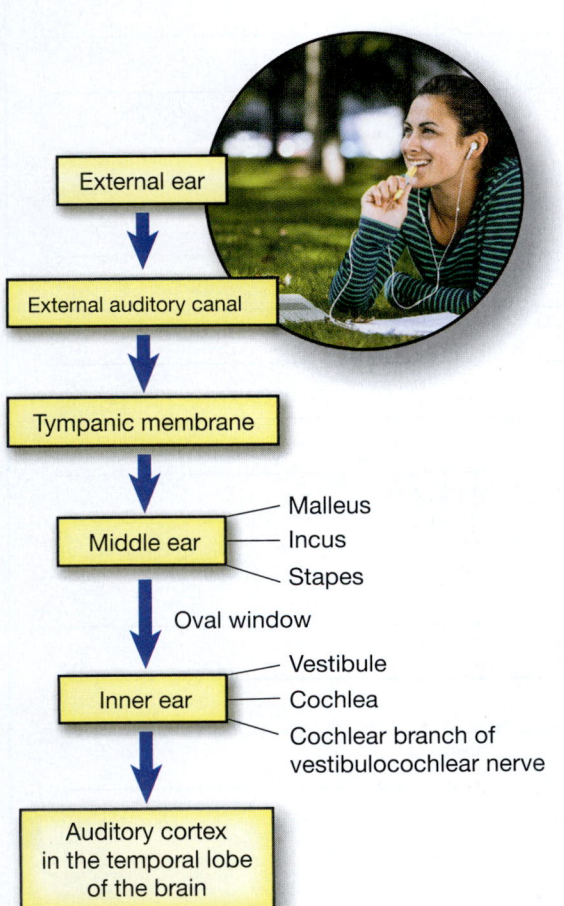

FIGURE 15-9 ■ The sense of hearing. Favorite music travels as sound waves through the external auditory canal. In the middle ear, the sound waves are converted into vibrations. In the inner ear, that motion is converted to nerve impulses that travel through the cochlear branch of the vestibulocochlear nerve (cranial nerve VIII) to the auditory cortex of the brain. The brain recognizes it as favorite music to be enjoyed!

Olfaction

The sense of smell begins with receptors in the nose that detect the molecules in odors that are in the inhaled air. This sensory information is relayed via the **olfactory nerve** (cranial nerve I) to the olfactory cortex in the brain to identify the smell.

Balance

The body's sense of balance includes maintaining body position while still or during movement. This is a coordinated effort between the inner ear and other body systems. The three **semicircular canals** of the inner ear are each oriented in a different plane: horizontally, vertically, and obliquely. As the head moves, hair cells (sensory receptors) in each semicircular canal send sensory information to the brain about the position of the head and neck. This sensory information is transmitted through the **vestibular branch** of the vestibulocochlear nerve (cranial nerve VIII). It travels to the brainstem and then to the cerebellum of the brain, where it is combined with other sensory information—awareness of body position (**proprioception**), visual information from the eyes, and sensory information from the nerves and muscles of the body—to establish the sense of balance.

Pronunciation/Word Parts

olfaction (ohl-FAK-shun)
 olfact/o- sense of smell
 -ion action; condition
The combining form **osm/o-** also means sense of smell.

olfactory (ohl-FAK-tor-ee)
 olfact/o- sense of smell
 -ory having the function of

vestibular (ves-TIH-byoo-lar)
 vestibul/o- entrance; vestibule
 -ar pertaining to

proprioception (PROH-pree-oh-SEP-shun)
 propri/o- one's own body
 -ception having a receptor

15.2 PRACTICE LAPS

Use the Answer Key at the end of the book to check your answers.

A. Give the Meaning of Combining Forms

Next to each combining form, write its meaning. The first one has been done for you.

Combining Form	Meaning	Combining Form	Meaning
1. **audit/o-**	*sense of hearing*	5. propri/o-	
2. cochle/o-		6. tympan/o-	
3. olfact/o-		7. vestibul/o-	
4. osm/o-			

B. Build Words

Read the definition of the medical word. Look at the combining form that is given. Select the correct suffix from the Suffix List, and write it on the blank line. Then build the medical word, and write it on the line. (Remember: You may need to remove the combining vowel. Always remove the hyphens and slash.) Be sure to check your spelling.

Suffix List

-ar (pertaining to)	-ic (pertaining to)	-ory (having the function of)
-ception (having a receptor)	-ion (action; condition)	

Definition of the Medical Word	Combining Form	Suffix	Build the Medical Word
Example: Pertaining to (an) entrance	**vestibul/o-**	*-ar*	*vestibular*

[You think pertaining to (-ar) + entrance (vestibul/o-). You change the order of the word parts to put the suffix last. You write vestibular.]

1. Pertaining to (a) spiral-shaped structure	cochle/o-		
2. Having the function of (the) sense of hearing	audit/o-		

continued on next page

Definition of the Medical Word	Combining Form	Suffix	Build the Medical Word
3. Having a receptor (that gives information about) one's own body (position)	propri/o-	_____	_____
4. Having the function of (the) sense of smell	olfact/o-	_____	_____
5. Pertaining to (the) eardrum	tympan/o-	_____	_____
6. Condition (of having the) sense of smell	olfact/o-	_____	_____

Vocabulary Review

Word or Phrase	Description	Combining Forms
Overview		
ears, nose, and throat	Interrelated group of anatomic structures of the **ears, nose,** and **throat,** located in the head and neck, that are considered together for the medical specialty of otolaryngology. They consist of external structures (ears, nose, mouth) and internal structures (middle ears, inner ears, nasal cavity, sinuses, oral cavity, pharynx, larynx). Some of these structures are also part of the gastrointestinal and respiratory systems. The function of the ears is the sense of hearing and helping to maintain balance. The function of the nose is olfaction, the sense of smell. In conjunction with other body systems, these structures also produce speech and function as part of the immune response.	**ot/o-** *ear* **nas/o-** *nose* **pharyng/o-** *pharynx; throat*
Anatomy of the Ears		
External Ear		
auricle	The visible external ear. Also known as the **pinna**.	**aur/i-** *ear* **auricul/o-** *ear* **ot/o-** *ear*
cerumen	Waxy, sticky substance secreted by glands in the external auditory canal. It traps dirt and has an antibiotic action against microorganisms.	
external auditory canal (EAC)	Passageway from the external ear to the tympanic membrane. It contains glands that secrete cerumen. The **external auditory meatus** is the opening to the external auditory canal.	**extern/o-** *outside* **audit/o-** *sense of hearing*
external ear	First part of the ear. It consists of the visible external structures of the auricle (pinna), helix, tragus, external auditory meatus, external auditory canal, and the bony mastoid process behind the ear. The external ear also includes the tympanic membrane at the end of the external auditory canal.	**extern/o-** *outside*
helix	Outer rim of tissue and cartilage that forms the *C* shape of the external ear and ends at the earlobe	
mastoid process	Bony projection of the temporal bone behind the external ear. It contains air cells that connect to the middle ear and to the eustachian tube.	**mast/o-** *breast; mastoid process* **mastoid/o-** *mastoid process*
tragus	Triangular cartilage anterior to the external auditory meatus	

Word or Phrase	Description	Combining Forms
tympanic membrane	Thin, pearly gray membrane at the end of the external auditory canal. It divides the external ear from the middle ear. Also known as the **eardrum**.	**tympan/o-** eardrum; tympanic membrane **myring/o-** eardrum; tympanic membrane
Middle Ear		
eustachian tube	Tube that connects the middle ear to the nasopharynx to allow air pressure in the middle ear and mastoid air cells to equalize with air pressure in the nose, throat, and outside of the body	
incus	Second bone of the middle ear. It is connected to the malleus on one end and to the stapes on the other end. Also known as the **anvil** because of its shape.	**incud/o-** anvil-shaped bone; incus
malleus	First bone of the middle ear. It is connected to the tympanic membrane on one end and to the incus on the other end. Also known as the **hammer** because of its shape.	**malle/o-** hammer-shaped bone; malleus
middle ear	Second part of the ear. It is a cavity (hollow area) in the temporal bone that contains the malleus, incus, and stapes bones. The middle ear is connected to the air cells of the mastoid process and to the nasopharynx by the eustachian tube.	
ossicles	The three tiny bones of the middle ear: malleus, incus, and stapes. These bones are connected to each other to form the **ossicular chain**.	**oss/i-** bone **ossicul/o-** ossicle; small bone
stapes	Third bone of the middle ear. It is connected to the incus on one end and fits into the membrane-covered opening of the oval window on the other end. Also known as the **stirrup** because of its shape.	**staped/o-** stapes; stirrup-shaped bone
Inner Ear		
cochlea	Spiral-shaped structure that sends sensory information to the brain about sound waves that enter the ear	**cochle/o-** cochlea; spiral-shaped structure
inner ear	Third part of the ear. It is a cavity that contains the vestibule, semicircular canals, and the cochlea, as well as the oval window and round window in the temporal bone between the middle and inner ear.	
labyrinth	All of the structures of the inner ear	**labyrinth/o-** labyrinth
oval window	Small, membrane-covered opening in the temporal bone between the middle ear and inner ear. It is connected to the stapes of the middle ear.	
round window	Small, membrane-covered opening in the temporal bone between the middle ear and inner ear	
semicircular canals	Three separate but intertwined fluid-filled canals in the inner ear that are each oriented in a different plane (horizontally, vertically, and obliquely). They send sensory information to the brain about the position of the head.	**circul/o-** circle
vestibule	Fluid-filled structure at the entrance to the inner ear. The superior part of the vestibule becomes the semicircular canals, and the inferior part becomes the cochlea. The vestibule has two small, membrane-covered openings in its bony wall: the oval window and round window.	**vestibul/o-** entrance; vestibule

Word or Phrase	Description	Combining Forms
External Nose and Nasal Cavity		
ala	Flared cartilage on the side of the nostril	
mucosa	Mucous membrane lining in the nasal cavity. It covers the turbinates and produces **mucus** that gives warmth and moisture to the air and traps foreign particles.	**mucos/o-** *mucous membrane*
naris	A nostril, one of the two external openings into the nasal cavity	
nasal cavity	Hollow area inside the nose whose walls are formed by the ethmoid and maxillary bones. It is lined with mucosa and is divided in the middle by the nasal septum. It contains the turbinates.	**nas/o-** *nose* **cav/o-** *hollow space* **rhin/o-** *nose*
nasal dorsum	Vertical ridge in the middle of the external nose. It is supported by the nasal bone.	**dors/o-** *back; dorsum*
nasal septum	Vertical wall of cartilage and bone that divides the nasal cavity into right and left sides	**sept/o-** *dividing wall; septum*
turbinates	Three long, scroll-like projections of bone (**superior, middle,** and **inferior turbinates**) that jut into the nasal cavity to slow down inhaled air. Also known as the **nasal conchae**. The turbinates are covered with **mucosa**.	**turbin/o-** *scroll-like structure* **super/o-** *above* **infer/o-** *below* **mucos/o-** *mucous membrane*
Sinuses		
ethmoid sinuses	Groups of small air cells within the ethmoid bone, located between the nose and the eyes	**ethm/o-** *sieve*
frontal sinuses	Hollow, air-filled cavities in the frontal bone, just superior and medial to each eyebrow	**front/o-** *front*
maxillary sinuses	Hollow, air-filled cavities in the maxilla (upper jaw bone) on either side of the nose. The maxillary sinuses are the largest of the sinuses.	**maxill/o-** *maxilla; upper jaw*
sinus	Hollow, air-filled cavity in a facial or cranial bone. A sinus is lined with mucous membrane that produces mucus. There are four pairs of sinuses (frontal, maxillary, ethmoid, and sphenoid). They are connected to each other and to the nasal cavity. Together, they are the **paranasal sinuses**.	**sinus/o-** *sinus* **nas/o-** *nose*
sphenoid sinuses	Hollow, air-filled cavities in the sphenoid bone, located posterior to the nasal cavity	**sphen/o-** *wedge shaped*
External Mouth and Oral Cavity		
hard palate	Structure that divides the oral cavity from the nasal cavity. It consists of the maxilla, palatine, and vomer bones. Together with the soft palate, it forms the roof of the mouth.	**palat/o-** *palate*
mentum	The chin. The anterior part of the mandible (lower jaw).	**ment/o-** *chin; mind*
mucosa	Mucous membrane that produces **mucus**. The **oral mucosa** lines the oral cavity. The **buccal mucosa** lines the cheek area of the oral cavity.	**mucos/o-** *mucous membrane* **or/o-** *mouth* **bucc/o-** *cheek*
nasolabial fold	Skin crease from the nose to the lip at the corner of the mouth	**nas/o-** *nose* **labi/o-** *labium; lip* **cheil/o-** *lip*

Word or Phrase	Description	Combining Forms
oral cavity	Hollow area inside the mouth that contains the tongue, hard palate, soft palate, uvula, teeth, and gums. It is lined with **oral mucosa**. In the cheek area, this is **buccal mucosa**. The hard and soft palate form the roof of the mouth. The mandible forms the floor of the mouth.	**or/o-** *mouth* **mucos/o-** *mucous membrane* **bucc/o-** *cheek*
philtrum	Vertical groove in the skin of the upper lip	
soft palate	Soft tissue extension of the hard palate at the back of the oral cavity. It ends with the fleshy **uvula** that hangs down in the back of the oral cavity.	**palat/o-** *palate*
submental lymph nodes	Lymph nodes beneath the chin. They contain special cells that are active in the immune response and attack bacteria and viruses in the oral cavity.	**ment/o-** *chin; mind*
temporoman-dibular joint (TMJ)	Movable joint where each side of the mandible (lower jaw) is attached to the temporal bone of the cranium	**tempor/o-** *side of the head; temple* **mandibul/o-** *lower jaw; mandible*
tongue	Large muscle in the oral cavity, the base of which is attached to the mandible	**gloss/o-** *tongue* **lingu/o-** *tongue*
Pharynx		
adenoids	Lymphoid tissue located in the roof and walls of the nasopharynx. The adenoids are part of the lymphatic system and function in the body's immune response.	**aden/o-** *gland* **adenoid/o-** *structure resembling a gland*
laryngopharynx	Area of the throat that is posterior to the larynx. It contains the lymphoid tissue of the lingual tonsils.	**laryng/o-** *larynx; voice box*
lingual tonsils	Lymphoid tissue located on either side of the base of the tongue in the laryngopharynx. The tonsils are part of the lymphatic system and function in the body's immune response.	**lingu/o-** *tongue* **tonsill/o-** *tonsil*
nasopharynx	Area of the throat that is posterior to the nasal cavity. The nasopharynx contains the lymphoid tissue of the adenoids and is connected to the middle ear by the eustachian tube.	**nas/o-** *nose*
oropharynx	Area of the throat that is posterior to the oral cavity. It contains the lymphoid tissue of the palatine tonsils.	**or/o-** *mouth*
palatine tonsils	Lymphoid tissue located on either side of the soft palate in the oropharynx. The tonsils are part of the lymphatic system and function in the body's immune response.	**palat/o-** *palate* **tonsill/o-** *tonsil*
pharynx	The throat. It is a shared passageway for food and air and is divided into three areas: the nasopharynx, oropharynx, and laryngopharynx. It contains lymphoid tissues of the adenoids and lingual and palatine tonsils.	**pharyng/o-** *pharynx; throat*
Larynx		
epiglottis	Lid-like structure that seals the larynx during swallowing	**glott/o-** *glottis of the larynx*
glottis	V-shaped structure in the larynx. It contains cartilage, ligaments, and the vocal cords.	**glott/o-** *glottis of the larynx*
larynx	Short, triangular structure that is visible on the anterior surface of the neck as the **laryngeal prominence** (Adam's apple). Internally, it contains the epiglottis, glottis, and vocal cords. Also known as the **voice box**.	**laryng/o-** *larynx; voice box*
vocal cords	Bands of connective tissue in the glottis that vibrate to produce sounds during speaking and singing	**voc/o-** *voice*

Word or Phrase	Description	Combining Forms
Physiology of the Ears, Nose, and Throat		
Sense of Hearing		
auditory cortex	Structure in each temporal lobe of the brain that interprets nerve impulses from the cochlea for the sense of hearing	**audit/o-** *sense of hearing*
cochlea	Hair cells (sensory receptors) in the cochlea detect vibrations from the fluid in the vestibule as loudness (intensity) and pitch (frequency) and change them into nerve impulses that travel on the cochlear branch of the vestibulocochlear nerve.	**cochle/o-** *cochlea; spiral-shaped structure*
cochlear branch	Part of the vestibulocochlear nerve that carries nerve impulses from the cochlea to the medulla oblongata of the brainstem	**cochle/o-** *cochlea; spiral-shaped structure*
external auditory canal	Carries sound waves from the external ear to the tympanic membrane	**extern/o-** *outside* **audit/o-** *sense of hearing*
external ear	Captures sound waves and funnels them into the external auditory canal where the sound waves are converted into the vibrations of the tympanic membrane	**extern/o-** *outside*
inner ear	The vibration of the stapes becomes vibrations of the membrane-covered oval window and the fluid in the vestibule of the inner ear. These vibrations are transmitted to the cochlea of the inner ear.	
middle ear	Malleus, incus, and stapes bones of the middle ear move in response to vibrations of the tympanic membrane. The stapes transmits these vibrations to the membrane-covered oval window between the middle and inner ear.	
oval window	Small, membrane-covered opening in the temporal bone between the middle and inner ear. It is connected to the stapes in the middle ear, and the stapes transmits its vibrations to the membrane of the oval window, which transmits vibrations to the fluid in the vestibule.	
round window	Membrane-covered opening in the temporal bone that divides the middle ear from the inner ear. The round window acts as a "safety valve," allowing vibrations in the vestibule to decrease as they cause the membrane to bulge into the middle ear.	
tympanic membrane	Changes sound waves into vibrations that cause movement of the bones of the middle ear	**tympan/o-** *eardrum; tympanic membrane*
vestibulocochlear nerve	Cranial nerve VIII. Carries nerve impulses from the cochlea (via the cochlear branch) for the sense of hearing. Carries nerve impulses from the semicircular canals (via the vestibular branch) to maintain balance.	**vestibul/o-** *entrance; vestibule* **cochle/o-** *cochlea; spiral-shaped structure*
Sense of Smell		
olfaction	The sense of smell. Receptors in the nose detect the molecules in odors and relay this information via the **olfactory nerve** (cranial nerve I) to the olfactory cortex in the brain where the smell is identified.	**olfact/o-** *sense of smell*
Balance		
balance	Includes maintaining body position (proprioception) and initiating movement. Balance is based on combined sensory information from the semicircular canals of the inner ear, visual information from the eyes, and sensory information from the nerves and muscles about the position of the body.	
proprioception	Awareness of the position of all parts of the body	**propri/o-** *one's own body*

Word or Phrase	Description	Combining Forms
semicircular canals	Canals in the inner ear that are oriented in three different planes. They contain hair cells (sensory receptors) that send sensory information to the brain about the position of the head and neck.	**circul/o-** *circle*
vestibular branch	Part of the vestibulocochlear nerve that carries nerve impulses from the semicircular canals to the brainstem and then to the cerebellum of the brain to maintain balance	**vestibul/o-** *entrance; vestibule*

Abbreviations Review

EAC	external auditory canal		**TM**	tympanic membrane
ENT	ears, nose, and throat		**TMJ**	temporomandibular joint

15.3 Diseases

Word or Phrase	Description	Pronunciation/Word Parts

Ears

Word or Phrase	Description	Pronunciation/Word Parts
acoustic neuroma	Benign (not cancerous) tumor of the vestibulocochlear nerve. Depending on the location of the tumor, it can cause pain, dizziness, or hearing loss. Treatment: Surgical removal	**acoustic** (ah-KOOS-tik) **acous/o-** *hearing; sound* **-tic** *pertaining to* **neuroma** (nyoor-OH-mah) **neur/o-** *nerve* **-oma** *mass; tumor*
cerumen impaction	Cerumen (earwax), epithelial cells, and hairs form a mass that occludes the external auditory canal. Treatment: Ear drops to soften the cerumen and irrigation with a saline solution and bulb syringe to wash it out; removal of cerumen with forceps (see Figure 15-10 ■).	**impaction** (im-PAK-shun) **impact/o-** *wedged in* **-ion** *action; condition*

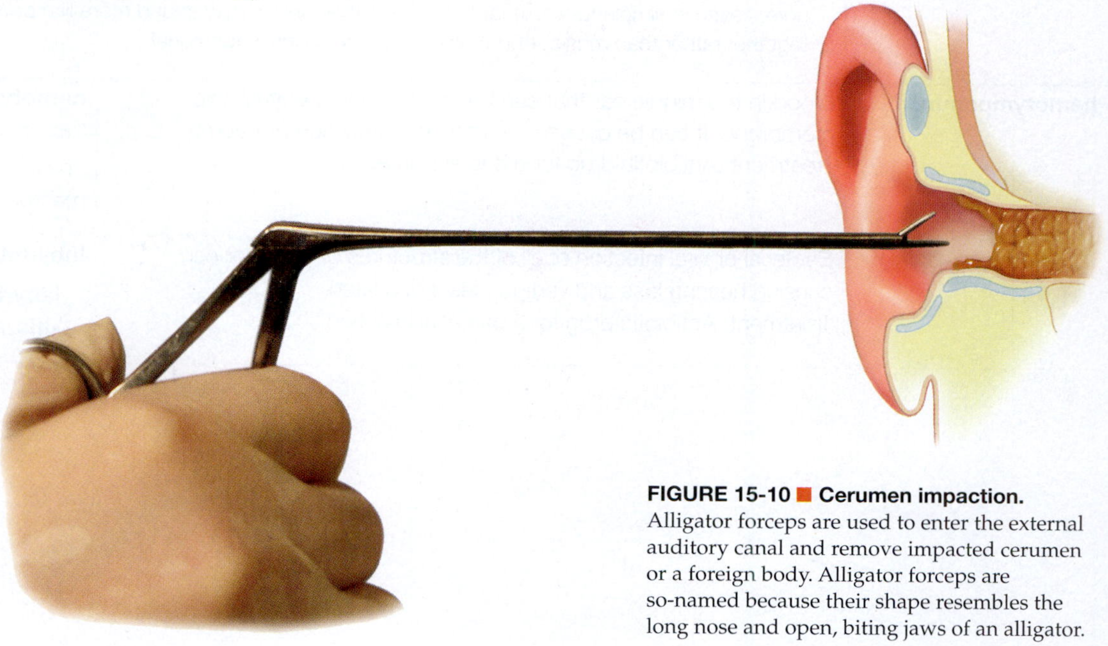

FIGURE 15-10 ■ **Cerumen impaction.**
Alligator forceps are used to enter the external auditory canal and remove impacted cerumen or a foreign body. Alligator forceps are so-named because their shape resembles the long nose and open, biting jaws of an alligator.

Word or Phrase	Description	Pronunciation/Word Parts
cholesteatoma	Benign, slow-growing tumor in the middle ear. It contains cholesterol deposits and epithelial cells. It can eventually destroy the bones of the middle ear and extend into the air cells of the mastoid process. The underlying cause is usually chronic otitis media. Treatment: Treat the underlying otitis media; surgical removal of the cholesteatoma	**cholesteatoma** (koh-LES-tee-ah-TOH-mah) *Cholesteatoma* is a combination of the word *cholesterol*, the Greek word *stear* (animal fat), and the suffix **-oma** (mass; tumor).

hearing loss	Temporary or progressive, permanent decline in the ability to hear sounds in one or both ears. Patients with a hearing loss are said to be **hearing impaired** or hard of hearing.
	• **Conductive hearing loss** occurs when sound waves cannot reach the inner ear because of a foreign body or infection in the external auditory canal, perforation of the tympanic membrane, fluid behind the tympanic membrane, degeneration of the bones in the middle ear, or otosclerosis (described later).
	• **Sensorineural hearing loss** occurs due to disease of the cochlea, damage to the inner ear from excessive noise, or changes due to aging that hinder the production or transmission of nerve impulses by the vestibulocochlear nerve.
	• **Mixed hearing loss** is a combination of both conductive and sensorineural hearing loss.
	• **Low-frequency hearing loss** is the inability to hear low-pitched sounds.
	• **High-frequency hearing loss** is the inability to hear high-pitched sounds.
	• **Presbycusis** is bilateral hearing loss due to aging. Also known as **presbyacusis**.
	• **Anacusis** is total deafness. Deaf-mutism is total deafness coupled with the inability to speak.
	Treatment: Correct the underlying cause; hearing aid; in some cases, a cochlear implant may be needed
		conductive (con-DUK-tiv)
		  conduct/o- *carrying; conveying*
		  -ive *pertaining to*
		
		sensorineural
		(SEN-soh-ree-NYOOR-al)
		  sensor/i- *sensory*
		  neur/o- *nerve*
		  -al *pertaining to*
		
		presbycusis
		(PREZ-bee-KYOO-sihs)
		
		presbyacusis
		(PREZ-bee-ah-KYOO-sihs)
		  presby/o- *old age*
		  -acusis *abnormal condition of hearing*
		
		anakusis (AN-ah-KYOO-sihs)

Dive Deeper

Tone deafness is not a type of hearing loss. It is the inability to identify differences in pitch between musical notes, even in simple tunes. In fact, the notes themselves may sound more like pots and pans banging together rather than music. About 5% of the population is tone deaf.

Word or Phrase	Description	Pronunciation/Word Parts
hemotympanum	Blood in the middle ear that can be seen behind the tympanic membrane. It can be caused by a bacterial infection or trauma. Treatment: Antibiotic drug for a bacterial infection	**hemotympanum** (HEE-moh-TIM-pah-num) The combining form **hem/o-** means *blood*.

labyrinthitis	Bacterial or viral infection of all of the structures of the inner ear, causing hearing loss and vertigo (described later).
	Treatment: Antibiotic drug for a bacterial infection
		labyrinthitis (LAB-ih-rin-THY-tihs)
		  labyrinth/o- *labyrinth*
		  -itis *infection of; inflammation of*

Word or Phrase	Description	Pronunciation/Word Parts
mastoiditis	Bacterial infection of the air cells in the bone of the mastoid process (see Figure 15-11 ■). This is caused by an untreated or chronic infection in the middle ear (otitis media). Symptoms include swelling and tenderness of the mastoid process behind the ear with drainage from the ear. Treatment: Antibiotic drug	**mastoiditis** (MAS-toyd-EYE-tihs) **mastoid/o-** *mastoid process* **-itis** *infection of; inflammation of*

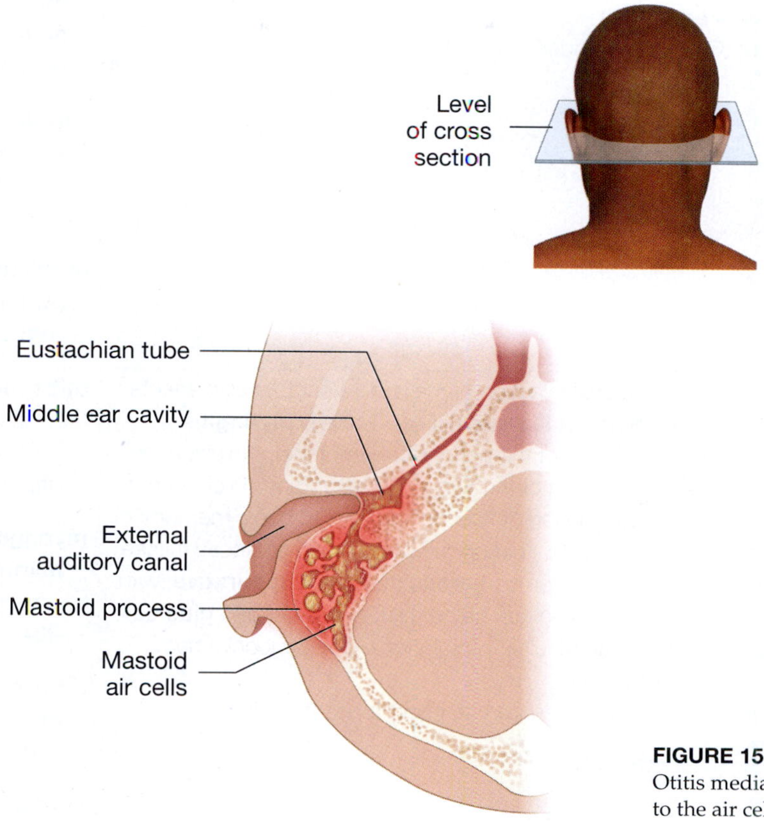

FIGURE 15-11 ■ **Mastoiditis.**
Otitis media in the middle ear can spread to the air cells of the mastoid process.

Word Alert
Sound-Alike Words

mastoiditis	(noun)	infection of the air cells in the bone of the mastoid process
		Example: The middle ear infection progressed to become mastoiditis.
mastitis	(noun)	infection of the mammary glands of the breast
		Example: Mastitis can develop in a mother who is breastfeeding her baby.

Word or Phrase	Description	Pronunciation/Word Parts
Meniere disease	Edema or fluctuating pressure of the fluid in the inner ear, causing episodes of tinnitus (described later), vertigo, hearing loss, and a feeling of fullness in the ear. It often affects just one ear. Treatment: Drug to treat the spinning sensation associated with vertigo	**Meniere** (men-YAIR)
motion sickness	Dizziness, nausea and vomiting, and a headache that is brought on by the irregular motions of riding in a car, boat, or airplane Treatment: Drug to treat motion sickness	

Word or Phrase	Description	Pronunciation/Word Parts
otitis externa	Bacterial infection of the external auditory canal. There is throbbing earache pain (**otalgia**) with a swollen, red external auditory canal and **serous** (clear) or **purulent** (with pus) drainage. It is caused by a foreign body in the ear or by the patient scratching or probing inside the ear. It also occurs in swimmers whose ear canals are rubbed by ear plugs and softened by continual exposure to water, and it is known as **swimmer's ear**. Treatment: Correct the underlying cause; antibiotic drug	**otitis externa** (oh-TY-tihs eks-TER-nah) 　**ot/o-** *ear* 　**-itis** *infection of; inflammation of* **otalgia** (oh-TAL-jah) 　**ot/o-** *ear* 　**alg/o-** *pain* 　**-ia** *condition; state; thing* **serous** (SEER-uhs) 　**ser/o-** *serum-like fluid; serum of the blood* 　**-ous** *pertaining to* **purulent** (PYOOR-yoo-lent) 　**purul/o-** *pus* 　**-ent** *pertaining to*
otitis media	Acute or chronic bacterial infection of the middle ear that also affects the tympanic membrane of the external ear. There is **myringitis** (redness and inflammation of the tympanic membrane), otalgia, a feeling of pressure, and bulging of the tympanic membrane. There can be an **effusion** (an accumulation of fluid behind the tympanic membrane) that creates an air-fluid level (fluid on the bottom and air above it) (see Figure 15-12 ■). This fluid can be **serous** (clear) or **suppurative** (with pus). In children, the effusion can be so thick that it is called **glue ear**. Chronic otitis media can result in perforation of the tympanic membrane (see Figure 15-13 ■). Treatment: Antibiotic drug; surgery to insert tubes to drain the middle ear	**otitis media** (oh-TY-tihs MEE-dee-ah) 　**ot/o-** *ear* 　**-itis** *infection of; inflammation of* **myringitis** (MEER-in-JY-tihs) 　**myring/o-** *eardrum; tympanic membrane* 　**-itis** *infection of; inflammation of* **effusion** (ee-FYOO-zhun) 　**effus/o-** *pouring out* 　**-ion** *action; condition* **suppurative** (SUH-poor-ah-TIV) 　**suppur/o-** *pus formation* 　**-ative** *pertaining to*

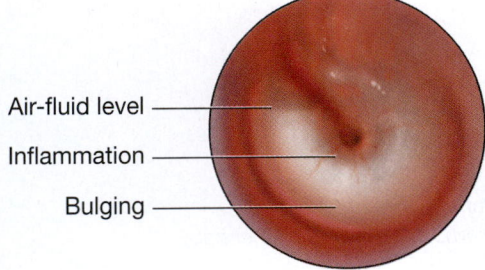

Air-fluid level
Inflammation
Bulging

FIGURE 15-12 ■ **Myringitis.**
The tympanic membrane is red and inflamed. There is dullness with no light reflex (see Figure 15-3 for comparison). There is a loss of normal landmarks (visibility of the malleus), and the entire tympanic membrane bulges out into the external auditory canal. Fluid from an effusion in the middle ear creates an air-fluid level that can be seen through the tympanic membrane.

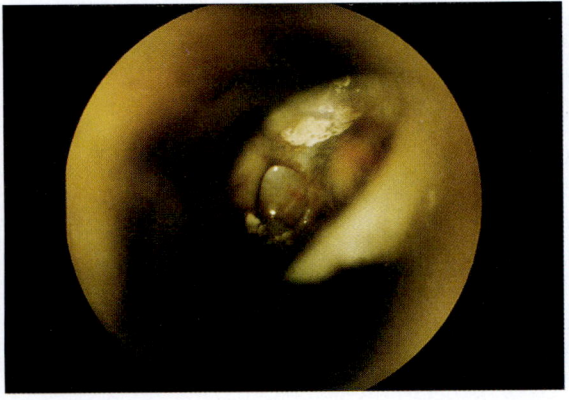

FIGURE 15-13 ■ **Perforated tympanic membrane.**
A perforated eardrum can be caused by chronic otitis media in the middle ear.

Word or Phrase	Description	Pronunciation/Word Parts
	## Across the Life Span **Pediatrics.** Otitis media is common in young children because the short eustachian tube is in a nearly horizontal position that allows bacteria and drainage from the nasopharynx to enter the middle ear. If otitis media is left untreated, the tympanic membrane can rupture or the bones of the middle ear can degenerate, resulting in permanent hearing loss. **Geriatrics.** Cerumen impaction occurs commonly in older adults because of dry skin, thick cerumen, growth of hair in the external auditory canal, and/or the presence of a hearing aid.	
otorrhea	Drainage of serous or purulent fluid from the ear. It can be caused by otitis externa or otitis media (when the tympanic membrane ruptures). It can also be caused by a fracture of the temporal bone of the cranium with leakage of cerebrospinal fluid into the ear. Treatment: Correct the underlying cause.	**otorrhea** (OH-toh-REE-ah) **ot/o-** *ear* **-rrhea** *discharge; flow*
otosclerosis	Abnormal deposits of bone in the middle ear, particularly between the stapes and the oval window. The stapes becomes immovable, causing conductive hearing loss. Certain families have a genetic predisposition to developing otosclerosis. Treatment: Hearing aid; stapedectomy	**otosclerosis** (OH-toh-skleh-ROH-sihs) **ot/o-** *ear* **scler/o-** *hard; sclera* **-osis** *abnormal condition; process*
ruptured tympanic membrane	Tear in the tympanic membrane due to excessive pressure or a middle ear infection. In pilots and deep-sea divers, unequal air pressure in the middle ear compared to the surrounding air or water pressure can rupture the tympanic membrane. Treatment: Tympanoplasty	
tinnitus	Sounds (such as buzzing, ringing, hissing, or roaring) that are heard constantly or intermittently in one or both ears, especially in a quiet environment. Also known as "ringing in the ears." It is caused by repeated exposure to excessive noise and is associated with hearing loss. It can also be related to the overuse of aspirin. Treatment: Soft background noise (hum of a fan or a device that generates "white noise") to mask the tinnitus and allow the patient to sleep	**tinnitus** (TIN-ih-tuhs)
vertigo	Sensation of motion and spinning when the head and inner ear move but the body is not moving, with a feeling that one's body or the environment is spinning or rotating. It is caused by a head cold, middle or inner ear infection, head trauma, degenerative changes of the semicircular canals, labyrinthitis, or Meniere disease. Treatment: Correct the underlying cause.	**vertigo** (VER-tih-goh)

Sinuses, Nose, and Nasal Cavity

allergic rhinitis	Allergic symptoms in the nose. In response to an inhaled antigen (pollen, dust, animal dander, mold), basophils and mast cells of the immune system release histamine. This causes nasal stuffiness; sneezing; **rhinorrhea** (clear mucus discharge from the nose); hypertrophy (enlargement) of the turbinates in the nose with their red, edematous, and swollen mucous membranes; and **postnasal drip (PND)**. When this occurs in the spring or fall and coincides with the blooming of certain trees and plants (grasses, maple trees, roses, goldenrod), it is known as **seasonal allergy** or **hay fever**. Treatment: Antihistamine drug, decongestant drug, corticosteroid drug	**allergic** (ah-LER-jik) **allerg/o-** *allergy* **-ic** *pertaining to* **rhinitis** (ry-NY-tihs) **rhin/o-** *nose* **-itis** *infection of; inflammation of* **rhinorrhea** (RY-noh-REE-ah) **rhin/o-** *nose* **-rrhea** *discharge; flow* **postnasal** (post-NAY-zal) **post-** *after; behind* **nas/o-** *nose* **-al** *pertaining to*

Word or Phrase	Description	Pronunciation/Word Parts
anosmia	Temporary or permanent loss of the sense of smell. It is most often caused by head trauma. Treatment: Correct the underlying cause.	**anosmia** (an-AWZ-mee-ah) **an-** *not; without* **osm/o-** *sense of smell* **-ia** *condition; state; thing*
epistaxis	Sudden, sometimes severe bleeding from the nose. It is due to irritation or dryness of the nasal mucosa with rupture of a small artery or it can be caused by trauma to the nose. Also known as a **nosebleed**. Treatment: Pack the nostril with gauze or use cautery to stop the bleeding.	**epistaxis** (EP-ih-STAK-sihs) The prefix **epi-** means *above; upon*. The suffix **-staxis** means *abnormal condition of hemorrhage*. Epistaxis: *Abnormal condition of hemorrhage (in a structure that is) upon (the face)*
nasal polyp	Benign, soft growth of the mucous membrane in the nose or sinuses. A single polyp may grow large enough to limit the flow of air or there may be several polyps. Treatment: Polypectomy	**polyp** (PAW-lip)
rhinophyma	Redness and hypertrophy (enlargement) of the nose with small-to-large, irregular lumps, usually seen in men. It is caused by the increased number of sebaceous glands associated with rosacea of the skin (described in Chapter 2, Dermatology). Treatment: Topical drug for rosacea	**rhinophyma** (RY-noh-FY-mah) **rhin/o-** *nose* **-phyma** *growth; tumor*
septal deviation	Lateral displacement of the nasal septum, significantly narrowing one nasal airway. This can be a congenital condition or it can be caused by trauma to the nose. Treatment: Surgical correction (septoplasty)	
sinusitis	Acute or chronic bacterial infection in one or more of the sinus cavities (see Figure 15-14 ■). There is headache, pain in the forehead or cheekbones over the sinus, postnasal drainage, fatigue, and fever. **Pansinusitis** involves all the sinuses or all of the sinuses on one side of the face. Treatment: Antibiotic drug; endoscopic sinus surgery	**sinusitis** (SY-nyoo-SY-tihs) **sinus/o-** *sinus* **-itis** *infection of; inflammation of* **pansinusitis** (PAN-sy-nyoo-SY-tihs) **pan-** *all* **sinus/o-** *sinus* **-itis** *infection of; inflammation of*

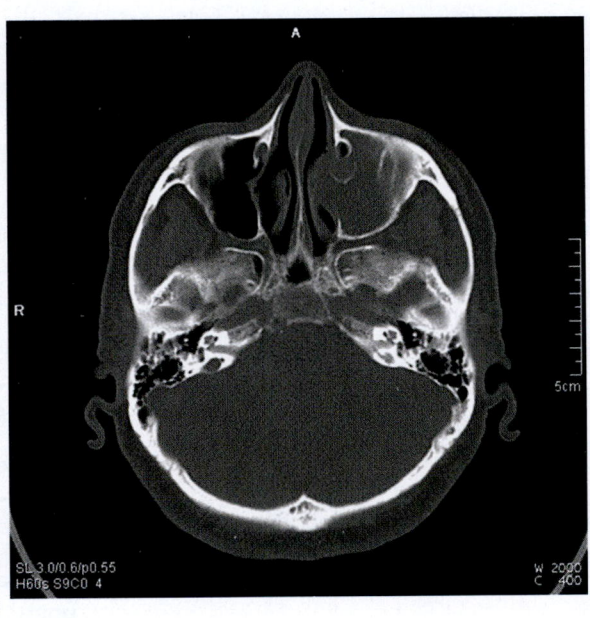

FIGURE 15-14 ■ Sinusitis.
This CT scan of the head shows the nose at the top of the image with the long, bony nasal septum inside the nasal cavity. The right maxillary sinus shows an open sinus cavity that is black. The left maxillary sinus shows severe swelling of the mucous membrane with no open sinus cavity. *Remember:* A CT scan is read as if you were at the patient's feet looking toward the head. Notice the small "R" on the left side of the image because the patient's right side is on your left side.

Word or Phrase	Description	Pronunciation/Word Parts
upper respiratory infection (URI)	Bacterial or viral infection of the nose that can spread to the throat and ears. The nose is also a part of the respiratory system, and this is an upper respiratory infection. Also known as a **common cold** or **head cold**. Treatment: Antibiotic drug for a bacterial infection; antibiotic drugs are not effective against viral infections.	

Oral Cavity and Pharynx

cancer of the mouth and neck	**Malignant** tumor (**carcinoma**) of the mucous membrane in the oral cavity, pharynx, or larynx. Smoking and using smokeless chewing tobacco can cause this.
	Treatment: Surgery to remove the tongue (glossectomy), larynx (laryngectomy), or jaw bone and neck muscles (radical neck dissection)
		cancer (KAN-ser)
		
		malignant (mah-LIG-nant)
		  malign/o- *cancer*
		  -ant *pertaining to*
		
		carcinoma (KAR-sih-NOH-mah)
		  carcin/o- *cancer*
		  -oma *mass; tumor*

cleft lip and palate	Congenital deformity in which the skin of the lip or the bones of the right and left maxilla fail to join in the center before birth. The resulting cleft can affect the nose, lip, teeth and gums, and hard and soft palate, and the cleft can be **unilateral** or **bilateral** (see Figure 15-15 ■). The child has difficulty speaking and eating.
	Treatment: Surgical correction
		cleft (KLEFT)
		
		unilateral (YOO-nih-LAT-eh-ral)
		  uni- *not paired; single*
		  later/o- *side*
		  -al *pertaining to*
		
		bilateral (by-LAT-eh-ral)
		  bi- *two*
		  later/o- *side*
		  -al *pertaining to*

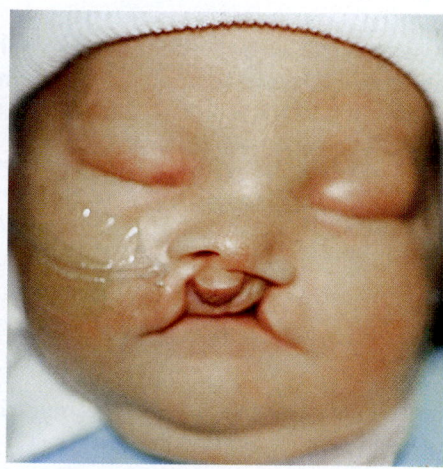

FIGURE 15-15 ■ Cleft lip and palate.
This infant has a bilateral cleft lip and palate. He has difficulty feeding from the breast or bottle because milk flows into the nasal cavity where it could be inhaled into the lungs. Note the feeding tube inserted in the right nostril and taped to the cheek; the tube goes to the stomach.

Clinical Connections

Surgery. A child with a cleft lip is born every 3 minutes somewhere in the world. These children may be shunned by their communities and even by their families. They often do not attend school because of being treated cruelly by the other children. Since its beginning 35 years ago, Operation Smile has provided free surgery to repair cleft lip to hundreds of thousands of children and adults around the world.

cold sores	Recurring, painful clusters of blisters on the skin of the lips or nose. They are caused by infection with **herpes simplex virus** type 1. After the initial infection, the virus remains dormant in a nerve until triggers of stress, sunlight, illness, or menstruation cause it to reappear. Also known as **fever blisters**. Treatment: Topical antiviral drug *Note:* Herpes simplex type 1 is different from herpes simplex type 2 (genital herpes), which is a sexually transmitted disease (described in Chapter 11, Male Reproductive Medicine).	**herpes simplex** (HER-peez SIM-pleks)

Word or Phrase	Description	Pronunciation/Word Parts
glossitis	Infection or inflammation of the tongue. It is caused by irritation from spicy or hot food, a food allergy, an infection, or vitamin B deficiency. Treatment: Correct the underlying cause.	**glossitis** (glaw-SY-tihs) **gloss/o-** *tongue* **-itis** *infection of; inflammation of*
leukoplakia	Thickened, irregular white patches on the tongue and mucous membrane of the oral cavity (see Figure 15-16 ■). If it is caused by chronic irritation from tobacco use, it can become cancerous. It can also be caused by irritation from an infection with the Epstein-Barr virus, an opportunistic infection seen in patients with AIDS. Treatment: Correct the underlying cause.	**leukoplakia** (LOO-koh-PLAY-kee-ah) **leuk/o-** *white* **plak/o-** *plaque* **-ia** *condition; state; thing*

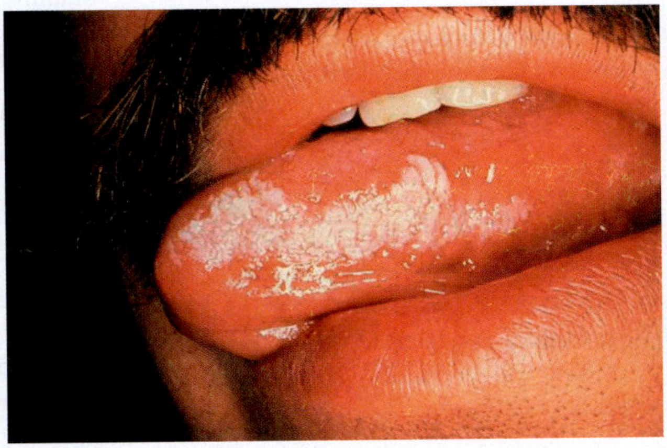

FIGURE 15-16 ■ Leukoplakia.
This white patch of leukoplakia on the tongue is in the mouth of a patient with AIDS. This is under the tongue, but leukoplakia can occur anywhere in the mouth.

Word or Phrase	Description	Pronunciation/Word Parts
pharyngitis	Bacterial or viral infection of the throat. When it is caused by the bacterium group A beta-hemolytic **streptococcus**, it is known as **strep throat**. It is important to diagnose strep throat and treat it with an antibiotic drug so that it does not cause the complication of rheumatic heart disease. Treatment: Antibiotic drug for a bacterial infection. A viral infection cannot be treated with an antibiotic drug.	**pharyngitis** (FAIR-in-JY-tihs) **pharyng/o-** *pharynx; throat* **-itis** *infection of; inflammation of* **streptococcus** (STREP-toh-KAW-kuhs) **strept/o-** *curved* **-coccus** *spherical bacterium* Streptococcus is a bacterium with the shape of spheres in a long, curved chain.
temporomandibular joint (TMJ) syndrome	Dysfunction of the movement of the temporomandibular joint. There is clicking of the joint, pain, muscle spasm, and difficulty opening the jaw. It is caused by clenching or grinding the teeth (often during sleep) or by misalignment of the teeth. Treatment: Dental bite guard worn at night; correction of misaligned teeth	**temporomandibular** (TEM-poh-ROH-man-DIH-byoo-lar) **tempor/o-** *side of the head; temple* **mandibul/o-** *lower jaw; mandible* **-ar** *pertaining to*

Word or Phrase	Description	Pronunciation/Word Parts
thrush	Oral infection caused by the yeast *Candida albicans*. It coats the tongue and mucosa of the oral cavity (see Figure 15-17 ■). Thrush is common in infants but is also seen in immunocompromised patients and patients with AIDS because their immune system cannot control its growth. It can also occur after an antibiotic drug kills bacteria in the mouth, allowing overgrowth of *Candida albicans*. Also known as **oral candidiasis**. Treatment: Oral antiyeast drug	**candidiasis** (KAN-dih-DY-ah-sihs) **candid/o-** *Candida; yeast* **-iasis** *process; state*

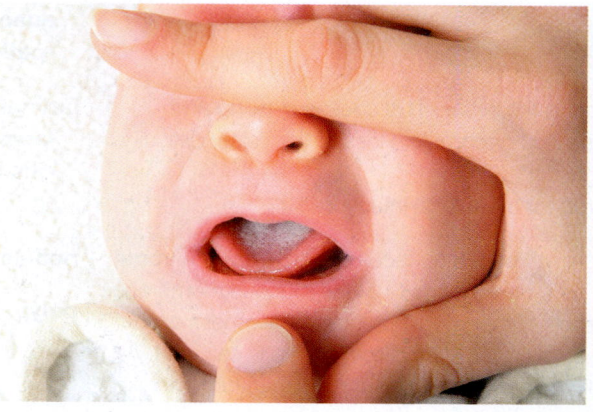

FIGURE 15-17 ■ Thrush.
The warm, moist environment of the mouth encourages the growth of this yeast-like fungus. It forms a thick white coating that resembles milk but cannot be wiped off.

tonsillitis	Acute or chronic viral or bacterial infection of the pharynx and palatine tonsils (see Figure 15-18 ■). There is a sore throat and difficulty swallowing, with mouth breathing and snoring. The tonsils hypertrophy (enlarge) and contain pus and debris. The adenoids may also hypertrophy and block the eustachian tubes. Treatment: Antibiotic drug for a bacterial infection; tonsillectomy	**tonsillitis** (TAWN-sil-EYE-tihs) **tonsill/o-** *tonsil* **-itis** *infection of; inflammation of*

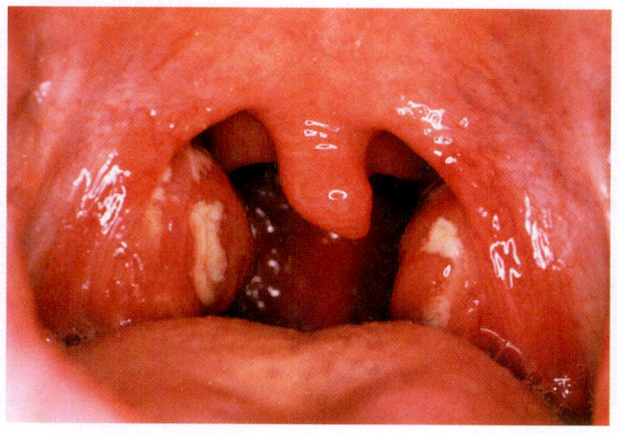

FIGURE 15-18 ■ Tonsillitis.
This patient has acute inflammation, infection, and hypertrophy of the palatine tonsils. There are also some areas of white pus, which indicate a bacterial infection. The uvula and posterior oropharynx are also inflamed.

Word Alert
Medical Word Spelling

tonsil	the lymphoid tissue in the throat	spelled with one *l*
tonsillitis	an inflammation or infection of the tonsils	spelled with two *l*'s
tonsillectomy	surgical removal of the tonsils	spelled with two *l*'s

Word or Phrase	Description	Pronunciation/Word Parts

Larynx and Neck

Word or Phrase	Description	Pronunciation/Word Parts
cervical lymphadenopathy	Enlargement of the lymph nodes in the neck. It is caused by infection, cancer, or the spread of a cancerous tumor from another site. Treatment: Correct the underlying cause.	**cervical** (SER-vih-kal) **cervic/o-** *cervix; neck* **-al** *pertaining to* **lymphadenopathy** (lim-FAD-eh-NAW-pah-thee) **lymph/o-** *lymph; lymphatic system* **aden/o-** *gland* **-pathy** *disease*
laryngitis	Bacterial or viral infection in the larynx. This causes swelling and inflammation with hoarseness or complete loss of the voice, difficulty swallowing, and a cough. Treatment: Antibiotic drug for a bacterial infection	**laryngitis** (LAIR-in-JY-tihs) **laryng/o-** *larynx; voice box* **-itis** *infection of; inflammation of*
vocal cord nodule	Small, benign, fibrous growth on the surface of a vocal cord. A **vocal cord polyp** is a larger, soft, benign growth of the mucous membranes that contains blood vessels. Either growth causes hoarseness and a change in the quality of the voice. A nodule or polyp is caused by strain from constant talking or singing or by chronic irritation from smoking or allergies. Treatment: Voice rest; surgical removal	**nodule** (NAW-dyool) **polyp** (PAW-lip)

15.3 PRACTICE LAPS

Use the Answer Key at the end of the book to check your answers.

A. Give the Meaning of Combining Forms

Next to each combining form, write its meaning. The first one has been done for you.

Combining Form	Meaning	Combining Form	Meaning
1. **acous/o-**	*hearing; sound*	11. hem/o-	
2. aden/o-		12. impact/o-	
3. alg/o-		13. labyrinth/o-	
4. allerg/o-		14. laryng/o-	
5. candid/o-		15. later/o-	
6. carcin/o-		16. leuk/o-	
7. cervic/o-		17. lymph/o-	
8. conduct/o-		18. malign/o-	
9. effus/o-		19. mandibul/o-	
10. gloss/o-		20. mastoid/o-	

Combining Form	Meaning	Combining Form	Meaning
21. myring/o-	_____	30. rhin/o-	_____
22. nas/o-	_____	31. scler/o-	_____
23. neur/o-	_____	32. sensor/i-	_____
24. osm/o-	_____	33. ser/o-	_____
25. ot/o-	_____	34. sinus/o-	_____
26. pharyng/o-	_____	35. strept/o-	_____
27. plak/o-	_____	36. suppur/o-	_____
28. presby/o-	_____	37. tempor/o-	_____
29. purul/o-	_____	38. tonsill/o-	_____

B. Build Words

Read the definition of the medical word. Look at the combining form that is given. Select the correct suffix from the Suffix List, and write it on the blank line. Then build the medical word, and write it on the line. (Remember: You may need to remove the combining vowel. Always remove the hyphens and slash.) Be sure to check your spelling.

Suffix List

-acusis (abnormal condition of hearing)
-al (pertaining to)
-ant (pertaining to)
-ative (pertaining to)

-coccus (spherical bacterium)
-ent (pertaining to)
-iasis (process; state)
-ic (pertaining to)
-ion (action; condition)

-itis (infection of; inflammation of)
-oma (mass; tumor)
-phyma (growth; tumor)
-rrhea (discharge; flow)
-tic (pertaining to)

Definition of the Medical Word	Combining Form	Suffix	Build the Medical Word
Example: Spherical bacterium (that is in a chain that is) curved	**strept/o-**	_-coccus_	_streptococcus_

[_You think_ spherical bacterium (-coccus) + curved (strept/o-). You change the order of the word parts to put the suffix last. You write streptococcus.]

1. Infection of (or) inflammation of (the) voice box	laryng/o-	_____	_____
2. Pertaining to cancer	malign/o-	_____	_____
3. Infection of (or) inflammation of (the) labyrinth	labyrinth/o-	_____	_____
4. Condition (of cerumen being) wedged in (the ear)	impact/o-	_____	_____
5. Infection of (or) inflammation of (the) tongue	gloss/o-	_____	_____
6. Mass (or) tumor (on a) nerve	neur/o-	_____	_____
7. Tumor (of the) nose	rhin/o-	_____	_____
8. Infection of (or) inflammation of (the) sinus	sinus/o-	_____	_____
9. Pertaining to pus formation	suppur/o-	_____	_____

continued on next page

Definition of the Medical Word	Combining Form	Suffix	Build the Medical Word
10. Infection of (or) inflammation of (the) tonsil	tonsill/o-	_____	_____
11. Discharge (or) flow (from the) nose	rhin/o-	_____	_____
12. Infection of (or) inflammation of (the) throat	pharyng/o-	_____	_____
13. Abnormal condition of hearing (in) old age	presby/o-	_____	_____
14. Discharge (or) flow (from the) ear	ot/o-	_____	_____
15. Pertaining to (an) allergy	allerg/o-	_____	_____
16. State of (a) yeast (infection)	candid/o-	_____	_____
17. Pertaining to hearing (or) sound	acous/o-	_____	_____
18. Pertaining to (the) neck	cervic/o-	_____	_____
19. Tumor (that is a) cancer	carcin/o-	_____	_____
20. Infection of (or) inflammation of (the) eardrum	myring/o-	_____	_____
21. Infection of (or) inflammation of (the) ear	ot/o-	_____	_____
22. Pertaining to pus	purul/o-	_____	_____

C. Define Abbreviations

1. PND _____

2. TMJ _____

3. URI _____

15.4 Laboratory, Diagnostic, and Radiologic Procedures

Word or Phrase	Description	Pronunciation/Word Parts

Hearing Tests

audiometry	Test that measures hearing acuity and documents hearing loss (see Figure 15-19 ■). The patient puts on headphones that are connected to an **audiometer**, which produces a series of pure tones, each at a different frequency (high or low pitch) and varying in intensity (loud or soft). The frequency is measured in **hertz (Hz)**. The intensity is measured in **decibels (dB)**. The patient presses a button to signal when the pure tone is heard. The result, displayed on a graph on the computer, is an **audiogram**. In **speech audiometry**, the patient hears spoken words and sentences. If he or she can repeat 50% of the words correctly, then this is the threshold of hearing ability for speech sounds. Both pure tone audiometry and speech audiometry are used to determine whether a patient needs a hearing aid.	**audiometry** (AW-dee-AW-meh-tree) **audi/o-** *hearing* **-metry** *process of measuring* **audiometer** (AW-dee-AW-meh-ter) **audi/o-** *hearing* **-meter** *instrument used to measure* **audiogram** (AW-dee-oh-GRAM) **audi/o-** *hearing* **-gram** *picture; record*

Word or Phrase	Description	Pronunciation/Word Parts

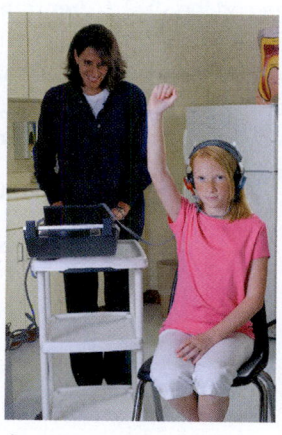
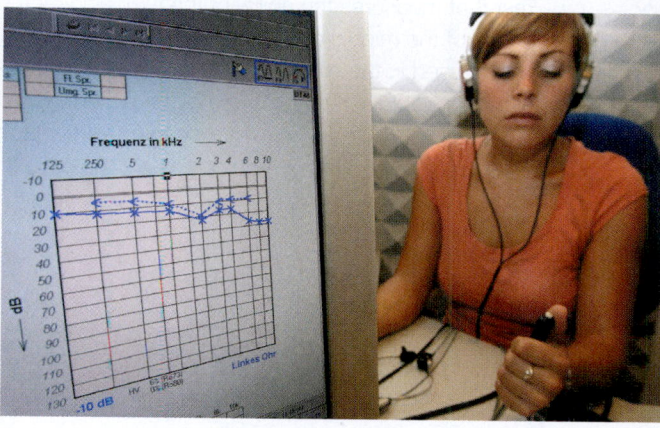

A.   B.

FIGURE 15-19 ■ Audiometry.
A. School hearing screening tests are usually done for students every other year, beginning in kindergarten. The school nurse, a speech-language pathologist, or an audiologist performs the test, using an audiometer. The hearing in each ear is tested with pure tone sounds at high and low frequencies, and the student raises his or her hand to indicate that the tone was heard. If any abnormality is noted, the child is sent for a comprehensive hearing evaluation.

B. This patient is undergoing audiometry. The test is performed in a soundproof booth, and headphones cover both ears to keep out outside noises. The hearing in each ear is tested separately, and the patient presses a button when she hears a sound. The audiogram results are displayed on a computer screen.

Word or Phrase	Description	Pronunciation/Word Parts
brainstem auditory evoked response (BAER)	Test that analyzes the brain's response to sounds. The patient listens as an audiometer produces a series of clicks. Electroencephalography (EEG) that records the brain waves is performed at the same time. A lesion or tumor in the auditory cortex of the brain or on the vestibulocochlear nerve will produce an abnormal EEG. Also known as an **auditory brainstem response (ABR)**.	
Rinne and Weber hearing tests	The Rinne tuning fork test evaluates bone conduction versus air conduction of sound in one ear at a time (see Figure 15-20 ■). A vibrating tuning fork is placed against the mastoid process behind one ear to test the bone conduction of sound. Then it is placed next to (but not touching) the helix of the same ear. If the sound is louder when the tuning fork is next to the ear, this is normal (because air conduction is normally greater than bone conduction); the test is said to be positive. If the sound is louder when the tuning fork touches the mastoid process, then the patient has a conductive hearing loss. A tuning fork of 256 Hz is used to test the hearing. This frequency corresponds to middle C on the piano. The Weber tuning fork test evaluates bone conduction of sound in both ears at the same time. The vibrating tuning fork is placed against the center of the forehead or on top of the head. In a normal test, the sound is heard equally in both ears.	**Rinne** (RIN-eh) **Weber** (VAY-ber)

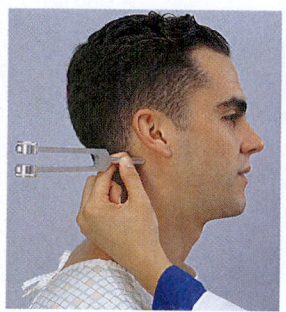
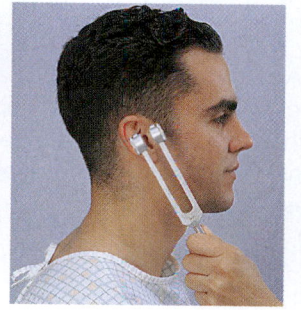

FIGURE 15-20 ■ Rinne test.
This hearing test uses a vibrating tuning fork to compare bone conduction of sound to air conduction of sound in the same ear.

Word or Phrase	Description	Pronunciation/Word Parts
tympanometry	Test that measures the ability of the tympanic membrane and the bones of the middle ear to move. Air pressure (rather than sound vibration) is used in the external auditory canal. If infection or disease has made the middle ear bones immovable, then the tympanic membrane will move very little. This resistance to movement is called **impedance**. The result, printed as a graph on the computer, is a **tympanogram**.	**tympanometry** (TIM-pah-NAW-meh-tree) **tympan/o-** *eardrum; tympanic membrane* **-metry** *process of measuring* **impedance** (im-PEE-dans) **tympanogram** (tim-PAN-oh-gram) **tympan/o-** *eardrum; tympanic membrane* **-gram** *picture; record*

Clinical Connections

Biology. Humans can hear sounds with a frequency as low as 20 Hz or as high as 20,000 Hz. In contrast, a dog can hear from 20 Hz to 45,000 Hz, and a porpoise can hear from 75 Hz to 150,000 Hz.

Laboratory and Radiologic Tests

culture and sensitivity (C&S)	Laboratory test to identify which bacterium is causing an ENT infection. A specimen of mucus or pus from the patient's nose, external ear, adenoids, tonsils, or throat (see Figure 15-21 ▪) is placed in a culture dish with disks of antibiotic drugs to see which drug the bacterium is sensitive to; this will be the antibiotic drug that is prescribed.	**culture** (KUL-chur) **sensitivity** (SEN-sih-TIV-ih-tee) **sensitiv/o-** *affected by; sensitive to* **-ity** *condition; state*

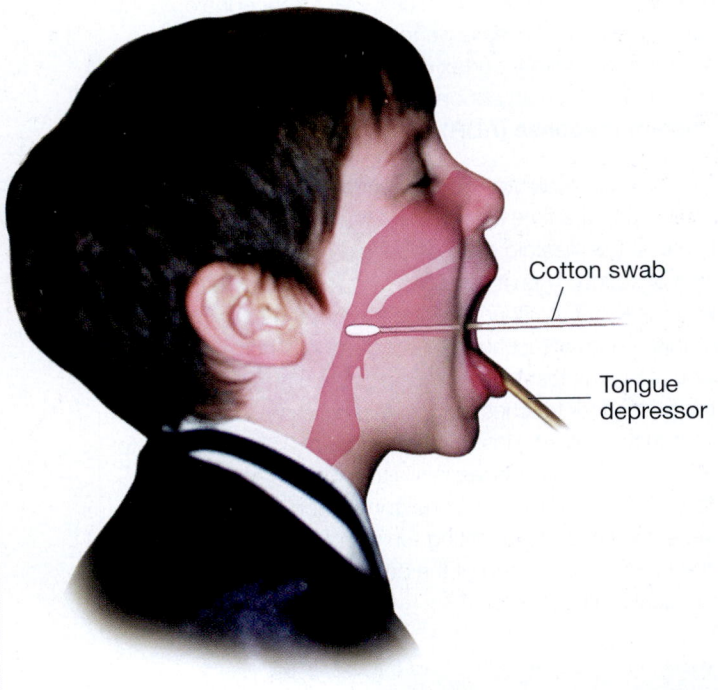

Cotton swab

Tongue depressor

FIGURE 15-21 ▪ Throat swab.
This child is having a swab taken of the oropharynx. The material on the swab will be sent to a laboratory for a culture and sensitivity test.

rapid strep test	Test kit for strep throat. A swab of mucus from the patient's throat is mixed with a solution of antibodies to group A streptococcus. A dipstick is immersed in the solution to give the test result. Unlike a standard culture and sensitivity test, the result of a rapid strep test is available in a few minutes so that the physician can immediately prescribe an antibiotic drug, if needed.	

Word or Phrase	Description	Pronunciation/Word Parts
RAST	Blood test that measures the amount of IgE produced when the blood is mixed with a specific antigen. It shows which of many substances the patient is allergic to and how severe the allergy is. RAST stands for *radioallergosorbent test*.	
sinus series	X-rays are taken from various angles to show all of the sinuses and confirm or rule out a diagnosis of sinusitis. Sinusitis shows as cloudy, opacified sinuses or thickened mucous membranes. Sometimes an air-fluid level can be seen within the sinus. If needed, a CT scan is done to show additional detail (see Figure 15-14).	

15.4 PRACTICE LAPS

Use the Answer Key at the end of the book to check your answers.

A. Give the Meaning of Combining Forms

Next to each combining form, write its meaning. The first one has been done for you.

Combining Form	Meaning
1. **audi/o-**	*hearing*
2. sensitiv/o-	
3. tympan/o-	

B. Build Words

Read the definition of the medical word. Look at the combining form that is given. Select the correct suffix from the Suffix List, and write it on the blank line. Then build the medical word, and write it on the line. (Remember: You may need to remove the combining vowel. Always remove the hyphens and slash.) Be sure to check your spelling.

Suffix List

-gram (picture; record) -meter (instrument used to measure)
-ity (condition; state) -metry (process of measuring)

Definition of the Medical Word	Combining Form	Suffix	Build the Medical Word
Example: Record (of the) tympanic membrane	**tympan/o-**	*-gram*	*tympanogram*

[*You think record (-gram) + tympanic membrane (tympan/o-). You change the order of the word parts to put the suffix last. You write tympanogram.*]

Definition of the Medical Word	Combining Form	Suffix	Build the Medical Word
1. Process of measuring (the) hearing	audi/o-		
2. Instrument used to measure (the) hearing	audi/o-		
3. State (of a bacterium being) sensitive to (an antibiotic drug)	sensitiv/o-		
4. Process of measuring (the) tympanic membrane	tympan/o-		
5. Record (of) hearing	audi/o-		

C. Define Abbreviations

1. ABR _____

2. BAER _____

15.5 Medical Procedures, Drugs, and Surgical Procedures

Word or Phrase	Description	Pronunciation/Word Parts

Medical Procedures

nose, sinus, mouth, and throat examinations	Procedures in which a nasal **speculum** is used to widen the nostril, while a penlight lights the nasal cavity. The frontal and maxillary sinuses are examined for tenderness by pressing with the fingertips on the forehead and cheekbones. A tongue depressor, penlight, and a laryngeal mirror are used to examine the oral cavity, pharynx, and larynx (see Figure 15-22 ■).	**speculum** (SPEH-kyoo-lum)

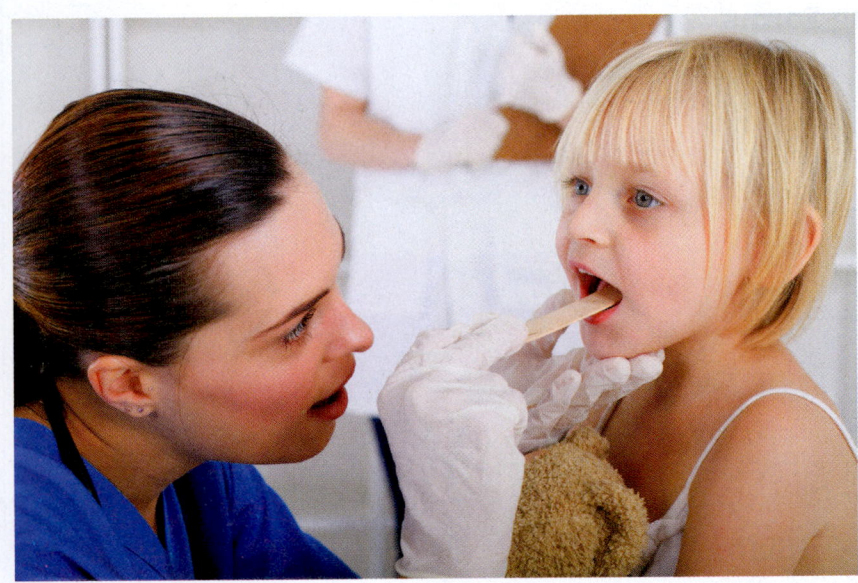

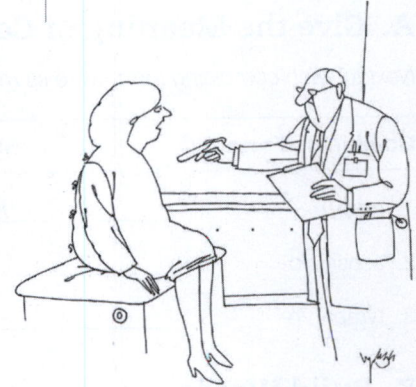

That's all you want me to say . . . Ah?

FIGURE 15-22 ■ Throat examination.
This pediatrician is examining this little girl's oropharynx by using a tongue depressor and having the child say "Ah."

otoscopy	Procedure to examine the external auditory canal and tympanic membrane (see Figure 15-23 ■). An **otoscope** provides light and magnification.	**otoscopy** (oh-TAW-skoh-pee) **ot/o-** *ear* **-scopy** *process of using an instrument to examine* **otoscope** (OH-toh-skohp) **ot/o-** *ear* **-scope** *instrument used to examine*

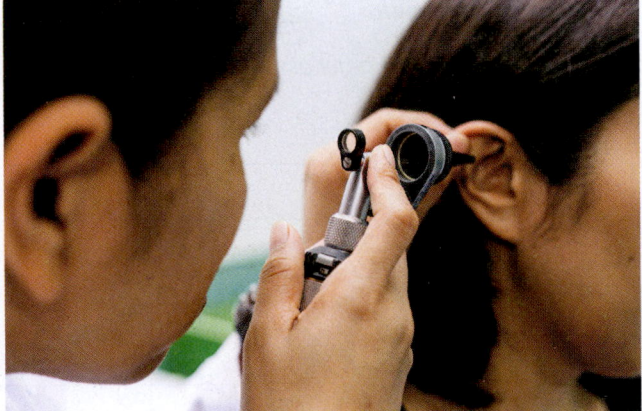

FIGURE 15-23 ■ Otoscopy.
The physician is using an otoscope to examine this patient's right external auditory canal and tympanic membrane. Before each use, a disposable black plastic tip (speculum) is placed over the part of the otoscope that enters the ear. For patients from 3 years old to adult, the physician gently pulls the helix backward and upward to straighten the external auditory canal and visualize the tympanic membrane. In infants younger than age 3, the helix is pulled backward and horizontally to straighten the external auditory canal.

Word or Phrase	Description	Pronunciation/Word Parts
Romberg sign	Procedure to assess balance. The patient stands with the feet together and the eyes closed. Swaying or falling to one side indicates a loss of balance and a possible inner ear disorder.	**Romberg** (RAWM-berg)

Category	Indication	Pronunciation/Word Parts

Drugs

antibiotic drug	Treats bacterial infections of the ears, nose, sinuses, or throat. *Note:* Antibiotic drugs are not effective against viral infections.	**antibiotic** (AN-tee-by-AW-tik) **anti-** *against* **bi/o-** *living organism; living tissue* **-tic** *pertaining to*
antihistamine drug	Blocks the effect of histamine released during an allergic reaction. Histamine causes symptoms of runny, itchy nose and nasal congestion.	**antihistamine** (AN-tee-HIS-tah-meen)
antitussive drug	Suppresses the cough center in the brain. Some of these drugs contain a narcotic drug.	**antitussive** (AN-tee-TUH-siv) **anti-** *against* **tuss/o-** *cough* **-ive** *pertaining to*
antiyeast drug	Treats yeast infections (oral candidiasis, thrush) of the mouth caused by *Candida albicans*. Solution is swished around the oral cavity and then swallowed.	**antiyeast** (AN-tee-YEEST)
corticosteroid drug	Treats severe inflammation of the ears, nose, or mouth. Topical ear drops, nasal spray, or an oral drug that works throughout the body.	**corticosteroid** (KOR-tih-koh-STAIR-oyd) **cortic/o-** *cortex; outer region* **-steroid** *steroid*
decongestant drug	Constricts blood vessels and decreases swelling of the mucous membranes of the nose and sinuses caused by colds and allergies. Topical nasal spray or oral drug.	**decongestant** (DEE-con-JES-tant) **de-** *reversal of; without* **congest/o-** *accumulation of fluid* **-ant** *pertaining to*
drug used to treat motion sickness	Decreases the sensitivity of the inner ear to motion and keeps nerve impulses from the inner ear from reaching the vomiting center in the brain	

Clinical Connections

Pharmacology. Aminoglycoside antibiotic drugs are known to damage the cochlea of the inner ear. This adverse drug effect is known as **ototoxicity**. Patients taking aminoglycoside drugs need to have audiometry done periodically to monitor their hearing.

A number of drugs are given by the **sublingual** route. The tablet is placed under the tongue and allowed to dissolve, and then the liquid drug is swallowed.

ototoxicity (OH-toh-tawk-SIS-ih-tee)
ot/o- *ear*
toxic/o- *poison*
-ity *condition; state*

sublingual (sub-LING-gwal)
sub- *below; underneath; less than*
lingu/o- *tongue*
-al *pertaining to*

Word or Phrase	Description	Pronunciation/Word Parts

Surgical Procedures

cheiloplasty	Procedure to repair the lip, usually because of a laceration. A cheiloplasty can be part of a larger surgical procedure to repair a cleft lip and palate (see Figure 15-24 ■).	**cheiloplasty** (KY-loh-PLAS-tee) **cheil/o-** *lip* **-plasty** *process of reshaping by surgery*

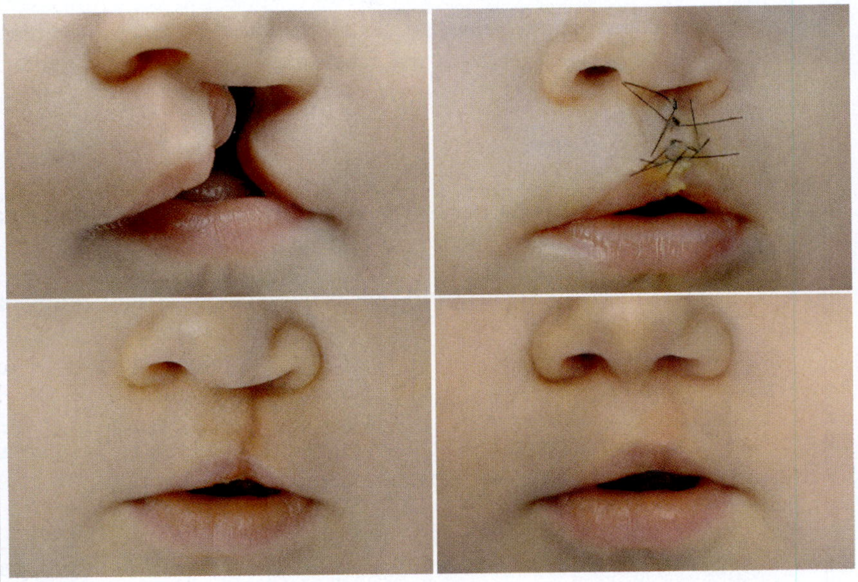

FIGURE 15-24 ■ Cleft lip repair.
This child had a cleft lip and cleft palate. A pediatric head and neck surgeon corrected the cleft palate and sutured the lip. Later, the sutures were removed. The final result is cosmetically pleasing.

cochlear implant	Procedure to insert a small, battery-powered implant beneath the skin behind the ear. Wires from the implant are placed through the round window and into the cochlea of the inner ear. When the implant "hears" a sound, it sends an electrical impulse to stimulate the cochlear portion of the vestibulocochlear nerve.	
endoscopic sinus surgery	Procedure that uses an **endoscope** (a flexible, fiberoptic scope with a magnifying lens and a light source) that is inserted through the nostril to examine the sinuses. **Endoscopy** is used to remove a polyp, treat sinusitis, or perform a biopsy.	**endoscopic** (EN-doh-SKAW-pik) **end/o-** *innermost; within* **scop/o-** *examine with an instrument* **-ic** *pertaining to* **endoscope** (EN-doh-skohp) **end/o-** *innermost; within* **-scope** *instrument used to examine* **endoscopy** (en-DAW-skoh-pee) **end/o-** *innermost; within* **-scopy** *process of using an instrument to examine*
mastoidectomy	Procedure to remove part of the mastoid process of the temporal bone because of infection	**mastoidectomy** (MAS-toyd-EK-toh-mee) **mastoid/o-** *mastoid process* **-ectomy** *surgical removal*

Word or Phrase	Description	Pronunciation/Word Parts
myringotomy	Procedure that uses a **myringotome** to make an incision in the tympanic membrane to drain fluid from the middle ear. For a chronic middle ear infection, a **pressure-equalizing (PE) tube** can be inserted through the incision to form a permanent opening into the middle ear (see Figure 15-25 ■). This procedure is a **tympanostomy**. 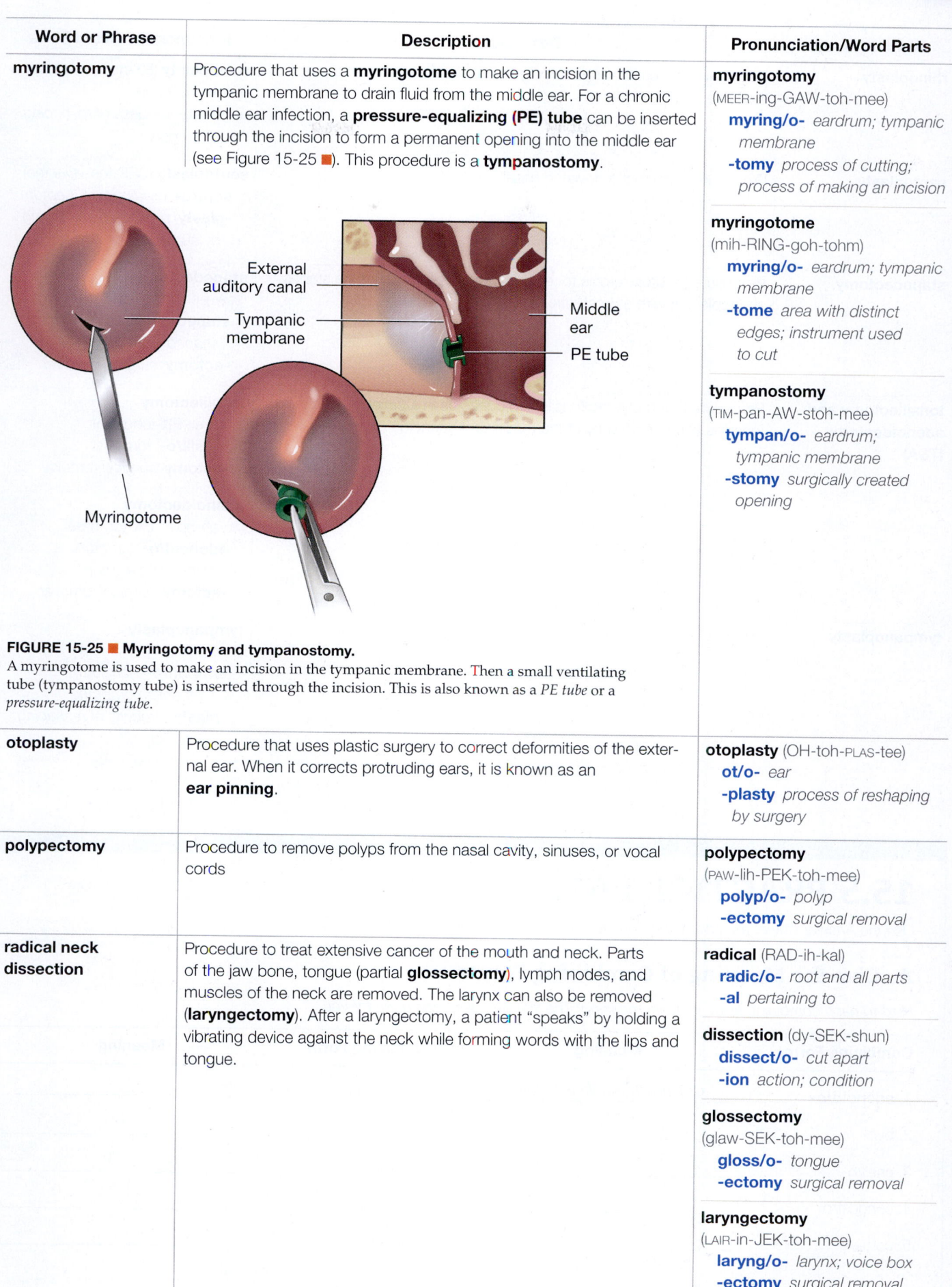 **FIGURE 15-25 ■ Myringotomy and tympanostomy.** A myringotome is used to make an incision in the tympanic membrane. Then a small ventilating tube (tympanostomy tube) is inserted through the incision. This is also known as a *PE tube* or a *pressure-equalizing tube*.	**myringotomy** (MEER-ing-GAW-toh-mee) **myring/o-** *eardrum; tympanic membrane* **-tomy** *process of cutting; process of making an incision* **myringotome** (mih-RING-goh-tohm) **myring/o-** *eardrum; tympanic membrane* **-tome** *area with distinct edges; instrument used to cut* **tympanostomy** (TIM-pan-AW-stoh-mee) **tympan/o-** *eardrum; tympanic membrane* **-stomy** *surgically created opening*
otoplasty	Procedure that uses plastic surgery to correct deformities of the external ear. When it corrects protruding ears, it is known as an **ear pinning**.	**otoplasty** (OH-toh-PLAS-tee) **ot/o-** *ear* **-plasty** *process of reshaping by surgery*
polypectomy	Procedure to remove polyps from the nasal cavity, sinuses, or vocal cords	**polypectomy** (PAW-lih-PEK-toh-mee) **polyp/o-** *polyp* **-ectomy** *surgical removal*
radical neck dissection	Procedure to treat extensive cancer of the mouth and neck. Parts of the jaw bone, tongue (partial **glossectomy**), lymph nodes, and muscles of the neck are removed. The larynx can also be removed (**laryngectomy**). After a laryngectomy, a patient "speaks" by holding a vibrating device against the neck while forming words with the lips and tongue.	**radical** (RAD-ih-kal) **radic/o-** *root and all parts* **-al** *pertaining to* **dissection** (dy-SEK-shun) **dissect/o-** *cut apart* **-ion** *action; condition* **glossectomy** (glaw-SEK-toh-mee) **gloss/o-** *tongue* **-ectomy** *surgical removal* **laryngectomy** (LAIR-in-JEK-toh-mee) **laryng/o-** *larynx; voice box* **-ectomy** *surgical removal*

Word or Phrase	Description	Pronunciation/Word Parts
rhinoplasty	Procedure that uses plastic surgery to change the size or shape of the nose	**rhinoplasty** (RY-noh-PLAS-tee) **rhin/o-** *nose* **-plasty** *process of reshaping by surgery*
septoplasty	Procedure to correct a deviated nasal septum	**septoplasty** (SEP-toh-PLAS-tee) **sept/o-** *dividing wall; septum* **-plasty** *process of reshaping by surgery*
stapedectomy	Procedure for otosclerosis to remove the diseased part of the stapes and replace it with a prosthetic device	**stapedectomy** (STAY-peh-DEK-toh-mee) **staped/o-** *stapes; stirrup-shaped bone* **-ectomy** *surgical removal*
tonsillectomy and adenoidectomy (T&A)	Procedure to remove the tonsils and adenoids in a patient with chronic tonsillitis and hypertrophy of the tonsils and adenoids	**tonsillectomy** (TAWN-sil-EK-toh-mee) **tonsill/o-** *tonsil* **-ectomy** *surgical removal* **adenoidectomy** (AD-eh-noyd-EK-toh-mee) **adenoid/o-** *structure resembling a gland* **-ectomy** *surgical removal*
tympanoplasty	Procedure to reconstruct a ruptured tympanic membrane	**tympanoplasty** (TIM-pah-noh-PLAS-tee) **tympan/o-** *eardrum; tympanic membrane* **-plasty** *process of reshaping by surgery*

15.5 PRACTICE LAPS

Use the Answer Key at the end of the book to check your answers.

A. Give the Meaning of Combining Forms

Next to each combining form, write its meaning. The first one has been done for you.

Combining Form	Meaning	Combining Form	Meaning
1. **adenoid/o-**	*structure resembling a gland*	6. dissect/o-	
2. bi/o-		7. end/o-	
3. cheil/o-		8. gloss/o-	
4. congest/o-		9. laryng/o-	
5. cortic/o-		10. lingu/o-	

Combining Form	Meaning	Combining Form	Meaning
11. mastoid/o-		18. sept/o-	
12. myring/o-		19. staped/o-	
13. ot/o-		20. toxic/o-	
14. polyp/o-		21. tuss/o-	
15. radic/o-		22. tonsill/o-	
16. rhin/o-		23. tympan/o-	
17. scop/o-			

B. Build Words

Read the definition of the medical word. Look at the combining form that is given. Select the correct suffix from the Suffix List, and write it on the blank line. Then build the medical word, and write it on the line. (Remember: You may need to remove the combining vowel. Always remove the hyphens and slash.) Be sure to check your spelling.

Suffix List

-ectomy (surgical removal)
-ion (action; condition)
-plasty (process of reshaping by surgery)
-scope (instrument used to examine)

-scopy (process of using an instrument to examine)
-stomy (surgically created opening)
-tome (area with distinct edges; instrument used to cut)
-tomy (process of cutting; process of making an incision)

Definition of the Medical Word	Combining Form	Suffix	Build the Medical Word
Example: Process of reshaping by surgery (on the) ear	**ot/o-**	*-plasty*	*otoplasty*

[You think process of reshaping by surgery (-plasty) + ear (ot/o-). You change the order of the word parts to put the suffix last. You write otoplasty.]

1. Process of making an incision (in the) eardrum	myring/o-		
2. Surgical removal (of a) stirrup-shaped bone	staped/o-		
3. Surgically created opening (in the) eardrum	tympan/o-		
4. Process of reshaping by surgery (on the) nose	rhin/o-		
5. Process of using an instrument to examine (the) ear	ot/o-		
6. Surgical removal (of a) polyp	polyp/o-		
7. Instrument used to examine within	end/o-		
8. Process of reshaping by surgery (on the) lip	cheil/o-		
9. Action (to) cut apart	dissect/o-		
10. Surgical removal (of the) tongue	gloss/o-		
11. Surgical removal (of the) tonsils	tonsill/o-		
12. Process of reshaping by surgery (on the) septum	sept/o-		
13. Instrument used to examine (the) ear	ot/o-		
14. Instrument used to cut (the) eardrum	myring/o-		

Abbreviations Summary

ABR	auditory brainstem response		**HEENT**	head, eyes, ears, nose, and throat
AD, A.D.	right ear (Latin, *auris dextra*)		**Hz**	hertz
AS, A.S.	left ear (Latin, *auris sinister*)		**PE**	pressure-equalizing (tube)
AU, A.U.	both ears (Latin, *aures unitas*); each ear (Latin, *auris uterque*)		**PND**	postnasal drip
			RAST	radioallergosorbent test
BAER	brainstem auditory evoked response		**T&A**	tonsillectomy and adenoidectomy
C&S	culture and sensitivity		**TM**	tympanic membrane
Db	decibel		**TMJ**	temporomandibular joint
EAC	external auditory canal		**URI**	upper respiratory infection
ENT	ears, nose, and throat			

According to the Institute for Safe Medication Practices (ISMP), these abbreviations for right ear (AD, A.D.), left ear (AS, A.S.), and both ears or each ear (AU, A.U.) can be misinterpreted, causing medication errors, and should not be used. However, because they are still used by some healthcare professionals, they are included in the Abbreviations Summary.

Word Alert

Abbreviations. Abbreviations are commonly used in all types of medical documents; however, they can mean different things to different people and their meanings can be misinterpreted. Always verify the meaning of an abbreviation.

- *C&S* means *culture and sensitivity*, but the sound-alike abbreviation *CNS* means *central nervous system*.
- *PE* means *pressure-equalizing (tube)*, but it also means *physical examination* and *pulmonary embolus*.
- *PND* means *postnasal drainage* or *postnasal drip*, but it also means *paroxysmal nocturnal dyspnea*.
- *TM* means *tympanic membrane*, but *TMJ* means *temporomandibular joint*.

It's Greek to Me! Did you notice that some words have two different combining forms? Combining forms from both Greek and Latin remain a part of medical language today.

Word	Greek	Latin	Medical Word Examples
ear	ot/o-	aur/i-, auricul/o-	otic; auricle, auricular
eardrum	tympan/o-	myring/o-	tympanic membrane; myringotomy
hearing	acous/o-	audi/o-, audit/o-	acoustic; audiogram, auditory canal
lip	cheil/o-	labi/o-	cheiloplasty; nasolabial
nose	rhin/o-	nas/o-	rhinoplasty; nasal
sense of smell	osm/o-	olfact/o-	anosmia; olfactory
tongue	gloss/o-	lingu/o-	glossectomy; sublingual

Career Focus

Meet David, an audiologist

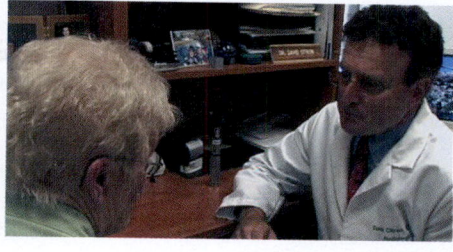

"Audiology is very exciting, not just because of all the changes in technology that have occurred, but also the fact that the profession is growing. One very large change is in the area of newborn hearing screening. Now we can screen babies right at birth. There are technologically advanced hearing aids. All of them are programmable by computer; we can individualize each person's hearing profile by programming the hearing aid to meet their specific needs. We tend to see a lot of people who have balance problems because one area of audiology deals with assessing and treating dizziness and vertigo. All audiologists need to have a doctoral degree and the reason for that is because of all the things we do—our scope of practice has grown so much."

- **Audiologists** are allied health professionals who perform hearing tests, diagnose hearing loss, and determine how patients can best use their remaining hearing. They also make and fit hearing aids. Audiologists work in schools, hospitals, physicians' offices, and their own private offices.
- **Otolaryngologists** or **otorhinolaryngologists** are physicians who practice in the medical specialty of otolaryngology. They diagnose and treat patients with diseases of the ears, nose, or throat. They are also known as ENT specialists. When otolaryngologists perform surgery, they are known as head and neck surgeons or **oral and maxillofacial surgeons**. Physicians can take additional training and become board certified in the subspecialties of pediatric otolaryngology, plastic surgery of the head and neck, or allergy and immunology. Malignancies of the ears, nose, and throat are treated medically by an **oncologist** or surgically by a head and neck surgeon or oral surgeon.

---

audiologist (AW-dee-AW-loh-jist)
  audi/o- *hearing*
  log/o- *study of; word*
  -ist *person who specializes in; thing that specializes in*

---

otolaryngologist
(OH-toh-LAIR-ing-GAW-loh-jist)
  ot/o- *ear*
  laryng/o- *larynx; voice box*
  log/o- *study of; word*
  -ist *person who specializes in; thing that specializes in*

---

otorhinolaryngologist
(OH-toh-RY-noh-LAIR-ing-GAW-loh-jist)
  ot/o- *ear*
  rhin/o- *nose*
  laryng/o- *larynx; voice box*
  log/o- *study of; word*
  -ist *person who specializes in; thing that specializes in*

---

maxillofacial (MAK-sih-loh-FAY-shal)
  maxill/o- *maxilla; upper jaw*
  faci/o- *face*
  -al *pertaining to*

---

surgeon (SER-jin)
  surg/o- *operative procedure*
  -eon *person who performs*

---

oncologist (ong-KAW-loh-jist)
  onc/o- *mass; tumor*
  log/o- *study of; word*
  -ist *person who specializes in; thing that specializes in*

Chapter Review Exercises

Dive In: Medical Language Exercises

Test your knowledge of the chapter by completing these review exercises. Use the Answer Key at the end of the book to check your answers. Note: Each of the numbered exercise headers corresponds to a numbered learning outcome at the beginning of the chapter.

15.1 Anatomy

MATCHING EXERCISE

Match each word or phrase to its location. Each location will have more than one matching word or phrase.

1. adenoids	_____ one of the sinuses
2. alae	_____ bone shaped like an anvil
3. cochlea	_____ spiral-shaped structure in the inner ear
4. ethmoid	_____ triangular cartilage by the external auditory meatus
5. helix	_____ outer C-shaped rim of ear tissue and cartilage
6. incus	_____ flared cartilage on the sides of the nostrils
7. malleus	_____ the chin
8. mentum	_____ first bone in the ossicular chain
9. naris	_____ fluid-filled structures in three different planes
10. nasal septum	_____ bone that fits into the oval window
11. nasopharynx	_____ divides the nasal cavity into right and left sides
12. ossicles	_____ entrance to the inner ear
13. semicircular canals	_____ slow down inhaled air
14. stapes	_____ two types are lingual and palatal
15. tonsils	_____ lymphoid tissue in the nasopharynx
16. tragus	_____ collective name for the bones of the middle ear
17. turbinates	_____ part of the throat that is posterior to the nose
18. vestibule	_____ external opening or nostril

CIRCLE EXERCISE

Circle the correct answer from the choices given.

1. The lingual tonsils are located in the (**laryngopharynx, nasopharynx, oropharynx**).
2. The visible external ear is called the (**adenoid, auricle, mastoid process**).
3. The middle ear is connected to the nasopharynx by the (**cochlea, eustachian tube, ossicles**).
4. The vertical groove in the skin of the upper lip is the (**buccal mucosa, nasolabial fold, philtrum**).

TRUE OR FALSE EXERCISE

*Indicate whether each statement is true or false by writing **T** or **F** on the line.*

1. _____ The semicircular canals help the body keep its balance.
2. _____ The eustachian tube connects the nasal cavity to the inner ear.
3. _____ The sinuses in the cheek on either side of the nose are the maxillary sinuses.
4. _____ The chin is also known as the *mentum*.
5. _____ The lingual tonsils are located on either side of the base of the tongue.
6. _____ The submental lymph nodes are located below the chin.
7. _____ The ossicular chain is located within the semicircular canals of the inner ear.

8. _____ The tympanic membrane divides the external auditory canal from the middle ear.

9. _____ Buccal means *pertaining to the cheek.*

10. _____ The epiglottis is located in the external ear.

PLURAL NOUN AND ADJECTIVE EXERCISE

Read the noun and write its plural form and/or adjective form on the line. Only write in the plural noun form if there is a blank line there for it. Be sure to check your spelling. The first one has been done for you.

Singular Noun	Plural Noun	Adjective	Singular Noun	Plural Noun	Adjective
1. **incus**	*incudes*	*incudal*	8. nose		_____
2. auricle		_____	9. ossicle	_____	_____
3. cochlea	_____	_____	10. pharynx		_____
4. larynx		_____	11. septum	_____	_____
5. malleus	_____	_____	12. stapes	_____	_____
6. meatus	_____		13. tonsil	_____	_____
7. naris	_____		14. vestibule		_____

DIVIDING WORDS EXERCISE

Separate these words into their component parts (prefix, combining form, suffix). Some words do not contain all three word parts. The first one has been done for you.

Medical Word	Prefix	Combining Form	Suffix	Medical Word	Prefix	Combining Form	Suffix
1. **mastoid**		*mast/o-*	*-oid*	7. nasopharynx		_____	_____
2. auditory		_____	_____	8. paranasal	_____	_____	_____
3. auricle		_____	_____	9. semicircular	_____	_____	_____
4. buccal		_____	_____	10. septal		_____	_____
5. epiglottic	_____	_____	_____	11. submental		_____	_____
6. maxillary		_____	_____	12. tympanic		_____	_____

SPELLING EXERCISE

Read each medical word pronunciation and write the medical word that it represents. Be sure to check your spelling. The first one has been done for you.

1. (MAS-toyd)   *mastoid*

2. (aw-RIH-kyoo-lar)   _____

3. (tim-PAN-ik)   _____

4. (yoo-STAY-shun)   _____

5. (TER-bih-nayt)   _____

6. (SFEE-noyd)   _____

7. (OR-oh-FAIR-ingks)   _____

RELATED COMBINING FORMS EXERCISE

Write the combining forms on the lines provided. (Hint: See the It's Greek to Me! feature box.)

1. Two combining forms that mean *eardrum.*   _____ _____

2. Two combining forms that mean *lip.*   _____ _____

3. Two combining forms that mean *nose.*   _____ _____

4. Two combining forms that mean *tongue.*   _____ _____

5. Three combining forms that mean *ear.*   _____ _____ _____

15.2 Physiology

MATCHING EXERCISE

Match each word or phrase to its description.

1. auditory cortex
2. cochlea
3. cranial nerve VIII
4. round window
5. proprioception
6. cranial nerve I
7. olfaction

_____ vestibulocochlear nerve

_____ in the temporal lobe of the brain

_____ olfactory nerve

_____ awareness of body position

_____ a "safety valve"

_____ sense of smell

_____ contains hair cells that detect loudness and pitch

CIRCLE EXERCISE

Circle the correct answer from the choices given.

1. The sense of balance is coordinated by all of the following *except* the (**eyes, muscular system, semicircular canals, vestibular nerve**).

2. The semicircular canals are oriented in all of the following planes *except* (**horizontal, oblique, vertical, vestibular**).

TRUE OR FALSE EXERCISE

*Indicate whether each statement is true or false by writing **T** or **F** on the line.*

1. _____ The external ear funnels sound waves into the inner ear.

2. _____ The pitch of the sound waves correlates to the location of stimulated hair cells in the cochlea.

3. _____ The temporal lobe is in the auditory cortex.

4. _____ Sound waves that reach the tympanic membrane are converted into nerve impulses.

DIVIDING WORDS EXERCISE

Separate these words into their component parts (combining form, suffix). The first one has been done for you.

Medical Word	Combining Form	Suffix	Medical Word	Combining Form	Suffix
1. **tympanic**	*tympan/o-*	*-ic*	4. proprioception	_____	_____
2. auditory	_____	_____	5. vestibular	_____	_____
3. cochlear	_____	_____	6. olfaction	_____	_____

SPELLING EXERCISE

Read each medical word pronunciation and write the medical word that it represents. Be sure to check your spelling. The first one has been done for you.

1. **(KOH-klee-ar)**   *cochlear*

2. (ves-TIH-byoo-loh-KOH-klee-ar) _____

3. (AW-dih-TOR-ee) _____

4. (PROH-pree-oh-SEP-shun) _____

RELATED COMBINING FORMS EXERCISE

Write the combining forms on the lines provided. (Hint: See the It's Greek to Me! feature box.)

1. Three combining forms that mean *hearing*.   _____ _____ _____

2. Two combining forms that mean *sense of smell*.   _____ _____

15.3 Diseases

MATCHING EXERCISE

Match each word or phrase to its description.

1. anosmia
2. cold sores
3. cholesteatoma
4. epistaxis
5. hemotympanum
6. otitis externa
7. otosclerosis
8. rhinophyma
9. suppurative
10. thrush
11. tinnitus
12. vertigo

_____ loss of the sense of smell

_____ ringing or buzzing in the ears

_____ tumor in the middle ear that can extend into the air cells of the mastoid process

_____ mouth infection with *Candida albicans*

_____ pertaining to pus

_____ blood in the middle ear that can be seen behind the eardrum

_____ bleeding from the nose

_____ enlarged, lumpy nose caused by rosacea

_____ swimmer's ear

_____ caused by herpes simplex virus type 1

_____ feeling as if the environment is spinning

_____ abnormal bone that forms and hardens between the stapes and oval window

TRUE OR FALSE EXERCISE

*Indicate whether each statement is true or false by writing **T** or **F** on the line.*

1. _____ Temporomandibular joint syndrome is caused by grinding of or misalignment of the teeth.
2. _____ Hemotympanum can be caused by infection or trauma.
3. _____ Sensorineural hearing loss is caused by a problem in the inner ear.
4. _____ Untreated middle ear infections can progress to otitis externa.
5. _____ An acoustic neuroma is a cancerous tumor of the vestibulocochlear nerve.
6. _____ A benign growth of the mucous membranes of the nose is known as *epistaxis*.
7. _____ Rhinorrhea is serous drainage from the middle ear.
8. _____ Buzzing or ringing sounds in the ear are known as *tinnitus*.
9. _____ Tone deafness is a type of conductive hearing loss.
10. _____ An effusion is fluid behind the tympanic membrane that creates an air-fluid level.
11. _____ Pansinusitis involves all of the sinuses or all of the sinuses on one side of the face.
12. _____ Smoking and using chewing tobacco can cause cancer of the mouth and neck.

CIRCLE EXERCISE

Circle the correct answer from the choices given.

1. All of the following contribute to the occurrence of a cerumen impaction *except* (**blood, earwax, epithelial cells, hairs, having a hearing aid**).
2. (**Anacusis, Otorrhea, Presbycusis**) is hearing loss due to aging.
3. Earache pain is also known as (**otalgia, otorrhea, otosclerosis**).
4. Which of these adjectives is related to pus? (**malignant, serous, suppurative**).
5. Allergic rhinitis is also known as all of the following *except* (**anosmia, hay fever, seasonal allergy**).
6. Glossitis is inflammation of the (**nose, tongue, sinuses**).
7. (**Leukoplakia, Polyp, Thrush**) is a thickened white patch in the mouth as seen in patients with AIDS.
8. Cervical lymphadenopathy is found in the (**inner ear, neck, tonsils**).

DIVIDING WORDS EXERCISE

Separate these words into their component parts (prefix, combining form, suffix). Some words do not contain all three word parts. The first one has been done for you.

Medical Word	Prefix	Combining Form	Suffix	Medical Word	Prefix	Combining Form	Suffix
1. **bilateral**	*bi-*	*later/o-*	*-al*	6. otorrhea		_____	_____
2. anosmia	_____	_____	_____	7. pansinusitis	_____	_____	_____
3. laryngitis		_____	_____	8. postnasal	_____	_____	_____
4. myringitis		_____	_____	9. presbyacusis		_____	_____
5. neuroma		_____	_____	10. rhinophyma		_____	_____

SPELLING EXERCISE

Read each medical word pronunciation and write the medical word that it represents. Be sure to check your spelling. The first one has been done for you.

1. **(ah-LER-jik)** _____*allergic*_____
2. (koh-LES-tee-ah-TOH-mah) _____
3. (OH-toh-REE-ah) _____

4. (TIN-ih-tuhs) _____
5. (HEE-moh-TIM-pah-num) _____
6. (ee-FYOO-zhun) _____

15.4 Laboratory, Diagnostic, and Radiologic Procedures

MATCHING EXERCISE

Match each word, phrase, or abbreviation to its description.

1. audiometer
2. BAER
3. C&S
4. CT scan
5. Rinne test
6. tuning fork

_____ tests bone conduction versus air conduction in one ear at a time
_____ a series of clicks and an EEG
_____ radiologic procedure to view the sinuses
_____ produces pure tones to test the hearing
_____ test to identify which bacterium is causing an infection
_____ used in a Weber hearing test

TRUE OR FALSE EXERCISE

Indicate whether each statement is true or false by writing **T** or **F** on the line.

1. _____ Speech audiometry uses spoken words and sentences to test the patient's hearing.
2. _____ The Rinne test evaluates bone conduction versus air conduction of sound.
3. _____ Impedance is resistance of the tympanic membrane to move when tested with air pressure.
4. _____ Air conduction of sound is always less than bone conduction of sound.
5. _____ The rapid strep test shows which allergens a patient is allergic to.

CIRCLE EXERCISE

Circle the correct answer from the choices given.

1. The process of measuring hearing acuity is (**an audiogram, an audiometer, audiometry**).
2. The frequency of a sound is measured in (**decibels, hertz, RAST**).

15.5 Medical Procedures, Drugs, and Surgical Procedures

MATCHING EXERCISE

Match each word or phrase to its description.

1. antiyeast drug
2. cheiloplasty
3. cochlear implant
4. myringotome
5. otoscopy
6. ototoxicity
7. rhinoplasty
8. Romberg sign
9. tympanostomy

_____ instrument used to cut the eardrum

_____ plastic surgery on the nose

_____ placed in the inner ear to correct total deafness

_____ treats oral candidiasis and thrush

_____ insertion of a PE tube into a permanent opening in the eardrum

_____ plastic surgery to repair the lip

_____ used to assess a patient's balance

_____ procedure to view inside the ear with a lighted instrument

_____ adverse drug effect from certain antibiotic drugs

CIRCLE EXERCISE

Circle the correct answer from the choices given.

1. A/An (**endoscope, otoscope, speculum**) is used to widen the nostril to examine the nasal cavity.
2. An (**antibiotic, antihistamine, antitussive**) drug is used to treat coughing.
3. A drug given by the sublingual route is (**placed in the external ear, placed under the tongue, sprayed in the nose**).
4. Endoscopy is used in all of the following ways *except* (**change the shape of the nose, perform a biopsy, remove a polyp**).
5. A (**rhinoplasty, septoplasty, stapedectomy**) is used to treat otosclerosis.
6. A (**PE tube, polypectomy, T&A**) is used to remove infected lymphoid tissue from the pharynx.

TRUE OR FALSE EXERCISE

*Indicate whether each statement is true or false by writing **T** or **F** on the line.*

1. _____ A tongue depressor, penlight, and laryngeal mirror are used to examine the oral cavity.
2. _____ A decongestant drug is used to treat severe inflammation in the nose.
3. _____ A cochlear implant is used to repair a cleft lip and palate.
4. _____ An otoplasty is also known as an *ear pinning*.
5. _____ A partial glossectomy is removal of the tongue to treat cancer of the mouth and neck.

DIVIDING WORDS EXERCISE

Separate these words into their component parts (prefix, combining form, suffix). Some words do not contain all three word parts. The first one has been done for you.

Medical Word	Prefix	Combining Form	Suffix	Medical Word	Prefix	Combining Form	Suffix
1. **antibiotic**	*anti-*	*bi/o-*	*-tic*	7. otoscopy		_____	_____
2. antitussive	_____	_____	_____	8. polypectomy		_____	_____
3. cheiloplasty		_____	_____	9. rhinoplasty		_____	_____
4. decongestant	_____	_____	_____	10. sublingual	_____	_____	_____
5. endoscope		_____	_____	11. tonsillectomy		_____	_____
6. myringotome		_____	_____				

SPELLING EXERCISE

Read each medical word pronunciation and write the medical word that it represents. Be sure to check your spelling. The first one has been done for you.

1. **(KY-loh-PLAS-tee)**   *cheiloplasty*
2. (oh-TAW-skoh-pee)   _____
3. (DEE-con-JES-tant)   _____
4. (EN-doh-SKAW-pik)   _____
5. (OH-toh-PLAS-tee)   _____

Immerse Yourself: Analyze Medical Reports

Electronic Patient Record #1

This is an excerpt from an Office Visit Note. Read the Note and answer the questions.

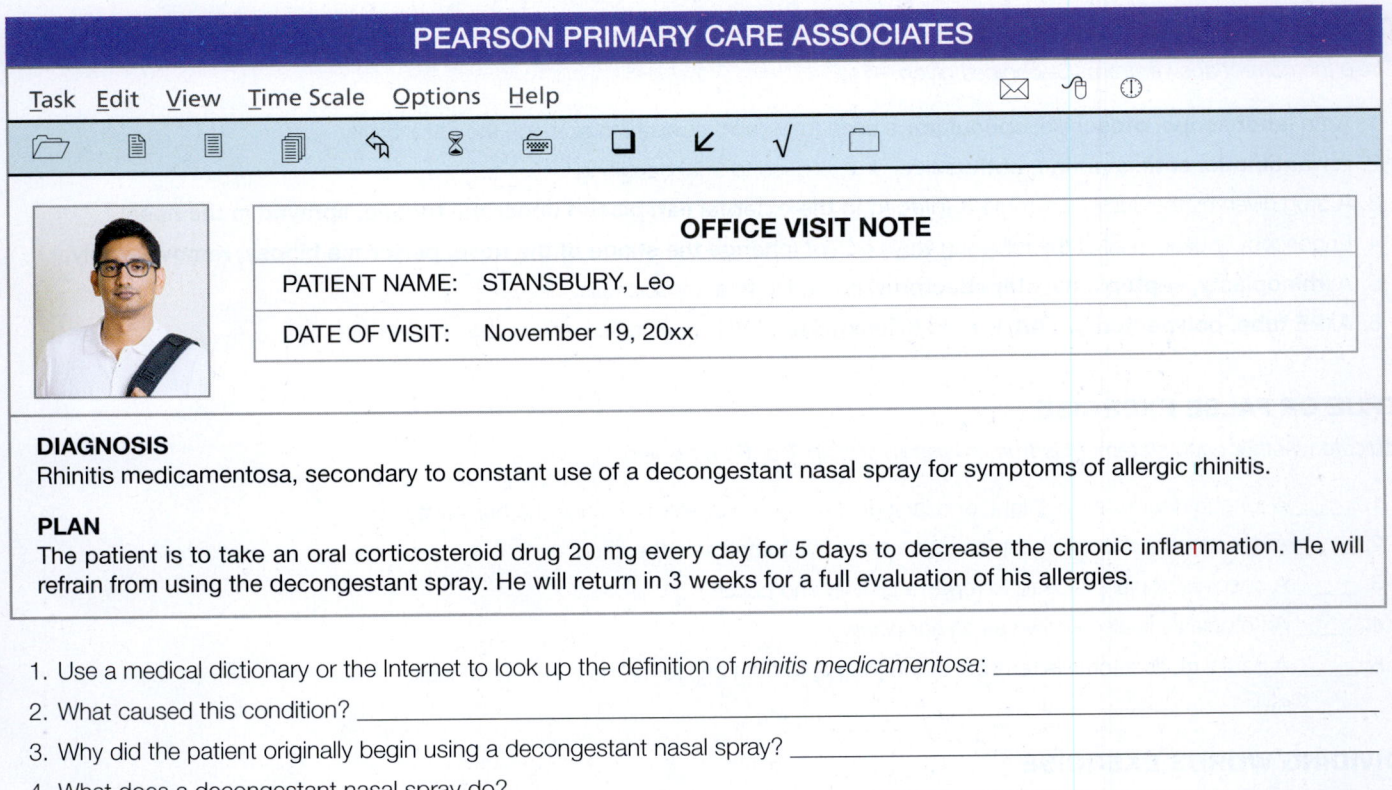

PEARSON PRIMARY CARE ASSOCIATES

Task   Edit   View   Time Scale   Options   Help

OFFICE VISIT NOTE

PATIENT NAME:	STANSBURY, Leo
DATE OF VISIT:	November 19, 20xx

DIAGNOSIS
Rhinitis medicamentosa, secondary to constant use of a decongestant nasal spray for symptoms of allergic rhinitis.

PLAN
The patient is to take an oral corticosteroid drug 20 mg every day for 5 days to decrease the chronic inflammation. He will refrain from using the decongestant spray. He will return in 3 weeks for a full evaluation of his allergies.

1. Use a medical dictionary or the Internet to look up the definition of *rhinitis medicamentosa*: _____

2. What caused this condition? _____

3. Why did the patient originally begin using a decongestant nasal spray? _____

4. What does a decongestant nasal spray do? _____

Electronic Patient Record #2

This is an Office Visit Note. Read the Note and answer the questions.

PEARSON FAMILY PRACTICE ASSOCIATES

Task Edit View Time Scale Options Help

OFFICE VISIT NOTE

PATIENT NAME:	ARQUETTE, Geanne
DATE OF VISIT:	November 19, 20xx

HISTORY:
This 32-year-old mother of two children had a slight fever, a sore throat, and a head cold that developed over a few days after both children had similar symptoms. She states that both children are in daycare and many children at the daycare center have been ill. A few days later, she also had the acute onset of severe pain and pressure over her right cheekbone and right forehead, but this subsided somewhat more recently. She continued to go to work but, within the last few days, has been experiencing increasing severe fatigue, is slightly dizzy at times, and has some pain in her ears.

PHYSICAL EXAMINATION:
On physical examination today, she has only a slightly increased temperature. She has slight pain on palpation of her forehead and cheekbone areas bilaterally. In both ears, the TMs are red and bulging outward.

ASSESSMENT:
1. Bilateral acute otitis media.
2. Previously acute but now subacute sinusitis.

PLAN:
An antibiotic drug 500 mg PO b.i.d. × 10 days. She is to call if she has any exacerbation of her symptoms.

Irene S. Klinitski, M.D.
_____
Irene S. Klinitski, M.D.

ISK: mtt
D: 11/19/xx
T: 11/19/xx

---

1. Divide *sinusitis* into its two word parts and give the meaning of each word part.

   Word Part   **Meaning**
   _____   _____
   _____   _____

2. Divide *bilateral* into its three word parts and give the meaning of each word part.

   Word Part   **Meaning**
   _____   _____
   _____   _____
   _____   _____

3. What does the abbreviation *TMs* stand for? _____

4. Which of the patient's symptoms began with an acute onset? _____

continued

5. What technique was used to do the physical examination of the sinuses? _____

6. What disease is now subacute? _____

7. What drug was prescribed for the patient? _____

8. Which of the four headings in this report gives the physician's diagnosis? _____

9. Which two pairs of sinuses are located beneath the forehead and cheekbones? _____

10. In Assessment #1, what abbreviation could be used instead of saying *bilateral*? _____

MyLab Medical Terminology™

MyLab Medical Terminology is a premium online homework management system that includes a host of features to help you study. Registered users will find:

- A multitude of quizzes and activities built within the MyLab platform

- Powerful tools that track and analyze your results—allowing you to create a personalized learning experience

- Videos and audio pronunciations to help enrich your progress

- Streaming lesson presentations (guided lectures) and self-paced learning modules

- A space where you and your instructor can check your progress and manage your assignments

Appendix A
Glossary of Medical Word Parts
Prefixes, Suffixes, and Combining Forms

Notes:

Rows shaded in orange contain **Prefixes**, abbreviated **P** in the Word Part Abbreviation column

Rows shaded in blue contain **Combining Forms**, abbreviated **CF**. The chapters where a combining form can be found are listed in the Chapter column (e.g., *C3* stands for *Chapter 3*).

Rows without shading contain **Suffixes**, abbreviated **S**.

A

Word Part	Meaning	Word Part Abbreviation	Chapter
a-	away from; without	P	
ab-	away from	P	
abdomin/o-	abdomen	CF	C1, C3, C5, C8, C12
ablat/o-	destroy; take away	CF	C5, C12
-able	able to be	S	
abort/o-	stop prematurely	CF	C12
abras/o-	scrape off	CF	C2, C14
absorpt/o-	absorb; take in	CF	C3, C10
-ac	pertaining to	S	
access/o-	contributing part; supplemental part	CF	C9
accommod/o-	adapt	CF	C14
acetabul/o-	socket of the hip joint	CF	C7
acid/o-	acid; low pH	CF	C10, C13
acous/o-	hearing; sound	CF	C15
acr/o-	extremity; highest point	CF	C12, C13
actin/o-	rays of the sun	CF	C2
act/o-	action	CF	C13
acu/o-	needle; sharpness	CF	C14
-acusis	abnormal condition of hearing	S	

Word Part	Meaning	Word Part Abbreviation	Chapter
-ad	in the direction of; toward	S	
ad-	toward	P	
-ade	action; process	S	
aden/o-	gland	CF	C3, C4, C6, C11, C12, C13, C15
adenoid/o-	structure resembling a gland	CF	C15
adhes/o-	stick to	CF	C3
adip/o-	fat	CF	C2
adnex/o-	accessory connecting parts	CF	C12
adolesc/o-	beginning of being an adult	CF	C11, C12
adren/o-	adrenal gland	CF	C13
adrenal/o-	adrenal gland	CF	C13
affect/o-	have an influence on; mood; state of mind	CF	C13
affer/o-	toward the center	CF	C9
ag/o-	lead to	CF	C13
-age	collection; group	S	
agglutin/o-	clumping; sticking	CF	C6
aggreg/o-	group crowded together	CF	C6
-al	pertaining to	S	
albin/o-	white	CF	C2
albumin/o-	albumin	CF	C10
alg/o-	pain	CF	C7, C8, C9, C15
alges/o-	sensation of pain	CF	C7, C8, C9, C10
align/o-	arranged in a straight line	CF	C7
aliment/o-	food; nourishment	CF	C3
-alis	pertaining to	S	
alkal/o-	base, high pH	CF	C10
all/o-	other; strange	CF	C2, C7
allerg/o-	allergy	CF	C6, C15
aller/o-	other work; strange activity	CF	C6
all/o-	other; strange	CF	C2, C7
alopec/o-	bald	CF	C2
alveol/o-	air sac	CF	C4

Word Part	Meaning	Word Part Abbreviation	Chapter
ambly/o-	dimness	CF	C14
ambulat/o-	walking	CF	C1, C10
amnes/o-	memory loss	CF	C9
amni/o-	amnion	CF	C12
-amnios	amniotic fluid	S	
amput/o-	cut off	CF	C7
amygdal/o-	almond shape	CF	C9
amyl/o-	carbohydrate; starch	CF	C3
-an	pertaining to	S	
an-	not; without	P	
ana-	apart; excessive	P	
anastom/o-	create an opening between two structures	CF	C3, C5, C12
-ance	state	S	
ancill/o-	accessory; servant	CF	C1
-ancy	state	S	
andr/o-	male	CF	C11, C13
aneurysm/o-	aneurysm; dilation	CF	C5, C9
angi/o-	blood vessel; lymphatic vessel	CF	C2, C5, C6, C9, C10, C14
angin/o-	angina	CF	C5
anis/o-	unequal	CF	C14
ankyl/o-	fused together; stiff	CF	C7
an/o-	anus	CF	C3
-ant	pertaining to	S	
antagon/o-	opposing effect	CF	C8, C13
ante-	before; forward	P	
anter/o-	before; front part	CF	C1, C8, C13, C14
anthrac/o-	coal	CF	C4
anti-	against	P	
aort/o-	aorta	CF	C5
apher/o-	withdrawal	CF	C6
apic/o-	apex; tip	CF	C5

Word Part	Meaning	Word Part Abbreviation	Chapter
apo-	away from	P	
append/o-	small structure hanging from a larger structure	CF	C3
appendic/o-	appendix	CF	C3
appendicul/o-	limb; small attached part	CF	C7
aque/o-	clear, watery fluid	CF	C14
-ar	pertaining to	S	
arachn/o-	spider; spider web	CF	C9
-arche	beginning	S	
areol/o-	small, circular area	CF	C12
-aris	pertaining to	S	
arter/o-	artery	CF	C5, C9
arteri/o-	artery	CF	C1, C4, C5, C9, C10
arteriol/o-	arteriole	CF	C5
arthr/o-	joint	CF	C1, C7
articul/o-	joint	CF	C7
-ary	pertaining to	S	
asbest/o-	asbestos	CF	C4
ascit/o-	ascites	CF	C3
-ase	enzyme	S	
aspir/o-	breathe in; suck in	CF	C4, C6, C11, C12
asthen/o-	lack of strength	CF	C8
asthm/o-	asthma	CF	C4
astr/o-	star-like structure	CF	C9
-ate	composed of; pertaining to	S	
-ated	composed of; pertaining to a condition	S	
atel/o-	incomplete	CF	C4
ather/o-	soft, fatty substance	CF	C5
atheromat/o-	fatty deposit; fatty mass	CF	C5
athet/o-	without position or purpose	CF	C8, C9
-atic	pertaining to	S	
-ating	pertaining to having	S	
-ation	being; having; process	S	

Word Part	Meaning	Word Part Abbreviation	Chapter
-ative	pertaining to	S	
-ator	person who does or produces; thing that does or produces	S	
-atory	pertaining to	S	
atri/o-	atrium; chamber that is open at the top	CF	C5
-ature	system composed of	S	
audi/o-	hearing	CF	C15
audit/o-	sense of hearing	CF	C9, C15
augment/o-	increase in degree or size	CF	C12
aur/i-	ear	CF	C15
auricul/o-	ear	CF	C15
auscult/o-	listening	CF	C1, C4, C5
aut/o-	self	CF	C2, C6, C7
autonom/o-	independent; self-governing	CF	C9
axi/o-	axis	CF	C7, C9
axill/o-	armpit; axilla	CF	C5

B

Word Part	Meaning	Word Part Abbreviation	Chapter
bacteri/o-	bacterium	CF	C10
balan/o-	glans penis	CF	C11
bar/o-	weight	CF	C3
bas/o-	alkaline; base of a structure	CF	C2, C6, C12
bi-	two	P	
bi/o-	living organism, living tissue	CF	C1, C2, C3, C4, C6, C8, C9, C10, C11, C12, C13, C14, C15
bifurcat/o-	divide into two branches	CF	C5
bil/i-	bile; gall	CF	C3
bili/o-	bile; gall	CF	C3
bilirubin/o-	bilirubin	CF	C12
-blast	immature cell	S	
blast/o-	embryonic; immature	CF	C9, C10, C14

Word Part	Meaning	Word Part Abbreviation	Chapter
blephar/o-	eyelid	CF	C2, C14
-body	structure; thing	S	
brachi/o-	arm	CF	C5, C8
brachy-	short	P	
brady-	slow	P	
bronchi/o-	bronchus	CF	C4
bronchiol/o-	bronchiole	CF	C4
bronch/o-	bronchus	CF	C4
bucc/o-	cheek	CF	C8, C15
buccin/o-	cheek	CF	C8
bulb/o-	bulb-like structure	CF	C11
bunion/o-	bunion	CF	C7
burs/o-	bursa	CF	C8

C

Word Part	Meaning	Word Part Abbreviation	Chapter
calc/i-	calcium	CF	C13
calc/o-	calcium	CF	C13
calcane/o-	calcaneus; heel bone	CF	C7
calcific/o-	hard from calcium	CF	C12
calcul/o-	stone	CF	C10
cali/o-	calyx	CF	C10
calic/o-	calyx	CF	C10
cancell/o-	lattice structure	CF	C7
cancer/o-	cancer	CF	C2, C3, C4, C8, C10, C11, C12
candid/o-	*Candida*; yeast	CF	C12, C15
capill/o-	capillary; hair-like structure	CF	C5
capn/o-	carbon dioxide	CF	C4
capsul/o-	capsule; enveloping structure	CF	C14
carbox/y-	carbon monoxide	CF	C4, C6

Word Part	Meaning	Word Part Abbreviation	Chapter
carcin/o-	cancer	CF	C2, C3, C4, C10, C11, C12, C13, C15
card/i-	heart	CF	C1
card/o-	heart	CF	C5
cardi/o-	heart	CF	C1, C4, C5, C8
carot/o-	loss of consciousness	CF	C5
carp/o-	wrist	CF	C7, C9
cartilagin/o-	cartilage	CF	C7
cata-	down	P	
catheter/o-	catheter	CF	C5, C10
caud/o-	tailbone	CF	C1
caus/o-	burning	CF	C9
cav/o-	hollow space	CF	C1, C7, C9, C12, C14, C15
cec/o-	cecum	CF	C3
-cele	hernia	S	
celi/o-	abdomen	CF	C3
cellul/o-	cell	CF	C1, C2, C3, C4
-centesis	procedure to puncture	S	
cephal/o-	head	CF	C1, C9, C12
-cephalus	head	S	
-ception	having a receptor	S	
-cere	waxy substance	S	
cerebell/o-	cerebellum	CF	C9
cerebr/o-	cerebrum	CF	C9
cervic/o-	cervix; neck	CF	C7, C12, C15
cheil/o-	lip	CF	C15
chem/o-	chemical; drug	CF	C3
chez/o-	pass feces	CF	C3
chir/o-	hand	CF	C7
chlor/o-	chloride	CF	C3
chol/e-	bile; gall	CF	C3
cholangi/o-	bile duct	CF	C3
cholecyst/o-	gallbladder	CF	C3

Word Part	Meaning	Word Part Abbreviation	Chapter
choledoch/o-	common bile duct	CF	C3
cholesterol/o-	cholesterol	CF	C5
chondr/o-	cartilage	CF	C1, C7
chorion/o-	chorion	CF	C12
choroid/o-	choroid	CF	C14
chrom/o-	color	CF	C6, C12, C13
chron/o-	time	CF	C1, C4, C10
cili/o-	hair-like structure	CF	C14
circa-	about	P	
circul/o-	circle	CF	C15
circulat/o-	moving in a circular route	CF	C5
circum-	around	P	
cirrh/o-	yellow	CF	C3
cis/o-	cut	CF	C2, C3, C6, C8, C9, C11, C12
-clast	cell that breaks down	S	
claudicat/o-	limping pain	CF	C5
clav/o-	clavicle, collarbone	CF	C5, C7
clavicul/o-	clavicle, collarbone	CF	C7
-cle	small thing	S	
cleid/o-	clavicle; collarbone	CF	C8
clinic/o-	medicine	CF	C11
clon/o-	identical group derived from one; rapid contracting and relaxing	CF	C9
-clonus	rapid contracting and relaxing	S	
-cnemius	leg	S	
coagul/o-	clotting	CF	C5, C6, C14
coarct/o-	narrowed	CF	C5
cocc/o-	spherical bacterium	CF	C4, C11
-coccus	spherical bacterium	S	
coccyg/o-	coccyx; tailbone	CF	C7
cochle/o-	cochlea; spiral-shaped structure	CF	C9, C15
cognit/o-	thinking	CF	C7, C9
coit/o-	sexual intercourse	CF	C11, C12

Word Part	Meaning	Word Part Abbreviation	Chapter
col/o-	colon	CF	C3, C10
coll/a-	fibers that hold together	CF	C2
-collis	condition of the neck	S	
colon/o-	colon	CF	C1, C3
colp/o-	vagina	CF	C12
comat/o-	unconsciousness	CF	C9
comminut/o-	break into small pieces	CF	C7
communic/o-	impart; transmit	CF	C1
communicat/o-	impart; transmit	CF	C1
compress/o-	press together	CF	C7
compromis/o-	exposed to danger	CF	C6
con-	with	P	
con/o-	cone	CF	C12
concept/o-	conceive; form	CF	C12
concuss/o-	violent impact	CF	C9
conduct/o-	carrying; conveying	CF	C5, C9, C14, C15
condyl/o-	rounded prominence	CF	C8
congenit/o-	present at birth	CF	C1, C7, C13
congest/o-	accumulation of fluid	CF	C5, C15
coni/o-	dust	CF	C4
conjug/o-	joined together	CF	C14
conjunctiv/o-	conjunctiva	CF	C14
constip/o-	compacted feces	CF	C3
constrict/o-	drawn together; narrowed	CF	C5
construct/o-	build	CF	C12
contin/o-	hold together	CF	C3, C10
contra-	against	P	
contract/o-	pull together	CF	C5, C8, C12
contus/o-	bruising	CF	C2, C8, C9
converg/o-	coming together	CF	C14
convolut/o-	coiled	CF	C10
convuls/o-	seizure	CF	C9

Word Part	Meaning	Word Part Abbreviation	Chapter
cor/o-	pupil	CF	C14
corne/o-	cornea	CF	C14
coron/o-	structure that encircles like a crown	CF	C1, C5, C7
corpor/o-	body	CF	C7, C10
cortic/o-	cortex; outer region	CF	C2, C4, C6, C7, C9, C10, C13, C14, C15
cosmet/o-	adorned; attractive	CF	
cost/o-	rib	CF	C1, C4, C7, C8
crani/o-	cranium; top part of the skull	CF	C1, C7, C9, C14
crin/o-	secrete	CF	C1, C11, C12, C13
-crine	pertaining to secreting	S	
-crit	separation of	S	
cry/o-	cold	CF	C2, C11, C12, C14
crypt/o-	hidden	CF	C11
culd/o-	cul-de-sac	CF	C12
cusp/o-	point; projection	CF	C5
cut/i-	skin	CF	C2
cutane/o-	skin	CF	C1, C2, C3, C5, C9, C10
cyan/o-	blue	CF	C1, C2, C4, C12
cycl/o-	ciliary body; circle; cycle	CF	C14
cyst/o-	bladder; fluid-filled sac; semisolid cyst	CF	C4, C10, C12, C14
cyt/o-	cell	CF	C1, C6, C9, C12, C13
-cyte	cell	S	

D

Word Part	Meaning	Word Part Abbreviation	Chapter
dacry/o-	lacrimal sac; tears	CF	C14
dactyl/o-	digit; finger; toe	CF	C7
-dactyly	condition of fingers or toes	S	
de-	reversal of; without	P	
defici/o-	inadequate; lacking	CF	C6, C11
deglutit/o-	swallowing	CF	C3

Word Part	Meaning	Word Part Abbreviation	Chapter
delt/o-	triangle	CF	C8
dem/o-	people; population	CF	C13
dendr/o-	branching structure	CF	C9
densit/o-	density	CF	C1, C7
dent/o-	tooth	CF	C1
depress/o-	press down	CF	C7, C12
derm/a-	skin	CF	C2
derm/o-	skin	CF	C1, C2
-derma	skin	S	
dermat/o-	skin	CF	C1, C2, C8
desicc/o-	dry up	CF	C2
-desis	procedure to fuse together	S	
dextr/o-	right; sugar	CF	C7, C13
di-	two	P	
dia-	complete; through	P	
diabet/o-	diabetes	CF	C9, C13, C14
diaphragmat/o-	diaphragm	CF	C4
diaphys/o-	shaft of a bone	CF	C7
diastol/o-	dilating	CF	C5
didym/o-	testis	CF	C11
-didymis	testis	S	
dietet/o-	diet; foods	CF	C1
different/o-	different; distinct	CF	C6
digest/o-	break down food; digest	CF	C1, C3
digit/o-	digit; finger; toe	CF	C11
dilat/o-	dilate; widen	CF	C4, C5, C12
dipl/o-	double	CF	C14
dips/o-	thirst	CF	C13
dis-	away from; lack of	P	
disk/o-	disk	CF	C9
dissect/o-	cut apart	CF	C5, C6, C12, C15

Word Part	Meaning	Word Part Abbreviation	Chapter
dissemin/o-	scattered throughout the body	CF	C6
dist/o-	away from the center or point of origin	CF	C1, C7, C10
diverticul/o-	diverticulum	CF	C3
donat/o-	gift; giving	CF	C6
dors/o-	back; dorsum	CF	C1, C9, C12, C15
-dose	measured quantity	S	
-drome	a running	S	
-duct	duct; tube	S	
duct/o-	bring; duct; move	CF	C8
duoden/o-	duodenum	CF	C3
dur/o-	dura mater	CF	C9, C12
dynam/o-	movement; power	CF	C2, C14
dys-	abnormal; difficult; painful	P	

E

Word Part	Meaning	Word Part Abbreviation	Chapter
-eal	pertaining to	S	
ec-	out; outward	P	
ecchym/o-	blood in the tissue	CF	C2
ech/o-	echo of a sound wave	CF	C5
eclamps/o-	seizure	CF	C12
-ectasis	condition of dilation	S	
ecto-	outermost; outside	P	
-ectomy	surgical removal	S	
ectop/o-	outside	CF	C5, C12
-ed	pertaining to	S	
-edema	swelling	S	
-ee	person who is the object of an action; thing that is the object of an action	S	
efface/o-	do away with; obliterate	CF	C12
effer/o-	away from the center	CF	C9

Word Part	Meaning	Word Part Abbreviation	Chapter
effus/o-	pouring out	CF	C4, C15
ejacul/o-	expel suddenly	CF	C11
ejaculat/o-	expel suddenly	CF	C11
elast/o-	flexing; stretching	CF	C2
electr/o-	electricity	CF	C2, C5, C6, C9, C10
elimin/o-	remove from the body	CF	C3
em-	in	P	
-ema	condition	S	
embol/o-	embolus; occluding plug	CF	C4, C6, C11, C12
embryon/o-	embryo; immature form	CF	C12
-emesis	abnormal condition of vomiting	S	
emet/o-	vomiting	CF	C3
-emia	condition of the blood; substance in the blood	S	
-emic	pertaining to a condition of the blood; pertaining to a substance in the blood	S	
emiss/o-	send out	CF	C9
emulsific/o-	liquid with suspended particles	CF	C3, C14
en-	in; inward; within	P	
-ence	state	S	
encephal/o-	brain	CF	C9
-encephaly	condition of the brain	S	
-ency	condition of being; condition of having	S	
endo-	innermost; within	P	
-ent	pertaining to	S	
enter/o-	intestine	CF	C1, C3
enucle/o-	remove the main part	CF	C11, C14
enur/o-	urinate	CF	C10
-eon	person who performs	S	
eosin/o-	eosin; red, acidic dye	CF	C6
ependym/o-	cellular lining	CF	C9
epi-	above; upon	P	
epilept/o-	seizure	CF	C9

Word Part	Meaning	Word Part Abbreviation	Chapter
epiphys/o-	enlarged end of long bone	CF	C7
episi/o-	vulva	CF	C12
-er	person who does or produces; thing that does or produces	S	
erect/o-	stand up	CF	C2, C11
erg/o-	activity; work	CF	C13
-ery	process	S	
erythemat/o-	redness	CF	C2
erythr/o-	red	CF	C6, C10
es/o-	inward	CF	C14
-esis	abnormal condition; process	S	
esophag/o-	esophagus	CF	C3, C5
esthes/o-	feeling; sensation	CF	C1, C2, C9, C12
esthet/o-	feeling; sensation	CF	C2, C9
estr/a-	female	CF	C12, C13
estr/o-	female	CF	C12, C13
ethm/o-	sieve	CF	C7, C15
eti/o-	cause of disease	CF	C1
-etic	pertaining to	S	
-ety	condition; state	S	
etym/o-	word origin	CF	C1
eu-	good; normal	P	
ex-	away from; out	P	
ex/o-	away from; external; outward	CF	C2, C14
exacerb/o-	increase; provoke	CF	C1
excori/o-	take out skin	CF	C2
excret/o-	removing from the body	CF	C10
express/o-	communicate	CF	C9
extens/o-	straightening	CF	C8
extern/o-	outside	CF	C1, C7, C8, C11, C12, C15
extra-	outside	P	
exud/o-	oozing fluid	CF	C2

F

Word Part	Meaning	Word Part Abbreviation	Chapter
faci/o-	face	CF	C9, C15
fallopi/o-	uterine tube	CF	C12
fasci/o-	fascia	CF	C8
fec/a-	feces; stool	CF	C3
fec/o-	feces; stool	CF	C3
femor/o-	femur; thigh bone	CF	C5, C7
fer/o-	bear	CF	C2, C10, C12
ferrit/o-	iron	CF	C6
fertil/o-	conceive; form	CF	C11, C12, C13
fet/o-	fetus	CF	C12
fibr/o-	fiber	CF	C4, C6, C8, C9, C12
fibrill/o-	muscle fiber; nerve fiber	CF	C5, C9
fibrin/o-	fibrin	CF	C6
fibul/o-	fibula	CF	C5, C7
filtr/o-	filter	CF	C10
filtrat/o-	filtering; straining	CF	C10
fiss/o-	splitting	CF	C2, C9
fixat/o-	make stable	CF	C7
flatul/o-	flatus; gas	CF	C3
flex/o-	bending	CF	C8, C12
fluoresce/o-	emit visible light	CF	C14
-flux	flow	S	
foc/o-	point of activity	CF	C9
foli/o-	leaf	CF	C2
folli/o-	sac-like structure	CF	C2, C11, C12, C13
follicul/o-	follicle	CF	C2
-form	having the form of	S	
format/o-	arrangement; structure	CF	C9
fove/o-	small, depressed area	CF	C14
fract/o-	bend; break up	CF	C1, C5, C7, C10, C14
fratern/o-	close relationship	CF	C12

Word Part	Meaning	Word Part Abbreviation	Chapter
-frice	cleaning agent	S	
front/o-	front	CF	C1, C7, C8, C9, C15
fulgur/o-	spark of electricity	CF	C2
fund/o-	fundus; part farthest from the opening	CF	C12, C14
fundu/o-	fundus; part farthest from the opening	CF	C14
fung/o-	fungus	CF	C2
fus/o-		CF	C4, C5, C6

G

Word Part	Meaning	Word Part Abbreviation	Chapter
galact/o-	milk	CF	C12, C13
ganglion/o-	ganglion	CF	C8
gangren/o-	gangrene	CF	C2
gastr/o-	stomach	CF	C1, C3, C5, C8
gemin/o-	group; set	CF	C1, C9
-geminy	action of pairing	S	
-gen	that which produces	S	
gen/o-	arising from; produced by	CF	C1, C4, C7, C10, C11, C12
-gene	gene	S	
gene/o-	gene	CF	C1, C12
gener/o-	creation; production	CF	C1, C7, C14
genit/o-	genitalia	CF	C1, C10, C11, C12, C13
ger/o-	old age	CF	C1
gestat/o-	conception to birth	CF	C12, C13
gigant/o-	giant	CF	C13
glandul/o-	gland	CF	C13
glauc/o-	silver gray	CF	C14
glen/o-	socket of a joint	CF	C7
gli/o-	supporting cells	CF	C9
-glia	group of cells that support	S	
glob/o-	comprehensive; shaped like a globe	CF	C4, C6, C9

Word Part	Meaning	Word Part Abbreviation	Chapter
globul/o-	shaped like a globe	CF	C6, C13
glomerul/o-	glomerulus	CF	C10
gloss/o-	tongue	CF	C3, C9, C15
glott/o-	glottis of the larynx	CF	C3, C4, C15
gluc/o-	glucose; sugar	CF	C3, C13
glyc/o-	glucose; sugar	CF	C13
glycos/o-	glucose; sugar	CF	C10, C13
gnos/o-	knowledge	CF	C1
gon/o-	ovum; spermatozoon	CF	C11, C12
gonad/o-	gonad; ovary; testis	CF	C12, C13
goni/o-	angle	CF	C7, C14
-grade	pertaining to going	S	
-graft	tissue for implant or transplant	S	
-gram	picture; record	S	
granul/o-	granule	CF	C6
-graph	instrument used to record	S	
-graphy	process of recording	S	
-gravida	pregnancy	S	
gustat/o-	sense of taste	CF	C3, C9
gynec/o-	female; woman	CF	C1, C11, C12, C13

H

Word Part	Meaning	Word Part Abbreviation	Chapter
habilit/o-	give ability	CF	C1, C8
hal/o-	breathe	CF	C4
hem/o-	blood	CF	C2, C4, C6, C7, C10, C12, C15
hemat/o-	blood	CF	C1, C3, C6, C9, C10
hemi-	one-half	P	
hemorrh/o-	flowing of blood	CF	C3
hemorrhoid/o-	hemorrhoid	CF	C3

Word Part	Meaning	Word Part Abbreviation	Chapter
hepat/o-	liver	CF	C1, C3, C5
heredit/o-	genetic inheritance	CF	C1
herni/o-	hernia; protruding part	CF	C3, C9
heter/o-	other	CF	C6
hiat/o-	gap; opening	CF	C3
hidr/o-	sweat	CF	C2, C12
hil/o-	indentation	CF	C4, C10
hirsut/o-	hairy	CF	C2, C13
home/o-	same	CF	C2, C10, C13
hormon/o-	hormone	CF	C13
humer/o-	humerus; upper arm bone	CF	C7
hy/o-	U-shaped structure	CF	C7
hyal/o-	clear, glass-like substance	CF	C10
hydatidi/o-	fluid-filled sacs	CF	C12
hydr/o-	fluid; water	CF	C3, C9, C10, C12
hyper-	above; more than normal	P	
hypo-	below; deficient	P	
hypophys/o-	pituitary gland	CF	C12
-hypophysis	pituitary gland	S	
hyster/o-	uterus; womb	CF	C12

I

Word Part	Meaning	Word Part Abbreviation	Chapter
-ia	condition; state; thing	S	
-iac	pertaining to	S	
-ial	pertaining to	S	
-ian	pertaining to	S	
-ias	condition	S	
-iasis	process; state	S	
-iatic	pertaining to a process or a state	S	

Word Part	Meaning	Word Part Abbreviation	Chapter
iatr/o-	medical treatment; physician	CF	C1, C3, C7, C8, C12
-iatry	medical treatment	S	
-ic	pertaining to	S	
-ical	pertaining to	S	
-ice	quality; state	S	
-ician	skilled expert; skilled professional	S	
-ics	knowledge; practice	S	
ict/o-	seizure	CF	C9
icter/o-	jaundice	CF	C2, C3, C14
-id	origin; resembling; source	S	
-ide	chemically modified structure	S	
idi/o-	individual; unknown	CF	C1
-il	small thing	S	
-ile	pertaining to	S	
ile/o-	ileum	CF	C3
ili/o-	ilium	CF	C5, C7
im-	not	P	
immun/o-	immune response	CF	C1, C6, C11
-immune	immune response	S	
impact/o-	wedged in	CF	C15
-in	substance	S	
in-	in; not; within	P	
incarcer/o-	imprison	CF	C3
incud/o-	anvil-shaped bone; incus	CF	C15
induct/o-	leading in	CF	C12
-ine	pertaining to	S	
infarct/o-	small area of dead tissue	CF	C5, C9
infect/o-	disease within	CF	C1, C3, C4
infer/o-	below	CF	C1, C14, C15
inflammat/o-	redness and warmth	CF	C7, C8, C12
infra-	below; beneath	P	
-ing	doing	S	

Word Part	Meaning	Word Part Abbreviation	Chapter
inguin/o-	groin	CF	C1, C3, C11
inhibit/o-	block; hold back	CF	C6, C13
inject/o-	insert; put in	CF	C8, C12
insemin/o-	sow a seed	CF	C12
insert/o-	introduce; put in	CF	C8
inspect/o-	looking at	CF	C1
insul/o-	island	CF	C13
insulin/o-	insulin	CF	C13
integument/o-	skin	CF	C1, C2
inter-	between	P	
intern/o-	inside	CF	C1, C8, C11, C12
interstiti/o-	spaces between tissue	CF	C10, C11
intestin/o-	intestine	CF	C1, C3
intra-	within	P	
intussuscept/o-	receive within	CF	C3
involut/o-	enlarged organ returns to normal size	CF	C12
iod/o-	iodine	CF	C13
-ion	action; condition	S	
-ior	pertaining to	S	
-ious	pertaining to	S	
ir/o-	iris	CF	C14
irid/o-	iris	CF	C14
isch/o-	block; keep back	CF	C5, C9, C12
ischi/o-	ischium	CF	C7
-ism	disease from a specific cause; process	S	
-ist	person who specializes in; thing that specializes in	S	
-istry	process related to a specialty	S	
-isy	condition of infection; condition of inflammation	S	
-ite	thing that pertains to	S	
-itian	skilled expert; skilled professional	S	
-ition	process of making	S	

Word Part	Meaning	Word Part Abbreviation	Chapter
-itis	infection of; inflammation of	S	
-ity	condition; state	S	
-ium	chemical element; structure	S	
-ive	pertaining to	S	
-ix	thing	S	
-ization	process of creating; process of inserting; process of making	S	
-izer	thing that affects in a particular way	S	

J

Word Part	Meaning	Word Part Abbreviation	Chapter
jaund/o-	yellow	CF	C2, C3, C14
jejun/o-	jejunum	CF	C3
jugul/o-	throat	CF	C5

K

Word Part	Meaning	Word Part Abbreviation	Chapter
kal/i-	potassium	CF	C10
kary/o-	nucleus of a cell	CF	C6
kel/o-	tumor	CF	C2
kerat/o-	cornea; hard, fibrous protein	CF	C2, C14
ket/o-	ketones	CF	C13
keton/o-	ketones	CF	C10
kilo-	one thousand	P	
-kinesis	abnormal condition of movement	S	
kin/o-	movement	CF	C3
-kine	movement	S	
kines/o-	movement	CF	C8
kyph/o-	bent; humpbacked	CF	C7

L

Word Part	Meaning	Word Part Abbreviation	Chapter
labi/o-	labium; lip	CF	C12, C15
laborat/o-	testing place	CF	C11
labyrinth/o-	labyrinth	CF	C15
lacer/o-	tearing	CF	C2
lacrim/o-	tears	CF	C7, C14
lact/i-	milk	CF	C12
lact/o-	milk	CF	C3, C12, C13
-lalia	abnormal condition of speech	S	
lamin/o-	flat area on a vertebra	CF	C9
langu/o-	words	CF	C1
lapar/o-	abdomen	CF	C1, C3, C12
laryng/o-	larynx; voice box	CF	C1, C3, C4, C15
lat/o-	dormant; hidden	CF	C4
later/o-	side	CF	C1, C7, C8, C12, C14, C15
lei/o-	smooth	CF	C12
lenticul/o-	lens	CF	C14
-lepsy	seizure	S	
leuk/o-	white	CF	C1, C6, C10, C12, C15
lev/o-	left	CF	C7
lex/o-	word	CF	C9
ligament/o-	ligament	CF	C7
ligat/o-	bind; tie up	CF	C12
limb/o-	border; edge	CF	C9
lingu/o-	tongue	CF	C3, C15
lip/o-	fat; lipid	CF	C2, C3, C5
lipid/o-	fat; lipid	CF	C5
-listhesis	abnormal condition of slipping	S	
-lith	stone	S	
lith/o-	stone	CF	C3, C10, C12
lob/o-	lobe of an organ	CF	C4, C12, C13
loc/o-	one place	CF	C6

Word Part	Meaning	Word Part Abbreviation	Chapter
locat/o-	place	CF	C7
log/o-	study of; word	CF	C2, C4, C5, C6, C7, C9, C11, C12, C13, C14, C15
-logy	study of	S	
lord/o-	swayback	CF	C7
lumb/o-	lower back	CF	C1, C7, C9
lumin/o-	lumen; opening	CF	C5
lun/o-	moon	CF	C2
luxat/o-	displacement	CF	C7
ly/o-	break down; destroy	CF	C9
lymph/o-	lymph; lymphatic system	CF	C1, C6, C9, C15
lys/o-	break down; destroy	CF	C10
-lysis	process to break down or destroy	S	
lyt/o-	break down; destroy	CF	C5, C6, C12
-lyte	dissolved substance	S	

M

Word Part	Meaning	Word Part Abbreviation	Chapter
macr/o-	large	CF	C6
macul/o-	small area; spot	CF	C14
magnet/o-	magnet	CF	C3, C9
mal-	bad; inadequate	P	
malac/o-	softening	CF	C7
malign/o-	cancer	CF	C2, C4, C9, C11, C12, C15
malle/o-	hammer-shaped bone; malleus	CF	C15
malleol/o-	malleolus	CF	C7
mamm/a-	breast	CF	C12
mamm/o-	breast	CF	C1, C12
man/o-	frenzy; thin	CF	C5, C9
mandibul/o-	lower jaw; mandible	CF	C3, C7, C15
manu/o-	hand	CF	C12
masset/o-	chewing	CF	C8

Word Part	Meaning	Word Part Abbreviation	Chapter
mast/o-	breast; mastoid process	CF	C7, C8, C11, C12, C13, C15
mastic/o-	chewing	CF	C3
mastoid/o-	mastoid process	CF	C15
matur/o-	mature	CF	C11, C12, C14
maxill/o-	maxilla; upper jaw	CF	C7, C15
mechanic/o-	physical force; tool	CF	C3
mediastin/o-	mediastinum	CF	C5
medi/o-	middle	CF	C1, C7, C8, C14
medic/o-	medicine	CF	C1
medull/o-	inner region; medulla	CF	C7, C13
mega-	large	P	
-megaly	enlargement	S	
mei/o-	decrease in number	CF	C11, C12
melan/o-	black	CF	C2, C3, C12, C13
melaton/o-	black	CF	C13
men/o-	month	CF	C12, C13
mening/o-	meninges	CF	C9
meningi/o-	meninges	CF	C9
menstru/o-	monthly discharge of blood	CF	C12
-ment	action; state	S	
ment/o-	chin; mind	CF	C9, C15
mesenter/o-	middle thing between the intestines	CF	C3
meso-	middle	P	
meta-	after; change; subsequent to; transition	P	
metabol/o-	transformation	CF	C4
-meter	instrument used to measure	S	
metr/o-	measurement; uterus; womb	CF	C10, C12
metri/o-	uterus; womb	CF	C12
-metry	process of measuring	S	
mi/o-	narrowing	CF	C14
micr/o-	one millionth; small	CF	C2, C6, C9, C13, C14
mictur/o-	making urine	CF	C10

Word Part	Meaning	Word Part Abbreviation	Chapter
mid-	middle	P	
-mileusis	process of carving	S	
mineral/o-	electrolyte; mineral	CF	C7, C13
mit/o-	thread-like strand	CF	C11, C12
mitr/o-	structure with two points	CF	C5
mobil/o-	movement	CF	C8
mon/o-	one; single	CF	C6
morph/o-	shape	CF	C6, C11
mot/o-	movement	CF	C8, C9, C14
motil/o-	movement	CF	C11
muc/o-	mucus	CF	C4
mucos/o-	mucous membrane	CF	C3, C10, C15
mult/i-	many	CF	C12, C13
muscul/o-	muscle	CF	C1, C7, C8
my/o-	muscle	CF	C5, C8, C9, C12
myc/o-	fungus	CF	C2
mydr/o-	widening	CF	C14
myel/o-	bone marrow; myelin; spinal cord	CF	C6, C7, C9
myelin/o-	myelin	CF	C9
myop/o-	near vision	CF	C14
myos/o-	muscle	CF	C8
myring/o-	eardrum; tympanic membrane	CF	C15
myx/o-	mucus-like substance	CF	C13

N

Word Part	Meaning	Word Part Abbreviation	Chapter
narc/o-	sleep; stupor	CF	C9
nas/o-	nose	CF	C1, C3, C4, C7, C14, C15
nat/o-	birth	CF	C1, C12
-nate	thing that is born	S	
ne/o	new	CF	C1, C2, C12, C14
nebul/o-	mist	CF	C4

Word Part	Meaning	Word Part Abbreviation	Chapter
necr/o-	dead body; dead tissue	CF	C2, C5, C7, C10
nephr/o-	kidney; nephron	CF	C10, C13
nerv/o-	nerve	CF	C1, C9
neur/o-	nerve	CF	C1, C8, C9, C10, C13, C15
neutr/o-	not taking part	CF	C6
-nine	pertaining to a chemical substance	S	
noct/o-	night	CF	C10
nod/o-	knob of tissue; node	CF	C13
nodul/o-	small, knobby mass	CF	C13
non-	not	P	
norm/o-	normal; usual	CF	C6
nosocomi/o-	hospital	CF	C1, C2
nuch/o-	neck	CF	C2, C9, C12
nucle/o-	nucleus of an atom or a cell	CF	C5, C6
null/i-	none	CF	C12
nutri/o-	nourishment	CF	C1
nutrit/o-	nourishment	CF	C1

O

Word Part	Meaning	Word Part Abbreviation	Chapter
o/o	egg; ovum	CF	C12
obstetr/o-	pregnancy and childbirth	CF	C1, C12
obstip/o-	severe constipation	CF	C3
obstruct/o-	blocked by a barrier	CF	C3, C4
occipit/o-	back of the head; occiput	CF	C7, C9
occupat/o-	work	CF	C8
ocul/o-	eye	CF	C9, C14
-oid	resembling	S	
-ol	chemical substance	S	
-ole	small thing	S	
olfact/o-	sense of smell	CF	C9, C15
olig/o-	few; scanty	CF	C9, C10, C11, C12

Word Part	Meaning	Word Part Abbreviation	Chapter
om/o-	mass; tumor	CF	C12
-oma	mass; tumor	S	
-omatosis	condition of masses; condition of tumors	S	
omphal/o-	navel; umbilicus	CF	C3
-on	structure; substance	S	
onc/o-	mass; tumor	CF	C1, C2, C9, C11, C12, C15
-one	chemical substance	S	
onych/o-	fingernail; toenail	CF	C2
oophor/o-	ovary	CF	C12
op/o-	vision	CF	C9, C14
operat/o-	perform a procedure; surgery	CF	C3
ophthalm/o-	eye	CF	C1, C14
opportun/o-	taking advantage of an opportunity; well timed	CF	C4, C6
-opsy	process of viewing	S	
opt/o-	eye; vision	CF	C9, C14
-opter	instrument used to measure	S	
-or	person who does or produces; thing that does or produces	S	
orbicul/o-	small circle	CF	C8
orch/o-	testis	CF	C11
orchi/o-	testis	CF	C11
orchid/o-	testis	CF	C11
orex/o-	appetite	CF	C3
organ/o-	living thing; organ	CF	C6
or/o-	mouth	CF	C3, C4, C15
orth/o-	straight	CF	C1, C4, C5, C7, C8
-ory	having the function of	S	
-ose	full of	S	
-osing	abnormal condition of making	S	
-osis	abnormal condition; process	S	
osm/o-	sense of smell	CF	C15
oss/i-	bone	CF	C7, C15

Word Part	Meaning	Word Part Abbreviation	Chapter
osse/o-	bone	CF	C17
ossicul/o-	ossicle; small bone	CF	C15
ossific/o-	changing into bone	CF	C7
oste/o-	bone	CF	C7
ot/o-	ear	CF	C1, C3, C15
-ous	pertaining to	S	
ov/i-	egg; ovum	CF	C12
ov/o-	egg; ovum	CF	C12
ovari/o-	ovary	CF	C12, C13
ovul/o-	egg; ovum	CF	C12
ox/i-	oxygen	CF	C4
ox/o-	oxygen	CF	C4
ox/y-	oxygen; quick	CF	C4, C6, C12, C13
oxygen/o-	oxygen	CF	C5

P

Word Part	Meaning	Word Part Abbreviation	Chapter
palat/o-	palate	CF	C7, C15
palliat/o-	reduce the severity	CF	C1
palpat/o-	feeling; touching	CF	C1
palpit/o-	quick throbbing	CF	C5
pan-	all	P	
pancreat/o-	pancreas	CF	C3, C13
papill/o-	elevated structure	CF	C2, C14
par-	beside	P	
par/o-	giving birth	CF	C12
para-	abnormal; apart from; beside; two parts of a pair	P	
parenchym/o-	functional cells of an organ	CF	
pareun/o-	sexual intercourse	CF	C11, C12
pariet/o-	wall of a cavity	CF	C4, C5, C7, C9, C12
part/o-	childbirth; labor	CF	C12, C13

Word Part	Meaning	Word Part Abbreviation	Chapter
parturit/o-	childbirth; labor	CF	C12
pat/o-	open	CF	C5
patell/o-	kneecap; patella	CF	C7
-path	person treating disease	S	
path/o-	disease	CF	C1, C6, C7
pathet/o-	suffering	CF	C9
-pathy	disease	S	
paus/o-	cessation	CF	C12
-pause	cessation	S	
pector/o-	chest	CF	C4, C5, C8
ped/o-	child	CF	C1, C7, C12
pedicul/o-	lice	CF	C2
pelv/o-	hip bone; pelvis; renal pelvis	CF	C1, C3, C7, C10, C12
pen/o-	penis	CF	C10, C11
pendul/o-	hanging down	CF	C12
-penia	condition of deficiency	S	
peps/o-	digestion	CF	C3
pepsin/o-	pepsin	CF	C3
pept/o-	digestion	CF	C3
per-	through; throughout	P	
percuss/o-	tapping	CF	C1, C4
peri-	around	P	
perine/o-	perineum	CF	C11, C12
peripher/o-	outer aspects	CF	C5, C9, C14
periton/o-	peritoneum	CF	C3
peritone/o-	peritoneum	CF	C3, C9, C10
perone/o-	fibula	CF	C5, C7, C8
-pexy	process of fixing in place	S	
phac/o-	lens	CF	C14
phag/o-	eating; swallowing	CF	C1, C3, C6, C13
-phage	thing that eats; thing that swallows	S	
phak/o-	lens	CF	C14

Word Part	Meaning	Word Part Abbreviation	Chapter
phalang/o-	digit; finger; toe	CF	C7
pharmac/o-	drug; medicine	CF	C1, C5
pharyng/o-	pharynx; throat	CF	C3, C4, C9, C15
-pharynx	pharynx; throat	S	
phas/o-	speech	CF	C9
phe/o-	gray	CF	C13
-phil	attraction to; fondness for	S	
phil/o-	attraction to: fondness for	CF	C4, C6
-phile	person who is attracted to or is fond of	S	
phim/o-	closed tight	CF	C11
phleb/o-	vein	CF	C5, C6
phob/o-	avoidance; fear	CF	C9, C14
phor/o-	bear; carry; range	CF	C2, C6, C10, C12, C14
phosphat/o-	phosphorus	CF	C11
phot/o-	light	CF	C2, C9, C12, C14
phren/o-	diaphragm; mind	CF	C4
phylact/o-	guarding; protecting	CF	C6, C12
-phylaxis	condition of guarding; condition of protecting	S	
-phyma	growth; tumor	S	
phys/o-	distend; grow; inflate	CF	C4
physi/o-	physical function	CF	C1, C5, C8
physic/o-	body	CF	C7, C8, C12
-physis	state of growing	S	
phys/o-	distend; grow; inflate	CF	C4
-phyte	growth	S	
pigment/o-	pigment	CF	C2
pil/o-	hair	CF	C2
pituit/o-	pituitary gland	CF	C13
pituitar/o-	pituitary gland	CF	C13
placent/o-	placenta	CF	C12
plak/o-	plaque	CF	C15
plas/o-	formation; growth	CF	C1, C11, C12

Word Part	Meaning	Word Part Abbreviation	Chapter
-plasm	formed substance; growth	S	
plasm/o-	plasma	CF	C6, C12
plast/o-	formation; growth	CF	C1, C2, C6
-plasty	process of reshaping by surgery	S	
pleg/o-	paralysis	CF	C1, C9, C14
pleur/o-	lung membrane	CF	C4
pne/o-	breathing	CF	C4, C12
-pnea	breathing	S	
pneum/o-	air; lung	CF	C4, C14
pneumon/o-	air; lung	CF	C1, C4
pod/o-	foot	CF	C7
-poiesis	process of formation	S	
-poietin	substance that forms	S	
polar/o-	negative state; positive state	CF	C5
poly-	many; much	P	
polyp/o-	polyp	CF	C3, C15
poplite/o-	back of the knee	CF	C5
por/o-	pores; small openings	CF	C7
port/o-	point of entry	CF	C5
post-	after; behind	P	
poster/o-	back part	CF	C1, C13, C14
potent/o-	capable of doing	CF	C9
pract/o-	medical practice	CF	C7
pre-	before; in front of	P	
pregn/o-	being with child	CF	C12
presby/o-	old age	CF	C14, C15
prevent/o-	prevent	CF	C1
priap/o-	persistent erection	CF	C11
prim/i-	first	CF	C12
pro-	before	P	
-probe	rod-like instrument	S	
proct/o-	rectum and anus	CF	C3

Word Part	Meaning	Word Part Abbreviation	Chapter
product/o-	produce	CF	C1, C11, C12
prolifer/o-	production of more of the same	CF	C12
pronat/o-	face down	CF	C8
propri/o-	one's own body	CF	C9, C15
prostat/o-	prostate gland	CF	C10, C11
prosth/o-	artificial part	CF	C7
prosthet/o-	artificial part	CF	C5
prote/o-	protein	CF	C6
protect/o-	defend; protect	CF	C2
protein/o-	protein	CF	C10
proxim/o-	near the center or point of origin	CF	C1, C10
prurit/o-	itching	CF	C2
psor/o-	itching	CF	C2
psych/o-	mind	CF	C1, C9
-ptosis	state of drooping; state of falling	S	
-ptysis	condition of coughing up	S	
pub/o-	hip bone; pelvis	CF	C7, C10
puber/o-	growing up	CF	C12, C13
pulmon/o-	lung	CF	C1, C4, C5
punct/o-	hole; perforation	CF	C6, C9
pupill/o-	pupil	CF	C14
purul/o-	pus	CF	C4, C15
py/o-	pus	CF	C4, C10, C12
pyel/o-	renal pelvis	CF	C10
pylor/o-	pylorus	CF	C3
pyr/o-	burning; fire	CF	C3

Q

Word Part	Meaning	Word Part Abbreviation	Chapter
quadr/o-	four	CF	C1
quadri-	four	P	

R

Word Part	Meaning	Word Part Abbreviation	Chapter
radi/o-	forearm bone; radius, x-ray	CF	C1, C4, C5, C7, C8, C10, C13
radic/o-	root and all parts	CF	C9, C10, C12, C15
radicul/o-	spinal nerve root	CF	C9
re-	again and again; backward; unable to	P	
recept/o-	receive	CF	C9, C12, C13
recess/o-	move back	CF	C14
rect/o-	rectum	CF	C3, C11, C12
recuper/o-	recover	CF	C1
reduct/o-	bring back; decrease	CF	C7, C12
regulat/o-	control	CF	C2
regurgit/o-	backward flow	CF	C3, C5
relax/o-	relax	CF	C8
remiss/o-	send back	CF	C1
ren/o-	kidney	CF	C5, C10, C13
resect/o-	cut out; remove	CF	C3, C4, C10, C11, C14
resist/o-	withstand the effect of	CF	C13
resuscit/o-	raise up again; revive	CF	C4, C5
retent/o-	hold back; keep	CF	C10
reticul/o-	small network	CF	C6
retin/o-	retina	CF	C13, C14
retro-	backward; behind	P	
rhabd/o-	rod shaped	CF	C8
rheumat/o-	watery discharge	CF	C5, C7
rhin/o-	nose	CF	C2, C15
rhiz/o-	spinal nerve root	CF	C9
rhytid/o-	wrinkle	CF	C2
rotat/o-	rotate	CF	C3, C8
rrhag/o-	excessive discharge; excessive flow	CF	C12
-rrhage	excessive discharge; excessive flow	S	
-rrhaphy	procedure of suturing	S	

Word Part	Meaning	Word Part Abbreviation	Chapter
rrhe/o-	discharge; flow	CF	C3
-rrhea	discharge; flow	S	
rub/o-	red	CF	C3
rrhythm/o-	rhythm	CF	C5
-rubin	red substance	S	

S

Word Part	Meaning	Word Part Abbreviation	Chapter
sacr/o-	sacrum	CF	C7
sagitt/o-	front to back	CF	C1, C7
saliv/o-	saliva	CF	C3
salping/o-	uterine tube	CF	C12
-salpinx	uterine tube	S	
saphen/o-	clearly visible	CF	C5
sarc/o-	connective tissue	CF	C2, C7, C8, C12
scapul/o-	scapula; shoulder blade	CF	C7
scient/o-	knowledge; science	CF	C11
scint/i-	point of light	CF	C3, C7
scintill/o-	point of light	CF	C9
scler/o-	hard; sclera	CF	C2, C5, C9, C10, C14, C15
scoli/o-	crooked; curved	CF	C7
scop/o-	examine with an instrument	CF	C3, C7, C10, C12, C14, C15
-scope	instrument used to examine	S	
-scopy	process of using an instrument to examine	S	
scot/o-	darkness	CF	C9, C14
scrot/o-	scrotum	CF	C11
seb/o-	oil; sebum	CF	C2
sebace/o-	oil; sebum	CF	C2
secret/o-	produce; secrete	CF	C10, C12
sect/o-	cut	CF	C2, C9
semi-	half; partly	P	

Word Part	Meaning	Word Part Abbreviation	Chapter
semin/i-	sperm; spermatozoon	**CF**	C11
semin/o-	sperm; spermatozoon	**CF**	C11, C12
sen/o-	old age	**CF**	C2
senil/o-	old age	**CF**	C9
sens/o-	feeling	**CF**	C2, C9
sensitiv/o-	affected by; sensitive to	**CF**	C2, C3, C6, C10, C15
sensor/i-	sensory	**CF**	C15
sept/o-	dividing wall; septum	**CF**	C4, C5, C15
septic/o	infection	**CF**	C6
ser/o-	serum-like fluid; serum of the blood	**CF**	C15
sex/o-	sex	**CF**	C11, C12
sial/o-	saliva; salivary gland	**CF**	C3
sigmoid/o-	sigmoid colon	**CF**	C3
-sin	substance	**S**	
sin/o-	channel; hollow cavity	**CF**	C5
sinus/o-	sinus	**CF**	C15
-sis	abnormal condition; process	**S**	
skelet/o-	skeleton	**CF**	C1, C7, C8
sol/o-	sun	**CF**	C2
somat/o-	body	**CF**	C9, C13
-some	body	**S**	
somn/o-	sleep	**CF**	C4, C9
son/o-	sound	**CF**	C3, C5, C9, C10, C11, C12, C13, C14
sorpt/o-	absorb	**CF**	C7
spad/o-	opening; tear	**CF**	C11
-spasm	sudden, involuntary muscle contraction	**S**	
spasmod/o-	spasm	**CF**	C10
spast/o-	spasm	**CF**	C3, C9
sperm/o-	sperm; spermatozoon	**CF**	C11
spermat/o-	sperm; spermatozoon	**CF**	C11
sphen/o-	wedge shaped	**CF**	C7, C15

Word Part	Meaning	Word Part Abbreviation	Chapter
sphenoid/o-	sphenoid bone; sphenoid sinus	CF	C13
-sphere	ball; sphere	S	
sphinct/o-	close tightly	CF	C3, C10
sphygm/o-	pulse	CF	C5
spin/o-	backbone; spine	CF	C1, C7, C9
spir/o-	breathe; coil	CF	C1, C2, C4, C7, C12
splen/o-	spleen	CF	C3, C6
spondyl/o-	vertebra	CF	C7
squam/o-	scale-like cell	CF	C2, C12
-stalsis	process of contraction	S	
staped/o-	stapes; stirrup-shaped bone	CF	C15
-stasis	standing still; staying in one place	S	
stat/o-	standing still; staying in one place	CF	C5, C13
-staxis	abnormal condition of hemorrhage	S	
steat/o-	fat	CF	C3
sten/o-	constriction; narrowness	CF	C5, C9
stere/o-	three dimensions	CF	C9, C12, C14
stern/o-	breastbone; sternum	CF	C7, C8
-steroid	steroid	S	
steroid/o-	steroid	CF	C7, C8, C11, C13
-sterol	lipid-containing compound	S	
steth/o-	chest	CF	C4, C5
stigmat/o-	mark; point	CF	C14
stimul/o-	exciting; strengthening	CF	C13
stomat/o-	mouth	CF	C3
-stomy	surgically created opening	S	
strept/o-	curved	CF	C15
stri/o-	parallel stripes	CF	C8
styl/o-	stake	CF	C7
sub-	below; underneath; less than	P	
suct/o-	suck	CF	C2
sudor/i-	sweat	CF	C2

Word Part	Meaning	Word Part Abbreviation	Chapter
super-	above; beyond	P	
super/o-	above	CF	C1, C14, C15
supinat/o-	lying on the back	CF	C8
supposit/o-	placed beneath	CF	C3
suppress/o-	press down	CF	C6
suppur/o-	pus formation	CF	C15
supra-	above	P	
surg/o-	operative procedure	CF	C1, C2, C3, C9, C11, C12, C15
suspens/o-	hanging	CF	C10, C12
sym-	together; with	P	
symptomat/o-	collection of symptoms	CF	C1
syn-	together	P	
syncop/o-	fainting	CF	C9
synerg/o-	joined, enhanced effect	CF	C8
synov/o-	joint membrane; synovium	CF	C7, C8
synovi/o-	joint membrane; synovium	CF	C7
synth/o-	put together	CF	C2
system/o-	body as a whole	CF	C2, C5, C6
systol/o-	contracting	CF	C5
-systole	process of contracting	S	

T

Word Part	Meaning	Word Part Abbreviation	Chapter
tachy-	fast	P	
tact/o-	touch	CF	C9, C12
tampon/o-	stop up	CF	C5
tars/o-	ankle	CF	C7
tax/o-	coordination	CF	C8
techn/o-	technical skill	CF	C1, C5, C7, C9
tele/o-	distance	CF	C5
tempor/o-	side of the head; temple	CF	C7, C8, C9, C15

Word Part	Meaning	Word Part Abbreviation	Chapter
ten/o-	tendon	CF	C8
tendin/o-	tendon	CF	C8
tens/o-	pressure	CF	C1, C5
termin/o-	boundary; end; word	CF	C1
test/i-	testis	CF	C11
test/o-	testis	CF	C11, C13
testicul/o-	testicle; testis	CF	C11, C13
tetr/a-	four	CF	C5
thalam/o-	thalamus	CF	C9, C13
theli/o-	cellular layer	CF	C2, C5
then/o-	thumb	CF	C8
therap/o-	treatment	CF	C1, C4, C7, C8
therapeut/o-	therapy; treatment	CF	C1, C12
-therapy	treatment	S	
therm/o-	heat	CF	C2, C14
thorac/o-	chest; thorax	CF	C1, C4, C5, C7
-thorax	chest; thorax	S	
thromb/o-	blood clot	CF	C5, C6
thym/o-	rage; thymus	CF	C6, C8, C13
thyr/o-	shield-shaped structure; thyroid gland	CF	C13
thyroid/o-	thyroid gland	CF	C1, C13
tibi/o-	shin bone; tibia	CF	C5, C7, C8
-tic	pertaining to	S	
-tion	being; having; process	S	
toc/o-	childbirth; labor	CF	C12, C13
tom/o-	cut; layer; slice	CF	C1, C3, C4, C6, C7, C9, C10
-tome	area with distinct edges; instrument used to cut	S	
-tomy	process of cutting; process of making an incision	S	
ton/o-	pressure; tone	CF	C9, C13, C14
tonsill/o-	tonsil	CF	C1, C15
topic/o-	specific area	CF	C2

Word Part	Meaning	Word Part Abbreviation	Chapter
-tor	person who does or produces; thing that does or produces	S	
tort/i-	twisted position	CF	C8
-tous	pertaining to	S	
tox/o-	poison	CF	C6, C12, C13
toxic/o-	poison	CF	C13, C15
trabecul/o-	mesh	CF	C14
trache/o-	trachea; windpipe	CF	C1, C4
tract/o-	pulling	CF	C4, C7, C9
trans-	across; through	P	
transmitt/o-	send across; send through	CF	C8, C9
transplant/o-	move and put in another place	CF	C3, C5, C6, C7, C10, C14
tri-	three	P	
trich/o-	hair	CF	C2
triglycerid/o-	triglyceride	CF	C5
-tripsy	process of crushing	S	
-triptor	thing that crushes	S	
trochle/o-	pulley-shaped structure	CF	C9, C14
-tron	instrument	S	
trop/o-	having an affinity for; stimulating; turning	CF	C12, C13, C14
troph/o-	development	CF	C8, C9
-trophy	process of development	S	
tub/o-	tube	CF	C4, C10, C11, C12
tuber/o-	nodule	CF	C4
tubercul/o-	nodule	CF	C4
tubul/o-	small tube	CF	C10
turbin/o-	scroll-like structure	CF	C4, C15
tuss/o-	cough	CF	C4, C15
-ty	quality; state	S	
tympan/o-	eardrum; tympanic membrane	CF	C15
-type	model of	S	

U

Word Part	Meaning	Word Part Abbreviation	Chapter
-ual	pertaining to	S	
-ula	small thing	S	
ulcerat/o-	ulcer	CF	C3, C14
-ule	small thing	S	
uln/o-	forearm bone; ulna	CF	C5, C7
ultra-	beyond; higher	P	
-um	period of time; structure	S	
umbilic/o-	navel; umbilicus	CF	C1, C3, C12
un-	not	P	
ungu/o-	fingernail; toenail	CF	C2
uni-	not paired; single	P	
ur/o-	urinary system; urine	CF	C1, C5, C10, C11, C12, C13
-ure	result of; system	S	
ureter/o-	ureter	CF	C10
urethr/o-	urethra	CF	C10, C11, C12
urin/o-	urinary system; urine	CF	C1, C10, C11, C12
uter/o-	uterus; womb	CF	C1, C12, C13
uve/o-	uvea	CF	C14

V

Word Part	Meaning	Word Part Abbreviation	Chapter
vaccin/o-	vaccine	CF	C6
vag/o-	vagus nerve; wandering	CF	C9
vagin/o-	vagina	CF	C1, C10, C12
valv/o-	valve	CF	C5
valvul/o-	valve	CF	C5
varic/o-	enlarged, tortuous vein; varix	CF	C5, C11
vas/o-	blood vessel; vas deferens	CF	C2, C5, C11
vascul/o-	blood vessel	CF	C1, C5, C6, C7, C9, C14
ven/i-	vein	CF	C6

Word Part	Meaning	Word Part Abbreviation	Chapter
ven/o-	vein	CF	C1, C3, C5, C9, C10
venere/o-	sexual intercourse	CF	C12
ventil/o-	air movement	CF	C4
ventr/o-	abdomen; front	CF	C1, C3, C9
ventricul/o-	ventricle	CF	C5, C9
verd/o-	green	CF	C3
vers/o-	travel; turn	CF	C1, C5, C8, C12
-verse	travel; turn	S	
vert/o-	travel; turn	CF	C8
vertebr/o-	vertebra	CF	C7
vesic/o-	bladder; fluid-filled sac	CF	C2, C10
vesicul/o-	fluid-filled sac	CF	C2
vestibul/o-	entrance; vestibule	CF	C9, C15
vir/o-	virus	CF	C2, C3, C4, C11, C14
viril/o-	masculine	CF	C13
vis/o-	sight; vision	CF	C9, C14
viscer/o-	large internal organs	CF	C4
vitre/o-	clear, gel-like substance	CF	C14
voc/o-	voice	CF	C15
volunt/o-	one's free will	CF	C8
vuls/o-	tear	CF	C8
vulv/o-	vulva	CF	C12

X

Word Part	Meaning	Word Part Abbreviation	Chapter
xer/o-	dry	CF	C2, C12, C14
xiph/o-	sword	CF	C7

Z

Word Part	Meaning	Word Part Abbreviation	Chapter
-zoon	animal; living thing	S	
zygomat/o-	cheekbone; zygoma	CF	C7

Appendix B
Glossary of Medical Abbreviations, Acronyms, and Short Forms

Notes:

*Abbreviations with an asterisk are those that have been flagged by The Joint Commission or the Institute of Safe Medication Practices as the source of errors. They should not be used. They are included here, however, because some practitioners and institutions still use them, and therefore you need to know what they mean.

†Many hospitals have removed this abbreviation from their official list because it has an undesirable meaning that is unrelated to the respiratory system.

A

A	blood type A in the ABO blood group	**ALP**	alkaline phosphatase
A&P	anatomy and physiology; auscultation and percussion	**ALS**	amyotrophic lateral sclerosis
AB	blood type AB in the ABO blood group	**ALT**	alanine aminotransferase; alanine transaminase
AB, Ab	abortion	**AMD**	age-related macular degeneration
ABD, abd	abdomen	**anti-CCP**	anti-cyclic citrullinated peptide
ABG	arterial blood gases	**AODM**	adult-onset diabetes mellitus
ABR	auditory brainstem response	**AP**	anteroposterior
ACE	angiotensin-converting enzyme	**AQI**	Air Quality Index
ACT	activated clotting time	**ARDS**	acute respiratory distress syndrome
ACTH	adrenocorticotropic hormone	**ARF**	acute renal failure
AD, A.D.*	right ear (Latin, *auris dextra*)	**ARMD**	age-related macular degeneration
ADA	American Diabetes Association; American Dietetic Association; Americans with Disabilities Act	**ART**	assisted reproductive technology
ADH	antidiuretic hormone	**AS, A.S.***	left ear (Latin, *auris sinister*)
ADHD	attention-deficit/hyperactivity disorder	**ASC**	ambulatory surgery center; atypical squamous cells
ADLs	activities of daily living	**ASCVD**	arteriosclerotic cardiovascular disease
AED	automatic external defibrillator	**ASD**	autism spectrum disorder
AFB	acid-fast bacillus	**AST**	aspartate aminotransferase; aspartate transaminase
AFP	alpha fetoprotein	**AU, A.U.***	both ears (Latin, *aures unitas*); each ear (Latin, *auris uterque*)
AGA	appropriate for gestational age		
AIDS	acquired immunodeficiency syndrome	**AUB**	abnormal uterine bleeding
AKA	above-the-knee amputation	**AV**	atrioventricular
AKI	acute kidney injury	**AVM**	arteriovenous malformation

B

B	blood type B in the ABO blood group	**BPH**	benign prostatic hyperplasia
BAEP	brainstem auditory evoked potential	**bpm**	beats per minute
BAER	brainstem auditory evoked response	**BPP**	biophysical profile
basos	basophils (short form)	***BRCA***	breast cancer (gene)
BE	barium enema	**BS**	breath sounds
BKA	below-the-knee amputation	**BSE**	breast self-examination
BM	bowel movement	**BSO**	bilateral salpingo-oophorectomy
BMD	bone mineral density	**BUN**	blood urea nitrogen
BP	blood pressure	**Bx**	biopsy
BPD	biparietal diameter (of the fetal head)		

C

C&S	culture and sensitivity	**CDE**	certified diabetes educator
C1	first cervical vertebra (atlas)	**CF**	cystic fibrosis
C1–C7	cervical vertebrae	**CGM**	continuous glucose monitoring
C2	second cervical vertebra (axis)	**CHF**	congestive heart failure
Ca	cancer; carcinoma (pronounced "c-a")	**CIN**	cervical intraepithelial neoplasia
Ca^{++}	calcium (an electrolyte); calcium ion	**CIS**	carcinoma *in situ*
CABG	coronary artery bypass graft (pronounced "cabbage")	**CK**	conductive keratoplasty
		CKD	chronic kidney disease
CAD	coronary artery disease	**CK-MB**	creatine kinase
CAPD	continuous ambulatory peritoneal dialysis	**Cl$^-$**	chloride (an electrolyte)
CAT, CT	computerized axial tomography	**CLO**	*Campylobacter*-like organism
cath	catheterize or catheterization (short form)	**CMG**	cystometrogram
CBC	complete blood count	**CNM**	certified nurse midwife
CBD	common bile duct	**CNS**	central nervous system
CBT	cognitive-behavorial therapy	**CO**	carbon monoxide
CC	Chief Complaint	**CO$_2$**	carbon dioxide
CCPD	continuous cycling peritoneal dialysis	**COPD**	chronic obstructive pulmonary disease
CCU	coronary care unit	**CP**	cerebral palsy
CD4	helper T cell	**CPAP**	continuous positive airway pressure (pronounced "SEE-pap")
CD8	suppressor T cell		
CDC	Centers for Disease Control and Prevention	**CPD**	cephalopelvic disproportion

CPK-MM	creatine phosphokinase–MM	**CTS**	carpal tunnel syndrome
CPR	cardiopulmonary resuscitation	**CV**	cardiovascular
CRF	chronic renal failure	**CVA**	cerebrovascular accident
CRNA	certified registered nurse anesthetist	**CVS**	chorionic villus sampling
CRPS	complex regional pain syndrome	**CXR**	chest x-ray
CSF	cerebrospinal fluid	**cysto**	cystoscopy (short form)
CT	computerized tomography		

D

D&C	dilation and curettage	**DM**	diabetes mellitus
Db	decibel	**DNR**	do not resuscitate
D.C.	Doctor of Chiropracty	**D.O.**	Doctor of Osteopathy
D.D.S.	Doctor of Dental Surgery	**DOE**	dyspnea on exertion
Derm	dermatology (short form)	**D.P.M.**	Doctor of Podiatric Medicine
DEXA	dual-energy x-ray absorptiometry	**DRE**	digital rectal examination
DI	diabetes insipidus	**DS**	Discharge Summary
DIC	disseminated intravascular coagulation	**DT**	delirium tremens
DIEP	deep inferior epigastric perforator	**DTRs**	deep tendon reflexes
DIP	distal interphalangeal (joint)	**DUB**	dysfunctional uterine bleeding
DJD	degenerative joint disease	**DVT**	deep venous thrombosis
DKA	diabetic ketoacidosis	**Dx**	diagnosis

E

EAC	external auditory canal	**EKG**	electrocardiogram; electrocardiography
EBV	Epstein-Barr virus	**ELISA**	enzyme-linked immunosorbent assay
ECG	electrocardiogram; electrocardiography	**EMG**	electromyogram; electromyography
ED	Emergency Department; erectile dysfunction	**EMR**	electronic medical record
EDB	estimated date of birth	**ENT**	ears, nose, and throat
EDC	estimated date of confinement	**EOM**	extraocular muscles
EDD	estimated date of delivery	**EOMI**	extraocular muscles intact
EEG	electroencephalogram; electroencephalography	**eos**	eosinophils (short form)
EGD	esophagogastroduodenoscopy	**epi's**	epithelial cells (in urine specimen; short form)
EHR	electronic health record	**EPR**	electronic patient record

ER	Emergency Room	**ESWL**	extracorporeal shock wave lithotripsy
ER+	estrogen receptor positive	**ESWT**	extracorporeal shock wave therapy
ERCP	endoscopic retrograde cholangiopancreatography	**ETT**	endotracheal tube
ESRD	end-stage renal disease		

F

FBG	fasting blood glucose	**FiO$_2$**	fraction (percentage) of inspired oxygen
FBO	foreign body object	**FSH**	follicle-stimulating hormone
FBS	fasting blood sugar	**FTI**	free thyroxine index
FEV$_1$	forced expiratory volume (in 1 second)	**FVC**	forced vital capacity
FH	Family History	**FX, Fx**	fracture
FHR	fetal heart rate		

G

G	gravida	**GH**	growth hormone
G/TPAL	gravida, term newborns, premature newborns, abortions, living children	**GI**	gastrointestinal
		GIFT	gamete intrafallopian transfer
GC	gonococcus (*Neisseria gonorrhoeae*)	**GTT**	glucose tolerance test
GCS	Glasgow Coma Scale (or Score)	**GU**	genitourinary; gonococcal urethritis
GDM	gestational diabetes mellitus	**GYN**	gynecology
GERD	gastroesophageal reflux disease		
GGTP, GGT	gamma-glutamyl transpeptidase		

H

H&H	hemoglobin and hematocrit	**HCV**	hepatitis C virus
H&P	History and Physical	**HDL**	high-density lipoprotein
HAI	healthcare-associated infection	**HEENT**	head, eyes, ears, nose, and throat
HAV	hepatitis A virus	**HER2**	human epidermal growth factor receptor 2
HbA$_{1C}$	hemoglobin A$_{1C}$	**Hgb**	hemoglobin
HBV	hepatitis B virus	**HIPAA**	Health Insurance Portability and Accountability Act
HCG	human chorionic gonadotropin	**HIV**	human immunodeficiency virus
HCO$_3^-$	bicarbonate (an electrolyte)	**HLA**	human leukocyte antigen
HCT	hematocrit	**HNP**	herniated nucleus pulposus

HoLEP	holmium laser enucleation of the prostate	**HSIL**	high-grade squamous intraepithelial lesion
hpf	high-power field	**HSV**	herpes simplex virus
HPI	History of Present Illness	**HTN**	hypertension
HPV	human papillomavirus	**Hz**	hertz
HRT	hormone replacement therapy		

I

I&D	incision and drainage	**IgG**	immunoglobulin G
I&O	intake and output	**IgM**	immunoglobulin M
IBD	inflammatory bowel disease	**IM**	intramuscular
IBS	irritable bowel syndrome	**INR**	international normalized ratio
ICP	intracranial pressure	**IOL**	intraocular lens
ICSI	intracytoplasmic sperm injection	**IOP**	intraocular pressure
ICU	intensive care unit	**IRDS**	infant respiratory distress syndrome
IDDM	insulin-dependent diabetes mellitus	**IRS**	insulin resistance syndrome
IgA	immunoglobulin A	**IUGR**	intrauterine growth retardation
IgD	immunoglobulin D	**IVF**	*in vitro* fertilization
IgE	immunoglobulin E	**IVP**	intravenous pyelogram; intravenous pyelography

K

K⁺	potassium (an electrolyte)	**KUB**	kidneys, ureters, bladder

L

L&D	labor and delivery	**LFTs**	liver function tests
L/S	lecithin/sphingomyelin (ratio)	**LGA**	large for gestational age
L1–L5	lumbar vertebrae	**LH**	luteinizing hormone
LA	left atrium	**LLE**	left lower extremity
LADA	latent autoimmune diabetes in adults	**LLL**	left lower lobe (of the lung)
LASIK	laser-assisted *in situ* keratomileusis (pronounced LAY-sik)	**LLQ**	left lower quadrant (of the abdomen)
LDH	lactate dehydrogenase	**LMP**	last menstrual period
LDL	low-density lipoprotein	**LOC**	level of consciousness; loss of consciousness
LEEP	loop electrosurgical excision procedure	**LP**	lumbar puncture

LPN	licensed practical nurse	**LUQ**	left upper quadrant (of the abdomen)
LSIL	low-grade squamous intraepithelial lesion	**LV**	left ventricle
LTBI	latent tuberculosis infection	**LVAD**	left ventricular assist device
LTK	laser thermal keratoplasty	**LVN**	licensed vocational nurse
LUE	left upper extremity	**lymphs**	lymphocytes (short form)
LUL	left upper lobe (of the lung)		

M

MCP	metacarpophalangeal (joint)	**mono**	mononucleosis (short form)
MD	muscular dystrophy	**monos**	monocytes (short form)
M.D.	Doctor of Medicine	**MRI**	magnetic resonance imaging
MDI	metered-dose inhaler	**MS**	multiple sclerosis
MDR-TB	multidrug-resistant tuberculosis	**MSH**	melanocyte-stimulating hormone
MI	myocardial infarction	**MUGA**	multiple-gated acquisition (scan) (pronounced "MUG-ah")
mL	milliliter (measure of volume)	**MVP**	mitral valve prolapse
mm Hg	millimeters of mercury		
MMSE	Mini-Mental State Examination		

N

N&V	nausea and vomiting	**NIDDM**	non-insulin-dependent diabetes mellitus
Na⁺	sodium ion (an electrolyte)	**NP**	nurse practitioner
NB	newborn	**NSAID**	nonsteroidal anti-inflammatory drug
NCD	neurocognitive disorder	**NSR**	normal sinus rhythm
NG	nasogastric	**NST**	nonstress test
NICU	neonatal intensive care unit; neurologic intensive care unit (both pronounced "NIK-yoo")		

O

O	blood type O in the ABO blood group	**OCD**	obsessive–compulsive disorder
O&P	ova and parasites	**OCG**	oral cholecystogram; oral cholecystography
O₂	oxygen	**OD**	overdose
OA	osteoarthritis	**OD, O.D.***	right eye (Latin, *oculus dexter*); Doctor of Optometry
OB	obstetrics	**OGTT**	oral glucose tolerance test
OB/GYN	obstetrics and gynecology	**ORIF**	open reduction and internal fixation

ortho	orthopedics (short form)		**OU, O.U.***	both eyes (Latin, *oculus unitas*); each eye (Latin, *oculus uterque*)
OS, O.S.*	left eye (Latin, *oculus sinister*)			
OSHA	Occupational Safety and Health Administration		**OXT**	oxytocin
OT	occupational therapist; occupational therapy			

P

P	para; pulse (rate)		**PMI**	point of maximum impulse
PA	posteroanterior; physician's assistant		**PMN**	polymorphonuclear (leukocyte)
PAC	premature atrial contraction		**PMS**	premenstrual syndrome
PAE	prostate artery embolization		**PND**	paroxysmal nocturnal dyspnea; postnasal drip
Pap	Papanicolaou test (short form)		**PO$_2$, pO$_2$**	partial pressure of oxygen
PAP	prostatic acid phosphatase		**polys**	polymorphonuclear leukocytes (short form)
PCO$_2$	partial pressure of carbon dioxide		**PPD**	packs per day (of cigarettes); purified protein derivative (TB test)
PCP	primary care physician			
PDT	photodynamic therapy		**PR**	pneumatic retinopexy
PE	Physical Examination; pressure-equalizing (tube)		**PR$^+$**	progesterone receptor positive
PEG	percutaneous endoscopic gastrostomy		**PRBCs**	packed red blood cells
PEJ	percutaneous endoscopic jejunostomy		**PRK**	photorefractive keratectomy
PERRL	pupils equal, round, and reactive to light		**PRL**	prolactin
PERRLA	pupils equal, round, reactive to light and accommodation		**pro time**	prothrombin time (short form)
			PROM	premature rupture of membranes
PET	positron emission tomography		**PSA**	prostate-specific antigen
PFT	pulmonary function test		**PT**	physical therapist; physical therapy; prothrombin time
pH	potential of hydrogen (acid or alkaline)		**PTCA**	percutaneous transluminal coronary angioplasty
Pharm.D.	Doctor of Pharmacy		**PTT**	partial thromboplastin time
PID	pelvic inflammatory disease		**PUD**	peptic ulcer disease
PK	pneumatic retinopexy		**PUL**	prostate urethral lift
PM&R	physical medicine and rehabilitation		**PUVA**	psoralen (drug and) ultraviolet A (light therapy)
PMDD	premenstrual dysphoric disorder		**PVC**	premature ventricular contraction
PMH	Past Medical History		**PVP**	photoselective vaporization of the prostate

Q

QCT	quantitative computerized tomography

R

R/O	rule out	**RML**	right middle lobe (of the lung)
RA	rheumatoid arthritis; right atrium; room air (no supplemental oxygen)	**RN**	registered nurse
		ROM	range of motion; rupture of membranes
RAIU	radioactive iodine uptake	**ROS**	Review of Systems
RAST	radioallergosorbent test	**RP**	retinitis pigmentosa
RBC	red blood cell	**RPR**	rapid plasma reagin (test for syphilis)
rehab	rehabilitation (short form)	**RRT**	registered respiratory therapist
REM	rapid eye movement	**RSI**	repetitive strain injury
RF	rheumatoid factor	**RUE**	right upper extremity
RICE	rest, ice, compression, and elevation	**RUL**	right upper lobe (of the lung)
RIND	reversible ischemic neurologic deficit	**RUQ**	right upper quadrant (of the abdomen)
RLE	right lower extremity	**RV**	right ventricle
RLL	right lower lobe (of the lung)		
RLQ	right lower quadrant (of the abdomen)		

S

S1	first sacral vertebra	**SLE**	systemic lupus erythematosus
S$_1$	first heart sound	**SNF**	skilled nursing facility
S$_2$	second heart sound	**SOB†**	shortness of breath
SA	sinoatrial	**SPEP**	serum protein electrophoresis (pronounced "S-pep")
SAB	spontaneous abortion	**SpO$_2$**	saturated partial oxygen
SAD	seasonal affective disorder	**SQ**	subcutaneous
SARS	severe acute respiratory syndrome	**SSEP**	somatosensory evoked potential
SBE	subacute bacterial endocarditis	**SSER**	somatosensory evoked response
SCC	squamous cell carcinoma	**SSRI**	selective serotonin reuptake inhibitor (drug)
SCI	spinal cord injury	**STD**	sexually transmitted disease
segs	segmented neutrophils (short form)	**STI**	sexually transmitted infection
SG, sp gr	specific gravity	**subcu, subQ***	subcutaneous (short form)
SGA	small for gestational age	**SUI**	stress urinary incontinence
SH	Social History		
SIADH	syndrome of inappropriate antidiuretic hormone		
SIDS	sudden infant death syndrome		

T

T&A	tonsillectomy and adenoidectomy	**TM**	tympanic membrane
T1–T12	thoracic vertebrae	**TMJ**	temporomandibular joint
T$_3$	triiodothyronine	**TNTC**	too numerous to count
T$_4$	thyroxine	**TPAL**	term newborns, premature newborns, abortions, living children
T$_7$	free thyroxine index (FTI)		
TAB	therapeutic abortion	**TPR**	temperature, pulse, and respirations
TAH-BSO	total abdominal hysterectomy and bilateral salpingo-oophorectomy	**TRAM**	transverse rectus abdominis muscle (flap) (pronounced "tram")
TB	tuberculosis	**TRUS**	transrectal ultrasound
TBI	traumatic brain injury	**TSE**	testicular self-examination
TEE	transesophageal echocardiogram; transesophageal echocardiography	**TSH**	thyroid-stimulating hormone
		TUMT	transurethral microwave therapy
TENS	transcutaneous electrical nerve stimulation	**TUNA**	transurethral needle ablation
TFTs	thyroid function tests	**TURBT**	transurethral resection of bladder tumor
THR	total hip replacement	**TURP**	transurethral resection of the prostate
TIA	transient ischemic attack	**TVH**	total vaginal hysterectomy
tib-fib	tibia-fibula (short form)		

U

UA	urinalysis	**URI**	upper respiratory infection
UGI	upper gastrointestinal (series)	**UTI**	urinary tract infection
UPEP	urine protein electrophoresis (pronounced "U-pep")	**UVB**	ultraviolet light B

V

V fib	ventricular fibrillation (short form)	**VDRL**	Venereal Disease Research Laboratory
V tach	ventricular tachycardia (short form)	**VEP**	visual evoked potential
V/Q	ventilation-perfusion (scan)	**VER**	visual evoked response
VBAC	vaginal birth after cesarean section (pronounced "V-back")	**VLDL**	very-low-density lipoprotein
		VMA	vanillylmandelic acid
VCUG	voiding cystourethrogram; voiding cystourethrography		

W

WBC white blood cell; white blood count

Z

ZIFT zygote intrafallopian transfer

Answer Key

Chapter 1 : Medical Language and Health Care Today

1.1 Practice Laps

A. Matching Exercise

3, 4, 6, 5, 7, 2, 1

B. True or False Exercise

1. T   3. T   5. T   7. T

C. Fill in the Blank Exercise

1. Reading
3. Thinking, analyzing, understanding
5. Speaking and pronouncing

1.2 Practice Laps

A. Give the Meaning of Combining Forms

1. breathe; coil
3. artery
5. living organism; living tissue
7. rib
9. skin
11. break down food; digest
13. feeling; sensation
15. intestine
17. side
19. breast
21. birth
23. pregnancy and childbirth
25. eating; swallowing
27. pressure; tension
29. thyroid gland
31. urinary system; urine
33. vagina

B. Matching Exercise

12, 5, 6, 9, 10, 8, 3, 11, 2 ,4, 7, 1

C. True or False Exercise

1. T   3. T   5. T

D. English Plural Noun Exercise

1. hormones   5. ovaries
3. arteries

E. Greek Plural Noun Exercise

1. irides   3. carcinomata

F. Latin Plural Noun Exercise

1. vertebrae   7. bacteria
3. bronchi   9. diagnoses
5. thrombi   11. apices

1.3 Practice Laps

A. True or False Exercise

1. T   3. F   5. F

B. Dividing Medical Words Exercise

1. cardi/o-   -logy
3. intestin/o-   -al
5. ven/o-   -ous
7. brady-   cardi/o-   -ia
9. tonsill/o-   -itis

C. Build Medical Words Exercise

Suffix that Begins with a Vowel

1. cardiac   3. intestinal   5. therapist

Suffix that Begins with a Consonant

7. arthropathy   9. cardiomegaly

D. Spell Medical Words Exercise

1. psychiatry   5. pelvic
3. tonsillitis   7. hypertension

E. Pronounce and Spell Exercise

1. abdominal   9. psychiatry
3. cardiology   11. tonsillectomy
5. digestive   13. pelvic
7. mammogram

1.4 Practice Laps

A. Label Structures

Body Directions

1. posterior (dorsal)
3. medial
5. proximal

Body Cavities

1. cranial cavity
3. thoracic cavity
5. abdominal cavity

Body Regions

1. right hypochondriac region
3. right lumbar region
5. right inguinal region
7. left lumbar region
9. hypogastric region

B. Give the Meaning of Combining Forms

1. back; dorsum
3. before; front part
5. tailbone
7. cell
9. cartilage
11. impart; transmit
13. structure that encircles like a crown
15. secrete
17. tooth
19. diet; foods
21. innermost; within
23. cause of a disease
25. outside
27. front
29. creation; production
31. arising from; produced by
33. knowledge
35. blood
37. medical treatment; physician
39. immune response
41. below
43. skin
45. intestine
47. side
49. lymph; lymphatic system
51. middle
53. birth
55. nerve
57. hospital
59. pregnancy and childbirth
61. eye
63. ear
65. child
67. drug; medicine
69. formation; growth
71. prevent
73. near the center or point of origin
75. lung
77. forearm bone; radius; x-rays
79. send back
81. skeleton
83. breathe; coil
85. operative procedure
87. boundary; end; word
89. chest; thorax
91. navel; umbilicus
93. urinary system; urine
95. abdomen; front

1.5 Practice Laps

A. Give the Meaning of Combining Forms

1. treatment
3. accessory; servant
5. reduce the severity
7. operative procedure

B. Define Abbreviations

1. diagnosis
3. electronic health record
5. primary care physician

Dive In: Medical Language Exercises

1.1 Medical Language

Circle Exercise

1. terminology
3. Arabic

True or False Exercise

1. F
3. T

Related Combining Forms Exercise

1. enter/o-, intestin/o-
3. dermat/o-, integument/o-

1.2 Medical Words: Singular and Plural Nouns and Word Parts

Matching Exercise

2, 1, 1, 2, 3, 3, 1

Matching Exercise

1, 10, 5, 4, 17, 9, 12, 15, 7, 6, 16, 20, 14, 3, 19, 18, 2, 8, 13, 11

Circle Exercise

1. -ae
3. intestine
5. phalanx
7. vertebrae
9. alveoli

True or False Exercise

1. F
3. F
5. T

Plural Noun Exercise

1. irides
3. ova
5. ovaries
7. bronchi
9. ganglia
11. arteries
13. testes

1.3 Divide, Build, Spell, and Pronounce Medical Words

Dividing Words Exercise

1.	langu/o-	-age	
3.	etym/o-	-logy	
5.	cardi/o-	-ac	
7.	muscul/o-	-ar	
9.	urin/o-	-ary	
11.	peri-	cardi/o-	-al
13.	anti-	bi/o-	-tic
15.	tonsill/o-	-ectomy	

Building Words Exercise

1.	-ive	digestive
3.	-ics	obstetrics
5.	-itis	tonsillitis
7.	-scopy	gastroscopy

Spelling Exercise

1. cardiac
3. mammography
5. tonsillitis
7. venous

Spelling and Pronunciation Exercise

1. cardiac
3. intravenous
5. tonsillitis

1.4 The Body in Health and Disease

Matching Exercise

4, 2, 7, 9, 5, 1, 3, 10, 11, 6, 8

Circle Exercise

1. etiology
3. remission
5. gastric
7. cardiac
9. urinary

True or False Exercise

1. F
3. T
5. T
7. F

Dividing Words Exercise

1.	ana-	tom/o-	-ical
3.		cephal/o-	-ad
5.	de-	gener/o-	-ative
7.	a-	symptomat/o-	-ic
9.		thorac/o-	-ic

Building Words Exercise

1.	-al	congenital
3.	-logy	symptomatology
5.	-ery	surgery
7.	-ary	integumentary
9.	-ics	obstetrics
11.	-ary	hereditary

Spelling Exercise

1. cardiac
3. mammography
5. tachycardia
7. urination

Spelling and Pronunciation Exercise

1. cardiac
3. tonsillitis
5. subcutaneous
7. hepatic
9. anatomy

1.5 Health Care Today

Matching Exercise

4, 5, 6, 1, 7, 2, 3, 9, 8

True or False Exercise

1. T
3. T
5. F
7. T
9. F

Fill in the Blank Exercise

1. It can be accessed by more than one healthcare professional at a time.

3. It can be retrieved quickly.

(Other correct answer: It provides seamless, immediate, and simultaneous access by several healthcare professionals to all parts of the record regardless of where those parts were created or stored.)

Dividing Words Exercise

1.	palliat/o-	-ive
3.	ambulat/o-	-ory
5.	techn/o-	-ician

Building Words Exercise

1.	-ion	inspection
3.	-ive	palliative
5.	-ion	palpation
7.	-ion	percussion

Define Abbreviations

1. Electronic patient record
3. Chief Complaint
5. Diagnosis

Immerse Yourself: Analyze Medical Reports

You Write the Report

1. gynecology
3. otolaryngology
5. dermatology
7. neonatology
9. orthopedics

Chapter 2 : Dermatology

2.1 Practice Laps

A. Label Structures

Skin and Subcutaneous Tissues

1. hair shaft
3. sebaceous gland
5. duct of sudoriferous gland
7. artery
9. sudoriferous gland
11. dermis

Nail

1. nail
3. lunula
5. nail bed

B. Give the Meaning of Combining Forms

1. follicle
3. skin
5. skin
7. skin

9. black
11. hair
13. sweat
15. hair

C. Build Words

1.	-al	ungual
3.	-gen	collagen
5.	-cyte	melanocyte
7.	-ous	sebaceous
9.	-ary	integumentary
11.	-in	melanin

2.2 Practice Laps

A. Give the Meaning of Combining Forms

1. defend; protect
3. same
5. control
7. heat

B. Build Words

1.	-al	nosocomial
3.	-tome	dermatome

2.3 Practice Laps

A. Give the Meaning of Combining Forms

1. rays of the sun
3. bruising
5. skin
7. blood
9. tearing
11. cancer
13. fingernail; toenail
15. itching
17. dry

B. Build Words

1.	-iasis	psoriasis
3.	-itis	dermatitis
5.	-osis	necrosis
7.	-plasm	neoplasm
9.	-cle	vesicle
11.	-rrhage	hemorrhage
13.	-ous	erythematous

C. Define Abbreviations

1. herpes simplex virus

2.4 Practice Laps

A. Give the Meaning of Combining Forms

1. skin
3. affected by; sensitive to

B. Define Abbreviations

1. culture and sensitivity
3. radioallergosorbent test

2.5 Practice Laps

A. Give the Meaning of Combining Forms

1. scrape off
3. living organism; living tissue
5. cold
7. feeling; sensation
9. fungus
11. light
13. operative procedure

B. Build Words

1. -opsy   biopsy
3. -ectomy   lipectomy
5. -graft   autograft
7. -tome   dermatome

C. Define Abbreviations

1. biopsy   3. photodynamic therapy

Dive In: Medical Language Exercises

2.1 Anatomy

Matching Exercise

5, 4, 9, 7, 6, 8, 1, 3, 2

Circle Exercise

1. nail bed   5. nail
3. hair

True or False Exercise

1. F   3. T

Dividing Words Exercise

1. dia-   phor/o-   -esis
3.   melan/o-   -cyte
5. ex-   foli/o-   -ation
7.   cut/i-   -cle
9. sub-   cutane/o-   -ous

Spelling Exercise

1. cutaneous   7. subcutaneous
3. melanocyte   9. lipocyte
5. diaphoresis

2.2 Physiology

Matching Exercise

4, 5, 6, 1, 2, 3

True or False Exercise

1. T   5. F
3. T

Dividing Words Exercise

1. sens/o-   -ation
3. home/o-   -stasis

Spelling Exercise

1. protection
3. thermoregulation

2.3 Diseases

Matching Exercise

6, 9, 1, 10, 12, 4, 11, 3, 5, 2, 8, 7

Circle Exercise

1. papule   7. eschar
3. cyst   9. jaundice
5. flat

True or False Exercise

1. F   5. F
3. T   7. T

Adjective Exercise

1. cancerous (or malignant)
3. diaphoretic
5. necrotic
7. vesicular

Dividing Words Exercise

1. dia-   phor/o-   -esis
3. an-   hidr/o-   -osis
5. extra-   vas/o-   -ation

Spelling Exercise

1. laceration   7. polydactyly
3. erythematous   9. psoriasis
5. neoplasm

English and Medical Word Equivalents Exercise

1. senile lentigo
3. decubitus ulcer (or pressure ulcer)
5. abrasion
7. onychomycosis
9. scabies
11. tinea capitis

2.4 Laboratory, Diagnostic, and Radiologic Procedures

Matching Exercise

3, 6, 2, 4, 1, 5

Spelling Exercise

1. Tzanck
3. sensitivity

2.5 Medical Procedures, Drugs, and Surgical Procedures

Matching Exercise

2, 6, 7, 5, 3, 4, 1, 8

Circle Exercise

1. debridement
3. intradermal
5. incisional biopsy
7. antifungal drugs

True or False Exercise

1. T
3. T
5. T

Dividing Words Exercise

1.	fulgur/o-	-ation
3. anti-	fung/o-	-al
5.	dermat/o-	-plasty
7.	rhytid/o-	-ectomy

Spelling Exercise

1. intradermal
3. cryosurgery
5. dermabrasion
7. transdermal

Immerse Yourself: Analyze Medical Reports

Electronic Patient Record

1. cellul/o- cell
   -itis   infection of; inflammation of
3. pruritus
5. welts
7. erythema nodosum

You Create The Electronic Health Record

1. herpes varicella-zoster   shingles   dermatome
3. laceration   anesthetic   sutures

Research Medical Words

1. condition of nail (biting)/eating
3. condition of hair pulling out (in a) frenzy

Chapter 3 : Gastroenterology

3.1 Practice Laps

A. Label Structures

Salivary Glands

1. oral cavity
3. teeth
5. submandibular gland
7. pharynx

Stomach

1. esophagus
3. pancreas
5. pylorus
7. rugae
9. cardia
11. omentum

Small and Large Intestines

1. liver
3. pancreas
5. ascending colon
7. descending colon
9. appendix
11. anal sphincter
13. jejunum
15. sigmoid colon

B. Give the Meaning of Combining Forms

1. abdomen
3. appendix
5. cecum
7. colon
9. intestine
11. stomach
13. liver
15. jejunum
17. mouth
19. pharynx; throat
21. pylorus
23. saliva
25. mouth

C. Build Words

1.	-eal	appendiceal
3.	-cyte	hepatocyte
5.	-ary	alimentary
7.	-ory	gustatory
9.	-ary	salivary
11.	-al	intestinal
13.	-er	sphincter

3.2 Practice Laps

A. Give the Meaning of Combining Forms

1. absorb; take in
3. pass feces
5. break down food
7. liquid with suspended particles

9. stomach

11. fat; lipid

13. pepsin

B. Build Words

1. -ion   deglutition

3. -ation   elimination

5. -in   gastrin

7. -gen   pepsinogen

9. -ase   lipase

3.3 Practice Laps

A. Give the Meaning of Combining Forms

1. appendix

3. abdomen

5. gallbladder

7. feces; stool

9. tongue

11. flowing of blood

13. yellow

15. navel; umbilicus

17. eating; swallowing

19. backward flow

21. fat

B. Build Words

1. -oma   carcinoma

3. -emesis   hematemesis

5. -ive   ulcerative

7. -cele   rectocele

9. -ation   constipation

11. -pathy   enteropathy

13. -itis   cholecystitis

15. -osis   polyposis

17. -oma   hepatoma

19. -lith   sialolith

C. Define Abbreviations

1. gastroesophageal reflux disease

3. inflammatory bowel disease

5. nausea and vomiting

3.4 Practice Laps

A. Give the Meaning of Combining Forms

1. bile; gall

3. bile; gall

5. skin

7. affected by; sensitive to

9. sound

11. vein

A. Build Words

1. -graphy   tomography

3. -gram   cholecystogram

5. -gram   cholangiogram

C. Define Abbreviations

1. barium enema

3. liver function tests

5. upper gastrointestinal

3.5 Practice Laps

A. Give the Meaning of Combining Forms

1. create an opening

3. weight

5. common bile duct

7. stomach

9. hernia

11. abdomen

13. nose

15. cut out; remove

17. placed beneath

19. move and put in another place

B. Build Words

1. -ectomy   gastrectomy

3. -tomy   lithotomy

5. -ectomy   polypectomy

7. -ation   transplantation

9. -ectomy   appendectomy

11. -ectomy   cholecystectomy

13. -plasty   gastroplasty

15. -ectomy   hemorrhoidectomy

C. Define Abbreviations

1. esophagogastroduodenoscopy

3. percutaneous endoscopic gastrostomy

Dive In: Medical Language Exercises

3.1 Anatomy

Matching Exercise

8, 10, 9, 7, 2, 1, 6, 3, 4, 5

Circle Exercise

1. fundus

3. duodenum

5. gallbladder

True or False Exercise

1. F

3. F

Plural Noun and Adjective Exercise

1.   mucosal

3.   anal

5.		cecal
7.		esophageal
9.	intestines	intestinal
11.		pancreatic
13.		pyloric
15.		salivary
17.		lingual

Dividing Words Exercise

1.	or/o-	-al
3.	bili/o-	-ary
5.	gastr/o-	-ic
7.	hepat/o-	-ic
9.	pharyng/o-	-eal
11.	sphinct/o-	-er

Spelling Exercise

1. abdominal
3. mucosal
5. uvula
7. jejunum
9. hepatic

3.2 Physiology

Matching Exercise

5, 7, 6, 3, 1, 4, 2, 8

Circle Exercise

1. fats
3. flatus
5. deglutition

True or False Exercise

1. T   3. F   5. F

Dividing Words Exercise

1.		absorpt/o-	-ion
3.	de-	fec/o-	-ation
5.		digest/o-	-ion
7.		lact/o-	-ase
9.		pepsin/o-	-gen

Spelling Exercise

1. mechanical
3. enzyme
5. glucose

3.3 Diseases

Matching Exercise

11, 2, 8, 4, 9, 3, 6, 12, 1, 14, 10, 5, 13, 7

Circle Exercise

1. tongue
3. intussusception
5. celiac disease
7. jaundice

True or False Exercise

1. F   7. F
3. T   9. T
5. T

Dividing Words Exercise

1.		carcin/o-	-oma
3.		appendic/o-	-itis
5.		diverticul/o-	-osis
7.		enter/o-	-pathy
9.		fec/a-	-lith
11.		hemat/o-	-emesis
13.		hepat/o-	-megaly
15.	poly-	phag/o-	-ia
17.	post-	operat/o-	-ive
19.		sial/o-	-lith

Spelling Exercise

1. hernia
3. cholecystitis
5. diverticulosis
7. gastroenteritis
9. hemorrhoid
11. jaundice
13. polyp

3.4 Laboratory, Diagnostic, and Radiologic Procedures

Matching Exercise

6, 1, 4, 8, 7, 5, 2, 3

True or False Exercise

1. T   5. T
3. F   7. T

Dividing Words Exercise

1.	sensitiv/o-	-ity
3.	intra-	ven/o-	-ous
5.	son/o-	-gram
7.	trans-	hepat/o-	-ic

Spelling Exercise

1. albumin
3. occult
5. endoscopic
7. cholecystogram

3.5 Medical Procedures, Drugs, and Surgical Procedures

Matching Exercise

5, 6, 7, 10, 3, 1, 8, 4, 9, 2

Circle Exercise

1. O&P
3. a surgical mesh
5. skin

True or False Exercise

1. T   3. T   5. T

Dividing Words Exercise

1. anti-   bi/o-   -tic
3. anti-   emet/o-   -ic
5.   bi/o-   -opsy
7.   col/o-   -stomy
9.   lapar/o-   -scope
11. per-   cutane/o-   -ous
13.   supposit/o-   -ory

Spelling Exercise

1. antacid   7. colostomy
3. antiemetic   9. herniorrhaphy
5. biopsy

Immerse Yourself: Analyze Medical Reports

Electronic Patient Record #1

1. an-   not; without
   orex/o-   appetite
   -ic   pertaining to
   dys-   abnormal; difficult; painful
   peps/o-   digestion
   -ia   condition; state; thing
   gastr/o-   stomach
   enter/o-   intestine
   -itis   infection of; inflammation of
3. food from the food truck

Electronic Patient Record #2

1. gastric
3. right lower quadrant
5. antacid
7. appendectomy
9. appendix
11. Pressing the hands on the right lower quadrant of the abdomen and then suddenly releasing the pressure; this will cause pain in a patient with appendicitis.
13. pancreas

You Create The Electronic Health Record

1. anorexia
3. gastroenteritis
5. colonoscopy
7. esophageal; hematemesis; cirrhosis; ascites
9. cholelithiasis; cholecystectomy

Chapter 4 : Pulmonology

4.1 Practice Laps

A. Label Structures

1. larynx   7. pharynx
3. cluster of alveoli   9. apex of lung
5. diaphragm   11. sternum

B. Give the Meaning of Combining Forms

1. air sac   9. pharynx; throat
3. bronchiole   11. lung
5. diaphragm   13. chest; thorax
7. nose

C. Build Words

1. -al   nasal
3. -ary   pulmonary
5. -ic   thoracic
7. -al   bronchial
9. -eal   laryngeal
11. -ar   alveolar

4.2 Practice Laps

A. Label Functions

1. bronchiole
3. carbon dioxide gas molecules
5. capillary wall

B. Give the Meaning of Combining Forms

1. carbon dioxide   7. oxygen; quick
3. breathe   9. breathe; coil
5. oxygen

C. Build Words

1. -ic   phrenic
3. -ism   metabolism

4.3 Practice Laps

A. Give the Meaning of Combining Forms

1. coal
3. cancer
5. embolus; occluding plug
7. cancer
9. air; lung
11. pus

B. Build Words

1. -osis   cyanosis

3. -ptysis   hemoptysis

5. -atic   asthmatic

7. -ectasis   atelectasis

9. -ism   embolism

C. Define Abbreviations

1. cystic fibrosis

3. dyspnea on exertion

5. latent tuberculosis infection

7. tuberculosis

4.4 Practice Laps

A. Give the Meaning of Combining Forms

1. artery

3. blood

5. forearm bone; radius; x-rays

7. cut; layer; slice

B. Build Words

1. -meter   oximeter

3. -ation   ventilation

C. Define Abbreviations

1. arterial blood gases

3. chest x-ray

5. pressure of the gas CO_2

4.5 Practice Laps

A. Give the Meaning of Combining Forms

1. listening

3. larynx; voice box

5. mist

7. air; lung

9. raise up again; revive

11. chest

13. trachea; windpipe

B. Build Words

1. -scope   laryngoscope

3. -tomy   thoracotomy

5. -ator   ventilator

7. -stomy   tracheostomy

C. Define Abbreviations

1. auscultation and percussion

3. endotracheal tube

5. room air

Dive In: Medical Language Exercises

4.1 Anatomy

Matching Exercise

6, 11, 2, 3, 5, 7, 8, 9, 1, 10, 4

Circle Exercise

1. lobe   **3.** hilum   **5.** epiglottis

True or False Exercise

1. F   **3.** F

Plural Noun and Adjective Exercise

1.   nasal

3. bronchi   bronchial

5.   hilar

7. lobes   lobar

9.   pharyngeal

11.   septal

13.   tracheal

Dividing Words Exercise

1. thorac/o-   -ic

3. epi-   glott/o-   -ic

5. pulmon/o-   -ary

7. re-   spir/o-   -atory

Spelling Exercise

1. tracheal   **5.** parietal

3. bronchiolar

4.2 Physiology

Circle Exercise

1. surfactant   **3.** carbon dioxide

True or False Exercise

1. T   **3.** T

Dividing Words Exercise

1. re-   spir/o-   -ation

3.   phren/o-   -ic

5.   metabol/o-   -ism

Spelling Exercise

1. cellular   **5.** exhalation

3. intercostal

4.3 Diseases

Matching Exercise

3, 6, 4, 1, 2, 7, 8, 5

True or False Exercise

1. T
3. F
5. T
7. T
9. F

Adjective Exercise

1. apneic
3. cancerous or malignant
5. dyspneic

Dividing Words Exercise

1. an-	ox/o-	-ia
3.	asthm/o-	-atic
5. circum-	or/o-	-al
7. em-	phys/o-	-ema
9. hyper-	capn/o-	-ia
11.	pleur/o-	-isy
13.	pneum/o-	-thorax

Spelling Exercise

1. infection
3. asthmatic
5. atelectasis
7. influenza
9. bronchopneumonia
11. orthopnea
13. cyanotic

4.4 Laboratory, Diagnostic, and Radiologic Procedures

Matching Exercise

7, 2, 8, 6, 9, 10, 3, 5, 1, 4

True or False Exercise

1. T
3. T

Dividing Words Exercise

1.	arteri/o-	-al
3. poly-	somn/o-	-graphy
5.	tom/o-	-graphy

Spelling Exercise

1. arterial
3. polysomography
5. radiography

4.5 Medical Procedures, Drugs, and Surgical Procedures

Matching Exercise

3, 7, 1, 6, 5, 4, 2

Circle Exercise

1. lung
3. productive coughs

True or False Exercise

1. F
3. T
5. T

Dividing Words Exercise

1. anti-	bi/o-	-tic
3. endo-	trache/o-	-al
5. in-	tub/o-	-ation
7. re-	spir/o-	-ator
9.	spir/o-	-metry

Spelling Exercise

1. cannula
3. auscultation
5. laryngoscope
7. bronchoscopy
9. tracheostomy

Immerse Yourself: Analyze Medical Reports

Electronic Patient Record #1

1. asthma
3. A stethoscope
5. a. ox/i-   oxygen
      -meter   instrument used to measure
   b. auscult/o-   listening
      -ation   being; having; process
7. metered-dose inhaler

Electronic Patient Record #2

1. shortness of breath
3. bronch/o-   bronchus
   -scopy   process of using an instrument to examine
5. a. culture and sensitivity
   b. chronic obstructive pulmonary disease
   c. left lower lobe
7. appendectomy
9. consolidative changes, density in the LLL, patchy infiltrate
11. barrel chest
13. right-sided pneumonia

Chapter 5 : Cardiology

5.1 Practice Laps

A. Label Structures

Heart

1. right pulmonary arteries
3. superior vena cava
5. right atrium
7. inferior vena cava

9. right ventricle

11. left pulmonary arteries

13. left pulmonary veins

15. mitral valve

17. septum

Arteries

1. ascending aorta
3. abdominal aorta
5. subclavian artery
7. brachial artery

9. renal artery
11. radial artery
13. femoral artery
15. tibial artery

B. Give the Meaning of Combining Forms

1. mediastinum
3. apex; tip
5. arteriole
7. atrium
9. divide into two branches
11. heart
13. loss of consciousness
15. clavicle; collarbone
17. point; projection
19. stomach
21. ilium
23. structure with two points
25. oxygen
27. fibula
29. back of the knee
31. lung
33. clearly visible
35. body as a whole
37. shin bone; tibia
39. valve
41. blood vessel; vas deferens
43. vein

C. Build Words

1. -ac   cardiac
3. -ary   axillary
5. -ar   jugular
7. -al   mitral

9. -al   atrial
11. -ic   aortic
13. -ature   vasculature
15. -ous   venous

5.2 Practice Laps

A. Label Functions

1. atrioventricular node
3. right atrium
5. bundle branches

7. left atrium
9. Purkinje fibers

B. Give the Meaning of Combining Forms

1. bend; break
3. pull together

5. outside
7. channel; hollow cavity

C. Build Words

1. -ic   ectopic
3. -ic   systolic

5.3 Practice Laps

A. Give the Meaning of Combining Forms

1. angina
3. soft, fatty substance
5. accumulation of fluid
7. narrowed
9. block; hold back
11. muscle
13. outer aspects
15. backward flow
17. hard; sclera
19. blood clot
21. blood vessel

B. Build Words

1. -megaly   cardiomegaly
3. -ation   coarctation
5. -oma   atheroma
7. -ose   varicose
9. -ion   claudication

C. Define Abbreviations

1. coronary artery disease
3. hypertension
5. mitral valve prolapse
7. premature ventricular contraction

5.4 Practice Laps

A. Give the Meaning of Combining Forms

1. heart
3. artery
5. echo of a sound wave
7. fat; lipid
9. physical function
11. distance
13. chamber that is filled; ventricle

B. Build Words

1. -graphy   venography
3. -gram   ventriculogram
5. -gram   angiogram

C. Define Abbreviations

1. electrocardiography
3. transesophageal echocardiography

5.5 Practice Laps

A. Give the Meaning of Combining Forms

1. destroy; take away
3. aneurysm; dilatation
5. apex; tip
7. clotting
9. muscle fiber; nerve fiber
11. artificial part
13. hard; sclera
15. contracting
17. blood clot
19. valve

B. Build Words

1. -al   apical
3. -osis   anastomosis
5. -ation   resuscitation
7. -ic   systolic
9. -tome   valvulotome
11. -plasty   valvuloplasty

C. Define Abbreviations

1. blood pressure
3. cardiopulmonary resuscitation
5. point of maximum impulse

Dive In: Medical Language Exercises

5.1 Anatomy

Matching Exercise

2, 9, 7, 6, 10, 4, 8, 5, 1, 3

Circle Exercise

1. aorta
3. foramen ovale
5. upper arm

True or False Exercise

1. F	9. T
3. F	11. T
5. F	13. T
7. F	15. F

Plural Noun and Adjective Exercise

1.   apical

3.	arteries	arterial
5.		cardiac
7.		pericardial
9.	valves	valvular
11.	veins	venous

Dividing Words Exercise

1.	arteriol/o-	-ar	
3.	bifurcat/o-	-ion	
5.	circulat/o-	-ory	
7.	de-	oxygen/o-	-ated
9.	pulmon/o-	-ary	
11.	tri-	cusp/o-	-id

Spelling Exercise

1. cardiovascular   5. thoracic
3. pericardium   7. vasoconstriction

5.2 Physiology

Matching Exercise

8, 9, 2, 6, 3, 1, 5, 4, 7

Circle Exercise

1. K^+
3. calcium

True or False Exercise

1. F   3. F

Dividing Words Exercise

1.	re-	polar/o-	-ization
3.	de-	polar/o-	-ization
5.	ectop/o-	-ic	
7.	systol/o-	-ic	

Spelling Exercise

1. Purkinje   5. ectopic
3. depolarization

5.3 Diseases

Matching Exercise

10, 6, 8, 3, 13, 11, 2, 15, 12, 7, 9, 4, 1, 5, 14

Circle Exercise

1. bradycardia   7. angina pectoris
3. aneurysm   9. heart attack
5. pulmonary edema

True or False Exercise

1. F	5. T
3. T	7. F

Adjective Exercise

1. bradycardic
3. arteriosclerotic
5. hypertensive

Dividing Words Exercises

1.	isch/o-	-emia
3.	ather/o-	-oma
5.	cardi/o-	-megaly
7. hyper-	cholesterol/o-	-emia
9.	infarct/o-	-ion
11.	phleb/o-	-itis

Spelling Exercise

1. murmur
3. anginal

5. atherosclerosis
7. cardiomyopathy
9. phlebitis
11. thrombophlebitis

5.4 Laboratory, Diagnostic, and Radiologic Procedures

Matching Exercise

5, 10, 9, 3, 8, 1, 7, 6, 4, 2

Circle Exercise

1. V_1–V_6
3. echocardiography
5. sound waves

Laboratory Test Exercise

CPT CODE		PANELS AND PROFILES	CPT CODE		PANELS AND PROFILES
80051		Electrolyte panel	85018		Hemoglobin (Hgb)
80053		Metabolic panel, comprehensive	83036		Hemoglobin A1c
80061	✓	Lipid panel	82728		Iron, total
80069		Renal function panel	83615		Lactate dehydrogenase (LDH)
		BLOOD TESTS	83721	✓	LDL lipoprotein
82040		Albumin	83655		Lead, blood
82247		Bilirubin, total	85730		Partial thromboplastin time (PTT)
86900		Blood type	85610		Prothrombin time (PT)
86140	✓	C-reactive protein (CRP)	84443		Thyroid-stimulating hormone (TSH)
82465	✓	Cholesterol, total	84436		Thyroxine (T4), total
82025		Complete blood count (CBC)	84478	✓	Triglycerides
82553	✓	Creatine kinase (CK-MB)	84480		Triiodothyronine (T3), total
82565		Creatinine, blood	84484	✓	Troponin
80162	✓	Digoxin drug level	84550		Uric acid
82947		Glucose, fasting	83719	✓	VLDL lipoprotein
82951		Glucose tolerance test	85025		White blood cell (WBC) count with differential
83718	✓	HDL lipoprotein			
85014		Hematocrit (HCT)			

5.5 Medical Procedures, Drugs, and Surgical Procedures

Matching Exercise

6, 3, 7, 4, 10, 8, 12, 1, 11, 5, 9, 2

Circle Exercise

1. diastolic
3. anastomosis
5. thrombolytic drug

True or False Exercise

1. T   3. T   5. T

Dividing Words Exercise

1. trans-	lumin/o-	-al
3.	aneurysm/o-	-ectomy
5. anti-	coagul/o-	-ant
7. de-	fibrill/o-	-ator
9.	resuscit/o-	-ation
11.	steth/o-	-scope

Proofreading and Spelling Exercise

1. sphygmomanometer
3. atheromatous
5. tachycardia
7. angioplasty
9. infarction

Immerse Yourself: Analyze Medical Reports

Electronic Patient Record #1

1. Blood pressure of 150/100
3. Resuscitated by the paramedics doing CPR

Electronic Patient Record #2

1. **a.** Coronary care unit
   b. Congestive heart failure
   c. Cardiopulmonary resuscitation
   d. Hypertension
3. **a.** CHF
   b. HTN
5. Right side
7. Congestive heart failure

You Write The Medical Report

1. angina pectoris, diaphoresis
3. arteriosclerosis, atherosclerosis, claudication, necrosis

Chapter 6 : Hematology and Immunology

6.1 Practice Laps

A. Label Structures

Cells and Structures

1. eosinophil
3. lymphocyte
5. monocyte

Lymphatic System

1. tonsils and adenoids
3. mediastinal lymph nodes
5. appendix and Peyer patches
7. cervical lymph nodes
9. spleen
11. red bone marrow

B. Give the Meaning of Combining Forms

1. alkaline; base of a structure
3. electricity
5. eosin; red, acidic dye
7. granule
9. blood
11. white
13. one; single

15. not taking part
17. oxygen; quick
19. small network
21. blood clot

C. Build Words

1. -blast   erythroblast
3. -cyte   leukocyte
5. -poiesis   hematopoiesis
7. -phil   neutrophil
9. -cyte   thrombocyte
11. -cyte   reticulocyte
13. -phil   basophil
15. -lyte   electrolyte

6.2 Practice Laps

A. Give the Meaning of Combining Forms

1. poison
3. other work; strange activity
5. clotting
7. fiber
9. blood
11. white
13. one millionth; small
15. disease
17. guarding; protecting
19. press down

B. Build Words

1. -stasis   hemostasis
3. -in   fibrin
5. -ity   immunity
7. -ic   systemic
9. -cyte   phagocyte

6.3 Practice Laps

A. Give the Meaning of Combining Forms

1. gland
3. color
5. cell
7. embolus; occluding plug
9. blood
11. white
13. large
15. one; single
17. normal; usual
19. attraction to; fondness for
21. infection

23. blood clot

25. blood vessel

B. Build Words

1. -ation   coagulation

3. -osis   thrombosis

5. -emia   septicemia

7. -pathy   coagulopathy

9. -emia   leukemia

11. -lysis   hemolysis

C. Define Abbreviations

1. acquired immunodeficiency syndrome

3. deep venous thrombosis

5. human immunodeficiency virus

6.4 Practice Laps

A. Give the Meaning of Combining Forms

1. different; distinct

3. blood vessel; lymphatic vessel

5. electricity

7. comprehensive; shaped like a globe

9. blood

11. lymph; lymphatic system

B. Build Words

1. -ation   agglutination   **3.** -crit   hematocrit

C. Define Abbreviations

1. activated clotting time   **5.** prothrombin time

3. hematocrit

6.5 Practice Laps

A. Give the Meaning of Combining Forms

1. breathe in; suck in   **15.** vein

3. self   **17.** protein

5. cut   **19.** spleen

7. cortex; outer region   **21.** blood clot

9. gift; giving   **23.** move and put in
                                        another place
11. pouring
                                   25. vein
13. block; hold back

B. Build Words

1. -ion   donation

3. -ity   immunity

5. -ectomy   splenectomy

7. -opsy   biopsy

9. -ation   transplantation

11. -ation   aspiration

Dive In: Medical Language Exercises

6.1 Anatomy

Matching Exercise

6, 5, 15, 7, 11, 10, 1, 3, 12, 2, 13, 4

Circle Exercise

1. erythroblast

3. eosinophils

5. neutrophil

True or False Exercise

1. T   **7.** T

3. T   **9.** T

5. T

Dividing Words Exercise

1. erythro-   -poietin

3. electr/o-   -lyte

5. hem/o-   -globin

7. lymph/o-   -cyte

9. neutr/o-   -phil

Spelling Exercise

1. electrolyte   **5.** agranulocyte

3. hemoglobin   **7.** lymphoid

6.2 Physiology

Matching Exercise

10, 3, 12, 4, 6, 14, 8, 7, 13, 9, 1, 11, 5, 2

Circle Exercise

1. fibrin   **5.** disease

3. thrombus

True or False Exercise

1. T   **5.** F

3. T

Dividing Words Exercise

1.   loc/o-   -al

3.   aller/o-   -gen

5.   hem/o-   -stasis

7.   immun/o-   -ity

9.   path/o-   -gen

11.   system/o-   -ic

Spelling Exercise

1. allergy

3. thrombocyte

5. pathogen

6.3 Diseases

Matching Exercise

3, 2, 7, 4, 9, 12, 13, 5, 6, 11, 10, 1, 14, 8

Circle Exercise

1. sepsis
3. red blood cells
5. intrinsic factor

True or False Exercise

1. T
3. T
5. T
7. F
9. T
11. F

Dividing Words Exercise

1. hypo-   chrom/o-   -ic
3.   embol/o-   -ism
5.   hem/o-   -rrhage
7.   leuk/o-   -emia
9. pan-   cyt/o-   -penia
11.   splen/o-   -megaly

Spelling Exercise

1. anemia
3. leukemia
5. coagulopathy
7. hemophilia

6.4 Laboratory, Diagnostic, and Radiologic Procedures

Matching Exercise

5, 2, 8, 1, 7, 9, 6, 3, 4

Circle Exercise

1. ferritin level
3. electrophoresis
5. Hgb

True or False Exercise

1. T
3. F
5. F

Laboratory Test Exercise

CPT CODE		LABORATORY TESTS	CPT CODE		LABORATORY TESTS
82040	✓	Albumin	82330		Calcium
82307		Blood alcohol	82375	✓	Carboxyhemoglobin
84520		Blood urea nitrogen (BUN)	82378		Carcincembryonic antigen (CEA)
82247		Bilirubin, total	82465		Cholesterol
87040		Blood culture	85025	✓	Complete blood count (CBC) with differential
86900	✓	Blood group	84144		Progesterone
82553		Creatine kinase (CK-MB)	85610	✓	Prothrombin time (PT)
82565		Creatinine, blood	84295	✓	Sodium
82575		Creatinine clearance	84403		Testosterone, total
80051	✓	Electrolyte panel	84443		Thyroid-stimulating hormone (TSH)
82670		Estradiol	84436		Thyroxine (T4), total
82947		Glucose	84478		Triglycenides
82951		Glucose tolerance test	84481		Triodothyronine (T3), free
85014	✓	Hematocrit (HCT)	84550		Uric acid
83036		Hemoglobin A1c	81001		Urinalysis
84702		Human chorionic gonadotropin (hCG)	87086		Urine culture
82728	✓	Iron, total	85048	✓	White blood cell (WBC) count
84132		Potassium			

6.5 Medical Procedures, Drugs, and Surgical Procedures

Matching Exercise

3, 5, 7, 2, 1, 8, 4, 6

Circle Exercise

1. iliac crest of the hip bone
3. immunity
5. polio

True or False Exercise

1. T
3. F
5. F

Dividing Words Exercise

1.   aspir/o-   -ation
3.   bi/o-   -opsy
5.   erythr/o-   -poietin
7.   phleb/o-   -tomy
9.   transplant/o-   -ation

Spelling Exercise

1. donation
3. phlebotomy
5. vaccination
7. thrombolytic

Immerse Yourself: Analyze Medical Reports

Electronic Patient Record #1

1. complete blood count (CBC)
3. platelets

Electronic Patient Record #2

1. b.
3. Enlarged lymph nodes in his neck on both sides (cervical lymphadenopathy)
5. He had HIV plus now he also has an opportunistic infection of *Pneumocystis jiroveci* pneumonia, which makes a diagnosis of AIDS
7. Kaposi sarcoma

Chapter 7 : Orthopedics: Skeletal System

7.1 Practice Laps

A. Label Structures

Head

1. temporal bone
3. sphenoid bone
5. nasal bone
7. zygomatic bone
9. mandible
11. parietal bone

Foot

1. tarsal bones
3. phalanges
5. talus

Entire Body

1. clavicle
3. humerus
5. costal cartilage
7. ulna
9. phalanges
11. patella
13. tibia
15. sternum
17. vertebra
19. sacrum
21. ischium
23. femur

B. Give the Meaning of Combining Forms

1. socket of the hip joint
3. joint
5. calcaneus; heel bone
7. wrist
9. cervix; neck
11. clavicle; collarbone
13. coccyx; tailbone
15. rib
17. digit; finger; toe
19. enlarged end of long bone
21. femur; thigh bone
23. front
25. humerus; upper arm bone
27. ilium
29. tears
31. lower back
33. breast; mastoid process
35. inner region; medulla
37. back of the head; occiput
39. bone
41. palate
43. kneecap; patella
45. fibula
47. hip bone; pubis
49. sacrum
51. skeleton
53. backbone; spine
55. breastbone; sternum
57. joint membrane; synovium
59. ankle
61. chest; thorax
63. forearm bone; ulna
65. sword

C. Build Words

1. -ic   thoracic
3. -ar   mandibular
5. -ic   pelvic
7. -ous   osseous
9. -al   vertebral
11. -ar   ulnar
13. -oid   ethmoid
15. -al   cervical
17. -al   humeral
19. -al   carpal
21. -eal   coccygeal
23. -ine   palatine
25. -eal   diaphyseal
27. -oid   xiphoid
29. -oid   hyoid

D. Define Abbreviations

1. cervical vertebrae 1–7
3. lumbar vertebrae 1–5
5. first sacral vertebra

7.2 Practice Laps

A. Give the Meaning of Combining Forms

1. changing into bone
3. bone

B. Build Words

1. -clast   osteoclast
3. -blast   osteoblast

7.3 Practice Laps

A. Give the Meaning of Combining Forms

1. arising from; produced by
3. arranged in a straight line
5. joint
7. present at birth
9. bend; break up
11. blood
13. left
15. study of; word
17. displacement
19. electrolyte; mineral
21. dead body; dead tissue
23. disease
25. watery discharge
27. crooked; curved
29. blood vessel

B. Build Words

1. -oma   chondroma
3. -ure   fracture
5. -itis   arthritis
7. -pathy   arthropathy
9. -oma   osteoma
11. -phyte osteophyte

C. Define Abbreviations

1. degenerative joint disease
3. rheumatoid arthritis

7.4 Practice Laps

A. Give the Meaning of Combining Forms

1. point of light
3. density

B. Build Words

1. -graphy   arthrography
3. -graphy   tomography

C. Define Abbreviations

1. bone mineral density
3. rheumatoid factor

7.5 Practice Laps

A. Give the Meaning of Combining Forms

1. steroid
3. other; strange
5. joint
7. self
9. body
11. make stable
13. redness and warmth
15. body
17. bring back; decrease
19. absorb
21. pulling

B. Build Words

1. -etic   prosthetic
3. -ectomy   bunionectomy
5. -metry   goniometry
7. -desis   arthrodesis
9. -ation   amputation
11. -ion   reduction
13. -scopy   arthroscopy
15. -esis   prosthesis
17. -centesis arthrocentesis

C. Define Abbreviations

1. extracorporeal shock wave therapy
3. range of motion

Dive In: Medical Language Exercises

7.1 Anatomy

Matching Exercise

13, 4, 12, 10, 18, 6, 15, 9, 7, 14, 3, 17, 1, 11, 2, 16, 5, 8

Circle Exercise

1. humerus
3. ankle
5. elbow
7. clavicle

True or False Exercise

1. T
3. F
5. T

Plural Noun and Adjective Exercise

1. ligaments	ligamentous	
3. bones	bony	
	osseous	
	osteal	
5.	clavicular	
7.	coccygeal	
9. femora	femoral	
11. humeri	humeral	
13.	ischial	

15.   mandibular
17.   nasal
19.   pelvic
21.   pubic
23. ribs   costal
25. scapulae   scapular
27.   spinal (or spinous)
29.   thoracic
31. ulnae   ulnar
33.   zygomatic

Dividing Words Exercise

1.   skelet/o-   -al
3.   articul/o-   -ation
5.   cav/o-   -ity
7.   clavicul/o- -ar
9. inter- cost/o-   -al
11. I   acrim/o-   -al
13.   mast/o-   -oid
15. meta- carp/o-   -al
17. peri- oste/o-   -al
19.   sphen/o-   -oid
21.   thorac/o-   -ic

Spelling Exercise

1. parietal   5. clavicular
3. musculoskeletal   7. xiphoid

7.2 Physiology

Circle Exercise

1. calcitonin   5. parathyroid hormone
3. osteocytes

True or False Exercise

1. F   3. T   5. F

Dividing Words Exercise

1.   oste/o-   -blast
3.   ossific/o-   -ation

Spelling Exercise

1. osteoclast   3. osteocyte

7.3 Diseases

Matching Exercise

12, 10, 7, 9, 15, 1, 11, 13, 14, 8, 5, 3, 6, 4, 16, 2

Circle Exercise

1. osteomyelitis   7. hairline
3. demineralization   9. crepitus
5. pectus excavatum

True or False Exercise

1. T   9. F
3. T   11. F
5. F   13. F
7. T

Dividing Words Exercise

1.   congenit/o- -al
3. a-   vascul/o-   -ar
5. de-   gener/o-   -ative
7. dis-   locat/o-   -ion
9.   kyph/o-   -osis
11.   oste/o-   -phyte

Spelling Exercise

1. arthritis   5. arthralgia
3. fracture

7.4 Laboratory, Diagnostic, and Radiologic Procedures

Circle Exercise

1. bone densitometry   3. rheumatoid factor

True or False Exercise

1. F   3. T   5. T

Spelling Exercise

1. tomography   5. densitometry
3. scintigraphy

7.5 Medical Procedures, Drugs, and Surgical Procedures

Matching Exercise

5, 3, 1, 2, 4, 6, 7

Circle Exercise

1. goniometer
3. arthrodesis
5. orthosis
7. inhibits osteoclasts

True or False Exercise

1. T   5. T
3. T

Dividing Words Exercise

1. non-   steroid/o-   -al
3. an-   alges/o-   -ic
5.   arthr/o-   -scope
7.   goni/o-   -meter
9.   orth/o-   -osis

Spelling Exercise

1. reduction
3. prosthesis
5. bunionectomy

Related Combining Forms Exercise

1. osse/o-, oss/i-, oste/o-
3. arthr/o-, articul/o-
5. fibul/o-, perone/o-

Immerse Yourself: Analyze Medical Reports

Electronic Patient Record #1

1. dextr/o- right; sugar
   scoli/o- crooked; curved
   -osis abnormal condition; process
3. orth/o- straight
   ped/o- child
   -ist person who specializes in; thing that specializes in
5. tibia
7. vertebrae
9. right

Electronic Patient Record #2

1. the operating room
3. an orthopedic device such as an artificial joint

Chapter 8 : Orthopedics: Muscular System

8.1 Practice Laps

A. Label Structures

Body Builder

1. temporalis muscle
3. trapezius muscle
5. triceps brachii muscle
7. brachioradialis muscle
9. gastrocnemius muscle
11. frontalis muscle
13. pectoralis major muscle
15. rectus abdominis muscle
17. tibialis anterior muscle

Dancers

1. rotation
3. slight flexion

5. plantar flexion
7. pronation

B. Give the Meaning of Combining Forms

1. abdomen
3. before; front part
5. cheek
7. clavicle; collarbone
9. triangle
11. fascia
13. stomach
15. inside
17. breast; mastoid process
19. muscle
21. small circle
23. fibula
25. skeleton
27. parallel stripes
29. side of the head; temple
31. tendon
33. shin bone; tibia

C. Build Words

1. -al fascial
3. -ion insertion
5. -ar muscular
7. -ar thenar
9. -er masseter
11. -oid deltoid
13. -al bursal
15. -ation striation
17. -ism synergism

8.2 Practice Laps

A. Give the Meaning of Combining Forms

1. fiber
3. fascia
5. muscle
7. send across; send through

B. Build Words

1. -cle fascicle

8.3 Practice Laps

A. Give the Meaning of Combining Forms

1. without position or purpose
3. lack of strength
5. cancer
7. pull together
9. skin
11. fiber

13. redness and warmth
15. side
17. muscle
19. rod shaped
21. joint membrane; synovium
23. tendon
25. twisted position
27. tear

B. Build Words

1. -itis   fasciitis
3. -al   lateral
5. -pathy   myopathy
7. -collis   torticollis
9. -al   medial
11. -clonus   myoclonus

C. Define Abbreviations

1. cumulative trauma disorder
3. Occupational Safety and Health Administration
5. repetitive strain injury

8.4 Practice Laps

A. Give the Meaning of Combining Forms

1. electricity

B. Define Abbreviations

1. creatine phosphokinase

8.5 Practice Laps

A. Give the Meaning of Combining Forms

1. steroid
3. living organism; living tissue
5. fascia
7. give ability
9. movement
11. muscle
13. relax
15. thymus

B. Build Words

1. -osis   orthosis
3. -rrhaphy   tenorrhaphy
5. -ity   mobility
7. -opsy   biopsy
9. -tomy   fasciotomy

C. Define Abbreviations

1. Americans with Disabilities Act
3. deep tendon reflexes
5. range of motion

Dive In: Medical Language Exercises

8.1 Anatomy

Matching Exercise

4, 8, 3, 6, 10, 11, 1, 12, 9, 13, 7, 5, 2

Circle Exercise

1. origin
3. musculature
5. deltoid

True or False Exercise

1. F
3. T
5. F
7. F
9. T

Plural Noun and Adjective Exercise

1. muscles   muscular
3. bursae   bursal

Dividing Words Exercise

1.   burs/o-   -al
3. inter-   cost/o-   -al
5.   anter/o-   -ior
7.   delt/o-   -oid
9.   masset/o-   -er

Spelling Exercise

1. fascia
3. sternocleidomastoid
5. oblique

8.2 Physiology

Matching Exercise

9, 4, 1, 8, 3, 7, 5, 10, 6, 2

True or False Exercise

1. T
3. T
5. T

Spelling Exercise

1. contraction
3. neurotransmitter

8.3 Diseases

Matching Exercise

10, 2, 4, 7, 9, 11, 8, 6, 5, 1, 3, 12

Circle Exercise

1. ataxia
3. athetoid
5. Duchenne
7. bursitis

True or False Exercise

1. F	7. T
3. F	9. T
5. F	11. F

Dividing Words Exercise

1.		contus/o-	-ion
3.	a-	vuls/o-	-ion
5.		burs/o-	-itis
7.	dys-	kines/o-	-ia
9.		tort/i-	-collis
11.	poly-	myos/o-	-itis

Spelling Exercise

1. atrophic	5. polymyositis
3. contusion	

English and Medical Word Equivalents Exercise

1. bursitis
3. torticollis
5. hyperextension-hyperflexion injury
7. medial epicondylitis

8.4 Laboratory, Diagnostic, and Radiologic Procedures

True or False Exercise

1. T	3. T

8.5 Medical Procedures, Drugs, and Surgical Procedures

Matching Exercise

6, 8, 9, 1, 5, 3, 2, 7, 4

Circle Exercise

1. fibromyalgia	5. exercise
3. thymectomy	

True or False Exercise

1. T	3. T	5. T

Dividing Words Exercise

1.	non-	steroid/o-	-al
3.		mobil/o-	-ity
5.	an-	alges/o-	-ic
7.		bi/o-	-opsy

Related Combining Forms Exercise

1. kines/o-, mobil/o-, mot/o-
3. ten/o-, tendin/o-

Proofreading and Spelling Exercise

1. orthopedics	7. inflammation
3. fascia	9. biopsy
5. fibromyalgia	11. tenorrhaphy

Immerse Yourself: Analyze Medical Reports

Electronic Patient Record #1 and #2

1. my/o-   muscle
   -pathy   disease
3. right quadriceps muscle biopsy
5. three
7. red-tan
9. b.
11. when the report comes back from the Armed Forces Institute of Pathology

Chapter 9 : Neurology

9.1 Practice Laps

A. Label Structures

Lobes of the Brain

1. frontal lobe	5. cerebellum
3. parietal lobe	

Midline Section of the Brain

1. pia mater
3. dura mater
5. subarachnoid space
7. white matter of the cerebrum

Meninges

1. cerebrum	7. pons
3. gyrus	9. corpus callosum
5. hypothalamus	11. cerebellum

B. Give the Meaning of Combining Forms

1. group; set
3. toward the center
5. spider; spider web
7. sense of hearing
9. hollow space
11. cerebrum
13. cortex; outer region
15. branching structure
17. dura mater

19. brain
21. feeling; sensation
23. face
25. front
27. sense of taste
29. meninges
31. one millionth; small
33. bone marrow; myelin; spinal cord
35. nerve
37. eye
39. few; scanty
41. wall of a cavity
43. outer aspects
45. spinal nerve root
47. feeling
49. backbone; spine
51. thalamus
53. vagus nerve; wandering
55. abdomen; front
57. sight; vision

C. Build Words

1.	-al	cerebral	15.	-on	neuron
3.	-al	neural	17.	-ory	olfactory
5.	-ar	ventricular	19.	-glia	neuroglia
7.	-eal	meningeal	21.	-al	occipital
9.	-ent	efferent	23.	-or	motor
11.	-al	peripheral	25.	-oid	amygdaloid
13.	-ory	sensory	27.	-cyte	astrocyte

D. Define Abbreviations

1. central nervous system

9.2 Practice Laps

A. Give the Meaning of Combining Forms

1. cell
3. myelin
5. receive

B. Build Words

1. -ite   dendrite
3. -ated   myelinated

9.3 Practice Laps

A. Give the Meaning of Combining Forms

1. fiber
3. memory loss

5. without position or purpose
7. burning
9. cerebrum
11. unconsciousness
13. bruising
15. cranium; top part of the skull
17. dura mater
19. seizure
21. feeling; sensation
23. arrangement; structure
25. blood
27. fluid; water
29. block; keep back
31. break down; destroy
33. meninges
35. myelin
37. sleep; stupor
39. neck
41. avoidance; fear
43. paralysis
45. point of light
47. darkness
49. old age
51. fainting
53. vein

B. Build Words

1.	-itis	neuritis
3.	-cele	meningocele
5.	-oma	hematoma
7.	-ic	epileptic
9.	-oma	neuroma
11.	-ity	senility
13.	-al	syncopal
15.	-ion	concussion
17.	-oid	athetoid
19.	-pathy	neuropathy
21.	-itis	meningitis
23.	-oma	scotoma

C. Define Abbreviations

1. amyotrophic lateral sclerosis
3. cerebral palsy
5. carpal tunnel syndrome
7. delirium tremens
9. intracranial pressure
11. multiple sclerosis

13. rapid eye movement

15. spinal cord injury

17. transient ischemic attack

9.4 Practice Laps

A. Give the Meaning of Combining Forms

1. axis

3. artery

5. electricity

7. brain

9. bone marrow; myelin; spinal cord

11. feeling

13. sleep

15. backbone; spine

B. Build Words

1. -graphy   tomography

3. -ion   conduction

5. -graphy   myelography

C. Define Abbreviations

1. alpha fetoprotein

3. cerebrospinal fluid

5. electroencephalography

7. somatosensory evoked potential

9. somatosensory evoked potential

9.5 Practice Laps

A. Give the Meaning of Combining Forms

1. cortex; outer region

3. aneurysm; dilation

5. living organism; living tissue

7. skin

9. seizure

11. study of; word

13. frenzy; thin

15. sleep; stupor

17. peritoneum

19. hole; perforation

21. three dimensions

23. touch

25. chamber that is filled; ventricle

B. Build Words

1. –tomy   rhizotomy

3. -ar   lumbar

5. -opsy   biopsy

7. -ion   traction

9. -ectomy   aneurysmectomy

C. Define Abbreviations

1. Glasgow Coma Scale

3. Mini-Mental State Examination

Dive In: Medical Language Exercises

9.1 Anatomy

Matching Exercise

7, 15, 9, 13, 12, 6, 3, 1, 10, 14, 8, 6, 5, 2, 11

Circle Exercise

1. cerebrum

3. \pia mater

5. left hemisphere of the cerebrum

7. oculomotor

9. ependymal cells

11. microglia

True or False Exercise

1. T	7. F
3. F	9. F
5. T	11. T

Plural Noun and Adjective Exercise

1.	nerves	neural
3.		cerebellar
5.	gyri	
7.		spinal
9.		thalamic

Dividing Words Exercise

1.		nerv/o-	-ous
3.		arachn/o-	-oid
5.	epi-	dur/o-	-al
7.	hypo-	thalam/o-	-ic
9.		neur/o-	-glia
11.		pariet/o-	-al

Spelling Exercise

1. cerebrum	5. subarachnoid
3. occipital	

9.2 Physiology

Matching Exercise

4, 2, 1, 5, 3

Circle Exercise

1. acetylcholine
3. it provides structural support for neurons

True or False Exercise

1. T
3. T
5. T

Dividing Words Exercise

1. neur/o-   -on
3. cyt/o-   -plasm
5. myelin/o-   -ated

Spelling Exercise

1. neuron
3. neurotransmitter

9.3 Diseases

Matching Exercise

5, 11, 10, 7, 2, 8, 9, 3, 6, 1, 4

True or False Exercise

1. T
3. F
5. T
7. T

Circle Exercise

1. shingles
3. subdural hematoma
5. paresthesias
7. delirium tremens

Dividing Words Exercise

1. mal-   format/o-   -ion
3. an-   esthes/o-   -ia
5. dys-   phag/o-   -ia
7. hemi-   pleg/o-   -ic
9. intra-   crani/o-   -al
11.   mening/o-   -cele
13.   radicul/o-   -pathy
15. tri-   gemin/o-   -al

Spelling Exercise

1. ischemia
3. cephalalgia
5. dyslexia
7. spina bifida

9.4 Laboratory, Diagnostic, and Radiologic Procedures

Matching Exercise

2, 6, 4, 1, 3, 5

True or False Exercise

1. T
3. T
5. T
7. T

Circle Exercise

1. carotid duplex scan
3. positron emission tomography

9.5 Medical Procedures, Drugs, and Surgical Procedures

Matching Exercise

1, 7, 2, 11, 3, 4, 8, 6, 5, 10

True or False Exercise

1. T
3. F
5. T

Circle Exercise

1. diskectomy
3. manometer
5. craniotomy

Dividing Words Exercise

1.   cortic/o-   -steroid
3.   aneurysm/o-   -ectomy
5.   bi/o-   -opsy
7. endo-   arter/o-   -ectomy
9. trans-   cutane/o-   -ous

Spelling Exercise

1. Babinski
3. anticonvulsant
5. craniotomy

Related Combining Forms Exercise

1. psych/o-, ment/o-
3. rhiz/o-, radicul/o-
5. epilept/o-, convuls/o-, ict/o-

Proofreading and Spelling Exercise

1. neurosurgery
3. meningioma
5. infarct
7. paralyzed
9. epilepsy

Immerse Yourself: Analyze Medical Reports

Electronic Patient Record #1

1. epilepsy
3. electroencephalography

   Electrodes are placed on the scalp and the computer records the patient's brain waves on the screen.

Electronic Patient Record #2

1. neur/o-   nerve
   log/o-   study of; word
   -ic   pertaining to

3. VER

5. paresthesias

7. **a.** light touch

   b. pinprick

   c. vibration

   d. position

   e. 2-point discrimination

9. Romberg

11. blockage of artery

13. remote memory intact; impairment of recent memory

15. coordination

17. multiple sclerosis

Chapter 10 : Urology

10.1 Practice Laps

A. Label Structures

Kidney

1. cortex

3. fibrous capsule

5. major calyx

7. ureter

Male Urinary System

1. ureter

3. penis

5. urethral meatus

7. prostatic urethra

B. Give the Meaning of Combining Forms

1. cortex; outer region

3. calyx

5. removing from the body

7. indentation

9. kidney; nephron

11. penis

13. prostate gland

15. kidney

17. ureter

19. urinary system; urine

21. bladder; fluid-filled sac

C. Build Words

1. -ory   excretory

3. -ar   hilar

5. -eal   caliceal

7. -ic   pelvic

9. -er   sphincter

11. -ic   prostatic

10.2 Practice Laps

A. Label Functions

1. glomerular capsule

3. renal arteriole

5. renal venule

7. distal convoluted tubule

B. Give the Meaning of Combining Forms

1. absorb; take in

3. away from the center or point of origin

5. urinate

7. filtering; straining

9. glomerulus

11. kidney; nephon

13. near the center or point of origin

15. produce; secrete

17. small tube

19. urinary system; urine

C. Build Words

1. -ation   urination

3. -ate   filtrate

5. -in   renin

7. -poietin   erythropoietin

9. -ule   tubule

11. -lyte   electrolyte

13. -ion   secretion

10.3 Practice Laps

A. Give the Meaning of Combining Forms

1. albumin

3. embryonic; immature

5. cancer

7. colon

9. hold together

11. urinate

13. glomerulus

15. blood

17. potassium

19. stone

21. kidney; nephron

23. night

25. protein

27. pus

29. hold back; keep

31. small tube

33. urinary system; urine

35. bladder; fluid-filled sac

B. Build Words

1. -itis   urethritis

3. -osis   necrosis

5. -ion   retention

7. -ptosis   nephroptosis

9. -itis   cystitis

11. -ic   chronic

C. Define Abbreviations

1. acute kidney injury

3. end-stage renal disease

5. urinary tract infection

10.4 Practice Laps

A. Give the Meaning of Combining Forms

1. acid; low pH

3. blood vessel; lymphatic vessel

5. bladder; fluid-filled sac; semisolid cyst

7. red

9. bend; break up

11. fluid; water

13. measurement; uterus; womb

15. bear; carry; range

17. affected by; sensitive to

19. cut; layer; slice

21. urinary system; urine

23. vein

B. Build Words

1. -ic   acidic

3. -ine   hyaline

5. -ine   alkaline

7. -cyte   erythrocyte

9. -ity   sensitivity

11. -gram   sonogram

C. Define Abbreviations

1. blood urea nitrogen

3. computerized tomography

5. intravenous pyelogram; intravenous pyelography

7. red blood cell

9. too numerous to count

11. urinalysis

13. white blood cell

10.5 Practice Laps

A. Give the Meaning of Combining Forms

1. sensation of pain

3. living organism; living tissue

5. body

7. bladder; fluid-filled sac; semisolid cyst

9. stone

11. kidney; nephron

13. hip bone; pubis

15. cut out; remove

17. sound

19. hanging

21. move and put in another place

B. Build Words

1. -ectomy   nephrectomy

3. -ization   catheterization

5. -ectomy   cystectomy

7. -scope   cystoscope

9. -ory   ambulatory

11. -scope   resectoscope

C. Define Abbreviations

1. continuous ambulatory peritoneal dialysis

3. extracorporeal shock wave lithotripsy

5. transurethral resection of the bladder

Dive In: Medical Language Exercises

10.1 Anatomy

Matching Exercise

4, 3, 7, 8, 5, 1, 6, 2

Circle Exercise

1. retroperitoneal space   5. medulla

3. urethra

True or False Exercise

1. T   3. T

Plural Noun and Adjective Exercise

1.   cortical

3. calices   caliceal

5. kidneys   renal

7.   pelvic

9. ureters   ureteral

Dividing Words Exercise

1.   urin/o-   -ary

3.   ren/o-   -al

5.   ureter/o-   -al

7.   prostat/o-   -ic

Spelling Exercise

1. prostatic   5. ureteral

3. genitourinary

10.2 Physiology

Matching Exercise

3, 4, 2, 5, 6, 1, 8, 7

Circle Exercise

1. protein metabolism   5. creatinine

3. reabsorption

True or False Exercise

1. T   3. T   5. F

Dividing Words Exercise

1.   mictur/o-   -ition

3.   electr/o-   -lyte

5. filtr/o-   -ate

7. home/o-   -stasis

9. tub/o-   -ule

Spelling Exercise

1. nephron

3. proximal

10.3 Diseases

Matching Exercise

11, 7, 10, 4, 13, 9, 12, 2, 8, 1, 3, 5, 6

Circle Exercise

1. a kidney stone

3. Drooping

5. blood

True or False Exercise

1. T   **7.** F

3. T   **9.** F

5. T   **11.** T

Dividing Words Exercise

1. cancer/o-   -ous

3. cali/o-   -ectasis

5. cyst/o-   -cele

7. necr/o-   -osis

9. nephr/o-   -ptosis

11. ur/o-   -emia

Spelling Exercise

1. colic

3. nephropathy

5. necrosis

7. cystitis

9. dysuria

10.4 Laboratory, Diagnostic, and Radiologic Procedures

Matching Exercise

4, 3, 5, 7, 6, 2, 8, 1

Circle Exercise

1. cystometer

3. dehydration

5. UA

7. sound waves

True or False Exercise

1. T

3. F

5. F

Dividing Words Exercise

1.   sensitiv/o-   -ity

3. de-   hydr/o-   -ation

5. intra-   ven/o-   -ous

7. re-   fract/o-   -meter

Laboratory Test Exercise

CPT CODE		LABORATORY TESTS	CPT CODE		LABORATORY TESTS
82040	✓	Albumin	85014		Hematocrit (HCT)
82307		Blood alcohol	83036		Hemoglobin A1c
84520	✓	Blood urea nitrogen (BUN)	84702		Human chorionic gonadotropin (hO3)
82247		Bilirubin, total	82728		Iron, total
87040		Blood culture	84132		Potassium
86900		Blood group	84144		Progesterone
82330		Calcium	85610		Prothrombin time (PT)
82375		Carboxyhemoglobin	84295		Sodium
82378		Carcinoembryonic antigen(CEA)	84403		Testosterone, total
82465		Cholesterol	84443		Thyroid-stimulating hormone(TSH)
85025		Complete blood count (CBC)	84436		Thyroxine (T4), total
82553		Creathe kinase, MB	84478		Triglycerides
82565	✓	Creatinine, blood	84481		Trilodothyronine (T3), free
82575	✓	Creatinine clearance	84550	✓	Uric acid
80051		Electrolyte panel	81001	✓	Urinalysis
82670		Estradiol	87086	✓	Urine culture
82947		Glucose	85048		White blood cell (WBC) count with differential
82951		Glucose tolerance test			

10.5 Medical Procedures, Drugs, and Surgical Procedures

Matching Exercise

4, 8, 6, 2, 5, 1, 7, 3

Circle Exercise

1. I&O
3. sound waves
5. fistula

True or False Exercise

1. F
3. T

Dividing Words Exercise

1. anti-   bi/o-   -tic
3.   cyst/o-   -ectomy
5.   cyst/o-   -scope
7. per-   cutane/o-   -ous
9. ultra-   son/o-   -ic

Spelling Exercise

1. resection
3. cystectomy
5. diuretic
7. nephrolithotomy

Immerse Yourself: Analyze Medical Reports

Electronic Patient Record

1. ur/o-   urinary system; urine
   log/o-   study of; word
   -ist   person who specializes in
3. hemat/o-   blood
   ur/o-   urinary system; urine
   -ia   condition; state; thing
5. UTI
7. catheterized
9. to know that the pain was not from appendicitis
11. to know that any blood in the urine was not from menstruation
13. to know that the pain was not from pregnancy

Related Combining Forms Exercise

1. cyst/o-, vesic/o-
3. lith/o-, calcul/o-

Research Medical Words

On-The-Job Challenge Exercise

Strangury is blockage or irritation at the base of the bladder with severe pain and a strong urge to urinate.

Sound-Alike Words Exercise

1. Kidney stone
   Heel bone in the foot
3. Outer layer of tissue of the kidney
   Outer layer of tissue of the adrenal gland

Chapter 11 : Male Reproductive Medicine

11.1 Practice Laps

A. Label Structures

1. vas deferens
3. corpus cavernosum
5. glans penis
7. ejaculatory duct
9. epididymis
11. scrotum

B. Give the Meaning of Combining Forms

1. glans penis
3. testis
5. stand up
7. genitalia
9. groin
11. testis
13. testis
15. perineum
17. scrotum
19. sperm; spermatozoon
21. sperm; spermatozoon
23. testis
25. tube
27. urinary system; urine

C. Build Words

1. -al   genital
3. -al   scrotal
5. -ad   gonad
7. -al   perineal
9. -ic   spermatic
11. -ic   prostatic
13. -ile   penile

11.2 Practice Laps

A. Give the Meaning of Combining Forms

1. beginning of being an adult
3. expel suddenly
5. sac-like structure
7. decrease in number
9. sexual intercourse
11. sperm; spermatozoon

B. Build Words

1. -ence   adolescence
3. -cyte   spermatocyte
5. -ion   erection

11.3 Practice Laps

A. Give the Meaning of Combining Forms

1. gland
3. cancer
5. spherical bacterium
7. hidden
9. testis
11. conceive; form
13. female; woman
15. cancer
17. few; scanty
19. testis
21. sexual intercourse
23. persistent erection
25. sperm; spermatozoon
27. development
29. varicose vein

B. Build Words

1.	-itis	prostatitis
3.	-ancy	malignancy
5.	-osis	phimosis
7.	-oma	seminoma
9.	-rrhea	gonorrhea

C. Define Abbreviations

1. acquired immunodeficiency syndrome
3. Centers for Disease Control and Prevention
5. gonococcus
7. sexually transmitted disease

11.4 Practice Laps

A. Give the Meaning of Combining Forms

1. shape
3. phosphate
5. sound

B. Build Words

| 1. | -ity | motility |
| 3. | -gram | sonogram |

C. Define Abbreviations

1. fluorescent treponemal antibody absorption
3. prostate-specific antigen
5. transrectal ultrasonography

11.5 Practice Laps

A. Give the Meaning of Combining Forms

1. male
3. living organism; living tissue
5. digit; finger; toe
7. remove the main part
9. prostate gland
11. urethra
13. virus

B. Build Words

1.	-opsy	biopsy
3.	-ectomy	orchiectomy
5.	-ectomy	vasectomy
7.	-scope	resectoscope
9.	-ectomy	prostatectomy
11.	-therapy	cryotherapy

C. Define Abbreviations

1. biopsy
3. holmium laser enucleation of the prostate
5. photoselective vaporization of the prostate
7. transurethral microwave therapy
9. transurethral resection of the prostate

Dive In: Medical Language Exercises

11.1 Anatomy

Matching Exercise

7, 4, 9, 6, 10, 11, 2, 3, 5, 1, 8

Circle Exercise

1. gonads
3. 23
5. foreskin

True or False Exercise

1. T
3. T

Plural Noun and Adjective Exercise

1.	corpora cavernosa	
3.		perineal
5.	testicles	testicular
7.		spermatic
9.		prostatic
11.		urethral

Dividing Words Exercise

1.	perine/o-	-al
3.	genit/o-	-al
5.	gon/o-	-ad
7.	semin/o-	-al

Spelling Exercise

1. epididymis
3. testicular
5. bulbouourethral

11.2 Physiology

Circle Exercise

1. meiosis
3. gamete
5. spermatocyte

True or False Exercise

1. T
3. F

Dividing Words Exercise

1. folli/o- -cle
3. mei/o- -osis
5. ejacul/o- -ation

Spelling Exercise

1. sexual
3. Spermatogenesis

11.3 Diseases

Matching Exercise

2, 4, 7, 9, 1, 8, 10, 5, 6, 3

Circle Exercise

1. chordee
3. infertility
5. impotence

True or False Exercise

1. T
3. T

Dividing Words Exercise

1. cancer/o- -ous
3. dys- pareun/o- -ia
5. epi- spad/o- -ias
7. hyper- plas/o- -ia
9. malign/o- -ancy
11. phim/o- -osis
13. priap/o- -ism
15. semin/o- -oma

Spelling Exercise

1. infertility
3. varicocele
5. adenocarcinoma
7. chordee
9. phimosis
11. gonorrhea

11.4 Laboratory, Diagnostic, and Radiologic Procedures

Matching Exercise

4, 7, 5, 1, 3, 6, 2

Circle Exercise

1. PSA
3. DNA analysis
5. TRUS

Dividing Words Exercise

1. phosphat/o- -ase
3. ultra- son/o- -graphy
5. morph/o- -logy

Spelling Exercise

1. hormone
3. motility

11.5 Medical Procedures, Drugs, and Surgical Procedures

Matching Exercise

6, 3, 2, 1, 4, 5

Circle Exercise

1. prepuce
3. vasovasostomy

True or False Exercise

1. F
3. T
5. F

Dividing Words Exercise

1. anti- bi/o- -tic
3. bi/o- -opsy
5. embol/o- -ization
7. trans- urethr/o- -al

Spelling Exercise

1. antiviral
3. aspiration
5. vasectomy

Immerse Yourself: Analyze Medical Reports

Electronic Patient Record #1

1. Congenital condition in which the opening of the foreskin is too small
3. His enlarged prostate gland blocks the prostatic urethra and the bladder cannot empty fully.
5. Holmium laser enucleation of the prostate

Electronic Patient Record #2

1. orchi/o- testis
-pexy process of fixing in place
3. back
5. suprapubic skin fold; scrotum
7. under the skin
9. before

You Create The Electronic Record

1. immunodeficiency; saliva; antiretroviral

Chapter 12 : Gynecology and Obstetrics

12.1 Practice Laps

A. Label Structures

External Female Genital Area

1. mons pubis
3. clitoris

5. vaginal introitus

7. vulva

9. anus

Uterus and Ovary

1. uterine tube

3. intrauterine cavity

5. myometrium

7. cervical canal

9. lumen of uterine tube

11. follicle at time of ovulation

13. fimbriae

15. uterine cervix

B. Give the Meaning of Combining Forms

1. hollow space

3. small, circular area

5. vagina

7. vulva

9. uterine tube

11. bending

13. milk

15. ovum; spermatozoon

17. inside

19. milk

21. lobe of an organ

23. breast

25. uterus; womb

27. muscle

29. ovary

31. egg; ovum

33. egg; ovum

35. produce

37. urethra

39. urinary system; urine

41. vagina

C. Build Words

1. -ary   mammary

3. -cyte   oocyte

5. -ar   areolar

7. -ity   cavity

9. -ar   vulvar

11. -al   adnexal

13. -al   labial

15. -ar   vulvar

D. Define Abbreviations

1. genitourinary

3. obstetrics

12.2 Practice Laps

A. Give the Meaning of Combining Forms

1. sex

3. beginning of being an adult

5. head

7. conceive; form

9. blue

11. embryo; immature form

13. female

15. fetus

17. close relationship

19. conception to birth

21. female; woman

23. block; keep back

25. decrease in number

27. monthly discharge of blood

29. birth

31. egg; ovum

33. oxygen; quick

35. childbirth; labor

37. placenta

39. growing up

41. childbirth; labor

43. navel; umbilicus

B. Build Words

1. -ation   ovulation

3. -ation   menstruation

5. -ation   lactation

7. -ion   conception

9. -ic   embryonic

11. -ization   fertilization

13. -al   placental

15. -ment   effacement

17. -ion   gestation

19. -cle   follicle

21. -ion   conception

23. -ion   dilation

C. Define Abbreviations

1. follicle-stimulating hormone

3. human chorionic gonadotropin

12.3 Practice Laps

A. Give the Meaning of Combining Forms

1. vagina

3. gland

5. bilirubin

7. *Candida*; yeast

9. head

11. press down

13. outside

15. fiber

17. conception to birth

19. fluid-filled sacs

21. redness and warmth

23. smooth

25. cancer

27. black

29. monthly discharge of blood

31. measurement; uterus; womb
33. neck
35. egg; ovum
37. cessation
39. bear; carry; range
41. formation; growth
43. pus
45. excessive discharge; excessive flow
47. connective tissue
49. childbirth; labor
51. tube

B. Build Words

1. -itis   vaginitis
3. -salpinx   hydrosalpinx
5. -ant   malignant
7. -itis   salpingitis
9. -form   hydatidiform
11. -salpinx   hemosalpinx
13. -oma   carcinoma
15. -cele   cystocele
17. -ory   inflammatory
19. -ion   abortion

C. Define Abbreviations

1. appropriate for gestational age
3. carcinoma *in situ*
5. dysfunctional uterine bleeding
7. human epidermal growth factor receptor 2
9. infant respiratory distress syndrome
11. large for gestational age
13. premenstrual dysphoric disorder
15. progesterone receptor positive
17. spontaneous abortion

12.4 Practice Laps

A. Give the Meaning of Combining Forms

1. wall of a cavity
3. cancer
5. color
7. cell
9. uterus; womb
11. new
13. receive
15. sound
17. dry

B. Build Words

1. -graphy   mammography
3. -centesis   amniocentesis
5. -logy   cytology
7. -tic   genetic

C. Define Abbreviations

1. alpha fetoprotein
3. biparietal diameter
5. cervical intraepithelial neoplasia
7. chorionic villus sampling
9. lecithin/sphingomyelin (ratio)
11. magnetic resonance imaging

12.5 Practice Laps

A. Give the Meaning of Combining Forms

1. bring back; decrease
3. stop prematurely
5. create an opening between two structures
7. increase in size or degree
9. cut
11. cone
13. cold
15. cell
17. cut apart
19. embolus; occluding plug
21. vulva
23. female
25. fundus; part farthest from the opening
27. uterus; womb
29. insert; put in
31. abdomen
33. bind; tie up
35. study of; word
37. breast
39. hand
41. many
43. none
45. ovary
47. hanging down
49. body
51. first
53. uterine tube
55. three dimensions
57. hanging
59. therapy; treatment
61. tube

B. Build Words

1. -tomy   amniotomy
3. -osis   anastomosis
5. -gen   estrogen

7. -ectomy   salpingectomy
9. -scopy   laparoscopy
11. -ectomy   oophorectomy
13. -scopy   colposcopy
15. -rrhaphy   colporrhaphy
17. -tomy   episiotomy
19. -scopy   culdoscopy
21. -plasty   mammoplasty
23. -ation   augmentation

C. Define Abbreviations

1. abortion
3. biophysical profile
5. bilateral salpingo-oophorectomy
7. deep inferior epigastric perforator (flap)
9. estimated date of birth
11. estimated date of delivery
13. gamete intrafallopian transfer
15. intracytoplasmic sperm injection
17. loop electrocautery excision procedure
19. nonsteroidal anti-inflammatory drug
21. therapeutic abortion
23. transverse rectus abdominis muscle
25. zygote intrafallopian transfer

Dive In: Medical Language Exercises

12.1 Anatomy

Matching Exercise

4, 8, 4, 1, 6, 7, 8, 7, 9, 1, 10, 4, 9, 1, 2, 8, 3, 5

Circle Exercise

1. clitoris   5. Bartholin's glands
3. endometrium

True or False Exercise

1. T   5. T
3. F   7. F

Plural Noun and Adjective Exercise

1. labia   labial
3.   cervical
5.   fundal
7. ova
9.   vaginal

Dividing Words Exercise

1.   vulv/o-   -ar

3.   genit/o-   -al
5.   o/o-   -cyte
7. intra-   uter/o-   -ine
9.   lob/o-   -ule

Spelling Exercise

1. Internal   3. uterine   5. perineum

Related Combining Forms Exercise

1. mast/o-, mamm/a-, mamm/o-
3. gynec/o-, estr/a-, estr/o-
5. oophor/o-, ovari/o-
7. colp/o-, vagin/o-

12.2 Physiology

Matching Exercise

13, 5, 10, 1, 7, 9, 12, 2, 6, 8, 11, 3, 4

Matching Exercise

6, 3, 8, 7, 4, 2, 5, 1

True or False Exercise

1. T   7. F
3. F   9. T
5. F   11. T

Circle Exercise

1. estradiol   5. mitosis
3. proliferative phase   7. parturition

Dividing Words Exercise

1.   sex/o-   -ual
3.   folli/o-   -cle
5. pre-   nat/o-   -al
7.   o/o-   -cyte
9.   concept/o-   -ion
11. post-   nat/o-   -al

Spelling Exercise

1. puberty   5. fertilization
3. oogenesis

12.3 Diseases

Matching Exercise

1, 7, 4, 8, 9, 13, 2, 6, 11, 12, 10, 3, 5

True or False Exercise

1. T   9. F
3. F   11. F
5. T   13. F
7. F   15. F

Circle Exercise

1.	breasts	7.	hemosalpinx
3.	ovarian	9.	prolapsed cord
5.	candidiasis	11.	dyspareunia

Dividing Words Exercise

1.		hem/o-	-rrhage
3.	an-	ovul/o-	-ation
5.	a-	men/o-	-rrhea
7.	pre-	menstru/o-	-al
9.	dys-	pareun/o-	-ia
11.		hem/o-	-salpinx

Spelling Exercise

1.	preeclampsia	5.	mastitis
3.	dysmenorrhea		

12.4 Laboratory, Diagnostic, and Radiologic Procedures

Matching Exercise

6, 3, 8, 5, 2, 4, 7, 1, 9

True or False Exercise

1.	F	3.	F

Circle Exercise

1. antibodies
3. alpha fetoprotein
5. estradiol hormone

12.5 Medical Procedures, Drugs, and Surgical Procedures

Matching Exercise

11, 9, 12, 4, 1, 10, 7, 2, 3, 5, 6, 8

True or False Exercise

1.	F	5.	T
3.	F	7.	T

Circle Exercise

1. speculum
3. BPP
5. breast

Dividing Words Exercise

1.	re-	construct/o-	-ive
3.		amni/o-	-tomy
5.	dys-	men/o-	-rrhea
7.	retro-	vers/o-	-ion

Spelling Exercise

1.	anastomosis	5.	amniotomy
3.	mastectomy		

Immerse Yourself: Analyze Medical Reports

Electronic Patient Record #1

1. Menorrhagia: A menstrual period with excessively heavy flow or a menstrual period that lasts longer than 7 days

   Oligomenorrhea: A menstrual period with very light flow or infrequent menstrual cycles (longer than 35 days before the next cycle begins) in a woman who previously had normal menstruation

   Dysmenorrhea: Painful menstruation

   Dyspareunia: Painful or difficult sexual intercourse or intercourse with postcoital pain.

3. No. Because she had a tubal ligation.
5. Procedure that uses a magnifying, lighted scope to visually examine the vagina and cervix
7. FHS: follicle-stimulating hormone

   LH: luteinizing hormone

Electronic Patient Record #2

1. AGA: appropriate for gestational age

   EDB: estimated date of birth

   EGA: estimated gestational age

   NICU: neonatal intensive care unit

   SAB: spontaneous abortion

3. gestat/o-   conception to birth

   -ion   action; condition

   -al   pertaining to

5. NSVD
7. version
9. molding
11. The anterior fontanel is on the top of the head. The smaller posterior fontanel is at the back of the head.
13. The mother had a temperature of 103.2 degrees. The newborn had a temperature of 101.2 degrees.

Proofreading and Spelling Exercise

1.	gynecologic	7.	amniocentesis
3.	uterus	9.	hysterectomy
5.	obstetrical		

You Create The Electronic Medical Record

1. failure of lactation
3. leukorrhea, yeast, antiyeast
5. infertility, salpingitis, polycystic, dyspareunia, laparoscopy, endometriosis

Chapter 13 : Endocrinology

13.1 Practice Laps

A. Label Structures

Endocrine Glands

1. thyroid gland
3. pancreas
5. ovary
7. hypothalamus
9. thymus

Thyroid and Parathyroid Glands

1. thyroid cartilage of the larynx
3. isthmus
5. left lobe of thyroid gland

B. Give the Meaning of Combining Forms

1. electrolyte; mineral
3. adrenal gland
5. lead to
7. before; front part
9. calcium
11. secrete
13. female
15. sac-like structure
17. gland
19. glucose; sugar
21. gonad; ovary; testis
23. hormone
25. insulin
27. iodine
29. inner region; medulla
31. black
33. ovary
35. pancreas
37. pituitary gland
39. body
41. exciting; strengthening
43. testis
45. rage; thymus
47. shield-shaped structure; thyroid gland
49. pressure; tone
51. urinary system; urine

C. Build Words

1. -in   insulin
3. -crine   endocrine

5. -cle   follicle
7. -ary   pituitary
9. -stasis   homeostasis
11. -gen   androgen
13. -ar   testicular
15. -ic   pancreatic
17. -ior   anterior

D. Define Abbreviations

1. adrenocorticotropic hormone
3. follicle-stimulating hormone
5. luteinizing hormone
7. prolactin
9. thyroid-stimulating hormone

13.2 Practice Laps

A. Give the Meaning of Combining Forms

1. opposing effect
3. same
5. block; hold back
7. exciting; strengthening

B. Build Words

1. -or   receptor
3. -ism   antagonism
5. -stasis   homeostasis

13.3 Practice Laps

A. Give the Meaning of Combining Forms

1. withstand the effect of
3. extremity; highest point
5. adrenal gland
7. calcium
9. color
11. diabetes
13. conceive; form
15. genitalia
17. glucose; sugar
19. female; woman
21. insulin
23. milk
25. month
27. mucus-like substance
29. childbirth; labor
31. pituitary gland
33. shield-shaped structure; thyroid gland
35. poison
37. uterus; womb

B. Build Words

1. -itis   thyroiditis
3. -ation   lactation
5. -rrhea   galactorrhea
7. -megaly   acromegaly
9. -al   congenital
11. -ty   puberty
13. -oma   carcinoma

C. Define Abbreviations

1. adrenocorticotropic hormone
3. adult-onset diabetes mellitus
5. diabetic ketoacidosis
7. follicle-stimulating hormone
9. insulin-dependent diabetes mellitus
11. latent autoimmune diabetes in adults
13. luteinizing hormone
15. prolactin
17. syndrome of inappropriate antidiuretic hormone

13.4 Practice Laps

A. Give the Meaning of Combining Forms

1. action
3. shaped like a globe
5. forearm bone; radius; x-rays
7. shield-shaped structure; thyroid gland

B. Define Abbreviations

1. antidiuretic hormone
3. fasting blood glucose
5. follicle-stimulating hormone
7. growth hormone
9. luteinizing hormone
11. radioactive iodine uptake
13. thyroid-stimulating hormone

13.5 Practice Laps

A. Give the Meaning of Combining Forms

1. cortex; outer region
3. living organism; living tissue
5. pituitary gland
7. sphenoid bone; sphenoid sinus
9. shield-shaped structure; thyroid gland

B. Build Words

1. -ectomy   lobectomy
3. -ectomy   hypophysectomy
5. -ectomy   adrenalectomy

Dive In: Medical Language Exercises

13.1 Anatomy

Matching Exercise

1, 10, 11, 7, 4, 9, 1, 6, 2, 6, 2, 5, 8, 3, 8

Circle Exercise

1. adrenal medulla
3. parathyroid glands
5. thymus
7. melatonin
9. OXT

True or False Exercise

1. F   5. T
3. T

Plural Noun and Adjective Exercise

1.	glands	glandular
3.	hormones	hormonal
5.		pancreatic
7.	medullae	medullary
9.	testes	testicular

Dividing Words Exercise

1.		anter/o-	-ior
3.		home/o-	-stasis
5.		hormon/o-	-al
7.		end/o-	-crine
9.	pro-	lact/o-	-in
11.		melaton/o-	-in
13.	para-	thyr/o-	-oid
15.		glyc/o-	-gen

Spelling Exercise

1. posterior   5. oxytocin
3. homeostasis   7. epinephrine

Related Combining Forms Exercise

1. andr/o-, viril/o-   3. galact/o-, lact/o-

13.2 Physiology

Matching Exercise

4, 1, 5, 2, 3

Circle Exercise

1. receptor   3. neurotransmitters

True or False Exercise

1. F   3. F

Dividing Words Exercise

1.	stimul/o-	-ation
3. syn-	erg/o-	-ism
5.	antagon/o-	-ism

Spelling Exercise

1. antagonism   **3.** synergism

13.3 Diseases

Matching Exercise

4, 10, 2, 8, 11, 3, 5, 1, 6, 9, 7

True or False Exercise

1. T   **5.** T

3. F

Circle Exercise

1. hypercalcemia   **5.** pregnancy

3. Graves disease   **7.** diabetes insipidus

Dividing Words Exercise

1.	lact/o-	-ation
3.	aden/o-	-oma
5.	gigant/o-	-ism
7. poly-	ur/o-	-ia
9.	thyroid/o-	-itis
11.	hirsut/o-	-ism

Spelling Exercise

1. microadenoma   **5.** thyroiditis

3. polydipsia

13.4 Laboratory, Diagnostic, and Radiologic Procedures

Matching Exercise

4, 9, 7, 8, 5, 2, 6, 1, 3

True or False Exercise

1. T   **3.** F

Circle Exercise

1. thyroid scan   **3.** blood calcium

Laboratory Test Exercise

CPT CODE		PANELS AND PROFILES
80047		Metabolic Panel, Basic
80050		General Health Panel
80051	✓	Electrolyte Panel
80053	✓	Metabolic Panel, Comprehensive
80055		Obstetric Panel
80061		Lipid Panel

80069		Renal Function Panel
80076		Hepatic Function Panel
80100		Drug Screening Panel
CPT CODE		**BLOOD TESTS**
80162		Digoxin Drug Level
82040		Albumin
82055		Blood Alcohol (ETCH)
82247		Blirubin, Total
82310	✓	Calcium, Total Blood
82375		Carboxyhemoglobin
82378		Carcincembryonic Angiten (CEA)
82435		Chloride
82465		Cholesterol
82553		Creatine Kinase, MB
CPT CODE		**BIOOD TESTS**
82565		Creatirine, Blood
82575		Creatirine Clearance
82670	✓	Estradiol
82947	✓	Glucose, Fasting
82951	✓	Glucose Tolerance Test (GTT)
83036	✓	Hemoglobin A1c
83540		Iron
83550		Iron, TBC
83655		Lead, Blood
83661		Fetal Lung Maturity (L/S Ratio)
83718		HDL Lipoprotein
83719		VLDL Lipoprotein
83721		LDL Lipoprotein
83735		Magnesium
84075		Alkaline Phosphatase
84132	✓	Potassium
84144	✓	Progesterone
84146	✓	Prolactin
84152		Prostate-Specific Antigen (PSA)
84155		Protein, Total
84295	✓	Sodium
84403	✓	Testosterone, Total
84443	✓	Thyroid-Stimulating Hormone (TSH)
84436	✓	Thyroxine (T_4), Total
84450		Aspartate Transaminase (AST)
84460		Alanine Transaminase (ALT)
84478		Triglycerides
84480	✓	Triiodothyririne (T_3), Total
84484		Troponin
84520		Blood Urea Nitrogen (BUN)
84550		Uric Acid
84702		Human Chorionic Gonadotropic (hCG), Serum

85004		White Blood Cell Gonadotropin (hCG), Serum
85014		Hematocrit (HCT)
85018		Hemoglobin (Hgb)
85025		Complete Blood Count (CBC)
85049		Platelet Count
85610		Prothrombin Time (PT)
85730		Partial Thromboplastin Time (PTT)
86038		Antinuclear Antibody (ANA)
86140		C-Reactive Protein
86592		Syphilis Blood Test (VDRL or RPR)
86701		HIV-1 Antibody
86762		Rubella Antibody
86812		Human Leukocyte Antigen (HLA) Typing
86900		Blood Type
86910		Blood Type for Paternity Testing
87340		Hepatitis B Surface Antigen
CPT CODE		**OTHER TESTS AND PROCEDURES**
36415		Venipuncture
81001	✓	Urinalysis, Automated
82270		Stool Occult Blood
87040		Blood Culture
87045		Stool Culture
87086		Urine Culture
87116		Acid-Fast Bacilli Culture
87177		Ova and Parasites
89220		Sputum Analysis
89300		Semen Analysis

13.5 Medical Procedures, Drugs, and Surgical Procedures

Matching Exercise

6, 4, 1, 2, 3, 5

Circle Exercise

1. iodine

3. myasthenia gravis

True or False Exercise

1. F

3. T

Dividing Words Exercise

1. anti-   diabet/o-   -ic

3.   bi/o-   -opsy

5.   thyroid/o-   -ectomy

7.   hypophys/o-   -ectomy

Spelling Exercise

1. biopsy

3. thyroidectomy

5. lobectomy

Immerse Yourself: Analyze Medical Reports

Electronic Patient Record #1

1. endo-   innermost; within

   crin/o-   secrete

   log/o-   study of; word

   -ist   person who specializes in

3. TSH

5. testosterone, thyroid hormone

7. hypothyroidism

9. surgical removal of an adenoma from the pituitary gland

Proofreading and Spelling Exercise

1. endocrinology   7. thyroidectomy

3. mellitus   9. thyromegaly

5. medulla

Chapter14 : Ophthalmology

14.1 Practice Laps

A. Label Structures

Lacrimal Glands

1. lacrimal gland   5. pupil

3. iris   7. nasolacrimal duct

Eye

1. sclera   9. choroid

3. conjunctiva   11. optic disk

5. cornea   13. fovea

7. iris   15. posterior cavity

B. Give the Meaning of Combining Forms

1. clear, watery fluid

3. before; front part

5. capsule; enveloping structure

7. choroid

9. conjunctiva

11. ciliary body; circle; cycle

13. fundus; part farthest from the opening

15. below

17. iris

19. side

21. small area; spot

23. narrowing

25. widening

27. eye

29. eye; vision

31. lens

33. pupil

35. above

37. pulley-shaped structure

39. clear, gel-like substance

C. Build Words

1. -al   scleral

3. -ary   pupillary

5. -ar   lenticular

7. -al   lacrimal

9. -ation   accommodation

11. -ary   ciliary

13. -al   lateral

15. -iasis   mydriasis

17. -al   iridal

14.2 Practice Laps

A. Give the Meaning of Combining Forms

1. bend; break up

3. vision

5. three dimensions

B. Build Words

1. -ion   vision

3. -ual   visual

14.3 Practice Laps

A. Give the Meaning of Combining Forms

1. scrape off

3. unequal

5. embryonic; immature

7. pupil

9. lacrimal sac; tears

11. diabetes

13. away from; external; outward

15. silver gray

17. iris

19. cornea; hard, fibrous protein

21. near vision

23. eye

25. vision

27. lens

29. light

31. retina

33. darkness

35. ulcer

37. dry

B. Build Words

1. -itis   iritis

3. -oma   scotoma

5. -ia   myopia

7. -ive   ulcerative

9. -ice   jaundice

11. -ptosis   blepharoptosis

C. Define Abbreviations

1. age-related macular degeneration

3. retinitis pigmentosa

14.4 Practice Laps

A. Give the Meaning of Combining Forms

1. blood vessel; lymphatic vessel

3. sound

B. Build Words

1. -in   fluorescein

3. -gram   sonogram

14.5 Practice Laps

A. Give the Meaning of Combining Forms

1. adapt

3. living organism; living tissue

5. capsule; enveloping structure

7. joined together

9. cortex; outer region

11. ciliary body; circle; cycle

13. remove the main part

15. fundus; part farthest from the opening

17. cornea; hard, fibrous protein

19. widening

21. eye

23. lens

25. light

27. air; lung

29. cut out; remove

31. heat

33. mesh

35. virus

37. clear, gel-like substance

B. Build Words

1. -meter   tonometer
3. -ectomy   vitrectomy
5. -mileusis   keratomileusis
7. -pexy   cryopexy
9. -plasty   blepharoplasty
11. -tomy   capsulotomy
13. -al   peripheral
15. -opter   phoropter
17. -metry   tonometry
19. -scopy   funduscopy

C. Define Abbreviations

1. conductive keratoplasty
3. intraocular lens
5. laser thermal keratoplasty
7. left eye
9. pupils equal, round, and react to light

Dive In: Medical Language Exercises

14.1 Anatomy

Matching Exercise

10, 6, 3, 7, 9, 4, 5, 8, 11, 1, 2

Circle Exercise

1. iris   3. optic disk   5. fundus

True or False Exercise

1. F   7. F
3. T   9. T
5. T

Plural Noun and Adjective Exercise

1. foveae   foveal
3. conjunctivae   conjunctival
5. irides   iridal
7. maculae   macular
9. sclerae   scleral

Dividing Words Exercise

1.   scler/o-   -al
3.   aque/o-   -ous
5.   cili/o-   -ary
7.   irid/o-   -al
9.   lenticul/o-   -ar
11.   op/o-   -tic
13.   super/o-   -ior

Spelling Exercise

1. mydriasis   5. ciliary
3. nasolacrimal

14.2 Physiology

Matching Exercise

4, 5, 1, 2, 3

Circle Exercise

1. cones   3. macula

True or False Exercise

1. T   3. T

Dividing Words Exercise

1.   vis/o-   -ion
3.   op/o-   -tic

Spelling Exercise

1. thalamus   3. vision   5. chiasm

14.3 Diseases

Matching Exercise

6, 10, 7, 5, 3, 11, 9, 1, 12, 2, 8, 4

True or False Exercise

1. T   7. T
3. T   9. F
5. T

Circle Exercise

1. nystagmus
3. glaucoma
5. dacryocystitis
7. diabetes mellitus

Dividing Words Exercise

1. hyper-   op/o-   -ia
3. a-   phak/o-   -ia
5.   blephar/o-   -itis
7. de-   gener/o-   -ation
9. hyper-   op/o-   -ia
11.   kerat/o-   -itis
13.   retin/o-   -pathy

Spelling Exercise

1. conjunctivitis
3. xerophthalmia
5. nystagmus
7. cataract
9. neovascularization

14.4 Laboratory, Diagnostic, and Radiologic Procedures

True or False Exercise

    1. T   **3.** T

14.5 Medical Procedures, Drugs, and Surgical Procedures

Matching Exercise

2, 6, 5, 1, 7, 3, 12, 8, 10, 9, 4, 13, 11

Circle Exercise

    1. accommodation

    3. slit lamp

    5. microkeratome

True or False Exercise

    1. T   **7.** T

    3. T   **9.** F

    5. T

Dividing Words Exercise

    1. anti-   bi/o-   -tic

    3. dys-   conjug/o-   -ate

    5.   mydr/o-   -iatic

    7.   phor/o-   -opter

Spelling Exercise

    1. visual   **5.** blepharoplasty

    3. ophthalmoscope   **7.** cryopexy

Proofreading Exercise

    1. visual   **7.** cataract

    3. conjunctiva   **9.** funduscopic

    5. macula

Related Combining Forms Exercise

    1. kerat/o-, corne/o-

    3. phac/o-, phak/o-, lenticul/o-

    5. op/o-, opt/o-, vis/o-

Immerse Yourself: Analyze Medical Reports

Electronic Patient Record

    1. fundus (or retina)

    3. scintillating scotoma temporary visual field defect of hemianopsia

    5. pupils equal, round, and reactive to light

    7. Blepharitis

    9. glaucoma

Chapter 15 : Otolaryngology

15.1 Practice Laps

A. Label Structures

Ear

    1. temporal bone

    3. incus

    5. tympanic membrane

    7. mastoid bone

    9. eustachian tube

    11. oval window

    13. vestibulocochlear nerve

    15. cochlea

Nose, Throat, and Mouth

    1. sphenoid sinus   **13.** frontal sinus

    3. adenoids   **15.** nasal cavity

    5. nasopharynx   **17.** oral cavity

    7. palatine tonsil   **19.** mandible

    9. lingual tonsil   **21.** trachea

    11. laryngopharynx

B. Give the Meaning of Combining Forms

    1. front

    3. gland

    5. hearing

    7. ear

    9. cheek

    11. lip

    13. back; dorsum

    15. outside

    17. anvil-shaped bone; incus

    19. labium; lip

    21. tongue

    23. lower jaw; mandible

    25. mastoid process

    27. chin; mind

    29. eardrum; tympanic membrane

    31. mouth

    33. ossicle; small bone

    35. nose

    37. sinus

    39. stapes; stirrup-shaped bone

    41. tonsil

43. eardrum; tympanic membrane

45. voice

C. Build Words

1. -al	nasal	**9.** -ar	cochlear		
3. -ar	mallear	**11.** -ory	auditory		
5. -ar	vestibular	**13.** -al	incudal		
7. -ic	tympanic	**15.** -ic	otic		

D. Define Abbreviations

1. external auditory canal

3. tympanic membrane

15.2 Practice Laps

A. Give the Meaning of Combining Forms

1. sense of hearing	**5.** one's own body	
3. sense of smell	**7.** entrance; vestibule	

B. Build Words

1. -ar   cochlear

3. -ception   proprioception

5. -ic   tympanic

15.3 Practice Laps

A. Give the Meaning of Combining Forms

1. hearing; sound

3. pain

5. *Candida*; yeast

7. cervix; neck

9. pouring out

11. blood

13. labyrinth

15. side

17. lymph; lymphatic system

19. lower jaw; mandible

21. eardrum; tympanic membrane

23. nerve

25. ear

27. plaque

29. pus

31. hard; sclera

33. serum-like fluid; serum of the blood

35. curved

37. side of the head; temple

B. Build Words

1. -itis   laryngitis

3. -itis   labyrinthitis

5. -itis   glossitis

7. -phyma   rhinophyma

9. -ative   suppurative

11. -rrhea   rhinorrhea

13. -acusis   presbyacusis

15. -ic   allergic

17. -tic   acoustic

19. -oma   carcinoma

21. -itis   otitis

C. Define Abbreviations

1. postnasal drip

3. upper respiratory infection

15.4 Practice Laps

A. Give the Meaning of Combining Forms

1. hearing

3. eardrum; tympanic membrane

B. Build Words

1. -metry   audiometry

3. -ity   sensitivity

5. -gram   audiogram

C. Define Abbreviations

1. auditory brainstem response

15.5 Practice Laps

A. Give the Meaning of Combining Forms

1. structure resembling a gland

3. lip

5. cortex; outer region

7. innermost; within

9. larynx; voice box

11. mastoid process

13. ear

15. root and all parts

17. examine with an instrument

19. stapes; stirrup-shaped bone

21. cough

23. eardrum; tympanic membrane

B. Build Words

1. -tomy   myringotomy

3. -stomy   tympanostomy

5. -scopy   otoscopy

7. -scope   endoscope

9. -ion   dissection

11. -ectomy   tonsillectomy
13. -scope   otoscope

Dive In: Medical Language Exercises

15.1 Anatomy

Matching Exercise

4, 6, 3, 16, 5, 2, 8, 7, 13, 14, 10, 18, 17, 15, 1, 12, 11, 9

Circle Exercise

1. laryngopharynx   **3.** eustachian tube

True or False Exercise

1. T   **5.** T   **9.** T
3. T   **7.** F

Plural Noun and Adjective Exercise

1. incudes   incudal
3. cochlea   cochlear
5. mallei   mallear
7. nares
9. ossicles   ossicular
11.   septal
13. tonsils   tonsillar

Dividing Words Exercise

1.   mast/o-   -oid
3.   aur/i-   -cle
5. epi-   glott/o-   -ic
7.   nas/o-   -al
9. semi-   circul/o-   -ar
11. sub-   ment/o-   -al

Spelling Exercise

1. mastoid   **5.** turbinate
3. tympanic   **7.** oropharynx

Related Combining Forms Exercise

1. myring/o-, tympan/o-   **5.** ot/o-, aur/i-, auricul/o-
3. nas/o-, rhin/o-

15.2 Physiology

Matching Exercise

3, 1, 6, 5, 4, 7, 2

Circle Exercise

1. vestibular nerve

True or False Exercise

1. F   **3.** F

Dividing Words Exercise

1. tympan/o-   -ic   **5.** vestibul/o-   -ar
3. cochle/o-   -ar

Spelling Exercise

1. cochlear   **3.** auditory

Related Combining Forms Exercise

1. acous/o-, audi/o-, audit/o-

15.3 Diseases

Matching Exercise

1, 11, 3, 10, 9, 5, 4, 8, 6, 2, 12, 7

True or False Exercise

1. T   **7.** F
3. T   **9.** F
5. F   **11.** T

Circle Exercise

1. blood   **5.** anosmia
3. otalgia   **7.** leukoplakia

Dividing Words Exercise

1. bi-   later/o-   -al
3.   laryng/o-   -itis
5.   neur/o-   -oma
7. pan-   sinus/o-   -itis
9.   presby/o-   -acusis

Spelling Exercise

1. allergic
3. otorrhea
5. hemotympanum

15.4 Laboratory, Diagnostic, and Radiologic Procedures

Matching Exercise

5, 2, 4, 1, 3, 6

True or False Exercise

1. T   **5.** F
3. T

Circle Exercise

1. audiometry

15.5 Medical Procedures, Drugs, and Surgical Procedures

Matching Exercise

4, 7, 3, 1, 9, 2, 8, 5, 6

Circle Exercise

1. speculum

3. placed under the tongue

5. stapedectomy

True or False Exercise

1. T   3. F   5. T

Dividing Words Exercise

1.	anti-	bi/o-	-tic
3.		cheil/o-	-plasty
5.		end/o-	-scope
7.		ot/o-	-scopy
9.		rhin/o-	-plasty
11.		tonsill/o-	-ectomy

Spelling Exercise

1. cheiloplasty   5. otoplasty

3. decongestant

Immerse Yourself: Analyze Medical Reports

Electronic Patient Record #1

1. condition of rebound nasal congestion from extended use of nasal decongestants

3. allergic rhinitis

Electronic Patient Record #2

1. sinus/o-   sinus

   -itis   infection of; inflammation of

3. tympanic membrane

5. palpation

7. antibiotic drug

9. frontal, maxillary

Credit

Index

A page number in italics refers to a figure (illustration or photograph). A page number followed by t refers to a table.